Pathology
in the
Tropics

Tribute
In memory of Mina

Pathology
in the
Tropics

G. M. EDINGTON

*C.B.E., M.B.E., M.D.(Glas.), F.R.C.Path, F.R.C.P.,
F.N.M.C.(Path.), D.C.P., D.T.M. & H., Hon.D.Sc.(Ibadan)*

*Professor and Head of Department of Pathology, Ahmadu Bello
University, Zaria, Nigeria. Formerly Professor and Head of Depart-
ment of Pathology, Deputy Vice-Chancellor and Ag. Vice-Chancellor,
University of Ibadan, Nigeria and Specialist Pathologist in charge
of the Medical Research Institute and Laboratory Services, Gold
Coast and Ghana*

H. M. GILLES

*K.O.S.J., B.Sc., M.D., F.R.C.P., F.F.C.M., F.M.C.P.H.(Nigeria),
D.T.M. & H.*

*Professor of Tropical Medicine, Liverpool School of Tropical Medicine,
University of Liverpool. Formerly Professor of Preventive and Social
Medicine, University of Ibadan, Nigeria. Consultant Physician,
United Liverpool Hospitals. Honorary Consultant in Malariology to
the Army*

Second Edition

EDWARD ARNOLD

ISBN: 0 7131 4239 1

PRINTED IN GREAT BRITAIN BY
WILLIAM CLOWES & SONS LIMITED
LONDON, COLCHESTER AND BECCLES

Foreword

By

Professor Sir Theo Crawford

B.Sc., M.D., F.R.C.P., F.R.C.P. (Glas.), F.R.C.Path.,
Department of Pathology, St. George's Hospital Medical School,
(University of London), Hyde Park Corner, London S.W.1

That good modern medical practice must be based on pathology and supported by an efficient pathology service is a truism nowhere more evident than in tropical countries. The great pioneers of tropical medicine in the nineteenth century had to double as pathologists: but with the growth of knowledge and the increasing complexity of modern laboratory work no man can encompass so broad a range of expertise. It is essential that students training to be doctors in tropical countries should understand fully the pathological basis of the diseases they will treat and it was no doubt for this end that *Pathology in the Tropics* was originally designed.

When the first edition appeared in 1969 it soon became clear that it would have a much wider readership than the one for which it was originally intended. It is invaluable for medical students and trainee pathologists in tropical countries who formerly had to make do with European or North American text-books; but it has found an important role also in pathology departments well outside the tropics. Modern high-speed travel and the population migrations which have been so widespread in recent years have disseminated 'tropical diseases' over most of the inhabited world, and certainly those of us who practice pathology in the United Kingdom must be ready at any time to encounter parasitic, genetic and other diseases, formerly regarded as confined to the tropics, amongst our biopsies or in our necropsy rooms. In these circumstances *Pathology in the Tropics* has proved a God-send to us, both for its succinct accounts of the important manifestations and for its convenient references to the literature for further study.

The production of such a book could hardly have been in better hands. Professor George Edington has devoted his working life to pathology, and to medical education in tropical West Africa. After many years in the Colonial Medical Service, including five years as pathologist in charge of the Medical Research Institute and laboratory services for Gold Coast and Ghana, he returned to England for a brief period to take up a consultant post in the

v

Liverpool region. But when the Chair of Pathology at Ibadan in Western Nigeria became vacant in 1958 the call of Africa proved too strong and he returned to spend the next 12 years establishing and running what was probably the most successful pathology unit in tropical Africa—and which in Edington's hands compared favourably with departments anywhere in the world. Professor Edington's final four years in Ibadan were spent as Deputy Vice-Chancellor and Acting Vice-Chancellor in his last year, a post which he filled with great distinction; and he has now moved to Ahmadu Bello University at Zaria in Northern Nigeria where he is again using his unique experience to develop a new department covering diagnostic work, teaching and research over the whole range of pathology.

The collaboration of Professor Edington with Professor Herbert Gilles is a most felicitous one. Dr. Gilles was for some years professor of preventive and social medicine at Ibadan. He brings to the team that detailed knowledge of community health, gained from personal experience of field work in tropical countries, which is essential for the effective application of laboratory medicine to health problems in a tropical environment. Dr. Gilles is now Professor of Tropical Medicine in Liverpool and his wide clinical experience is reflected in the well-balanced clinico-pathological correlations that are achieved throughout the book.

It is a real privilege to have been invited to write a Foreword to launch this second edition on its way.

London, 1974   T.C.

Preface to Second Edition

The generous reception accorded in the first edition has made it necessary for us to prepare a second edition much earlier than we had planned. The rapid advances in knowledge of pathology in the tropics obviated against reprinting the first edition. We are grateful to the many reviewers and others for their helpful criticism and we have attempted to correct the errors and omissions they brought to our attention. We have maintained our original intention to concentrate on the pathology of the diseases which occur exclusively in the tropics and those which are world-wide but which present in the tropics with unusual manifestations or frequencies. Short accounts of diseases of the eye and skin have been added and the auto-immune diseases have been mentioned including the part that immunological surveillance may play in malignant disease. Malignant disease in children has been mentioned and the description of lymphoreticular tumours expanded. Because of the possible importance of the Epstein–Barr virus in certain forms of neoplasia a description of the pathology of infectious mononucleosis is given. Lassa fever and Marburg disease are included in the virus diseases and the Australia antigen is discussed when the pathology of the liver is considered, as is also alphafetoprotein. In few areas in the tropics is an electron microscope available and we have found it of value to embed material locally for later examination in more sophisticated centres. A short description of the method employed is given in the Appendix.

G.M.E.
H.M.G.

Preface to First Edition

One of the great difficulties encountered in teaching pathology in the tropics is the lack of a suitable textbook. It was our original intention therefore to produce a companion to the standard textbooks of pathology orientated to the undergraduate student in the tropics. However, on the advice of several colleagues and following our own inclination, many of the subjects in the following text have been described in much more depth than would be required of the undergraduate, who will therefore require some measure of direction in his reading. Recognizing also the scarcity of library facilities in many areas a reasonably extensive bibliography has been included. It is hoped, therefore, that this publication will be found to be of some value, not only to the medical student but to young pathologists and research workers in the tropics, to those pathologists, trained in the Western tradition, who may be visiting tropical areas in a temporary capacity and also to pathologists in Europe and America working in areas where substantial immigration from the tropics has occurred.

The study of pathology is still in its infancy in many tropical areas. The basic patterns of many common disease processes have still to be defined. The present accepted descriptions of many diseases in temperate climates will be found to be modified in the tropics by environmental factors (including parasitic infections and dietary deficiencies), by the altered immunological status of the host and by inherited haemoglobin or enzymatic abnormalities. We have tried in the first chapter to outline some of these problems.

It is assumed that the reader has a knowledge of general pathology. In the following chapters we deal with the diseases which occur exclusively in the tropics and those which are world wide but which present in the tropics with unusual manifestations or frequencies. In the latter group only the pathological and/or epidemiological aspects of interest to workers in the tropics are usually discussed. Cosmopolitan diseases which are rare or present in the tropics in the classical manner and are well described in standard textbooks are not discussed in any detail if at all. We have attempted to indicate areas in which information is lacking and, at times, perhaps rashly, have recorded our own impressions and opinions. Excluding the skin manifestations of the common tropical diseases, dermatological pathology has not been dealt with and only the pathology of a few neonatal conditions has been described.

Pathology does not imply purely a morphological study but includes abnormalities of function and we have, therefore, attempted to correlate the effect of the physiological requirements of the various parasites on the nutritional and immunological responses of the host. It must be remembered, however, that multiple infections and infestations are usual and the part that any one parasite plays in the morbid processes in the host may be extremely difficult, if not impossible, to evaluate—malaria in stable areas being the best example.

Epidemiology has been described at some length, as a knowledge of this subject is a pre-requisite to prevention which should be the prime aim of teachers in every branch of medicine. The disappearance of yaws from vast areas of the world illustrates this point and is the reason why it is somewhat cursorily treated in the text.

Considerable attention has also been directed to geographical pathology as this may provide clues as to aetiology in populations with differing nutritional, social, economic and other environmental factors. Caution, however, should be exercised in placing too much reliance on geographical studies as they depend upon the recording of clearly definable facts in a known population or a representative sample of it and at present accurate morbidity and mortality statistics are all too rare in most areas. It is also well known that disease patterns may vary in similar peoples living within a few hundred miles of each other and this must be remembered when generalizations are made regarding incidence rates in continents or even in individual countries. Nevertheless, we believe that extended geographical studies will prove of value in helping to elucidate some of the aetiological problems which are at present obscure in many tropical and non-tropical conditions. Particular attention has been paid to the geographical study of malignant disease.

In the Appendix are included a number of diagnostic techniques which have been found to be of value in tropical practice and are not readily available in standard textbooks of pathology. Special attention has been given to the diagnosis of the abnormal haemoglobin diseases and to blood transfusion techniques as it was considered they might be of value to practitioners working in isolation and divorced from sophisticated laboratory services. Details of serological and immunological techniques (many of which are highly specialized) have not been included but relevant references to which interested readers may refer have been included in the text.

No attempt has been made to include a table of normal values as these will be found to vary in different geographical areas. Relative references when available have been given.

G.M.E.
H.M.G.

Acknowledgements

Our first and most sincere thanks must go to Mary Jane Edington without whose encouragement, patience and perseverance neither the first nor the second edition of this book would have been possible.

We owe much to many friends and colleagues, and acknowledgement is made below and in the text. If we have unwittingly omitted any authority we crave their indulgence and pardon.

We thankfully acknowledge the assistance and advice of the following friends and colleagues: Dr. O. O. Akingkube; Mr. J. P. Brady; Dr. S. G. Browne, Professor D. F. Cappell; Dr. B. Clark; Dr. B. Greenwood; Professor C. V. Harrison; Professor H. Lehmann; Dr. L. Luzzatto; Dr. B. O. Osunkoya; Dr. H. A. Reid; Air Vice-Marshall Stamm; Professor D. Weatherall; Professor A. O. Williams; Dr. Sheila Worlledge.

We wish to record our gratitude to the many persons who supplied illustrations all of whom are acknowledged in the text, in particular, however, we wish to thank the American Registry of Pathology, Armed Forces Institute of Pathology for allowing us liberal use of the photographs from Ash and Spitz, *Pathology of Tropical Diseases*.

We are especially grateful to Mr. H. Hague and Mrs. M. Amosu, Miss Joan Morris, Miss Jean Hankinson, Mrs. T. Odelola and Mr. A. J. Okeoma.

Finally we wish to pay thankful tribute to the patience and efficiency of our secretaries. We must also thank Edward Arnold Ltd., for dealing effectively with many editorial problems.

Contents

Foreword by Professor Sir Theo Crawford   v

1   The Tropical Environment   1

2   Protozoal Diseases   10

3   Helminthic Diseases   91

4   Rickettsial and Viral Diseases   212

5   Diseases Caused by Fungi   264

6   Bacterial Diseases   296

7   Spirochaetal Diseases   340

8   The Circulatory System   348

9   The Respiratory System   390

10   The Haemopoietic System   404

11   The Alimentary System   513

12   The Nervous System   601

13   The Urinary and Reproductive Systems   616

14   The Endocrine Glands   653

15   Disorders of Nutrition   668

16   Miscellaneous Disorders   690

   Appendix   753

   References   783

   Index   915

I

The Tropical Environment

Tropical countries are faced with many problems of community-wide endemic and sometimes epidemic diseases which may have serious physical and economic effects on the population. In addition, individuals are exposed to diseases that are common to temperate and tropical climates alike. As a background to these diseases both in the individual and in the community, there are nutritional, social, environmental, and genetic factors which directly or indirectly influence the progress of the disease patterns themselves and are usually more adverse in the tropics. As far as the pathologist is concerned multiple infections and infestations, genetic and nutritional abnormalities are frequently present in one individual, and in some instances it is difficult if not impossible to assess the importance that any one of these plays in the clinico-pathological or post-mortem findings.

The interplay between diet, environment, social, cultural and genetic background in the tropics has been emphasized by many workers. Studies of village communities in Ghana (Colbourne *et al.* 1950); the Gambia (McGregor and Smith, 1952); Nigeria (Gilles, 1967); Egypt (Weir *et al.* 1952); Taiwan (Bergner *et al.* 1964); Thailand (Harinasuta *et al.* 1967); India (Pathanayak *et al.* 1967); and other areas of the tropics have demonstrated that the burden of disease is heavy and complex. It is known that a prodigious wastage of life occurs in young children in the tropics within four years of birth. The reasons for this high death rate are multiple and not at all easy to dissociate. In areas where thiamine deficiency is common, it has been shown that there is a relatively high mortality due to infantile beriberi between 2 and 5 months of age, compared with similar areas where dietary lack of thiamine does not occur (Aykroyd and Krishnan, 1941). For many years the importance of malnutrition has been emphasized; thus, for example, Wills and Waterlow (1958) have suggested that the death rate at ages 1–4 years might be used as an index of the nutritional state of a country, a suggestion supported recently by Uttley (1963). Yet in areas where malnutrition is uncommon, infant mortality remains very high (McGregor *et al.* 1961).

Urbanization and industrialization

One of the most significant changes taking place in the tropics is the migration of people from rural to urban areas where industrial and commercial enterprises are developing. The proximity of slums and shanty towns to modern buildings and large departmental stores commonly occurs. The effects of urbanization are most vividly seen in mportant ports such as Lagos, Hong Kong, Singapore, and Calcutta (WHO, 1967).

Most emerging nations are giving priority to industrialization, thus byssinosis, until recently an industrial hazard of Lancashire, is now spreading to cotton- and flax-growing countries such as Egypt, the Sudan, and the Indian subcontinent. Manuwa (1971) has emphasized the changing pattern of disease in Nigerian cities and its implications for the problem of occupational health, while Phoon *et al.* (1973) has studied the health problems of children in high rise apartments in Singapore.

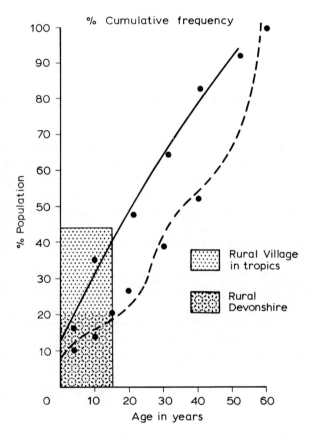

FIG. 1.1. Age distribution in a rural village in the tropics and in England.

Demography

The figures relating to the age distribution of village populations in many areas of the tropics reveal that young persons under 14 years of age make up over 40 per cent of the population in marked contrast to the situation pertaining in the developed countries of the world (Fig. 1.1).

Examination of the age and sex pyramid of tropical rural populations (Loraine, 1974), reveals several striking features (Fig. 1.2): (*a*) a broad base reflecting a high fertility rate and a high wastage of child life, (*b*) a relative absence of adolescents as a result of migration to the cities, (*c*) a small number of persons over 60 years of age. This demographic pattern is fairly widespread throughout the rural tropics but as might be expected it is not universal and important variations occur, especially in urban areas or as a result of differing social, cultural, and religious habits. The incidence of twinning is extremely high in some areas of the tropics and this is especially so in Nigeria, Taiwan, and Egypt. A stochastic computer simulation model has been used to study the demography of the Yanomanö Indians of Venezuela and Brazil, whose organization is typical of many primitive societies (MacCluer *et al.* 1971).

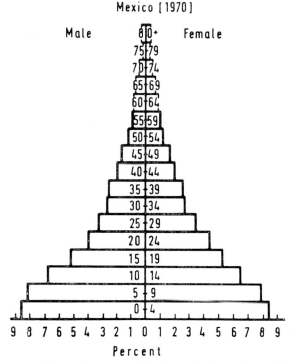

FIG. 1.2. Sex and age pyramid of a tropical rural population.

Mortality

Great caution must be exercised in accepting and interpreting death rates in the tropics. Most observers would agree however that although discrepancies occur not only between village and village but also from year to year, childhood mortality in many areas of the tropics is still very high. Table 1.1 compares the neonatal, infantile and childhood rates reported from various tropical countries. Improvement of health services have undoubtedly already lowered these mortalities in many of them, but in most there are still remote rural areas where the position has not materially altered. An inter-American investigation of mortality in childhood was carried out by PAHO (1971); while Aug *et al.* (1974) reviewed the hospital mortality in a Singapore Paediatric Unit.

TABLE 1.1. *Neonatal, infantile, and child mortality up to 4 years of age in some tropical countries and in the United Kingdom*

	Neonatal Rate/1000	Infantile Rate/1000	Child (3 months– 4 years) Rate/1000	Source
Ruwan Sanyin	—	170·0	380	Gilles (1975)
Akufo	50	109·0	430	Gilles (1967)
Imesi	78	295·0	277	Morley (1963)
Gambia	54	134·0	400	McGregor *et al.* (1961)
Senegal	—	172·0	344	Senecal *et al.* (1962)
Guinea	—	217·0	415	Senecal *et al.* (1962)
Egypt	—	215·0	—	Weir *et al.* (1952)
Mombasa	—	147·0	—	Rosenwald (1963)
Haiti	—	176·9	—	WHO (1967)
Chile	—	114·2	—	Plank and Milanesi (1967)
Colombia	—	83·3	—	WHO (1967)
Aden	—	92·8	—	WHO (1967)
India	—	72·8	—	WHO (1967)
Singapore	—	29·9	—	WHO (1967)
United Kingdom	—	19·9	—	WHO (1967)

Cropping system

Land use has a direct bearing on the economic and dietary patterns of rural village communities. The data on percentage cultivated land under each crop in a West African village is illustrated in Fig. 1.3. Differing land-use patterns will naturally be found in groundnut or palm kernel growing areas; where cotton or jute is the main cash crop, where rice, plantain, sweet potatoes, or red beans are the staple diet.

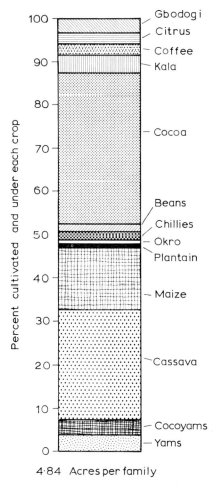

FIG. 1.3. Cropping pattern in a West African village.

Nutrition

Clinical evidence of malnutrition especially in children is widespread throughout the tropics. The predominant nutritional deficiencies vary greatly from area to area and are discussed in some detail in Chapter 15. It is important to remember that tropical diets may be poor in some nutrients and rich in others. Thus in many parts of Africa the low protein intake is in marked contrast with the high iron and vitamin A intakes that are found. Seasonal variations in diet are important and must be taken into consideration in the final assessment.

The serum protein pattern of many tropical—especially African—populations differs markedly from that in Europe and America. (Satokar and Lewis, 1954; Holmes *et al.* 1955; Bakker *et al.* 1957; Gilles and McGregor, 1961). The serum contains less albumin and more γ-globulin than the serum of Europeans, thus giving lower values for the A/G ratio. The causes of this difference have been the subject of considerable discussion during the last few years. The consensus of opinion is that the high γ-globulin levels are related to the development of malaria immunity (see Chapter 2) as well as a response to the many other infective agents that are prevalent in the tropics.

Parasitic infections

Polyparasitism is extremely common and many species of parasites may cohabit in the same host. In both rural and many urban environments, the water used for drinking, washing, and other domestic purposes is a source of guinea-worms and schistosomiasis. The food eaten, both meat and vegetables, is a source of tapeworm, roundworm and whipworm. Where freshwater fish or crustacea are consumed liver or lung flukes predominate. The soil is infected with hookworm and strongyloidiasis while biting insects convey malaria, trypanosomiasis, onchocerciasis or filariasis. Dogs, cats and other animals in the houses and yards predispose to zoonotic parasitic infections such as toxocariasis, and assist the mechanical spread of intestinal helminths.

Communicable diseases

Communicable diseases are widespread in the tropics and occur at a much earlier age than in Europe and America, they are particularly prevalent and an important cause of morbidity and mortality in the pre-school child.

In India, tuberculosis still kills half a million people a year and there are over 5 million cases; cholera and smallpox are major problems; there are 2·5 million cases of leprosy, and other diseases such as trachoma, diphtheria, poliomyelitis, rabies and haemorrhagic fever are common (Pathanayak *et al.* 1967). Measles is endemic in many areas and in West Africa it is considered one of the most killing diseases of the pre-school child (Morley, 1963; Senecal *et al.* 1962). Pneumonia and bronchopneumonia, tetanus, whooping cough and other infections are rampant.

Diarrhoeal diseases represent a major public health problem in many developing countries. Although widespread in the tropics they affect most severely the pre-school child—the critical period being 1–4 years of age. Some of the acute diarrhoeas are specific infective diseases, e.g. shigellosis and salmonellosis, another and major proportion have no demonstrable infectious agent. The death rates from diarrhoeal diseases are impressive enough in themselves—thus in three Guatemalan villages over a 10-year period they ranged from 12 to 36 per cent in the age groups 0–4, with a maximal mortality in the second year of life (Gordon *et al.* 1964). For school children and adults the rates are a fraction of those during the earlier years of life. In addition diarrhoeal disease has an indirect effect on the mortality of children after the neonatal period by contributing to death from kwashiorkar (Behar *et al.* 1958), marasmus (McLaren, 1966a), and from such infectious diseases as measles (Morley *et al.* 1963).

Non–infective diseases

Important non-infective diseases, e.g. endomyocardial fibrosis, add to the complexity of the environment; some malignant conditions, although cosmopolitan, occur predominantly in tropical countries, e.g. primary liver-cell carcinoma and chorioncarcinoma; these and other diseases are described in detail in subsequent chapters.

Haematology

In Table 1.2 the haemoglobin levels in a village in the tropics are compared with the haemoglobin values found in a town of rural England.

TABLE 1.2. *Mean adult haemoglobin values in an African village (Akufo) and in Wensleydale (rural Yorkshire, U.K.)*

	Akufo		Wensleydale	
Age	M.	F.	M.	F.
15–24	11·6	11·2	14·1	11·9
25–34	13·0	11·0	14·3	12·7
35–44	13·2	11·1	14·3	12·7
45–54	12·6	12·0	14·1	13·1
55+	11·6	10·7	13·9	13·0

The average haemoglobin levels of the population averaged 2 g per cent below those considered normal in Europe and America. This difference is observed at all ages and in both sexes. The possible causes of anaemia in this village were numerous. Hookworm infection was almost 100 per cent in those over 5 years of age; *P. falciparum* malaria is practically constantly found in children from 3 months of age to 5 years. The serum albumin level of children and adults is low. Bacterial and viral infections are common especially in childhood. Thirty per cent of the population are heterozygote for haemoglobin S or C and 2·5 per cent are either homozygous or doubly heterozygous for S or C. Folic-acid deficiency was noted in most pregnant women. Which of these various factors is predominant in producing anaemia in the various age groups still requires careful analysis. It has been suggested that the low values for haemoglobin concentration are caused by high plasma volumes and do not necessarily indicate that the subjects are anaemic (Edozien, 1965). Similar findings and similar difficulties in disentangling the multifactorial aspects of anaemia in the tropics have been reported from other areas and are fully discussed in Chapter 10.

Genetics

In recent years interest in genetics has been greatly stimulated in the tropics and subtropics by the discovery that high gene frequencies for some genetic traits are maintained by providing a protection to the carrier against falciparum malaria (Allison, 1954). The genetic markers vary in importance from one area to the other; thus while haemoglobin S is the most important abnormal haemoglobin in Africa, it is superseded by haemoglobin E and thalassaemia in South East Asia. It appears likely that neutropenia is a normal genetically determined characteristic of many indigenous African peoples (Shaper and Lewis, 1971). The relative importance of these genetic abnormalities is dealt with in Chapter 10.

Cultural and other factors

It is well known that infant feeding and child care show striking variations in different cultures; very early childbearing and other adverse factors make childbearing in the tropics inefficient and dangerous for both mother and fetus (Thompson and Baird, 1967a, b, c). Political upheavals revive old health problems; thus in Zaire, trypanosomiasis which, until recently, was fairly well controlled, is rampant once again. The social factors which influence the behaviour in the presence of sickness of people belonging to different ethnic groups cannot be ignored in the tropical context (Maclean, 1965). Finally, the population pressure, most evident in the Indian sub-continent, upsets the delicate balance between food supply and demand.

The situation described in the preceding pages has been observed in various parts of the tropical world. Whether the basic diet is cassava, rice, plantain, sweet potatoes, or red beans; whether the main communicable diseases are tuberculosis, schistosomiasis, or trachoma; whether kwashiorkor, vitamin-A deficiency, or marasmus are the main nutritional diseases; or whether the important genetic factors are haemoglobin S, haemoglobin E, or thalassaemia—the association and dissociation of these various factors as a cause of mortality presents a puzzling problem to the pathologist in the tropics.

Socio-Economic development schemes

The construction of dams in Africa, South-East Asia, the Middle East and South America has resulted in increased production of electricity, agricultural products, and fish in the man-made lakes. Health hazards associated with these very beneficial schemes have until recently been ignored (Sornmani *et al.*, 1973), and this has been particularly the case regarding the spread of schistosomiasis. Studies of these health problems are vital and are now being carried out in anticipation of such schemes (Kitikoon *et al.*, 1973).

2

Protozoal Diseases

The major protozoal diseases of man constitute one of the most important groups of infections in tropical countries. Thus it was estimated that in 1960 the annual number of cases of malaria throughout the world was 140 million with 980,000 deaths (Bruce-Chwatt, 1967; WHO, 1974). Although the world-wide malaria eradication campaign has freed many millions of people, malaria is still widely distributed throughout the tropics (Gilles, 1974). The following protozoal diseases are described in this chapter: (i) malaria, (ii) the trypanosomiases, (iii) the leishmaniases, (iv) amoebiasis, (v) giardiasis, (vi) trichomonads, (vii) isosporiasis, (viii) toxoplasmosis, (ix) sarcosporidiosis, (x) *Pneumocystis carinii*, and (xi) balantidiasis.

MALARIA

Human malaria is a disease of wide distribution caused by sporozoa of the genus *Plasmodium*. It is found in regions lying roughly between latitudes 60° N and 40° S. There are four species of the parasite that infect man: *P. falciparum*, *P. vivax*, *P. malariae*, and *P. ovale*. The differentiation of the species depends on the morphology and staining of the parasites and associated changes in the containing cells. The most common and important infections are those caused by *P. falciparum* and *P. vivax*. Mixed infections occur. It is of interest to note that certain simian malarias can rarely be transmitted to man (Coatney, 1968; Fong *et al.*, 1971).

The arthropod hosts are females of certain species of *Anopheles* mosquito. The predominant malaria vectors are *A. gambiae*, *A. funestus*, *A. darlingi* and *A. punctulatus* (Gordon and Lavoipierre, 1962).

Clinically malaria is characterized by fever, splenomegaly, varying degrees of anaemia, and various syndromes resulting from the involvement of individual organs. In addition, the indirect effects of malaria in populations in which it is endemic are arousing more and more interest. The alteration of the immunological status of the host by the hypertrophy or 'blockade' of the reticulo-endothelial system is being associated with an increased frequency of certain types of malignant lymphomas, with a lowered frequency of autoimmune disease, a decreased antibody response to certain infections and with a syndrome termed 'idiopathic tropical splenomegaly'. In addition *P. malariae* infection is associated with a specific type of renal lesion manifesting itself clinically as the nephrotic syndrome. These are discussed in their appropriate context. In this chapter malaria will be dealt with under the following headings: (1) Life cycle, (2) Epidemiology, (3) Immunity, (4) General pathology, (5) Pathology of individual organs, and (6) Diagnostic pathology.

Life cycle

The complete life cycle of the human malaria parasite embraces (1) a period of development within the mosquito, and (2) a period of infection in man.

After ingestion of human infected blood a period of development lasting 10–14 days occurs in the mosquito resulting in the production of *sporozoites*. A bite infects the human host with these forms which remain in the circulating blood for 30 minutes or less, then enter tissue cells notably in the liver, where the *pre-erythrocytic cycle* takes place.

During the succeeding 7–9 days the sporozoites develop in the parenchmal cells of the liver. This stage of development is known as the pre-erythrocytic cycle. The cryptozoic schizonts thus formed rupture and release numerous merozoites most of which enter the circulation to invade the erythrocytes, thus starting the erythrocytic cycle. Attempts have been made to investigate the metabolism of this stage of the parasite's existence. Tissue culture techniques have been utilized and the influence of various types of media on the development of the parasite in the parenchymal cells has been studied. Information on this stage of parasitic development is as yet, however, scanty and inconclusive. As in the short sporozoite phase no symptoms of malaria are experienced during the pre-erythrocytic cycle. Although Shortt and his colleagues demonstrated pre-erythrocytic schizogony in human malaria in 1948, it is interesting to note that neither cryptozoic nor metazoic schizonts (exo-erythrocytic schizonts) have been reported in infections in man in areas of intense malaria transmission, despite search for these forms in liver biopsy and necropsy material. The liberation of the merozoites from the liver cells and their entry into the blood stream initiates the erythrocytic cycle. The plasmodium first appears in red cells as a small speck of chromatin surrounded by scanty cytoplasm, and soon becomes a ring-shaped trophozoite. As the parasite develops, pigment particles appear in the cytoplasm, and the chromatin is more prominent. Chromatin division then proceeds and when complete there is formed the mature schizont containing daughter merozoites. The parasitized red blood cell now ruptures, releasing merozoites the majority of which re-enter erythrocytes to re-initiate erythrocytic schizogony. In *P. falciparum* infection the erythrocytic cycle takes 36–48 hours (subtertian); in *P. vivax* and *P. ovale* infections 48 hours (tertian); and *P. malariae* 72 hours (quartan). The powers of invasion of the species of plasmodia differ considerably. *P. vivax* develops most easily in the youngest erythrocytes, so that at any one time not more than 2 per cent of red cells are invaded. *P. malariae* develops chiefly in the older red cells, the infection rate seldom exceeding 2 per cent. *P. falciparum* invades all ages of erythrocytes indiscriminately and infection rates up to 15 per cent or more of red cells have been noted.

Much information is available regarding the metabolism of the malaria parasite from the moment it first invades the red blood cell to its subsequent development into a schizont. Both the metabolic pathways and nutritional requirement have been most extensively studied in avian malaria (*P. lophurae*), (Trager, 1964). The malaria parasite appears to possess the same mechanism for the breakdown of glucose as its vertebrate host. The chief source of parasite protein is the haemoglobin of the erythrocyte. Electron microscopy studies have demonstrated that the parasites engulf portions of the red cell cytoplasm by invaginating their limiting membranes— a process known as 'phagotrophy' (Rudzinska and Trager, 1957). The ultrastructure of red cells infected by *P. falciparum* in man was studied by Miller (1972). All available studies suggest that the nucleic acid metabolism of malaria parasites is similar to that of other organisms; morover it has been shown that malarial parasites have a very high lipid content. Several substances are needed for the extra-cellular survival of *P. lophurae*, e.g. pyruvate; diphosphopyridine nucleotide; adenosine triphosphate; malate; coenzyme A; leucovorin; red cell extract and gelatin (Trager, 1958). These are probably also necessary for the development of the malaria parasites of man. A detailed review of the metabolism of the malaria parasite and its host was carried out by Fletcher and Maegraith (1972).

In response to some unknown stimulus a number of the merozoites released after erythrocytic schizogony develop into male and female forms known as *gametocytes*. Gametocytes are believed to be inert in man. They provide the reservoir of infection enabling mosquitos to perpetuate the malaria cycle, and remain within the red cell for the duration of their survival, i.e., up to 120 days.

A certain proportion of the merozoites liberated from the cryptozoic schizonts of the pre-erythrocytic phase, do *not* enter the blood stream but re-enter the parenchymal cells of the liver to produce the secondary or meta-cryptozoic schizonts which are responsible for the persistence of the *exo-erythrocytic cycle*. (EE) The re-appearance of malaria after clinical cure results from the parasite's ability to persist in the tissues in this (EE) form. The eventual discharge of merozoites from these EE forms into the blood stream, results in reinvasion of red blood cells so producing a relapse. The exo-erythrocytic cycle occurs in *P. vivax*, *P. ovale* and *P. malariae* infections. *P. vivax* can usually produce relapses up to 3 years after infection; while *P. malariae* has occasionally relapsed 10, 20, or even 30 years after a primary infection. Patients suffering from *P. ovale* malaria have recently been seen in Europe and the United States of America. All the infections were contracted in West Africa and relatively long periods of latency were noticed. The infections were of considerable severity but spontaneous recovery was the rule (Zuidema and Meuwissen, 1966). The mechanism of malaria relapse was studied by Contacos and Collins (1973). In *P. falciparum* malaria the liver phase is said not to persist, it follows therefore that when adequate treatment for the erythrocytic cycle is given relapses do not occur. It is therefore rare for *P. falciparum* infections to relapse after 1 year of freedom from exposure to infection, although a few authentic cases with long intervals prior to relapse have been described (Verdrager, 1964). Enzyme typing of malaria parasites (Carter and Voller, 1973) has demonstrated variations in *P. falciparum* in Gambia (Carter and McGregor, 1973).

Malaria pigment is derived from the haemoglobin of the invaded red cell and is composed of haem plus denatured protein (Deegan and Maegraith, 1956). It is discussed in some detail later.

Epidemiology

The effect that malaria exerts on any population is largely governed by its epidemiological pattern. In this respect we shall consider two epidemiological extremes—stable and unstable malaria. The salient differences are shown below (MacDonald, 1957).

Stable malaria	Unstable malaria
1. Transmission occurs throughout the year. Fairly uniform intensity of transmission. Pattern repeats itself annually with astonishing regularity, showing little variation over several years.	Transmission seasonal—intensity of transmission variable. Liable to flare up into dramatic epidemics.
2. Potent resistance in the community due to prevailing intense transmission.	General lack of immunity in the community due to the low level of transmission, which only occasionally becomes intense.
3. Main impact of disease in young children.	Impact of disease on all age groups.
4. Difficult to eradicate.	Eradicated with greater ease than stable malaria.
5. Classical areas where it occurs— West Africa, Lowlands of New Guinea.	Classical areas—high plateau of Ethiopia or Highlands of New Guinea.

The natural history of 'stable' malaria can be divided for convenience into several distinct and successive stages of the host–malarial parasite relationship (Gilles, 1967). There is a first phase of transient resistance to infection immediately after birth and this lasts for a few months. Four main hypotheses have been formulated to explain this relative resistance of the new-born infant to malarial infection (Gilles, 1957). These are (1) transplacental acquisition of humoral immunity from the mother, (2) low levels of para-amino benzoic acid in exclusively maternal milk diets, (3) selective vector biting, and (4) the presence of a high concentration of fetal haemoglobin. It is now quite clear that the most important factor in producing this early resistance to infection is the passive transfer of protective antibodies from the mother contained in the 7S γ-globulin fraction (IgG) of the serum. This explains why the first infection with *P. falciparum* in infants born of immune mothers is generally associated with a low grade parasitaemia and very mild clinical symptoms (Garnham, 1949).

The second phase coincides with the period when inherited antibodies are exhausted and acquired immunity has not yet developed. This stage starts at 6 months and lasts up to 3 to 5 years. It is during this period that the clinical effects are severe with a mortality estimated at between 5–15 per cent.

From 5 years onwards the effects of acquired immunity become increasingly apparent, clinical manifestations become progressively milder and a considerable degree of antiparasitic immunity occurs with suppression of the high levels of parasitaemia associated with the second phase. The duration of each stage in the sequence is dependent on local conditions, being most compressed (as short as 3 years) in areas where transmission is perennially intense, availability of antimalarial drugs is negligible, and no attempts at malaria control have been made. It is more widely spread (up to 8 years) in developed urban areas. It follows that in older children and adults morbidity due to malaria is low and its mortality negligible.

The level of endemicity of malaria in a community is measured by clinical and by entomological techniques. The former determine parasite rates in random blood samples and spleen indices. In areas of stable malaria a close correlation exists between parasite and spleen rates (Fig. 2.1); this close correspondence is however occasionally absent, e.g. in New Guinea (Metselaar, 1956).

The epidemiology of *P. malariae* infection is described on p. 627.

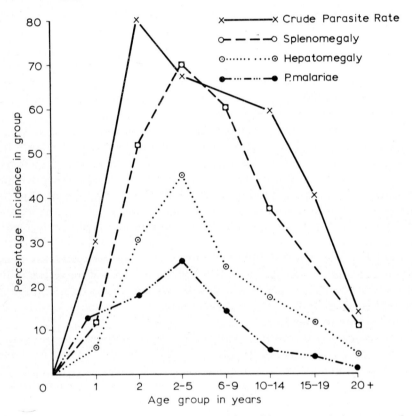

FIG. 2.1. Prevalence of malaria splenomegaly and hepatomegaly in an area of stable malaria (rural village population 1500 persons).

Immunity

This can be considered under four main headings: (a) Cellular, (b) Humoral, (c) Inherited factors in the blood, and (d) Racial.

Cellular

The response of phagocytic cells in malaria was shown in early histological studies and for many years resistance to the disease was considered to be exclusively cellular in nature. The reticulo-endothelial system undergoes intense proliferation during malarial infection and the macrophages of the spleen, liver, and bone marrow have been shown to phagocytose parasitized and unparasitized erythrocytes, isolated parasites and malarial pigment. In areas of stable malaria, large amounts of this pigment are continuously being engulfed by the reticulo-endothelial system over periods of years and the part that this possible 'blockade' plays in the immunological mechanism of the host, both in the fields of infection and malignancy, has still to be elucidated. It has been shown that peripheral blood lymphocytes from patients partially immune to P. falciparum transform to blast forms when cultured in vitro with P. falciparum extracts. Lymphocytes from uninfected persons were unaffected (Kass et al. 1971). Phillips et al. (1970) focus attention on possible cell-mediated immune mechanisms in P. Knowlesi malaria.

Humoral

Recent studies have demonstrated and stressed the importance of humoral immunity. Several workers have demonstrated that the concentration of gamma globulin in the serum of the new-born African infant is considerably higher than corresponding values reported from Europe. It was further shown that, in 'stable' areas, malarial infection contributes significantly to the maintenance of high γ-globulin levels in all subjects after the first year of life, (Gilles and McGregor, 1959 and 1961; McGregor and Gilles, 1960); and moreover that γ-globulin prepared from the sera of adults immune to malaria has a consistent therapeutic effect when administered to West African children suffering from heavy P. falciparum infection. Serum from the cord blood of infants born of immune mothers has a similar effect. It is now generally accepted that acquired malarial immunity is basically dependent upon the presence of circulating antibody which is associated with the 7S γ-globulin fraction (IgG) of serum (Cohen et al. 1961; Edozien et al. (1962). Greenwood (1974) has discussed the possible role of a B-cell mitogen in the hypergammaglobulinaemia associated with malaria and trypanosomiasis. An indirect fluorescent antibody technique has been evolved which has demonstrated the presence of malarial antibodies in the sera of infected persons (Tobie and Coatney, 1961; Voller and Bray, 1962); while Desowitz and Saave (1965) showed that an indirect haemagglutination test could serve as a measure of protective immunity. The fluorescent antibody technique has also revealed that a number of different species of mammalian plasmodia possess common antigens (Collins *et al.* 1966). This is of interest in view of the finding that East African strains of *P. falciparum* were found to be responsive to treatment with 'immune' West African γ-globulin (McGregor *et al.* 1964). In contrast Sadun *et al.* (1966) reported that gamma globulin from West Africa failed to show marked protective activity in chimpanzees infected with a drug-resistant strain of falciparum malaria from South East Asia. McGregor *et al.* (1966) used antigens prepared from the blood of children to demonstrate, by gel-diffusion techniques, the existence of precipitating antibodies in the serum of immune patients.

McGregor and Wilson (1971) and Wilson *et al.* (1973) described three main types of *P. falciparum* antigens, L (labile), R (resistant), and S (stable) by investigating their storage properties. Butcher and Cohen (1972) showed that chronic malarial infection lead to synthesis of antibodies with wide cross-reactivity, and felt that this may be encouraging from the point of view of malaria vaccine production.

It is probable that the two mechanisms of defence in malaria, the cellular (through the reticulo-endothelial system) and the humoral (through the 7S γ-globulin (IgG) are inter-dependent (McGregor, 1974).

Inherited factors in the blood

It has been postulated that the following hereditary red cell traits protect against the lethal effects of malaria: (1) haemoglobin S, (2) haemoglobin C, (3) haemoglobin E, (4) thalassaemia, (5) glucose-6-phosphate dehydrogenase deficiency. The only convincing evidence to date concerns sickle-cell haemoglobin, and possibly G-6-Pd deficiency (p. 465).

Racial

It has long been known that Negroes in the U.S.A. had a vivax infection rate lower than that of whites and that it was more difficult to infect them with this species in the course of malarial therapy. The most evident consequence of resistance to *P. vivax* in Negroes occurs in West Africa, where, in many regions, it cannot be found in the indigenous population; yet the parasite is common in the inhabitants of the Eastern Congo and East Africa. Whether this *racial* difference is related to the genetic conditions mentioned above or not, is unknown.

General pathology

The pathological changes occurring in malaria can be described as those caused by the parasite itself, those due to the reaction of the host, and finally by the effect of the infection on individual organs.

(a) The role of the malaria parasite

It has already been shown that the developing trophozoite depends upon the host for its nutritional requirements. It follows, therefore, that the development of the parasite must in part depend on successful competition with the host for certain substances required equally by both. The possible effects of this on the host/parasite relationships are discussed later.

Changes in the red cell, and particularly changes in its surface have been described in malaria. Thus a reduction in the electrical charge on the surface of both parasitized and unparasitized erythrocytes has been demonstrated in bird malaria. The ultrastructure of the red cell infected with *P. malariae* has been described by Smith and Theakston (1970). All parasitized cells were covered with small symmetrical tubercules. Such appearances have not been described previously in the red cells of man and no attempt was made to interpret the findings. Direct observation of the circulation in severe malaria has shown that, at a certain stage of the infection, a substance, which has been identified as fibrin, appears as a fine precipitate around the erythrocytes. The appearance of this substance is followed by clumping of the erythrocytes into what is described as a 'sludge', which interferes with the passage of blood through the finer blood vessels. It was also noted that red cells coated with the precipitated 'fibrin' become sticky to macrophages, the appearance of the precipitate coinciding with avid phagocytosis of both parasitized and unparasitized cells. Sheagren *et al.* (1970) have shown by utilizing the rate of clearance of ^{125}I labelled microaggregated human serum albumin that in acute malaria enhanced phagocytosis is present.

The cause of the pyrexia in malaria is obscure and various factors including sensitivity to the released merozoites, the sudden release of potassium, haemozoin, and cell debris have all been considered in this connection. Dunn (1969) has shown in Rhesus monkeys that red blood cell sodium is significantly increased in *Plasmodium knowlesi* infection. Cellular potassium is decreased in proportion to the elevation of sodium. It is also possible that pyrexia develops as a sensitivity reaction to parasite protein which is released together with the residual body (Peters, 1965). No satisfactory evidence has as yet been produced to show that the parasite produces a toxin, although studies have demonstrated the presence of a factor circulating in the blood of monkeys infected with *P. knowlesi* malaria which can at times inhibit the respiration and oxidative phosphorylation of normal mitochondria (Maegraith, 1966; Fletcher and Maegraith, 1972).

The production of malaria pigment—(haemozoin)

It is usually stated that, in malaria, two types of pigment are found, namely haemozoin formed by the parasite, and haemosiderin formed in the reticulo-endothelial cells of the host by the breakdown of haemoglobin liberated from the erythrocyte during the haemolytic process. Haemosiderin deposition in the organs is therefore a non-specific finding in malaria and it is discussed when the changes in the individual organs are considered.

It has been shown that as the parasite grows in the erythrocyte, there is a drastic reduction in the haemoglobin content and pigment (haemozoin) appears in the parasite itself. Haemozoin is an iron porphyrin proteinoid complex formed by the trophozoite from the breakdown of the haemoglobin of the host cell (Sherman *et al.* 1965). It is a grey black pigment (dark brown on microscopy) insoluble in acids, and it is seen as granules or masses in the developing trophozoites and schizonts and, following release on red cell rupture, in the monocytes and other reticulo-endothelial cells of the host. It does not give the Prussian blue reaction; it can be removed from tissue sections by a saturated alcoholic solution of picric acid and it cannot be differentiated from formalin pigment by histochemical methods. If the presence of malaria is suspected in biopsy or necropsy material a non-form-alin-containing fluid should therefore be used for fixation prior to embedding or sectioning. The character and amount of pigment produced vary with the species of parasite. Pigment is not considered an important factor in tissue injury. The method of disposal of haemozoin by the host has not been determined. It is thought unlikely that its iron-containing portion is made available for haemoglobin synthesis. It has been shown that chloroquine-resistant trophozoites of *P. berghei* do not form typical grains of haemozoin (Peters *et al.* 1965); in contrast pigment formation is normal in chloroquine-resistant parasites of *P. falciparum* (Mcnamara *et al.* 1967). Peters *et al.* (1973) have carried out a series of studies on the dynamics of drug resistance in *P. berghei* malaria.

(b) Host reaction

It is not easy to relate the presence of the malaria parasite within the erythrocyte to the varied remote pathological processes in the host. Thus, general circulatory disturbances resulting in the development of malarial shock and its associated phenomena have been described in *P. falciparum* infections (algid malaria). Of a more local nature, we have the failure of renal blood flow with consequent urinary suppression and uraemia, and the changes in the liver circulation partly due to dynamic interference with intralobular blood flow, leading in some patients to relative centrilobular haemostasis (Maegraith, 1966). The deficient circulation of the blood is further embarrassed by the 'stickiness' of the parasitized red cells and the late-developing 'sludging' of the circulating erythrocytes. The patho-physiology of severe malaria is therefore basically the result of a regional upset of the microcirculation, especially in the brain, liver, lungs and kidneys. This failure of the microcirculation causes damage to the vascular endo-thelium with resulting oedema of the target organs. Parasitised red blood cells lose their deformability and 'log-jam' the microcirculation. Micro-vascular coagulation may be an important pathogenic factor in some cases of severe falciparum malaria, though it might be a protective mechanism, preventing haemorrhage from damaged microvessels (Reid and Nkrumah 1972). Other important factors of the pathophysiology of malaria have been fully described by Maegraith and Fletcher (1972). The effects of these many dynamic changes will become evident when the pathology of the individual organs is described.

Little is known of the possible relationship between nutritional status of the host, concurrent infections with other organisms, and malaria. With regard to the nutrition of the host, it has been stated that malaria may become virulent and epidemics are more likely in malnourished populations. This would not be in accordance with our experience in an area of 'stable' falciparum malaria where death from cerebral malaria or malarial anaemia usually occurs in the well-nourished child and very rarely, if at all, in the marasmic or kwashiorkor patient. This observation has been confirmed by Hendrickse et al. (1971). It is interesting to speculate whether the deficiency of essential amino acids and other factors in these children might inhibit the development of severe infection, as has been shown to occur in rat malaria (Platt, 1958).

Apart from malnutrition, the pre-school child in the tropics is attacked by a bewildering variety of infections with protozoa, helminths, bacteria, and viruses. The 'crowding out' of an antibody response has long been known to occur if an antigen is injected into an animal when active production of another antibody is taking place. It is possible, therefore, that the immune response to malarial infection might be temporarily suppressed during the periods of heavy infection with other organisms. The converse has already been demonstrated, namely that the proportion of antibody responders following tetanus toxoid inoculation is significantly lower in malarious than in non-malarious African children (McGregor and Barr, 1962). Greenwood et al. (1972) have shown that children with acute malaria had a diminished antibody response to the O antigen of S. typhi and to tetanus toxoid. Their cellular immune responses were normal.

The possible effect of other infections on morbidity and mortality in children in areas of stable malaria is discussed later.

Pathology of the individual organs

In the non-immune, death from malaria is almost always due to *P. falciparum* infection; deaths from *P. vivax* infection occasionally occur but there is little information on their pathology in the literature. It is doubtful if *P. malariae* or *P. ovale* ever directly cause fatalities. This last statement may, however, require modification as it is possible that *P. malariae* may be concerned in the production of renal disease causing death in cardio-renal failure in older children and young adults. This parasite has also been implicated as a possible factor in the idiopathic tropical spleno-megaly syndrome (p. 492).

With these two exceptions the following description of the pathology of malaria in the various organs refers mainly to the changes seen in *P. falciparum* infections. The pathological changes seen are of three types, namely: (1) acute lesions responsible for death in the non-immune, (2) changes occurring in the organs of the partially immune child who has died from other causes, and (3) changes occurring in the organs of individuals suffering from untreated repeated attacks of malaria.

In spite of the many forms of pernicious malaria described in the literature, death from *P. falciparum* in individuals living in areas of stable malaria, in which most of our experience has been gained, is either due to cerebral malaria or malarial anaemia, whereas deaths in non-immune U.S. Army personnel in Vietnam were associated with acute renal insufficiency, cerebral malaria and pulmonary oedema (Canfield, 1969).

Death has been reported however in association with medical shock (algid malaria), renal failure with or without haemoglobinuria, severe diarrhoea (choleraic malaria), hepatic failure (bilious remittent fever), and hyperpyrexia (Maegraith, 1948).

In an area of stable malaria it is relatively easy at autopsy to decide if malaria is the direct cause of death, but it is almost impossible in some children to assess the importance of malaria as an indirect causal factor. At necropsy, in these children, malarial pigment is normally found in large amounts in the cells of the reticulo-endothelial system and parasites may be found in smears from the brain and spleen. Frequently bronchopneumonia, protein malnutrition, ascariasis and malaria infection of varying severity may be present in one subject. With such findings it is difficult to assess the relative importance of these conditions in causing death. This problem does not arise in older children and adults, as the amount of haemozoin present in the organs is small or there may be none. In general it can be said that we have never attributed death to malaria in the absence of evidence of a heavy parasitaemia or of cerebral lesions which will be described later.

An attempt has therefore been made to differentiate the lesions seen in these varying manifestations of malaria when the changes in the individual organs are discussed below.

The central nervous system

The most severe lesions in the central nervous system are seen in cerebral malaria due to *P. falciparum* infection. Although changes have been reported in the spinal cord and peripheral nerves the most marked changes are seen in the brain itself. Headache, irritability, hyperpyrexia, convulsions and coma are concomitant clinical findings, and electroencephalogram abnormalities have been recorded (Nouhouayi, 1967).

The meninges are grossly congested, the smaller vessels being packed with parasitized cells. A perivascular lymphocytic infiltration has been described but this is rare in our experience. The brain itself may show gross congestion only, but it is usually leaden in colour—the smaller vessels of the grey matter being packed with red cells containing pigmented parasites in all stages of development. Gross congestion of the vessels is invariable, and in the majority of instances numerous petechial haemorrhages are evident in the white matter of the cerebrum, brain stem and cerebellum (Fig. 2.2).

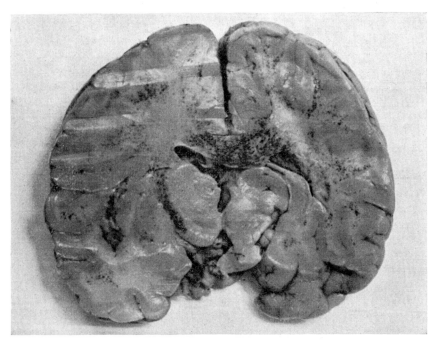

FIG. 2.2. Cerebral malaria. Showing numerous petechial haemorrhages scattered throughout the white matter of the brain. (*By courtesy Ann. trop. Med. Parasit.*)

Haemorrhages are not usually seen in the grey matter although they can occur there; this lesser liability to haemorrhage is thought to be due to the greater number of capillaries and anastomatic channels in this area of the brain as compared with the white matter. Histologically the capillaries and arterioles are packed with parasitized cells, and ring haemorrhages are a striking feature. These consist of a central 'blocked' vessel (most frequently an arteriole), containing an agglutinated mass of parasitized erythrocytes surrounded by brain tissue, and then by a ring of extravasated red blood cells (Fig. 2.3). Although parasites are said not to be found in these haemorrhages they are present at the periphery in some of our material.

In older haemorrhages necrosis of the midzonal brain tissue occurs, and there is a peripheral reaction of small glial cells—the so-called malarial granuloma. Healing is said to cause subsequent scarring possibly with residual brain damage; this, however, has not yet been convincingly proved.

Death can occur in cerebral malaria with few parasites in the majority of the cerebral vessels. In these cases parasitized erythrocytes have been seen in the central vessels or in the erythrocytes in the ring haemorrhage, and a history of treatment prior to death has usually been obtained.

In deaths due to malarial anaemia there is pallor of the brain and its coverings, the vessels are empty and pigment has not been seen in the endothelial cells of the vessels.

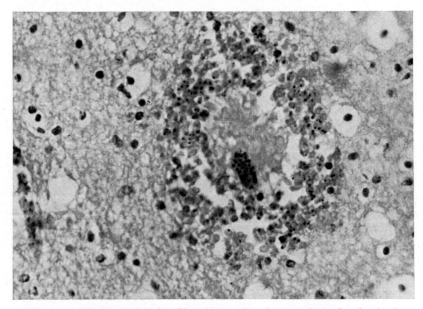

FIG. 2.3. Cerebral malaria. Showing a ring haemorrhage in the brain. Blocked capillaries can be distinguished in lesions (× 320).

The actual mechanism of the changes seen in the brain is controversial but the lesions can best be described as vascular and haemorrhagic leading to degeneration of brain cells and tissue, and subsequently a cellular reaction. Maegraith (1948) has emphasized that similar lesions may be seen in hyperthermia, mechanical interference with blood flow, and in certain types of narcotic poisoning. He has postulated that anoxia and probably hypoglycaemia are important underlying factors. It would appear to us that his explanation of the initial lesion being sludging of blood and stasis, with local anoxaemia causing changes in the endothelial cells, would adequately explain the histological changes and clinical symptoms. These changes are followed by loss of intravascular fluid causing further slowing of the blood stream, haemorrhage eventually occurring through the damaged vessel wall. It is conceivable, however, that the sludging is secondary to damage of the mitochondria in brain capillary endothelium and consequent loss of fluid into the pericapillary tissues. It has recently been postulated that intravascular coagulation may play an important role in the pathogenesis of cerebral lesions and a precipitous fall in plasma fibrinogen, suggesting intravascular coagulation, has been demonstrated in two patients with cerebral malaria (Devakul et al. 1966). We have also demonstrated strands of fibrin by Gram Weigert's stain in the brain capillaries in patients dying of cerebral malaria (Figs. 2.4 and 2.5).

Degeneration of brain cells and tissue occurs in areas of local ischaemia, and in these areas subsequent chromatolysis and neuronal degeneration have been described. It is postulated that eventually a glial reaction occurs with healing by scar tissue formation.

Changes in the reticulo-endothelial system and blood-forming organs

The changes in the reticulo-endothelial system are discussed when the individual organs are considered and are, briefly, those due to immunological processes with changes in the serum protein values, and those due to the presence of a haemolytic anaemia.

Anaemia

Most of the factors responsible for malarial anaemia are ill understood. Nevertheless, the following points are established: (1) parasitized and unparasitized cells are phagocytosed and destroyed; (2) anaemia is not necessarily related to the degree of parasitaemia; (3) transfused cells in a malarial patient may be destroyed more rapidly than in a normal recipient; (4) there is a fall in complement during the acute attack; (5) in animals malarial antigens alone, in the absence of infection, may adversely affect the

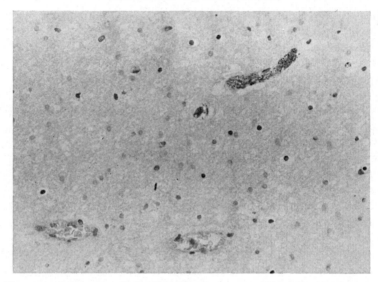

FIG. 2.4. Cerebral malaria. A capillary is shown containing pigmented parasites and strands of fibrin. Two larger cerebral vessels contain normal red cells and no fibrin (Gram-Weigert × 135).

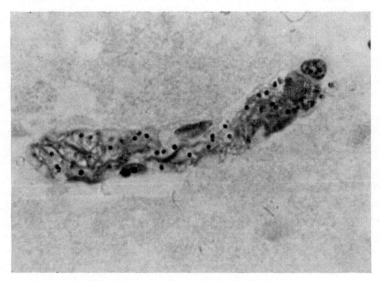

FIG. 2.5. Cerebral malaria. Capillary in centre of cerebral haemorrhage showing strands of fibrin and malarial pigment (Gram-Weigert × 250).

red cells (Zuckerman, 1963); (6) fluorescent antibody techniques will differentially stain malarial parasites, Schuffner's dots, and Maurer's clefts (Tobie and Coatney, 1961; Voller and Bray, 1962); (7) corticosteroid therapy may prove of value in blackwater fever; and (8) there may be a marrow–peripheral blood barrier (Thonnard-Neumann, 1944).

In the acute stage there may be few changes in the morphology of the red cell other than those changes initiated by the parasite itself. In other instances, however, anaemia may be marked and the findings in the peripheral blood thus depend upon the duration and stage of the infection. It must be remembered that malaria is a potent cause of severe anaemia in children from the age of 6 months to at least 3 years in areas of stable malaria and it may be sufficiently acute and severe as to cause death.

The anaemia is haemolytic and in the acute attack there may be a sudden and dramatic fall in the haemoglobin values of the blood. It is usually normocytic and normochromic, or hypochromic but macrocytic if there is a marked reticulocytosis or if folic-acid deficiency eventuates—a not uncommon complication in tropical areas. The causes of folic acid deficiency in such patients are multiple: (1) inadequate dietary folate; (2) reduced absorption of folic acid; (3) increased utilization due to haemolysis and fever of malaria; and (4) possible drug inhibition by antimalarial chemotherapy (Strickland and Nostinazi, 1970). The peripheral blood film shows many parasites, polychromasia, anisocytosis, poikilocytosis, target cells, basophilic stippling and, in severe cases, Cabot's rings, Howel Jolly bodies, and nucleated red cells. A reticulocytosis may be present but this is more usual as a result of treatment. The indirect Coombs test is negative but occasionally a direct antiglobulin test of immunoglobin (Ig) G type may be positive (Adner et al. 1968). Leucocytosis may occur early and be followed by leucopenia and monocytosis. Even with a leucopenia, however, the polymorphonuclear leucocyte count shows a shift to the left. Rarely there may be haemozoin in the polymorphonuclear leucocytes, but it is very commonly present in the monocytes. The platelets are diminished (Sodeman and Jeffery, 1966) and there is a depletion of the labile coagulation factors (V and VIII) and accumulation of fibrinogen degradation products in the blood (Dennis et al. 1966). Dennis et al. (1967) have shown in United States army personnel suffering from drug-resistant P. falciparum malaria that there is accelerated intravenous coagulation with thrombocytopenia and a prolonged prothrombin time. There was a decrease in multiple coagulation factors and in plasminogen deficiency. An accumulation of fibrinogen breakdown products in the blood was noted. On the other hand it has been shown that significant thrombocytopenia can occur without evidence of intravascular coagulation. Heparin therefore should only be utilized in therapy after clotting factors have been shown to be depleted.

There are probably two mechanisms responsible for the thrombocytopenia:
  (1) consumption coagulopathy and
  (2) phagocytosis by the reticulo-endothelial system. There is also, of
      course, the possibility of failure of release from the marrow (Beale
      et al. 1972).

A severe haemorrhagic diathesis may occur due to a defibrination syndrome
perhaps due to the stimulation of fibrinolytic activity secondary to the generalized intravascular coagulation. There is excessive breakdown of haemoglobin
to its component parts, globin, bilirubin and iron moieties; the iron and globin are stored and re-utilized. The pre-hepatic haemobilirubin, which is
alcohol soluble and of large molecular weight (unconjugated), increases in the
blood, giving a positive indirect van den Bergh reaction. There is increased
secretion of cholebilirubin in the bile with production of excess urobilinogen
in the faeces, and increased absorption by the blood and thus increased
urobilinogen in the urine. If liver function is interfered with, as in the
bilious remittent type of pernicious malaria, there may be an increase
of cholebilirubin (water soluble, conjugated bilirubin) in the blood, giving
a biphasic van den Bergh reaction, and bile may be present in the urine.
This, in our experience, is rare. In contrast to blackwater fever there is
usually an absence of significant amounts of haemoglobin and methaemalbumin in the serum.

In addition to haemozoin which has been previously discussed, haemosiderin, a dark yellow trivalent iron-containing pigment, is formed in the
reticulo-endothelial system from the breakdown of haemoglobin contained
in red cell debris liberated during schizogony, from senescent and parasitized
cells, and from unparasitized cells haemolysed or phagocytosed during the
acute attack. It is deposited mainly in the spleen, liver and marrow. This
pigment can be differentiated from haemozoin in tissue in that it gives a
positive Prussian blue reaction. It may, however, be absent in malaria in man
and it has been noted to vary inversely with the amount of haemozoin
produced in laboratory animals (Allen et al. 1960). These findings suggest
that the haemosiderin formed by the reticulo-endothelial system from the
breakdown of haemoglobin is immediately available and is re-utilized in the
synthesis of the large amounts of haemoglobin necessitated by the haemolytic
process.

Bone marrow

The bone marrow is greyish red, soft and hyperaemic and is increased in
the long bones. In the acute stage its vessels are full of parasitized erythrocytes and haemozoin is present in the reticulo-endothelial cells and monocytes. There is a marked normoblastic hyperplasia even in the absence of a
reticulocytosis in the peripheral blood and there is also myelocytic prolifer-

ation (Russell *et al.* 1963). Some authors, however, have demonstrated a temporary inhibition of the marrow during parasitaemia (Srichaikul *et al.* 1967). Megaloblastic change may result if folic-acid deficiency occurs.

The spleen

In the acute attack the spleen is enlarged, and tense, and the cut surface is slaty greyish red with the malpighian corpuscles prominent. The consistency may be soft if a terminal bronchopneumonia is present. Histologically the blood vessels, Billroth cords, and sinusoids are filled with parasitized red cells. Parasitized and unparasitized cells and haemozoin are seen in the pulp histiocytes and sinusoidal lining cells. Pigment may be found lying free in the pulp and sinusoids, and in our experience it is also found in the germinal follicles. A splenic smear reveals developing forms of parasites and haemozoin lying free and contained in monocytes. Degeneration of the endothelial cells of splenic vessels may occur causing thrombosis, haemorrhage and infarction.

With increasing immunity the spleen becomes at first jet black with much pigment in the cords, but gradually the congestion decreases and the pigment disappears first from the sinusoids and last from the cords with parasitized cells becoming scanty. The spleen diminishes in size, the capsule becomes greyish, fibrotic, and wrinkled, perhaps with some evidence of old-standing perisplentitis, and some fibrosis is seen in the pulp.

In a proportion of adults in stable areas, however, the spleen does remain palpable—more frequently in females. At present the reason for this persisting splenomegaly is obscure, but it is probably related to an inadequate or altered immunological response to the infection. It is not clear if this type of splenomegaly is in any way related to idiopathic tropical splenomegaly which is discussed separately in Chapter 10.

Rupture of the spleen is a not uncommon complication of malaria and usually occurs through the hilar region. It should be emphasized that, if such an accident occurs and splenectomy is performed for this or any other reason in an immune individual living in an area of stable malaria, continuous suppressive antimalarial therapy must be considered to prevent the possible development of a severe malarial infection. We have seen death from cerebral malaria in only one Nigerian adult and this occurred in a patient suffering from chronic lymphatic leukaemia in whom splenectomy had been performed sometime previously, and in whom the possible consequent development of a severe malarial infection had not been considered.

The liver

The pathological changes in the liver vary according to the immunological status of the individual and the mode of death. In cerebral malaria the liver is enlarged and tense and its colour varies from dark red to slaty grey. If, however, anaemia has been gross the liver is enlarged and pale yellowish grey in colour.

Histologically the striking feature in the acute stage is the gross congestion of the sinusoids and centrilobular veins by parasitized erythrocytes. The Kupffer cells are hypertrophied and contain parasitized and unparasitized red blood cells, remnants of parasites and granules and masses of haemozoin, with haemosiderin inconstantly present. The parenchymal cells may contain haemosiderin but never haemozoin. One of the most striking and constantly reported features has been degeneration and necrosis in the centrilobular regions in the absence of heart failure—a feature which has not been noticeable in our experience of autopsies on children dying of cerebral malaria in West Africa (Edington, 1954). Various theories have been advanced to explain these centrilobular changes, but it would appear that, as they can occur without evidence of heart failure and, in blackwater fever, with relatively few parasites present, as well as in other acute infective processes, they are most probably due to local stagnation of circulation in the central lobular zones which depends to some extent on hypersentivity of the sympathetic nervous system (Skirrow and Maegraith, 1964). A mild lymphocytic infiltration may be present in the portal tracts. Voller *et al.* (1970) have reported a sinusoidal lymphocytosis similar to that which occurs in the tropical splenomegaly syndrome (p. 492) in a small proportion of rhesus monkeys infected with malaria. If death has been due to anaemia the centrilobular veins and sinusoids are dilated and contain few cells, the Kupffer cells showing a picture similar to that already described.

In that age group in which immunity to *P. falciparum* is developing the liver at autopsy is usually enlarged, pale or congested, and the greyish-black portal tracts stand out prominently. Histologically a considerable degree of sinusoidal congestion may be present varying according to the degree of anaemia and the ultimate cause of death.

Haemozoin is now concentrated in the Kupffer cells in the periportal regions and also is found in histiocytes or lying free in the portal tracts, in contrast to the diffuse distribution in the Kupffer cells seen throughout the lobule in the acute phase. Such a histopathological picture of pigment at the periphery of the lobule and in the portal tracts is constantly seen in the young school child in areas of stable malaria, and it is indicative of a degree of immunity. In these children the parasite densities are decreasing and the pigmented parasites and released pigment in the portal and hepatic blood appear to be contained at the periphery of the lobule, the Kupffer cells in the centrilobular regions being relatively free from pigment.

With increasing immunity the amount of haemozoin in the hepatic reticulo-endothelial cells gradually decreases, until with established immunity none may be detectable. The portal tracts may show a more marked cellular infiltration in these older children—mainly lymphocytic—and mild fibrosis has been reported. This, however, is inconstant and malaria is not now considered a possible aetiological agent in the cirrhosis of the liver which is so commonly seen in many parts of the tropics.

From the foregoing it will be obvious that there may be derangement of liver function tests. In the acute attack there may be bromsulphthalein retention, positive flocculation tests and some evidence of biliary obstruction (this last finding, however, being uncommon). The chronic bilious remittent type of *P. falciparum* malaria is, as previously mentioned, rare in our experience.

Lowering of the albumin and fibrinogen levels in the blood are also found in malaria.

The kidneys

Excluding the lesions seen in the nephrotic syndrome associated with *P. malariae* infection and blackwater fever, which are dealt with separately, the descriptions of pathological lesions seen in the kidney in malarial infections would appear to be variable. Similarly the number of patients showing proteinuria in recorded series has varied from 1 to 75 per cent.

In our experience, in cerebral malaria the striking feature is gross congestion of the vessels with parasitized erythrocytes—especially in the capillaries of the glomerular tuft. Acute renal failure with oliguria and urea retention, has, however, been described (Jackson and Woodruff, 1962; Reid *et al.* 1967) and the pathogenesis of this lesion is discussed when the pathology of blackwater fever is considered. Renal failure of short duration has been observed in patients with heavy infection of *P. falciparum*. This was associated with a low urine sodium, a retained ability of tubular reabsorption of water, a decrease in endogenous creatinine and *p*-amino-hippurate clearances. Renal biopsy showed focal vacuolization of the proximal convoluted tubules but no other abnormalities (Sitprija *et al.* 1967).

Acute diffuse glomerulo-nephritis has been described in association with *P. falciparum* malaria. This is a rare complication, but cannot be entirely dismissed at present as we have seen haemozoin in the mesangial cells of the glomeruli in two patients with a proliferative nephritis. Berger *et al.* (1967) have reported the occurrence of the nephrotic syndrome due to a proliferative glomerulonephritis in 2 per cent of non-immune military personnel suffering from *P. falciparum*. Further investigations are required to determine the significance of these findings. Pigment has been described in vessels, free in the interstitial tissue, occasionally in the epithelial cells of the tubules, and within phagocytes in the capsular spaces. It has also been described in both the epithelial and endothelial cells of the glomeruli. Hyaline, epithelial, and granular casts may be present in the tubules. Scattered small haemorrhages may be seen in the cortex and medulla.

Macroscopically, in the acute stage, the kidneys are usually slightly enlarged and usually congested. Punctate haemorrhages may be present in the pelvis, the cortex, and medulla.

In the chronic stages the description of the kidney has varied from the large white to the small granular contracted kidney and it is considered that these descriptions most probably refer to renal conditions associated with *P. malariae* infections. Certainly in an area of stable malaria there is no convincing evidence to date that *P. falciparum* is involved in chronic renal disease.

In acute diffuse glomerulo-nephritis the incidence and densities of *P. falciparum* infection are similar to those found in comparable age groups of the population and the incidence of chronic glomerulo-nephritis in post mortem material would not suggest that a parasite as commonly found as *P. falciparum* was playing a part in its aetiology.

To sum up, excluding renal disease associated with *P. malariae* infection and blackwater fever, in malaria tubular necrosis may occasionally occur and a proliferative nephritis may rarely occur. The renal lesions responsible for the variable proteinuria which occurs are obscure and may be related to capillary basement membrane changes in the glomeruli. Blackwater fever and the nephrotic syndrome associated with *P. malariae* are discussed on p. 463 and p. 627 respectively.

Adrenals

Changes in the adrenals are variable. Degenerative and necrotic changes in the inner zone of the cortex with loss of lipid have been described. The more usual finding, however, is gross congestion and haemorrhage which could explain the clinical manifestations associated with algid malaria. The pathological changes in the adrenals are associated with disturbances of physiological function, such as depression of the secretion of adreno-cortical hormones, disturbances of water–salt balance and variations in secretion of adrenalin. An Addisonian-like syndrome with asthenia, hypotension, peripheral vascular collapse and digestive disturbances has been described but this is rare in our experience.

Overt symptoms of malaria in the immune adult are said to be precipitated by surgical operations, anaesthesia, or any other form of stress. In our experience in an area of stable malaria no convincing evidence in support of this finding has been obtained. The administration of steroids in animal malaria results in a marked increase in parasitaemia possibly due to suppression of the immunological response, and this has also been shown to occur in human malaria. Although steroid therapy has been given fairly frequently in Ibadan without antimalarial cover, no exacerbation of clinical malaria has been observed.

The lungs

It is difficult to assign pathological changes in the lungs purely to malaria. There is no doubt, however, that clinical bronchitis and its complications are common in children with malaria. In the acute stages the smaller vessels are packed with parasitized erythrocytes and small haemorrhages may be present. Pneumonitis and bronchopneumonia are frequently concomitant findings. It is sometimes difficult to assess the relative responsibility of bronchopneumonia and malarial infection as the ultimate cause of death.

Deaton (1970) has described two patients dying of pulmonary oedema even although antimalarial therapy had cleared the parasitaemia and vigorous therapy was undertaken. The findings in the lung at autopsy in one case showed only pulmonary oedema with acute and subacute passive congestion. No parasitized erythrocytes were seen and no lesions were noticed in the heart of C.N.S. to account for death. The microscopy of the kidney was not reported. Overhydration did not appear to be a factor. Hyaline membrane formation, thickened alveolar septa and areas of alveolar haemorrhage have been noted in the lungs. The basic lesion appeared to be injury to the capillaries of the lung with congestion and leakage of oedema fluid. Giant nuclear masses have been reported in the lungs in malignant malaria (Goodall, 1974).

The cardiovascular system

In the acute stages there is the usual picture of vessels congested with parasitized erythrocytes in the heart. Small subendocardial haemorrhages may occur but are rare. In the more chronic stages fatty degeneration of the myofibrils and brown atrophy have been described but there is no evidence that malarial heart disease is an entity.

In severe malarial anaemia in children, the findings in the heart are not striking, the general effects being those of increase in blood volume and anoxia. The relative acuteness of the illness operates against the occurrence of dilatation or hypertrophy or marked changes in the myofibrils of the heart. Interstitial oedema is a frequent finding.

Gastro-intestinal tract

Congestion with capillary stasis, necrosis and haemorrhages can occur in the acute stages, and in the algid type of malaria extensive desquamation of the epithelium occurs. This type of malaria is rare in our experience, but there is no doubt that gastroenteritis is a common complication of malaria in children and that it clears rapidly on antimalarial therapy. Olson and Johnston (1969) have noticed impaired xylose absorption in acute falciparum malaria and jejunal biopsy revealed minimal vascular congestion and oedema of the lamina propria. These findings were thought to suggest that there may be decreased splanchnic blood flow, a finding which has been observed in simian-malaria models.

Malaria and pregnancy

Malaria surveys carried out in village communities, especially in Africa, have consistently revealed a higher parasitaemia in pregnancy and especially so in primigravidae (Gilles, 1967). An attenuation of malaria immunity during pregnancy has been postulated (Bruce-Chwatt, 1952) and it has been noted that splenomegaly is more frequently recorded in pregnant and non-pregnant women than in men in areas of stable malaria—a finding also suggestive of altered immunity in the adult female (Schofield, 1964).

Malaria in unstable areas is an important direct cause of maternal and fetal mortality. In our experience in stable areas, malaria is not a direct cause of maternal death, but anaemia in pregnancy is certainly a common cause of death, and malaria is considered to be indirectly related to the anaemia. Thus, Rosenberg et al. (1973) demonstrated rising titres of IgM antibodies to red cells and autoimmune anaemia in patients with falciparum malaria. Moreover, during pregnancy there is an increase in the frequency and severity of overt attacks of malaria (Gilles et al. 1969; Kortmann, 1972). Abortion and premature labour may be precipitated by the pyrexial episodes while the severe anaemia can cause stillbirths, and intra-uterine and neonatal deaths (Lawson and Stewart, 1967). The effect of placental parasitization on birth weight has been extensively studied (Archibald, 1956; Cannon, 1958) and a relationship has been established between the low birth weight of the African neonate and malarial infection of the placenta (Bruce-Chwatt, 1959). Placental parasitization is also responsible for stillbirths, and intra-uterine and neonatal deaths.

Developing trophozoites are numerous in the intervillous spaces and are found in the greatest numbers next to the trophoblast of the stratum spongiosium, and haemozoin may be seen within the fibrin masses, in some instances surrounding degenerate villi. It would appear that the 'stickier' parasitized cell tends to 'sludge' in the eddies of the slow-moving placental stream and, as pigment is seen in the fibrin, most probably favours fibrin deposition on the villi thus hastening the degenerative processes, interfering with the nutriment of the fetus and causing stillbirths and premature labour. There is an increase of cells—mainly histiocytes—in the maternal sinuses of the placenta (Blacklock and Gordon, 1925). The maternal blood in the intervillous spaces is high in glucose content—favouring the development of the parasite. Neither pigment nor parasites have been seen in the fetal vessels and congenital malaria only occurs in the neonates of unprotected susceptible immigrants from non-malarious areas, or in neonates of indigenous mothers in areas of unstable malaria.

Malaria and blood transfusion—see p. 481.

Diagnostic pathology

Malaria is one of the commonest causes of anaemia in young children living in 'stable' areas. The mechanism of the anaemia has already been discussed. With severe lysis, there may be haemoglobin and methaemalbumin in the plasma, and the plasma potassium may be raised. Sodium and chloride concentrations are low when vomiting and diarrhoea accompany the malaria attack. The blood sugar concentration varies in relation to the stage of infection, the most pronounced and progressive fall of blood sugar occurring shortly before death in association with very low liver glycogen content. The chemical findings in malaria are dependent on the state of the liver, kidney, and the water–electrolyte balance of the body.

A decrease in albumin concentrations and a rise in globulins, especially IgG and IgM immunoglobulins, occurs in acute malaria. Hepatic function tests are often abnormal (Deller *et al.* 1967). The urinary changes are variable. In the mild attacks of *P. falciparum* malaria, albuminuria with casts may be found. With advancing severity bilirubin may appear, the amount of urine decreases and complete suppression may occur. In this context it is important to record daily the fluid output and to measure the specific gravity of the urine and the plasma urea concentration. The urinary findings in the nephrotic syndrome associated with *P. malariae* will be described in Chapter 13.

The certain diagnosis of malaria is parasitological and is made by examining thick blood films stained with Field or Giemsa stains. Although species diagnosis can be made on thick films it is usually made on thin films stained with Leishman or Giemsa stains and depends on the characteristics mentioned in Table 2.1. As a rule only ring forms and gametocytes are found in the peripheral blood in falciparum malaria unless the infection is severe, in which case, schizonts also appear. In cases of vivax, malariae and ovale malaria all forms of the asexual parasites are found.

Zaman (1972) has used impregnated filter paper strips for staining malaria parasites; while Janis (1971) described a technique based on the fact that acridine orange selectivity stains nucleic acid. Sadun (1972) has reviewed the research and development of serologic tests for malaria while Eden *et al.* (1973) have looked into the feasibility of computer screening of blood films for the detection of malaria parasites.

BABESIOSIS

Piroplasms are widely distributed in cattle and dogs, their presence may present a hazard to splenectomized persons or to those whose splenic or immunological function is deficient (Garnham *et al.* 1969).

TABLE 2.1. *Differentiation of malarial parasites*

A. Thin film

	P. falciparum	*P. vivax*	*P. malariae*	*P. ovale*
Number and stages of parasites	Up to 15% or more of red cells infected—small rings and game-tocytes. Rarely schizonts	Rarely above 2% of red cells infected—all stages of parasite development seen	Usually less than 2% of red cells infected—all stages seen	As *P. vivax*
Trophozoites	Delicate, much smaller than diameter of red cell which is *not* enlarged. Maurer's dots	Amoeboid. Parasite fills red cells. Red cell enlarged. Erythrocytes dotted with Schuffner's dots	Not amoeboid. Band forms present. Parasites do not fill red cells. Red cell not enlarged. No Schuffner's dots	Not amoeboid. Red cell often oval, fimbriated and enlarged. Schuffner's dots present
Schizonts	Does not fill red cell—5–30 merozoites. Only seen in fulmin-ating cases	Fills enlarged red cell. 12–24 merozoites	Smaller than in *P. vivax*, 6–12 merozoites. Pigment abundant	6–12 merozoites. Pigment not so abundant as *P. malariae*
Gametocytes	Crescentic shape	Round or oval—pigment irregularly scattered	Round and compact—pigment abundant and peripherally placed	As *P. vivax*

B. Thick film

	P. falciparum	*P. vivax*	*P. malariae*	*P. ovale*
Number and stages of parasites	Often numerous. Usually all ring forms	Few. All stages seen	Few. All stages seen	Few. All stages seen
Trophozoites	Ring forms with single or double dot	Ring forms and larger amoeboid forms with dispersed granular pigment	Ring forms and older stages with relatively abundant pigment. Solid and regular	as *P. vivax*
Schizonts	Generally not present in peripheral blood. If present associated with very *numerous* typical ring forms	Pigment granular and clumped. Other stages of parasite development also present	Pigment compact clump—other stages of parasite development also present	As *P. vivax*
Gametocytes	Same as thin film	Same as thin film	Same as thin film	Same as thin film

TRYPANOSOMIASES

The trypanosome species pathogenic for man can be classified into two groups: (1) those transmitted through the bite of a blood-sucking fly, i.e. *Trypanosoma gambiense* and *T. rhodesiense*, which cause African Trypanosomiasis, and (2) those transmitted by faecal contamination from an arthropod vector, e.g. *T. cruzi*, which causes South American Trypanosomiasis (Chagas' disease). *T. rangeli* is often found in human blood in South America but is believed to be non-pathogenic.

A. AFRICAN TRYPANOMIASIS

Life cycle

In man *T. gambiense* and *T. rhodesiense* are morphologically identical, varying in length from 10 to 30 μm with a pointed anterior end and blunt posterior. The cytoplasm stains blue with a Romanowsky stain, there is a large oval centrally placed nucleus, a small posteriorly placed kinetoplast, and an undulating membrane projecting beyond the anterior end of the body. Other morphological forms in blood are also seen. *T. gambiense* and *rhodesiense* have a similar life cycle. When blood containing trypanosomes is ingested by a suitable species of *Glossina* the trypanosomes reach the intestine of the fly and undergo cyclical development, eventually developing into infective metacyclic forms in the salivary glands. These are introduced when saliva is injected into the wound produced during the act of feeding. Multiplication of the trypanosomes occurs in the blood. The entire cycle of development in the fly, after feeding on blood containing trypanosomes, is about 3 weeks. Electron microscope studies have resulted in advances in knowledge of the morphology of trypanosomes (Vickerman, 1962, and Boisson *et al.* 1965). Culture media most suitable for the several species of African pathogenic trypanosomes have been reviewed by Lehmann (1961a, b). Williamson (1963) has reviewed the information available on their physiology and chemical composition. Parasites can now be preserved at low temperatures and this has facilitated the maintenance of strains for experimental work (Lumsden, 1964). An excellent book on the African trypanosomiases in now available (Mulligan, 1970).

Epidemiology

The distribution of human trypanosomiasis in Africa is related to the presence of *Glossina* species capable of transmitting the infections. It extends from the southern limits of the Sahara to latitude 20° S. In West Africa and up to the western Rift valley, the disease is caused mainly by *T. brucei gambiense* transmitted by *G. palpalis* or *G. tachinoides*, while to the east of longitude 30° E, *T. gambiense* is replaced by *T. brucei rhodesiense* and transmission is by *G. morsitans*, and *G. pallidipes* (Vaucel *et al.* 1963).

The maintenance of human trypanosomiasis in Africa depends on the interrelations of three elements—the vertebrate host, the parasite, and the vector responsible for transmission (Willett, 1965). Sleeping sickness is essentially a disease of rural populations and its prevalence is largely dependent on the degree of contact between man and tsetse, this is particularly so with Gambiense sleeping sickness. Thus at the height of the dry season, riverine species of fly are often restricted to isolated pools of water which are essential to the local human population for so many of their activities, e.g. collecting water and firewood, washing, fishing, and cultivation. The sacred groves of some religions may also provide foci of intimate man/fly contact. Over recent years there has been an increasing incidence and dispersion of *T. rhodesiense* sleeping sickness on the north-east shores of Lake Victoria, associated with increased fishing activity and increasing and irregular settlement of the tsetse-fly belt of south-east Uganda (Robertson, 1963). The incidence and geographical distribution of *T. rhodesiense* sleeping sickness in the Lambwe Valley of Kenya is described by Watson (1973).

In general, in endemic conditions, the incidence of sleeping sickness is greater in males. In contrast to this usual picture Hutchinson (1953) found that in the Gambia, the women and older girls were most affected because they were exposed while working in the rice fields. In epidemic conditions no clear sex difference in incidence occurs and the proportion of children infected rises sharply. Congenital infections do occur (Burke, 1973) but are rare. Adverse environmental climatic conditions can effect the mean period between emergence of the young fly (pupa) and the taking of the first blood meal as well as the period of development of trypanosomes in the vector; these factors can influence the chance of transmission of the disease (Wijers, 1958). No animal reservoir for *T. gambiense* has yet been proved but *T. rhodesiense* has been isolated from bush-buck (Heisch *et al.* 1958) and from hartebeest (Geigy *et al.* 1972) and so a reservoir in wild animals—long suspected—has now been proved. Domestic ungulates too can serve as hosts, e.g. oxen (Mwambu, 1973). A recent review of the epidemiology of African sleeping sickness with particular reference to the relationship between the disease and the total environment was produced by Baker (1974). Serum IgM levels can be used as an aid to the detection of trypanosomiasis at community level (Binz and Watson, 1973).

Immunology

The evolution of resistance in human populations constantly exposed to infection has not been properly studied, although there is some indication of greater resistance in persons in endemic areas than in those never exposed to infection (Soltys, 1963). Species specificity exists to a remarkable degree in trypanosomiasis—thus man is highly resistant to infection by animal trypanosomes. The main body of the work on immunity in trypanosomiasis has been done in animals. Thus a racial non-specific resistance has been demonstrated in the N'Dama cattle of West Africa by Chandler (1958), although Desowitz (1959) believes that this racial resistance to trypanosomes is due to acquired immunity. Studies by various workers have shown that protective antibodies act by rendering the parasite susceptible to phago-cytosis or lysis or both. The antigenic structure of trypanosomes has been reviewed by Weitz (1963). The surface of variant antigens elicit agglutin-ating, neutralizing and precipitating IgM antibodies, which are specific for each parasitaemic population. Common antigens elicit IgG antibodies as detected by fluorescent, complement fixation and indirect agglutination tests. The pathology of sleeping sickness is probably related to immune—hypersensitivity reactions mediated by cells or by antigen—antibody complexes (De Raadt, 1974).

Pathology of Gambian trypanosomiasis

This can be conveniently described in three stages: (1) the invasion of the dermis by metacyclic trypanosomes and their subsequent multiplication with the production of a local chancre, (2) widespread dissemination of the trypanosomes by the lymphatics and blood stream with the most marked changes in the reticulo-endothelial system, and (3) central nervous system involvement.

In the early stages of the disease, the patient may complain of few symptoms or there may be persistent headache, febrile attacks, transient orbital or joint swellings with enlargement of the lymphatic glands, especially those in the posterior cervical triangle (Winterbottom's sign). A papular lesion may be present at the site of the tsetse bite. Somewhat later there is disturbance of vision, lassitude, and delayed pain sensation with deep hyperaesthesia (Kérandel's sign). The spleen and liver may be enlarged and palpable. Circinate eruptions are usual. During this stage the trypano-somes are present in the blood and reticulo-endothelial system. They utilize oxygen, glucose, amino acids, and heme. The erythrocyte of the host is in some way affected in that it becomes more fragile and a progressive microcytic anaemia develops with a corresponding erythroblastic reaction in the marrow. The infection also causes immunosuppression; the ability of the host to raise antibodies to other antigens is impaired, rendering it susceptible to intercurrent infections (Goodwin, 1974; Greenwood et al. 1973).

There is a fall in albumin and a rise in globulin in the plasma. This is mainly due to an increase in γ-globulin, which is greater than would be expected from increased antibody production alone, and altered reactivity of the reticulo-endothelial system or impaired liver function have been somewhat vaguely suggested as possible factors in this increase.

Changes in liver function tests, reversible on therapy, do occur in the early and late stages of both gambiense and rhodesiense infections (Robertson and Jenkins, 1959).

The changes in the plasma proteins have been shown to cause a marked increase in the erythrocyte sedimentation rate and autoagglutination is a constant finding. The shortened life span of the erythrocyte contributes to the rise in serum potassium which occurs and the metabolism of the parasite causes a marked hypoglycaemia.

There is a mild leucocytosis with an absolute increase in monocytes and lymphocytes.

Excluding lymph nodes the morbid anatomical changes have not been satisfactorily described at this stage but changes in the liver, spleen and central nervous system must have occurred. A mild myocarditis would also be expected.

In the later stages, occurring anything from 6 months to years after the original infection, mental and nervous changes become clinically obvious. Multiple sclerosis may be simulated. Manic depressive symptoms or a gradual mental deterioration resulting in marasmus and death may occur. Intercurrent infection is common.

The cerebrospinal fluid is under increased pressure and the cell count is raised, lymphocytes and monocytes predominating. Eosinophils, trypanosomes, and the morula cells of Mott may be present.

The morula cell is thought to be a plasma cell whose cytoplasm has undergone degenerative changes. It contains numerous rounded eosinophilic bodies and resembles the mulberry (Fig. 2.6). It is an IgM producing cell (Greenwood, 1973). This cell is not specific for trypanosomiasis but may be found in other chronic cerebral infections. The total protein is increased, the changes being mainly in the β- and γ-globulin fractions.

The reticulo-endothelial system

In the early stages the lymphatic glands are enlarged, soft, and contain numerous trypanosomes. They show lymphatic and histocytic proliferation. Histiocytes contain erythrocytes, cellular debris, and fragmented trypanosomes. Small haemorrhages and later fibrosis occurs and no trypanosomes are found. In the spleen which may terminally be only slightly enlarged the Malphigian corpuscles are inconspicuous. There is proliferation of histiocytes and sinusoidal lining cells, with erythrophagocytosis a feature, and haemosiderin deposits may be detectable. Areas of focal necrosis and fibrosis are described. Trypanosomes may be detected in the bone marrow, which shows mild myeloid and erythroid hyperplasia.

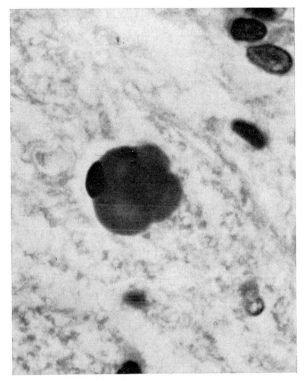

FIG. 2.6. African trypanosomiasis. Morula cell of Mott in brain tissue.
(× 1000)

Other organs

The liver shows non-specific toxic changes. The Kupffer cells may be hyperplastic and contain red blood cells and haemosiderin. In the heart a mild pericardial effusion and haemorrhages in the endo- and epicardium occur. Histologically there may be evidence of a mild long-standing myocarditis.

In the lungs evidence of a long-standing vasculitis with areas of fibrosis and collapse may be seen. Similar vascular lesions may cause renal damage.

The central nervous system

The most marked changes are seen in the brain late in the disease. There is a chronic meningo-encephalitis. The dura may be adherent to the skull and the pia arachnoid. The brain is congested and the convolutions flattened. Small haemorrhages may be present in its substance. The III and IV ventricles and basal cisterns are dilated and the lining ependyma thickened and roughened.

Histologically the meninges are thickened and infiltrated with lymphocytes, histiocytes, morula cells, and occasionally eosinophils and polymorphonuclear leucocytes. A similar infiltrate is seen in the Virchow Robin spaces (perivascular cuffing) (Fig. 2.7). Trypanosomes may be present in the infiltrate and in the substance of the brain itself but are rarely recognized in our experience. Focal collections of glial cells and lymphocytes may be present in the parenchyma of the frontal lobe, hypothalamic region, pons

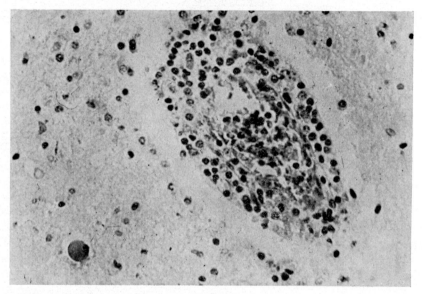

FIG. 2.7. African trypanosomiasis. Brain. Perivascular cuffing. (H and E × 135).

and medulla. Demyelinization of nerves may occur. Similar lesions may occur in the spinal cord with inflammatory changes in the spinal root ganglia.

Segmental loss of myelin with an accumulation of macrophages has been described in cranial, spinal root, and peripheral nerve tissue in association with a vasculitis and Wallerian degeneration may occur (Janssens et al. 1956). Degeneration of nerve-cell bodies may occur secondarily to the destruction of the nerve fibre. The pathological lesions of the nerves appear to occur intermittently and it has been suggested that they are due to a local endotoxin liberated on the death of the trypanosome.

The eye

Ocular symptoms may be due to central nervous system involvement and external ophthalmoplegia, ptosis, papilloedema and optic atrophy are late manifestations of the infection (Reid, 1966). Interstitial keratitis and iridocyclitis also occur in the late stages. Optic atrophy may also be a complication of therapy.

Pathology of rhodesiense trypanosomiasis

Clinically *T. rhodesiense* infections are much more acute than those caused by *T. gambiense* and run a more rapid and fatal course. A chancre may occur at the site of the bite; this local reaction is commoner in Caucasians and more prominent in *T. rhodesiense* than in *T. gambiense* infections. Irregular febrile attacks with peripheral oedema and mild glandular enlargement occur. Signs of cardiac involvement may be noticed and wasting is prominent. The typical sleeping sickness syndrome is usually absent but mental symptoms and acute mania occur. Trypanosomes are abundant in the blood and appear early in the cerebrospinal fluid.

In general it can be said that the pathology of this infection resembles that of *T. gambiense* with the following modifications.

In the brain the lesions are less florid and may be confined to a histocytic infiltration of the membranes. Effusions in the pleural, pericardial, and peritoneal cavities are common (Hawking and Greenfield, 1941). Cardiac involvement may be severe (Manson-Bahr and Charters, 1963). There may be marked infiltration of the interstitial tissue of the heart by histiocytes, lymphocytes, plasma cells, and polymorphonuclear leucocytes. Focal infiltrates occur in the endocardium and occasional giant cells may be noted. Trypanosomes may or may not be present in the pericardial fluid.

Diagnostic pathology

Microscopical examination of blood, lymph fluid, serous fluids, or C.S.F. with or without concentration techniques may reveal the organism in fresh or suitably stained preparations. *In-vitro* culture of trypanosomes has proved sensitive and reliable (Weinman, 1963) as has the complement-fixation test (De Raadt, 1967). A fluorescent antibody test for the serodiagnosis of African trypanosomiasis has been developed by Sadun *et al.* (1963) and recently modified by Bailey *et al.* (1967). Other tests which can be used both for diagnosis and to differentiate human from animal trypanosomes are— the blood incubation infectivity test (Rickman and Robson, 1970); a newer fluorescent antibody technique (Latif and Adam, 1973); and techniques of biochemical taxonomy (Kilgour and Godfrey, 1973; Editorial, 1974). A raised serum bilirubin level, excess urobilinogen, and bilirubinuria, is common in early acutely febrile rhodesiense cases (Robertson and

Jenkins, 1959) but they are not raised in the late stages of the disease. The bromsulphalein excretion test is also abnormal in the acutely febrile early stage associated with a precipitous fall in the serum albumin. In the late stages of both gambiense and rhodesiense infections the total plasma proteins are high and the γ-globulin grossly increased except in wasted patients in whom the total serum proteins and especially albumin are low. The lymphocytes and protein content of the C.S.F. are invariably raised and sugar low when the central nervous system is involved. Lucasse (1965) and Mattern et al. (1965) applied the fluorescent antibody test to the C.S.F. of patients with sleeping sickness, they found antibodies in all the samples which showed pathological changes. The test was sensitive, specific, and suitable for the early detection of involvement of the nervous system. A raised IgM level is also found in the C.S.F. and has proved a very useful diagnostic sign of the disease.

The serum levels of IgM, IgA, and IgG are raised in both *T. gambiense* and *T. rhodesiense* infections (Mattern et al. 1967; Cunningham et al. 1967). High levels of M-antiglobulins (rheumatoid-factor-like globulins) can occur in African trypanosomiasis, and a heterophile antibody, which may provide a means of differential diagnosis between Gambian and Rhodesian sleeping sickness, is present in sera from *T. rhodesiense* patients (Brown et al. 1967). EEG sometimes shows a disturbed wave pattern, and air encephalography dilatation of the ventricles when brain involvement has occurred.

B. SOUTH AMERICAN TRYPANOSOMIASIS (CHAGAS' DISEASE)

Life cycle

The adult trypanosomes, which measure about 20 μm in length with a central nucleus and very large posterior kinetoplast, are found in the blood. When ingested by blood-sucking reduviid bugs, after a period of development in the invertebrate host's intestinal canal lasting 8–10 days, trypanosomes, known as 'metacyclic' forms re-appear in the hindgut and are passed with the faeces of the insect. Infection of man takes place when faecal matter is rubbed into scratch wounds and the wound caused by the bite of the insect. Certain trypanosomes leave the blood stream and invade various organs especially the myocardium. Here they assume a leishmanoid appearance and rapid multiplication by binary fission takes place forming nests of Leishman–Donovan bodies. At a later stage these leishmanoid forms elongate and are eventually transformed into trypanosomes, which make their way through the tissues and into the blood stream. *T. cruzi* can be grown in tissue culture (Neva et al. 1961).

Epidemiology

Chagas' disease extends from Northern Argentina and Chile to the Southern half of the United States. The most important vector bugs belong to the genera *Triatoma*, *Panstrongylus*, and *Rhodnius*. These reduviid bugs are largely disseminated throughout the rural areas of Latin America where the mud huts of the agricultural workers are their favourite habitats. The usual mode of transmission is by rubbing infected faeces into cuts or abrasions or into the intact skin or mucous membrane. Transmission occurs predominantly at night since reduviid bugs attack only in darkness. The disease is observed at any age, although children are mainly affected. Other methods of infection are via a damaged placenta, by blood transfusion, and laboratory transmission from infected syringes or blood. Dogs and cats are important domestic reservoirs of *T. cruzi* and there are in addition about 150 species of sylvatic reservoirs among which the armadillo and the opossum are well known. In Bolivia and south western Peru guinea-pigs are the most important animal reservoir (Torrico, 1959). Marked differences exist in the severity and clinical manifestations of the disease in different areas of South America, and strain differences alone are unlikely to be the reason (Zeledon, 1974). *R. rattus* has also been shown to be an important reservoir of *T. cruzi* in the province of Panama (Edgcomb and Johnson, 1970). Little is known about immunity to Chagas' disease. Cross-immunity between five different strains of *T. cruzi* in guinea-pigs was demonstrated by direct and indirect immunofluorescence techniques (Essenfeld and Fennell, 1964).

Infections with another trypanosome, *T. rangeli*, have been found in various animals, and human infections with this trypanosome have also been reported (Penalver *et al.* 1956). In contrast to *T. cruzi* the transmission of this disease is by the actual bite of the reduviid bug rather than through its excreta.

Pathology

Chagas' disease may present in congenital, acute, or chronic forms.

The congenital form presents as a meningo-encephalitis with fundal changes and hepatosplenomegaly. It is uncommon.

Probably only about 1 per cent of individuals infected show clinical signs in the early stages, but as many as 30 per cent may suffer symptoms in the chronic stage (Rosenbaum, 1964). For interested readers the pathology of American trypanosomiasis has been extensively reviewed by Koberle (1968).

Acute stage

This is most frequently seen in children and the mortality may be 10 per cent. Adolescents and adults are usually less severely affected. A local inflammatory swelling occurs in the skin at the site of inoculation (chagoma) and is usually situated in the head and neck region. This is followed by a regional lymphangitis with nodular swellings along the course of the vessels.

Unilateral conjunctivitis, oedema of the eyelids and adenitis of the lachrymal gland occur if the trypanosomes have entered through the conjunctiva (Romana's sign). Subcutaneous swellings may be present on the upper trunk region. Fever, facial or generalized non-pitting oedema, lymphadenopathy, hepatosplenomegaly, meningoencephalitis, and signs of acute myocarditis may occur. Disturbances of conduction producing A-V blocks of all kinds, from first-degree block to complete heart block occur (Anselmi and Moleiro, 1974). Transient skin rashes are not unusual. The thyroid swelling and consequent myxoedema described by Chagas are now thought to be incidental findings due to concomitant endemic goitre (Ash and Spitz, 1945). Chapino (1973) has reported on 20 cases in children observed in Cochabamba in Bolivia in whom the cardiac manifestations were frequently accompanied by shock.

Trypanosomes are present in the peripheral blood and may be found in the cerebrospinal fluid. Serum aspartate aminotransferase values are increased in the blood and there is lowering of the serum albumin with raised α- β-, and γ-globulins. There is a tendency to leucopenia.

At the site of inoculation leishmanial forms cause a local inflammatory reaction with infiltration of lymphocytes, histiocytes and plasma cells. A spreading gelatinous oedema may be present in the tissues and the nodules described clinically are secondary chagomas. There is histiocytic proliferation in the lymphatic glands and leishmanial forms of the parasite may be

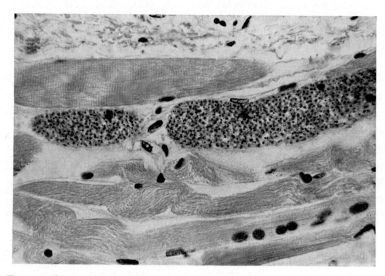

Fig. 2.8. Chagas' disease. Oesophagus. Pseudocysts containing leishmanial forms in muscle of upper oesophagus (H and E × 320). (*By courtesy of Professor F. Koberle.*)

found intra- or extracellularly. Flagellate forms are said to be present in the medullary zones.

It is said that the organisms affect particularly striated muscle, the myocardium and brain tissue but, in view of the changes described later in the chronic stages, they must be widely disseminated in the body unless an immunological mechanism is postulated in the aetiology of lesions in the chronic stage.

Pseudocysts containing numerous leishmanial forms are formed in *striated muscle*. Smooth muscle may also be affected (Fig. 2.8). It should be noted that in leishmaniasis in contrast the organisms are usually found in the reticulo-endothelial system. The structure of the muscle fibre is not radically altered, the cross-striations usually being preserved and the nucleus preserving its integrity by light microscopy. There is no surrounding cellular

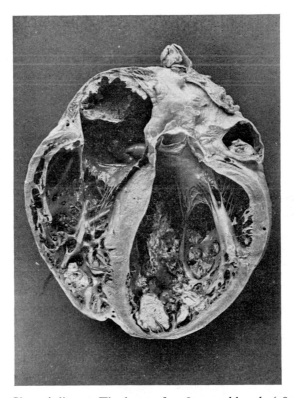

FIG. 2.9. Chagas' disease. The heart of a 28-year-old male (580g). The dilatation of the right atrium and both ventricles is marked. Note the marked thinning of ventricular walls, especially at the apices. Numerous mural thrombi are present. (*By courtesy of Professor F. Koberle.*)

infiltrate. With rupture of the pseudocyst and release of the contained organisms, a marked inflammatory reaction, however, occurs with infiltration of plasma cells, lymphocytes and monocytes.

The heart, at necropsy, may show a sero-fibrinous pericarditis. It is enlarged and dilated. The myocardium is pale and of soft consistency and may contain streaks of yellow material. Punctate haemorrhages occur in the myo-, epi-, and endocardium. Mural thrombi may be present at the apex of the left ventricle (Fig. 2.9).

Histologically pseudocysts are usually found in the myofibrils (Fig. 2.10), but are said to be uncommon in ganglion cells. There is an intense interstitial inflammatory reaction in which leishmaniform bodies may or may not be present. The infiltrate consists of lymphocytes, plasma cells, histiocytes, and monocytes. Polymorphonuclear leucocytes are rarely seen. The absence of organisms in a number of the lesions has suggested that there may be an underlying toxic or immunoallergic mechanism in their causation. Focal areas of myocytolysis and fragmentation and degeneration of muscle fibres occur. A necrotizing arteritis and perineural inflammation has been described. Focal inflammatory lesions with or without nests of organisms may be seen in the vicinity of degenerating ganglion cells.

The brain is oedematous and congested and pseudocysts may be found in the ganglion and neuroglial cells. Leishmanial forms may be found in the parenchyma especially in the region of capillaries in the forebrain, cere-

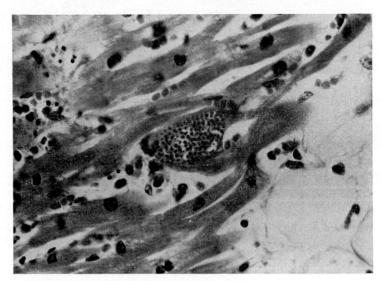

FIG. 2.10. Chagas' disease. Section of heart muscle, showing a pseudocyst. Fatty infiltration and small foci of necrosis are evident (H and E × 320).

bellum, and brain stem surrounded by neuroglial and plasma cells. Neighbouring ganglion cells may be damaged with consequent disorganization of axis cylinders. The meninges may be infiltrated by lymphocytes, monocytes, and histiocytes, and perivascular cuffing may be noted in adjacent vessels. The spinal cord may also be affected.

Other organs

Serous effusions may be present in the pleural and peritoneal cavities. The liver and spleen show degenerative and congestive changes. Petechial haemorrhages are seen in muscle and histologically are due to the lesions caused by the trypanosomes as previously described. Granulomatous lesions and a necrotizing arteritis may be found in the muscular layer of the intestinal tract with associated degenerative changes in Auerbach's plexus (Koberle, 1963).

In the lungs bronchopneumonia is a usual complication most probably precipitated by granulomatous lesions in the walls of the bronchioles.

It is possible that lesions also occur in the adrenal as an Addisonian-like syndrome has been described in the chronic stages.

Chronic stage

The acute stage may merge imperceptibly into the chronic, with signs of central nervous system or cardiac involvement being the most usual presentations clinically. This, however, is not the common natural history of the disease and clinical manifestations of the chronic stage usually present 10–20 years after a minor or unnoticed primary infection.

The fundamental lesion of the chronic stage is destruction of ganglion cells in the peripheral autonomic or central nervous system and occurs in the heart, bronchi, and intestinal canal as well as in the medulla and cerebellum. The mechanism of this destruction is debatable and has been attributed to the effects of a toxin liberated from dead or dying trypanosomes or to an immunoallergic reaction specifically directed against ganglion cells (Jaffe et al. 1961; Kozma, 1962). It is interesting to note that the presence of a neurotropic endotoxin has also been postulated in African trypanosomiasis (Janssens et al. 1956).

Clinically chronic meningo-encephalitis may occur. Dilatation of the bronchi, oesophagus, stomach, duodenum, appendix, colon, gall bladder, bile ducts, urinary bladder, and ureters due to these lesions has been described, the most common being megaoesophagus and megacolon.

The heart, however, would appear to be the most frequently affected organ and the clinical and pathological features are dealt with in some detail below (Andrade and Andrade, 1967).

Chagas' cardiopathy may occur in almost one-third of the population in endemic areas. Males in the 15- to 50-year-old age group are affected more frequently than females and manual workers are more frequently affected than sedentary. The condition may be unsuspected and sudden death, frequently precipitated by emotional stress, is common. In others palpitation and dyspnoea are usual complaints, and terminally, congestive cardiac failure and oedema occur. The heart is enlarged. Signs of relative mitral or tricuspid valve incompetence may be present. Right bundle branch, atrio-ventricular and left bundle branch block are common and occur in that order. The electrocardiographic alterations may simulate infarction of the myocardium involving the anterior wall and septum. Embolic episodes are not uncommon.

The heart

Residual pericardial thickening may be present. The most important and common finding is hypertrophy and dilatation of the heart, often markedly affecting the pulmonary conus. Weights of over 1000 g, with an average of 525 g, have been recorded. The hypertrophy and dilatation is global and valvular lesions are absent. Thinning of the apical myocardium in the ventricles (most usually the left) is a characteristic lesion and aneurysmal formation in the apical region of the left ventricle is found in approximately 50 per cent of subjects and is considered to be due to haemodynamic factors. Mural thrombi in the right auricle and apical regions of the ventricles are common. Patchy white fibrotic lesions may be seen in the myocardium, most frequently in the left ventricle. Patchy greyish-white endocardial thickenings may be present. There is a marked accentuation of the trabecular pattern in the ventricles, and in many instances this pattern with the thinning of either the left or right ventricular walls and apical dilatations give a picture quite distinct from that seen in idiopathic cardiomegaly described in Africa. The coronary arteries are dilated and, although minimal atheroma may be present, no evidence of occlusion has been demonstrated by dissection or injection techniques.

Histologically a marked reduction in the ganglion cells in the sino-auricular node has been demonstrated (Koberle, 1963).

Degenerative changes in the nerves in the subendocardium, myocardium, and interstitial tissue, with an associated inflammatory change, may be evident. A careful search may reveal the presence of pseudocysts in a relatively small proportion of hearts. There may be a mild focal infiltration of inflammatory cells. Focal areas of myocytolysis, focal necrosis, fibrosis, and hyaline change occur. Non-specific changes occur in the myofibrils (vacuolization, fragmentation, and bizarre nuclear forms). Patchy areas of fibroelastosis may occur on the endocardial surface and thrombi may be incorporated into the wall.

To summarize: there are lesions in the myocardium suggestive of a burnt-out myocarditis and also lesions suggestive of relative ischaemia. There would also appear however to be another factor involved shown by the thinning of the muscle and aneurysmal dilatations which are uncommon in other idiopathic cardiomyopathies and are most probably due to haemodynamic factors consequent upon damage to the nervous tissue of the conducting system—the heart to all intents and purposes being denervated. (Koberle, 1974).

Other organs

Embolic lesions may be present most usually in the brain, spleen or kidney, in addition to the changes of chronic venous congestion. Lesions may also be present in the intestine and lungs—bronchicctasis occasionally being a complication. A careful histopathological study is indicated in all patients dying of chronic Chagas' disease to elucidate the extent of the lesions.

Diagnostic pathology

Trypanosomes may be demonstrated in wet and stained blood films; in lymph gland juice, or in C.S.F., and may be cultured on N.N.N. medium. A complement-fixation test (Guenerio–Machado test)—employing antigen from flagellates cultivated *in vitro*—is widely used and is the most sensitive means of diagnosis (Hawking, 1964). Maekelt (1963) reviewed the various procedures used in the diagnosis of American trypanosomiasis and discussed their value in the different stages of the disease. Immuno-fluorescence has been used in the diagnosis of Chagas' disease and Biagi *et al.* (1964) prefer this technique to the complement-fixation test. Animal inoculation is another useful method of diagnosis.

LEISHMANIASES

The leishmaniases occur over wide areas of the globe from China across Asia, India, Persia, and Afghanistan, the Caucasus, the Middle and Near East, the Mediterranean basin, East and West Africa, the Sudan, and South America. It is convenient to subdivide the leishmaniases into three clinical types: the visceral, the cutaneous, and the muco-cutaneous. This classification is however an oversimplification of a complex situation as evidenced by the data given in Table 2.2.

Life cycle

There are two phases in the life cycle of *Leishmania*: an aflagellate (leishmanial) rounded form which occurs in man and in animal reservoir hosts; and a flagellate (leptomonad) form which is found in the vector sandfly and in culture media. The

TABLE 2.2. *Parasites causing leishmaniasis in man* (after Preston and Dumonde, 1975)

Distribution	Leishmanial 'species' (geographical variant)	Clinical manifestations		Tendency for infection to generalize or persist
		Localized and self-healing	Generalized and/or non-healing	
Africa[1]; India[1]; C. Asia[2]; China[2]; Middle East[3]; Mediterranean[3]	L. donovani*	Primary leishmanioma	RES (Kala Azar)	Usual
	L. infantum*		Mucocutaneous	Infrequent
			PKADL	Infrequent
South and Central America	L. chagasi	Primary leishmanioma	RES	Usual
Asia; Mediterranean	L. tropica	Ulcer (Oriental Sore)	Lupoid ulcers ('recidiva')	Infrequent
Africa (Ethiopia)	L. aethiopica**	Ulcer	DCL ('diffusa')	Infrequent
Mexico; Guatemala; British Honduras	L. m. mexicana	L. mexicana complex† Ulcer (Chiclero's Ulcer)	Persistent ulcers if on ear	Usual (≃70 per cent)
Venezuela	L. m. pifanoi	Ulcer	DCL	Only 20 cases reported
Amazon basin	L. m. amazonensis	Ulcer	DCL	Infrequent
Brazil; Bolivia; Paraguay; Columbia; Venezuela	L. b. brasiliensis	L. brasiliensis complex† Ulcer	Persistent multiple ulcers	?
			Mucocutaneous (espundia)	20–30 per cent
Guyana; N. Brazil	L. b. guyanensis	Crater-like ulcer (pian bois)	Persistent multiple ulcers	?
Panama	L. b. panamensis	Crater-like ulcer	Persistent multiple ulcers	?
Peru	L. peruviana	Ulcer (uta)	Not observed	—

Abbreviations: Res, 'reticuloendothelial' (mononuclear phagocyte) system; DCL, diffuse cutaneous leishmaniasis; PKADL, post-kala-azar dermal leishmanoid. This is a sequel of visceral leishmaniasis following specific treatment.

References: ** Bray, Ashford and Bray (1973); †Lainson and Shaw (1972).

* Age incidence of *visceral leishmaniasis:* 1, 5–25 yr; 2, all ages; 3, < 5 yr (da Silva, 1957).

former is oval (2 × 3 μm) and consists of cytoplasm, a round nucleus, and a small, more deeply staining, rod-shaped kinetoplast or rhizoplant and a vacuole (see Fig. 2.11). It is known as the Leishman–Donovan (L–D) body. In man leishmanias multiply by binary fission. They are most commonly found in the large mononuclear cells of the reticulo-endothelial system, especially in the liver, spleen, and bone marrow; leishmanial forms are also found in the leucocytes of the circulating blood.

When the appropriate sandfly feeds on an infected person, it ingests the parasites with the blood meal. These develop in its gut into the flagellate (leptomonad) forms, which migrate forwards, multiply, and form a mass which may block the pharynx of the sandfly. When the sandfly next feeds, some of the leptomonads become

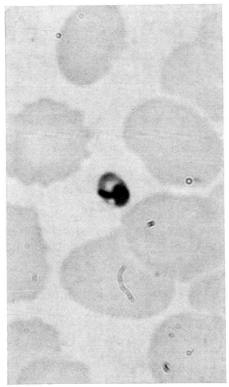

Fig. 2.11. Leishmaniasis. Leishman–Donovan (L–D) body, showing round nucleus and small, deeply-staining, rod-shaped kinetoplast (× 1575).

dislodged and are injected into the new host in the process of feeding; they again assume the leishmanial form. They are phagocytosed by macrophages, multiply by simple division and cause the cells to rupture. They are then carried in the circulation to the sites already referred to where they give rise to the characteristic lesions. Following specific treatment in some cases they pass from their visceral habitat— liver, spleen, etc. back to the skin, giving rise to the condition described as post-kala-azar dermal leishmaniasis.

The above life history applies to *L. donovani* which is the causative organism of visceral leishmaniasis. In cutaneous and muco-cutaneous leishmaniasis, the multiplication of the leishmanial forms takes place in the skin and the appropriate sandfly vectors become infected by feeding on a cutaneous lesion.

It is easy to maintain leishmania strains (leptomonad form) in culture, and many satisfactory media containing blood have been described. It has been pointed out that strains change after various periods in culture, particularly in their infectivity for laboratory animals. The leishmanial form, which in nature lives as an intracellular parasite in the mammalian host, has usually been cultivated successfully only in association with the living host cell. Recently, however, growth and multiplication of leishmania in a cell-free medium has been achieved. Electron microscopic studies of both the intra-cellular leishmanial and extracellular leptomonad forms have been made and they have provided valuable information on the morphology of the leishmanias (Jadin and Creemers, 1966; Sanyal and Sen Gupta, 1967). Comparative studies on the isoenzymes and DNA of leishmanial parasites have recently been carried out by Chance *et al.* (1973).

Epidemiology

The epidemiology of the leishmaniases whether visceral, cutaneous or muco-cutaneous is in every case determined by a reservoir of infection (animal, man or both) from which local Phlebotomine sandflies infect themselves by ingesting leishmanial forms from blood or infected tissues. The climatic conditions of the various foci of leishmaniasis range from arid to tropical humid and the terrain and altitude are equally variable (Adler, 1964). Modes of transmission other than by sandflies, e.g. marital (Symmers, 1960), blood transfusion (Andre *et al.* 1957), and intra-uterine infection (Low and Cook, 1926), are of no epidemiological significance. With the possible exception of Indian kala-azar it is increasingly being recognized that in most endemic foci the leishmaniases are zoonoses. The importance of this cosmopolitan disease has been well recognized by WHO (1971).

A. VISCERAL LEISHMANIASIS

There are three distinct types of visceral leishmaniasis: (*a*) Indian kala-azar, (*b*) kala-azar associated predominantly with a canine reservoir, and (*c*) African kala-azar. Kalar-azar is essentially a rural disease, and *L. donovani* is now accepted as the cause of all forms of kala-azar. Post-kala-azar dermal leishmaniasis occurs as a sequel of visceral leishmaniasis.

(*a*) *Indian kala-azar* is unique in so far as man is the only known natural host of the infection. The vector, *P. argentipes*, breeds in close proximity to human habitations and feeds readily on man. All age groups are susceptible with a peak incidence at 10–20 years. Devastating epidemics may occur. The lesions of *post-kala-azar dermal leishmaniasis* are of epidemiological importance since they contain numerous L–D bodies in the dermis and are readily accessible to sandflies; they are a feature of Indian kala-azar but are also seen elsewhere.

(*b*) *Kala-azar predominantly associated with a canine reservoir*. In the Mediterranean basin, Portugal, North Africa, the Caucasus, China, Brazil and other parts of South America, the domestic dog, fox and jackal are very important reservoirs of human infection (Deane and Deane, 1964; Busuttil, 1974).

Visceral leishmaniasis associated with a canine reservoir is predominantly a disease of children under 10 years. The most important vector sandflies are *Phelebotomus chinensis* in China, *P. longipalpis* in Brazil, and *P. perniciosus* in the Mediterranean. An outbreak of visceral leishmaniasis in Italy with many peculiar features has been reported by Pampiglione *et al.* (1974). Adults were the chief sufferers.

The course of the disease was most unusual in its rapidity (7 patients died within two months of the onset), in enlargement of liver rather than spleen, in the absence of leucopenia in nearly half the patients, and in the comparative rarity of the organism either in biopsies or at necropsy. Moreover, the liver showed extensive granulomas, haemorrhages or necrosis— rare changes in the ordinary forms of kala-azar. Other strange and interesting features were the serological reactions, which indicated that leishmaniasis had swept through valleys near Bologna causing many occult or subclinical infections and leaving the population largely immune. Surveys showed that the chief vector of Italian kala-azar—*P. perniciosus*—was rare or absent, and that the dog was apparently not a reservoir.

(*c*) *African kala-azar*. The epidemiology of the disease in the Sudan and Kenya presents unique features differing from those described above. There is a primary stage in the skin (leishmanoma) which lasts for some time before the symptoms of kala-azar develop, and this is of prime epidemiological importance; in this area rodents may form a reservoir of infection (Manson-Bahr and Southgate, 1964). There is a definite relationship between the proximity of homes to termite hills and the incidence of kala-azar (Southgate and Oriedo, 1962). The most important vectors are *P. martini* in Kenya and *P. orientalis* in the Sudan where the disease attacks all age groups but is commoner in adults than in children (Sati, 1962). The human distribution is affected by immunity as well as by relative exposure to infection (Southgate and Oriedo, 1967).

Immunity

Cellular reactions in the visceral leishmaniases consist of a proliferation of histiocytes and secondary infiltration by lymphocytes and plasma cells, which is generalized throughout the viscera particularly the spleen, liver, bone marrow and lymphatic glands (Adler, 1964). In addition circulating antibodies demonstrable by complement fixation have been recorded (Sen Gupta and Adhikari, 1952). A pronounced hyperglobulinaemia with an inversion of the globulin/albumin ratio is a feature of visceral leishmaniasis. Patients cured of kala-azar by chemotherapy are immune to subsequent reinfection. Taub (1956) demonstrated a substance in newborn children which destroyed leptomonads of *L. donovani*; the factor then seemed to disappear until the age of $5\frac{1}{2}$ years and was commonly present above 6 years old. It was described as heat labile, non-dializable, and probably an euglobulin. In East Africa Manson-Bahr (1961) showed that subjects who have received an intradermal inoculation of a rodent strain of leishmania are immune to subsequent challenge with a human strain of *L. donovani*. Subclinical infections occur, as evidenced by the presence of a positive leishmania test in individuals who have never had overt signs of disease. Liver biopsies in these patients have shown typical leishmanoid forms in granulomas of the liver (Manson-Bahr, personal communication).

Pathology

The three forms of kala-azar due to *L. donovani* are Indian, visceral with a canine reservoir, and African. In spite of differences in their severity, response to therapy and age distribution, they are manifestations of a common disease process. The pathological changes, with the exception of the primary skin lesion in African and post-kala-azar dermal leishmaniasis in the Indian form, are indistinguishable and are described below. The incubation period is usually a few months but may be as short as 10 days or as long as 9 years. A primary papular lesion occurs at the site of the bite in African kala-azar but is rare in the other forms. In the acute stages intermittent or remittent fever, malaise and headache may be complained of. Hepatosplenomegaly, lymphadenopathy and albuminuria occur.

In the established disease the patient becomes anaemic and cachectic. The hair is dull and dry and vitamin deficiencies may be apparent. Haemorrhagic manifestations due to thrombocytopenia and agranulocytosis have been observed. Secondary infection and cancrum oris may occur in children.

There is progressive anaemia of a hyperchromic macrocytic or normochromic normocytic type. Leucopenia with a reduction in the polymorphonuclear leucocytes and thrombocytopenia are usual. The erythrocyte sedimentation rate is raised and auto-agglutination of erythrocytes may be marked. The reticulocyte count is usually low. The overall findings are those of 'hypersplenism' (p. 490). Occasionally a leukaemoid reaction may be seen in the peripheral blood. Prothrombin is decreased and the coagulation time may be prolonged and this may be of importance if surgical biopsy procedures are contemplated. There is hypoalbuminaemia with a rise in gamma globulin of a slow-moving variety which contains a large proportion of 7S (IgG) component (Sen Gupta, 1965). There is also evidence of adrenocortical dysfunction, sodium and chloride excretion being raised, and the 17-ketosteroids may be low in the urine.

The reticulo-endothelial system

The parasite shows a predilection for this system. In the acute stages the *lymphatic glands* are enlarged, congested and there is marked proliferation of histiocytes and lymphocytes. The histiocytes contain parasites best shown by a Giemsa stain although they can be identified readily on routine H-E staining. They appear as oval bodies about 2–3 μm in length and have a pink staining outline with pale cytoplasm. The eccentric spherical nucleus is about 1 μm in diameter and the rod-shaped rhizoplast may or may not be detectable. Gland puncture is a simple and consistently effective method of diagnosis.

In the chronic stages fibrosis of the capsule and portions of the gland occur. Compact sheets of histiocytes and multinucleated cells may be found in the sinuses. Intracellular parasites can be detected but are not numerous.

The retropharyngeal and tonsillar lymphoid tissue may be affected and leishmania may be found in oral and nasal secretions.

The spleen

In the acute stage the spleen is grossly enlarged and the pulp histiocytes and sinusoidal lining cells are packed with parasites. Areas of necrosis and infarction and sheets of plasma cells may be present. Follicular lesions occur but are unusual and foci of extramedullary erythropoiesis may be noted. In the chronic stages splenomegaly persists. The capsule and supporting trabeculae become thickened and fibrous. Fibrotic areas may be scattered throughout the parenchyma. Parasitized histiocytes are present in the pulp and sinusoids. If splenic puncture is contemplated prior investigation of the platelet level and clotting factors should be undertaken.

The bone marrow

The bone marrow is hyperplastic in the acute stages and numerous histiocytes contain the parasites (Fig. 2.12). In the chronic stages there is depression of myeloid elements and megakaryocytes may also be decreased.

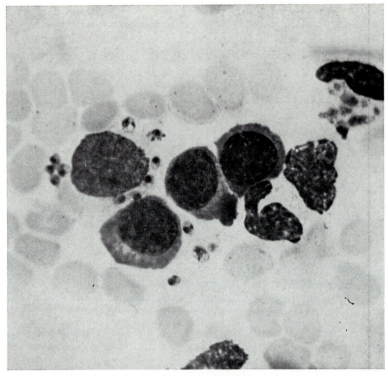

FIG. 2.12. Leishmaniasis. Bone marrow. Histiocyte containing numerous Leishman–Donovan (L–D) bodies (× 750).

There is an increase of fibrous tissue but intracellular parasites can still be detected. Marrow puncture is a valuable diagnostic procedure.

The liver

The Kupffer cells are packed with parasites and there may be parasites within histiocytes in the portal tracts in which there may also be focal collections of lymphocytes and plasma cells. The parenchymal cells show non-specific degenerative changes and glycogen is diminished. Leishman bodies have actually been described in them (Meleney, 1925). An intra-lobular fibrosis has been described but cirrhosis if present, must be considered an incidental finding.

The gastro-intestinal tract

Histiocytes containing parasites may be seen in the lamina propria of the duodenum and jejunum. The villi are enlarged and swollen and ulceration can follow. Parasites have been detected in the faeces. No information is available on the possibility of these lesions leading to a secondary malabsorption syndrome. Leishmanial enteritis has been reported as a terminal event from the Sudan (Sati, 1962), and parasites were found in large numbers in smears from the small intestine.

Other organs

Lesions have been described in the testes, lungs, adrenals, pancreas, skin, thymus, parotid gland, kidneys, heart, and meninges. Essentially the lesions consist of parasites within histiocytes with a variable lymphocytic and plasma cell infiltration (Andrade and Andrade, 1966).

Blockage of the glomerular capillaries occurs and parasites have been seen in the urine. Albuminuria is a marked feature of the disease.

Myocarditis is a rare complication. Histiocytes containing organisms, lymphocytes, plasma cells, and polymorphonuclear leucocytes have been seen in the interstitial tissue with associated degenerative changes and fragmentation of the myofibrils (Meleny, 1925). Parasitized histiocytes may be present in the alveolar walls of the lungs and the interstitial tissue of the testes. In the adrenals lesions have been noted in both the medulla and cortex.

Post-kala-azar dermal leishmanoid

In Indian kala-azar this condition occurs in 1–2 years following treatment. About 20 per cent of patients are affected. In African kala-azar it appears in about 2 per cent of cases as the visceral disease subsides. Hypopigmented or erythematous macules or nodular lesions occur on the face, trunk and anus (Sen Gupta and Bhattacharjee, 1953). Superficial ulceration is not common but if it occurs it may be a source of infection.

The hypo-pigmented macules show decreased pigment in the basal layer and there are focal granulomatous lesions in the subpapillary layer of the dermis consisting of histiocytes and lymphocytes in avascular tissue. Few organisms are present. Adnexal structures may be surrounded but sweat glands tend to escape.

In the erythematous lesions there is confluent granulomatous infiltration in the dermis and moderate numbers of parasites are present. In the nodular lesions the epidermis is thinned and atrophic with loss of rete pegs. There is usually a subpapillary zone free from infection. There are numerous vascular granulomata with occasional giant cells present in the dermis. Parasites are relatively numerous. A xanthomatous form also occurs. The electron micrograph morphology of the L–D body occurring in a nodular lesion of a dermal leishmanoid has recently been described (Sanyal and Sen Gupta, 1967).

B. CUTANEOUS LEISHMANIASIS

Several varieties of cutaneous leishmaniases have been described from the Old and New World. These include (1) oriental sore, (2) chiclero ulcer, (3) uta, (4) leishmaniasis tegumentaria diffusa, (5) Ethiopian (cutaneous) leishmaniasis, (6) lupoid leishmaniasis.

1. **Oriental sore** (tropical sore; bouton d'Orient; Aleppo, Baghdad, or Delhi boil; Pendah sore).

Epidemiology

This cutaneous infection is widely distributed in the Indian sub-continent, the Middle East, Ethiopia, Southern Russia, the Mediterranean countries, Nigeria, China, and the Sudan. The most important vectors are *P. papatasii* and *P. sergenti*. The disease is most commonly seen in children and in highly endemic areas most of the adult population have been infected in childhood. The parasite responsible is *L. tropica* of which two varieties are recognized on clinical and epidemiological grounds. *L. tropica* var. *major* is an infection of rodents occasionally transmitted to man which produces a disease with a short incubation period, rapid course of under 6 months, much inflammatory reaction, and the 'moist' lesion it produces contains few parasites; while *L. tropica minor* is an infection of dogs only occasionally of man, characterized by a 'dry' lesion containing many parasites with a long incubation period, course of over 1 year and a mild inflammatory reaction (Manson-Bahr, 1963).

Immunity to *L. tropica* follows spontaneous cure and experimental attempt at reinfection gives negative results; moreover 98 per cent of cases of oriental sore show a delayed hypersensitivity test (Montenegro reaction) in response to the intradermal inoculation of dead and washed leptomonads (Adler, 1964). Infection of *L. tropica* var. *major* protects against *L. tropica* var. *minor* but not vice versa (Kozhevnikov, 1958).

Pathology

The viscera are not affected in oriental sore and the parasite is found in the reticulo-endothelial cells in the dermis, in lymphatic channels and rarely in the regional lymph nodes. The lesions are found in the exposed parts of the body, the extremities, and face. In the 'moist' type they commence as bluish red nodules. Bullae are formed and ulceration and extension of the lesion with associated regional lymphatic enlargement occur fairly rapidly but are self-limiting and heal by scarring within the year. The scars may cause considerable disfigurement.

Histologically there is evidence of acute and chronic inflammation.

Histiocytes containing parasites are scanty. The reaction in the lymphatic glands is usually non specific.

In the dry type due to *L. tropica minor* the age and site distribution are similar to that described above. The lesions may be single or multiple and commence as firm papules which enlarge; scabs occur on the surface and in some months an indurated crusted ulcer forms. They vary in size from 1 to 5 cm, run a chronic course and lymphatic nodules are few.

The histopathology depends upon the stage of the disease (Kurban *et al.* 1966). In the early stages there is a massive infiltration of the dermis by histiocytes containing numerous leishman bodies and monocytes. The epidermal changes are variable and include hyperkeratosis, parakeratosis, follicular plugging, basal-cell degeneration and either atrophy or acanthosis with pseudo-epitheliomatous hyperplasia. Occasionally intradermal abscesses may be seen. Intracellular leishman bodies have been described in the prickle-cell layer of the epidermis. In the late stages tuberculoid follicles are found and leishmania are scanty and may only be present in 50 per cent of patients. There is usually an absence of necrosis and Langhans giant cells and plasma cells are scanty. Schaumann and asteroid bodies are not seen.

2. Chiclero ulcer (forest yaws; bubas)

The cutaneous leishmaniases of the New World—chiclero ulcer, Uta, and leishmaniasis tegumentaria diffusa—are scattered in Central and South America over an area extending from 22° N to 30° S of the equator. They are characterized epidemiologically by the fact that they are (1) zoonoses, and (2) predominantly non-urban diseases, usually confined to the forest regions or jungles. Convit and Pinardi (1974) have suggested that the various cutaneous forms of leishmaniases in South America are conditioned by the various types of response of the human host towards the leishmanial parasite.

Epidemiology

L. m. mexicana is the cause of 'chichlero's ulcer' in Mexico and neighbouring countries. The infection is virtually restricted to people who habitually live and work in the forests with the result that women and children are rarely affected. It is an 'occupational disease' of the chicleros who spend a considerable time in the forests bleeding the 'sapodella' trees for chewing-gum latex. The disease is almost always limited to a single dermal lesion usually in the ear (Lainson and Strangways-Dixon, 1963). Forest rodents are the important animal reservoirs and man is an accidental host (Lainson and Strangways-Dixon, 1964). Transmission of *L. m. mexicana* is by

Phlebotomus pessoanus in British Honduras (Strangways-Dixon and Lainson, 1966).

With *L. m. mexicana* a solid and long-lasting immunity is developed from the first infection and the development of this immunity occurs very early in the course of the disease (Lainson and Strangways-Dixon, 1963).

Pathology

L. m. mexicana causes cartilage invasion of the pinna with lupus-like lesions which ulcerate and can cause considerable deformity on healing. The lesions are known as chiclero ulcers or Bay sores. Histologically they reveal the usual histiocytic infiltration with parasites present with later follicular formation. Parasites are usually scanty. The condition is usually self-limiting and metastasis to the mucous membranes does not occur.

3. Uta

L. peruviana causes cutaneous lesions on exposed sites such as the face, arm and leg—and the disease is known as uta in Peru.

The mucous membranes or viscera are not usually affected. The lesion commences as a small papule which eventually ulcerates in 6 months or so and a round or oval punched-out ulcer with raised indurated margins is formed. It is not painful. Secondary bead-like nodules may be seen along the draining lymphatic channels. These may break down and ulcerate. The regional lymphatic glands may be enlarged, but this is usually due to secondary infection rather than to the presence of leishmania (Thornburg *et al.* 1952). Superficially in the ulcer there is an exudate of neutrophil polymorphonuclear leucocytes superimposed on a chronic inflammatory process consisting of plasma cells, lymphocytes, and monocytes. Histiocytes are scanty but may be found at the periphery of the lesion or around the adnexal structures. Follicles, giant cells, and Russell bodies may be present. The epidermis shows acanthosis and pseudoepitheliomatous hyperplasia. Leishmania are usually scanty in these later lesions, but are present in large numbers in the nodular lymphatic swellings.

4. Leishmaniasis tegumentaria diffusa

L. m. pifanoi is said to cause disseminated cutaneous leishmaniasis in Bolivia and Venezuela. It commences as a localized nodular lesion which ulcerates, satellite lesions appear and dissemination occurs with the formation of macules, plaques, and papules until practically the whole dermis is involved. The viscera are not affected. Histologically the lesion consists of masses of histiocytes packed with leishmania. The leishmania intradermal test (Montenegro) is always negative (Convit and Kerdel-Vegas, 1965).

5. Ethiopian cutaneous leishmaniasis

Price and Fitzherbert (1965) described an antimony-resistant cutaneous leishmaniasis endemic in Ethiopia. They subdivided it into a *lepromatoid type*, very similar to that described above and the histological features of which are similar to those of lepromatous leprosy except for the presence of lcishmania.

In addition they noted an *intermediate group* characterized histologically by the appearance of tuberculoid follicles with scanty parasites alongside histiocytic areas rich in parasites; and a *tuberculoid* type. An accompanying lymphangitis and elephantiasis sometimes occur. The Montenegro test closely follows the histological appearance. It is negative in the 'pseudo-lepromatous' type and positive in the tuberculoid type (Bryceson and Leithead, 1966).

Cutaneous leishmaniasis of the Ethiopian highlands is caused by *L. aethiopica* (Bray *et al.* 1973). The epidemiology is a 'web' of causation involving the *Phlebotomus longipes* group, rock hyraxes (the animal reservoir), *leishmania* and man (Bray, 1974).

6. Lupoid leishmaniasis

Lupoid leishmaniasis or leishmaniasis recidiva is a relapsing form of cutaneous leishmaniasis which is especially common in the Middle East. The lesion looks like lupus vulgaris, spreads slowly over large areas of the body, may last for many years, and the histological picture resembles that of tuberculosis. Organisms are difficult to detect.

C. MUCO-CUTANEOUS LEISHMANIASIS (Espundia)

Espundia is widely distributed through South and Central America.

Epidemiology

Muco-cutaneous leishmaniasis is caused by *L. b. braziliensis* and the sand-flies *P. whitmani*, *P. passoai*, and *P. migonei* are proven vectors of the disease. The most important animal reservoir of infection is the spiny rat. The infection is often confined to the skin but metastases to mucous membrane often occur through the blood stream. The parasite has a predilection for the naso-pharynx. It appears that clinical immunity to heterologous strains of leishmania docs occur, an obscrvation in kccping with the finding that although *L. b. braziliensis*, *L. tropica* and *L. m. mexicana* can easily be distinguished from each other serologically they share certain common antigens. It seems, moreover, that chiclero's ulcer, oriental sore, and uta produce low levels of circulating antibody in the serum despite the fact that they result in life-long immunity in most patients, while patients suffering from muco-cutaneous leishmaniasis possess high levels of circulating antibody (Bray and Lainson, 1965). Lainson and Shaw (1972) have described a *L. braziliensis* complex capable of producing cutaneous lesions which can be self-healing or persistent and the gradation between the cutaneous and mucocutaneous varieties is sometimes imperceptible.

Pathology

There would appear to be severe and mild forms. It has been suggested that the latter, which is usually confined to dermal lesions with the mucosa only involved in a small percentage of cases, is due to a variant of *L. b. brasiliensis—L. b. guyanensis*. The condition occurs at any age and in either sex. The mucous membrane of the nasal cavity may be affected *ab initio*, by direct extension, or by secondary lymphatic or blood-borne spread from a primary skin lesion (Convit *et al*. 1957). There may be an interval of many years between the primary and muco-cutaneous lesions. Secondary lesions occur in the larynx, pharynx, and oral cavity, and in the skin of the limbs. The dermatological lesions resemble those described in *oriental sore*. Fibrous, pendulous, or hyperplastic polyps occur in the nasal cavities and latterly fungating eroding indurated ulcers may destroy the nasal cartilage and similar fungating lesions occur in the tongue, buccal mucosa, and larynx. The regional lymph glands are involved and keratitis has been described (Jaffe, 1954). Scrapings from the mucosa may reveal the presence of parasites. The histological features are variable. There is an intense infiltrate of chronic inflammatory cells with a variable number of histiocytes containing leishmania present. Tuberculoid follicles are seen in the later stages when organisms are scanty. A somewhat similar condition has been described in the Sudan and Asia but visceral involvement is usual in these types.

A table summarizing the immunological response in various types of leishmaniasis is given in Table 2.3.

Diagnostic pathology

L. donovani can be demonstrated in Giemsa-stained smears from the peripheral blood (usually very scanty), spleen, liver, lymph nodes, or bone marrow, and culture of material obtained from the above sources, or by inoculation into hamsters. Leucopenia is a common finding. Tests based on increase in serum gamma globulin are at best only indicative but not diagnostic of the disease (e.g. Napier, Chopra, etc.). The complement-fixation test is very useful in the diagnosis of early cases (Sen Gupta and Adhikari, 1952). The indirect fluorescent antibody technique has been suc-

TABLE 2.3. *Leishmaniasis in man: resistance and the immunological response* (by courtesy of Dr. Patricia Preston)

Pattern of infection	Clinical manifestations	Parasite load	Immunological response		
			Hypersensitivity		Circulating antibody
			Immediate (types 1, 2)	Delayed (type 4)	
Subclinical	None	±	?	++	?
Self-healing	Leishmanioma ulcer	+	+ (types 1, 2)*	++	+
Non-healing: 'anergic'	Disseminated, nodular (DCL, some PKADL)	+++	?	−	+
	Disseminated, visceral (kala-azar)	+++	?	−	++/+++
Non-healing: 'allergic'	Localized, ulcerative (mucocutaneous: espundia, L. donovani; recidiva; persistent multiple ulcers; some PKADL)	±	+ (types 1, 2)†	++/+++	+/++

* Type 1 in cases of *L. mexicana* and *L. braziliensis* complex (Shaw, pers. comm.). Type 2 in cases of *L. braziliensis* complex (Serekii, 1941; Rotberg, 1951); *L. tropica* Iraq (Bray, Rahim and Tajeldin, 1967).
† Type 1 in espundia and persistent multiple ulcers of *L. braziliensis* complex (Shaw, pers. comm.). Type 2 in 'recidiva' (Sagher, 1947; Poray *et al.* 1967).
DCL: diffuse cutaneous leishmaniasis.
PKADL: Post kala-azar dermal leishmanoid.

cessfully used in the sero-diagnosis of kala-azar (Duxbury and Sadun, 1964); negative results were reported from *L. tropica* patients.

The diagnosis of infection with *L. tropica* is made by examining microscopically material obtained by puncture of the undivided edge of the ulcer after appropriate staining. Culture of the material in N.N.N.-type medium should also be done. Biopsy of skin under the edge of the ulcer can provide proof of infection. Histologically the organism may be confused with *H. capsulatum* which, however, stains well with methenamine silver and thus allows differentiation. The Montenegro (leishmanin) test is positive in 95 per cent of patients with *L. tropica*; in contrast it is negative in the active stages of Indian kala-azar.

L. mexicana can be demonstrated in material obtained from the initial ulcers or from the lesions in the mucous membrane, or cultured material or N.N.N. medium. The Montenegro skin test is positive in 92 per cent of patients (Lopes and Laender, 1945) but negative in the disseminated form of leishmaniasis due to *L. pifanoi*.

AMOEBIASIS

Amoebiasis is caused by the protozoon *Entamoeba histolytica*. The parasite lives in the large intestine as an amoeba; it may cause ulceration of the intestinal mucosa. Secondary lesions may occur, most commonly in the liver but other tissues can be affected, e.g. lungs, brain, genital organs, and skin. Amoebiasis has a worldwide distribution but clinical disease occurs most frequently in tropical and sub-tropical latitudes. In temperate climates the infection is usually non-pathogenic and so symptomless.

Life cycle

The amoeba multiplies by binary fission. It lives in the lumen of the large intestine where under suitable conditions it invades the mucous membrane and submucosa. If red blood cells are available, the amoeba will ingest them. When diarrhoea occurs, amoebae are expelled to the exterior as such, and then are found in the freshly passed fluid stools. Amoebae are very sensitive to environmental changes, and so are short lived outside the body. When there is no diarrhoea and other conditions are favourable for encystation, the amoebae cease feeding, become spherical, secrete a cyst wall and the nucleus divides twice to form the characteristic mature four-nucleate cyst.

There are two other characteristic structures, a glycogen vacuole which acts as a carbohydrate reserve, and chromatoid bodies which are a ribosome store. Cysts kept cool and moist remain viable for several weeks.

The cyst is the infective form, and when ingested hatches in the lower part of the small intestine or upper part of the large intestine and a four-nucleate amoeba emerges from the cyst. After a series of nuclear and cytoplasmic divisions, each multinucleate amoeba gives rise to eight uninucleate amoebae, which establish themselves and multiply in the large intestine.

The sizes of the cysts produced by individual strains vary from 7 μm to 15 μm in diameter; they can be divided into two groups, those strains producing cysts over 10 μm and those below 10 μm in diameter (Hoare, 1949). The strains producing small cysts are now held to belong to a separate species, *E. hartmanni*. Infections with *E. hartmanni* are symptomless.

Experimental infection of rats and kittens has proved useful for assessing the virulence of various strains of *E. histolytica*. But in spite of much effort, the basis for pathogenicity has not been unequivocally determined (Neal, 1966).

In order to establish itself in the intestine *E. histolytica* requires an association with bacteria but it is still not clear how the amoebae invade the intestinal mucosa (Neal, 1960 and 1972; Rao and Padma, 1971). *In-vitro* cultivation has been achieved in a variety of media in the presence of bacteria, and it has been demonstrated that trophozoites possess proteolytic enzymes capable of digesting the epithelium of the large intestine. Thus, gelatinases, hyaluronidase activity and other proteolytic enzymes have been demonstrated in strains of *E. histolytica*, but the presence of these substances has not specifically been correlated with the pathogenicity of a strain (Jarumilinta and Maegraith, 1961). Within the true *E. histolytica* group of amoebae some differences have been found by DNA base composition and genome size (Gelderman *et al.* 1971) as well as by immunofluorescence (Nayebi, 1971). The ultrastructure of trophozoites grown axenically has been described by Feria-Velasco and Trevino (1972).

E. histolytica infection may extend directly from the large intestine to surrounding structures within the abdomen, or it may be spread by artificial and natural orifices to the surrounding skin. More commonly the infection spreads extra-intestinally by blood-borne embolism, especially to the liver by the portal circulation; from here it again can extend directly to neighbouring structures, e.g. pleura and lung or the pericardium. Alternatively embolic spread may occur to the brain or other organs.

Epidemiology

Infection with *E. histolytica* occurs throughout both temperate and tropical climates, although the incidence of overt disease is high only in the tropics and subtropics. The disease is spread by cyst passers, who may be divided into two main groups—(a) convalescents who have recovered from an acute attack, and (b) individuals who can recall no clinical evidence of infection. The latter possibly are the more common source of infection, even in countries with high standards of hygiene. Bad sanitation is more important than climate in the predominance of overt infection in the tropics. Carrier rates of *E. histolytica* among symptomless subjects have varied between 20 per cent and 80 per cent in some communities (Stamm, 1966; Editorial, 1968). The parasite can be transmitted by direct contact through the contaminated hands of cyst carriers, e.g. in institutions; it is also transmitted indirectly by means of contaminated food, such as raw vegetables fertilized with fresh human faeces; and through the intermediary of food handlers and flies. Infected water has occasionally been held responsible for the transmission of large outbreaks of the disease.

Although several animals harbour *E. histolytica*—monkeys, dogs, pigs, rats, cats—they are thought to be of no epidemiological importance in human infections. Amoebiasis is not infrequently a house or family infection. Among other factors influencing the epidemiology of the disease we have to consider the following: age and sex, race, immunity, and diet.

Age and sex

Any differences that have been reported in the incidence of the disease between males and females are probably related to exposure rather than a true sex susceptibility to the infection (Abioye and Edington, 1972; Da Silva, 1970; Rivera, 1972). The disease seems to appear in fulminating form in pregnant and puerperal women. This may be a corticosteroid effect (Eisert *et al.* 1959; Kanani and Knight, 1969). Amoebiasis in childhood is not uncommon and may be severe, especially in the malnourished, or following measles (Lewis and Antia, 1969). It usually occurs in the age group nil to 6 years, as those between the ages of 7–16 years seem to enjoy a greater immunity to ill effects from *E. histolytica* infection than others (Wilmot, 1962). Invasive amoebiasis in children and young infants may be commoner than is supposed (Larracilla *et al.* 1971).

Race

All races are susceptible to the disease. Although the infection is often milder in Europeans, this is probably related to sanitary standards, diet, and freedom from debilitating disorders, rather than to a genuine racial factor. Reports from Madras indicate that amoebiasis was twenty times more frequent in Hindus than in Muslims, while in Durban the incidence and severity of amoebic dysentery is greater in Africans than in Indians or Europeans (Wilmot, 1962).

Immunity

There is no evidence that amoebiasis confers any protective immunity and the infection can persist for many years after its establishment. Krupp (1966) has demonstrated by immunoelectrophoresis that antigenic differences occur among different strains of amoebae. Immunity in relation to amoebiasis has been fully reviewed by Tharaveny (1969).

Diet

Experimental and clinical observations have demonstrated that diet can enhance or diminish the incidence and severity of amoebic infection. Despite these observations the role of dietetic factors is not at all clear and the conclusions offered on it are conflicting; (Artigas and Beaver, 1961). The general condition of patients also plays an important role; thus, severe cases of amoebiasis were often seen among soldiers on active service. Biagi and Beltian (1969) showed that dietary cholesterol, testosterone, progesterone and cortisone all enhance the virulence of amoebiasis in experimental animals while Ross and Knight (1973) showed that protein deficient rats showed a greater susceptibility to infection and caecal ulceration than controls.

Pathology

The large intestine is usually the primary site of amoebic infection and in order of frequency, the regions affected are the caecum, flexures, descending colon, and rectum. The appendix is sometimes involved and rarely the ileum may be invaded.

Macroscopically the large intestine may be studded with discrete ulcers with pointing overhanging edges, the intervening mucosa being relatively normal (Fig. 2.13). These 'vertical' deep ulcers are in contrast to the superficial shallow, spreading ulcers seen in bacillary dysentery. At necropsy, however, the lesions are usually much more extensive. The ulcers spread laterally in the submucosa and become confluent. Large areas of mucosa are lost and greenish shaggy sloughs may involve the muscle coat and extend even to the serosa. In other cases a stringy, seaweed-like slough may cover most of the mucosa leaving only occasional islands of recognizable tissue (Ash and Spitz, 1945). In patients whose host/parasite balance has been altered either

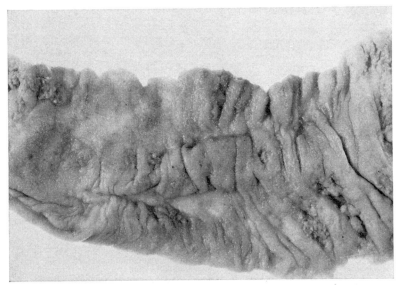

FIG. 2.13. Amoebic dysentery. Colon showing amoebic ulceration.

by drugs, concurrent disease, or pregnancy the whole of the mucosa may be sloughing, dark, and gangrenous and the underlying amoebic infection may be difficult to detect. The wall of the bowel is thickened and friable (Payet *et al.* 1957).

Microscopic pathology

It has always been thought that the trophozoites migrated into the lumina of the crypts of Lieberkuhn and destroyed the mucosal cells by proteolytic action. Recently, however, Prathap and Gilman (1970) have claimed that it is the interglandular surface epithelium that is the site of initial penetration. Colonies may establish themselves in the mucosa with remarkably little reaction on the part of the tissues. The muscularis mucosae is somewhat resistant to this enzyme and the infection may be confined to the mucosa —small, pin-point, flask-shaped ulcers with overhanging edges result. Penetration of the basement membrane and muscularis is usual in lesions seen at necropsy. The amoebae spread laterally beneath the muscularis and intestinal epithelium, forming large 'flask-shaped' or 'water-bottle' ulcers. These ulcers have overhanging edges and consist of a flask-shaped zone of necrosis surrounded by a low-grade inflammatory reaction with lymphocytes and macrophages predominant (Fig. 2.14). A variable fibroblastic reaction

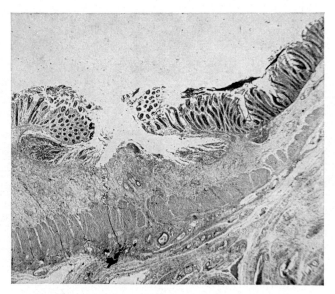

FIG. 2.14. Amoebic dysentery. Section of flask-like amoebic ulcer of colon, illustrating the overhanging edges. (H and E × 48)

is present. Amoebae are present at the periphery of the lesion in the submucosa and muscle layers (Fig. 2.15). They may also be seen in the necrotic tissue itself. They are present singly or in small groups and are round, or oval, bodies slightly larger than the macrophages and have a clear zone surrounding them. They stain positively by a periodic acid Schiff technique. The presence of secondary bacterial infection determines the presence or absence of acute inflammatory cells. Prathap and Gilman (1970) have described the histological changes seen in rectal biopsies from 53 patients with proven acute intestinal amoebiasis. The normal lamina propria contains a moderate number of plasma cells, lymphocytes and eosinophils. Neutrophils are rare. An occasional lymphoid follicle may be seen. They classified the lesions seen as non-specific, mucopenic depression with micro-ulceration, early invasive lesion with superficial ulceration and late invasive lesion with deep ulceration (Gilman and Prathnap, 1971).

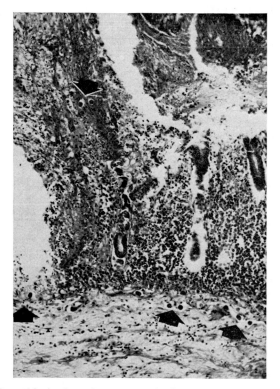

FIG. 2.15. Amoebiasis. Amoebae are seen in the necrotic mucosa and beneath the muscularis mucosa (H and E × 100).

The non-specific lesion consisted of mucosal thickening with a mild to moderate infiltration of neutrophils in an oedematous, congested lamina propria. Lymphoid tissue showed reactive hyperplasia. Amoebae rarely were present in the surface exudate. The lesion described as mucopenic depression with micro-ulceration consisted of small focal superficial ulcers with a decrease in mucosal thickness and mucin depletion. Epithelial cells might contain neutrophils and mitotic figures were numerous. Amoebae were confined to the luminal surface. In the early invasive lesion with superficial ulceration amoebae were seen in the epithelium adjacent to the basement membrane and in the lamina propria with destruction of overlying structures. The crypts were rarely involved. The late invasive lesion was the classical 'flask ulcer' described above.

Immediate complications of intestinal amoebiasis (excluding the liver)

The deep penetrating ulcers are sometimes the seat of considerable haemorrhage or perforation, the latter leading to peritonitis and paralytic ileus. Peritonitis is the commonest local complication and the commonest cause of death from amoebic complications in Durban. The bowel becomes thin and porous with slow seepage of intestinal contents and this is a more usual cause of peritonitis than perforation of a deep penetrating ulcer (Powell and Wilmot, 1966). A series of 73 cases of amoebic peritonitis have been described from Bombay, India (Kapoor *et al.* 1972). Infection of the appendix associated with contiguous caecal and mesenteric lesions may simulate an appendix abscess and caeco-caecal intussusception has been described. Stricture may occur. Lesions in the rectum and anus may track in the deeper tissues, with resulting rectal and anal fistulae. Ulceration of the skin of the anus and abdominal wall occurs and cervical and vaginal ulceration have been noted in association with ulceration in the inguinal region (Mulas and Rodriguez, 1964; Norwich and Lieberman, 1969). Venereal skin infection and urethral amoebiasis following rectal intercourse have been described (Mylins and Ten Seldam, 1962; Sasea and Amin, 1962).

Lesions have also very rarely been described in the joints, salivary glands, stomach, spleen, suprarenals, kidneys, bladder, testes, ovaries, and fallopian tubes. Cerebral abscess has been recorded in the absence of liver lesions, but in general haematogenous spread from intestinal lesions to other organs excluding the liver is rare.

The amoeboma

In areas of stasis in the large bowel mainly the caecum, rectum, sigmoid, and transverse colon, a progressive low-grade inflammatory reaction with marked fibroblastic proliferation may occur in a secondarily infected amoebic abscess. The lesion consists of a core of necrosis with acute and chronic inflammatory cells surrounded by proliferating fibroblasts and a variable number of newly formed blood vessels. The amoebae are found in the central zone of fibrosis and in the necrotic tissue. A considerable mass may form and simulate a neoplasm. The regional lymph nodes are enlarged and hyperplastic. The granuloma of the bowel wall may arise at the site of an amoebic ulcer (Powell, 1974). Stool examination may be negative and radiological examination indeterminate (Recio, 1965). The presence of an unidentified intra-abdominal mass should always call for a serologic test for amoebiasis—either the F.A.T. test, gel diffusion or indirect haemagglutination test.

Ulcerative post-dysenteric colitis

This complication often follows a severe attack of amoebic dysentery; it occurs in patients who have passed sloughs of colonic mucosa in the acute attack. Amoebae are no longer present (as a result of treatment) but residual damage such as to cause diarrhoea to continue is evident. At endoscopy the mucosa is red and oedematous but ulceration is usually absent; although occasionally superficial mucosal erosions and large ulcers persist. The course is not unlike that of chronic non-specific ulcerative colitis but whereas the amoebic gel diffusion test is invariably negative in the latter, it is 100 per cent positive in patients with post-dysenteric colitis.

Amoebiasis and the liver

Amoebae may be seen in the portal venules in intestinal amoebiasis, by which route they are carried to the liver. They may also enter the lymphatics but must be destroyed in the lymphatic glands with little reaction as few if any enter the blood stream via the thoracic duct. There are, however, no records of amoebae being detected in the abdominal lymphatic glands.

The presence of the amoebae in the liver may be responsible for a diffuse hepatitis or a liver abscess or abscesses may form. Although there is no doubt that, in some individuals with evidence of intestinal amoebiasis, a clinical syndrome of fever with an enlarged, tender liver and a mild leucocytosis which responds dramatically to treatment with emetine hydrochloride occurs, the majority of observers would agree that conclusive pathological proof of chronic diffuse amoebic hepatitis as an entity is lacking. Excluding the reports of one group of workers who have described the presence of amoebae in the liver (Doxiades et al. 1961), the pathological findings have been non-specific in this condition. There is infiltration of the portal tracts of the liver with chronic inflammatory cells and the Kupffer cells are hypertrophied.

Liver abscess is the most common extra-intestinal complication of intestinal amoebiasis. The abscess is usually single but multiple abscesses are not uncommon. The right lobe of the liver is most frequently affected, especially the posterior portion of the dome. The left lobe may, however, be solely involved. Bile would appear to destroy the amoebae as the gall bladder is never affected. In over 50 per cent of patients with amoebic infections of the liver there may be no evidence of amoebic infection on stool examination. The amoebae cause lysis of the parenchymal cells of the liver primarily in the periportal region. An extending necrosis follows and the abscess cavity may reach a diameter of 12 cm. The cavity contains sterile, chocolate-coloured fluid, the result of the lysis of liver cells, granular debris, and few inflammatory cells. Amoebae may or may not be present in the pus. Histologically the wall of the abscess consists of necrotic tissue and compressed liver parenchyma containing a variable infiltrate of monocytes, plasma cells, lymphocytes, and fibroblasts. Amoebae may be seen in the area of coagulative necrosis or in the least affected compressed liver tissue (Fig. 2.16).

Secondary infection by various organisms may occur, especially following surgical intervention (pyogenic organisms, *Esch. coli*, *B. pyocyaneus* and even *S. typhi* have been described). If this occurs the pus becomes yellow,

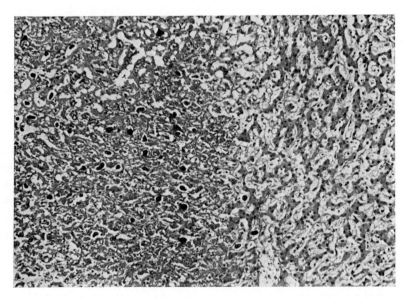

FIG. 2.16. Amoebic liver abscess. Section of liver, showing numerous amoebae in a necrotic abscess. Note the absence of an inflammatory reaction (PAS × 100).

cream, or green in colour and amoebae become even more difficult to identify.

Vakil *et al.* (1970) have reported atypical manifestations of amoebic abscess of the liver in a considerable number of patients, viz: jaundice of both the hepatocellular and cholestatic types; neurological manifestations of hepatic precoma and coma, presentation as a localized mass in the epigastrium; presentation with fever malaise and leucocytosis with few signs or symptoms pointing to liver involvement and lastly those patients admitted with the provisional diagnosis of 'acute abdomen'.

Liver-function tests are not diagnostic. The successful introduction of hepatic photo-screening techniques employing radioactive colloidal gold (^{198}Au) or ^{131}I Rose Bengal has allowed earlier diagnosis and more accurate location of the abscess in sophisticated centres (Sheehy *et al.* 1968). The plasma cholinesterase is low and anaesthesia may be a hazard (Mullan and Williams, 1965). The serum alkaline phosphatase and transaminases may be increased. The serum bilirubin is rarely greater than 2 mg per 100 ml (Salako, 1967). A degree of anaemia is common and deficient absorption of vitamin B_{12} has been reported (Devakul *et al.* 1967). Leucocytosis, rarely above 25,000 per mm^3, is usual but not invariable. The ESR is nearly always raised and usually over 50 mm in the hour.

Complications of liver abscess

The right lobe of the diaphragm is usually raised and direct extension of the abscess to the pleural cavity or base of the right lung is not uncommon. Movement of the diaphragm is restricted. Less commonly than right-sided pulmonary involvement the abscess may rupture into the stomach, intestine, peritoneal cavity, hepatic vein or even through the chest wall. Rarely haematogenous spread from the abscess to the left lung may occur. Caval thrombosis is a rare complication.

Pericarditis has been reported in 7·5 per cent of patients with hepatic abscesses (Psulley, 1965). The parietal pericardium is thickened and there is thick, greenish-yellow purulent material between the layers whose surfaces are yellowish-grey and granular. Histologically there may be amoebae in the amorphous necrotic material surrounded by their characteristic clear zone, if viable at the time of fixation, and scanty monocytes and lymphocytes are present. The pericardium shows layers of coagulative necrosis, granulation tissue, and fibrosis, the underlying myocardium on the epicardial surface being relatively unaffected. When death occurs in these patients with suppurative pericarditis it is due to cardiac tamponade or constrictive pericarditis. Patients with only a serous pericardial effusion have also been described (McLeod *et al.* 1966).

Amoebiasis and malignancy

Carcinoma of the colon has been observed following amoebiasis and carcinoma and lymphoreticular tumours have been described in association with the condition. However, as large bowel cancer is rare in many parts of the tropics where the incidence of amoebiasis is high, these isolated reports must be regarded as fortuitous and a causal association between amoebic infection of the large bowel and malignant change cannot be accepted. Cutaneous amoebiasis of the perianal region or vulva may mimic carcinoma (Ten Seldam, 1970); three cases of amoebiasis of the cervix uteri closely resembled tumours (McClatchie and Sambhi, 1971).

DIAGNOSTIC PATHOLOGY

A. AMOEBIC DYSENTERY

The clinical diagnosis of amoebiasis has to be confirmed by identification of *E. histolytica*. During an attack of amoebic dysentery the motions are loose, offensive, and contain mucus and blood; faecal elements are always present (Stamm, 1965). On microscopical examination motile amoebae, some with engorged red cells, will be found in the freshly passed stool or in specimens removed at sigmoidoscopy or proctoscopy (Fig. 2.17).

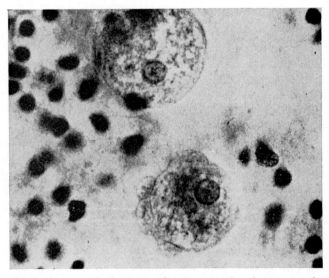

FIG. 2.17. Acute amoebic dysentery. Stool smear, showing two trophozoites of *E. histolytica*. A small, centrally-placed nucleolus can be seen in the nucleus, the chromatin of which is scanty and largely concentrated on the nuclear membrane (× 400).

In asymptomatic infections, and during remission, the stool is semiformed and contains *E. histolytica* cysts. They can be seen to contain one or more bar-shaped chromatoid bodies and staining with iodine reveals one to four nuclei and a glycogen mass. Repeated stool examinations (six to ten) should be made before absence of infection can confidently be assumed. Concentration techniques for cysts are available, and cultural methods may assist diagnosis in scanty infections.

Sigmoidoscopy

Amoebic ulceration is commonly found in the rectum and sigmoid, so that sigmoidoscopic examination often affords valuable information. Usually, small yellow ulcers with surrounding hyperaemia are seen, while in between the ulcers the mucous membrane is not inflamed. In chronic cases, amoebic lesions may appear as 'pin-point craters' irregularly disposed.

Radiology

This is useful for the differential diagnosis of other ulcerative conditions of the bowel and for assessing the effect of treatment on amoebomas.

Serology

Until recently immunological methods for the diagnosis of intestinal and extra-intestinal amoebiasis have been equivocal. Complement-fixation precipitin, intradermal, and fluorescent antibody tests have all been used with varying success. Newer techniques with improved antigens have given good results. Since serology as a diagnostic technique is more useful in extra-intestinal than in intestinal amoebiasis, it will be dealt with below.

B. EXTRA-INTESTINAL AMOEBIASIS

The diagnosis of extra-intestinal amoebiasis can be difficult and atypical clinical presentations especially of amoebic liver abscess are not uncommon. Concomitant amoebic dysentery may be present in 5–10 per cent of patients. *E. histolytica* frequently are not found in the stools, and a polymorphonuclear leucocytosis may not be present. Diagnostic aspiration may produce the typical 'chocolate coloured' or 'anchovy sauce' pus and immediate direct examination of the abscess contents may reveal amoebae. Rarely, culture in media pre-conditioned with suitable bacteria such as *Esch. coli* or *Clostridium welchii* reveals amoebae missed on direct examination. Results of liver-function tests are very variable, serum phosphatase and serum glutamic pyruvic transaminase values may be raised. In broncho-pulmonary amoebiasis amoebae may be detected in the sputum by experienced observers.

Radiology

Liver abscess may cause a raised right diaphragm which shows restricted movement. Though the normal shape of the right dome may be preserved, localized bulging or 'humping' is sometimes seen. A small pleural effusion is frequently recorded while basal atelectasis usually linear in appearance also occurs. Diagnostic methods, other than simple radiography, that have been used include aspiration with air or lipiodol replacement, splenic venography, and the induction of a pneumoperitoneum (Ellman *et al.* 1965). Isotope scanning of the liver and ultrasonic sounding have also been used for defining liver abscesses (de Dominicis *et al.* 1966). Amoebic lung abscesses are usually thick-walled and occur mainly in the anterior basal segment of the right lower lobe; consolidation with or without abscess formation may also occur.

Serology

The need for a reliable laboratory test for the diagnosis of extra-intestinal amoebiasis has long been felt. A recent review of the serological diagnosis of amoebiasis was carried out by Wery-Paskoff *et al.* (1974). The following tests have been used with success:

1. *Complement-fixation test* (Fulton *et al.* 1951; Robinson, 1972)

Recent results of this test using improved antigens in the diagnosis of amoebiasis in an endemic area have revealed that it was positive in 100 per cent of patients suffering from amoebic liver abscess; and in 16 per cent of cases with intestinal amoebiasis. Controls gave negative results in all cases. A correlation of antibody titre with the type of amoebic involvement revealed that the titres were very low in intestinal amoebiasis and high in amoebic hepatitis and amoebic abscesses of the liver. The complement fixation titres drop more rapidly in treated cases than do haemagglutination titres.

2. *Amoebic gel-diffusion precipitin test* (Powell *et al.* 1965)

This test is positive in 96 per cent of patients suffering from amoebic liver abscess. On the other hand, it has also been found positive in 15 per cent of Africans in hospital with diseases other than amoebiasis.

3. *Indirect haemagglutination test* (Kessel *et al.* 1965)

This test is positive in 100 per cent of amoebic liver abscess patients; 98 per cent of dysentery cases; and 66 per cent of asymptomatic carriers. The test remains positive for many years following the initial infection, although the titre of reactivity may drop gradually.

4. *Fluorescent antibody test* (Jeanes, 1966; Parelkar and Stamm, 1973)

The indirect fluorescence method has also been used. More positives are obtained from acute than from chronic cases of intestinal amoebiasis, while all extra-intestinal cases give positive results. Positive results have however also occurred in individuals with no conventional evidence of amoebic infection. It is too soon to assess the possible value of this serological test in the diagnosis of amoebiasis.

5. *Latex agglutination test* (Morris *et al.* 1970)

A simple latex agglutination test taking only minutes to perform seems promising, and a commercial kit is available. Stamm *et al.* (1973) have recently evaluated the test.

Other amoebae

Primary amoebic meningoencephalitis is a recently discovered human disease caused by amoebae quite different from those traditionally regarded as parasitic in man, Carter (1972) and Willaert (1974) have comprehensively reviewed the subject. The amoebae (*Naegleria* and *Hartmanella*) are usually free-living in water, decaying organic matter etc. Swimming pools would appear to be a potent source of infection. They are small and have a distinctive nucleus. They grow readily on simple media. The amoebae invade the nasal mucosa and reach the meninges and brain along the olfactory nerve filaments. The C.S.F. shows some increase of protein and large numbers of pus and some red blood cells. An acute inflammatory exudate is found in the subarachnoid space. Thrombosis, necrosis of blood vessels and focal haemorrhages occur. The inferior aspect of the olfactory bulbs is particularly heavily involved. The amoebae can be recognized microscopically in fresh specimens of cerebrospinal fluid in a cell-counting chamber. They only appear as 'smudges' on stained films. Cultural methods can be utilized. Histologically in the brain there is a dense infiltration of the subarachnoid space by neutrophils, macrophages and amoebae. The amoebae are palely stained, rounded cells with rather granular cytoplasm and a small usually eccentric nucleus containing a conspicuous karyosome (Symmers, 1969).

Infection of the human gut may occur with other amoebae namely *E. coli*, *Dientamoeba fragilis*, *Endolimax nana*, and *Iodamoeba butschlii*. There is controversy, however, concerning the actual pathogenicity of these organisms. Derrick (1948) described a fatal case of generalized amoebiasis in a Japanese prisoner-of-war which he attributed to an overwhelming infection with *I. butschlii*. Human infection with *Entamoeba polecki** is common in parts of New Guinea where pigs and man live in close association (McMillan and Kelly, 1970).

FLAGELLATE AND OTHER INTESTINAL PROTOZOA

A number of flagellate protozoa commonly parasitize the human intestine and genito-urinary tract, e.g. *Trichomonas hominis, Chilomastix mesnili, T. vaginalis,* and *Giardia lamblia*. The ones with real claims to pathogenicity are *G. lamblia* and *T. vaginalis* which are found both in the tropics and in temperate countries. Barnes and McKay (1962) from New Guinea have described a case of *C. mesnili* infection of the genito-urinary tract with painful micturition and haematuria, while *T. vaginalis* urethritis is common in males.

GIARDIASIS

Heavy infection with *G. lamblia* is often accompanied by diarrhoea or steatorrhoea. Brandborg *et al.* (1967) have demonstrated invasion of the mucosa in 6 of 10 patients by suction biopsies from the duodenum and proximal colon, and have emphasized that the organism may be an important pathogen of man. Any lingering doubts about its pathogenicity have been laid to rest by recent reports of epidemics at a ski resort, among passengers returned from a Mediterranean cruise and among people who have travelled in the U.S.S.R. (*Lancet*, 1974). Electron microscopy has demonstrated *Giardia* within mucosal cells (Morecki and Parker, 1967).

Life cycle

The trophozoite lives in the upper part of the small intestine particularly the duodenum and jejunum. In appearance it resembles a half-pear split longitudinally measuring 12–18 μm in length. It reproduces itself by a complicated process of binary fission. The cysts—which are the infective forms—occur in the faeces, often in enormous numbers. They are oval in shape, contain at first two nuclei which divide, giving rise to four in the mature cyst. Cultivation in artificial media has been achieved. The trophozoites are found among the mucus threads adherent to the mucous membrane of the small intestine, causing pathological changes such as a partial villous atrophy and an apparent increase in the size and number of the goblet cells.

---

* *Entamoeba polecki*, a parasite of pigs, has very occasionally been reported as an infection in man (Levin and Armstrong, 1970). This infection should be suspected if intestinal amoebiasis is resistant to treatment. Differentiation from the trophozoite of *E. histolytica* can be difficult. The cysts of *E. polecki* however are consistently uninucleate. The nucleus is smaller than that seen in the uninucleate cysts of *E. histolytica* which is one-third to half the diameter of the cyst. The cyst of *E. polecki* may contain as many as 30 chromatoid bars whereas *E. histolytica* usually contains fewer than 10.

Epidemiology

The infection is transmitted by the ingestion of cysts, as a result of insanitary habits or contaminated food. It is common in children and in adults sometimes causing symptoms of malabsorption in both due to mechanical irritation rather than invasion of the mucous membrane. *G. lamblia* is harboured by many animals but these play little part in the epidemiology of human infections. Giardia infections may persist for years and the parasite may invade the biliary tract. Symptomatic giardiasis is being increasingly recognized among travellers (Walzer *et al.* 1971; Steiner *et al.* 1971 and Babb *et al.* 1971). During a 10-year study in India 23 per cent of 300 patients with non-dysenteric diarrhoea were found to be infected with *Giardia* (Antia *et al.* 1966); Symposium, 1970). A 248-page monograph written in Rumanian has been devoted to giardiasis (Lucian, 1971). Of great interest is the relationship between Giardia infection and immunoglobulin deficiency syndromes (Ament and Rubin, 1972; Brown *et al.* 1972).

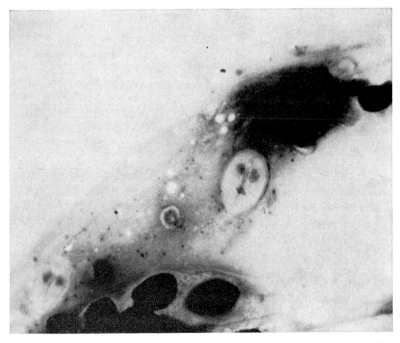

FIG. 2.18. Giardiasis. Jejunal biopsy material. The paired nuclei, axostyle, and parabasal body are clearly seen (× 750). (*By courtesy of Dr. John H. Yardley.*)

Pathology

G. lamblia usually is present as an apparently incidental finding in healthy individuals. In others mild symptoms of abdominal discomfort and morning diarrhoea may be present. A sprue-like condition can occur in children (Cortner, 1959) and occasionally in adults chronic diarrhoea, steatorrhoea, and the malabsorption syndrome are also seen (Yardley *et al.* 1964). Death has been attributed to giardiasis in a subject with acute, non-specific ulceration of the small intestine (McGrath *et al.* 1940), but this must be an exceedingly rare occurrence.

Jejunal biopsies (Yardley *et al.* 1964) have shown focal acute inflammatory lesions superimposed on a non-specific chronic inflammatory infiltrate in the mucosa. In addition the villi are shortened and thickened and there is an increased number of epithelial cells in mitosis (Alp and Hislop, 1969). The familiar dorsal view of the organism is uncommon in biopsy material (Fig. 2.18). The parasites are seen as thin, basophilic, sickle-shaped bodies about the size of the nuclei of epithelial cells lying outside the mucosa itself (Fig. 2.19).

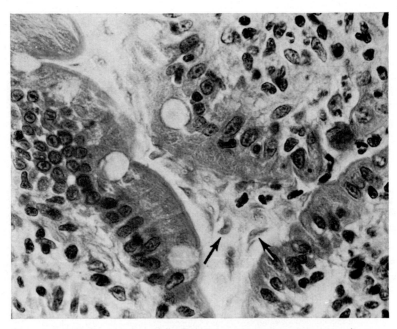

FIG. 2.19. Giardiasis. Jejunal biopsy, illustrating giardia near the base of the villi and closely applied to the epithelium. Polymorphonuclear leucocytes are invading the epithelium and are present in the lumen between the villi (H and E × 450). (*By courtesy of Dr. John H. Yardley.*)

Diagnostic pathology

Diagnosis of the infection is made by finding cysts of the parasite in formed stools and vegetative forms in fluid stools. Fat absorption may be impaired and additional evidence of malabsorption—as described in sprue (p. 528)—may be present. An ingenious method of sampling the upper small bowel with a recoverable nylon yarn swallowed in a weighted capsule has been found useful (Beal *et al.* 1970).

TRICHOMONAS HOMINUS AND T. VAGINALIS

T. hominis inhabits the caecum and large intestine. The body is pear-shaped, 10–15 μm in length. The single ovoid nucleus is situated in the rounded anterior end and there are three flagella. There is no cystic phase. The presence of these flagellates in diarrhoeic stools has no pathogenic significance. *T. vaginalis* is found in the vagina and male urethra. It is larger than *T. hominis*, reaching 27 μm in length, and usually has five anterior flagella. No cysts are known. The flagellate is commonly found during the reproductive period in women, and men play an important part in the transmission of the infection. The incidence of infection in the vagina may be high and the presence of the parasite is associated with lowered vaginal acidity.

In the female vaginitis is usual and an anterior urethritis may occur. Posterior urethritis is rare and the bladder is never affected.

The vagina is inflamed and tender. Erosions may be present which histologically show a superficial coagulum containing trichomonads and cellular elements of the blood. In the submucosa there is a non-specific chronic inflammatory reaction with a variable number of neutrophil polymorphonuclears present. Trichomonads may or may not be seen. Secondary infection is usual in these cases.

In the male urethritis is not uncommon and the infection may spread to the bladder and prostate gland. The condition is usually mild unless secondary infection occurs.

Diagnosis is made by finding the flagellate in vaginal and prostatic secretions or in the urine. *T. vaginalis* may be identified in the moist slide by dark ground or phase contrast microscopic examination. Inoculation of a vaginal swab into culture medium incubated at 37 °C for 24–48 hours will give better results. The organism may also be identified in cervical smears stained by the Papinicolaou method.

ISOSPORIASIS

The coccidia *Isosopora belli* and *I. hominis* are widely distributed in the tropical world. No pathological accounts are available and the pathogenicity of these organisms is mild and controversial (Limbos *et al.* 1965). Brandberg *et al.* (1970) described the life cycle of *I. belli* and the literature has been reviewed by Jarpa Gana (1966) who also described a personal series of 57 patients most of whom had symptoms with diarrhoea, weight loss and fever. High prevalence rates have been reported from Rumania, Holland and Chile.

TOXOPLASMOSIS

Toxoplasmosis is caused by the coccidian parasite *Toxoplasma gondii*. It is a disease with a world-wide distribution.

Life cycle

The life cycle of *T. gondii* is similar to that of coccidian parasites and its taxonomic status is now considered to be a coccidian parasite related to the genus *Isopora* (Hutchison *et al.* 1970). When extracellular, the organism is crescent shaped, about 6 μm long. The cytoplasm stains blue with Giemsa and the eccentric nucleus red. In the intracellular stages *T. gondii* appears singly or in clusters within the reticulo-endothelial cells. Aggregations of the organisms may form pseudocysts. The cystic form of the parasite reaches 100 μm in diameter. Reproduction of the organism is by binary fission. Toxoplasma trophozoites and cysts characterize acute and chronic infections respectively, but cysts may form early in the acute stage and trophozoites may remain active for years in some chronic infections. Zaman and Colley (1972) described the fine structure and host–parasite relationship of *T. gondii* during penetration of macrophages.

Epidemiology

The method of transmission of *T. gondii* from person to person is un-known except in congenital infections. Surveys of various populations have shown that a high incidence of asymptomatic infection occurs in the warm to hot humid areas, and a low incidence in the cold areas and hot dry areas. Serological tests in Singapore have shown that the Chinese—beef and pork eaters—have a lower frequency of antibodies to toxoplasmosis than Malays and Indians (Zaman and Goh, 1969). In general there does not appear to be any difference in infection rate between urban and rural populations, between sexes or between races in the same environment. *T. gondii* is widely distributed in the animal kingdom, being particularly common in cats, dogs, and rabbits (Hutchison *et al.* 1972). However, in spite of the circumstantial evidence indicating a possible transmission between animals and man, it is probable that both may become infected from a common source or sources (Hartley, 1966). Ingestion of raw beef and pork meat are a recognized mode of infection and it has been demonstrated that infection was particularly high in a tuberculosis hospital in France, where the children were fed raw or underdone meat (Desmonts *et al.* 1965). High infection rates have also been found in sewage workers, rabbit trappers, laboratory workers, and nurses. The role of droplet infection, mechanical subcutaneous inoculation by biting, or blood-sucking arthropods in the transmission of toxoplasmosis has yet to be proved. Zigas and Benfante (1972) have reviewed the whole subject and evaluated current progress in human toxoplasmosis. Roever-Bennet (1972) has reviewed the status of toxoplasmosis in seven African countries and it is clear that *T. gondii* is widely distributed in large parts of Africa, in man as well as animals.

Immunity

Toxoplasmosis is prevalent in many species of mammals and birds and rarely does any harm. Only occasionally is illness produced and in man this may vary in severity from slight glandular enlargement to a fatal meningo-encephalitis. It has been suggested that resistance to *Toxoplasma* is due to persistent latent infection (Beattie, 1963).

Pathology

The infection may be congenital or acquired.

Acquired toxplasmosis

Clinically the types of acquired toxoplasmosis can be classified as follows:

(1) asymptomatic; (2) acute; (3) glandular; (4) chronic.

Most infections, as shown by population surveys, must have been asymptomatic. Acute fulminating fevers are uncommon and are characterized by fever, erythematous or petechial skin rashes, and signs of central nervous system and cardiac involvement. A similarity to typhus fever has been noted. Excluding the asymptomatic type the glandular type is most common and is difficult to distinguish from infectious mononucleosis. The Paul–Bunnell test is, however, negative. The symptoms in the chronic form are variegated and the condition is difficult to diagnose. Vague gastro-intestinal symptoms, muscular and joint pains, and signs of generalized or focal central nervous system involvement, are described. Pain in the eye, blurring of vision and even blindness may be complained of. In the majority of instances these eye complaints are, however, unassociated with other symptoms of toxoplasmosis.

The parasites proliferate in the cells of the reticulo-endothelial system and parenchymal cells of practically every organ.

The most severe lesions are seen in striated muscle, the central nervous system, and heart. The lungs, liver, pancreas, spleen, testes, kidneys, hypophysis, and adrenal may also be affected and generalized lymphadenopathy is a feature of the more subacute form of the disease. The essential lesion in the acute form of the disease is a small area of focal necrosis surrounded by a variable cellular inflammatory reaction depending upon the tissue affected (Remington *et al.* 1960). Organisms may or may not be present singly, in pairs or rosettes. They are crescentic, measuring 3–5 · 3 μm. One end is pointed and the other blunted and contains the nucleus. There is no kinetoplast. In the great majority of instances they are not detected in routine paraffin embedded sections probably because of shrinkage, and celloidin embedding is preferable (Wilder, 1952). They stain well with H and E and are PAS-positive and Gram-negative. Pseudocysts within cells without surrounding reaction are usually present. They are about 30 × 100 μm in size and contain numerous basophilic nuclei with no septa apparent. A reticulin stain may outline the wall (Kass *et al.* 1952) which is also PAS-positive. The mechanism of the tissue reaction is not entirely clear. It may follow rupture of the pseudocyts or be a reaction to the dissemination of free toxoplasma organisms prior to its formation (Kass *et al.* 1952).

Changes in the individual organs

A focal embolic encephalomyelitis has been described in the *brain* but the usual changes are scattered small areas of focal necrosis surrounded by macrophages, lymphocytes and, occasionally, multinucleated giant cells. The Virchow–Robin space may be infiltrated with lymphocytes and plasma cells. Small pseudocysts may be seen in some foci and in others free toxoplasmas but usually there are no organisms. Pseudocysts may be present in the parenchymal cells with no surrounding reaction apparent. Granulomatous lesions simulating space occupying lesions have been described (Bobowski and Reed, 1958; Koeze and Klinson, 1964). Intracranial calcification is rare. The predominant cell in the C.S.F. may be the monocyte and toxoplasmas may be seen. Dubin *et al.* (1971) describe a patient with systemic lupus erythmatosis who was treated with systemic corticosteroids and cyclophosphamide. Neurologic signs and symptoms developed and death ensued. Autopsy revealed the presence of cerebral toxoplasmosis which was the cause of death. Schuman *et al.* (1967) have associated toxoplasma infection with tumours of the central nervous system, specifically astrocytomas. This deserves further study.

Jasim and Taha (1971) have reported that 4 · 9 per cent to 22 · 8 per cent of skin tests have been positive in the populations examined in Iraq and described four cases of toxoplasmic lymphadenitis in males aged 20–38 years.

In the *myocardium* pseudocysts are generally seen within the myofibrils and there are scattered foci of necrosis surrounded by monocytes and lymphocytes, with neutrophils and eosinophils present in variable numbers (Sexton *et al*. 1953). An associated pericarditis may be present. Hypertrophy and dilation of the heart with patchy areas of fibrosis in the myocardium in the absence of an inflammatory infiltrate have been described from Chile (Arribada and Escobar, 1968).

In the *lungs* non-specific broncho-pneumonic changes may be found. An interstitial pneumonitis with proliferation of the alveolar lining cells, many containing parasites, and a gelatinous exudate in the alveoli are diagnostic if observed.

In *striated muscle* there is necrosis of individual fibres with sarcolemmal proliferation and infiltration around these necrotic areas by macrophages, lymphocytes and occasionally neutrophils. Once again pseudocysts may be seen in the muscle cells without a surrounding inflammatory reaction. Polymyositis due to toxoplasmosis is rare but does occur (Chandar *et al*. 1968).

Lesions in the *eye* are usually unilateral but may be bilateral, and pathologically are most commonly diagnosed as tuberculosis or as a granulomatous lesion of unknown aetiology (Wilder, 1952). The retina, choroid, and frequently the sclera, are involved. There is necrosis of the retina and choroid with a surrounding zone of epitheloid cells and giant cells, some containing melanin pigment. Lymphocytes and plasma cells with varying numbers of eosinophils and neutrophils are also seen. Rounded structures containing amorphous eosinophilic material, possibly degenerate pseudocysts, may also be present in the necrotic material. It should be noted that in ocular toxoplasmosis the dye test may be of low titre and rise rapidly after enucleation (Jacobs *et al*. 1954).

The *glandular* is the most frequent form of clinical presentation in the acquired type of infection. The nodes show follicular hyperplasia with central chromatolysis. There is histiocytic proliferation in the sinusoids and islands of large eosinophilic histiocytic reticulum cells may be scattered throughout the gland. Foci of necrosis may be present. Parasites are rarely seen histologically (Saunders and Thatcher, 1963) although invariably isolated on animal inoculation. Similar lesions may be seen in the spleen. Specific lesions in the bone marrow have not been described, but the occasional presence of leukaemoid reaction in the peripheral blood suggests that they occur.

Focal necrotic lesions with an inflammatory infiltrate may also be present in the liver, pancreas, testes, kidney, hypophysis, and adrenal.

As previously stated the signs and symptoms in the chronic stage are vague and the pathology, excluding the eye lesions, has not been well described. A chronic myocarditis and chronic lesions in the muscles have been noted, and a local hypersensitivity to released toxoplasma from ruptured cells is the suggested mechanism. A chronic local lesion with localized lymphadenitis has occurred in a laboratory worker following a finger prick with infected material (Ström, 1951).

Congenital toxoplasmosis

The infection is acquired from the mother and toxoplasma may be isolated from the placenta or vaginal discharge (Mellgren *et al.* 1952). The symptomatology and pathology depend upon the gestational period at which the fetus is infected and may be classified as acute, subacute, and chronic. Elliott (1970) has described the placental findings in a third-month abortion. The placenta was avascular with stromal fibrosis and necrotizing inflammation in the villi. Numerous large multinucleated giant cells were present with nodular accumulations of histiocytes beneath the syncytial layer. Encysted and free forms of toxoplasma were found in these areas of histiocytic inflammation. The parasites were also found in villi and in the syncytial trophoblastic layer without an inflammatory reaction.

In the acute form death may occur *in utero* or the neonate may suffer from jaundice, skin rashes, hepatomegaly, lymphadenopathy, and meningo-encephalitis. This type is rarely seen and the pathology in the organs is similar to that described in the adult.

In the subacute form there has been a subsidence of the acute lesions and the child presents with cerebral calcification, chorioretinitis, which is usually bilateral in contrast to the acquired form, hydrocephaly or micro-cephaly and various signs of central nervous system involvement.

The chronic form may be asymptomatic or exhibit mild symptoms of the subacute stage. Relapses may occur and meningo-encephalitis or chorioretinitis may be seen in older children.

In the brain miliary granulomata may be scattered throughout. The ependyma is affected and the infiltrating cells are monocytes, plasma cells and eosinophils. The meningeal reaction is less marked than the peri-ventricular. The lesions become calcified in the cortical layers and may be seen radiologically as bilateral rounded shadows 1–3 mm in diameter. Cysts may be present in healthy tissue. Signs of hydrocephalus and thinning of the skull may occur. The protein in the cerebrospinal fluid is increased and may be xanthochromatic with an increase of lymphocytes and monocytes, and organisms may be isolated.

Bilateral chorioretinitis is usually present in the eye and shows as yellow-ish-white foci in the fundus with a similar histopathology as already described. They may heal with residual scarring and optic neuritis may occur.

As in the adult form lesions may be present in the myocardium, skeletal muscle, and abdominal viscera.

Diagnostic pathology

In the blood there may be a leucocytosis or leucopenia. An eosinophilia has been described (Cathie, 1954). There may be a mild degree of anaemia and a leukaemoid reaction and atypical lymphocytes may be seen.

Toxoplasma may be isolated from blood, cerebrospinal fluid, saliva, sputum, lymph nodes, skin, liver, and muscle by intraperitoneal injection of the biopsy or other material into mice, guinea-pigs, or hamsters. Mice are most suitable as they do not suffer from toxoplasmosis as a laboratory infection (Kass *et al.* 1952).

Histological examination of muscle (especially the gastrocnemius) or liver may reveal the presence of specific lesions, but the examination of lymph nodes usually fails to reveal the organisms although the pathology itself may point to a diagnosis. A portion of the biopsy should therefore not be put in fixative but should be refrigerated, and kept in a solution of penicillin and streptomycin, 100 units/ml of each in normal saline, prior to animal inoculation.

A number of serological tests have been described for the detection of antibodies to *T. gondii*; the cytoplasm-modifying test of Sabin–Feldman (dye-test) (Sabin and Feldman, 1948) is the one most widely used. It is a sensitive test which shows the presence of antibody in many of the normal adult population and the most convincing method of diagnosing active toxoplasmosis is by the demonstration of at least a fourfold rise in titre, coupled with the isolation of toxoplasma in tissues or body fluids by inoculation of mice.

Other serological tests in common use are: (1) complement-fixation tests, (2) direct agglutination test, (3) haemagglutination test, (4) fluorescent antibody test (Fulton, 1963; Fletcher, 1965). Recently a toxoplasma neutralization test (Nikkels, 1965) and a micro-agglutination test have been described. A review of the seroepidemiology of toxoplasma infection in man was given by Fleck (1972).

It has been suggested that tests for toxoplasmosis should be performed in cases of lymphadenopathy of uncertain aetiology, choroidoretinitis, and neonatal illness with hydrocephalus, meningeal symptoms, or generalized illness with hepatosplenomegaly (Fleck and Ludham, 1965).

SARCOSPORIDIOSIS

Sarcosporidia are a group of muscle-inhabiting, spore-forming protozoa and the species have been placed in a single genus (*Sarcocystis*). Some protozoologists consider them fungi. They are parasites of pigs, mice, sheep, cattle, horses, and birds and are rarely found in man. The sarcosysts (Meischer's tubes) are elongated tubular bodies which distend the muscle fibres. The life cycle is unknown. The human parasite is called *S. lindemanni* and the probable mode of transmission is by ingestion of infected food or drink contaminated with the faeces of the above animals. Human infections are accidental and diagnosis is made by finding Meischer's tubes in sections of muscle; in one case the parasites were found in the heart (Gilmore *et al.* 1942).

PNEUMOCYSTIS CARINII

P. carinii causes an interstitial plasma cell pneumonia in premature or debilitated infants usually in the first three months of life. Sporadic cases occur in patients with gamma globulin abnormalities, blood dyscrasias or on steroid or radiation therapy (Barnett *et al.* 1969). It is a parasite of dogs, rats, sheep and other animals. The mode of transmission is unknown.

The parasites are small unicellular roundish organisms about 5 μm in diameter and can be stained by Giemsa, a periodic acid Schiff technique or methenamine silver.

In the lungs masses of pneumocystis are found in the foamy semi-liquid substance which fills the alveoli and bronchioles. Laryngeal and tracheal swabs are said to be negative. The parasites have been seen in lymph nodes and in the spleen. Cytomegalic inclusion disease has been noted not infrequently with the infection.

Barton and Campbell (1967) have described the ultra-structure. Whitcomb *et al.* (1970), in serial pulmonary function studies, considered that the infection might lead to pulmonary fibrosis.

BALANTIDIASIS

Balantidiasis in man has been recorded from most parts of the world, and is caused by infection with the ciliate protozoon, *Balantidium coli*, which is a common parasite of the pig.

Life cycle

The large ovoid cysts are passed in the faeces and contain the parasite which may be seen moving actively. The enclosed balantidium then loses its cilia, and sometimes two individuals are found in the same cyst. *B. coli* reproduces asexually by transverse fission. Transmission of infection takes place by ingestion of cysts, but the subsequent life cycle is not known. There are many methods of culturing the organism; usually human serum diluted with saline is used (Arean and Koppish, 1956). For their nutrition balantidia depend mostly on starches and red blood cells.

Epidemiology

B. coli has been found in the intestinal contents of man and a large number of animals—wild boars, sheep, horses, rats, frogs, monkeys, etc., but domestic pigs are much the most important reservoir hosts. Infection in man is comparatively rare despite man's close contact with pigs in many countries, and in more than 50 per cent of human cases there may be no history of contact with pigs.

It is possible that man is most often infected by fingers, food, drinking water, or soil contaminated by pig faeces containing balantidia, usually in the encysted form. Flies or handling of the intestines of infected animals are other possible modes of transmission. Furthermore, the possibility of infection from green vegetables grown in soil fertilized by pig excrement must be borne in mind, especially as cysts may remain viable for weeks in moist faeces.

The reported incidence in man is very variable (0·1–5·1 per cent) and depends on whether freshly collected specimens of faeces are examined or not. Epidemics have been reported from mental institutions, and in New Guinea a high incidence of infection has been recorded (Van der Hoeven and Rijpstra, 1957).

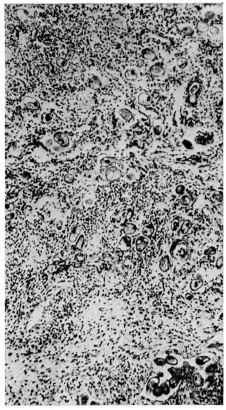

FIG. 2.20. Balantidiosis. Section shows parasites in large numbers throughout all the intestinal coats. The exudate consists of lymphocytes and polymorphonuclear and eosinophil leucocytes. Note the well-marked, kidney-shaped nucleus (× 135).

Pathology

B. coli can cause severe ulcerative lesions of the large intestine. These may involve the whole length from the caecum to rectum, but the recto-sigmoid segment is most commonly and severely involved. The distal portion of the ileum is rarely involved (Arean and Koppisch, 1956). Macroscopically the lesions resemble those of amoebic dysentery. The earliest lesions are small flask-shaped ulcers which may expand and coalesce. The edges are ragged, swollen, and undermined and the base is covered with necrotic greyish-green or black slough. The whole thickness of the wall may be affected and perforation with peritonitis may occur. Acute and chronic appendicitis are rare complications.

The organism passes through the epithelial basement membrane and muscularis mucosae to reach the submucosa. In the experimental animal an infiltrate of eosinophils, monocytes, and lymphocytes has been described. In man, however, necrosis and lymphocytic infiltration is usual with a varying infiltrate of neutrophils. The edges of the ulcer are undermined and there is a surface layer of fibrin, erythrocytes, leucocytes, and cellular debris. Balantidia are found at the periphery of the lesion and in the muscular coat and may be surrounded by a clear space with little cellular reaction (Fig. 2.20). Although balantidia have been noted in lymph notes, neither inflammatory lesions in mesenteric lymph nodes nor in the liver have been reported, but the organisms have been detected in one instance in the heart.

Diagnostic pathology

The stools are bloody and mucoid. Examination of faeces will reveal the typical large ovoid cysts 45–60 μm in length containing the parasite. The trophozoites may also be seen in freshly collected stools. The protozoon is oval in shape and of variable size—30–200 μm in length by 40–60 μm in breadth. The body is clothed with a thick covering of cilia arranged in longitudinal rows. Both the direct and indirect fluorescent antibody techniques have recently been applied in the diagnosis of *B. coli* (Zaman, 1965).

3

Helminthic Diseases

Introduction

The helminthic diseases, whether soil-transmitted, vector borne, or resulting from particular social habits, provide some of the great public health
problems of the tropics. The disease processes brought about may be of a
general or local nature, and are either the results of reactions by the human
host to the worm or are due to the worms depriving the body of essential
nutrients. Raised levels of serum IgG have been described in the human
helminthiases (Kojima *et al.* 1972). The immunology of parasitic infection
was reviewed by Bryceson (1974).

A. NEMATODES

Many of the roundworms are important agents of human disease and in
this section the following conditions are described: (1) hookworm infection,
(2) ascariasis, (3) toxocariasis, (4) strongyloidiasis, (5) trichuriasis, (6)
enterobiasis, (7) trichinellosis, (8) angiostrongyliasis, (9) gnathostomiasis,
(10) trichostrongyliasis, (11) the filariases, (12) dracontiasis, (13) cutaneous
larva migrans and (14) intestinal capillariasis.

HOOKWORM INFECTION

The geographical distribution of the two hookworms, *Ancylostoma duodenale* and *Necator americanus* used to be regarded as relatively distinct, the former being more prevalent in the Old World in Europe, the Middle East, etc.,
and the latter in the New World in America and tropical Africa. During the
past few decades both parasites have become widely distributed throughout
the tropics and subtropics, and rigid demarcations are no longer tenable.
When a parasite is universally distributed it is always difficult to be sure to
what extent it is responsible for disease in the community, and what significance to attach to its presence in an individual. A variable proportion of
any population where hookworm is endemic develops serious disease as
a consequence of infection, and hookworm anaemia may be considered to
represent a breakdown of adaptation.

Life Cycle

The life histories of *A. duodenale* and *N. americanus* are identical. The adult worms are small (8–10 mm long) and live in the upper part of the small intestine, mainly in the jejunum, attaching themselves to villi which are sucked into their buccal cavities.

The egg (about 60 μm) is passed in the faeces containing a segmented ovum. When deposited on warm, moist soil, a larva rapidly develops in the egg and hatches after one or two days. The newly hatched 'rhabditiform' larva passes through a 7- to 10-day free-living cycle in the soil, moulting twice, and becoming the sheathed 'filariform' larva which is infective to man. In a suitable environment—warm, damp soil—these larvae can survive several months. Man is infected by the larvae penetrating his skin, they then migrate by way of the venous system to the right ventricle of the heart and to the lungs into the alveoli. From the alveoli the larvae are passively carried upwards to the trachea and larynx into the oesophagus to the stomach and small intestine which they reach 3–5 days after they have penetrated the skin. After a further 4–5 weeks the worms become sexually mature and may live from 1 to 9 years. It has been shown that whereas migrating larvae of *Necator* grow and develop in the lungs, those of *Ancylostoma* do not; they undergo the same early development in the intestinal mucosa. One female *Ancylostoma* produces about 30,000 eggs and one female Necator about 9000 eggs per day. *A. ceylanicum* causes infection in man around Calcutta (Chowdhury and Schad, 1972).

Epidemiology

Although man is the only important source of human hookworm infection, the epidemiology of the disease is dependent upon the interaction of three factors—the suitability of the environment for the eggs or larvae; the mode and extent of faecal pollution of the soil; and the mode and extent of contact between infected soil and skin.

Thus survival of hookworm larvae is favoured in a damp, sandy or friable soil with decaying vegetation, and a temperature of 24–32 °C. Larvae move very little horizontally but can migrate upwards as much as 1 metre. *A. duodenale* eggs resist dessication more than those of *Necator*, while the development of hookworm larvae in the eggs and subsequent hatching can be retarded in the absence of oxygen. Insanitary disposal of faeces or the use of human faeces as soil fertilizer are the chief sources of human infection in countries where individuals are bare-footed. Thus, it is to be expected that hookworm infection will have a higher prevalence in agricultural than in town workers—and that in many tropical countries it is an occupational disease of the farming community. Experiments have shown that although *Necator* infection is acquired almost exclusively by the percutaneous route, *Ancylostoma* infection may be contracted either percutaneously or orally—the latter mode of entry gives special point to the reports of contamination of vegetables by these larvae.

Contrary to the general belief, Schad *et al.* (1973) have shown that larvae of

A. duodenale do not always develop directly to adulthood upon invasion of man. Thus, in West Bengal, India, arrested development appears to be a seasonal phenomenon which results in (*a*) reduction of egg output wasted in seeding an inhospitable environment and (*b*) a marked increase in eggs entering the environment just before the monsoon begins. Kochar *et al.* (1974) have investigated the relationship of some key behavioural and social factors to the levels of hookworm infection by studying the defaecation behaviour of a population in Rural Bengal, India.

Immunity

Providing people are equally exposed to hookworm infection, both sexes and all ages are susceptible. In communities in which the parasite has long been endemic, the inhabitants develop a host/parasite balance in which the worm load is limited, thus although the infection rate in some rural areas of the tropics may be 100 per cent only a small proportion develop hookworm anaemia. It is not known whether those heavy infections resulting in anaemia are dependent upon repeated exposure to a high intensity of infection, or whether they represent a failure of immunity. Many workers have reported that in their experience the heaviest worm loads are seen at the ages at which infection is first acquired—whether in infancy, later childhood, or, in the case of newcomers to endemic areas, in adult life. Moreover there seem to be clinical differences in the reactions of the host to a first infection in contrast to chronic infections—eosinophilia and malabsorption, which are usually features of the former, are often absent in the latter. In dogs, the appearance of immunity coincides with the disappearance of eosinophilia and malabsorption (Otto, 1941).

There is little direct evidence about the effects of host immunity on hookworm in man. de Hurtado and Layrisse (1968) felt that the response of the skin to a hookworm larva antigen was both specific and sensitive and thus reliable enough for the screening of infected populations. On the other hand, Ball *et al.* (1971) suggest caution in the interpretation of both positive and negative responses to immediate and delayed hypersensitivity skin reactions. The results of repeated infections with *Nematospiroides dubius* of a population of mice, reproduced features common to highly endemic human hookworm infection notably its stability and the occurrence of very heavy infections at first exposure and in a small proportion of repeatedly infected animals. Exposure of mice to heavy infection during the period required for resistance to develop consistently resulted in a heavy worm load, and provides a possible explanation for early heavy infections in man (Bartlett and Ball, 1972).

Soulsby and Gilles (1974) carried out gel diffusion precipitation and indirect haemagglutination tests on sera of individuals aged from 6 months to

60 years in a *Necator americanus* endemic area. Children younger than 24 months showed either no, or a low, antibody response to hookworm antigen. Adults showed higher and at times high titres. On electrophoresis, a change in the location of haemagglutins in the serum was noted in patients with hookworm anaemia as compared to normal blood donors. Good reviews on the immune response to nematode infections have been submitted by Jarrett and Urquhart (1971) and Ogilvie and Jones (1971).

Pathology

The site of entrance through the skin of the filariform larvae is often characterized by a dermatitis known as 'ground or coolie itch'. There is intense itching, oedema and erythema and later a papulo-vesicular eruption which lasts up to 2 weeks. In endemic areas these symptoms either pass unnoticed or are rare.

The pathogenicity of the migratory stages of hookworms is mild compared with that of *Ascaris*, although pulmonary reactions to *Ancylostoma* infection have been noted. In the stage of migration through the lungs minute haemorrhages may occur with eosinophilic and leucocytic infiltration, but once again these seem rare in the tropics. When an individual is first infected eosinophils may account for 30 per cent or more of the total white cells. The pathological changes that follow the invasive phase are due to (i) anaemia, (ii) hypoalbuminaemia, and (iii) possibly disturbances in gastro-intestinal function.

Anaemia

The main feature of the established adult infection is the production of anaemia. The pathogenesis of the anaemia caused by hookworm is dependent upon three parameters: ($1°$) the iron content of the human diet; ($2°$) the state of the iron reserves; ($3°$) the intensity and duration of infection. These factors will vary in different tropical countries but must always be taken into account for a proper evaluation of a particular situation. Thus in Nigeria, where the iron intake is high, 21–30 mg daily, people whose only pathological source of bleeding is hookworm infection show no evidence of iron deple-tion, as evinced by a low serum iron concentration or an iron-deficiency anaemia, unless they harbour more than 800 worms (Gilles *et al.* 1964). Whereas in Mauritius (Stott, 1961), where the total iron content of the food is only between 5–10 mg daily, it was found that even moderate hookworm loads could cause sufficient blood loss to precipitate anaemia (Table 3.1).

In human hookworm infection the loss of red cells into the gut is propor-tional to the worm load and has variously been reported as between 0·03 and 0·05 ml of blood per worm per day for *N. americanus* and between 0·16 and 0·34 ml for *A. duodenale*. The volume of blood sucked does not alter

TABLE 3.I. *Relationship between hookworm anaemia, worm load and iron intake in various parts of the world*

Author	Country	Threshold of worm load	Dietary iron mg/day
Carr	Mexico	0	
Stott	Mauritius	0	5–10
Sturrock	Tanzania	40	
Layrisse and Roche	Venezuela	♀80	12–30
		♂200	
Hill and Andrews	U.S.A.	200	
Darling *et al.*	Fiji	300	
Gordon	Sierra Leone	800	
Gilles *et al.*	Nigeria	800	>30

significantly with the development of anaemia, though the quantity of red cells of course decreases. The concept of persistent bleeding ulcers left behind by migrating worms has little histological support in human infections and bleeding usually stops immediately after complete worming. These findings are not unexpected when it is considered that there is a complete turnover of the jejunal epithelium every six to twenty-four hours. Nor is any concrete proof available to date in support of the toxic theory of the causation of hookworm anaemia. It is important to recognize that part of haemoglobin iron which the hookworm ingests and excretes while in the duodenum and upper jejunum is reabsorbed from the gut. This proportion increases as the patient becomes depleted of iron and amounts to between 40 and 60 per cent as measured by double isotope studies (Roche *et al.* 1959).

In some parts of the tropics, e.g. India and Colombia, there occurs a superadded folic acid megaloblastic anaemia which is often masked by the severe iron-deficiency anaemia and which only becomes overt after a partial haematological response to iron therapy (Borrero *et al.* 1961; Daftary and Bhende, 1956). The pathogenesis of folic-acid deficiency in severe hookworm infection may be due to a variety of factors: defective folic-acid absorption, deficient folic-acid in the diet, and increased demands. The classical anaemia of uncomplicated hookworm disease is however a hypochromic mycrocytic anaemia. The distribution of haemoglobins phenotypes is similar in patients with hookworm anaemia as in the general population (Table 3.2).

Hypoalbuminaemia

In addition to anaemia, loss of protein is another important manifestation of hookworm infection. When hypoalbuminaemia occurs it is due to a

TABLE 3.2. *Haematological findings and ova counts in* 183 *male Nigerian patients with hookworm anaemia*

No. of patients	Haemoglobin (g/100 ml)	Mean cell haemoglobin concentration (%)	Serum iron (μg/100 ml)	Ova/g of faeces	Hb genotype (%)		
					AA	AS	AC
183 (Mean)	3·2	20	20	46,000	72	22	6
(Range)	1·3–6·0	17–30	4–70	22,000–116,000			

combined loss of blood and lymph and the protein loss is well in excess of the red blood cells loss. There is nearly always also a limited capacity for albumin synthesis, the latter being brought about by a variety of factors such as anaemia, which affects the liver-cell function; coincidental disease of the liver, e.g. tuberculosis; loss of appetite; and possibly failure to reabsorb amino acids from the albumin passing into the gut. Kobayashi (1929) found that the serum albumin concentration was often low in hookworm anaemia and Salah (1938) attributed the severe oedema to hypoalbuminaemia rather than to the heart failure that may be present. Brumpt and Ho Thi Sang (1955) found that, in their patients, oedema did not respond to mercurial diuretics, even after their anaemia had been corrected, but subsided rapidly when they were wormed. They suggested that oedema might be due to hypoproteinaemia following loss of plasma proteins in the stools. Hookworm disease can therefore be added to the list of causes leading to a protein-losing enteropathy

Gastrointestinal function

Various types of digestive disorders have been attributed to hookworm disease. They range from epigastric disorders to dirt eating. Duodenitis and peptic ulceration have both been suspected of being the result of hookworm infection. The prevalence of duodenal ulceration in our 183 male patients with hookworm anaemia was similar to that encountered in the general out-patients population of University College, Ibadan. Pimparkar *et al.* (1970) found that gastric acid secretion was low, both at the basal state and after maximal stimulation with histamine, as compared with normal controls, moreover fibrogastroscopy did not reveal any gross abnormality. Barium meal X-rays reveal non-specific changes of disordered motor function and any appearances consistent with a diagnosis of duodenitis are unrelated to hookworm disease (Rowland, 1966).

There is some disagreement in published reports about the effects of hookworm on the mucosa of the duodenum and jejunum (Banwell, 1962; Salem and Truelove, 1964; Sheehy *et al.* 1962). The experience of the majority of workers is that uncomplicated hookworm anaemia is generally not associated with gross malabsorption, and that intestinal morphology as determined by peroral mucosal biopsies, is within normal range. Recently Da Costa (1971) could find no clinical evidence of malabsorption in Jamaican patients, nor was there any significant difference in the rate of small-intestinal dioxyribonucleic acid (DNA) loss when compared with normal controls. It is more than likely that some investigators reporting abnormalities have in fact studied patients with hookworm infection and pre-existing intestinal disease, especially when anaemia and the presence of hookworm ova in the stools have been the criteria of selection, without consideration of the number of worms present. It is possible however that there may be true differences between patients, depending upon such factors as duration of infection, race and presence of other parasites, e.g. strongyloidiasis or giardiasis.

Diagnosis

There are several different techniques available for the diagnosis of hookworm infections—the direct smear which may or may not be quantitated; some form of salt flotation; some form of faecal concentration procedure; and faecal culture (coproculture) for species diagnosis. These have been thoroughly and critically reviewed recently by Davis (1972). The ordinary direct saline smear is an examination of 2–3 mg of faeces; quantitative approaches to this examination has been made frequently, notably by Beaver, but provide no more than a rough estimate of worm burden because of the inherent insensitivity of the technique (WHO, 1965). Another form of direct smear, the cellophane thick smear or Kato technique, samples 50–60 mg of faeces, is simple to perform, of wide application and gives better quantitative estimates of egg output and hence worm load.

While brine flotation (with sodium chloride, magnesium sulphate or zinc sulphate) uses 1 g of faeces and is sensitive for nematode egg recovery, sub-sampling from the surface is unreliable for quantitative estimates and trematode eggs shrink; it is essentially a variant of a concentration method. Lane's direct centrifugal flotation (DCF) modification gives quantitative estimates but has the disadvantage of requiring special centrifuge buckets.

The various types of formalin–ether or acid–ether techniques are all concentration methods and the purpose is to recover small numbers of eggs; they are not useful for quantitative studies.

Stoll's dilution egg-counting technique, probably more widely used than any other, uses 4 g faeces. It depends essentially on the formulation of a homogenous suspension of eggs in the diluent with examination of sub-samples representing 5 or 10 mg of faeces. It has the advantage that numerous replicates are possible and thus some stability of the mean egg count is established. It has the disadvantage that light infections are not detected as the technique has a lower limit of sensibility of about 200 eggs per gram of stool. It should not be used for diagnostic work and its utility lies in the epidemiological field where egg outputs and hence worm loads in different populations can be compared. It is useful for roughly estimating the degree of reduction of egg output in patients not parasitologically cured after treatment.

Techniques of coproculture are rightly assuming much greater significance in both epidemiological and clinical studies of hookworm and other nematodes, since they possess sensitivity unequalled by any egg recovery method and, moreover, are species specific. Although laboratory culture methods for recovery of hookworm larvae from faecal samples or soil have long been known to parasitologists, it was not until Harada and Mori (1951) introduced the concept of filter paper culture in test tubes that their utility became widely appreciated. Improvements in the original technique such as the adoption of polyethylene tubes for culture (Sada *et al.* 1965) and the use of the ancyloscope or the steromicroscope have made this method indispensable for the study of hookworm.

ASCARIASIS

Ascaris lumbricoides, the large intestinal round worm has a world wide distribution the incidence of which is largely determined by local habits in the disposal of faeces. Its highest prevalence is in the hot humid climates of Asia, Africa, and tropical America.

Life cycle

The adult worms live in the small intestine. Their colour is brownish-yellow and they may reach a length of 40 cm. The female is prolific, laying up to 200,000 eggs a day. The typical egg has a yellowish-brown mamillated appearance.

The eggs are passed in the faeces and providing the environment is suitable a larva develops within the egg and becomes infective in about 10 days. After eggs containing larvae are swallowed by man, the young worms hatch, are set free in the small intestine and begin their migration. This takes them through the wall of the small intestine, and by way of the hepatic portal system to the liver. They are then carried by the blood stream to the right heart and to the lungs, where they remain for several days, after which they migrate passively up the bronchi and trachea to the pharynx. They are now swallowed and re-enter the small intestine where they become sexually mature in about 2 months. Although it lives in the gut, whether it leads an aerobic or anaerobic existence is still controversial (Editorial, 1970). Present evidence would suggest that the *ascaris* is an aerobic parasite specifically adapted to live at low oxygen tension (Smith, 1969). The effect that the presence of *Ascaris* in the intestine of man, by perhaps altering the oxygen tension, has on the intestinal flora is unknown.

A. lumbricoides in the gut is largely motionless and lives in the contents of the small intestine away from the mucosa. Aerobic respiration is therefore low and accounts for only a small part of the energy required by the parasite. Large amounts of glycogen are known to be stored in the tissues of the worm and ascorbic acid is also present. Since complex media are necessary to cultivate nematode parasites, it has been difficult to draw any definite conclusions about their nutrition. There is evidence, however, that the presence of *Ascaris* in the intestine of children leads to impairment of protein digestion and absorption (Venkatachalam and Patwardhan, 1953).

The migratory phase of larval development in the liver and lungs requires 8–15 days and is associated with fever, allergic dermatitis, eosinophilia, and pneumonitis or pneumonia; a focal granulomatous tissue reaction occurring around dead or dying larvae or ova has been described in man and animals. These and other manifestations of the larval and adult stages of the parasite will be discussed fully later.

Epidemiology

Infection is spread by faecal pollution of the soil. The eggs are swallowed as a result of ingestion of soil or contact between the mouth and various inanimate objects carrying the adherent eggs. Contamination of food or drink by dust or handling is also a source of infection. Eggs of *Ascaris* pass unaltered through the intestine of coprophagous animals and can thus be transported to locations other than human defaecation sites. The well protected eggs withstand drying and can survive for very lengthy periods.

Although all age groups show infection in endemic areas, the incidence and intensity are highest in the younger age groups. Infants may be parasitized soon after birth by ova on the mother's fingers. In human subjects the observed differences in incidence and intensity at different ages are probably due to differences in behaviour and occupational activities between children and adults as well as to the development of acquired resistance. Ascaris infections in children can lead to marked nutritional impairment when a high parasite load is associated with a low protein intake (Tripathy *et al.* 1971; Lysek, 1974).

Ascaris eggs are resistant to cold and to disinfectants in the strengths in normal use. They are killed by direct sunlight and by temperatures above 45°C. Under optimum conditions eggs may remain viable for as long as 1 year. *A. suum*, which infects pigs, is morphologically identical and can mature in man but cross infection has not been proved. In epidemiological studies, serological tests (e.g. larval microprecipitation test) are useful to detect early infections as well as the lung manifestations of the larval stages of *Ascaris* infection (Lejkina, 1965).

Immunity

Most of the work upon which present knowledge of the immunology in *Ascaris* and other nematode infections is based comes from experimental animal infections.

It has been shown that susceptibility to infection is greatest in the young animal and declines with advancing age, reaching a peak at the onset of sexual maturity. This difference has been termed 'age resistance' and has been attributed to the changing physiological pattern from youth to age, involving the antibody-forming mechanism, endocrine balance, and mucus production in the alimentary tract (WHO, 1964).

Circulating antibodies in the serum can be demonstrated to play a definite role in the mechanism of immunity, and protection has been induced by the passive transfer of immune serum to susceptible experimental hosts. Using a microprecipitation test to detect antibodies in humans, it has been shown that antibodies to *Ascaris* are present in the blood during the early period of infection, but they disappear by the time the worms have reached sexual maturity (Lejkina, 1965).

Pathology

The pathology of ascariasis can broadly be divided into the stage of larval migration and the stage of the established infection. A retrospective study of the American Armed Forces Institute of Pathology material revealed 35 fatal ascaris infections (Piggott *et al.* 1970).

Larval migration

As the first stage larvae penetrate the intestinal wall haemorrhages may occur in the mucosa. The most usual clinical and pathological effects are, however, seen in the lungs. Ascaris pneumonia may occur 4–16 days after infection and larvae may be found in the sputum. The combination of fever, cough, expectoration, eosinophilia and pulmonary infiltration on radiological examination constitutes 'Loeffler's syndrome'. Death has been ascribed to ascaris pneumonia. Portions of larvae have been noted in the bronchioles with a marked patchy infiltration of polymorphonuclear and eosinophil leucocytes with scattered Charcot–Leyden crystals. These crystals are found in a number of conditions and can be formed *in vitro* within minutes from man's eosinophils lysed with a surface-active agent. The crystals are colourless and have the appearance of two hexagonal pyramids placed base to base. They measure 20–40 μm in length and are 2–4 μm at the broadest portion (El Hashmi, 1971). Accompanying granulomatous lesions may be present in the liver (Beaver and Danaraj, 1958). Histological descriptions of the acute pulmonary lesions are few and they rarely become chronic. Ossifying pulmonary granulomatoses due to the presence of the larvae have been described in one patient.

Hepatomegaly has been described during the stage of migration and focal areas of necrosis infiltrated with eosinophils and neutrophils may be present in the liver. The larvae are rapidly destroyed and are not usually present in the lesions, which are rare in our experience. Larvae have been described in other organs of the body. Lesions have been described in the optic thalamus, spinal canal, pituitary gland, epididymis, and myocardium. Aberrant larvae have also been implicated as a cause of meningitis in children. They are, however, very rarely seen in these situations and when present care must be taken to differentiate them from the larvae of toxocara, which are much more commonly found in ectopic lesions.

It is difficult to assess the importance of this larval migratory stage as a cause of morbidity and mortality in tropical areas. In a busy outpatient paediatric practice milder forms of the syndrome could quite easily be missed. It is our impression that it rarely, if ever, causes mortality. In older children and adults who, in the majority of instances, appear to be living in harmony with the parasite, the larval stage with reinfection would appear to be silent. The most obvious cause of mortality and morbidity occurs in children in the presence of the adult worms once the infection is established. It would appear, however, to be a problem of some magnitude among the Arab population of Eastern Saudi Arabia (Gelpi and Mustafa, 1968).

Established infection

In the intestinal canal a tangled mass of worms frequently causes obstruction in children (Crane *et al.* 1965). Volvulus and gangrene of the bowel, intussusception, and appendicitis also occur. Ascaris infection has also been implicated as a causative factor in intestinal perforation usually following a non-specific ulcer in the lower end of the ileum. This condition has, however, also been seen in the absence of ascariasis and we are not convinced that a causal relationship is proven. The adults do, however, perforate through postoperative suture lines and their presence in the peritoneal cavity has been recorded (Qassab and Al-Khateeb, 1966). In addition, ova in this position may set up a granulomatous peritonitis (Areán, 1958). The presence of the ova in the intestinal canal itself causes no lesions. Intestinal ascariasis has been said to cause a mesenteric lymphadenitis but definite proof is lacking. Gastro-intestinal discomfort and vomiting are not infrequent complications. The presence of worms in the vomitus is frequently noted and blockage of the larynx or trachea by aspiration is a not uncommon cause of asphyxia in children.

Outside the intestinal lumen the worms do not survive for long. Death of the adult releases products of protein breakdown and in a sensitized patient an acute necrotizing inflammation can occur.

Pancreatitis has been described in childhood and has been thought to be due to a number of factors: (i) regurgitation of bile within the pancreatic duct due to blockage of the ampulla of Vater, (ii) the presence of enteric organisms carried into the pancreatic duct by the worm itself, or (iii) an acute necrotizing process surrounding the disintegrating products of the worm (Fig. 3.1).

The adult worms may enter the common bile duct and even intrahepatic ducts with the development of obstructive jaundice. Pyogenic cholangitis, cholangitis, acute cholecystitis, and perforation of the bile ducts are also complications (Hsu, 1962; Yue, 1974). The formation of biliary calculi containing fragments and multiple ova of ascaris has been described by a number of authors (Raney *et al.* 1970). The adults have been reported as being discharged from a periumbilical abscess and from umbilical fistulae (Jelliffe, 1952). Ascarides may be found in the liver itself and the ova and

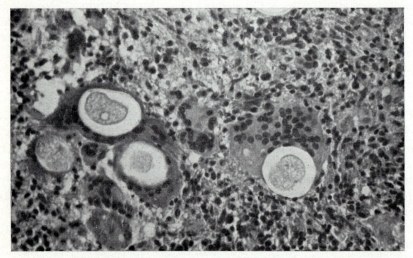

FIG. 3.1. Granulomatous peritonitis due to the ova *A. lumbricoides.* Note the giant cells engulfing the ova and the surrounding chronic inflammatory (H and E × 450).

fragments of the adults cause a necrotic lesion surrounded by eosinophils, and neutrophils, later to be replaced by chronic inflammatory cells, giant cells, and proliferating fibroblasts. *Ascaris* ova alone may cause these lesions in the liver (Khaleque and Alam, 1963), and also acute abscesses and haemorrhage (Rosenbaum and Johnston, 1966). Both the adults and the ova soon disintegrate and may not be detectable in the lesions. Although it has been said that *A. lumbricoides* is second only to *E. histolytica* as a cause of liver abscesses (Reay *et al.* 1964) this is not so in our experience. Adult worms have also been described in the Eustachian tube, paranasal sinuses, and even within the cavity of the heart itself.

Diagnostic pathology

The microscopical diagnosis of ascariasis can be confirmed by examination of faeces samples. Because of their characteristic morphology and colour the ova can be found relatively easily in 'direct smears'. Concentration and quantitative techniques are available.

Many serological tests have been employed in the diagnosis of *Ascaris* infection. They include: complement fixation, ring precipitation, larval precipitation, agar diffusion, haemagglutination, or immuno-electrophoresis. None of these is at present regarded as very satisfactory for diagnostic purposes.

Occasionally, round worms are recognized during barium meal examination (Middlemiss, 1961). In patients with acute intestinal obstruction X-ray of the abdomen reveals the masses of worms.

In the early phases of *Ascaris* infection a moderate eosinophilia is present, pulmonary infiltration may be revealed radiologically, while larvae may occasionally be found in the sputum, together with eosinophils and Charcot–Leydon crystals.

TOXOCARIASIS (Visceral Larva Migrans)

Evidence has now accumulated that human disease due to larval migration of *Toxocara canis* and *T. catis* constitutes an important public health problem, and although the majority of reports to date have emanated from the more developed countries (Beaver *et al.* 1956; Woodruff, 1964), the authors believe that it is merely a question of time before these infections are widely reported from the tropics as a major cause of some of the otherwise unexplained clinical syndromes seen in these areas. Many aspects of toxocariasis have been described by Woodruff (1970).

Life cycle

T. canis and *T. cati* are parasites of dogs and cats and their presence in the human host is an abnormal migration of their larval phase.

Under favourable conditions, the eggs passed in the dog's faeces become infective in 2–3 weeks. From the swallowed eggs emerge the contained second stage larvae which penetrate the intestinal walls and reach the liver. The majority of larvae remain in the liver but others may pass on to the lungs or other organs of the body including the central nervous system and the eye. Occasionally the larvae complete their cycle of development in the human host resulting in infection with adult *T. canis* or *T. cati*. Wiseman and Lovell (1969) have reported such a case in which a child of 14 months vomited adult *Toxocara cati* with no haematological or serological evidence of toxocaral infection. It is possible, therefore, that if larvae rather than eggs are ingested they may develop to maturity in the intestines without a circulatory or tissue phase of migration.

Rodan and Buckley (1969) have recorded the case of a boy aged 4 years who vomited a specimen of *Toxocara cati* without other symptoms apart from epigastric pain. A cat in the household was the probable source of infection. The specimen was a male measuring 36 mm long by 1 mm in maximum diameter; oesophagus 2·65 × 0·4 mm with posterior ventriculus; cervical alae broad 1·5 × 0·3 mm, spicules 1·9 mm long; cuticular striations 12–16 μm apart; tail 0·2 mm long typically probular; caudal papillae not well defined.

Epidemiology

Infection is acquired by ingesting soil which has been contaminated usually by dogs' faeces. Young children are particularly susceptible to toxocariasis because of their habit of eating dirt, and of handling soiled fur of puppies and then putting the fingers in the mouth. The severity of the disease depends upon the numbers of worms that have invaded the body and the duration of infection. Ehrenford (1957) has shown that puppies are more infected than adult dogs and that the incidence among bitches is lower at all ages. The majority of cases have been reported from the Eastern half of the United States (Beaver 1959) but the disease has been recognized in the Philippines, Mexico, Hawaii, Turkey, Puerto Rico, and other countries. Wiseman and Woodruff (1971) have shown that the prevalence of infection in dogs is high in the humid areas of Ibadan and Dar-es-Salaam (36 and 28 per cent respectively), 12 per cent in the dry area of Masailand and 6 per cent in Nairobi. Toxocara skin tests in the population showed a relatively high frequency in Ibadan and Dar-es-Salaam with a low frequency in Nairobi. It is possible that nematode larvae other than *Toxocara* may be involved in visceral larva migrans (Otsuru *et al.* 1965). Viral encephalitis due to larval migration has been reported (van Thiel, 1960) and the transmission of poliomyelitis virus by larvae of toxocara has been postulated (Woodruff, 1968). The fluorescent antibody titres, reagin levels and IgE have been estimated in experimental infections (Hogarth Scott *et al.* 1969).

Pathology

The migrating larvae, which may live for some years in experimental animals, stimulate an inflammatory reaction in their wake.

As almost any organ in the body can be affected the symptomatology is protean and depends upon the site and number of larvae and the sensitivity of the host. Pulmonary symptoms are most usual but cardiac, renal, neurological, and ocular symptoms may be complained of and the liver and spleen are usually enlarged. An eosinophilia is usual and the plasma globulins are increased. Tropical eosinophilia may be closely simulated.

Isolated lesions without systemic manifestations may occur and an erroneous diagnosis of retinoblastoma has been made in children (Wilder, 1950; Nichols, 1956; Ashton, 1960).

The initial lesion is composed of fibrinoid material and eosinophils stimulated by the presence of the larva. Later, epithelioid cells and fibroblasts with a varying number of giant cells, lymphocytes and plasma cells form a granuloma. A fibrous capsule eventually encloses the larva.

Other nematode larvae may occasion similar histological changes, namely *Ascaris lumbricoides*, *A. suis*, *Ancylostoma caninum*, *Necator americanus*, and *Strongyloides stercoralis* (Huntley *et al.* 1965). The larval toxocara are smaller than the others, *T. canis* being 18–20 μm and *T. cati* 12–16 μm in width. A transverse section at mid-intestinal level showing the maximal width, lateral alae, excretory cell, and intestine is adequate for diagnostic purposes (Nichols, 1956).

Macroscopically no lesions may be noted or small, greyish, pin-point lesions may be scattered throughout the affected organs.

Histologically the liver is invariably affected and the lungs, eyes (choroid and retina), brain, heart, kidney, and striated muscle are frequently involved. Toxocara larval papillitis has been described both in a child (Bird *et al.* 1970), in whom enucleation allowed histological proof of the presence of a *T. canis* larva in the optic disc, as well as in an adult (Phillips and McKenzie, 1973). It has been suggested that lesions in muscles may be concerned in the aetiology of tropical myositis (O'Brien, 1963) but definite proof is lacking.

Diagnostic pathology

One of the most prominent diagnostic features of visceral larva migrans is a high, stable persistent eosinophilia not uncommonly reaching levels of 50–60 per cent. In some cases the levels have been suggestive of eosinophilic leukaemia. Hyperglobulinaemia is a less constant and less specific feature of the syndrome. Serum anti-γ-globulin factors have, however, been demonstrated in young children with visceral larva migrans (Huntley *et al.* 1965). The feasibility of identifying *Toxocara* larvae in tissue sections was demonstrated by Nichols' (1956) and provides the most certain means of making a definitive diagnosis. Serodiagnostic methods (Sadun *et al.* 1957) and the fluorescent antibody test have also been used (Mitchell, 1964; Hogarth-Scott, 1966). The sensitivity and specificity of these have yet to be fully evaluated. A modified haemagglutination test has also been used (Aljeboori and Ivey, 1970). Liver biopsy has proved valuable in some instances and, if the lungs are affected, larvae and eosinophils may be found in the sputum.

STRONGYLOIDIASIS

Strongyloides stercoralis is a common intestinal parasite of man with a geographical distribution similar to that of the hookworm.

Life cycle

The life cycle is complicated. The females (about 2 mm long and 50 μm broad) live in the duodenal and jejunal mucosa. They produce ova containing rhabditiform larvae which are released in the lumen of the small intestine. The larvae are easily found in the freshly passed faeces of man. Outside the host, if the environment is suitable, they become the infective, filariform larvae, which infect man by penetrating the intact skin.

In addition to this direct development, the rhabditiform larvae can, under certain conditions of moisture and temperature, undergo a separate, free-living reproductive generation in the soil. They develop into free-living male and female larvae the latter of which lay fertilized eggs from which rhabditiform larvae are produced. These either become filariform and infect man or become free-living unisexual worms capable of continuing the cycle in the soil.

If conditions are not suitable for these two types of development, *Strongyloides* provides for itself a further safeguard. The rhabditiform larvae can develop into filariform larvae in the intestine of the host. These infective forms then either penetrate the bowel or the perianal skin, thus producing auto-infection. The long-standing infections which continue in the absence of reinfection, are maintained in this way.

Having penetrated the bowel mucosa or the skin the filariform larvae travel by way of the venous system to the lungs. In the alveoli they may mature, the fertilized females producing eggs and rhabditiform larvae in the lungs. Alternatively they may migrate up the bronchioles to the larynx and eventually reach the duodenum and jejunum where they invade the mucosa. In the mucosa the female deposits eggs containing the rhabditiform larvae and the cycle recommences. Little is known of the metabolic requirements of the parasite and the effects of these on the host.

Epidemiology

The epidemiological features of strongyloides infection are very similar to those already described for hookworm, the infection usually being acquired through the skin. The resistance of *S. stercoralis* larvae in the soil is very low and optimal conditions of warmth, oxygen, light, and moisture are required for survival of its free-living soil-inhabiting reproductive generation. This may explain, in part, the remarkable patchy distribution of infection which is observed not only on a broad geographical basis but also within relatively small areas, and which has led to the belief that various strains of *S. stercoralis* occur, each adapted to a different set of environmental circumstances.

The most important epidemiological difference between hookworm and *S. stercoralis* is the phenomenon of auto-infection through the perianal skin or bowel or bowel mucosa. This mode of infection seems particularly common in south-eastern Asia and Ethiopia. *S. stercoralis* infection can be very chronic and persist for several years; in one case 36 years elapsed between contact and diagnosis (Brown and Perna, 1958).

Immunity

Little is known about immunity to *S. stercoralis* infection in man. Resistance to reinfection has been shown with various species of *Strongyloides*, and precipitation has been observed around the orifices of larvae in immune serum. It seems that steroid therapy, immunosuppression and debilitating diseases may in some patients with *S. stercoralis* infection cause the parasite to become a dangerous pathogen (Willis and Nwokolo, 1966; Rivera *et al.* 1970 and Adam *et al.* 1973). The conditions leading to auto-infection are unknown and may be morphological, immunological, or related to the nutritional status of the host.

Pathology

Clinically there may be an itchy erythematous rash at the site of penetration of the filariform larvae. As the larvae pass through the lungs pulmonary symptoms of varying severity occur and larvae may be detected in the sputum. Eosinophilia is described in this stage which is generally mild or symptomless. The more severe effects are seen with auto-infection.

Generally the established infection causes few symptoms (Janssens, 1965) and larvae are not uncommonly found in the faeces in individuals in the tropics undergoing routine medical examination. Mild abdominal symptoms and diarrhoea may be complained of. In a number of individuals, however, strongyloidiasis can produce a severe and even fatal illness (Poltera, 1974). From a study of post mortem findings these would appear to occur with auto-infection (Bras *et al.* 1964; Wilson and Thompson, 1964; Kyle *et al.* 1948; Hartz, 1946).

The filariform larvae which have developed prematurely in the bowel, invade the bowel wall and/or the perianal skin and urticarial lesions, weals and linear lesions reminiscent of creeping eruption have been described in the perianal region and elsewhere on the trunk. The migration may cause a recurrent form of Loeffler's disease with pulmonary symptoms and eosinophilia with, in addition, diarrhoea and hepatomegaly (Poltera, 1972; Nwokolo and Imohiosen, 1973). The malabsorption syndrome with dependant oedema and ascites and acute small bowel obstruction have been described, the youngest patient being aged 6 months (Walker-Smith *et al.* 1969). The obstruction in this case was due to ileus and oedema of the wall of the small bowel. Lympadenitis was considered to be due to the presence of larvae and *Esch. coli*. An *Esch. coli* septicaemia with meningitis has been reported as a complication (Brown and Perna, 1958). Duodenal aspiration may show the presence of adults or larvae and jejunal biopsy shows marked inflammatory changes in the lamina propria. The villi are shortened and blunt (Figs. 3.2 and 3.3).

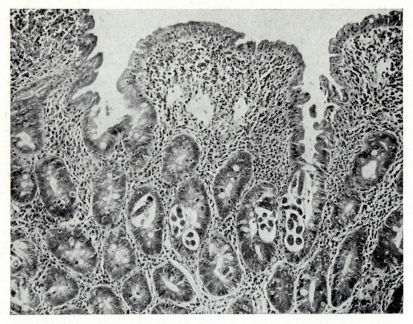

Fig. 3.2. Strongyloidiasis. Jejunal biopsy, showing blunting of the villi (subtotal villus atrophy), dilated lymphatics, and an inflammatory exudate in the lamina propria. Larvae and ova are present in the crypts (H and E × 130). (*By courtesy of Dr. John H. Yardley.*)

Adult worms, ova, and larvae may be present in the mucosa or crypts. The villi may return to normal with treatment (Beker *et al.* 1963).

In subjects dying of the infection the macroscopic findings are non-specific. The stomach and duodenum may be inflamed and congested. A duodenal stricture has been described. The small intestine may be collapsed or distended (Alcorn and Kotcher, 1961). Any portion of the intestine may be thickened and oedematous. Small ulcers may be present in the lower ileum and large bowel (Rivas Gomez and Aleman, 1967) and focal abscesses have been noted. Da Costa (1971) noted that small intestinal deoxyribonu-cleic acid (DNA) loss rates were high in patients with hyperinfestation. Following treatment the rates returned to normal. It was suggested that the high epithelial cell turnover in these patients might result in an excessive loss of endogenous substances which might be an important mechanism in causing malnutrition and hypoproteinaemia in patients with *S. stercoralis* hyperinfestation. Hyperinfection has been seen in malignant lymphomas, systemic lupus erythematosus and leprosy.

The ileum, appendix and the colon are sites of larval reinvasion. Oval

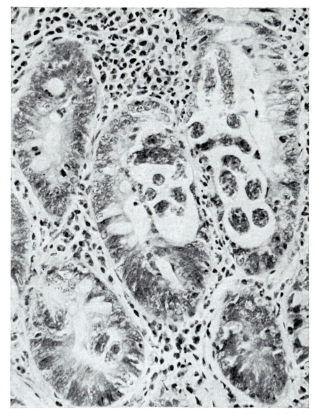

FIG. 3.3. Strongyloidiasis. High-power view of Fig. 3.2, demonstrating larvae and ova in the crypts of lieberkuhn. There is focal loss of lining epithelial cells and mitoses are numerous (H and E × 320). (*By courtesy of Dr. John H. Yardley.*)

tuberculoid foci in all coats may be seen with coagulation necrosis at the centre. Occasionally degenerating larvae may be seen in these lesions. A granulomatous colitis may be present in the large bowel and clinically steatorrhoea hypocalcaemia and hypoproteinaemia may result. The mesenteric glands are enlarged and hyperaemic. Any such findings at post mortem should raise the suspicion of strongyloides superinfection and microscopic examination of the intestinal contents should be undertaken; a portion of the duodenum in addition to other tissues should be preserved for histopathological examination (De Paola, 1962).

The lungs may show abscess formation and terminal bronchopneumonic or mild inflammatory changes. The liver is enlarged and congested and small, pin-point, yellow granulomas may be seen. Fatty change will be evident if the subject is malnourished.

Histologically the adults, ova, and larvae are usually found in the mucosa of the duodenum or in the crypts. There is little reaction to the adults but a mild eosinophilia and lymphocytic infiltration may be present. On section the cuticle shows well marked cross-striations best shown by Giemsa's stain.

Larvae may be found in any part of the bowel wall and in the pyloric and abdominal lymphatic glands. They have also been described in the lymphatics and portal venous channels. The surrounding tissue reaction may be slight but granulomatous lesions with eosinophils and scanty giant cells and even necrosis have been described. Ulceration, if present, is usually acute and non-specific.

In the lungs larvae are found in the interstitial tissue and an associated lobular pneumonia may be present. Adult worms have also been found associated with chronic inflammatory lesions. Larvae and granulomatous lesions have been noted in the liver. Rarely the kidney may be involved and larvae have been seen in the urine. In one instance scattered larvae were noted in the heart, with a surrounding lymphocytic reaction. They have also been isolated from pleural and pericardial effusions and found in the lymphatics of the gall bladder, in the pancreas, adrenal, thyroid, and parathyroid glands.

Diagnostic pathology

Examination of a fresh stool sample by the 'direct smear' technique will reveal free and active larvae, which makes the diagnosis of infection with *S. stercoralis* easy. If the faeces is not fresh, then the larvae must be differentiated on morphological grounds from hookworm rhabditiform larvae which under optimal environmental conditions can hatch out in the faeces in a relatively short time (Siffert, 1972). In some cases repeated stool examination may be negative when the larvae are easily demonstrated in the jejunal fluid. *S. stercoralis* can sometimes be diagnosed by examination of the sputum. There usually is an eosinophilia ranging from 8–60 per cent in the invasive stages of the disease. Serological tests have been used but are of little value in the diagnosis of human strongyloidiasis.

In many parts of the tropics *S. stercoralis* exists as a relatively harmless parasite in the majority of infected patients. Blood losses may, however, occur in heavy infections and recent studies have demonstrated that absorption of fat is impaired. A malabsorption syndrome (Toh and Chow, 1969) akin to sprue may be produced and absorption tests have revealed abnormalities in glucose tolerance and in ^{131}oleic acid excretion. Irritability or deformity of the deodenum has been reported on radiological examination, as well as changes in the ileum and jejunum with atrophy of villi (Beker *et al.* 1963). The 'string test' referred to under giardiasis (p. 81) has been found very useful in obtaining *Strongyloides* larvae from the jejunum.

When *S. stercoralis* results in the malabsorption syndrome, the typical clinico-pathological findings of this condition are found (p. 526), and jejunal biopsy may be diagnostic.

TRICHURIASIS

This infection is due to the whipworm—*Trichuris trichiura*—the distribution of which is cosmopolitan, although it is more prevalent in the warm humid tropics.

Life cycle

The sexually mature worms, which are about 5 cm long, have a whip-like shape and live in the caecum and upper colon of man. After fertilization the eggs are passed in the faeces within 4 weeks of infection and embryonic development takes place in the soil. Under favourable conditions of moisture and temperature the larvae develop inside the eggs within 2–5 weeks. The embryonated eggs are infective.

When the eggs are ingested by man the larvae escape into the upper small intestine and migrate directly to the caecum where they become adults within 1–3 months.

Epidemiology

Soil pollution is the determining factor in the prevalence and intensity of infection in a community, and clay soils are more favourable than sandy soils. Transmission occurs through the insanitary habit of promiscuous defaecation; infection usually results from the ingestion of infective ova from contaminated hands, food, or drink. Although trichuris infection of domestic and other animals occurs, it is unlikely that animal reservoirs play a part in the epidemiology of human infection. Coprophagous animals can transport trichuris eggs to locations other than human defaecation sites, since the eggs are passed unaltered through their intestine. Malnutrition may be the principal cause of increased pathogenicity of *T. trichiura* (Marques *et al.* 1962).

Nothing is known concerning immunity to trichuriasis. The higher prevalence in children is probably due to greater exposure to infection.

Pathology

The whip-like anterior portion attaches itself to the mucosa of the lower ileum and large intestine and the worm obtains its nourishment either by liquifying the mucosal cells by its secretions or by sucking blood. In the majority of cases they produce no symptoms and the amount of blood lost is small. Heavy infections of over 1000 worms may cause bloody diarrhoea with anaemia and prolapse of the rectum with whipworms adherent to the mucosa, which may be haemorrhagic and ulcerated (Jung and Jelliffe, 1952; Ramsey, 1962). The serious massive infections appear to occur more often in undernourished children, and massive trichuriasis may play a role in the pathogenesis of protein/calorie malnutrition in some areas. Appendicitis and peritonitis with the presence of the worms in the peritoneal cavity have been described. Very rarely regurgitation of the adults into the lungs has been noted. An eosinophilia is usual and a hypochromic anaemia with hyperplasia of the bone marrow occurs in massive infections.

Diagnostic pathology

Direct smear examination of faeces will reveal the characteristic lemon-shaped ova. An egg count on an ordinary wet faecal smear (containing about 2 mg of faeces) of more than 100 ova is indicative of a heavy infection. Concentration and quantitative techniques can be applied. Light infections resulting in egg counts below 10,000/g are not likely to produce symptoms and make up the great majority of infections.

Eosinophilia (10–20 per cent) is usually present especially in massive infections. An associated microcytic hypochromic anaemia may be seen and the mucoid sticky stools may contain a preponderance of eosinophil cells and Charcot–Leyden crystals. Sigmoidoscopy reveals mucus and the worms attached to the mucosa of the rectum and sigmoid colon; the mucosa is hyperaemic, oedematous, friable, and bleeds easily.

ENTEROBIASIS

This infection is due to the pinworm—*Enterobius vermicularis*, is prevalent throughout the world and is probably less common in the tropics than in countries of the temperate zone.

Life cycle

The female worm is about 8–13 mm long while the male worm—which is rarely seen—is only 2–5 mm. They both live in the caecum, where copulation takes place. The gravid females then migrate to the colon and rectum and at night pass through the anus to deposit their eggs on the perianal skin and genitocrural folds. Within a few hours larvae develop within the eggs which are now infective. Upon ingestion by man, the larvae hatch in the duodenum and mature in the caecum. The life cycle from egg to adult lasts 3–7 weeks. The survival of the ova depends upon temperature and humidity; viability being greatest in cool, moist surroundings.

Epidemiology

The highest incidence of enterobiasis is in school children from 5–15 years. It is very prevalent in crowded districts with faulty hygiene, in institutional groups, and among members of the same family.

The ova from the perianal region are transferred to night clothes, towels, and bedding, and infection may follow when these are handled. Infective ova may be present in the dust and infection can therefore take place by inhalation. The intense pruritus around the perianal regions results in scratching and the hands, specially beneath the finger nails, become contaminated and ova are transferred directly to the mouth or indirectly through food and other objects which have been handled. Occasionally the larvae after hatching in the perianal regions re-enter the anus and migrate to the caecum where they mature (retroinfection). There may be a racial susceptibility to infection; thus Puerto Rican children living in crowded conditions in New York had a lower incidence of infection than white, non-Puerto Rican children (Most *et al.* 1963).

Pathology

Clinically the infection may be symptomless or there may be mild gastro-intestinal discomfort and pruritus ani. Appendicitis is a complication and intestinal obstruction due to masses of the worms has been reported, but is exceedingly rare.

Vaginitis and pelvic complaints may occur in girls and prostatitis is a rare complication in males. Adult worms have also been reported to cause aural and nasal irritation.

The worms are found in the caecum and large intestine and less commonly in the lower ileum. The female attaches itself to the mucosa and may penetrate into the glands and stroma. The lesions so caused have been best described in appendices removed surgically in children in which parasitic invasion of the wall is common (Richmond and Guthrie, 1964). Sinuous tracks are formed containing eosinophils, necrotic debris and Charcot–Leyden crystals (best demonstrated by Giemsa stain). Portions of the worm are seen centrally and the lateral cuticular crests persist for some time (Fig. 3.4).

In other areas there may be a variable surrounding infiltration of lymphocytes and eosinophils with epithelioid cells and occasional giant cells present. Secondary infection and abscess formation can occur but would appear to be rare in the appendix. These have been described in the large intestine where multiple petechiae and mucosal and submucosal ulcers may be found.

Larvae and adults may invade the genital tract of females, causing a vaginitis, and granulomatous lesions have been described in the uterus, Fallopian tubes, and peritoneum (Beddoe, 1956). The lesions are similar to those described in the appendix but, in addition, ova may be present. In rare instances secondary infection with abscess formation occurs (Croce *et al.* 1956).

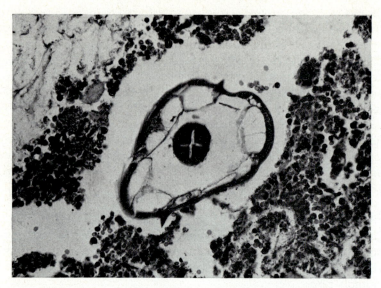

Fig. 3.4. Enterobiasis. Transverse section of enterobius in appendix, showing cephalic alae and muscular oesophagus (H and E × 30).

An eosinophilic abscess has been described in the prostate gland (Symmers, 1957).

Secondary ischio-rectal abscesses may follow the perianal eczema, due to the scratching, caused by irritation set up by the migrating females.

Diagnostic pathology

Adult female worms may be found in the faeces or perianal skin. The method of choice for making a diagnosis is the Scotch adhesive tape swab applied to the perianal region in the morning before bathing or defaecation. Ova are identified by their asymmetrical shape and well-developed embryo when the tape is mounted on a slide for examination. The Scotch tape can be also applied to that part of the person's clothing which has been in contact with the perianal region. At least three examinations should be carried out before a negative diagnosis is made. Enterobiasis is very infectious and if one person is infected in a household all other members of the family should be suspect.

TRICHINELLOSIS (Trichinosis)

Trichinellosis is a disease caused by the encysted larvae of *Trichinella spiralis*. This parasite is more prevalent in temperate than in tropical countries and is mainly confined to those countries where pork is eaten.

Life cycle

The adult worms are found in the small intestine of a number of carniverous animals including the pig, bush-pig, rats, hyenas, and other hosts. Their life span in the intestine is approximately 8 weeks.

After fertilization, the female worms bury themselves in the intestinal mucosa and each produces about 1500 larvae. The larvae migrate via the intestinal lymphatics to the thoracic duct and into the blood stream, whence they are distributed to the muscles. Here they develop and become encysted between the muscle fibres in 5–7 weeks. Calcification occurs in about 18 months but the encysted larvae remain alive for many years. When flesh containing encysted larvae is ingested by a suitable host the larvae are released by the action of digestive juices on the capsule and the cycle is repeated in the new host. In susceptible animals the larvae grow into sexually differentiated adults which on mating produce larvae which then invade striated muscle. In man, infection terminates at the cystic stage. Encysted larvae are known to utilize glycogen, protein, and lipids which they derive from the muscles that they have invaded.

Epidemiology

Trichinellosis in man results from eating raw or inadequately cooked pork or pork products, e.g. sausage meat. In Kenya the bush-pig is a common source of infection. Pigs become infected chiefly from eating uncooked slaughter-house refuse containing infected meat scraps; occasionally rats, which have a high, natural infection rate of trichinosis, can be a source of infection when they are eaten by pigs.

Serological tests have shown that in many communities the incidence of infection is appreciably higher than the number of clinically diagnosed cases, and it is obvious that many light infections pass unnoticed (Harvey and Kershaw, 1964). In recent years small and large epidemics have occurred (Kershaw et al. 1956). Congenital trichinosis has been reported.

In experimental animals acquired immunity to trichinosis has been produced in a variety of ways, but whether recovery from a light infection confers resistance to subsequent reinfection in man is not yet certain.

Anti-adult and anti-larval antibodies have been demonstrated in the γ-globulin fraction of serum of trichinosis animals, and a whole variety of immunological methods have been used for diagnostic and epidemiological purposes. High-quality antigens are, however, essential for these purposes.

Pathology

The symptomatology and pathology depend upon the intensity of infection. Beeson's four cardinal features of the disease are: fever, orbital oedema, myalgia, and eosinophilia (Beeson, 1941). In the early, migratory phase there are gastro-intestinal disturbances, fever, and urticaria. A typhoid-like fever may then ensue with manifestations of ocular, cardiac, respiratory, muscular, and central nervous system involvement.

The larvae may invade the lungs, pleura, pancreas, gall bladder, kidney, central nervous system, heart, muscles, and subcutaneous tissues.

Death may occur in this stage and focal necroses with an intense eosinophilic infiltration are found in the affected tissue. In the heart a focal interstitial myocarditis occurs around the migrating larvae which, however, never encyst in this situation (Semple *et al.* 1954).

An acute, non-suppurative meningitis with perivascular lymphocytic and monocytic infiltration, focal granulomatous lesions, and capillary thrombosis may be found in the central nervous system. Cavernous sinus thrombosis and sixth nerve palsy have also been described. Larvae are usually scanty but may be found occasionally in the cerebrospinal fluid (Meltzer and Bockman, 1957). Larvae may invade the eye muscles and lesions may be present in the choroid and retina. Oedema with chemosis of the conjunctiva is a common finding.

In the intestine there is a catarrhal enteritis with petechial haemorrhages, oedema and slight ulceration. In the lungs there are foci of monocytic and eosinophilic infiltration, pulmonary oedema, and bronchopneumonia. Pulmonary infarction and embolism may occur.

The skeletal muscles are preferentially invaded, and an acute interstitial inflammation results. There is basophilic degeneration of muscle fibres and

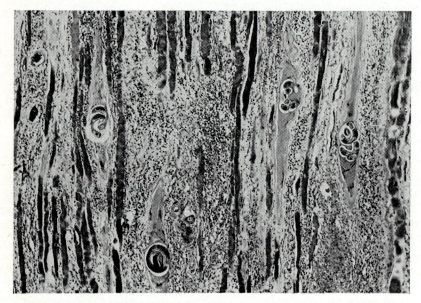

Fɪɢ. 3.5. Trichinellosis. Encysted larvae of *T. spiralis* in human muscle
(× 30).

the initial infiltrate of neutrophils and eosinophils is replaced by lymphocytes, plasma cells, monocytes, epithelioid cells, fibroblasts and even giant
cells. The larvae are gradually enclosed in hyaline connective tissue and
a lemon-shaped cyst is formed (Fig. 3.5). Calcification commences at
about 6 months following invasion either at the poles of the capsule or in the
larva itself. Newly-formed cysts are invisible to the naked eye but appear as
tiny white spots in muscle when calcification occurs. They are seldom
detected on radiological examination. The striated muscles which are most
active are usually those most heavily parasitized, e.g. diaphragmatic,
abdominal, intercostal, lingual, and laryngeal. It has recently been shown,
however, that in monkeys and baboons the lowest mean densities were found
in the diaphragm and it was pointed out that the limited human autopsies in
the literature do not confirm the belief that the diaphragm is the most
heavily infected muscle in man (Nelson et al. 1963). During the acute stages
there is a fall in the albumin/globulin ratio due to an increase in γ-globulin
and the fibrinogen level may be low. The erythrocyte sedimentation rate is
low. There is a mild leucocytosis with a marked rise in eosinophils by the
sixth week of infection which falls to normal by the end of 1 year.

Diagnostic pathology

One of the most constant, single, diagnostic aids in trichinosis is a rising
eosinophilia 10–40 per cent; parasitological diagnosis is based on the
finding of the encysted larval worms in a thin piece of muscle biopsy
compressed between two glass slides and examined under a low magnification of the microscope. In light infections when direct examination is
negative the biopsy specimen should be incubated overnight in an acid–
pepsin mixture and the centrifuged deposit examined for larvae (Editorial,
1954).

Recently, intradermal and serological tests have been widely used
(Kagan, 1960). They include (i) complement fixation, (ii) bentonite agglutination, (iii) latex agglutination, (iv) cholesterol agglutination, (v)
fluorescent antibody.

(i) Complement fixation test

This test can provide a diagnosis in the first week of the disease—the
specificity of the test is high.

(ii) Bentonite ⎫
(iii) Latex ⎬ *agglutination test*
(iv) Cholesterol ⎭

All these three are excellent tests for diagnosing recent infections, but are
unreliable in chronic infections.

(v) Fluorescent antibody test

This test is sensitive and specific for trichinosis. It becomes positive in human beings when tested 48 days after infection. The test can be carried out with drops of human serum or blood which are placed on filter paper and dried. They can then, if required, be sent through the post or stored (Sadun *et al.* 1962).

(vi) Intradermal

This test is not as specific as the serological tests mentioned above and gives 15 per cent of false-negative results in acute cases.

The reliability of all the above tests depends upon a high-quality antigen.

ANGIOSTRONGYLIASIS

Eosinophilic meningo-encephalitis due to *Angiostrongylus cantonensis* is an increasing public health problem in the Pacific area. The first cases in the tropics were recognized in New Caledonia in 1950 and the infection has since been reported from Hawaii, Tahiti, the other Pacific Islands, Indonesia, and Thailand.

Life cycle

A. cantonensis is essentially a parasite of rats and only occasionally infects man. The eggs hatch in the faeces of the rat in which they are expelled, and the infective larvae invade certain snails or slugs. These are later eaten by rats, which thereby become infected. The life cycle in man is unknown, but young adult worms have been found in the cerebrospinal fluid and the brain where they measured 8–12 mm in length. Experimental infections of monkeys with larvae of *A. cantonensis* have produced a clinical laboratory picture resembling very closely human eosinophilic meningo-encephalitis. The larvae can survive temperatures as low as 6 or 7° C.

Epidemiology

Human infection results from the accidental ingestion of infected snails, slugs, and land planarians (worm-like creatures) found on unwashed vegetables, such as lettuce (Deschiens and Courdurier 1966). Freshwater prawns may become infected from snails and slugs washed into rivers and estuaries during rainy weather. This was thought to be the main source of local, human infection in Tahiti (Alicata, 1962; Alicata and Brown, 1962). Eating raw or pickled snails of the genus *Pila* is considered the mode of infection in Thailand; the percentage of positive snails for *A. cantonensis* infections varies from 1·8 to 72 per cent (Punyagupta, 1956). The peak incidence of eosinophilic meningitis occurs in the cooler, rainy months between July and November; during this period lettuces and strawberries are most consumed, and when unwashed lead to infection (South Pacific Commission, 1965). In Thailand males are affected twice as frequently as females, the highest attack rate occurring in the second and third decade (Punyagupta *et al.* 1967). It has been suggested that *A. cantonensis* originated in the islands of the Indian Ocean—Madagascar, Mauritius, Ceylon—and then spread eastward to South East Asia and so to the Pacific area, and the giant African snail *Achatina fulica* might have been instrumental in the spread of the parasite. In Malaysia, the shelled slug *M. malayanus* has been shown to shed infective third-stage larvae, but no human cases have yet been reported (Lim Boo Liat, 1967).

Pathology

Clinically infection may cause a meningo-encephalitis with eosinophils, eosinophilic material, giant cells, and even young adult worms in the C.S.F. (Rosen *et al.* 1962; Jindrak and Alicata, 1965). The protein is raised and the sugar content lowered.

The main changes at autopsy, in the few which have been performed as the disease is seldom fatal, have been in the brain.

The dura may be adherent to the leptomeninges which are thickened and congested. Small areas of softening may be present in the white or grey matter of the cerebral hemispheres or cerebellum. Histologically the meninges and subarachnoid spaces are infiltrated with plasma cells, lymphoctyes, eosinophils, multinucleated giant cells, and scanty neutrophil polymorphonuclear leucocytes. Charcot–Leyden crystals may be present and the nematode has been seen in the subarachnoid space. Living or dead worms have been found in the substance of the brain surrounded in some instances by little cellular reaction—in others by eosinophilic material, eosinophils, phagocytes, lymphocytes, Charcot–Leyden crystals, and foreign-body giant cells. Blood vessels in the vicinity show perivascular cuffing by lymphocytes and phagocytes containing pigment, probably lipofuscin. Areas of necrosis with an associated lymphocytic and glial reaction may be seen in the absence of parasitic material. The nematodes measure 0·16–8 mm and careful sectioning of the brain is required to find them. Their appearance on transverse section is shown in Figs. 3.6 and 3.7.

Diagnostic pathology

C.S.F. examination reveals increase in protein, but the striking feature is the large numbers of eosinophils (60–80 per cent)—worms are sometimes found in the C.S.F. and can be identified as *A. cantonensis*.

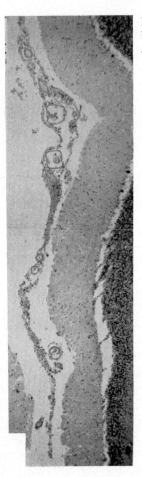

FIG. 3.6. Angiostrongyliasis. Cerebellar cortex with bodies of nematodes in the pia mater. (*By courtesy Ann. trop. Med. Parasit.*)

FIG. 3.7. Angiostrongyliasis. The parasite in the pons varolii; granular brown pigment is present in the intestinal cells. (*By courtesy Ann. trop. Med. Parasit.*)

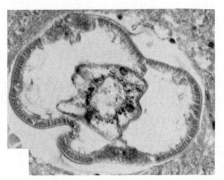

GNATHOSTOMIASIS

The normal hosts for *Gnathostoma spinigerum* are domestic and wild felines, dogs, and foxes. Human infections have, however, been reported from Israel, the Sudan, India, and the Far East. The majority of human cases to date have occurred in Thailand.

Life cycle

The life cycle in the definitive animal hosts is well known, and involves two intermediate hosts—a Cyclops and a fish or an amphibian. Man is an unnatural host and the immature worms may locate either in the internal organs or near the surface of the body, but as the larvae rarely develop into adults the life cycle in man is not known. Adults have, however, been reported in the intestine and ova passed in human faeces.

Epidemiology

Gnathostoma infection in human beings is not uncommon in Thailand and a substantial animal reservoir of *G. spinigerum* has been reported. The parasite has been isolated from cats, dogs, domestic pigs, freshwater fish, eels, snakes, frogs, leopards, and fish-eating birds (Daengsvang *et al.* 1964). Human infection usually results from eating fermented fish, which is a Thai delicacy much liked by women. Other ways for man to acquire the infection are by eating other forms of fish, frogs, and possibly snakes infected with encysted larvae. Little is known about human immunity to gnathostomiasis.

Pathology

Clinically, gnathostomiasis may present as 'creeping eruption' (p. 144). The immature larva stimulates an inflammatory reaction as it migrates and burrows through the tissues. Lesions are found in the internal organs and near the surface of the body. Transitory swellings consisting of eosinophils, histiocytes and plasma cells in oedematous tissue surrounding the parasite occur, and are sometimes associated with fever, abdominal and chest pain, dry cough, and blood eosinophilia (Punyagupta and Juttijudata, 1967). Secondary infection with abscess formation has been reported in the subcutaneous tissues in most parts of the body and many viscera, including the eye, may be affected. Haemoptysis, haematuria, angioneurotic oedema, or gastro-intestinal disorders may be the presenting symptoms. Eosinophilic meningitis due to *G. spinigerum* has also been reported. Bunnag *et al.* (1970) have described the neuropathological findings in nine autopsies performed on patients dying of eosinophilic myeloencephalitis due to gnathostomiasis. Clinically headache, severe sharp shooting pains in the trunk, limbs or perinaeum, and sensory disturbance preceded paralysis of both lower limbs. Hemiplegia occurred in one patient. Oedema of the eyelids and impairment of visual acuity might occur. The C.S.F. showed an eosinophilic pleocytosis and might be xanthochromic. The protein content was within normal limits. Necrotic areas were present in the spinal cord forming linear serpiginous tracks approximately 1 mm in diameter. The external surface of the brain might show generalized flattening of the gyri, some exudate or blood and even subarachnoid haemorrhage. A living worm was seen moving over the brain in one case. In the brain itself there were multiple areas of haemorrhage. Microscopically the typical lesion was a focus of acute softening with degeneration of surrounding neurones, lymphocytes and plasma cells with a variable number of eosinophils surrounding these areas. The meninges were thickened and oedematous and infiltrated with chronic inflammatory cells. The early onset of nerve root pain was considered to be due to the parasite entering the cord via the nerve trunks and passing upwards to the brain itself. The mortality rate is high and at autopsy immature adult specimens of *G. spinigerum* have been recovered from the brain. Severe agonizing pain over the trunk and extremities followed by paralysis and coma occurs (Bunnag *et al.* 1967). Prasasmith (1974) has described a case of neuro-otological gnathostomiasis.

Diagnostic pathology

Diagnosis in human infections depends on finding the immature worms and identifying them. Cutaneous tests with antigens from larval or adult worms as well as the precipitin test have been used for diagnosis (Tada *et al.* 1966). Eosinophilia is present.

Trichostrongyliasis

Species of *Trichostrongylus* are commonly parasitic in the digestive tract of herbivorous animals and only occur as incidental infections of man. The maturing or adult worms attach themselves to the mucosa of the small intestine and mild anaemia from haemorrhage may occur in very heavy infections.

FILARIASES

Under this generic title are grouped a variety of diseases which bear little relation to each other pathologically although they are produced by nematode worms all belonging to the superfamily Filarioidea. The following conditions will be described:

Disease	Filarial worm
1. Filariasis	*Wuchereria bancrofti* or *Brugia malayi*
2. Loiasis	*Loa loa*
3. Onchocerciasis	*Onchocerca volvulus*
4. Streptocerciasis	*Acanthocheilonema streptocerca*
5. Dirofilariasis	*Dirofilaria conjunctivae*

The pathogenicity of two other filarial worms, *Acanthocheilonema, perstans* and *Mansonella ozzardi,* has not been fully determined, and will only be briefly mentioned. The morphological differences of the various filarial worms are given in Table 3.3.

Filariasis (Bancroftian and Malayan)

Filariasis results from infection with the parasitic nematodes *Wuchereria bancrofti* and *Brugia malayi.*

TABLE 3.3

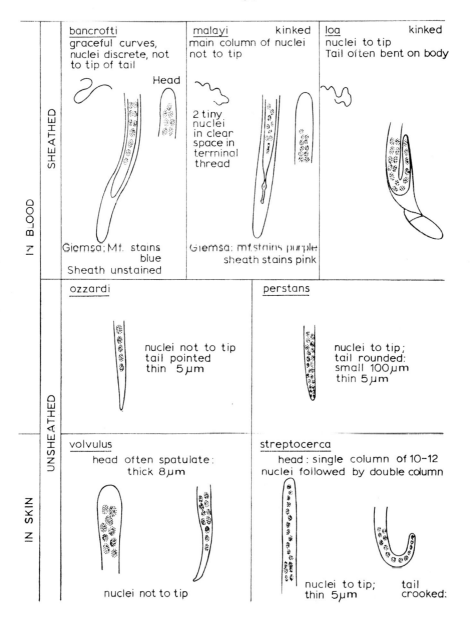

bancrofti
graceful curves,
nuclei discrete, not
to tip of tail

Head

Giemsa; Mf. stains
blue
Sheath unstained

malayi   kinked
main column of nuclei
not to tip

2 tiny
nuclei
in clear
space in
terminal
thread

Giemsa; mf.stains purple
sheath stains pink

loa   kinked
nuclei to tip
Tail often bent on body

IN BLOOD — SHEATHED

ozzardi

nuclei not to tip
tail pointed
thin 5 μm

perstans

nuclei to tip;
tail rounded:
small 100 μm
thin 5 μm

IN SKIN / UNSHEATHED

volvulus
head often spatulate:
thick 8 μm

nuclei not to tip

streptocerca
head: single column of 10–12
nuclei followed by double column

nuclei to tip;   tail
thin 5 μm   crooked:

Life cycle

The features of the life cycles of these two filariae are practically identical. The adult worms live in the lymphatic system where the female worms, which are viviparous, produce sheathed microfilariae which are about 200–300 μm long. The microfilariae make their way to and circulate in the blood stream where they are ingested by a mosquito. After ingestion the microfilariae escape from the sheath, penetrate the gut wall of the insect and pass to the thoracic muscles where they undergo development. After 2 or more weeks the infective larvae reach the proboscis and enter another vertebrate host when the mosquito is biting. It is not certain how they reach the lymphatics after the insect bites. Many species of mosquitoes, belonging to the genera *Culex*, *Aëdes*, *Anopheles*, and *Mansonioides*, can act as intermediate hosts of *W. bancrofti* and *B. malayi*.

The microfilariae of *B. malayi* can be distinguished from those of *W. bancrofti* on morphological grounds and by their staining reaction to Giemsa (see Table 3.3). The adult worms are also morphologically different (Rao and Maplestone, 1940). The best medium for the *in vitro* cultivation of *microfilaria bancrofti* consists of 0·2 ml inactivated human serum, 2 ml of mosquito extract in Ringer glucose (pH 7·0) at a temperature of 27 °C (Weinstein, 1958).

Microfilariae of both *W. bancrofti* and *B. malayi* appear in the peripheral blood at distinct times of the day—a characteristic referred to as periodicity. The controlling mechanism for this periodicity has never been satisfactorily explained. It does not appear to depend on the parasympathetic system nor is the microfilaria count influenced by alteration in the corticosteroid level in the blood of man, or by a general anaesthetic (Hawking, 1965).

Epidemiology

Whereas *W. bancrofti* has so far been found only in man, *B. malayi* is a parasite of both man and animals. The geographical distribution of the parasites is determined largely by climate and the distribution of their mosquito vectors (Edeson and Wilson, 1964; South Pacific Commission, 1965). Recent studies of filariasis have been reported from Zaire (Fain *et al.*, 1974) and the Sudan (Abdalla, 1974).

Wuchereria bancrofti

Two biologically different forms of *W. bancrofti* exist—the nocturnal periodic form, in which the microfilariae appear in the peripheral blood between 10 p.m. and 2 a.m., and is predominantly an infection of urban communities, transmitted by the domestic night-biting mosquito, *Culex pipiens fatigans*. It has an almost world-wide distribution, occurring in Central and South America, West, Central and East Africa; Egypt, and South East Asia. The other form, which is diurnally subperiodic, i.e. microfilariae are present in appreciable numbers throughout the 24 hours but show a consistent minor peak diurnally (usually sometime in the afternoon), is restricted to Polynesia and is transmitted mainly by day-biting mosquitoes (Saugnain and Outin-Fabre, 1972).

Brugia malayi

Human infection with *B. malayi* has only been recognized in Asia, where it is predominantly an infection of rural populations, in contrast to the usual distribution of *W. bancrofti*. It has a tendency to occur in small endemic foci which have been found in countries extending from the west coast of India to New Guinea, the Philippines and Japan. There are two forms of *B. malayi*, the periodic in which the microfilariae show a markedly nocturnal periodicity in the blood (10 p.m.–2 a.m.), and the subperiodic form in which the microfilariae tend to be present throughout the 24 hours with a minor nocturnal peak from 10 p.m.–6 a.m. (Turner and Edeson, 1957). The former is transmitted by the *Mansonia* mosquitoes of open swamps which bite mainly at night, while the latter is transmitted by the *Mansonia* of swamp forest, mosquitoes which will bite in shade at any time. The periodic form is found mainly in man, and animal infections are rare. In contrast the subperiodic form is found in many animals (primates, carnivores, rodents, etc.) as well as man.

Timor microfilaria

This new microfilaria was recently discovered by David and Edeson (1965) in the Portuguese island of Timor. There is no animal reservoir and the vector is unknown. The periodicity and symptomatology are similar to that of the periodic form of *W. bancrofti*. Recently another new microfilaria has been discovered in Madagascar and named *W. bancrofti* var. *Vauceli*.

Symptoms attributable to filariasis can present many years after a relatively brief period of exposure to infection (Trent, 1963), although severe disabling symptoms or deformity are usually due to long periods of exposure and reinfection. Males are usually more frequently affected than females. This higher incidence of microfilaraemia in males is probably due to a greater chance of infection; it is possible, however, that a hormonal influence may be responsible (Chatterjee and Chowdury, 1964). Most surveys for either form of *W. bancrofti* have shown low microfilaria rates in children below the age of 5 years, probably because *W. bancrofti* takes a long time to produce a patent microfilaraemia. In contrast (Wilson, 1961) has shown that high microfilariae rates occur in children under 5 years with both the periodic and the subperiodic form of *B. malayi*; in fact a low infection rate among children under 5 years usually implies low transmission for *B. malayi* in the area surveyed. A methodology for community diagnosis and a mathematical model have been devised (Southgate, 1974a and b).

Pathology

In general the pathological lesions produced by *W. bancrofti* and *B. malayi* are similar and the following description applies to both species.

When differences do exist they are mentioned in the appropriate section of the text. The pathology is described according to the stage of the disease namely acute, subacute and chronic. Chyluria, hydrocoele, and elephantiasis are dealt with separately (Nelson, 1966).

Acute stage

The acute stage may manifest itself clinically as little as two months after infection. On the other hand, individuals living in endemic areas may never exhibit this stage and evidence of chronic infection may occur many years later, if at all. Microfilariae may be detected in the blood in the course of surveys or on routine investigations in patients with no symptoms directly related to the filarial infection.

Epididymitis is frequently the first and only symptom but transient erythematous lesions with lymphadenopathy and mild pyrexia are common and it should be noted that microfilariae are not demonstrable in the peripheral blood at this stage and biopsy may be the only certain diagnostic method. The regions most frequently affected are the lymphatics of the spermatic cord (funiculitis), the upper arm (epitrochlear and axillary glands) and the inguinal glands in *W. bancrofti* infections, and the pelvic, inguinal, and popliteal regions in *B. malayi*. Adult worms are not infrequently present in the breast in the female (Cooray, 1960). An acute funiculoepididymitis and periorchitis associated with secondary bacterial infection and septicaemia causing death have been reported (Lichtenberg, 1957). A non-filarial endemic funiculitis has been reported however in Ceylon and Egypt (Power, 1946). Acute scrotal lymphangitis and inguinal lymphadenitis with infective cellulitis and even massive scrotal gangrene occur.

The *histological lesions* produced in the lymphatic system are those of oedema, eosinophilic infiltration, congestion and the presence of a variable number of monocytic cells. Adult worms may or may not be detected within the lymphatics or medullary sinuses of the lymph nodes (Fig. 3.8). If present they may be surrounded by a deposit of fibrinoid material. On cross-section the worms have a smooth, pink cuticle and a double uterus containing embryos measuring 20–30 μm in diameter. The lymph nodes, which are discrete and freely moveable, are hyperplastic with mitotic figures in the germinal centres and a marked increase of eosinophils in the sinuses. The lymphatic channels show retrograde lymphagiectasis and contain a thin, pink-staining albuminous fluid.

In the testes there is infiltration of the septa and lobules by lymphocytes, plasma cells, and eosinophils, which may be found in sheets. The veins show an eosinophilic endophlebitis and there is perivascular cuffing in the tunica albuginia (Hartz, 1950).

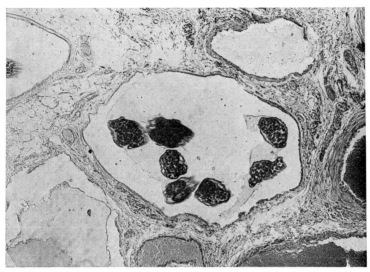

FIG. 3.8. Bancroftian filariasis. Adult filarial worms in a dilated lymph channel. Note the large vascular channels at the edge of the section (× 30).

In the blood there is a mild leucocytosis with a relative lymphocytosis and mild eosinophilia (much more marked in *B. malayi* infections). Those lesions are suggestive of a supersensitive reaction to the toxic or metabolic products of the worm and this would explain the fleeting and reversible character of their clinical manifestations (Michael, 1944; Zuckerman and Hibbard, 1945; Rifkin and Thompson, 1945; Wartman, 1947).

When mature, fertilized females release microfilariae which enter the blood stream through the thoracic duct, their periodicity depends upon the species. The microfilaria were at one time considered to be relatively harmless but have recently been implicated as an aetiological agent in tropical eosinophilia (Gault *et al.* 1960), causing lesions in the lung and granulomatous lesions in other organs, including the liver (Burganinon, 1937) and spleen. An eosinophilic myocarditis has also been attributed to their presence in the heart.

Subacute stage

Clinically exacerbations due to a hypersensitivity reaction or to associated infection may cause recurrent symptoms of pyrexia and lymphangitis; even abscess formation and synovitis have been described.

In this stage death and disintegration of the adult worms occur. The walls of the lymphatics become thickened and the disintegrating adults are surrounded by granulomatous tissue consisting of epithelioid cells, foreign-body giant cells, fibroblasts and variable numbers of eosinophils, lympho-cytes, and plasma cells. Eventually calcification of the adult worm may occur—usually commencing centrally—due to the deposition of alkaline soaps in the ischaemic area. An associated phlebitis and angiitis especially in the cord and epididymus may occur. The walls of the blood vessels are infiltrated with chronic inflammatory cells with associated intimal thickening and thrombus formation. A similar inflammatory infiltrate may affect the dilated lymphatic channels—the composite pathological changes being those of a retrograde thrombolymphangitis with associated vascular changes which may occur some distance distally from the site of the disintegrating parasites.

In the regional lymphatic glands there is an increase of epithelioid cells and eosinophils. Small follicles with Langhans-type giant cells may be present. Similar lesions may be seen in the spleen and microfilariae may be noted (Dhayagude and Amin, 1942).

Chronic stage

Elephantiasis of the limbs, scrotum or vulva, chyluria and chylous ascites are common complications. Das and Sen (1968) have described chylous arthritis of the knee joint in systemic filariasis. The histopathology was that of an acute inflammation. The lipid content of the joint fluid was high. Varicose groin glands, varicocoeles, and hydrocoele may also develop. Infection may supervene in any of these lesions and multiple discharging sinuses may be formed—especially in the scrotum—the so-called lymph scrotum. Extensive involvement of the abdominal lymphatic glands by adults and microfilaria has been considered a causal factor in peritonitis.

Fibrosis and obliteration of lymphatic glands, blockage of lymphatic channels by granulomatous lesions or by fibrin thrombi in various stages of organization and, occasionally, superadded venous thrombosis, are the causal factors in this stage. The site of the obstructive fibrotic lesions determines the clinical presentation outlined above.

Chyluria

This can be defined as a pathological condition characterized by the passage of chylomicrons in the urine (Cahill, 1965). It is common in Bancroftian filariasis due to the periodic (nocturnal) form but rare with the subperiodic (diurnal) variety; chyluria due to B. malayi infection has not been observed. Signs and symptoms of chronic filarial infection may or may not be present but microfilariae of W. bancrofti are usually present in the peripheral blood. It may occur with no history of past infection and may be asymptomatic clinically. A mild hypochromic anaemia and hypo-protein-aemia are usually found. Urinary complications due to infection may occur.

Lymphangiography reveals an abnormally early excretion of lipiodol in the urine and Cahill (1965) considered that this indicates abnormal lymphatic communications between the abdominal and renal lymphatics. Akisada and Tani (1970) by lymphography have demonstrated lymphatico-pelvic fistulae. Abnormalities of the para-aortic nodes or of the thoracic duct were considered responsible for the reflux of lipiodol into the collecting lymphatics of the kidney.

Hydrocoele

Although hydrocoele occurs in areas where filariasis is unknown and has been attributed to trauma in young and infection in older men (Wallace, 1960), studies in endemic areas of Bancroftian filariasis have shown an association between the two conditions (Hawking, 1940; Galindo et al. 1962). Bhatnagar et al. (1970) have shown that hydrocele has no effect on the testicular substance apart from an increase in fibrous tissue in the tunica and the peritubular and inter-tubular tissues. Spermatogenesis is unimpaired. It should be noted that other parasitic agents have also been implicated as causative agents in hydrocoele in the tropics, viz.: *Mansonella ozzardi*, *Loa loa*, and *O. volvulus*. Hydrocoele has not been described as occurring in *B. malayi* infections.

Elephantiasis

This condition may be congenital (primary) or the result of acquired obliterative disease of the lymphatic system (secondary). Primary lymphoedema has been well described by Kinmonth et al. (1957) and will not be further considered here.

Secondary lymphoedema is the end result of recurrent lymphangitis, regardless of the primary aetiological agent, and although *W. bancrofti* (Fouques et al. 1972) and *B. malayi* infections are probably the most important cause of elephantiasis in tropical areas other factors must not be overlooked (Price, 1974).

In Ibadan, Nigeria, for instance, Ngu and Konstam (1964) found that the most important causes of lymphoedema of the lower limb were tuberculous-inguinal adenitis, chronic pyogenic infection, and malignant infiltration of the regional lymphatic glands. No case was attributed to filariasis. Price (1972) in contrast to the finding of Ngu and Konstam considered that in Ethiopia the pathology of elephantiasis of the lower limbs was due to the constant absorption of an irritant substance through the bare feet of patients during walking—silica and aluminium being implicated, as birefringent crystals were seen in the inguinal lymphatic glands. In Tanzania, it was considered that *A. perstans* might be the aetiological agent in patients suffering from elephantiasis in the absence of *W. bancrofti* infection (Jordan *et al.* 1956). *A. streptocerca* in the Congo, *O. volvulus*, and *Loa loa* have also been considered causal factors in this condition (Browne, 1960). Lymphogranuloma venereum is also a common cause of elephantiasis of the vulva in females and schistosomiasis has been recorded as a cause of elephantiasis of the penis. It should not, therefore, be taken for granted that every patient presenting with elephantiasis in the tropics is suffering from filariasis and a careful investigation is indicated to exclude other causes— these include blood smears, the Frei, Heaf, and filarial antigen tests, biopsy, and lymphangiography.

In elephantiasis the skin of the affected part becomes smooth and tense— later dry, scaly, fissured, and verrucous. It should be noted that in *B. malayi* infections, the lower leg (below knee) is usually affected, with involvement of the popliteal and femoral glands, whereas in Bancrofti infections the whole limb is usually affected. Other common sites in Bancroftian filariasis are the vulva, scrotum, upper arm, and breast.

The retention of fluid with a high protein content in the tissue spaces due to obliteration of the lymphatics stimulates the production of fibrous tissue and the oedema is of a solid non-pitting character. The tissues below the deep fascia are unaffected (Paul, 1963).

Histologically in the early stages there is atrophy of the epidermis, dilatation of lymphatics in the dermis with surrounding plasma cells, lymphocytes, and occasional eosinophils. The blood vessels are compressed. Interstitial oedema and fibrous tissue proliferation occur. Eventually there is excessive hyperkeratosis and acanthosis with scarring and loss of elastica in the dermis, leading to nodular and fissured lesions. Occasionally, giant-cell systems may be present. An increase in acid-mucopolysaccharide, mast-cell populations, and histamine content have been noted in lymphoedematous tissues (Chowdury, 1967).

Diagnostic pathology

The finding of microfilariae in the blood provides the certain diagnosis of filarial infection. Thick blood films should be taken at the appropriate times (e.g. at night for microfilaria bancrofti) and fresh coverslip preparations examined. Simultaneously, dried, stained specimens should be made and identification of the microfilariae made according to the diagnostic criteria given in Table 3.1. Microfilariae may also be found in fluids obtained from hydrocoeles, varices, pleura, joints, and in ascitic fluid. Eosinophilia is usually present. It is important to realize that microfilariae may be absent in the very early or late stages of the infection—thus in only 4 per cent of patients with elephantiasis and 30 per cent with hydrocoeles were microfilariae found in the blood (Jordan, 1960). Occasionally the adult filarial worms may be found in biopsy of lymph glands (Wartman, 1947), or by X-ray when calcified.

Techniques are available for concentrating blood microfilariae (Knott, 1939; Bell, 1967). Partono and Cross (1973) have evaluated these concentration methods against the thick smear for demonstrating microfilariae in the blood; while Yong (1973) has evolved an indirect fluorescent antibody technique using micro fragments of *W. bancrofti*.

Serodiagnostic methods for the diagnosis of filariasis have been widely used. The subject was fully reviewed by Kagan (1963). There is a range of variation in the results obtained and these variations derive partly from differences in technique of antigen preparation. These immuno-diagnostic methods are group specific (i.e. positive in any filarial infection) and on the whole still unsatisfactory with the possible exception of the filarial complement-fixation test (FCFT). Recently Ciferri *et al.* (1965) attempted to evaluate intracutaneous tests in bancroftian filariasis with an antigen prepared from *Onchocerca* compared with one prepared from *Dirofilaria immitis* (canine filaria). A logarithmic relationship appeared to exist between the weal area and nitrogen content of injected antigen; it appeared, however, that onchocercal extracts elicited more specific reactions in persons infected with Onchocerciasis. According to Smith *et al.* (1971) the value of the skin test with *D. immitis* seems limited to two situations. (1) A large reaction may help to confirm a clinical diagnosis of filariasis when parasites cannot be found and (2) the frequency distribution of skin reaction sizes in local populations may help, where blood surveys are impossible, to indicate areas in which some filarial infection is being transmitted.

LOIASIS

This is an infection due to the filarial worm *Loa loa* and is characterized by transient subcutaneous swellings.

Life cycle

The adult worms live in the connective tissue of man and the females, which are about 70mm long, produce microfilariae which pass into the blood stream. The microfilariae are sheathed and about 300 μm in length; they appear in greatest numbers in the blood during the day. When the circulating microfilariae are taken up by suitable species of *Chrysops*, they pass from the stomach to the thoracic muscles and after a period of development, lasting about 12 days, present in the proboscis; when the fly next feeds on a human host the larvae penetrate the skin and migrate in the connective tissues. They reach maturity in about a year.

Epidemiology

Loiasis is found in the equatorial rain forest belt of Africa stretching from the Gulf of Guinea in the West to the Great Lakes in the East.

Various species of *Chrysops* are the only known vectors of loiasis and they breed in densely shaded, slow-moving streams and swamps. The adults live in the tree tops, the females coming down to attack man at ground level or to lay their eggs on the mud and decaying vegetation of stagnant waters. The males do not feed on blood. *Chrysops* are attracted by movement, light and smoke from wood fires; they bite in daylight and seem to prefer dark to white skins. In man all ages and both sexes are affected although overt infection in young children is uncommon probably due to the long incubation period of the filarial worm. The ecology of human loiasis in Nigeria was described by Ogunba (1972).

Pathology

The pathology has been inadequately studied. There may be a weal at the site of the bite of the *Chrysops*. It is not known if symptoms occur as the worms grow to maturity. The adults pass through the connective tissue and are attracted to the surface of the body by heat. Fugitive swellings (Calabar swellings) or the outline of the worm itself may be seen on any part of the body, the most dramatic being its appearance beneath the conjunctiva. The histopathology of ocular loiasis in Uganda was described by Poltera (1973). The swelling is due to a transient inflammatory oedematous allergic reaction to the presence of the worm. Clinically, vague symptoms of mild fever, generalized muscular pains, paraesthesia, pruritis, urticaria, anorexia, and loss of weight may be complained of. An eosinophilia is usual. Pain, conjunctivitis, and lachrymation may be present if the eye is affected. The Calabar swellings are painless non-pitting subcutaneous swellings about 5 cm in diameter which disappear spontaneously in a few days. Occasionally the parasite may become encapsulated and secondary infection with abscess formation single or multiple may occur.

A suppurative arthritis has been attributed to loiasis as have also hydrocoele and unilateral oedema of the lower limb. The parasite has been found in the C.S.F. associated with a meningo-encephalitis. The lesions caused by the microfilariae are unknown but fibrosis and eosinophils in the spleen have been attributed to their presence, and occasionally microfilariae, presumably loa, with a surrounding cellular reaction, have been seen in the heart in Ibadan. It is of interest to note that a cardiomyopathy with eosinophilia has been ascribed to *Loa loa* infection (Gerbaux *et al.* 1957) and the possible relationship of filariasis to endomyocardial fibrosis is discussed on p. 358. Following therapy the microfilariae are said to be destroyed in the liver and this may be followed by generalized allergic manifestations.

Diagnostic pathology

Microfilariae may be found in the peripheral blood taken preferably around mid-day and they can be differentiated on morphological grounds from other sheathed microfilariae (see p. 123). Concentration techniques are useful to detect scanty infections (Bell, 1967). The adult worms may be seen wriggling under the conjunctiva. A high eosinophilia (60–80 per cent) is usually present. The filarial complement-fixation test gives the highest incidence of positive results with loiasis (Ridley, 1956), and is particularly useful in early infections before microfilariae have appeared in the blood, or in unisexual infections when microfilariae are absent. Intradermal tests are available but have the same limitations in their use as in the other filarial infections.

ONCHOCERCIASIS

This infection is caused by the nematode *Onchocerca volvulus* and is characterized by the development of skin changes, subcutaneous nodules and ocular lesions.

Life cycle

The adult worms are found in subcutaneous nodules and tissue spaces. The females which are ovoviviparous measure about 50 cm in length while the males are only 2–4 cm long. Worms of both sexes are found coiled together in nodules and larvae are present in large numbers near the coiled gravid female. The developed larvae (microfilariae) vary greatly in size (150–350 μm) and are unsheathed.

Microfilariae are ingested when the vector—a *Simulium* fly—feeds on an infected individual. The microfilariae develop in the thoracic muscles of the fly after escaping from its stomach, and after a series of moults become infective larvae on reaching the proboscis. When the *Simulium* next bites an individual the larval forms of *Onchocerca* are injected under the skin. The development in the fly takes about 15 days and the common vectors are *S. damnosum* and *S. naevi* (in Africa), and *S. metallicum*, *S. callidium*, and *S. ochraceum* (in Central America). The microfilariae introduced by the fly mature in the subcutaneous tissues. In some instances a fibrous tissue reaction around the adults causes the formation of nodules. After about a year the female worm produces microfilariae. The microfilariae remain in the skin and do not enter the peripheral blood. In Central America *O. volvulus* is called *O. caecutiens*, which is a morphologically similar nematode. Survival *in vitro* of microfilariae of *O. volvulus* has been achieved in a medium containing salt solution, ascitic fluid, embryo extract, and penicillin, at 38 °C and pH 7·2.

Epidemiology

Onchocerciasis has a focal distribution in both African and tropical America. It is endemic in West Africa, in Equatorial and East Africa, and in the Sudan. It occurs in central America and in parts of Venezuela and Colombia (WHO 1966; Villegas et al. 1972; Editorial, 1974). Although *O. volvulus* has been found in primates, in most endemic areas the infection is maintained by man-to-man transmission. *Simulium* can breed at high altitudes (2000 ft — 610 metres — or more) and the larvae and pupae are found attached to submerged vegetation and stones in highly oxygenated waters.

They are also found at sea level along the banks of very large rivers such as the Niger. The larvae of *S. naevi* have been found adherent to the carapace of certain aquatic crabs.

The period of greatest transmission is in the rainy season coinciding, as might be expected, with the period of maximal *Simulium* breeding. The disease is widespread and males are infected more frequently than females but this is probably an occupational hazard. The incidence of infection increases with age and in an endemic area 75 per cent of persons might be infected by middle age (Woodruff *et al.* 1966a, b). No clear relationship is necessarily found between the number of microfilariae in the skin and the extent or degree of the lesions (Reber and Hoeppli, 1964). Comparisons between African and Central American onchocerciasis reveal certain epidemiological and clinical differences. Thus in some parts of Africa there is a tendency for the microfilariae to be most numerous in the most dependent parts of the body (Kershaw *et al.* 1954; Woodruff *et al.* 1963); while in Guatemala microfilariae are abundant in the upper parts of the body (De Leon and Duke, 1966). A relationship seems to exist between the site of biting of the vector and the localization of nodules (Lagraulet *et al.* 1964). As would be expected, in Africa the majority of nodules are found in the lower parts of the body, whereas in Central America as many as 70 per cent are found on the head. Bony lesions of the occipital region of the skull produced by these nodules are found in 5 per cent of patients.

In Central America infection is acquired at an early age and in the Cheapas State of Mexico 50 per cent of children are infected by the age of 14 years (Nunez, 1963). Both in Mexico and Guatemala 'eresipela de la costa' is found in children and young persons and 'mal del morado' in the older age groups. Both these syndromes, the features of which are described below, are associated with high microfilaria densities. Moreover, in Guatemala very much more severe corneal and iris lesions are encountered than is usual in Africa.

Onchocercal blindness

In Africa, it is generally agreed that anterior segment lesions are due to *O. volvulus*. Anderson and Fuglsang (1973) have pointed out that as many as 50 per cent of cases of microfilaria in the anterior chamber might be missed in surveys based on a single routine examination and that ocular massage and head manoeuvres considerably decrease this figure.

Considerable disagreement however exists as to whether choroido-retinal lesions are a direct complication of ocular onchocerciasis or not. The major cause of disagreement has been the demonstration that in the forest belt of Africa the incidence of ocular complications is low in contrast to the savannah regions where it is high, despite a high prevalence of onchocerciasis in both areas. It was pointed out by Budden (1963) that there are distinct epidemiological differences between forest and savannah onchocerciasis. Thus in the savannah areas transmission is seasonal, man/fly contact probably more intimate, and the host resistance may be lower because of the shorter transmission season. There is no evidence that vitamin A is involved (Woodruff et al. 1963) and though vitamin B-complex deficiency has been postulated (Choyce, 1964) no proof has been produced that this plays any part in the onchocercal blindness of the savannah areas. The consensus of opinion is that the differences in the incidence of ocular onchocercal complications between the savannah and forest onchocerciasis in Africa are due to differences in intensity and duration of infection. Quere et al. (1963) believe that ocular lesions are invariably associated with onchocerciasis and that anterior and posterior lesions are part of an unified sequence of inflammatory processes; while Waddy (1966) has observed that high blindness rates are associated with communities in which infection is common in childhood and that a glance at the children's legs in a village could enable one to make a fairly close estimate of the local blindness rate. Onchocercal blindness is rare before the age of thirty. Berghout (1973) found an unexpectedly high prevalence of glaucoma in patients with onchocerciasis in Ghana; she ascribes the presence of juvenile glaucoma to onchocercal infection.

In contrast to the situation in Africa there is general agreement about the nature of the ocular complications in Central America which are predominantly found in the anterior segment of the eye, blindness being due to the end results of onchocercal kerato-iridoyclitis with the typical occluded and down-drawn pupil described by Pacheco-Luna (1921). In Guatemala more severe corneal and iris lesions are encountered than in Africa. In this context it is interesting to note that De Leon and Duke (1966) believe that the Guatemalan and African strains of O. volvulus are different parasites and it is possible that they may possess different propensities for producing eye lesions. In a series of meticulous studies ranging over several years (1966–1973) Duke and his colleagues have detailed the various factors that influence the transmission of onchocerciasis (Duke et al. 1973). Anderson et al. (1974) have recently carried out very careful comparative studies of onchocerciasis in rain-forest and sudan-savanna.

Little is known about immunity in onchocerciasis. It has been observed, however, that in Tanzania, microfilarial densities do not increase significantly beyond the age of twenty. Whether this is due to the development of partial immunity or some other factors has yet to be determined. Choyce (1972) has suggested, though not proved, that the ocular changes of onchocerciasis are conditioned by the immunological state of the patient or population at risk.

Pathology

Adult worms may wander freely in the subcutaneous tissues and microfilariae may be found in the skin in the absence of nodules. However, the adults are usually found inextricably wound together in subcutaneous fibrous nodules varying in size from 1 to 6 cm in diameter. Their distribution differs in South America and Africa, being more frequent in the upper trunk, upper limbs, and suboccipital regions in the former and in the lower limbs and pelvic girdle in the latter. They are firm and mobile on palpation. On section the nodules consist of firm, white fibrous tissue with cystic areas filled with yellowish necrotic or greyish viscid material containing microfilariae and portions of adults. Secondary infection with abscess formation is a complication. Occasionally, adults may affect the larger joints with the occurrence of synovitis and arthritis. Microfilariae may be detected in the joint fluid.

Histological examination

The adults stimulate an inflammatory and fibroblastic reaction in the surrounding tissues and, although it has been stated that this reaction does not occur until death of the worm, we could not subscribe entirely to this as numerous microfilariae are frequently seen in the fibrous tissue surrounding the adults, and the uterus of the female contains embryos with well-stained nuclei, suggesting viability. Transverse or oblique sections of numerous adult male and female worms are usually seen, however, and it is of course possible that the death of one of these may have stimulated the host reaction. The male is smaller than the female on cross-section. The female contains a double uterus containing microfilariae. A thin outer cuticle encloses a thicker muscular layer which bounds an internal coelomic cavity. In the female this cavity contains large uterine and ovarian sacs full of developing embryos (Fig. 3.9) but in the inconspicuous male the genitalia are much less in evidence. The narrow tubular gut is wedged between the genitalia. The cuticle and outer coat of the genital sacs stain red with van Gieson's stain and PAS techniques, and neither elastic tissue nor reticulin is present. In the uterus each microfilaria is ensheathed in a thin PAS-positive membrane. The cells lining the alimentary tube contain much haemosiderin. With death of the worm the embryos undergo necrosis with blurring of the nuclei, and later a homogeneous basophilic or eosinophilic material is formed. Eventually most of the worm is absorbed and only fragments of the cuticle may remain (Israel, 1959).

Calcification may occur in the nodule and in the scrotum a number of these superficial nodules may give rise to calcinosis circumscripta of the scrotal wall (Browne, 1962).

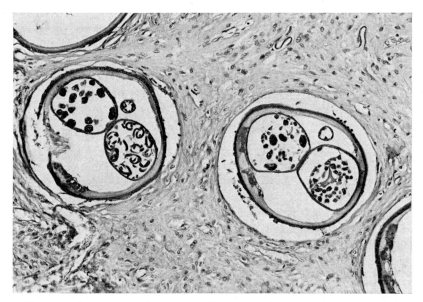

FIG. 3.9. Onchocerciasis. Section through onchocercal nodule, showing adult worms and microfilariae (× 30).

The adults may be intimately and individually surrounded by cellular fibrous tissue with a varying number of lymphocytes, eosinophils, plasma cells, and polymorphonuclear leucocytes. Disintegrating worms may be surrounded by lakes of purulent debris or in other areas by large numbers of macrophages—many of them foamy and containing lipid material. Giant cells, cholesterol clefts, and frank fat necrosis may be seen. Palisading of epithelioid cells round the worms and giant-cell granulomata occur. Numerous microfilariae may be seen in the broad peripheral area of fibrous tissue. With dense collagenosis and death of the adults, microfilariae are usually absent.

The dermal lesions of onchocerciasis

Numerous microfilariae may be found in the dermis without a surrounding inflammatory reaction (Hawking, 1952) and clinically the condition may be symptomless and the skin macroscopically normal. Following therapy an inflammatory exudate has been noted around the microfilariae and intense pruritus may be experienced. It is therefore likely that the microfilariae do not produce skin lesions whilst alive but only following death, when their products stimulate a cellular response. Neutrophil polymorphonuclear leucocytes infiltrate around the parasite and are quickly succeeded by eosinophils, lymphocytes, plasma cells, and fibroblasts. Clinically, dermatitis occurs in the form of lichenoid lesions, xeroderma, or 'lizard skin'. The skin becomes thickened, wrinkled, and inelastic, resembling the skin of the aged, and the term presbydermia has been used. Cutaneous depigmentation over bony prominences and in the pretibial inguinal and pectoral regions may occur (Browne, 1960). Papillomata have been noted in association with the dermal lesions.

Histological examination

In the earlier lesions the microfilariae are seen lying free in the connective tissue and lymphatics of the dermis. They are most numerous in the dermal papillae, which are oedematous and hyperaemic. Later there is loss of papillae, with atrophy and hyperkeratosis of the epidermis. Clumps of melanin pigment may be present in the dermis, which shows loss of elastica with fibrosis and perivascular lymphocytic infiltration with occlusion of the smaller blood vessels (Rodger, 1962). With depigmentation there is absence of melanin, flattening of the rete pegs, hyperkeratosis, and fibrosis of the dermis with increase in elastic tissue. Repigmentation may occur with therapy (Browne, 1960).

Onchocerciasis, elephantiasis, 'hanging groin' and hydrocoele

Microfilariae have been noted in the lymphatics of the dermis. In addition the onchodermatitis may produce intense irritation with secondary lesions and infection due to scratching. Enlargement of regional lymphatic glands occurs. An elephantoid condition of the face has been described in South America. Elephantiasis, especially of the fundus of the scrotum but also of the lower limbs, penis, labia, anal region, and occasionally of the axillary region, has been described (Cherry, 1959). Following sclerosing hypertrophic lymphadenopathy of the inguino-crural glands 'hanging groin' or adenolymphocoele occurs. The affected lymphatic glands are grey-white due to excessive fibrosis, and surrounded by gelatinous loose connective tissue containing distended, hypertrophied lymphatic channels.

There may be lymph varix. The changes in the glands are not thought to be due to the presence of adult worms or microfilariae, although they have been noted (Hughes, 1954), but to attacks of recurrent bacterial infection from the skin lesions. In the inguinal region the enlarged femoral and inguinal glands sag down in the inelastic oedematous, thinned connective tissue drawing a sac of irregularly atrophic and thickened skin, thus forming the so-called 'hanging groin' lesion in males or the 'pseudo-Hottentot apron' in females. These conditions are found in older patients in areas where the intensity of infection is high, and poor environmental hygienic factors are concerned in their aetiology.

Microfilariae have been noted in hydrocoele fluid but the causal relationship between this condition and onchocerciasis is debatable. Adult worms have been seen in the testis and its secondary membranes (Hughes, 1954). *Onchocerca volvulus* microfilariae have been found in the urine (Fuglsang and Anderson, 1973; Buck, 1974).

Ocular lesions in onchocerciasis

It is common to observe numerous living microfilariae in the anterior chamber of the eye in the absence of ocular symptoms. It is likely that lesions follow death of the embryo. Healthy microfilariae have been seen in all tissues of the eye, including the optic nerve. It is therefore reasonable to suppose that pathological changes due to their death could occur in all tissues and theoretically anterior and posterior segment lesions should occur. The absence of these lesions in South America is difficult to explain.

An inflammatory reaction occurs around the dead microfilariae with secondary perivascular lymphocytic infiltration and vascular changes. Fluffy opacities occur in the cornea due to these lesions which during resolution give the snow-flake appearance (Budden, 1958). Later an iritis may develop and with secondary glaucoma be a potent cause of blindness. In the posterior segment choroidoretinitis, optic neuritis, and atrophy occur, the exact mechanism of these lesions being controversial (Rodger 1959).

Two other conditions of interest are *Erisipela de la Costa* and *Mal morado*.

Erisipela de la Costa

This manifestation of onchocerciasis is found in Guatemala and Mexico, usually in heavily infected persons under 20 years of age. It is characterized by an erythematous area, usually in the face or upper trunk.

Mal del morado

This is a purplish eruption affecting the head, neck, arms or pectoral regions, which may be papular or in plaques. It is again seen in heavily infected persons but in contrast to *Erisipela de la Costa* it occurs in the age groups over 40 years.

Diagnostic pathology

Microfilariae of *O. volvulus* are identified by examination of skin or conjunctival snips (see p. 759). They are most easily found in samples of skin taken from the region of the nodule. Alternatively, the skin snip is teased, immersed in saline, and the deposit examined after centrifugation (Buck, 1974). Excision of nodules for histological examination will reveal the adult worms, while aspiration of fluid from nodules will occasionally show microfilariae. Microfilariae may also be seen in the anterior chamber of the eye with an ophthalmoscope or slit lamp. Buck *et al.* (1972) found micro-filariae in the urine in as many as 31·4 per cent of infected persons. A moderate eosinophilia is usually present. Very occasionally microfilaraemia due to *O. volvulus* has been described (Fain *et al.* 1974).

Various serological tests have been used with variable success in the diagnosis of onchocerciasis—these include complement fixation; intra-dermal; precipitin (Biguet *et al.* 1964); immunofluorescence (Lucasse and Hoeppli, 1963); and a haemagglutination reaction (Rose *et al.* 1966).

STREPTOCERCIASIS

This infection (due to *Acanthocheilonema streptocerca*) has been reported from West Africa and the Congo. The most important vector in *Culicoides grahami*. The adults inhabit the subcutaneous tissues in the shoulder girdle region and the micro-filariae are most commonly found in the skin overlying that area, and in the skin of the chest, upper arms, and forearms (Kershaw *et al.* 1954).

The infection is generally considered to be harmless but it has been considered a factor in elephantiasis in the Congo and an itching reddish-brown papulo-vesicular eruption cured by Banocide has been reported in a European (Duke, 1957).

Diagnosis is made by finding the typical microfilariae (see p. 123) in skin snips. Serological and skin filarial tests may be positive.

Dirofilariasis

Various species of *Dirofilaria* have been reported from the Mediterranean basin, the Balkans, South America, Turkey, Africa, and the United States. They include *D. conjunctivae, D. repens, D. magalhaesi,* and *D. louisanensis.* Moorhouse *et al.* (1973) has described four human cases from Queensland, Australia, caused by the dog heartworm, *D. immitis.* The life cycle of these parasites in man is not fully known and it seems probable that mosquitoes or fleas are the natural intermediate hosts (Faust, 1957; Sams and Beck, 1959).

The adults do not develop normally in man. The immature worms cause painful transitory erythematous nodules which are most frequently seen in the upper arm and trunk (Welty *et al.* 1963). A granulomatous reaction with eosinophils is stimulated by the presence of the worm.

Adults have been detected in man in the digital artery, the eyelid, left ventricle, inferior vena cava, and in the subcutaneous tissues (De Carneri *et al.* 1973). They have been reported as causing infarcts of the lung (Harrison and Thompson, 1965); or may radiologically present as solitary 'coin' lesions (Beskin *et al.* 1966).

In sections of the lung the worm measures up to 190 μm in cross-section. The surface of the cuticle is cross-striated and consists of three layers lined by large muscle cells enclosing the gut and reproductive organs. Broad lateral cords are present. An associated infarctive lesion surrounded by eosinophils is usual. Neafie and Piggot (1971) have reported the findings in eight cases of pulmonary diro-filariasis. The microscopic appearances were uniform. A rounded focus of coagula-tion necrosis with a border of fibrous tissue and granulomatous inflammation is characteristic and usually contains segments of the worms. They can be identified as of the genus *Dirofilaria* because of their thick, multilayered cuticle, prominent transverse striations, internal longitudinal cuticular ridges and abundant somatic muscle. Broad lateral cords are characteristic of the mature well-preserved adult *D. immitis* found in dogs and they have also been described in the larval and adolescent stages. This feature was of little value in identifying the worms in this study. No sexually mature adult worms of *D. immitis* have yet been found in the lungs of man—nor have the microfilariae ever been demonstrated in man's peripheral blood. Dobson and Welch (1974) have described cases of eosinophilic meningitis due to *D. immities* which were diagnosed by immunofluorescence and Arthus hypersensitivity.

The dog heartworm has only recently been recognized as a cause of pulmonary coin lesions. In the differential diagnosis carcinoma, tuberculosis, fungal infections and hamartomas has to be considered.

Dipetalonema perstans

D. perstans has an extensive distribution throughout Africa, Tropical America, and the Caribbean. Marinkelle (1973) has recently described the first finding of *D. perstans* in Colombia. The adults have been reported in the liver, pleura, pericardium, mesentery, perirenal and retroperitoneal tissues. The microfilariae are nocturnally subperiodic and are unsheathed (Table 3.1). The intermediate vectors are *Culicoides austini* and *C. graham* in Africa. The detailed epidemiology has not been studied but it is known that many individuals in some African villages may harbour the parasite.

In the majority of individuals the infection apparently causes no ill effects. Janssens feels, however, that there may be certain persons in whom this infection does produce clinical illness (Janssens, 1964). A tropical eosinophilia-like syndrome has been reported (Gelfand and Bernberg, 1959), and Calabar swellings as well as generalized symptoms including neurological and psychic disturbances were attributed to this infection in twenty-seven of sixty-one white American missionaries affected (Adolph, *et al.* 1962), and in one patient by Gelfand and Wessels (1964). Upper abdominal pain has been associated with hepatomegaly and the presence of numerous microfilariae in the sinusoids of the liver (Garratt, 1945). The microfilariae, which are 100 μm × 4·5 μm, are found in the blood (see p. 123). A significant eosinophilia may be present (Wiseman, 1967). Acute encephalomyelitis with repeated demonstration of *P. perstans* microfilariae in the spinal fluid has been described (Dukes *et al.* 1968).

Mansonella ozzardi

This filarial worm is confined to the New World and is found in South America and in certain foci in the Carribbean. The adult worms are embedded in visceral adipose tissue. The vectors are *Culicoides* spp.

Adults have been identified in the mesentery and peritoneum. It has been reported to be a cause of moderate fever, inguinal adenitis, severe headache with dizziness and erythematous skin eruptions which may be accompanied by oedema and eosinophilia. A feeling of cold in the legs and arthralgia are almost always present in affected persons over the age of 16 years (Undiano, 1966).

Diagnosis is made by finding the unsheathed microfilariae in the peripheral blood (see p. 123). The size of the microfilaria is 170–240 μm long, while the adult male and female worms measure respectively 3·2 cm and 6·5–8 cm.

Protothecosis

A unique infection of the foot of an African by an acholuric alga *Prototheca segbwema* has been described in a number of papers by Davies and others (Davies and Wilkinson, 1967). The lesion on the foot resembled the 'mossy foot' of elephantiasis and organisms were detected in the enlarged femoral glands. It stains deeply in histological sections by the periodic acid schiff method and can be grown on Sabourand's glucose agar.

DRACONTIASIS

Synonym: Dracunculiasis.

The Guinea-worm—*Dracunculus medinensis*—has been known since ancient times. It occurs in local distributions in Africa, the Middle East, India, Pakistan, the Caribbean islands, Guyana, and Brazil.

Life cycle

The sexually mature female is up to 1 m long and 2 mm in diameter; the uterus, which occupies most of the body, contains millions of embryos. The male is small and its fate after copulation is not known.

When the gravid female is ready to discharge the larvae, the cephalic end of the worm approaches the skin, and secretes a substance which causes a blister to form. When the surface of the blister comes in contact with water, the anterior end of the vagina protrudes and the uterus expels the embryos into the water until the supply is exhausted. The female worm then shrivels and dies.

The larvae liberated in water must be taken up by suitable species of *Cyclops*, in which they develop into infective forms in about 3 weeks. Man becomes infected by drinking water containing infected *Cyclops*. These are digested by the gastric juices and the freed larvae penetrate the wall of the digestive tract and eventually migrate to the subcutaneous tissues. The female worm requires about 1 year before it is ready to discharge her embryos.

Epidemiology

Contamination of water with larvae from infected persons takes place when such persons draw drinking water from shallow ponds or wells. The water in these ponds, being stagnant with a high organic content, favours the presence of the vector species of *Cyclops*. In the dry season in some areas these ponds are much frequented since they often provide the only readily accessible source of water, thus creating a high cyclops/man contact ratio. In other places, transmission may occur during the rains when surface pools exist which disappear in the dry season. Infection can also be contracted when drinking water while bathing in contaminated pools or during ritual washing of the mouth in the performance of religious ablutions.

It has been suggested that gastric acidity may be responsible for resistance to infection in some exposed persons but this hypothesis has been repudiated (Gilles and Ball, 1964). Little is known about immunity to Guinea-worm infection.

Pathology

The incubation period is symptomless. Occasionally just prior to the blistering and extrusion of embryos generalized symptoms of an allergic nature may be complained of—or these may also occur during surgical removal of the worm.

The mature female is usually present in the connective tissues of the limbs and trunk. It most commonly presents on the surface of the body in the feet, ankles, and lower limbs, but may present on the trunk (especially the back in water carriers), arms, and rarely the head and neck. The female secretes a toxic substance which causes a local inflammatory lesion infiltrated with eosinophils, monocytes and polymorphonuclear leucocytes. A vesicle develops in the epidermis which ruptures on contact with water, and allows the embryos to escape. Secondary infection of this lesion with ulceration is common and a spreading cellulitis may occur involving subcutaneous and deeper tissues with consequent fibrosis and deformities.

The mature female, however, may never reach the surface of the body and may be absorbed without a marked reaction on the part of the host or calcification of the worm may occur and be detected on radiological examination (Reddy et al. 1968). Secondary infection once again, however, may occur and we have seen severe infections in joints especially the knee joint and a toxin liberated from the worm may be the cause in some instances. The aspirated fluid is usually brownish in colour and contains pus cells and fragments of the worm, and in the wall of the cavity a foreign-body giant cell reaction is usual. In some cases the aspirated fluid is sterile and at arthrotomy the entire adult worm is seen in the joint (Reddy and Sivaramappa, 1968). A coiled-up worm has also been seen in an abscess cavity in the pericardium, causing constrictive pericarditis (Kinare et al. 1962). An eosinophilia may occur in the early stages of infection prior to the liberation of the embryos or with damage to the parasite. Paraplegia as well as quadriplegia due to an extradural Guinea-worm abscess have been described (Reddy and Valli, 1967; Donaldson and Angelo, 1961), as well as scrotal, vesical, and renal lesions.

Diagnostic pathology

A microscopical diagnosis can be made by placing a few drops of water on the Guinea-worm blister. This stimulates the discharge of embryos which can be seen on examination of the water under a 16 mm objective. Calcified female Guinea-worms are often incidentally seen on radiological examination. An increase in γ-globulin has been reported (Jain and Gupta, 1966) and intradermal tests have been used (Ramsay, 1935).

CUTANEOUS LARVA MIGRANS (*'Creeping eruption'*)

This is caused by the invasion of the skin by larvae of various species of animal nematodes. The species most frequently involved are *A. caninum* and *A. braziliense*, found mainly in dogs and cats respectively; however, *Uncinaria stenocephala* of dogs, *Aceylanilum* of dogs and cats, *Bunostomum phlebotomum* of cattle, *Strongyloides* spp. of various animals, and man, and *Necator americanus* of man, have also been reported as causing creeping eruption.

The infection is usually acquired by contact with infected ground polluted by animal faeces and, less commonly, from clothing which has been spread out on the ground after laundering.

The skin lesion in creeping eruption typically involves the epidermis. At the site of penetration a small papule forms which later becomes vesicular. As the larva migrates it causes a linear erythematous reaction along its track, which progresses at a rate of 2–3 cm daily and is often serpiginous. The lesions progress faster and are relatively wide if *Strongyloides* species are responsible. The older parts of the lesion become crusted in 2 or 3 days and disappear in about 2 weeks. When large numbers invade the same limited area, the individual reactions become confluent, producing a central area of vesicular eruption with individual trails recognizable only at the margins. Secondary bacterial infection is common. Active migration may continue for weeks or months, associated with severe pruritus. There is evidence that some of the larvae producing the skin lesion later migrate to the lungs causing pulmonary infiltration. It is difficult to obtain larvae in skin biopsies, and when they are found in sectioned skin it is not possible to make a specific diagnosis because the microstructure in histological sections of only a few of the most common species has been described* (Beaver, 1964).

CAPILLARIASIS

Human intestinal capillariasis is a new helminthic disease caused by the nematode *Capillaria philippinensis*. It occurs in a limited area of Central Luzon adjacent to the South China Sea and, so far, has not been reported from other areas. There are over 200 nematodes of the genus *Capillaria* but only a few have been found in man and only *C. philippinensis* has caused an appreciable health problem (Watten *et al.* 1972). More than 1000 cases with over 100 deaths have been confirmed. Patients with intestinal capillariasis have abdominal pain, diarrhoea, muscle wasting, and oedema often leading to debility and death in two to four months. Clinical studies have shown the presence of a severe protein-losing enteropathy and malabsorption of fats and sugars. Effective treatment has consisted of fluid and electrolyte replacement and prolonged antihelminthic therapy with thiabendazole (Whalen *et al.* 1969). The

---

*Some of the parasitological techniques used for the laboratory diagnosis of the protozoal and helminthic diseases are described in the appendix. A plate showing the morphological appearances of helminth ova is also given.

nematode *C. philippinensis* (Blackwood *et al.* 1968) is clearly related to *T. trichiura* and *T. spiralis*.

The egg is 45 × 21 μm, has a peanut shape with bipolar but not protuberant plugs and a pitted shell. The mode of transmission is probably by the ingestion of three species of marine fish. An autoinfective cycle has been shown to occur in man (Cross *et. al.* 1972).

OESOPHAGOSTOMA

An abdominal abscess containing sterile cloudy fluid has been caused by a species of oesophagostoma in East Africa. The same parasite may cause colonic abscesses (Marshall and Deneka, 1969).

B. TREMATODES

The most widespread and important trematode infection is schistoso-miasis, and there are three main species of schistosome which infect man —*Schistosoma haematobium*, *S. mansoni*, and *S. japonicum*, all of which inhabit the blood. The other trematodes all gain entrance to man through the digestive tract and are conveniently divided into (*a*) *intestinal flukes* which cause fasciolopsiasis, heterophiasis, and metagonimiasis, (*b*) *liver flukes* resulting in clonorchiasis, opisthorchiasis, fascioliasis, and dicro-coeliasis, and (*c*) *lung flukes* which give rise to paragonomiasis in man.

SCHISTOSOMIASES

The above term implies the pathological conditions resulting from infection by blood-flukes of the genus *Schistosoma*, which are parasitic in man in various parts of the world. The three most important species which infect man are: *S. haematobium*, *S. mansoni*, and *S. japonicum*, and only the patho-logical effects of these infections will be described in detail. Other rarer parasites of man include *S. intercalatum* (Wright *et al.* 1972), *S. bovis*, *S. matthei*, *S. curassoni* (Payet *et al.* 1966), and possibly *S. capense*.

S. haematobium is widely distributed throughout tropical and subtropical Africa. It is also prevalent in the islands of the Indian Ocean, in Madagascar, and a small focus exists in a village outside Bombay. The disease is characterized by haematuria.

S. mansoni has a more focal distribution in tropical and subtropical Africa. It occurs in Israel and in the Yemen. It is also present over wide areas of Central and South America, the Caribbean islands, and Surinam where *S. haematobium* has not established itself. The disease is characterized by dysenteric symptoms and in severe cases by fibrosis of the liver with enlarge-ment of the spleen and ascites (Sormani, 1969). An *S. japonicum* Mekong strain was recently described from Khong Island (Sormani *et al.* 1973; Kitikoon *et al.* 1973). A species like *S. japonicum* has been described from Northern Thailand.

S. japonicum is confined to the Far East and is found extensively through-out the Yangtse basin. It is also present in Japan, Taiwan, the Philippine Islands, and parts of Burma and Thailand. Recently a case has been described from Malaysia (Murugasu and Dissanaike, 1973), and a report of the position in mainland China was given by Cheng (1971). The disease is characterized by visceral lesions with dysenteric symptoms, hepatic fibrosis, splenomegaly, and ascites.

The clinical and pathological manifestations of schistosomiasis are governed by the species of parasites, the intensity of infection, including the frequency and severity of exposures, and the immunological and perhaps the nutritional status of the individual. After a description of the life cycle, the epidemiology of the three species of schistosomes is reviewed and is followed by an account of the general pathological effects produced by these trematodes. The detailed pathology of the individual species of schistosomes is then described and the section ends with an account of diagnostic methods applicable to *S. haematobium*, *S. mansoni*, and *S. japonicum*.

Life cycle

The cycle of development of the three common species of schistosomes which infect man is as follows. The adult worms live in the portal vessels and in the inferior mesenteric veins. *S. haematobium* normally migrates when mated to the vesical plexus, the males carrying the females in their gynaecophoric canals; *S. mansoni*

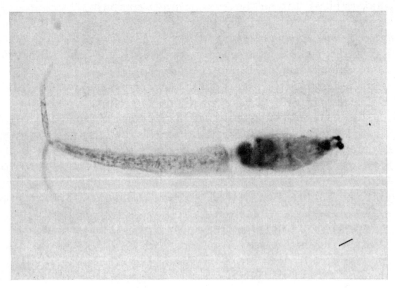

Fig. 3.10. Schistosome cercariae have a characteristic forked tail.

to the veins draining the wall of the large intestine, while *S. japonicum* invades the branches of the superior mesenteric veins draining the mesentery and small intestine, as well as the inferior mesenteric veins draining the large bowel, and in these sites the eggs are laid. Smith *et al.* (1969) have described the structure of the integument of *S. mansoni* by histochemical and electron microscopical studies.

The eggs pass through the tissues and enter respectively the bladder (*S. haematobium*), the large intestine (*S. mansoni*), and the small and large bowel (*S. japonicum*), and so are passed to the exterior in the urine and faeces. The eggs if deposited in fresh water give rise to miracidia which must penetrate a suitable snail host within 1 or 2 days. In the snail vigorous multiplication and cyclical development take place to form cercariae some 4 or more weeks after invasion. The fully developed cercaria emerges from the snail and enters the water. Man is infected while wading, bathing, or drinking water infected by the cercariae, which rapidly penetrate his intact skin or mucous membrane. The cercaria (Fig. 3.10) casts its forked tail in penetrating, becoming a schistosomule (young schistosome) and migrates by an indirect route possibly through the lungs and the diaphragm to the portal vein, where it becomes mature. The adult males are from about 10 mm to 15 mm long; the body is infolded ventrally to form the gynaecophoric canal in which the female is enclosed during copulation or after sexual maturity is reached. The females are about 14–26 mm long and darker in colour than the males (Fig. 3.11). *S. japonicum* takes 25–28 days from cercarial penetration to oviposition, *S. mansoni* about 30 days, and *S. haematobium* 10–12 weeks. Mating takes place in the portal vessels and the paired males, carrying the females in their gynaecophoric canals, migrate to the sites where eggs are laid. It is estimated that the female *S. japonicum* lays 50–300 ova daily, the female *S. mansoni* 1–4 ova daily, while the *S. haematobium* female lays 20–30 ova daily.

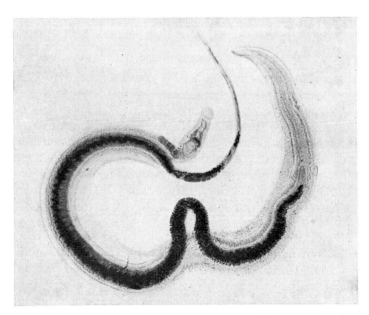

FIG. 3.11. Adult male and female schistosome worms in copula.

Adult schistosomes may survive and continue to pass eggs 20–30 years after initial infection; this extreme longevity is noteworthy. The eggs of *S. haematobium* are characterized by their terminal spines; the eggs of *S. mansoni* have lateral spines; while those of *S. japonicum* have a rudimentary knob-like lateral spine (see p. 761).

Many attempts have been made to induce growth in young schistosomes (schistosomulae) as well as to maintain adult schistosomes in the laboratory, in order to study the metabolic requirements of these flukes. Our knowledge, however, remains rudimentary and conclusions have been conflicting. Thus, some workers have suggested that protein and other non-dializable components of serum are of little significance in the survival of the worms and that they are capable of an anaerobic existence; while others have succeeded in maintaining schistosomes in a medium containing twenty-six amino acids, a series of enzymes, co-enzymes, nucleic-acid derivatives, vitamins, glucose, and glutamates in a balanced salt solution. Degradation of glucose supplies a large part of the energy of schistosomes and they can utilize five times their weight of sugar in 24 hours, some of it being stored as glycogen, some giving rise to lactic acid and a part being transaminated. Schistosomes seem to prefer basic amino acids and basic sugars. They can also digest globin from which individual amino acids and peptides are released (Ross and Bueding, 1950; Cheever and Weller, 1958).

Schistosomes excrete a pigment which is brown-yellowish in colour, and occurs as small granules or clumps mainly within the cytoplasm of the cells of the reticulo-endothelial system of the host. It is probably a complex porphyrin compound made up of a haemoglobin derivative (haematin) coupled with a nitrogenous moiety. It is the residue of metabolism of the hosts red blood cells by the adult worms and is evidence of their presence. The pigment can be differentiated from malarial pigment both electronmicroscopically and chemically (Moore *et al.* 1975; Homewood and Moore, 1975). Ultrastructure studies have revealed interesting properties of the schistosome integument (Smith *et al.* 1969; Silk *et al.* 1969).

Epidemiology

The epidemiology of schistosomiasis is characterized by a complexity seldom paralleled by that of other infectious diseases. Eight major factors are involved, namely: (1) man's insanitary habits; (2) man's association with water; (3) the relative efficiency of the molluscan intermediate host; (4) animal reservoirs of schistosomes; (5) diet; (6) age of the human host; (7) intensity of infection; and (8) immunity. Since these factors are extremely variable there is no constant pattern of transmission and the epidemiology may, and often does, vary from locality to locality (Olivier and Ansari, 1967; Gilles *et al.* 1973).

Man's insanitary habits

The habits and customs of the population play a large role in the maintenance of the disease, thus indiscriminate defaecation and urination constitute the basic elements. Other factors such as population density and certain religious practices (ablutions) also help to promote the spread of infection.

Man's association with water

The transmission of schistosomiasis is strongly influenced by water-use practices. Many schemes for the development and conservation of water resources have been put into use in recent years, and there is every indication that in the tropical and subtropical countries such schemes will continue to increase. They result in more intensive farming, greater human contact with surface water, and an increase in water-borne diseases. Moreover, the network of canals designed to carry water to reclaimed land creates ideal habitats for vector snails capable of transmitting schistosomiasis. All these factors facilitate the completion of the schistosome life cycle.

Intermediate snail hosts

S. *haematobium* is transmitted by snails of the genus *Bulinus; S. mansoni* by snails of the genus *Biomphalaria, Australorbis* and *Tropicorbis*; and S. *japonicum* by snails of the genus *Oncomelania, Katayama* and *Schistosomophora*, which are amphibious. Several factors play a part in supporting snail colonies of the various genera. Among the most important are, the temperature, salinity and velocity of the water, and the presence of aquatic vegetation. Marked seasonal fluctuations in numbers of snails have been recorded, and, in general, workers have noted a drop in snail density during the main rainy periods followed by an upsurge in numbers and the production of large numbers of young snails during the drier, warmer months which immediately follow (Webbe, 1965). Work has been done in various parts of the world on the relative susceptibilities of these molluscan intermediate hosts to schistosome infections under carefully standardized conditions, as well as the effects of infection upon the snails. It has been demonstrated that susceptibility of the snails to infection with S. *mansoni* varies a great deal and that such differences in susceptibility may be regulated genetically. Similarly the larval stages of S. *mansoni* have been shown to develop without any tissue reaction in highly susceptible snails, whereas in partially resistant snails they are destroyed by phagocytic action. These studies are providing a better understanding of snail/parasite relationships and the opportunity of estimating transmission potential.

Animal reservoirs of schistosomes

The evidence to date supports the suggestion that man is the only true host of S. *haematobium* and that the few records of the parasite from animals represent incidental infections.

It is probable that baboons are capable of maintaining and transmitting S. *mansoni*, but no evidence has yet been found that S. *mansoni* infection was being maintained in a baboon community in the absence of infection contracted from man.

Although rodents can maintain the animal schistosome *S. rhodaini* in isolated foci in Africa, they seem to be of no importance as reservoirs of human schistosomes.

In contrast *S. japonicum* has a great number of mammals, chiefly domestic, as its normal hosts and these play an important role in the dissemination of the disease. In order of epidemiological importance these are the dog, the cow, the cow, the rat, the pig, the water-buffalo, and the goat—nevertheless 75 per cent of transmission results from man. A Taiwan strain of *S. japonicum* has been described which is purely zoophilic and does not develop in man.

Diet

The role of nutrition in human host/schistosome relations is undoubtedly complex. It is possible, however, that the wide range of symptomatology seen in different parts of the world may be due in part to variation in the diet of the people (de Witt *et al.* 1964). Thus it has been shown that in nutritionally deficient mice *S. mansoni* cercariae are able to penetrate and migrate, but the development of the worms to adulthood is retarded. Similarly, although the rate of infection is higher in animals maintained on a diet deficient in certain amino acids and vitamins, the stunted worms only rarely reach sexual maturity. Finally, it has been found that the therapeutic activity of antimonials against *S. mansoni* in mice may be increased up to sixteen times by modifying the diet of the host.

Studies in Puerto Rico have yielded evidence that improvement of the diets of humans infected with *S. mansoni* may have marked beneficial effects on the outcome of therapy. Similarly from Africa it has been shown that a difference in dietary habits can influence the outcome of antimony treatment (Bell, 1964). Identification of the factor or factors responsible could be of considerable practical importance in the epidemiology of the disease.

Age of the human host

It has been shown in many surveys from different parts of the world that in endemic areas the heaviest worm burdens and largest number of eggs occur in the second decade of life of the local population. During the third and subsequent decades the load of infection drops significantly and the incidence of the disease in endemic areas diminishes. The precise reasons for this are not clear but may be related to diminished exposure to infection, diminished intensity of infection, and the development of immunity. Immigrants to an endemic area are susceptible at any age and exhibit a marked sensitivity to their initial infection.

Intensity of infection

By using egg-counting techniques it has been shown that in the age groups showing the highest prevalence of *S. haematobium* and *S. mansoni* infection, the egg loads in the urine and faeces respectively are also the highest. Thus the median egg load in a group of persons provides for epidemiological studies an additional parameter to that of the prevalence of infection (Jordan, 1966; Bradley, 1965). It has been suggested that there are 3 phases in an age—cohort's experience of endemic infection: acquisition and increase of infection, a phase of decreasing worm load combined with concomitant immunity, and a steady state phase, with loss of immunity and reinfection balancing, in later life (McCullough and Bradley, 1973; Bradley and McCullough, 1973). Jordan *et al.* (1974) have questioned whether these authors' data provide additional evidence for the occurrence of concomitant immunity.

A close correlation has been shown to exist between intensity of infection and the pathogenicity of the disease (Edington *et al.* 1970). A direct relationship has recently been demonstrated between intensity of infection and lesions of the urinary tract in *S. haematobium* infections (Forsyth and Macdonald, 1965a, b; Lucas *et al.* 1966). It also appears that a lower prevalence of hydronephrosis occurs in girls than in boys. Comparative studies of egg load in livers at autopsy are now being carried out in *S. mansoni* infections in Africa and South America and the results may prove very revealing. Recently a mathematical model for the study of the epidemiology of schistosome infections has been described (Macdonald, 1965). Among the factors involved in the dynamics of infection are: multiplication of the parasites, the rate of contamination of water, the degree of exposure of human beings to the water, the snail density, and the longevity of the worm (Nasell and Hirsch, 1973).

Immunity

There is evidence of the development in man of some degree of resistance against reinfection but there is as yet no demonstrable relationship between the antibodies detectable by present serological methods and such resistance. Clarke (1966) has shown that the Africans in Rhodesia have a higher degree of both natural and acquired resistance than the Europeans; that resistance to *S. haematobium* does not protect against *S. mansoni* infection, and that the degree of resistance to both parasites is dependent on the nature and extent of exposure to infection.

For several years investigations have been proceeding to gain some understanding on the nature of the stimulus responsible for inducing resistance in schistosomiasis and the stage of the life cycle which is mainly responsible for stimulating the immune mechanism. Most of the studies on immunity in schistosomiasis have been carried out in animals infected with *S. mansoni* and extreme caution is needed before the many interesting results obtained can be applied to man, especially as immunological differences are known to occur between the various experimental animals (Smithers, 1962; Lichtenberg, 1967). Reagin-like antibodies have been demonstrated in monkeys infected with *S. mansoni* and *S. japonicum* (Ogilvie, 1964; Hsu *et al.* 1966); but their role in the development of immunity has not been determined. Smithers and Terry (1967) have demonstrated that powerful resistance may be induced by adult Schistosome worms. It is postulated that there is a host-like antigen in the worm's integument which acts as a disguise protecting the worm against the host's normal immune response (Clegg *et al.* 1970; 1971*a* and *b*).

The immuno pathogenesis of schistosomiasis was critically reviewed by Warren (1972). In this stimulating paper he describes a chain of events which traverses the realms of pathophysiology, immunology and molecular biology.

It has been suggested that constant exposure of man to cercariae from animal schistosomes may result in partial immunization of the human host to *S. haematobium* and *S. mansoni* infections. Nelson and his colleagues in a series of meticulous studies have developed the whole theme of heterologous immunity in schistosomiasis (Massoud and Nelson, 1973).

The pathogenesis of schistosomiasis

The pathological changes vary according to the species but are best generally described in Table 3.4, compiled by a WHO Scientific Group on Research in Bilharziasis (1967).

The stages of invasion and maturation

This is common to all the species of schistosomes. The severity of the clinical manifestations is greatest in *S. japonicum* infection and least in *S. haematobium*, with *S. mansoni* occupying an intermediate position. The severity of the symptoms varies markedly in this stage from individual to individual and is considered to be related more to the degree of sensitization of the patient than to the intensity of the infection. The more severe clinical manifestations are related to oviposition and to the metabolic processes of the live miracidium. A reaction to the immature worm also occurs (Areán, 1966).

The patient may exhibit a localized itching erythematous or papular rash at the site of entry of the cercariae (cercarial dermatitis or swimmers' itch). This would appear to be unusual in *S. japonicum* infection (Billings *et al.*

TABLE 3.4. *A classification of the course of bilharziasis—based on parasitological, clinical, and pathological aspects*

Stage	Parasitological	Clinical	Pathological
1. Stage of invasion	A. Penetration B. Migration	Cercarial skin reaction if present Fever, cough if present Katayama syndrome	Papular dermatitis Inflammatory reactions in lungs and liver
2. Stage of maturation	Completion of maturation and early oviposition with migration to definitive sites	Acute febrile illness, not always recognized or present	Hyperergic reactions, generalized and local, to products of eggs and/or young schistosome
3. Stage of established infection	Intensive oviposition accompanied by a corresponding egg excretion	Stage of early chronic disease, characterized for instance by haematuria, or intestinal and other digestive manifestations	Local inflammatory reactions to ova resulting mainly in granuloma formation. Fibrosis is not a predominant feature
4. Stage of late infection	Prolonged infection (often with reduced or discontinued egg extrusion)	Stage of chronic disease, e.g. cor pulmonale, fistula obstructive uropathy, renal failure, and portal hypertension	Progressive formation varying with intensity of infection and possibly other factors, of fibrous tissue, with its consequences and sequelae according to the organs involved

1946). Mild bronchitic symptoms, pyrexia, and eosinophilia are usual and may mimic tropical eosinophilia, but are evanescent in character. In more severe cases there may be chills, headache, and generalized lymphadenopathy with enlargement of the spleen and liver. Urticarial skin rashes with oedema of the face and eyelids and even angioneurotic oedema may occur. In a few patients with *S. japonicum* infection signs of severe central nervous system involvement with a normal cerebrospinal fluid have been recorded

(Carrol, 1946). Following these initial symptoms ova usually appear in the stools in the case of *S. japonicum* and *S. mansoni* infections in a few days but a longer period, usually 3 months, may elapse before they are detected in the urine in *S. haematobium* infections. An outbreak of Katayama syndrome —fever, eosinophilia and other symptoms— associated with *S. haematobium* has been described from Rhodesia (Clarke *et al.* 1970) and various clinical types of early infection are associated with *S. mansoni* in Brazil (Neves, 1970).

The manifestations of both these stages are rarely recognized in children in holoendemic areas. The immediate diagnosis is difficult, as the complement-fixation test is usually negative and the intradermal reaction to cercarial antigen always negative in these stages.

The stages of established infection and late effects

The severity and types of lesions are dependent on the factors previously mentioned, the most important being the species of schistosome and intensity of infection. Irrespective of the species, however, the pathological changes depend upon the host's local reaction to the presence of ova in the tissues. The characteristic morphology of the various ova should be demonstrable in tissue sections, and ova of *S. mansoni* contain an alcohol/ acid-fast substance in the capsule and miracidium which can be demonstrated by Ziehl–Neilsen's method of staining which helps to differentiate them from the ova of *S. haematobium*. Muller and Taylor (1972) stated that egg shells of *S. mansoni*, *S. intercalatum*, *S. rhodaini* and *S. mansoni/S. rhodaini* hybrid in sections of tissues of laboratory hosts were Ziehl–Neilsen positive whereas those of *S. haematobium*, *S. matthei* and *S. bovis* were negative. In most instances living ova may pass through the tissues with little cellular reaction, the clinical effects being consequently mild. In other instances, however, the ova are retained in various sites and a varying inflammatory reaction occurs. The tissues become congested and oedematous and around the ovum (more frequently in *S. japonicum* infection) a rim of fibrinoid material may be seen (Hoeppli, 1932) which is thought to represent antigen–antibody complexes. It occurs most frequently in young patients with heavy infection of recent origin and is seen around intact eggs containing mature miracidia (Lichtenberg *et al.* 1966). The predominantly inner antigenic zone of the material deposited around the ovum contains diastase-resistant, PAS-positive, acid-fast, autofluorescent material identical to the eggshell substance and high concentrations of sulphydryl-disulphide-rich protein also abundant in the miracidial cephalic glands. Other components of the inner zone are also traceable to the eggshell and the cephalic glands. The outer zone, previously noted to contain high concentrations of antibody, was observed to abound in tryptophan-rich protein. Integrating these facts with the biology of the schistosome egg, it was concluded that at maturation, the miracidial cephalic glands produce an antigenic, cystine- and cysteine-rich protein which leaks through the eggshell (and possibly catalyses eggshell lysis), evokes an immune response in the host, and preci- pitates with a tryptophan-rich host globulin to produce the Hoeppli pheno- mena. Thus, the formation of the Hoeppli phenomenon is contingent upon a high degree of host sensitization (Smith and Lichtenberg, 1967). Usually surrounding the ovum there is necrosis and infiltration of epithelioid cells, plasma cells, and lymphocytes, with eosinophils present in varying propor tions—the most severe reaction being an eosinophilic abscess. Charcot– Leyden crystals may be present. With the death of the ovum within 3 weeks foreign-body giant cells appear. The epithelioid cells increase in number and reparative fibrosis occurs. These lesions are usually referred to as pseudo- tubercles. Macroscopically, in the early stages they appear as yellow grains surrounded by a hyperaemic zone, and later with healing they become white. Eventually the egg remnants may disappear or become calcified and dense collagen is formed. The mechanisms governing the extent of the fibrosis and calcification are, however, ill understood as they vary widely from patient to patient, but would appear to some extent to be related to intensity of infection. Many of the irreversible lesions are due to the mech- anical effects of these fibrotic lesions—stenosis of the portal vein, ureters, pulmonary arteries, etc. Recent post-mortem studies have shown that the extra vesical pathological lesions are directly related to the intensity of infection as shown by the ova load per gram of bladder tissue demonstrated by the digest method (p. 766) (Edington et al. 1970). This most probably accounts for the differing estimates of the morbidity and mortality caused by the infection in various parts of Africa. Although in this study the frequency of schistosomiasis was 20 per cent and hydroureter and hydronephrosis were relatively common complications, the mortality was negligible. It was of interest to note that 30–40 per cent of males were infected at the age of 50 years, although the number of eggs in the bladder were less than those noted in the 20–39-year-old age group.

The pathology of S. haematobium infection

As S. haematobium mainly affects the urinary tract, in contrast to S. japonicum and S. mansoni which involve the intestine, it will be discussed separately.

The stage of established infection and oviposition is characterized by fever, headache, muscular pains, anorexia, dysuria, and terminal haema- turia, the presence and severity of these symptoms depending upon the intensity of infection, which can be assessed by the numbers of ova in the urine. An initial eosinophilia is usual, with a rise in serum α_2 and γ-globulin. It should be noted that rectal snips yield eggs in 70 per cent of these patients.

The liver and spleen are not usually palpable unless one is working in an area of stable malaria. An anaemia of normocytic orthochromic type is usual. Pyelography and micturating cystography may be normal but ureteric reflux and filling defects in the bladder have been described in high incidence in children living in holoendemic areas of schistosomiasis in East and West Africa. The ultimate prognosis in these children has still to be assessed. Calcification of the bladder may be seen at a relatively early stage of infection and it is outlined by linear, lamellated, wavy calcifications (Makar, 1957).

The later changes of *S. haematobium* infection are described when the pathology of the individual organs is considered below.

The bladder

Many lesions occur in the bladder and these can be described as acute, polypoid, fibrous plaques and 'ground glass' lesions, sandy patches, ulceration, stricture, leukoplakia and cystitis glandularis, fibrosis and calcification of the bladder wall and bladder neck obstruction. As the bladder may appear normal macroscopically even in fairly severe infections, at post mortem mucosal snips should be taken and press preparations examined microscopically if *S. haematobium* infection is suspected.

In the acute stage the bladder may only be hyperaemic, with or without petechial haemorrhages. Ova retained in the epithelium or in the vesical

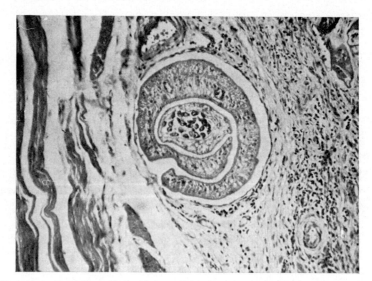

FIG. 3.12. *S. haematobium*. Male and female adult schistosomes in a vein in submucosa of the bladder (H and E × 130).

tissues, most usually in the subepithelial layer, cause the formation of the pseudotubercles already described and the bladder may be studded by these small, yellow seed-like bodies surrounded by a zone of hyperaemia, later resembling white sago grains. They are most frequently present in the area of the trigone, with the base and lateral walls next most commonly affected. Adult schistosomes are frequently present in the neighbouring vesical veins (Fig. 3.12). Nodular or polypoid lesions may be formed by coalescence of the tubercles, hyperplasia of the mucosa, and early fibrosis and hypertrophy of muscle. In the early stages these are hyperaemic and mulberry like. These active proliferating papillomatous or granulomatous lesions are responsible for the bladder-filling defects seen radiologically in the early stages. Later the ova become calcified, atrophy of the mucosa with underlying fibrosis of

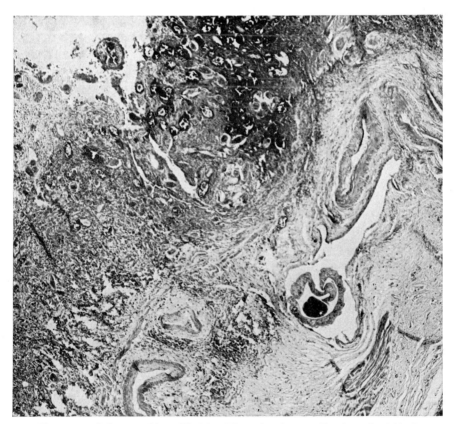

FIG. 3.13. *S. haematobium*. Bladder. There is a large collection of calcified ova in the submucosa of the bladder with a marked infiltrate of chronic inflammatory cells. Sections of adult male and female schistosomes can be seen in a vein. There is marked fibrosis of the bladder wall (H and E × 100).

the connective tissue occurs and the lesions shrink and are represented by
white fibrous plaques on the mucosal surface (Fig. 3.13). With less severe
proliferation the bladder mucosa may eventually present a flat, ground-glass
appearance due to widespread atrophy of the epithelium with underlying
fibrosis. In addition to the mulberry-like multiple granulomatous polyps
described, a fibro-calcific type also commonly occurs. This is a small,
usually solitary, lesion with the raised surface resembling macroscopically
the sandy patch. The central core of dense fibrous tissue contains dilated
capillaries and calcified ova. The epithelium is denuded. A third type of
polyp (the villous) is less common and has thickened club-shaped fronds
covered with hyperplastic epithelium. These polyps rarely resemble the
classical polyp with its delicate fronds covered by transitional epithelium.

The most common lesion however in vesical schistosomiasis is the so-
called 'sandy patch'. This is a late lesion and is most often seen in the trigone
area in which the mucosa is roughened, raised and greyish-golden-brown in
colour. The overlying epithelium may be irregularly thickened or atrophic
and areas of squamous metaplasia have been described. In the submucosa
and muscularis, pseudotubercles and foreign-body granulomas may be seen
surrounding ova in various stages of disintegration or calcification, but the
predominant feature is fibrosis, with calcified ova scattered in variable
numbers in the dense collagenous tissue. In many instances the cellular
reaction has disappeared or scanty lymphocytes and plasma cells may be
present. In other instances there may be a fairly heavy lymphocytic
infiltration, and the presence of lymph follicles has been described.

The epithelium of the bladder may undergo a number of changes, varying
from marked hyperplasia to atrophy. Foci of leukoplakia may be present.
At the edges of nodules or polyps the mucous membrane is folded, forming
shallow pits or pseudoglands, the lumina of which may become occluded by
hypertrophy of the epithelium, with the formation of broad epithelial pegs
which may become detached from the surface, giving the appearance of
isolated islets of epithelium in the submucosa—the so-called Brunn's nests.
These down-growths may become vesicular and lined by tall columnar
epithelium (cystitis glandularis) and in the presence of a lymphocytic
infiltration, may resemble cystitis cystica. It should be noted that cystitis
cystica and glandularis are non-specific pathological findings and are seen
in chronic bladder infections with obstruction or stone formation. The
aetiology of these changes are ill-understood (Parker, 1970). Squamous
metaplasia may occur in these lesions.

Intractable ulceration of the mucosa and bladder wall has been described
but would appear to vary in different endemic areas, being common in
Egypt and uncommon in Rhodesia and West Africa. Bacterial infection may
spread rapidly to the ureters, kidneys, peritoneum and periurethral regions,

and between the bladder and bowel, with consequent multiple abscesses, septicaemia, and death. The urethra may be directly involved, with consequent stricture formation, and an elephantoid condition of the penis has been described.

It has been postulated that there is an increased incidence of urinary bacterial infection in vesical schistosomiasis and that the incidence of S. typhi urinary carrier rate is high (Weir et al. 1952). In Egypt, schistosomiasis does seem to predispose to a high S. typhi urinary carrier rate (Hathout, 1966), but in Nigeria this has not been found to be the case (Pi-Sunyer et al. 1965). From a consideration of the pathology, however, it would seem reasonable to accept that a severely affected bladder would have less resistance to infection if once established, and every precaution should be taken to eliminate the risk of infection if instrumentation has to be resorted to.

It must be emphasized that in vesical schistosomiasis all types of lesions may be seen in one bladder and all areas in the bladder wall may be affected. In the most severe cases the whole thickness of the bladder wall may undergo fibrosis and calcification—in others focal muscular hypertrophy and diverticula may be found. With fibrosis of the bladder, the trigone and bladder neck are pulled forward anteriorly with consequent bladder-neck obstruction, a late complication which is seen frequently in Egypt, with all the consequent effects of urinary retention, including multiple sinuses in the scrotum and perineum. Atala et al. (1969) have undertaken a detailed study of bladder-neck obstruction in Egypt and concluded that in many cases the fibrotic obstruction occurred in the posterior urethra and that urethroscopy was the most satisfactory method of definitive diagnosis.

The ureters

The lower thirds of the ureters are frequently bilaterally affected, as they have a common blood supply with the bladder. In addition there may be secondary changes in the ureters induced by the bladder lesions. In the acute stages in up to 20 per cent of children in endemic areas uretero-vesical incompetence with reflux, and in a lesser proportion hydronephrosis, can be demonstrated. It is probable that these changes are due to oedema and congestion, perhaps with pseudotubercle formation in the region of the vesical portion of the ureter, with consequent distortion. Pseudotubercles with all the consequential changes described in the bladder may occur in the ureteric wall. Mucoid degeneration of Brunn's nests may occur just as in the bladder, with the formation of ureteritis glandularis, including polypi and ureteritis cystica. Stricture and/or dilatation of the ureter eventually result. Fibrosis of the bladder may also result in stenosis of the ureteric orifices. It has been stated that in 70 per cent of patients the ureters are affected. Linear calcification in the uretral wall may occur, usually at the lower end, and is said to be pathognomonic. On the other hand, punctate spots of calcification may be seen (uretritis calcinosa), the calcification arising in the contents of uretritis cystica. Occasionally also calcification may arise in a polyp (Maged and Soliman, 1968). From any of the above-mentioned lesions obstructive hydroureter with tortuosity and hydronephrosis leading to impaired renal function with renal failure may occur. Obstructive renal failure is an entity and even anuria can occur (Dukes and Mynors, 1970; Ghoneim et al. 1971). If infection occurs, pyonephrosis and acute pyelonephritis are common complications. Owing to the anatomical configuration of the urinary tract these lesions are more common in males. Although it has been stated that neoplasm of the ureter and renal pelvis may result from these lesions this has not been our experience.

The kidney

Lesions directly due to the parasite are not commonly seen in the kidney, but occasionally ova are found in the renal parenchyma or in the submucous tissue of the calyces and renal pelvis. Interstitial nephritis has been described in a few patients. Rarely, adult worms may enter the interlobular veins and after their death cause an acute eosinophilic necrotizing lesion (Areán, 1966). Calcification of the renal capsule has been reported in one case. Ova were noted histologically. The renal parenchyma was not affected (Atala and Zaher, 1969).

Hydronephrosis, pyonephrosis, and acute pyelonephritis due to vesical and ureteric lesions are, however, not uncommon and may cause death (Edington, 1957). The occurrence of chronic pyelonephritis is, however, more controversial and the part that S. haematobium plays in the aetiology of hypertension in endemic areas has still to be assessed, although preliminary surveys would suggest that it is not great. Ezzat et al. (1974) have reported an association between S. haematobium infection and heavy proteinuria. Calculi have been described in the urethra, bladder, ureter, and kidney. The relationship between S. haematobium infection and urinary calculi is discussed on p. 636.

Granulomatous lesions may rarely occur in the urethral wall, leading to strictures in the bulbous portion. Lymphoedema of the penis and scrotum has been reported, and Zaher and El Deef (1969) have described urethritis cystica of the posterior portion of the urethra in Egypt.

The reproductive organs

The frequency and severity of the lesions in the reproductive organs will depend upon the intensity of infection. In males the prostate and seminal vesicles will be affected in all severe infections if digest studies are undertaken. All types of lesions occur but in general in our experience they are mild. Ova may be seen in the seminal fluid. The importance of schistosomiasis as an aetiological agent in prostatitis is still undecided. It may be important in severe infections, and Khafagy and Khalil (1970) have demonstrated the presence of local bilharzial antibodies in the prostatic fluid of 12 of 15 patients suffering from active urinary schistosomiasis and chronic prostatitis.

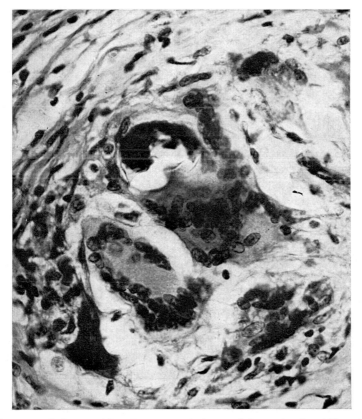

FIG. 3.14. *S. haematobium*. Pronounced giant-cell formation in a bilharzial tubercle (seminal vesicle, H and E × 375).

Although the seminal vesicles are frequently and heavily infected severe lesions are unusual in our experience and are usually inactive with fibrosis and mild lymphocytic infiltration present. These findings are in keeping with those reported by previous authors and recently reviewed by Gelfand *et al.* (1970). Although calcification of the seminal vesicles and ova in the seminal fluid have been reported clinically, it is felt that only in very rare cases is *S. haematobium* infection likely to produce lesions leading to infertility. A few ova will be detected on digest in the testes and epididymus. Very rarely granulomatous lesions may be seen in the testes. Ova have been reported in hydrocele fluid.

In the female in severe infections ova will be noted in digest studies as follows: cervix (100 per cent); vagina (100 per cent); uterus (66 per cent); ovaries (30 per cent); and Fallopian tubes (30 per cent) (Edington *et al.* 1972). Lesions are most frequently seen histologically in the cervix and vagina and very much less frequently in the uterus, ovaries or Fallopian tubes. With regard to the cervix, it is seldom markedly affected but induration, erosions, granulomata, nodules and polypoid lesions may occur— or the infection may be an incidental finding (Boulle and Notelovitz, 1964; Williams, 1967). Contact bleeding may occur and carcinoma may be suspected clinically. Cellular atypia and ova have been noted in cervical smears in South Africa but the condition was not considered precancerous (Berry, 1966). Youssef *et al.* (1970) however found in Egypt that of 121 patients with schistomiasis of the cervix 15 or 16 have an associated invasive squamous cell carcinoma which was highly differentiated. In our experience carcinoma of the cervix is usually poorly differentiated. Whilst therefore we would agree with the South African workers that the presence of ova in carcinoma of the cervix may merely be an incidental finding, it should be remembered that in areas of intense infection the findings may differ and caution should be shown in interpreting histological findings in the absence of controlled studies or of a knowledge of the intensity of infection. In addition ova have been noted incidentally in association with choriocarcinoma, cystadenocarcinoma and a cystic teratoma of the ovary (Paradinas, 1971) and tuberculous endometritis.

Although the vagina is frequently infected the lesions are usually inert.

In the Fallopian tubes the ova are found in the wall, the mucosa being relatively undamaged, and although salpingitis, salpingo-oöphoritis and ectopic tubal pregnancy have been described in haematobium infection (El Bedri, 1958) it is not considered a common cause of infertility in females. Lesions are rarely seen in the body of the uterus although ova have been reported in endometrial curettings.

The gastro-intestinal tract

Rectal involvement occurs in approximately 70 per cent of infections (Fig. 3.15) and the remainder of the large intestine and appendix are not infrequently affected. The infection is usually of light intensity but rectal snips followed by compression preparations usually reveal the presence of ova. Gross lesions are rare but granular areas in the mucosa resembling

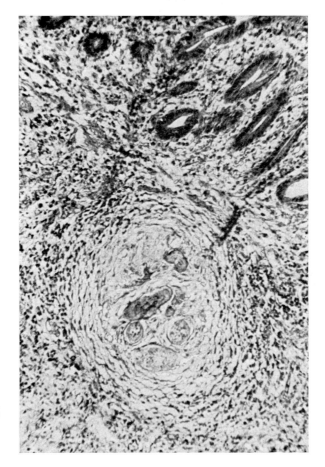

FIG. 3.15. *S. haematobium*. A schistosome tubercle in the submucosa of the
rectum (H and E × 150).

sandy patches are common. Acute intestinal obstruction following intussusception due to granulomatous lesions in the large intestine have been
described (Gelfand and Hammalr, 1966) and polypoid lesions may occur.

The appendix is infected and bilharzial appendicitis is probably an
entity. In endemic areas routine necropsy examination of appendices has
revealed a lower incidence of infection than that found in surgical appendicectomy specimens, the incidence in our material being 3 and 7 per cent
respectively. Asymptomatic infection of the appendix is therefore not uncommon and the possibility of schistosomal lesions in surgically removed

appendices being merely coincidental must be entertained (Edington *et al.* 1974).

The presence of ova with pseudotubercle formation or scarring has been noted in the stomach, small intestine, peritoneum, mesentery, and pancreas, but these lesions are not common.

The liver

The liver is much more severely affected in *S. japonicum* and *S. mansoni* infections. In *S. haematobium* infection, however, lesions are usually present in the liver and are represented by pseudotubercles in the parenchyma adjacent to the portal tracts. Small focal scars result. The lobular architecture is not disturbed and, although piece-meal parenchymal necrosis has been described, this is not so in our experience and it is considered that *S. haematobium* infection is unlikely to be an aetiological agent in the production of cirrhosis (Edington 1967). Schistosomal pigment may be present in the Kupffer cells or portal tracts of the liver. The death of adult worms in the portal veins has been considered a cause of pyelophlebitis. This, once again, we have never seen. In surveys in endemic areas liver function tests have been shown to be essentially within normal limits. Eggs may be seen on liver biopsy. Bilharzial cholecystitis with the formation of calculi in the biliary tract has been reported in one patient from South Africa (Botha, 1963).

The lung

There is no doubt that in *S. haematobium* infection pseudotubercles are frequently seen in the lung, usually at the periphery and adjacent to the pulmonary arterioles. Necrotizing lesions of the arterioles with healing may cause an obliterative endarteritis (Damluja *et al.* 1964). This obstruction to the vascular bed causes raised pulmonary arterial pressure, with hypertrophy and eventual failure of the right ventricle. This type of cor pulmonale can occur in haematobium infection but its exact incidence is debatable and this subject is dealt with more fully when *japonicum* and *mansoni* infections are discussed. It is of interest that in spite of the high incidence of schistosomiasis in Egypt, in 5314 hospital admissions in Cairo due to respiratory disease only 90 were considered to be due to parasitic infection ($1 \cdot 7$ per cent). Twenty-nine were due to amoebiasis and only 24 to pulmonary schistosomiasis (Abdel-Hakim, 1965). Localized broncho-pulmonary lesions consisting of numerous schistosomal tubercles in varying stages of fibrosis and simulating a neoplasm are rare, and it has been thought that these lesions may be caused by the presence of adult worms in the pulmonary arterial tree (Abdel-Hakim and Elwi, 1963). A granulomatous lesion in the larynx has also been reported.

The reticulo-endothelial system and blood-forming organs

In the early stages an eosinophilia is usual and following repeated small haemorrhages a normocytic orthochromic anaemia occurs. Schistosomal pigment may be found in the Kupffer cells of the liver and sinusoidal lining cells and histiocytes in the spleen. It is evidence of the presence of living adult worms and is present in greater amounts in *japonicum* and *mansoni* infections. Lesions in the spleen are not common in haematobium infections and the splenomegaly and hypersplenism syndromes described in the other two infections are rare. Isolated pseudotubercles may occasionally be observed.

Other organs

There is literally no organ in the body exempt from possible lesions. Granulomatous and warty vegetating lesions containing eggs occur in the skin and occasionally associated malignant change has been noted (El-Zawahry, 1965). Although changes in the central nervous system occur most frequently in *japonicum* infections they also occur in *haematobium*. Bird (1965); Odeku *et al.* (1968) and Sennara (1969) have described the cerebral and spinal granulomatous lesions which can occur in *S. haematobium* infections. Cerebral- and spinal-granulomatous lesions occur and an acute transverse myelitis has been described, in which the lesions are predominantly foci of cellular necrosis with ova inconstantly present. The cord may be affected in the absence of bladder or rectal lesions and an eosinophilia may be the only indication of parasitic infection. The complement-fixation test is, however, positive. The cerebrospinal fluid may show an increase of mononuclear cells and lymphocytes with a rise in the protein content. The level of glucose is normal. Rarely the joints may be affected. Pseudotubercles and ova have also been noted in the wall of the gall bladder and have been associated with cholecystitis. Very occasionally adult worms have been described in the coronary arteries and ova in the myocardium (Faust, 1948).

S. haematobium and carcinoma of the bladder

In areas where *S. haematobium* infection is intense the incidence of vesical cancer is high—the most striking figures being given by the late Manuel Prates in Mozambique (Prates and Torres, 1965).

In these areas vesical cancer occurs in younger age groups than would be expected in Europe or North America, there is no great preponderance of the male sex and the most common type of tumour is the squamous-cell carcinoma, in contrast to the transitional cell type which predominates in the United States and Europe. The frequent association of calcification of the bladder with carcinoma is also noteworthy. It is considered therefore that there is evidence of an association between *S. haematobium* infestation and cancer of the bladder (Gelfand *et al.* 1967).

Before considering possible causal agents a brief classification of epithelial tumours of the bladder is given below.

Classification of epithelial tumours of the bladder

Epithelial tumours of the bladder may be defined according to their growth pattern and their histology. The most common growth patterns are (1) papillary, (2) papillary and infiltrating, and (3) sessile, nodular, and infiltrating.

The papillary carcinoma is uncommon in bilharzial areas although it accounts for up to 80 per cent of vesical carcinomas in the United States and Europe. The non-infiltrating type has to be differentiated from the benign papilloma in which the epithelial cells are indistinguishable from the normal bladder transitional cell epithelium, are regularly arranged, normally differentiated, and three to five layers of cells thick. The basement membrane should be intact. More than five layers of cells with increased mitotic activity and lack of differentiation justifies the diagnosis of carcinoma. The sessile, nodular, and infiltrating or nodulo-ulcerative types, are more commonly seen in bilharzial areas than the papillary.

Histologically, epithelial tumours of the bladder are usually described as:

(1) Papilloma (benign).   (4) Adenocarcinoma.
(2) Transitional-cell carcinoma.   (5) Undifferentiated carcinoma.
(3) Squamous-cell carcinoma.   (6) Combined.

Excluding the papilloma and the undifferentiated carcinoma, carcinomas are usually classified into three grades according to their degree of differentiation, the most highly differentiated being Grade I.

Villous papilloma of the bladder is said to be rare in many areas in Africa. Transitional-cell carcinoma is the most common form of bladder tumour seen in North America and Europe.

In contrast, in areas of bilharziasis, squamous-cell carcinomas account for up to 60 per cent of all bladder tumours instead of the usual figure of 10 per cent, or less, found in North America and Europe. In addition, in endemic areas, ova of *S. haematobium* are commonly present in such tumours. It should be noted that squamous metaplasia is not uncommon in anaplastic tumours and these should not be classified as squamous-cell carcinomas.

It must also, however, be pointed out that squamous-cell carcinomas of the bladder accounted for about one-third of vesical carcinomas in Jamaica where bilharziasis is not present and was considered to be associated with urethral stricture. A high incidence of this type of tumour has also been noted in Uganda, where the incidence of schistosomiasis is said to be low. Although the trigone is most frequently affected in schistosomiasis, tumours usually arise in the bladder neck, lateral walls, or fundus.

Adenocarcinomas

Adenocarcinomas form a low percentage of vesical cancer (0·4–2 per cent) and they may arise from mucus-secreting glands, present in small numbers at the base of the bladder, or from remnants of the urachus at the dome. Metaplasia of the bladder mucosa to a glandular type may also occur and may present in the combined type of tumour.

Undifferentiated carcinoma

This tumour forms a considerable percentage of bladder cancers. There is a marked tendency to metaplasia, resulting in the production of squamous or glandular epithelium, and if this occurs the tumour should be classified as combined.

Pathogenesis of vesical carcinoma in haematobium infections

Various theories have been advanced regarding the possible mechanism of schistosomal vesical carcinogenesis—the most obvious being chronic irritation of the epithelium of the bladder by the passage of ova during muscular contraction or following its reaction to the inflammatory processes stimulated by their retention. The presence of a miracidial toxin has also been considered.

It has recently been shown that β-glucuronidase, an enzyme concerned in the metabolism of tryptophan, is increased in the urine in a number of urinary tract lesions, including bilharziasis. This enzyme may hydrolyse innocuous tryptophan metabolites in the vesical urine, with the release of carcinogenic substances (Fripp, 1965). It has also been shown that in areas of Africa there is a high intake of 5-hydroxy-tryptophane due to a high dietary intake of plantains and bananas, with a consequently increased urinary excretion of 5-hydroxy-indole-acetic acid. The output of other urinary enzymes has also been shown to be altered in haematobium infections, alkaline phosphatase being increased and acid phosphatase decreased.

Any theory of the mechanism of vesical carcinogenesis in haematobium infection must satisfactorily explain that (a) many infected individuals never develop vesical cancer, (b) in some areas of haematobium infection it has been impossible to demonstrate a high incidence of vesical cancer, and (c) the infection is not associated with malignant change in other organs.

No single factor considered above would satisfy these criteria. It is considered that the development of vesical cancer in haematobium infections is multifactorial and depends upon an intense infection with severe pathological changes associated with chemical changes in the urine and some urinary stasis in the bladder.

The pathology of *S. mansoni* and *S. japonicum* infections

The stage of established infection and oviposition is characterized by fever, headache, and diarrhoea. An eosinophilia is usual and the liver and spleen are usually enlarged and tender. Anorexia and weight loss are usual. There may be pulmonary, cerebral or other extra-abdominal symptoms. A severe form of dermatitis, 'Kabure', seen in workers in rice fields in Japan has been shown to be due to an avian schistosome (grey starling). The cercariae cause a severe monocytic and eosinophilic reaction in the dermis.

In contrast to *S. haematobium* infections the genito-urinary tract is rarely affected.

The gastro-intestinal tract

Ova are discharged from the mesenteric venules through the mucosa into the intestinal lumen. The number of ova produced by *S. japonicum* is much greater than that by *S. mansoni*. As in the bladder some of the ova, varying in their proportions in individuals, are retained in the tissues and an eosinophilic reaction occurs with the formation of eosinophilic abscesses. In the large intestine the mucosa is reddened and granular with pin-point, yellowish elevations surrounded by a hyperaemic zone. Shallow ulcers may form which are more extensive in *japonicum* than in *mansoni* infections. The inflammatory reaction in the submucosa causes epithelial hyperplasia, with the formation of sessile or pedunculated polyps. Polypoid lesions of the colon have been reported to occur in 17–20 per cent of Egyptian patients with schistosomiasis (Lehman *et al.* 1970) and excessive protein loss has been described. The severity of the loss depended on the extent of the polyposis and mucosal disease but not on the intensity of infection as measured by the 24-hour excretion of schistosome eggs (Facid *et al.* 1974). It should be noted, however, that Cheever and Andrade (1967) found no evidence of colonic polyposis in 502 subjects suffering from *S. mansoni* infection in Brazil. The muscular layer and serosa are freqently affected and the pseudotubercles may be associated with a focal exudative peritonitis and intestinal adhesions. Inflammatory masses may be produced in the intestinal wall—the so-called bilharzioma. With progressive fibrosis the intestinal wall may become rigid, with narrowing of the lumen and stenosis. The mesentery is infected and thickened and thrombosis of the veins may occur. Granulomatous lesions may be present in the retroperitoneal and mesenteric lymph nodes and masses of the mesenteric glands may simulate a neoplasm—the so-called pseudotumour. Caecocolic intussusception, intestinal obstruction, and rectal prolapse have been described. With secondary infection ischiorectal and anorectal abscesses and fistulae may form and fibro-epithelial polyps are not uncommon in the anal region.

Infection of the appendix is common and rarely the small intestine may be more affected than the large.

Pyloric obstruction has been described in *japonicum* infection (Nai-Kuang and Pen-Ching, 1957) and lesions may be found in the stomach, peritoneum, and pancreas.

It has been suggested that the chronic colitis seen in japonicum infections may be a pre-malignant condition and following polyp formation adenocarcinomatous change, which may be unifocal or multifocal, occurs (Ch'en et al. 1965; Dao et al. 1956).

The liver

As the ova in these infections are released in the portal venous system the liver is invariably affected, the degree of involvement depending upon the intensity of infection. Because of the greater oviposition in *japonicum* infections the liver is affected earlier and more severely than in *mansoni*.

Grossly the liver may be small, enlarged, or normal in size. The capsule may show a fine or coarse nodularity and is often bosselated (Areán, 1966). The left lobe may be disproportionately enlarged (Cheever and Andrade, 1967).

In the most severe infections the 'clay pipe-stem cirrhosis' described by Symmers in 1904 is produced (Brown, 1974). The use of the term cirrhosis should be discarded for reasons which are discussed later. The liver is of firm consistency and the cut surface appears to have white clay pipe-stems thrust through its parenchyma at various angles, against a background of pinkish-brown to grey relatively normal liver tissue. These white areas, which may be round, oval, or stellate, are due to the terminal fibrotic reaction originally caused by the presence of the ova in and around the portal venous radicles. Dilated portal veins may be noted in some scars and in others they may be obliterated. Focal nodular hyperplasia may be seen in the subcapsular region and a fine periportal type of fibrosis has been described in Egypt (Hashem, 1947).

Histologically the ova are present in the portal and periportal regions and all types of reaction may be present, from the acute eosinophilic to the dense collagenous. In *S. japonicum* infections the ova may appear conglutinated by a transparent substance, probably of parasitic origin, and large acute abscesses may form, with prolonged delay in the formation of pseudotubercles and fibrous tissue formation (Arean, 1964). The ova are trapped in the intrahepatic portal venules and occasionally reach the sinusoids. Adult worms may be seen occasionally in the vessels. The branches of the portal vein in the portal tracts are severely affected due to the destruction of the vascular wall and the reaction stimulated by the ova. Whether this is the sole mechanism involved in the pathogenesis of the lesion is debatable, the presence of dead worms producing necrotizing lesions and immune mechanisms have been postulated as factors or cofactors. The vessel may be completely occluded by a granulomatous reaction with destruction of the elastic and muscle layers. Sclerosis and endarteritis of the branches of the portal vein are usual (Fig. 3.16). Intrahepatic thrombophlebitis may occur. Portal vein branches in portal tracts, especially in the periphery of the liver, are blocked. An increase in the number and size of the intrahepatic arterial branches explains the normal hepatic blood flow seen in many patients with the disease (Andrade and Cheever, 1971). The lumina of other veins may be obliterated by loose fibrous tissue containing thin-walled vascular channels—the end result of a thrombotic process. Similar channels may also be seen in the fibrosed portal tracts, in areas reminiscent of cavernous haemangioma—the so-called angiomatoids. Their formation and function is not clear and whether they are evidence of previous thrombotic episodes or

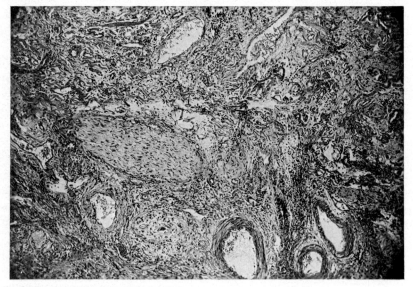

FIG. 3.16. *S. mansoni.* Portal area, showing hypertrophy of nerves, sclerosis of hepatic arteries, and portal vein replaced by vascularized connective tissue (H and E × 130). (*By courtesy of Dr. V. M. Arean.*)

are abnormal communications between the portal and hepatic circulations has still to be elucidated (Aidaros and Soliman, 1961). Hypertrophied nerve trunks and bile ducts may be seen in the distorted portal tracts. Schistosomal pigment may be seen in histiocytes or lying free in the fibrous tissue, as well as in the proliferating and hypertrophied Kupffer cells. The intrahepatic arterioles may also be affected and show medial hypertrophy and intimal proliferation.

The parenchymal cells are usually unaffected, although, due to the widespread vascular damage, anoxic episodes can occur. Focal atrophy, fatty change, and haemorrhage have been described, probably accounting for the nodular hyperplasia which may be seen in the subcapsular region at the periphery of the vascular tree. Acute massive necrosis may be precipitated by haemorrhage from an oesophageal varix, cardiac failure, or portal-vein thrombosis (Andrade, 1965).

Schistosomiasis, cirrhosis, and carcinoma of the liver

If cirrhosis of the liver is defined as 'diffuse destruction of the normal architecture of the liver associated with nodular regeneration of hepatic parenchyma in the presence of widespread fibrosis' it can be deduced from the above description that schistosomiasis does not cause cirrhosis of the liver, and there is much evidence to show that there is no correlation between the incidence of schistosomiasis and cirrhosis of the liver in many populations. The present body of opinion discounts *S. haematobium* and *S. mansoni* as causative agents in cirrhosis of the liver, but *S. japonicum* may be implicated in Japan (Miyake, 1967).

It must be realized that schistosomiasis occurs in many developing countries where malnutrition in childhood, infectious hepatitis, the presence of possible hepatotoxic agents, and a relatively high incidence of cirrhosis of the liver are common. The presence of scanty ova in a cirrhotic liver in these areas must not be taken as proof of aetiology and controlled studies must be undertaken to prove or disprove their significance. The present body of opinion discounts schistosomiasis as a causative agent in cirrhosis of the liver.

The term pipe-stem cirrhosis is therefore considered unsuitable and pipe-stem fibrosis is to be preferred, or schistosomal hepatic fibrosis as suggested by Hashem (1947).

Carcinoma of the liver has been mentioned in association with *S. japonicum* infection but there is no evidence which proves a causal relationship between *S. mansoni* and *S. haematobium* infection and carcinoma of the liver.

Clinically the pathological changes in the liver induce presinusoidal portal hypertension with the development of a collateral circulation, ascites, and hypoproteinaemia.

The patient is usually below the age of 30 years with an enlarged palpable liver. There is an absence of jaundice or hepatocellular failure and the striking feature is portal hypertension with the development of a porto-systemic collateral circulation. There is gross splenomegaly. Gynaecomastia and other signs of parenchymal liver cell damage, including altered liver function tests, are usually lacking.

Haematemesis from oesophageal varices may precipitate hepatic anoxia, liver failure and coma.

Sudden cardiac failure or portal vein thrombosis may, once again, cause liver failure to dominate the clinical picture. Splenic vein thrombosis may also occur.

Liver biopsy is often unrewarding as the penetrating needle usually glances off the firm fibrous tissue. Splenoportography, hepatic-vein catheterization, or surgical wedge biopsy are more useful procedures. It is generally considered that the presence of numerous ova in the periportal fibrous tissue are necessary for a final diagnosis of pipe-stem fibrosis of the liver to be made (Fig. 3.17).

In cirrhosis and pipe-stem fibrosis the portal vein pressure is high but in

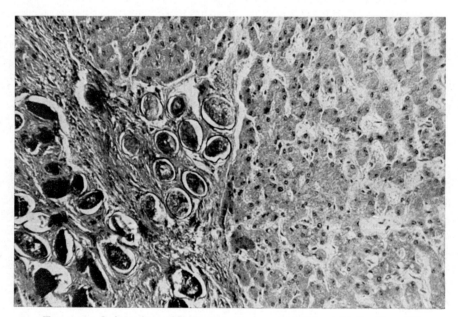

FIG. 3.17. *S. japonicum.* Numerous ova in a portal tract in the liver (H and E × 180).

the latter the pressure of the so-called 'occluded suprahepatic vein' is normal while it is high in the former.

The reticulo-endothelial system

The spleen becomes enlarged and tender in the stage of established infection—usually due to congestive changes—schistosomal tubercles may be found but are not a striking feature. Infarcts may be present and thrombosis of the splenic vein has been described. Histologically there is fibrous thickening of the septa, hyperplasia of the histocytic reticulum cells, and disappearance of the lymphoid follicles. Schistosomal pigment may be present but is never great in amount. There is gross congestion of the sinuses with scattered areas of fresh and old haemorrhage. Sidero-fibrotic nodules (Gandy–Gamna bodies) are not uncommonly found. Ova with an accompanying reaction have been described in abdominal lymphatic glands. When periportal hepatic fibrosis is established gross splenomegaly may result with signs of 'hypersplenism'. Erythropoiesis may be depressed, with anaemia, leucopenia, and thrombocytopenia occurring. Dwarfism has been attributed to these infections and growth abnormalities have been relieved by splenectomy. A prolonged fever associated with salmonellosis has been described in hepatosplenic schistosomiasis due to *S. mansoni*. It is of interest that Andrade and Abreu (1971) have noted an association of follicular lymphoma of the spleen in patients with hepatosplenic schistosomiasis mansoni. It was present in 8 of 863 surgically removed spleens and superficial lymph nodes were not enlarged. One patient developed a reticulo-sarcoma. Abdel-Moneim (1972) has analysed 128 cases of rupture of the spleen in Egypt. The vast majority occurred in patients with normal spleens despite the large number of villagers who have hepatosplenomegaly due to schistosomiasis. It was concluded that rupture of the spleen in patients with schistosomiasis and chronic malaria is rare.

The lungs

Lesions in the lungs may occur during the stage of invasion—a larval pneumonitis during cercarial migration—or an allergic arteriolitis with clinical attacks of bronchial asthma on reinfection.

In japonicum and mansoni infections, the lungs are not usually severely affected until, as would be expected, a portosystemic collateral circulation due to pipe-stem fibrosis is established, allowing ova released in the portal veins direct access to the systemic venous circulation. Although ova are more frequently found in the lungs in haematobium infections, the more severe pathological effects are seen in the late stages of japonicum and mansoni infections (Fig. 3.18). The pulmonary lesions can be classified into (1)

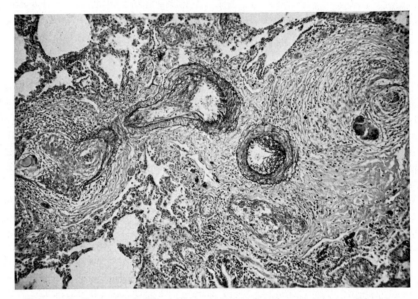

FIG. 3.18. *S. mansoni*. The pulmonary arteries show severe proliferative endarteritis. Towards the left the vessel is occluded by a granulomatous process with remnants of eggs. Extravascular pseudotubercles can be seen and there is an angiomatoid area below the cross section of the narrowed pulmonary artery (Weigert's reticulin stain × 130). (*By courtesy of Dr. V. M. Arean.*)

localized, (2) interstitial, (3) widespread arterial involvement with right ventricular hypertrophy (cor pulmonale), and (4) the cyanotic syndrome.

The localized lesion consisting of numerous pseudotubercles has already been described (p. 164). In addition a focal acute necrotizing pneumonia can occur and is thought to be caused by the presence of dead adult worms in the pulmonary artery (Shaw and Ghareeb, 1938). Necrosis of the arterial wall with an acute necrotizing pneumonia occurs. With healing, remnants of the calcified worm are found in a focus of scar tissue. In laboratory animals treatment has been known to cause embolization of adult worms to the lungs and this has been a suggested mechanism of the localized lesions in man. In man following treatment, however, a diffuse miliary infiltration of the lungs and patchy consolidation have been described and would be best classified as the interstitial form.

Interstitial pulmonary schistosomiasis. Not infrequently pseudotubercules may be detected in the interstitial tissue following the course of the smaller pulmonary arteries. Healed focal lesions in the arterioles may or may not be detected and the heart is not involved.

Cor pulmonale. There would appear to be at least two types of lesions caused by the presence of the ova in the pulmonary circulation. The first is the granulomatous type of lesion caused by the presence of the ova themselves and the second is a necrotizing arteriolitis caused by products released by the miracidia and thought to be associated with immune mechanisms (Faria 1954; Chaves, 1966; Briers, 1974). In the granulomatous lesion the ova set up an intense eosinophilic reaction in the smaller pulmonary arterioles and cause vascular occlusion and thrombosis. Pseudotubercles are formed and the thrombi become organized and recanalized, leading to angiomatoid lesions. The wall of the vessel may be focally destroyed with consequent pseudoaneurysm formation. The surrounding adventitia is affected and adjacent veins may become thrombosed. Newly-formed blood vessels may communicate with the arterial angiomatoid lesions with the formation of arteriovenous fistulae. Endarterial polypi representing organized mural thrombi may be seen.

The second type of lesion appears to be unrelated to the ova and is a fibrinoid necrosis involving the intima or entire arteriolar wall, with a surrounding lymphocytic and monocytic infiltration. This leads to an obliterative endarteritis, with concentric or eccentric intimal proliferation and a cellular or acellular fibrosis with elastosis. The lesions are similar to those seen in idiopathic hypertension. The obstructive vascular lesions cause pulmonary hypertension with consequent atheroma and superadded secondary changes in the arteries (medial hypertrophy and subendothelial fibrosis). Eventually hypertrophy of the right ventricle ensues with dilatation of the pulmonary valve.

Clinically, the patients are predominantly young males who complain of dyspnoea, praecordial and chest pain, and swelling of the lower limbs. Clubbing of the fingers is rare and cyanosis uncommon, as the pulmonary capillaries are unaffected. Haemoptyses are rare. Radiological studies show marked enlargement and dilatation of the right ventricle and a fine nodular mottling may be present in the lungs. The electrocardiogram shows right axis deviation and right ventricular hypertrophy. The examination of the sputum for the presence of ova may be a helpful diagnostic feature. De Leon and Tavera (1968) have reported on 10 cases of pulmonary schistosomiasis in the Philippines due to *S. japonica* infection. Ova were not found in the sputum. It was thought they were walled off by parenchymal tissue. Needle biopsy of the lung was thought to be the only possible method of diagnosis. In these patients the diagnosis was unsuspected during life and only discovered at necropsy. It is of interest that two of the patients had lymphosarcoma, and schistosomiasis was suggested as an aetiological agent.

The cyanotic syndrome. A chronic form of pulmonary disease with cyanosis and finger clubbing which occurs in the absence of pulmonary hypertension has been described in South America and attributed to mansoni infection (Faria *et al.* 1959). The ova are thought to involve the smaller pulmonary veins causing arteriovenous fistulae with consequent oxygen unsaturation of the arterial blood. Others have, however, considered that the shunts may not be directly related to pulmonary schistosomiasis but to other factors. Oxygen unsaturation of the arterial blood can occur in cirrhosis with portal hypertension, but in patients with the cyanotic syndrome liver fibrosis is minimal and portal hypertension has not been noted (Wessel *et al.* 1965).

The central nervous system

Convulsions, epileptiform seizures, aphasia, and transverse myelitis occur. Cerebral symptoms are more common in japonicum infection and cord symptoms in mansoni. In the established condition small tubercles may be found in the meninges and in the white and grey matter of the brain and cord. Areas of softening due to thrombosis can occur. The lesions usually contain large numbers of ova in necrotic material surrounded by eosinophils, neutrophils, and multinucleated giant cells, with a peripheral area of epithelioid cells and lymphocytes. Fibroblastic proliferation and hyperplasia of glial cells with neuronal degeneration occur. Adult worms are not usually seen in the brain substance. The protein and cells in the cerebrospinal fluid are increased. Eosinophils, if present, are a suggestive diagnostic sign. Marcial-Rojas and Fiol (1963) reported two cases of transverse myelitis due to *S. mansoni* infection and reviewed the world literature on the neurologic complications of schistosomiasis in 95 patients. *S. japonicum* was the most frequent infecting parasite, followed by *S. mansoni* and lastly *S. haematobium*. Epilepsy, transverse myelitis, hemiplegia and aphasia, flaccid paralysis and a brain tumour syndrome could all occur. Bracken *et al.* (1948) described the pathology in three American soldiers who died in the acute stage of *S. japonicum* infection in the Philippines. Acute necrotizing tubercles associated with viable ova were found in the brain, meninges, mesenteric lymph nodes, skin myocardium, and adrenal medulla.

Genito-urinary system

In the male, mansoni infection may very rarely affect the bladder, prostate, testes, and kidney. However, Da Silva *et al.* (1970), in patients with no clinical evidence of renal disease, found electron-dense deposits in basement membranes and laminated bodies near the mesangial cells. The deposits were shown to be IgG by immunofluorescence. The glomeruli were normal on light microscopy. It was considered that the changes described were due to the deposition of immunocomplexes on the glomerular capillary walls. Renal glomeruli are frequently damaged in patients with hepatosplenic schistosomiasis. There would appear to be a spectrum of changes that include mesangial cell proliferation, deposition of mesangial matrix, glomerulosclerosis and glomerulo-nephritis (Andrade et al. (1971). Ova have been noted in the urine (Arean, 1956). In the female in mansoni infection the ovaries, tubes, cervix, and rarely the vulva, may be affected. In the Fallopian tube the ova are more frequently found in the mucosa than in the walls in contrast to S. haematobium (Arean, 1956). There are isolated reports of S. japonicum affecting the female genitalia and transplacental infection of the fetus has been recorded once (Sutherland et al. 1965). The gynaecological lesions caused by the migration of ova and adult worms of S. mansoni through the pelvic plexus have been reported by many authors. Lesions have been described in the ovaries, fallopian tubes, cervix, uterus, vulva, vagina and labia major (Chaves and Palitot, 1964).

Other organs

Literally any organ or tissue in the body can be involved and lesions have been described in the heart, adrenal, thyroid, pancreas, gall bladder, and bone marrow. Endocrine disturbances manifested by intolerance to cold, loss of body hair, and libido; sterility and dwarfism have been described in the late stages of the infection (Hsuech and Wu, 1963). Impaired glucose tolerance has been described (Sukkar et al. 1974)

Clinical and diagnostic pathology

Eosinophilia is usual during the early invasion and toxaemic stages, in all types of schistosomiasis, but it is very inconstant thereafter. The rate of leucocyte excretion in patients with urinary schistosomiasis is increased; it is unrelated to bacteriuria but directly proportional to the rate of egg excretion (Dukes et al. 1967). Urinary leucocytes in S. haematobium infections may be largely eosinophils derived from the perioval inflammatory lesions in the bladder and the conventional report of 'pus cells' in the urines of patients with vesical schistosomiasis may be misleading, since in many such instances the urines on culture are found free from bacteria (Powell et al. 1965). A decrease in serum albumin, an increase of a_2- and γ-globulins, positive flocculation tests, elevated serum transaminase and alkaline phosphatase activity, and slightly increased bromsulphthalein retention have all been reported in S. japonicum infections in the acute stages of the disease. A significant lowering of serum cholinesterase levels has been reported from Egypt, and there was an indication that the fall in cholinesterase ran parallel with the degree and length of the disease process. The following schematic representation covers the main diagnostic criteria for schistosomiasis.

A. *Direct diagnosis*   1. Eggs in excreta   ⎰ (i) Urine
   (finding eggs)   ⎨ (ii) Stool
                                                  ⎱ (iii) Sputum (occasionally)

                          2. Eggs in body   ⎧ (i) Rectal biopsy
                                                 ⎪ (ii) Vesical biopsy
                                                 ⎨ (iii) Liver biopsy
                                                 ⎪ (iv) Others, e.g. appendix; genitalia
                                                 ⎩ (v) Digestion of organs

B. *Indirect diagnosis*   1. Endoscopy
                          2. X-rays
                          3. Immuno-diagnostic methods

A. **Direct diagnosis**

S. haematobium is the easiest infection to diagnose by finding the characteristic eggs with terminal spines on direct examination of the urine. Live eggs are always accompanied by microscopic or macroscopic haematuria. They can be recognized by seeing the wriggling movement of the contained miracidium, the flickering of the flame cells, or by the hatching test. Dead eggs, on the other hand, are opaque and granular and give a negative hatching test. The peak output of eggs occurs around noon, when the load may be twenty times as high as in the early morning. In light infections, concentration of urine followed by a special staining technique may have to be employed. Eggs of *S. haematobium* are also found in the faeces and they are frequently present in the rectal mucosa, where they are found on rectal biopsy. These eggs are usually dead or calcified.

S. mansoni and *S. japonicum* eggs are difficult to find on direct smear examination of the faeces except in very heavy infections and concentration techniques are usually necessary. The eggs are recognized by their typical lateral spine in *S. mansoni* and rudimentary lateral knob in *S. japonicum*. Live eggs have the same characteristics as described for *S. haematobium*. They are frequently found in rectal biopsy material, as are eggs of *S. japonicum*. It is not uncommon for *S. mansoni* eggs to be found in the urine. Liver-biopsy specimens can be examined as fresh preparations or after conventional sections are cut. Adult worms are sometimes seen lying in vessels in transverse sections of papillomata of the bladder, in rectal polyps, or in ectopic sites.

B. **Indirect diagnosis**

Cystoscopy in *S. haematobium* infections reveals the typical bladder changes already described; while sigmoidoscopy may reveal polypi in *S. mansoni* and *S. japonicum* infections. Ova are trapped in the mucosa and submucosa of the large intestine and cause a granulomatous reaction. *S. mansoni* ova become calcified much less frequently than do those of *S. japonicum*.

In *S. japonicum* infections sigmoidoscopy may reveal scars, clusters of grape-like granulomas, brownish discrete depressions—'pock marks'— and polypoid growths which may lead to intestinal obstruction of the large intestine in the rectal and sigmoid regions.

Carcinomatous changes in association with the chronic lesions of *S. japonicum* in the large intestine have been described.

Calcification of the bladder revealed by radiology is diagnostic of *S. haematobium* infections, while intravenous and retrograde pyelography may show dilatation of ureters and back-pressure kidney effects. Barium enema may reveal polypi in *S. mansoni* and *S. japonicum* infections. Several immunological methods can be used for the diagnosis of schistosomiasis. They are positive in all types of human schistosomiasis and are therefore group specific. They have been used for the diagnosis of individual cases as well as for epidemiological surveys. The details of performing the tests can be found in the relevant references, a short account of their significance follows (Kagan and Pellegrino, 1961):

1. *Intradermal test* (Pellegrino *et al.* 1957)

The test is performed on the back, adequate antigen concentration must be used and the antigen of *S. mansoni* has now been standardized by the WHO. Though the test sensitivity varies with the patient's age and sex, the criteria for its interpretation may be adjusted so as to get positive results in about 90 per cent of patients with schistosomiasis. False-positive reactions do not exceed 5 per cent. The test is positive before eggs appear in the excreta and hence its usefulness in diagnosing early infection. It is not quantitative.

2. *Complement-fixation test* (Chaffe *et al.* 1954)

This is a very reliable test in children and is quantitative. The test sensitivity is about 90–95 per cent and its specificity close to 100 per cent. It is the method of choice for the diagnosis of individual cases.

3. *Circumoval test* (Oliver-Gonzalez *et al.* 1955)

This test is positive in about 70 per cent of schistosome-infected patients; false-positive results are obtained in 7 per cent of cases. It displays few advantages over the tests already described.

4. *Immunofluorescence test* (Sadun *et al.* 1961)

This test is positive in about 85 per cent of schistosome-infected patients, and about 5 per cent false-positive results occur. It is valuable for epidemiological surveys since blood may be collected by finger puncture in filter paper. In some areas, however, specificity can be low and this test requires further study before final evaluation.

5. *Slide flocculation test* (Anderson, 1960)

Positive reactions are obtained in about 95 per cent of schistosome-infected patients, with 6 per cent false-positive results. This serological method, being easily performed, is valuable in epidemiological surveys.

6. *Plasma-card test* (Sadun *et al.* 1963)

This test is positive in about 86 per cent of schistosome-infected patients, with 6 per cent false-positive results. It can be easily carried out under field conditions and is useful in epidemiological surveys.

FASCIOLOPSIASIS

This infection is caused by the large, fleshy fluke—*Fasciolopsis buski*—which is found mainly in China, but also in India, Indo-China, Thailand, Malaya, Indonesia, Taiwan, and Europe (Viranuvatti *et al.* 1953). It is estimated that 10 million people are infected with *F. buski* in the Far East (Cross, 1969).

Life cycle

F. buski is normally an intestinal parasite of the pig and of man and inhabits the small intestine. The eggs are passed in the faeces and the miracidium is released and swims in water until it penetrates a suitable mollusc host of the genus *Segmentina*—where it develops into a sporocyst, redia, and cercaria. When the cercariae leave the snail they encyst on aquatic plants. When the encysted cercariae are ingested by man, the cyst wall is dissolved in the duodenum and the liberated larvae attach themselves to the mucosa, where they develop into adult worms whose nourishment is derived from the duodenal secretions. The egg output per worm is very high, averaging 25,000 eggs per day.

Epidemiology

Man is infected when he eats raw water-plants contaminated with encysted cercariae. The commonest source of infected edible water plants are the water caltrops and water chestnuts which are often cultivated in ponds fertilized by human faeces (Sadun and Maiphoon, 1953). In China these tubers are eaten raw and fresh from July to September and, as they are peeled with the teeth, an easy entry of the cercariae to the mouth is provided. Pigs are an important animal reservoir, infecting the stagnant ponds in which edible water plants grow.

Pathology

In the majority of instances the infection is symptomless. Foci of inflammation may occur at the site of attachment of the worm in the small intestine.

With heavy infections (1000–2000 flukes) abdominal pain with alternate diarrhoea and constipation may occur. Intestinal stasis, ulceration and even obstruction have been described. Anaemia with a variable eosinophilia and oedema of the face, abdominal wall, genitalia and lower limbs sometimes with ascites occur in severe cases and death may occur from exhaustion.

Diagnostic pathology

The diagnosis can be made by finding the characteristic operculated ova in the faeces, there may be a leucocytosis and eosinophilia. Occasionally, adult flukes are vomited or found in the faeces.

HETEROPHYIASIS AND METAGONIMIASIS

These conditions are due to infection by two very minute flukes— *Heterophyes heterophyes* and *Metagonimus yokagawai*. In the tropics the former is found in Egypt, Tunisia, South China, India, and the Philippines, while the latter occurs in the Far East and Indonesia.

Life cycle

The life cycle and pathogenesis of both flukes is similar. The adults live in the upper part of the small intestine embedded in mucus or in the mucosal folds. The eggs containing miracidia are passed in the faeces and, on ingestion by suitable snails, develop into sporocysts, rediae and cercariae. The cercariae then leave the snails and enter the appropriate fish, in which they encyst into infective metacercariae. When the fish are eaten raw or partially cooked the metacercariae are liberated and the larvae develop into adult worms in the small intestine.

The first snail intermediate hosts for *H. heterophyes* are brackish-water snails (e.g. *Pirenella conica*), while the second intermediate hosts are mullets; for *M. yokogawai* the hosts are snails of the *Semisulcospira* species and salmanoid and cyprinoid fishes.

The pathogenicity of parasitic infection is very low, unless aberrant ova enter the circulation when the spinal cord may be affected (Africa *et al.* 1935; 1937).

Epidemiology

In addition to man other mammals are also infected and, like clonorchis infection, heterophiasis is acquired by eating raw or partially cooked infected fish.

Pathology

Little is known about the pathological effects. Ova have, however, been seen in the myocardium and mitral valve, with consequent sclerosis and heart failure supervening (Africa *et al.* 1937). Sheir and Aboul-Enein (1970) have discussed the demographic, clinical and therapeutic appraisal of over 200 cases of heterophyiasis causing dyspepsia and gastroentero-colitis.

Diagnostic pathology

Diagnosis is made by finding the characteristic ova in the faeces. There may be eosinophilia.

CLONORCHIASIS

The causative parasite of clonorchiasis is the oriental liver fluke *Clonorchis sinensis* which is mainly found in the Far East. Endemic foci occur in Japan, South Korea, South Eastern China, Taiwan, and Vietnam. It is an important infection in Korea (Soh, 1969); while the prevalence in Hong Kong is 25 per cent. Most of these infections are probably from Mainland China (Huang *et al.* 1969).

Life cycle

The adult *C. sinensis* is a flat, transparent fluke which inhabits the bile ducts and sometimes the pancreatic ducts of man and other fish-eating mammals. It is from 10 to 25 mm long and 3 to 5 mm in breadth (Fig. 3.19).

Self-fertilization is the common means of fecundation and the ova are carried down the common bile duct to the duodenum and are passed in the faeces. On reaching water the ova are ingested by a suitable snail (e.g. genus *Bithynia*) and hatch in the snail's digestive tract. The enclosed miracidia develop in the snail host into sporocysts and rediae within which cercariae develop. These eventually break out of the mother redia and escape from the snail into the water.

The cercariae with unforked tails penetrate the scales of one of several freshwater fishes (e.g. Cyprinoid) and encyst in their flesh, skin, and gills. Here they develop into numerous encysted metacercariae which are the infective forms, and which remain viable for 2 months after the death of the fish.

When ingested by man the metacercariae are freed by the action of the gastric and duodenal juices, and the larvae migrate to the common bile duct and then into the smaller biliary radicles where they mature into adults.

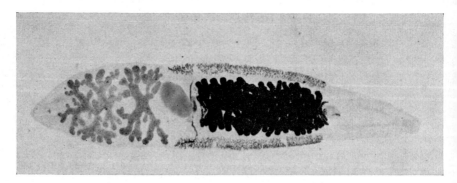

FIG. 3.19. Clonorchiasis. Adult *Clonorchis sinensis*.

Epidemiology

Man and other mammals are infected by eating raw or undercooked fish containing metacercariae. Fish ponds fertilized with fresh human faeces are a common source of infection. Infected fish exported to other countries can result in the spread of the disease to areas where the parasite is not normally found. As with paragonomiasis many animals harbour *C. sinensis*, but their importance in the epidemiology of the human disease has yet to be fully assessed.

Clonorchiasis is rare in infants under 1 year of age, it begins, however, at about 2 years rising to 65 per cent in those aged 21–30 years and to a peak of 80 per cent in those dying between the ages of 51–60 years (Hou and Pang, 1964). Males are more frequently infected than females, but there are no social differences in the prevalence of the disease because of the universal custom of eating raw fish. The life span of the worm is 25–30 years. Ouchterlony gel diffusion has been used to study the antigens of clonorchis (Sun and Gibson 1969).

Pathology

The effects of clonorchiasis depend upon the intensity and duration of the infection and the degree of liver damage derived from the presence of the worms and associated factors. Although alcoholism and malnutrition have been mentioned in this connection by far the most important are the presence of secondary infection and the possibility of malignant change.

C. sinensis has been noted in the liver in 65 per cent of post-mortem examinations undertaken in Hong Kong (Hou and Pang, 1964). The majority of infections are asymptomatic, or mild abdominal discomfort and digestive disturbances may be complained of. In some patients intermittent or remittent fever, anorexia, epigastric pain, and jaundice occur and are evidence of recurrent pyogenic cholangitis; in others, symptoms of carcinoma of the liver may supervene. A severe form of suppurative pancholangitis with coma, fever, jaundice, rigors, and marked hypoglycaemia has been described (McFadzean and Yeung, 1965).

The flukes mature in the smaller biliary passages of the liver and with light infections all that may be noted at autopsy is undue prominence of the medium-sized portal tracts, with some dilatation of the bile ducts containing the transparent reddish parasites. With heavier infections localized dilatations of the intrahepatic bile ducts, especially in the left lobe of the liver, occur and may be seen as pale-blue cystic structures on the serous surface. Focal dilatations and cystic areas, containing clear bile—or cloudy if infection has occurred—and adult worms, surrounded by relatively normal liver tissue, are seen on section. Generalized dilatation of the ducts is unusual unless the common bile duct has been obstructed by stone, tumour, or inflammatory stricture (Hou, 1955). If secondary bacterial infection has occurred multiple abscesses may be seen in the liver substance. Even with heavy infestation and secondary infection the surrounding liver tissue may show no evidence of nodular fibrosis and hyperplasia. The part that clonorchiasis plays in the production of cirrhosis is debatable, although portal and biliary cirrhosis have been described in association with the infection.

The adults are unable to exist in the gall bladder and are only found there in heavy infections as hard, friable, dark bodies.

Microscopic pathology

The presence of the flukes in the bile ducts causes desquamation and proliferation of the epithelial lining cells with excessive mucin formation (Fig. 3.20). The epithelium is thrown into adenomatous folds with a variable amount of connective-tissue stroma present. The adenomatous change is proportional to the degree of infestation and is caused by the mechanical irritation of the worm and the chemical irritation due to its metabolic processes when alive or degradation products when dead. There may be no

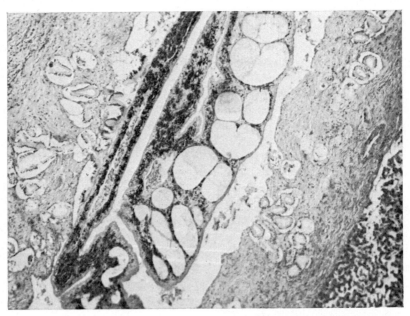

FIG. 3.20. Clonorchiasis. *Clonorchis sinensis* in bile duct. Note the loss of bile duct epithelium in areas and the glandular elements in the fibrous sub-mucosa (H and E × 30). (*By courtesy of Professor R. Gibson.*)

surrounding cellular reaction in the wall of the bile duct and ova are not usually seen at this stage. As the condition becomes more chronic the walls of the bile ducts are infiltrated with leucocytes including eosinophils, their vascularity is increased and the smaller portal vessels may become fibrosed with associated dilatation of the portal vein and increase of pressure (Hoeppli, 1933). Blockage of intrahepatic ducts, with desquamation of the tall columnar epithelium, and cystic dilatation occurs. Pigment stones containing dead worms, ova, and inflammatory products may be found in brownish-green amorphous material—the so-called biliary mud. Secondary infection, usually due to *Esch. coli*, causes cholangitis, cholangio-hepatitis, pylephlebitis, and multiple abscesses.

The pancreas

Worms are frequently present in the pancreatic duct and may give rise to clinical symptoms of acute pancreatitis with raised serum amylase or urinary diastase levels (McFadzean and Yeung, 1966). Adenomatous hyperplasia of the lining epithelium and periductal fibrosis occurs. Squamous-celled metaplasia of the ductular epithelium is common. Pancreatic necrosis is, however, said to be rare.

Clonorchiasis and carcinoma of the liver

The adenomatous hyperplasia of the bile duct epithelium would appear to be associated with the development of multifocal adenocarcinoma of the liver (Hou, 1956). The highest recorded incidence is in males from the age of 36 years onwards.

Macroscopically the tumours may be seen as greyish or pinkish lesions in or surrounding bile duct walls in the infected liver. The surrounding liver tissue is in most instances relatively normal. According to Hou (1956) the lesions can be classified as follows:

(*a*) Cancer arising from the lining epithelial cells of the bile duct
    (i) A polypoid adenocarcinoma.
    (ii) An anaplastic carcinoma.
(*b*) Cancer arising from adenomatous tissue within the wall of the bile duct.
(*c*) A mixture of types (*a*) and (*b*).

The tumours do not show a uniform histopathological pattern but are predominantly adenocarcinomas in various stages of differentiation. Mucin may be abundant or scanty and there is an absence of glycogen and bile pigment. Areas of necrosis are frequent and squamous metaplasia occurs in a small percentage. The anaplastic type resembles primary liver-celled carcinoma but is not common.

Metastases may be found in regional lymphatic glands, diaphragm, lungs, suprarenal, omentum, heart, kidney, bone, brain, and gall bladder.

This type of hepatic tumour differs markedly from the common primary liver-celled carcinoma seen in other parts of the tropics, where there is a close association with cirrhosis (p. 589) and there is some evidence that clonorchiasis may cause tumours in the livers of animals. It is therefore not unreasonable to conclude that clonorchiasis can be responsible for the occurrence of a primary adenocarcinoma of the liver in man (Yamagati *et al.* 1964).

Diagnostic pathology

A definitive diagnosis is made by finding the typical operculated ova by 'direct smear' examination of the faeces or duodenal aspirate.

There is usually a leucocytosis (23,000–48,000) with eosinophilia. In severe cases with secondary infection of the bile ducts there may be severe hypoglycaemia with blood sugars of 22–45 mg per cent; bilirubin levels of 3–10 mg per cent; and the alkaline phosphatase may be raised 20–76KA units.

Serological and intradermal tests have been disappointing because trematodes possess group antigens. The indirect haemagglutination test is reported to be more sensitive than the others (Pacheco *et al.* 1960).

OPISTHORCHIASIS

This disease is due to two parasitic trematodes—*Opisthorchis felineus* and *O. viverrini*. In the tropics the former is prevalent in the Philippines, India, Japan, and Vietnam, while the latter has been reported from north and north-east Thailand and Laos. Opisthorchiasis is an important problem in Thailand (Harinasuta, 1969) and in the Ukraine (Gritsay and Yabukov, 1970).

Life cycle

The life cycle and pathogenesis of these two human hepatic trematodes are similar to that of *C. sinensis* (Fig. 3.21). The adults inhabit the distal bile ducts and the ova

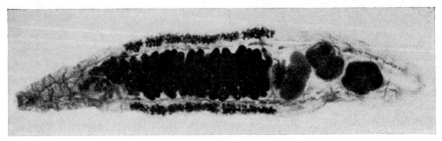

FIG. 3.21. Opisthorchiasis. Adult opisthorchis worm.

are passed out in the faeces—after ingestion by the appropriate snails (e.g. *Bithynia*) the miracidia develop into cercariae which in turn penetrate the flesh of suitable species of freshwater fishes (e.g. Cyprinoid family) in which they encyst and develop into metacercariae. When the metacercariae are ingested by a suitable host—man, domestic, wild, and fur-bearing animals—they encyst in the duodenum and migrate to the distal bile ducts particularly those of the left lobe of the liver. The entire life cycle takes about 4 months. The adult measures 10 mm long by 2 mm broad.

Epidemiology

Man and reservoir hosts are infected by the consumption of raw or insufficiently cooked fish. Snails and fish are infected by faeces deposited on the sandy shores and washed into the streams. The chief reservoir of *O. felineus* is the cat (Erhardt *et al.* 1962).

In north-east Thailand 90 per cent of people over the age of 10 are infected with *O. viverrini* and it is estimated that over 3·5 million persons in Thailand harbour the parasite. The source of infection is a popular dish called 'Keompla', consisting of raw fish, roasted rice, and vegetables seasoned with garlic, lemon juice, fish sauce, and pepper. Chinese residents of Thailand who do not eat raw fish are free from infection (Harinasuta and Vajrasthira, 1960). The largest number of human infections occur during the latter portion of the rainy season and the first part of the dry season, i.e. from September to February (Sadun, 1955).

Pathology

The pathological findings are similar to those found in clonorchiasis. The liver is usually enlarged. The bile ducts also are usually enlarged, dilated and cystic. The portal tracts may be fibrosed but true cirrhosis is only a coincidental finding. Secondary bacterial infection is common with cholangitis, hepatitis, and liver abscess occurring as complications. Cholecystitis and empyema of the gall gladder may also occur. Stone formation is said to be unusual.

Histologically there is proliferation of the epithelial cells lining the bile ducts with the formation of adenomatous polypi and glandular acini. A mild periductal inflammatory reaction with subsequent fibrosis is usual. The pancreatic ducts may be similarly affected.

There is a high incidence of cholangiocellular carcinoma of the liver in opisthorchiasis which is considered to be related to the epithelial changes occurring in the ducts due to the presence of the parasite (Tansurat, 1966).

Diagnostic pathology

This is made by finding the ova on 'direct smear' examination of faeces or duodenal aspirate. They are indistinguishable from those of *C. sinensis*.

Percutaneous transhepatic cholangiography reveals four types of radiological patterns (1) a single cystic cavity, (2) mulberry-like dilatation of the intrahepatic bile ducts (3) a combination of (1) and (2), and (4) dilatation of intrahepatic bile ducts (Viranuvatti *et al.* 1967).

FASCIOLIASIS

This infection is caused by the trematode—*Fasciola hepatica*: 'sheep-liver fluke'—which has a world-wide distribution in ruminants being especially prevalent in the sheep rearing areas of the world. In some areas, e.g. Hawaii, the causative agent of fascioliasis is *F. gigantica* (Alicata, 1953; Hammond, 1974).

Life cycle

The adult worm, which is large (30 mm long and 13 mm broad) flat, and leaf-shaped, lives in the bile ducts or liver parenchyma, of sheep, cattle, goats, and other animals and man. The eggs are passed in the faeces and hatch in a moist environment. The released miracidia then enter the appropriate species of snails (*Lymnaea*), and develop successively into sporocysts, rediae, and cercariae. The cercariae then leave their snail host and encyst on various grasses and water plants. When this water vegetation is ingested by the appropriate hosts, the larvae excyst in the intestine, penetrate the mucosa, enter the liver through the portal circulation, and eventually reach the bile ducts, where they mature in about 3 months.

F. hepatica obtains its nourishment from the biliary secretions and can absorb simple carbohydrates.

Epidemiology

Man usually contracts infection by eating lettuce or water cress contaminated by sheep or other animals' faeces. The highest incidence of infection occurs in low, damp pastures where the grasses and the water are infected with encysted cercariae. Little is known about immunity in human infections, but it has been demonstrated that immunization of rabbits with proteins of *F. hepatica* prior to infection produces inhibition of development of the parasites although the numbers were not significantly reduced (Urquhart *et al.* 1954).

Pathology

During the stage of migration there may be pain in the upper right abdomen with mild fever. The syndrome may mimic hepatitis but an eosinophilia is usual and small necrotic foci or microabscesses infiltrated with eosinophils and leucocytes have been described in the liver (Belding, 1965).

A condition known as halzoun occurs in the Middle East in those who eat raw liver of the sheep or goat. Pharyngeal pain, epistaxis, haemoptysis, and dysphagia occur, and there may be aural symptoms and oedema of the face and neck. The symptoms are due to infection of the pharynx by young specimens of *F. hepatica*. The leeches *Limnatis nilotica* (Watson and Kerim, 1956) and *Dinobdella ferox* (Keegan *et al.* 1970) can cause a similar condition. Halzoun has also been reported in India. It is caused by eating raw bladders of catfish infected with the fluke *Isoparorchis hypselobagri* superficially resembling *Fasciolopsis* (Chandler, 1955).

Schacher *et al.* (1969) have reported the finding of living nymphs of *Linguatula serrata* in two Lebanese patients who were suffering from halzoun contracted from eating raw liver of domestic herbivores.

In the stage of established infection ova are present in the duodenal contents or faeces. The adults are usually present in the biliary passages but are occasionally found in ectopic situations. Subcutaneous abscesses in the thorax and epileptiform convulsions have been recorded.

Clinically the infection may be silent or there may be wasting and signs and symptoms of chronic liver disease, with portal hypertension a late manifestation. Mild anaemia, sometimes macrocytic with a variable eosinophil count, is usual.

The adult causes desquamation and adenomatous hyperplasia of the epithelium of the biliary ducts. Pericholangitis (neutrophils and eosinophils) and cystic dilatation of the ducts occur. Cholangitis and cholecystitis with cholelithiasis may be complications. There is fibrosis of the portal tracts and the adjacent liver tissue is compressed and inflammatory cells may be present (Biggart, 1937). Hepatomegaly is common. Biopsy of the liver may show marked infiltration with eosinophils (Facey and Marsden, 1966). Although cirrhosis of the liver is mentioned as a complication of fascioliasis we consider this as yet unproven. The portal fibrosis may lead to portal hypertension, with splenomegaly and ascites. In contrast to clonorchiasis and opisthorciasis, malignant change has not been recorded.

The ova may be found in various tissues and cause a focal inflammatory reaction with subsequent fibrosis.

Diagnostic pathology

The finding of the typical operculated eggs in the faeces ($150 \times 90 \mu$m) is diagnostic, but unfortunately these do not appear till about 3 months after infection. Duodenal intubation may reveal the ova in biliary secretions at an earlier stage of the disease (Lavier and Deschiens, 1956). There may be a leucocytosis ($12,000-40,000/$mm^3) and an eosinophilia of 40–85 per cent.

Intracutaneous and serological tests are useful but not specific or sensitive enough (Pautrizel *et al.* 1962); the haemagglutination test is reputed to be the most sensitive (Pautrizel *et al.* 1960). Serodiagnosis is more specific using subcuticular antigen which only cross-reacts with *F. gigantica* (Taillez and Korach, 1970).

DICROCOELIASIS

The small trematode *Dicrocoelium dendriticum* may be seen in the intrahepatic bile ducts. It is about 10 mm in length. The eggs (40 × 30 μm) are ingested by various species of land snails and develop into cercariae; these are eaten by ants in which the cercariae develop into metacercariae. Man is accidentally infected following ingestion of ants.

Fibrous thickening of the portal tracts has been described (Roche, 1948), and progressive jaundice has been reported (Mandoul *et al.* 1966).

PARAGONIMIASIS

Human infection is due to the lung fluke—*Paragonimus westermani*— which has a wide geographical distribution. It occurs focally throughout the Far East, South East Asia, the Pacific Islands, West Africa, and parts of South America. A new species, *P. africanus*, which is considered to be the local causative agent of paragonimiasis has been described from the Cameroons (Vogel and Crewe, 1965). Other species responsible for human infections are *P. siamensis* and *P. heterotremus* (Miyazaki and Vajrasthira, 1967).

Life cycle

The adult worm is a reddish-brown, oval fluke (about 12 mm long 6 mm wide and 5 mm thick) which lives mainly in cavities in the lungs (Fig. 3.22). From these pulmo-

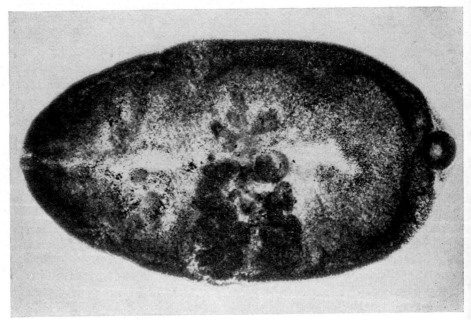

FIG. 3.22. Paragonimiasis. Adult *Paragonimus westermani*.

nary pockets the ova escape through the bronchioles and are discharged in the sputum or in the faeces if the sputum is swallowed. In other anatomical sites the ova reach the outside world only when abscesses are formed and rupture.

The contained miracidia hatch in water and enter a suitable species of snail (e.g. *Melania* spp.) in which they develop into cercariae. The cercariae emerge from the snail and penetrate the flesh of certain freshwater crabs and crayfish where they encyst. Man and susceptible animals are infected by eating these raw or partially cooked crustaceans.

After ingestion, the larvae excyst and penetrate the wall of the jejunum into the peritoneal cavity. They then pass through the diaphragm into the pleural cavity and finally burrow into the lungs where, enclosed in a cystic cavity, they grow to adult worms 5–6 weeks after ingestion.

Epidemiology

Transmission is maintained by faecal and sputum pollution of water in which the appropriate snails and vector crustacans live, and by the custom of eating uncooked crabs and crayfish soaked in alcohol, vinegar, brine, or wine. Infection can also occur during the preparation of such food, when encysted cercariae can be left on the knife or other utensils.

Although in most areas infection is higher in males than in females (Sadun *et al.* 1960; Kulka and Barabas, 1955), in the Cameroons women are infected three times as often as men. The peak age of incidence is between 11 and 35 years of age. Walton and Chyu (1959) reported that in a measles epidemic in Korea 80 per cent of *Paragonimus* infections were produced by the administration of the fluid extract of crushed crabs given medicinally to the patients.

Although a considerable domestic and wild animal reservoir of *Paragonimus* infection exists, the part it plays in the epidemiology of human disease has yet to be fully determined. The infection may persist for many years after leaving endemic areas. Little is known about immunity in man to *Paragonimus* infection. As the peak incidence is in young adults it may imply that resistance develops with age.

Pathology

Clinically the first symptoms are usually cough, expectoration of bloody sputum, and, later, signs of bronchiectasis or lung abscess. Cerebral symptoms occur in about 25 per cent of patients (Chang *et al.* 1958) and many other organs may be affected—abdominal viscera including intestine, spermatic cord, epididymis, scrotum, vaginal wall, lumbar and gluteal muscles, spinal canal, and the subcutaneous tissues of the thoracic and abdominal wall, and extremities. The pathogenesis and pathology of paragonimiasis have been reviewed by Lin and Lei (1963).

Respiratory system

The pathology in the lungs can be roughly divided into three stages—the stage of infiltration, the encysted stage, and the stage of healing or cicatrization. Secondary infection with abscess formation may supervene. The parasite tunnels in the parenchyma of the lung, usually at the periphery (Fig. 3.23). There is a leucocytic reaction around the parasite. Subpleural reddish-brown and later slate-blue cysts are formed, consisting of a wall of fibrous tissue enclosing adults and ova with an associated infiltration of eosinophils and polymorphonuclear leucocytes. Charcot–Leyden crystals may be present. The cystic lesions may communicate with one another and almost invariably with a bronchus. Absorption of the worm with collapse of the cyst walls and reparative fibrosis and calcification may occur. Areas of atelectasis and compensatory emphysema surround the cysts. Secondary infection may cause a lung abscess distal to the lesion or in the cyst itself. Fibrous thickening of the pleura with adhesions and even empyema occur.

The radiological findings may be divided into (*a*) pleural, and (*b*) parenchymatous. Thus there may be pleural thickening and obliteration of the costophrenic angle; while the parenchymatous lesions can be conveniently divided into four stages. Firstly, an infiltrative stage seen radiologically as a temporary cloudy opacity when the parasite first arrives in the lung. This is followed by a nodular stage of long duration corresponding to the formation of cystic cavities. Thirdly a fibrotic stage, with extension of

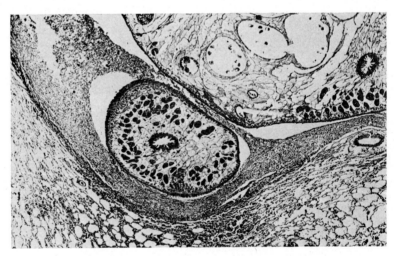

FIG. 3.23. Paragonimiasis. Lung. *P. westermani*. Note the reaction around the worm. A few ova can be seen in the uterus of the uppermost worm. (*By courtesy of Ash and Spitz.*)

the above changes and pleural involvement, occurring with the death of the parasite, and finally a stage of calcification with small calcified spots either solitary or grouped. Ova may be reaspirated and disseminated in the smaller bronchioles, where they stimulate an eosinophilic inflammatory reaction with, later, small pseudotubercle formation. Tuberculosis is a not uncommon coincidental finding in paragonimiasis.

Central nervous system

Cerebral lesions, clinically presenting as space-occupying lesions, and due to the presence of the adults, are not uncommon. The temporal and occipital lobes are most frequently involved. Burrows and, later, cysts, are found which contain usually a single disintegrating adult, ova and inflammatory cells. There is marked gliosis in the wall (Klemme, 1966; Kim and Walker, 1961). Calcification occurs and may be detected radiologically (Kim and Bahk, 1964). Changes in the cerebrospinal fluid occur. Ova have been present in about 10 per cent of cerebral cases, the cell count is raised, as is the protein, and Pandy's test is positive. The spinal cord is rarely involved but a transverse myelitis has been described.

Abdominal paragonimiasis

Free adults have been noted in the abdominal cavity with an associated fibrinous exudate containing ova and eosinophils. Adhesions with symptoms of intestinal obstruction or appendicitis may occur. Abscesses due to the presence of adult worms have been noted in the omentum, liver, spleen, adrenals, kidneys, and bladder. Ova have been seen in the urine. Ulceration of the intestine with the presence of ova in the faeces is a not uncommon finding.

Other organs

Nodules and abscesses containing adults may be found in the muscles and subcutaneous tissues of the abdomen and thighs. A psoas abscess has been recorded and lesions may occur in the vagina in females and the scrotum in males.

Diagnostic pathology

The infected sputum is characteristically sticky and bloody, usually of a dark, brownish-red colour. The characteristically shaped eggs are usually found in the sputum or in the faeces on 'direct smear' examination or by concentration techniques. In the first year of infection eggs are seldom found but there is usually an eosinophilia of about 20–30 per cent.

Precipitin reactions with crude and fractionated antigens, intradermal tests, and complement-fixation tests have all been used for diagnostic and epidemiological purposes. Cross-reactions with other trematodes limit the usefulness of these tests, although the weal is larger and more closely defined with the homologous antigen (Watten *et al.* 1960).

C. CESTODES

The cestodes, or tapeworms, are widely distributed throughout the world and the important diseases that they give rise to are (1) taeniasis, (2) cysticercosis, (3) hydatid disease, and (4) diphyllobothriasis.

TAENIASIS

Taeniasis may occur in all countries where beef or pork are eaten. The beef tapeworm—*Taenia saginata*—has a cosmopolitan distribution and is particularly common in the Middle East, Kenya, and Ethiopia. The pork tapeworm—*T. solium*—is also widely distributed and its larval stage, *Cysticercus cellulosae*, produces cysticercosis in man.

Life cycle

The life cycles and pathogenesis of *T. saginata* and *T. solium* are similar, with the exception of the classical intermediate hosts which are cattle and pigs respectively.

The adult worms live in the small intestine of man only. The respective intermediate hosts become infected by swallowing eggs or mature segments passed in the faeces. The embryos hatch, penetrate the intestinal wall and are carried by the blood stream to the skeletal muscles, as well as to the tongue, heart, diaphragm, and liver.

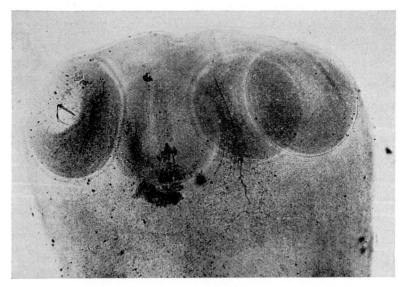

FIG. 3.24. *T. saginata.* Lateral view of scolex, showing suckers.

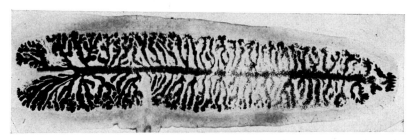

Fig. 3.25. *T. saginata*. Gravid proglottis showing numerous lateral
branches of uterus.

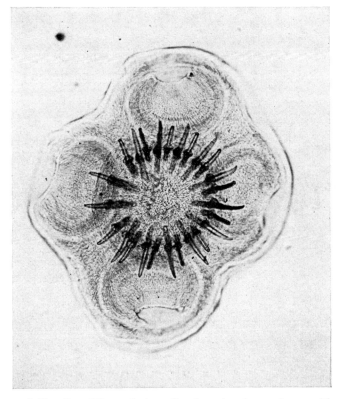

Fig. 3.26. *T. solium*. The end view of scolex, showing suckers and hooks.

The sites of predilection appear to vary in different areas, and in these sites the larvae invaginate, grow and encyst to become the infective *C. bovis* and *C. cellulosae* in about 10 weeks.

The encysted bladder-like larval forms are pearly-white in colour and contain the invaginated heads of the future adult worms. The cysts of *C. bovis* live for about 9 months, while those of *C. cellulosae* remain viable for 3–6 years.

When infected beef or pork is ingested by man, the cysts are dissolved by the gastric juices; the worms pass to the small intestine, and the heads evaginate and attach themselves to the intestinal wall, where they develop into adult worms and within 2 to 3 months gravid segments are discharged.

The adult *T. saginata* is from 4–10 m long, the head contains four suckers but no hooks (Fig. 3.24), and the uterus has eighteen to thirty compound lateral branches on each side (Fig. 3.25); while *T. solium* is only 2–8 m long, the head contains four suckers as well as a double crown of large and small hooks (Fig. 3.26), and the uterus has only seven to twelve lateral branches on each side (Fig. 3.27). Each mature segment of either worm contains a set of male and female reproductive organs. The ova of *T. saginata* and *T. solium* are morphologically indistinguishable from each other.

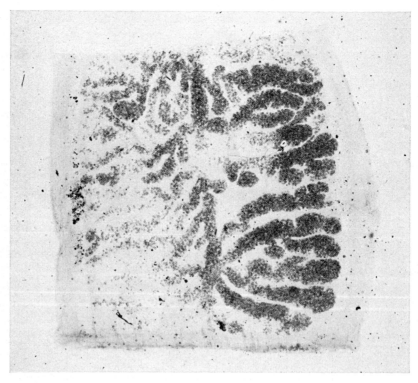

FIG. 3.27. *T. solium.* Gravid proglottis, showing few lateral branches of uterus.

Tapeworms absorb protein and B-complex vitamins from the intestinal mucosa of the host (Chandler, 1943), and are nutritionally dependent on man's carbohydrate diet for growth and reproduction. Starvation of the host reduces the number of tapeworms, retards growth and curtails the production of ova in experimental infections (Burlingame and Chandler, 1941).

Epidemiology

The world incidence of *T. saginata* is much higher than that of *T. solium* and it is estimated that in some parts of Kenya infection rates of taeniasis in man may approach 100 per cent and that 30 per cent of cattle may harbour cysticerci (Nelson *et al.* 1965).

T. saginata is uncommon in young children and the incidence increases with age (Doby *et al.* 1957). The sexes are equally susceptible—man acquires infection by eating raw or partially cooked beef, while cattle are infected while grazing on pastures, fertilized by human faeces, which are flooded with sewage-laden water. The role of birds in the transmission of the disease is not clear (Silverman, 1955). The epidemiology and other aspects of beef tapeworm infection have been reviewed by Pawlowski and Schultz (1972).

T. solium is spread by the insanitary disposal of faeces, thus providing the pigs with a ready opportunity for infection when they ingest human excreta. Man is infected when eating uncooked or insufficiently cooked pork.

Pathology

The presence of the worms (*T. saginata* or *T. solium*) in the intestinal tract may produce no symptoms. Epigastric pain and vague abdominal discomfort are not, however, unusual findings and there may be a mild eosinophilia or lymphocytosis.

In rare instances the proglottides may cause appendicitis. A tangled mass of worms can cause intestinal obstruction, and intestinal perforation with secondary peritonitis has been reported. We have seen *T. solium* expelled through a stab wound of the abdomen with little upset to the patient. Pancreatic necrosis and cholecystitis due to the presence of the worms in the pancreatic or cystic ducts may occur. Rarely, in patients with a long-standing infection, prolonged watery diarrhoea may result, fatally.

Diagnostic pathology

'Direct smear' examination of the faeces rarely reveals the typical taenia ova; the intact segments which usually are passed can be compressed between two glass slides and the branches of the uterus at their origin from the main uterine stem can be counted and a differentiation easily made between *T. saginata* (twenty to thirty-five and *T. solium* (seven to twelve). Sexual characteristics other than the number of uterine branches, can also be used to distinguish *T. saginata* and *T. solium* (Proctor, 1972). The haemagglutination test is positive in about 50 per cent of patients (Machnica-Roguska and Zwierz, 1966).

CYSTICERCOSIS

The adult *T. solium* is a parasite of man alone and the worm lives in the small intestine while the larval worm encysts in pork flesh as *Cysticercus cellulosae*. The pig acts as the classical intermediate host. Man can become infected with the larval worm, and this condition is known as cysticercosis.

Epidemiology

Direct infection of man by larval worms of *T. solium* can occur by ingestion of water and food contaminated by faeces or flies or by unclean hands transferring eggs from the adult worm carrier. Moreover, autoinfection can occur by a person carrying eggs from the anus to the mouth on the fingers or by massive regurgitation of ova from the small intestine into the stomach.

The liberated larvae penetrate the intestinal mucosa and are then carried by the blood stream to various parts of the body where they encyst, the commonest sites being the subcutaneous tissues, skeletal muscles, and the brain. The cysticercus takes about 4 months to develop and becomes enveloped in a fibrous capsule, which eventually calcifies and may be seen radiologically. *C. cellulosae* are small, oval or spherical, whitish bodies with an opalescent transparency and denser spot on one side where the scolex tapeworm head) is invaginated (Fig. 3.28). The life span of the cysticercus varies from a few months to 35 years (Dixon and Lipscomb, 1961); while the

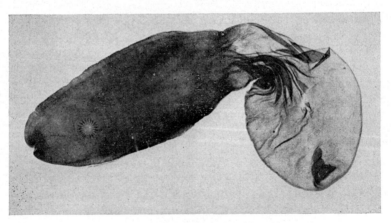

FIG. 3.28. Cysticercosis. *Cysticercus cellulosae.*

geographical distribution of cysticercosis is necessarily similar to that of *T. solium*. A monograph on the morphology and pathogenicity of *C. cellulosae* and *C. bovis* has appeared (Slais, 1970). A recent survey of the problem in Ruanda was carried out by Vanderick and Mbonyingabo (1972).

Pathology

In the migrating phase mild muscular pains and fever may be complained of. The cysticerci are well tolerated in the tissues whilst alive and symptoms may not appear until several years after infection, indeed the infection may be silent and may be detected as an incidental finding at necropsy. The clinical symptoms depend upon the site and the numbers of the cysticerci in the viscera; the organs affected are, in decreasing order of frequency, the cerebrum, meninges, skeletal muscles, cerebellum and heart. Infection may also be encountered in the eye, liver, lung, pancreas, parotid gland and peritoneum (Dixon and Lipscomb, 1961). Eosinophilia is inconstant.

The central nervous system

The clinical effects are not usually seen until several years after infection, when death of the parasite evokes a toxic inflammatory reaction. The symptomatology is protean and may include signs of increased intracranial pressure, visual and psychic disturbances, epileptiform fits, personality changes, and motor and sensory paralysis.

The cysts, which vary in size up to 20 mm, are found most frequently in the meninges of the cortex and in the frontal and parietal lobes and along the line of the middle meningeal arteries and its branches. The ventricular system may be affected and cysts may be found floating freely in the fluid. Hydrocephalus may be a sequel. Degenerative changes within the cyst may render microscopic diagnosis difficult, and confusion with *Coenurus cerebralis* is possible. Purulent meningitis and meningo-encephalitis are complications. The cyst with its one scolex is usually circular in the cerebral tissue and the death of the larvae stimulates an inflammatory reaction consisting of microglial cells and lymphocytes surrounded by sclerosed neuroglia which may extend for some distance from the cyst itself. Periarteritis and endarteritis in associated vessels occur. Calcification may or may not occur and usually commences in the scolex. X-ray of the skull may be of no help in diagnosis. Encephalomalacia with abscess formation is a complication. Infection of the spinal cord can occur but is rare (Singh *et al.* 1966).

Other organs

Either the muscles of the eye or the eye itself may be affected. Invasion occurs through the retinal or uveal vessels. The cyst may be in the vitreous humour—a sausage-shaped light-grey body 6–14mm in size—or in the substance of the tissues, and provoke a surrounding inflammatory reaction with conjunctivitis, uveitis, retinitis and choroidal atrophy as complications.

The cyst in the muscles, heart, or other organs is oat-shaped and in the superficial tissues forms smooth, firm, palpable nodules from 0·5 to 2cm in length. The larva is surrounded by three layers, (1) an inner cellular layer consisting of eosinophils, lymphocytes and plasma cells or later by histio-cytes, foam cells and giant cells, (2) a central layer of fibroblasts and scanty chronic inflammatory cells, and (3) an outer layer of vascular granulation tissue. Eventually, when calcification occurs, as is usual in muscle, the parasite is surrounded by dense fibrous tissue, with atrophy of the immediate surrounding parenchymal or muscular tissue.

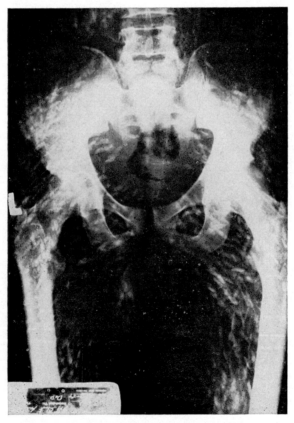

FIG. 3.29. X-ray of pelvis showing numerous calcified cysticercae in muscle. (By courtesy of Mr. Petana.)

Diagnostic pathology

Diagnosis is made on clinical grounds, either because of epileptiform symptoms in persons exposed to infection or by the presence of palpable subcutaneous cysts. The calcified cysts in the muscles of the body are detected radiologically (Fig. 3.29); calcification in the brain occurs much later and in only about 30 per cent of patients with epileptiform symptoms. Eosinophilia occurs in about 10 per cent of persons in the earlier stages of cerebral cysticercosis (Dixon and Hargreaves, 1944). There are no specific C.S.F. changes. Excision of the larva and its microscopical examination may reveal a typical cysticercus. Intradermal and precipitin tests have been used (Biagi and Tay, 1958); the haemagglutination test has given 85 per cent of positive reactions in proved cases of cysticercosis.

HYDATID DISEASE

This disease can be caused by any one of three species of the genus *Echinococcus*—*Echinococcus granulosus*, *E. multilocularis*, and *E. oligaettas*. Since the epidemiological and pathological features of these three tapeworms are very similar, a detailed description of only *E. granulosus* is given here.

Hydatid disease—caused by the larval form of *E. granulosus*—has a cosmopolitan distribution, being particularly prevalent in the sheep and cattle raising areas of the world. There are estimated to be 600–800 new cases of hydatid disease annually in Chile (Neghme and Silva, 1968) and the case histories of 144 infected Chilean children are documented (Neira *et al*. 1968).

Life cycle

The adult *Echinococcus* is a small tapeworm about 5 mm in length which inhabits chiefly the upper part of the small intestine of canines, especially dogs and wolves.

When the ova, which are passed in the faeces, are swallowed by man or other intermediate hosts (e.g. sheep, cattle, horses, etc.) the enclosed embryo is liberated in the duodenum. It penetrates the intestinal mucosa, reaches the portal circulation, and is usually held up in the liver within 12 hours to develop into a hydatid cyst. If the embryo passes the liver filter, it enters the general circulation, and thus reaches the lungs and other parts of the body. It then develops into a hydatid cyst wherever it eventually comes to rest. Two main varieties of cysts occur—the unilocular and the multilocular. The unilocular hydatid cyst develops a wall with two layers; the outer layer is thick, laminated, and elastic, while the inner layer is made up of a protoplasmic matrix containing many nuclei. Around the cyst there is a connective-tissue capsule formed by the tissues of the host. From the inner or germinal layer bulb-like processes arise which are termed *brood capsules* (Fig. 3.30). By a process of localized proliferation and invagination of the wall of the brood capsules numerous *scolices* (tapeworm heads) are produced. Each scolex is borne on a pedicle and has suckers and two rows of hooklets. Some of the brood capsules separate from the walls and settle to the bottom of the cyst as a fine granular sediment, 'hydatid sand'. As the

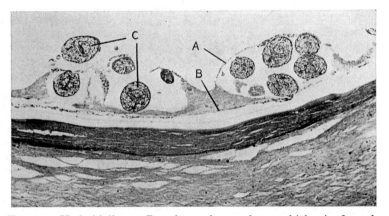

FIG. 3.30. Hydatid disease. Brood capsules are shown which arise from the single layer (A) arising from the germinal membrane (B) invaginated scolices (C) arise as buds from the inner surface of the brood capsule. The thick, laminated outer layer and the fibrous capsule formed by the host are well shown. (*By courtesy of Ash and Spitz.*)

hydatid cyst enlarges invaginations of the wall may give rise to daughter cysts and from them granddaughter cysts may arise in a similar manner.

In some cases in which no effective encapsulation occurs the daughter cysts develop as a result of evaginations of the cyst wall producing the *multilocular* or *alveolar* hydatid cyst. This variety of hydatid cyst is due to *E. multilocularis*. When the hydatid is eaten by definitive hosts—dogs, foxes, wolves, and certain other carnivorous animals—the numerous larvae develop into sexually mature worms in a few weeks. Dogs are usually infected when they eat the infected viscera of sheep or cattle. The cultivation *in vitro* of *E. granulosus* from onchosphere to cystic larva has been achieved (Heath and Smyth, 1970).

Epidemiology

Infected ova may live for weeks in shady environments but they are quickly destroyed by sunlight and high temperatures. Man acquires hydatid disease when he swallows infected ova as a result of his close association with dogs, and the insanitary habit of not washing his hands before ingesting food. Although infection is usually acquired in childhood, clinical symptoms do not appear until adult life. The dog-faeces contaminating fleeces of sheep can also be an indirect source of human infection. It has been shown that in Kenya hydatid cysts are present in more than 30 per cent of cattle, sheep, and goats, though the disease in man occurs infrequently, except in the areas of Turkana (Babero *et al.* 1963). Canines are heavily infected while light infections have been recorded in wild carnivores, e.g. jackals and hyenas. The main cycle of transmission in Kenya is between dogs and domestic livestock. Turkana tribesmen are the most heavily infected people in

Kenya because of the intimate contact between children and the large number of infected canines in the area—here dogs are used to clean the face and anal regions of babies. It has been demonstrated that hydatid fluids contain some protein components derived from the host (Kagan and Norman, 1963).

The current prevalence and distribution of hydatidosis with special reference to the Americas has been reviewed by Williams *et al.* (1971). Libyan arabs are sometimes infected by the hot wind from the desert bringing dust containing hydated ova from the faeces of dogs and jackals Fossati, 1970).

Pathology

When the ingested ovum reaches the duodenum the hexacanth embryo is released and penetrates the intestinal wall, to enter the portal circulation and thus reach the liver, the right lobe of which is the common site for a hydatid cyst to form. Cysts are usually single but may be multiple and involve the left lobe. Larvae may pass through the liver and the following organs may be affected in order of frequency: lungs (71%), muscle and cellular tissues (5%); brain (5%); spleen (2·5%); kidneys (2%); other abdominal organs (5%); bone (0·5%) and infrequently the heart, thyroid (Porges, 1971) and other organs.

In the stage of migration there may be a mild reaction with fever and urticarial skin reactions. There is an eosinophilic reaction to the larva itself which subsides as the host's fibrous tissue capsule thickens. In man the hydatid cyst may be (*a*) the classical unilocular, (*b*) the osseous or, (*c*) the alveolar. The *alveolar* multiloculated cyst is usually found in the liver and macroscopically is sponge-like in appearance. In the brain it resembles a bunch of grapes. The small cysts are usually sterile, consisting of an external laminated membrane and containing glairy, greenish fluid. They are separated from each other by the connective tissue of the host in which areas of necrosis and calcification are found. A number of the cysts must, however, be fertile as metastases are the rule.

The *classical unilocular* hydatid may be sterile but is usually fertile and surrounded by the terminal fibrosis of the host tissues following a granulomatous reaction. Rupture of fertile cysts, depending on their site, causes dissemination of daughter cysts and scolices with the formation of secondary metastatic hydatids. The escape of the cyst fluid and 'hydatid sand' may cause a severe allergic reaction with urticarial lesions, pruritus, fever, abdominal pain, dyspnoea, cyanosis, delirium, and syncope, in addition to a marked eosinophilia.

In bone the usual fibrous capsule of the host is not formed and instead of the usual rounded form of the hydatid, the cyst assumes an irregular branching shape as it penetrates the bony canals. Erosion of bone occurs and the medullary cavity is eventually invaded, where the cyst assumes its normal spherical form. The more highly vascularized areas, the epiphyses of long bones and the centres of the vertebral bodies, ilium and ribs, are most frequently affected. Radiologically they appear as rounded areas of rarefaction. Spontaneous fractures are not uncommon.

Hydatid disease of the liver

Although the infection is usually contracted in childhood a hydatid cyst of the liver may not produce symptoms until adult life and an interval of over 30 years has been known to exist between primary infection and manifestation of symptoms. The cyst is usually single in the right lobe and about 7 cm in diameter. Macroscopically it is surrounded by greyish-white fibrous and compressed liver tissue, contains a glairy fluid and thin, white daughter cysts may be identified. Exogenous cysts if present are usually bile stained. Secondary infection may occur and salmonellae and pyogenic organisms have been isolated. Rupture may occur from secondary infection, trauma or operative interference. The possible severe allergic manifestations have already been referred to and secondary abdominal echinococcosis is a grave complication. Rupture may also occur into the gall bladder, biliary tree, pleural cavity, or hepatic vein, with secondary metastases in the lungs. In a number of instances coincident hydatid disease and primary liver-cell carcinoma has ben recorded but no causal relationship has been suggested.

The alveolar type of cyst which usually occurs in the liver has been referred to above.

Hydatid disease of the lung

The cyst is most frequently found in the lung in children. Rupture may be caused by coughing, infection, or muscular strain. A chronic pulmonary abscess may result if infection is present and, if the cyst ruptures into the bronchi, scolices may be present in the sputum. Rupture may also occur into the mediastinum or pleural cavity (Rakower and Milwidsky, 1964) with secondary dissemination. Pneumothorax and haemothorax are other possible complications.

Hydatid disease of the central nervous system

In the brain the cysts are usually single and present as a space-occupying lesion. Rupture may disseminate the lesions to the subarachnoid space in the cord. The cord may also be affected by extension of a hydatid from the vertebrae or paravertebral tissues (Rayport et al. 1964). Scolices may occasionally be seen in the cerebrospinal fluid. The hydatids are usually fertile and, if suspected, angiography should be employed as a diagnostic procedure in preference to ventriculography which may puncture the cyst and disseminate the infection. Embolic secondaries have been reported from primary hydatid cysts in the lungs, liver, and heart.

Hydatid disease of the heart

This may be an unsuspected finding at autopsy (Chapadeiro et al. 1965). The cysts may, however, rupture into the percardium or into the right or left side of the heart with consequent pulmonary metastases or systemic embolism causing infarction, thrombosis, or aneurysmal formation (di Bello, 1955). Di Bello et al. (1970) reported the rupture of a hydatid cyst of the heart which caused constrictive pericarditis.

Hydatid disease of other organs

The cysts are usually single in the spleen or kidney and in the latter organ may rupture into the renal pelvis, with the consequent finding of jelly-like hydatid material in the urine associated with renal colic and dysuria (Musacchio and Mitchell, 1966). Echinococcus of the orbit has been described from Kenya (McClatchie and Manku, 1967). Bickers (1970) has described the cysts in the ovaries, broad ligament and uterus. One patient discharged *Echinococcus* cysts via the uterus and vagina. Pregnancy was obstructed in one patient.

It is of interest that Cameron and Stavely (1957) detected blood-group P substance in hydatid cyst fluids and a potent P_1 antibody has been detected in patients with the condition.

Diagnostic pathology

If the hydatid cysts rupture, their contents—hooklets, scolices, etc.—may be found in the faeces, sputum, or urine (Fig. 3.31). Eosinophilia is present but is usually moderate in degree (300–2000/mm^3) and there may be hypergammaglobulinaemia.

Radiological examination will reveal the presence and location of hydatid cysts. Recently, radioisotope scanning has been used for the detection of the sites of local lesions. Selective angiography is valuable in the diagnosis of hydatid disease of the liver (McLoughlin and Hobbs, 1970).

Intradermal and serological tests have greatly increased the chances of diagnosis.

In patients known to have hydatid disease the sensitivity of the *intradermal Casoni test* has varied from 57 to 100 per cent. A positive test may persist for 5 years or more after excision of a cyst. It has recently been suggested that the crude sterile hydatid fluid used in Casoni antigen may contain too much nitrogen to give specific results. An intradermal test antigen made up from an extract of lyophilized cyst material of *E. multilo-*

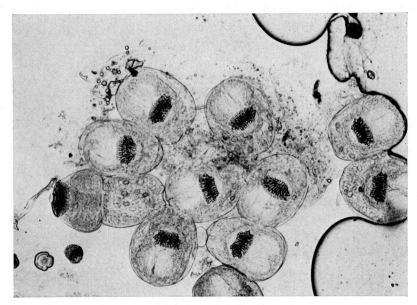

FIG. 3.31. Hydatid disease. Hydatid sand. Note hooklets.

cularis from experimental secondary infections in gerbils seems preferable (Kagan *et al.* 1966).

The *complement-fixation test* is positive in 70 per cent of patients and may persist for 2 years after elimination of the infection (Nobili *et al.* 1966).

The *indirect haemagglutination test* (Arabatzis and Papapanagrotou, 1963) is positive in 90 per cent of cases and only 2 per cent of control sera give measurable titres. Other serological tests used are the bentonite flocculation test (Norman *et al.* 1959), 71 per cent sensitive; the latex flocculation test; precipitin tests; and conglutination tests. A comparative evaluation of tests used in the diagnosis of hydatid cysts revealed the Casoni test to be the most sensitive (Roy *et al.* 1970).

It has been suggested that separation of the hydatid cyst from host tissue in the lung is so complete that little to no antigen escapes from the cyst to stimulate antibody production in the host. Moreover cysts in the lungs are frequently found to be infertile, which may be a contributory factor to the lack of antigenicity.

The indirect immunofluorescent reaction has also been successfully used in the diagnosis of hydatid disease (Moroni and Sorice, 1966). It appears to give satisfactory results (Gore *et al.* 1970). It is suggested that a scolex antigen is most satisfactory and such a preserved antigen has been prepared (Beggs and Fischman, 1970).

DIPHYLLOBOTHRIASIS

Infection by the fish tapeworm—*Diphyllobothrium latum*—is more common in the temperate zones than in the tropics, where it has only been reported from the Philippines, Madagascar, Botswana, Uganda, and southern Chile.

Life cycle

The adult, which may be 10 m long, lives in the ileum of man or of other mammals, and may have as many as 4000 segments. The gravid segments disintegrate and the ova are passed in the faeces. On reaching water the ciliated embryo escapes and is swallowed by the first intermediate host—a freshwater crustacean (*Cyclops* or *Diaptomus* species—in which it develops as a *procercoid*. When the infected crustaceans are swallowed by various freshwater fishes—salmon, pike, etc.—further development takes place in the musculature of these second intermediate hosts to form *plerocercoids* (Belding, 1965). When man and other animals eat raw fish the plerocercoid is liberated and attaches itself to the small intestine where it grows into an adult in about 6 weeks.

Epidemiology

Man is infected by eating raw or insufficiently cooked fish; the latter acquire their infections in waters contaminated by faeces containing ova of *D. latum*. As with the other tapeworms the adult fish tapeworm is long-lived.

Although infected dogs show immunity to superinfection this is not so in man.

Pathology

In the majority of infections no ill effects ensue. In a small proportion of patients, however, functional, nervous, and gastro-intestinal disturbances and evidence of vitamin deficiency and anaemia may occur. The anaemia may be non-specific and due to iron deficiency or it may be of a true Addisonian type with the infection merely a coincidental factor.

In less than 1 per cent of infected patients a megaloblastic anaemia due to the presence of the parasite may develop. It resembles pernicious or Addisonian anaemia both clinically and haematologically but tends to occur in a younger age group with both intrinsic factor and free hydrochlorlic acid sometimes present.

The tapeworm probably competes with the host for the available B_{12} in the diet or may, in some way, interfere with the secretion of intrinsic factor. The former explanation is the more likely as *D. latum* contains about fifty times as much B_{12} per gram of tissue as is found in most other tapeworms. In addition the nearer the worm is to the jejunum the greater is the likelihood of megolablastic anaemia.

Diagnostic pathology

If segments are passed in the faeces or vomitus, diagnosis can be made by seeing the typical rosette-shaped uterus when the segment is crushed between two glass slides; more commonly, however, 'direct smear' examination of the faeces will reveal the characteristic operculate ova.

DWARF TAPEWORM INFECTIONS

Three dwarf tapeworm infections can occur in man due to *Hymenolepis nana, H. diminuta,* and *Drepanidotaenia lanceolata* respectively. They all occur in the tropics and subtropics.

Life cycle

The adult of *H. nana* measures about 20mm in length and contains 100–200 segments; it lives in the upper ileum attached to the intestinal mucosa by its globular head. The gravid segments rupture in the intestine and the eggs containing an infective embryo are passed in the faeces. When ingested by man, the embryo penetrates a villus and develops into a cysticercoid larva. On maturity it ruptures the villus, returns to the intestine and attaches itself to the mucosa, giving rise to segments. About a month is required from the time of infection to the first appearance of ova in the faeces.

The adult of *H. diminuta* also inhabits the small intestine and is larger than *H. nana*. The ova containing the embryo are passed in the faeces and it undergoes a cycle of development in rat fleas and other insects. When man ingests food contaminated with these insects, the liberated larva attaches itself to the intestine.

D. lanceolata is an infection of birds and man has only very rarely been accidentally infected.

Epidemiology

H. nana is a common tapeworm of man in the south-eastern United States, parts of South America, and India. Man becomes infected by ingesting the ova in food or water that has been contaminated by human or rat faeces. The infection can also be transmitted directly from hand to mouth. Owing to the unhygienic habits of children *H. nana* is more prevalent in them, with the highest incidence occurring between 4 and 9 years (Keller *et al.* 1932). Although rats and mice are commonly infected, man is the chief source of human infections, infection being spread directly from patient to patient without utilizing an intermediate host.

H. diminuta is an infection of rats and mice, man being an incidental host. The principal source of infection is food contaminated by rat and mice droppings on which the intermediate insect hosts also thrive. When man eats food containing these insect vectors he gets accidentally infected. Human infection is chiefly in children who ingest rat fleas.

Pathology

In the majority of infected individuals the infection is silent. Abdominal pain and diarrhoea can occur and epileptiform convulsions, headache and/or strabismus have been ascribed to the absorption of toxic products of the worm.

Diagnostic pathology

A moderate eosinophilia (4–16 per cent) occurs in both *H. nana* and *H. diminuta* infections. Diagnosis is made by finding the characteristic ova in the faeces.

COENURUS CEREBRALIS

Multiceps multiceps is a canine tapeworm, the larval stages of which—*Coenurus cerebralis*—occasionally infect man. Larvae of other species of *Multiceps* have also been incriminated as causing cerebral and other manifestations in man. The adult lives in the dog's intestine and ova are passed in the faeces. Contamination of food or water may take place. The condition has been described from the Congo, Europe, Africa, and the U.S.A. Templeton (1968) recorded 14 cases in Uganda, mostly children. All presented with a solitary subcutaneous lump usually on the chest wall. Strangely enough C.N.S. involvement has not yet been reported from Africa although the majority of cases reported in world literature are from tropical Africa.

In the intestine of man the hexacanth embryo penetrates the intestinal wall and develops in tissues into the cystic form which is known as a *coenurus* (Fig. 3.32). The brain is the organ of predilection and the globular cyst containing multiple tapeworm heads (scolices) develops in about 3 months. The wall of the cyst is delicate and semi-transparent and on its inner aspect the numerous tapeworm heads develop and can be seen through the cyst wall as small opaque nodules. In contrast to the echinococcus cyst, daughter cysts are not formed. *Coenurus* cysts have also been found in the eyeball (Raper and Dockeray, 1956) and subcutaneous tissues (Fain, 1956).

Excluding Africa and the few instances in which coenuri have been described beneath the conjunctiva or in the eyeball the larvae would appear to develop mainly

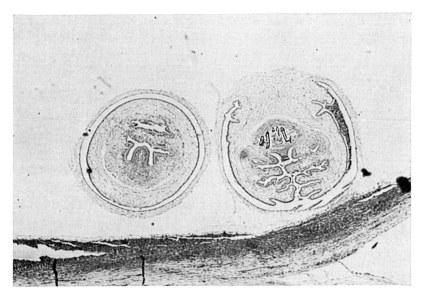

FIG. 3.32. Coenurus. Section shows two scolices in cyst excised from biceps muscle (× 30).

in tissue of the central nervous system. They have been described in the lateral ventricles and in the brain substance of the cerebellum and frontal and occipital lobes (Wainright, 1957). The clinical signs are those of a space-occupying lesion of the brain and there may or may not be changes in the cerebrospinal fluid. The protein may be raised and the lymphocytes and monocytes increased (Watson and Laurie, 1955). Scolices may be present. Man is infected by ingestion of food or water contaminated with dog's infected faeces; diagnosis is made by recovering when possible the larvae from infected tissues. Wilson (1972) described the first reported case from Ghana.

DIPYLIDIASIS

This is an accidental infection of man with the dog tapeworm—*Dipylidium caninum*. The adults live in the small intestine and the gravid segments are passed in the faeces. The ova which are liberated are then eaten by fleas and lice. Man becomes infected by swallowing infected fleas or lice from dogs or cats, in the case of children, by fondling these household pets. Mild abdominal symptoms may be complained of.

The dog tapeworm has a cosmopolitan distribution and diagnosis is made by finding the characteristically ivory-coloured gravid segments passed in the faeces or occasionally by finding the typical ova.

SPARGANOSIS

The larvae of several species of *Diphyllobothrium* are found in man and are known as spargana. Both *Sparganum mansoni* and *S. proliferum* produce sparganosis.

Life cycle

The adults are found in the intestines of carnivorous mammals, e.g. dogs, cats, and wild felines. The ova, passed in the faeces, on reaching water hatch in less than 3 weeks and release a ciliated embryo. When this is ingested by several species of *Cyclops*, it develops into a procercoid larva. When the infected *Cyclops* is ingested by man, frogs, snakes, birds, or mammals, the larvae penetrate the intestinal wall and develop into the infective plerocercoid larva (sparganum) in the muscular tissues and other parts of the body. These spargana are elongated, white ribbons measuring several centimetres in length (1–25 cm) and a few millimetres in breadth. When these plerocercoid larvae are eaten by suitable hosts the worms mature into adults in the intestine. The larval *S. proliferum* has the ability to proliferate after initial localization; thus branched proliferating processes may separate from the parent worm and develop into separate organisms. In some patients the spargana were recovered by the thousands in various parts of the body (Tashiro, 1924).

Epidemiology

Sparganosis has been reported in man from many tropical countries such as South East Asia, Africa, Madagascar, China, and South America. Man is an intermediate host and humans are infected either by ingestion of infected *Cyclops* containing the procercoid stage, by ingestion of raw infected flesh of amphibia, reptiles, birds, and mammals, or from the direct transference of infective larvae into cutaneous lesions when fresh flesh of infected vertebrates is applied as a poultice on injured surfaces (Faust, 1929).

Pathology

The condition usually manifests itself clinically by eosinophilia and localized swelling (Foster et al. 1965). The mass may enlarge in a linear fashion and a sensation of a wriggling movement may be experienced. Any tissue in the body may be affected, including the heart and brain, although spargana are usually located in the sub-cutaneous tissues (Swartzwelder et al. (1964). Orbital lesions are also common. The parasite is surrounded by fibrinoid material and eosinophils with radiating epithelioid cells and fibroblasts at the periphery. Charcot–Leyden crystals may be present (Weinstein et al. 1954). The parenchyma of the larva is essentially devoid of structures except for scattered calcareous, laminated basophilic bodies and longitudinal bundles of smooth muscle. There is an external eosinophilic wavy cuticle that rests on a subcuticular layer of radially orientated cuboidal cells with pyknotic nuclei and pale acidophilic cytoplasm. Later a cavity is formed lined by fibrous tissue in which there may be haemosiderin deposits and a sparse cellular infiltrate. Secondary infection with abscess formation is a complication (Cox, 1965). The prognosis is usually good, excluding S. proliferum infection in which thousands of larvae may be distributed throughout the body.

Diagnosis is made by finding the typical plerocercoid larvae in the affected tissues. Eosinophilia is common and usually marked.

4

Rickettsial and Viral Diseases

RICKETTSIAL DISEASES

The rickettsiae that affect man are pleomorphic coccobacillary intracellular organisms living and multiplying in arthropod tissues. In zoological status they are classified as bacteria. The rickettsial diseases of man are divided into five main groups, as shown in Table 4.1.

TABLE 4.1. *Classification of rickettsial diseases* (Horsfall and Tamm, 1965)

Disease	Causative agent	Vector	Animal reservoir
A. TYPHUS GROUP			
(i) Epidemic	*Rickettsia prowazeki*	*Pediculus humanus*	None
(ii) Brill–Zinsser disease	*R. prowazeki*	*P. humanus*	None
(iii) Murine	*R. mooseri*	*Xenopsylla cheopis*	Rat
B. SPOTTED FEVER GROUP			
(i) American spotted fevers	*R. rickettsi*	Various species of ticks	Many species of small mammals
(ii) Fievre boutonneuse	*R. conori*		
(iii) Siberian tick typhus	*R. siberica*		
(iv) Queensland tick typhus	*R. australis*		
(v) Rickettsialpox	*R. akari*	Mite	
C. SCRUB TYPHUS	*R. tsutsugamushi*	Trombiculid mites	Small mammals, mice, and field rats
D. TRENCH FEVER	*R. quintana*	*P. humanus*	None
E. Q FEVER	*Coxiella burneti*	None (Ticks)	Cattle, sheep, goats, and wild animals

Most of the rickettsial diseases have a world-wide distribution, and are not confined to the tropics. Their epidemiology and pathology are fully described in standard textbooks. We shall therefore only consider in detail in this section *scrub typhus*, which occurs throughout much of the Far East.

In the second part of this chapter, we describe the arboviruses as well as other viral diseases which though cosmopolitan in distribution are of special importance in the tropics.

Epidemic louse-borne typhus

This disease is commoner in cold climates than in the tropics. Man is the main reservoir of infection although in Tunisia serological evidence has been obtained that the rat may also be a reservoir of epidemic typhus in that country (Juminer, 1960). In Ethiopia, it has lost its overwhelming dominance and epidemic typhus is now the least common of the rickettsial infections (Reiss-Gutfreund, 1967). A small outbreak occurred in Uganda in 1972 (Sezi et al. 1972); while two substantial epidemics occurred in 1973 and 1974 in Burundi and Rwanda (WHO, 1974).

Murine typhus

Flea-borne (murine) typhus is widely distributed and occurs wherever the rat lives in close association with man, irrespective of climate. In a recent serological survey carried out in the Ivory Coast, varieties of murine typhus had an overall frequency of 4·5 per cent but were more prevalent among adults (6 per cent) and also more frequent in the coastal regions (7 per cent) (Gidel et al. 1966).

Tick typhus

An outbreak of tick typhus occurred in the coastal plain of Israel recently (Gutman et al. 1973).

Q fever

The recognition and epidemiology of this zoonosis have been thoroughly reviewed by Derrick (1964). Q fever infection has been reported in man as well as in animals such as cattle, sheep, goats, and fowls, and occurs in all five continents. Sporadic and epidemic outbreaks have been described from the Congo, Cameroons and Madagascar (Guoud, 1964) and serological evidence of its existence has been obtained in Nigeria (Collard and Udeozo, 1959), and in Saudi-Arabia (Gelpi, 1966).

Q fever in the acute form is rarely fatal but fatalities may occur more frequently in equatorial Africa (Babudieri, 1953). Death is usually due to lobar pneumonia but the exudate is mononuclear in character. Granulomatous lesions consisting of lymphocytes, polymorphs, eosinophils, and giant cells may be seen in the liver. Granulomatous lesions and colonies of rickettsial may be seen on the valves in endocarditis (Andrews and Marmion, 1959). Lesions may also be present in the spleen, testes, kidney, and brain.

Scrub typhus

Synonyms. Mite-borne typhus; tsutsugamushi disease; Japanese river or flood fever; tropical typhus; rural typhus.

This is an acute febrile disease characterized by fever, a cutaneous rash which appears on the fifth day and an eschar at the site of attachment of the trombiculid mites which transmit the disease. The causative organism is *Rickettsia tsutsugamushi* (*R. orientalis*).

Epidemiology

The disease occurs in Japan, East and South East Asia, and in the Southwest Pacific islands. The two most important vectors of scrub typhus are *Trombicula akamushi* and *T. deliensis*. The disease may be encountered in grassy fields, along the river banks, in abandoned rice fields, in forest or jungles, and in the neglected shrubby fringes between field and forest. The different epidemiological patterns of the disease are related to the influence of climatic variations on the life cycle of the trombiculid mite vectors. The seasonal occurrence of tsutsugamushi disease in Japan corresponds exactly with the time of appearance of each species of vector, *T. akamushi* in summer; *T. scutellaris* in autumn and winter; and *T. pallida* in winter and early spring (Tamiya, 1962). While the terrain of *T. akamushi* is limited to places along the rivers, other vectors seem to extend far beyond river banks. In Malaya, scrub typhus occurs throughout the year (Audy and Harrison, 1951). Cardigan *et al.* (1972) emphasized that there is a jungle cycle with a high risk to man in addition to the acquisition of disease in grasslands and scrub areas. Man is only an accidental host, while field-mice, rats, possibly other small mammals, and ground-frequenting birds are the natural hosts responsible for the continuing transmission of *R. tsutsugamushi* from infected to uninfected mites (Mackie *et al.* 1946; Trishnananda *et al.* 1966). The mites function both as vector and reservoir since transovarial transmission of rickettsial infection occurs.

The presence of scrub-typhus infection in rodents or trombiculid mites in unusual habitats in West Pakistan—e.g. alpine terrain at 10,500 ft., semidesert, and desert 'oasis greenhouse'—has been reported by Traub *et al.* 1967). Walker *et al.* (1973) have isolated *R. tsutsugamushi* from the blood and tissues of over 30 species of mammals in Malaysia.

Pathology

Scrub typhus can present in the classical manner with a primary ulcer or eschar and a high mortality in the untreated case, or in a mild and even subclinical form with no eschar and minimal mortality. The former is usually acquired in forest areas while the mild or subclinical types are contracted in rice fields or grass scrub foci (Trishnananda *et al.* 1965).

Autopsy changes are not striking. Usually the eschar is found with enlargement of the regional lymph nodes or generalized lymphadenopathy.

The body cavities contain an amount of serofibrinous fluid while the lungs show a haemorrhagic pneumonia with secondary bronchopneumonic changes. There is hepatosplenomegaly with congestion of the parenchymatous organs. No rash is usually seen.

Microscopic examination reveals that, as in other rickettsial diseases, the basic pathological lesions are found in the vascular system. There is a disseminated focal vasculitis and a perivasculitis of the smaller vessels with accumulations of monocytes, plasma cells, and lymphocytes. The most striking vascular changes are found in the heart, lungs, brain, and kidneys. An acute focal and diffuse non-suppurative myocarditis is characteristically

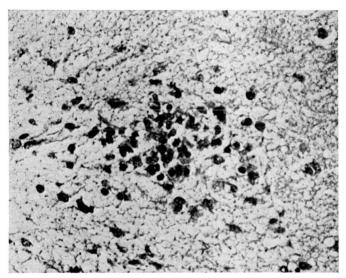

FIG. 4.1. Scrub typhus. 'A typhus nodule' in the cerebral cortex.
(*By courtesy of Ash and Spitz.*)

present. The lungs show an interstitial and lobular pneumonia. In the brain there may be a true lymphocytic meningitis and encephalitis with perivascular cuffing and formation of glial nodules (Fig. 4.1). The kidneys show focal interstitial lesions, while in the spleen and lymph nodes there is a monocytic infiltration of the pulp and sinuses and necrosis of the follicles.

Diagnostic pathology

A diagnosis of scrub typhus can be made by recovering *R. tsutsugamushi* from the blood of a patient during the febrile period by culture in living-tissue culture media or in the yolk-sac membrane of developing chick embryos. Intraperitoneal inoculation of blood or of tissue into white mice results in fatal illness, and on autopsy there is a white peritoneal exudate with numerous organisms in the peritoneal cells. The organism can also be recovered from human tissue taken at post mortem.

The most widely used serological test for the diagnosis of scrub typhus is the Weil–Felix reaction. Agglutinins for Proteus OXK but not for Proteus OX19 or OX2 appear in the patient's serum about the tenth day of the disease reaching a maximum titre by the end of the third week after which they rapidly decline. Serial examination reveals a four-fold or greater rise in titre. The complement-fixation test has also been used for diagnostic and sero-epidemiological surveys (Shishido, 1964). Indirect immuno-fluorescence employing smears of rickettsiae as antigen can be used for the specific diagnosis of scrub typhus (Elisberg and Bozeman, 1966). Gan *et al.* (1972) have shown that the filter paper technique of collecting blood specimens for scrub typhus indirect fluorescent antibody titre, works as well as serum. The technique is reliable and reproducable.

The results obtained by Weil–Felix tests from patients with the various forms of typhus are summarized in Table 4.2.

TABLE 4.2. *Weil–Felix reaction in typhus fevers*

TABLE	STANDARD STRAINS		
Typhus Fever	OX19	OX2	OXK
Mite-borne	−	−	+ + +
Tick-borne	− to + +	− to + +	−
Louse-borne —	+ + + to −	+ + to −	−
Flea-borne —			

In the majority of cases of louse-borne and flea-borne typhus OX19 is agglutinated to a high titre; while in tick-borne typhus OX19 and OX2 are only agglutinated to a low titre.

VIRAL DISEASES

THE ARBOVIRUSES

The arthropod-borne viruses (arboviruses) may cause various syndromes in man or, alternatively, may present as atypical or subclinical infections only recognizable by antibody studies. The majority are zoonoses and about 70 out of the 200 different arboviruses identified are known to cause disease in man. The definitive diagnosis depends upon isolation of the virus from patients early in the infection, with demonstration of a rise in titre of antibodies to the particular agent in at least two sera taken during the acute and convalescent stages of the disease.

Three main groups of arboviruses have been serologically defined as Groups A, B, and C, and the important viruses within these groups are listed in Table 4.3. Since the majority produce non-fatal infections there is little information on the pathology of these diseases, and in this section we shall therefore limit ourselves to some of the arboviruses the pathological features of which have been adequately described.

TABLE 4.3. *Some clinically recognized arboviruses in the tropics* (Horsfall and Tamm, 1965)

Group A	Group B	Group C	Other (grouped and ungrouped)
Chikungunya	Yellow fever	Apeu	Bunyamwara group
Mayaro	Dengue	Caraparu	Bwamba group
O'Nyong-Nyong	St. Louis encephalitis	Itaqui	Phlebotomus fever group
Venezuelan equine encephalitis	Japanese encephalitis	Madrid	Simber group—Oroponche
Western equine encephalitis	Murray Valley encephalitis	Marituba	Tacaribe group—Junin
Eastern equine encephalitis	West Nile	Murutucu	Vesicular stomatitis group
	Ilhéus	Nepuyo	Colorado tick fever
	Spondweni	Oriboca	Crimean-Central Asian haemorrhagic fever
	Uganda S-H336	Ossa	
	Wesselsbron		Kemerovo
	Tick-borne encephalitis		Rift Valley fever
	Kyasanur Forest disease		California group
			Guama group
			Nakiwogo
			Nairobi sheep disease

Because infection usually produces prolonged immunity, attack rates in all age groups indicate the introduction of a new arbovirus, while disease confined to children implies reintroduction of virus or overflow from a continuous animal cycle to susceptible humans. Mosquitoes are the most common vectors of arboviruses, ticks the next most common, and *Phlebotomus* and *Culicoides* the least frequently involved (WHO, 1967; Metselaar *et al.* 1974). A computer-simulated model has been designed to express in quantitative terms the factors which play a role in the transmission cycle of an arbovirus (De Moor and Steffens, 1970). Parker *et al.* (1972) have reviewed the current epidemiological literature on viruses of the California arbovirus group.

ARBOVIRUSES: GROUP A

All the viruses in this group (about seventeen) have a number of general properties common to each other and to the rest of the arboviruses. The natural vectors or suspected vectors for all the known Group A viruses are mosquitoes. Clinically recognizable diseases of man have been described for (i) *Chikungunya virus* which occurs in Africa, Thailand, Cambodia, and India (Ross, 1956; Hammon *et al.* 1960; Moore *et al.* 1974). Chikungunya virus in Uganda is probably due to an intensive epizootic in forest monkeys transmitted by *Ae. africanus* with incidental leakage to man by inefficient vector systems which alone could not maintain an outbreak (McCrae *et al.* 1971). Mouse embryo cell cultures have been used for the primary isolation of chikungunya virus (David-West, 1972); (ii) *Mayaro virus* which is found in Trinidad, Brazil, and Bolivia (Anderson *et al.* 1957; Schmidt *et al.* 1959); (iii) *O'Nyong-Nyong virus* which produced an explosive epidemic disease in East Africa (Haddow *et al.* 1960); (iv) *Venezuelan equine encephalitis virus.* This is an epizootic of horses which affects man, and human outbreaks with fatalities have occurred in Venezuela, Colombia, and Panama (PAHO, 1963). Scherer (1972) has reported on ecological studies of Venezuelan encephalitis virus in Mexico. The subject was reviewed in the *Lancet* (1973).

WESTERN EQUINE ENCEPHALITIS VIRUS (WEE)

This virus causes an encephalitis of variable severity. Fatal human cases are more common in children than in adults. It occurs in North America, Brazil, Guyana, Argentina, Mexico, and Eastern Europe. *Culex tarsalis* is the principal vector (Hammon *et al.* 1941).

Pathology

The brain and cord are oedematous. Small areas of focal necrosis with destruction of neurones are found in the basal nuclei, midbrain, and cerebellum. Microscopic haemorrhages are seen in the pons, medulla, and basal ganglia. Perivascular cuffing is also observed (Quong, 1942; Finley *et al.* 1955). Specific diagnosis is based on isolation of the virus or on serological tests.

EASTERN EQUINE ENCEPHALITIS VIRUS (EEE)

Eastern equine encephalitis virus produces a severe form of encephalitis in man, with highest epidemic attack rates in children. It is found in North,

Central, and South America, including the Caribbean. The vector is a mosquito. The first isolation of (EEE) virus was reported from Trinidad by Corniou *et al.* (1972) from a patient with encephalitis.

Pathology

Oedema and generalized congestion of the visceral organs are found at autopsy. There is a diffuse meningo-encephalitis with destruction of neurones, polymorphonuclear infiltration, and marked perivascular cuffing. Involvement of the basal nuclei and brain stem is very marked (Farber *et al.* 1940).

ARBOVIRUSES: GROUP B

The diseases most important to man result from infections with arboviruses of this group, most of which have mosquitoes as their vectors, with the exception of a subgroup which are tick-borne. Antigenic cross-reactivity is marked in the group B viruses, so that in areas where there is a high endemicity, e.g. tropical Africa, serological diagnosis may be difficult, and the most rapid and definitive diagnostic method of active infection is by virus isolation. Many infections are symptomless and pathological data consequently are scanty. Clinically recognizable disease has been described for the following viruses in this group: (i) *Murray Valley encephalitis virus* which occurs in Australia and New Guinea producing a high attack rate in children and with clinical and pathological manifestations similar to Japanese virus infection (Robertson, 1952); (ii) *West Nile virus* has been isolated in Africa, the Near East, and India. It produces a dengue-like syndrome (Taylor *et al.* 1956; Klingberg *et al.* 1959); (iii) *Ilhéus virus* is found in South and Central America and Trinidad (Spence *et al.* 1962; Causey *et al.* 1961); (iv) *Spondweni, Uganda S-M336* and *Wesselsbron* viruses respectively occur in South Africa and Nigeria (Kokernot *et al.* 1957; Macnamara *et al.* 1959), Uganda and South Africa (Dick and Haddow, 1952; Smithburn *et al.* 1957), and in South Africa and Portuguese East Africa (Smithburn *et al.* 1957; Kokernot *et al.* 1960). Gordon Smith *et al.* (1974) have shown that the general trend of arbovirus infections in Sarawak—mostly Japanese B encephalitis and dengue—was of highest infection rates in coastal, estuarine and inland forest areas. Urban areas had the lowest rates.

YELLOW FEVER

Yellow fever is an acute infectious disease of sudden onset and variable severity caused by a virus transmitted by mosquitoes. It is characterized by fever, jaundice, haemorrhagic manifestations, and albuminuria. Recovery leads to lasting immunity.

Epidemiology

Yellow fever is endemic in large areas of South America and tropical Africa (WHO, 1972 and 1973). Epidemics occur from time to time, such as that in the Sudan and Ethiopia (Serie, 1963), Senegal (Chambon *et al.* 1967), and Nigeria (Monath *et al.* 1974; Lee *et al.* 1974).

There are two main epidemiological forms of yellow fever: (1) *Urban type*. The mosquito vector is *Aëdes aegypti*, which is primarily a domestic mosquito which breeds in or near houses, with the female preferring to lay her eggs in water collecting in artificial containers such as old tins, etc.

The virus cycle is Man–Mosquito–Man; this method of spread requires large numbers of susceptible hosts and hence tends to occur in large towns. Villages, with frequent passage of people from one village to another, will also be suitable for this type of spread. Urban type yellow fever can be effectively controlled by anti-mosquito measures.

(2) *Jungle type*. This may occur either in endemic or epizootic forms. In the endemic form, the disease, which is primarily one of monkeys, is almost constantly present, and sporadic cases of human infection occur from time to time. The primary spread of the virus is from monkey to monkey, via *A. africanus*: this mosquito lives in the tops of trees, and only occasionally will bite man, for example when a tree is felled.

However, there is another way in which the yellow fever virus can be transmitted from the monkey to man: certain monkeys have the habit of raiding crops, particularly bananas; another mosquito, *A. simpsoni*, occurs on the edges of forests, and becomes infected by biting infected raiding monkeys, and then later bites the farmer when he collects his crops. *A. simpsoni* thus acts as a so-called 'Link-host'. Monath and Kemp (1973) have emphasized the importance of non-human primates in the epidemiology of yellow fever in Nigeria.

In South America the principal vectors belong to *Haemagogus* species. An interesting geographical study of yellow fever in Latin America was published by Ward in 1972. 'Jungle' yellow fever can occur as an epizootic among monkeys in regions where the disease has been absent for some years, resulting in a high mortality among the indigenous monkeys. Such an epizootic brings with it, of course, the chance of human outbreaks of the disease. There is evidence to suggest that the presence of extensive immunity to other Group-B viruses modifies the severity and spread of yellow fever (Macnamara *et al.* 1959).

The virus

Unmodified yellow fever virus attacks the cells of all three embryonic layers (pantropic). All strains show some degree of neurotropism, but the severity of the illness is largely due to the degree of viscero-tropism shown; i.e. the degree of affinity shown for the abdominal viscera, particularly the liver. The degree of virulence shown by the virus can be modified by serial passage through mouse brain, or by culture in chick embryos or in tissue culture.

The virus actually multiplies in the mosquito host: after biting an infected person or monkey, the mosquito itself becomes infective after an interval of about 12 days (extrinsic incubation period) and remains infective for the rest of its life. Mosquitoes are the only insects able to transmit infection.

Pathology

The virus enters the body by the bite of an infected mosquito and then passes to the regional lymphatic glands, where it multiplies. After some days it enters the blood and the most severe pathological effects are seen in the liver, kidney, and lymphoreticular tissue, including the bone marrow. Petechial haemorrhages in the skin, epistaxis, haematemesis (black vomit), and melaena are common manifestations of the disease and at autopsy haemorrhages may be found in any organ in the body. These symptoms may occur early and may be due to the direct effect of the virus on capillary endothelium or to the marked prothrombin deficiency which occurs with hepatic involvement. A leucocytosis may occur in the early stages but is followed by a leucopenia which is correlated with lymphocytic depletion in the spleen and degenerative lesions in the bone marrow.

A progressively increasing albuminuria is usual and is correlated with the pathological changes of an acute tubular necrosis. As these changes occur early in yellow fever it is most probable that the virus itself damages the tubular cells. This, however, has never been proven and death in the first 6 days of the infection is usually considered hepatic in origin, with renal lesions predominating after this stage (Elton *et al.* 1955). Bile pigment, bile salts and casts are also usually present in the urine in the early stages. Proteinuria, haemoglobinuria, and oliguria may progress to anuria, uraemia, coma and death. At autopsy the kidney is swollen with cortical pallor and medullary congestion. Depending upon the duration of the illness the changes in the epithelial cells of the proximal tubules may vary from fatty change in the early to coagulation necrosis in the later stages. Basophilic concretions containing calcium and disintegrated products of haemoglobin may be present as casts in the tubules.

In the heart, in addition to endocardial, myocardial or epicardial haemorrhages, fatty change is usual and may account for Faget's sign—a relatively slow pulse in spite of a raised temperature.

There may also be haemorrhages in the pancreas and lungs and a mild perivascular mononuclear cuffing has been described in the brain. By far the most striking and characteristic changes, however, occur in the liver. At post mortem the liver is yellowish in colour and of soft consistency. In experimentally induced yellow fever in monkeys the earliest histopathological change is said to be a hyaline necrosis of the Kupffer cells (Smetana, 1962). This is rarely seen in man and the usual lesion is 'midzonal' necrosis of the parenchymal cells of the liver (Fig. 4.2). Frequently, however, almost

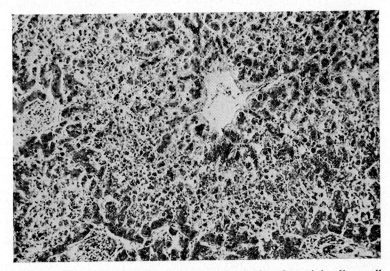

FIG. 4.2. Yellow fever. Mid-zonal necrosis—a rim of surviving liver cells can be seen around the central vein and portal tracts. Note the 'pepper and salt' distribution. Fatty change can be seen in the liver cells. (*By courtesy of Ash and Spitz.*)

the complete lobule may be involved, but a rim of surviving liver cells around the portal tracts and centrilobular veins usually points to the diagnosis. The liver cells undergo a patchy eosinophilic hyaline necrosis, the nucleus disappears and a dense acidophilic mass remains— this is the Councilman body, which is not pathognomonic for yellow fever and may be seen in other forms of hepatitis. The patchy or focal degeneration of individual liver cells in the cords gives the so-called 'salt and pepper' appearance of the liver on examination with a low-power objective. A number of Kupffer cells may appear to have engulfed degenerative parenchymal cells and show this Councilman change (Bugher, 1951). The reticulin pattern is usually normal and post-necrotic cirrhosis is not considered to be a sequel of yellow fever. Fatty change is usual in the hepatocytes. In addition to enlarged eosinophilic nucleoli, acidophilic intranuclear inclusions (Torre's bodies) may be present. Bile-duct proliferation does not occur and bile retention is most unusual, as is a cellular inflammatory infiltration. Liver biopsy will show the characteristic changes only in the acute stage of the illness. Ballooning and feathery degeneration of the hepatocytes are prominent in biopsy material in addition to the eosinophilic necrosis around which there may be an infiltration of cells with strap-like nuclei and occasional mononuclear cells. Iron pigment can be detected in Kupffer cells and traces of lipofuscin in both Kupffer and parenchymal cells. Glycogen is very much reduced. Later probably from the twelfth day onwards the changes are those of a non-specific hepatitis with eosinophilic and ochre bodies in the sinusoids (Francis *et al.* 1972). To sum up: the diagnostic features which we have found useful in diagnosing yellow fever from the examination of the liver are:

(1) A rim of surviving liver cells around the portal tracts and centrilobular veins.
(2) The presence of the Councilman lesion and enlarged eosinophilic nucleoli in the nuclei of surviving liver cells.
(3) The absence of both bile retention and evidence of an inflammatory reaction.

The severe liver damage influences the prothrombin content of the blood and hypoglycaemia is usual. Pneumonia, parotitis, cutaneous infections, and renal abscesses are frequent complications. In the adrenal, necrosis of the cortical cells of the outer fascicular zone has been described.

Diagnostic pathology

Virus isolation from the blood up to the fourth day of the disease is the diagnostic procedure of choice (Macnamara, 1954). Isolation of virus is by intracerebral inoculation of mice. Demonstration of a rising titre of antibodies in the serum during the course of the illness may be used bearing in mind that there may be cross-reaction with other viruses of the Group-B arbovirus group. Neutralization, complement fixation, or haemagglutination inhibition tests are also employed, depending on the particular circumstances and the likelihood of previous exposure to other Group-B viruses. To confirm that the infection is due to yellow fever, the rise in HI, CF, and N antibodies should be greater for yellow fever virus than for other group B arboviruses. Histology of the liver in fatal cases establishes the diagnosis. Occasionally virus can be isolated from this organ (Anderson and Wattley, 1955).

DENGUE VIRUSES

Synonyms. Break-bone fever; haemorrhagic fever.

Dengue viruses produce, in general, a non-fatal, short, febrile illness, characterized by severe myalgia and joint pains. The occurrence of haemorrhagic phenomena with a significant mortality, especially in childhood, has been a feature of recent epidemics in South East Asia. There are four main serotypes of Dengue viruses, numbers 1, 2, 3, and 4.

Epidemiology

A. aegypti is the established mosquito vector of the dengue viruses responsible for dengue fever which is distributed throughout large areas of the world. In recent years, epidemics of dengue with haemorrhagic phenomena—*South East Asian haemorrhagic fever*—have been reported from widely spaced regions—in Calcutta, the Philippines, Thailand, Malaysia, and Singapore (Chauduri *et al.* 1964; Hammon *et al.* 1961; Rudnik *et al.* 1965; Goldsmith *et al.* 1965), and dengue viruses have been isolated from *A. aegypti* during these epidemics (Halstead *et al.* 1963). The epidemics have an urban distribution with cases clustered in the crowded, poorer, central districts of cities. The disease is usually seen in races of oriental origin, and haemorrhagic fatal manifestations are confined to persons under 15 years of age with a peak incidence in the 3–6 year group.

A fatal case of dengue haemorrhagic fever in an American child has recently been described from Thailand (Russell *et al.* 1967). In 1972, 23,831 cases were reported from Thailand with a fatality rate of 2·9 per cent (WHO, 1974). Some outbreaks of haemorrhagic fever have been caused by the arbovirus *Chikungunya* (Group A). On the whole the syndrome associated with *Chikungunya* infection is milder than haemorrhagic dengue. The subject of mosquito-borne haemorrhagic fever of South and South East Asia has been admirably reviewed by Johnson *et al.* (1967). The pathogenic mechanisms in dengue haemorrhagic fever were described by an international study group. It has been postulated that the dengue shock syndrome occurs as a result of a second infection with a heterologous dengue virus and that an immunological mechanism is involved in the pathogenesis of the syndrome (WHO, 1973).

Pathology

Neither the gross nor microscopical findings in fatal cases of *South East Asian haemorrhagic fever* are pathognomonic, although haemorrhages beneath the capsule of the liver and in the endocardium of the left ventricle are suggestive of the condition. Very rarely the virus may be isolated from liver tissue. Clear or blood-stained effusions are usual and focal or subserous haemorrhages may be found in any organ. A protein-rich gelatinous, retroperitoneal oedema has been described.

In the reticulo-endothelial system there are necroses and marked lymphoid depletion in the spleen and lymphnodes. Erythrophagocytosis and phagocytosis of lymphocytes with proliferation of reticulum cells and giant cells have been described. There is an increase of megakaryocytes in the cords of the spleen, lungs, and glomeruli of the kidney. In the lungs there is an interstitial pneumonitis consisting of lymphocytes, histiocytes and plasma cells. In the liver focal necroses occur and acidophilic bodies 8–12 μm in diameter may be seen lying free in the sinusoids (Nelson, 1960; Bhamarapatvi *et al.* 1967). Haemorrhagic necrosis of the adrenal and focal necroses in the pituitary have been noted but are uncommon. Central nervous system involvement is rare. The kidneys are swollen with a pale cortex and congested medulla. Proteinaceous material and red blood cells may be present in Bowman's space and the tubular lumina. The features of acute tubular necrosis may be present (Tan *et al.* 1967).

During the febrile stage there is leucopenia and thrombocytopenia, later followed by a leucocytosis. The viraemia is brief and the virus may be isolated by intracerebral inoculation in suckling mice. The prothrombin time is prolonged and clot retraction is poor. The marrow is hypocellular and maturation arrest of megakaryocytes has been described. The transaminases may be raised indicating liver damage. Albumin, red cells and casts are present in the urine in the early stages; later oliguria or anuria may occur. Definitive laboratory diagnosis is determined by virological and serological tests. A disappearance of B_{1C}-globulin occurs both in the acute and convalescent phase of the disease (Tuchinda and Jayavasu, 1967).

ST. LOUIS ENCEPHALITIS VIRUS

Infection with this virus usually runs a benign course with fever and headache lasting a few days. The disease is found mostly in the United States (Eherenkranz *et al.* 1963), but cases have been reported from Trinidad, Panama, and Jamaica (Anderson *et al.* 1957; Galindo *et al.* 1959; Irvine *et al.* 1963). The virus also occurs in many countries of South America. Wild birds and bird-feeding mosquitoes maintain the infection while man is the incidental dead-end host. *Culex* mosquitoes are the important vectors.

Pathology

In the elderly a more severe illness may occur resulting in an encephalitis with permanent sequelae. A leucocytosis is found and the cerebrospinal fluid shows a raised pressure and a moderate increase in cells and protein.

At autopsy the brain and spinal cord are congested and may exhibit small haemorrhages. Neuronal damage occurs mainly in the mid-brain stem (Shinner, 1963).

The virus is rarely recovered from blood and the diagnosis rests on a rise in titre of specific antibodies.

JAPANESE ENCEPHALITIS VIRUS

Synonyms. Type B encephalitis; JE.

The majority of infections are inapparent or mild. The disease occurs in China, Korea, Japan, Malaya, Singapore, and India. The virus is spread from rural to urban areas by viraemic birds (Scherer *et al.* 1959). There are two peaks of incidence—under 9 years and over 60 years (Matsuda, 1962). The most efficient vectors are *Culex tritaeniorhynchus* and *C. gelidus* and the preferred vertebrate hosts are birds and domestic animals, e.g. pigs; man being only an incidental host. The highest infection rates in man appear in populations which have close contact with both pigs and ricefields. Rodents are also susceptible to JE virus (Williams and Imlarp, 1972).

Pathology

Frank encephalitis with serious sequelae, e.g. mental, motor, and cerebrellar impairment, usually occurs in young children. A leucocytosis with a moderate neutropenia is found and the cerebrospinal fluid shows a rise in protein content and a mononuclear pleocytosis. The brain is oedematous and congested; there is a generalized degeneration of neurones with necrosis and perivascular cuffing. The Purkinje cells are destroyed and severe involvement of the spinal cord, similar to that in poliomyelitis, occurs (Zimmerman, 1946). The specific diagnosis is made by virus isolation or serological tests.

TICK-BORNE ENCEPHALITIS VIRUSES

This group includes (i) Tick-borne encephalitis, (ii) Louping ill, (iii) Omsk haemorrhagic fever, (iv) Kyasanur Forest disease, (v) Negishi virus, (vi) Pavassan virus, (vii) Langats virus. Most of these viruses are commoner in the temperate than in tropical climates.

TICK-BORNE ENCEPHALITIS (TBE)

Synonyms. Russian spring-summer encephalitis; Far Eastern encephalitis; Central European tick-borne encephalitis.

Tick-borne encephalitis occurs in the U.S.S.R., Central Europe, and the Far East. Man acquires the infection when bitten by infected ticks or by drinking unpasteurized goat's milk. The principal vector ticks are *Ixodes persucaltus* and *I. ricinus*. The disease may be inapparent, mild, or fatal and at autopsy the usual changes of encephalitis are seen in the brain but the involvement of the spinal cord is often also severe.

KYASANUR FOREST DISEASE

The virus of Kyasanur Forest disease has only been found in Mysore State, India. The disease occurs more frequently in the dry season and in persons working in the forest (Anderson, 1963). The principal vector is the tick *Haemaphysalis spinigera*. Small mammals and monkeys have been shown to be reservoir hosts (Boshell, 1969).

Pathology

Headache, fever, myalgia, gastrointestinal haemorrhage, bronchiolitis, and mild encephalitis make up the clinical picture; leucopenia thrombocytopenia, impaired liver function and albuminuria may occur (Chatterjea *et al.* 1963). In the cerebrospinal fluid there may be a pleocytosis and increased protein.

The pathological findings have been described by Iyer *et al.* (1959). There is a moderate parenchymal degeneration of the liver and kidneys, massive or patchy haemorrhagic consolidation of the lungs, and a moderate to marked prominence of the reticulo-endothelial tissue of the spleen and liver, with evidence of active erythrophagocytosis. Varying amounts of recently altered blood are found in the intestines without any gross lesions to account for it. The brain reveals no gross or microscopical abnormalities. Virus can be isolated from the liver, spleen, kidney, lung, heart, and skeletal muscles, but not from the brain.

GROUP C VIRUSES

The Group-C viruses have only been isolated from Brazil, Trinidad, Panama, and the U.S.S.R., while antibodies in man have been reported from Africa (Casals and Whitman, 1961; Causey, 1966). The illness they produce is mild and no deaths have been recorded.

OTHER VIRUSES

Many other viruses, some grouped, and others as yet ungrouped are known to produce disease in man. The illness is usually mild and large segments of the population show neutralizing antibodies to the various viruses resulting from sub-clinical infections.

(i) BUNYAMWERA GROUP

Bunyamwera virus has been isolated in Uganda, South Africa, and Nigeria (Smithburn *et al.* 1946; Bearcroft *et al.* 1963); *Ilesha virus* in

Nigeria; *Germiston virus* in South Africa; and *Guaroa virus* in Colombia and Brazil. Neutralizing antibodies against the various members of the Bunyamwara group have been found in residents of Uganda, South Africa, Mozambique, Nigeria, Ghana, Liberia, Ethiopia, Brazil, Colombia, and the Amazon Valley.

(ii) BWAMBA GROUP

Bwamba virus was isolated from Uganda (Smithburn *et al.* 1941) and neutralizing antibodies have been detected from Uganda, Tanganyika, Mozambique, Nigeria, and other parts of Africa. No fatal cases have been reported.

(iii) PHLEBOTOMUS FEVER GROUP

The diseases caused by viruses in this group are non-fatal and no patholo- gical accounts are available. The vectors are various species of *Phlebotomus* and the distribution of the disease is limited between the latitudes 25° and 45° N. There are two types of viruses the Sicilian and the Neapolitan.

(iv) SIMBUM GROUP—OPORONCHE VIRUS

Oporonche virus disease occurs in Trinidad and Brazil. It is a non-fatal illness with a symptomatology similar to that of the other arboviruses.

(v) TACARIBE GROUP—JUNIN VIRUS (Argentinian haemorrhagic fever)

Argentinian haemorrhagic fever is caused by the Junin virus (Arribalzaga, 1955) and Bolivian haemorrhagic fever by the Machupo virus (MacKenzie *et al.* 1963; Johnson *et al.* 1965). Severe and sometimes fatal disease is characterized by fever myalgia, haemorrhagic manifestations and renal involvement. Machupo virus has been isolated from small rodents (*Calomys callosus*), and elimination of these dramatically interrupted a continuing human epidemic.

Pathology

Laboratory investigations show a marked leucopenia, thrombocytopenia, a raised blood urea, albuminuria, and casts in the urine. At autopsy marked congestion and oedema of all the viscera especially of the liver and kidney is seen. Microscopically there is, in the kidneys, a granular degeneration of the epithelial cells of the convoluted tubules with hyaline and blood casts and intratubular haemorrhages. The hepatic cells also show granular degeneration and oedema around the central vein (Pirosky *et al.* 1959). The pathology of Bolivian haemorrhagic fever has been well described by Child *et al.* (1967). Congestion and interstitial haemorrhages occurred in various organs especially the gastro-intestinal and central nervous systems. Focal coagulative necrosis may occur in the liver and acidophilic bodies in the Kupffer cells and free in the sinusoids were constant findings. Phagocytosis was widespread in the reticulo-endothelial system and an interstitial pneumonia was usual.

(vi) RIFT VALLEY FEVER VIRUS

This virus causes a non-fatal disease in man, characterized by fever, myalgia, severe headache, epistaxis, and occasionally ocular complications. It is widespread in Central and South Africa. The vectors are mosquitoes and the cycle is maintained through wild and domestic animals. Man in infected through contact with sick animals by inhalation of virus; thus the disease is not uncommon in farmers, shepherds, butchers, and veterinarians (Miller et al. 1963).

OTHER VIRAL INFECTIONS

Of the many other viral infections that occur in the tropics the following are of particular importance and are described in some detail:— (1) Lassa fever, (2) rabies, (3) smallpox, (4) chickenpox, (5) trachoma, (6) lympho-granuloma venereum, (7) measles, (8) Margburg disease, (9) herpes simplex, (10) infectious mononucleosis, (11) poliomyelitis and other enteroviruses, (12) slow virus infections (WHO, 1974).

LASSA FEVER

In 1969 a new virus disease was reported from Lassa in North Eastern Nigeria (Frame et al. 1970). It caused the death of two missionary nurses and the grave illness of a third. The third patient was flown to the United States where she recovered. Plasma from this patient was effective in the treatment of a patient who acquired the infection whilst working with tissue cultures and mice infected with the virus (Leifer et al. 1970). The character-istics of the virus have been described by Buckley and Casals (1970) and Buckley et al. (1970). It was shown to be a new member of the recently proposed arenovirus group which includes lymphocytic choriomeningitis and the Tacaribe group viruses (Henderson et al. 1972) which are lipid solvent-sensitive, ribonucleic acid-containing viruses.

The typical disease picture in the original cases includes: high fever, toxicity, headache, vomiting, diarrhoea, severe pharyngitis with white patches in the pharynx, soft palate and tonsillar pillars, cough, epigastric pain and tenderness and bleeding tendency. Cervical lymphadenopathy, pleural effusion, myocarditis and renal failure were also described. A further outbreak of the condition in Jos, Nigeria, in 1970, was reported by Troup et al. (1970) and it was suggested that the prognosis might not be so grave as originally considered and that Lassa fever might include a spectrum of disease ranging from the asymptomatic through a mild disease to a serious and fatal illness. A further outbreak has been reported from Liberia (Editorial, 1972) and all evidence would suggest that the infection is widespread throughout West Africa. Transmission of infection can occur from person to person probably through the respiratory tract. Dr. J. M. Troup performed the two autopsies on which our knowledge of the pathology is based. An accident during these examinations led to her death from the condition she was investigating. Tribute to Dr. Troup has been paid in an article by Edington and White (1972). Apart from direct transmission from a patient and inoculation at post mortem the exact mode of transmission is unknown. Respiratory and urine droplet spread may be a likely method. *Mastomys natalensis*, the common domestic and peridomestic rodent of West Africa is a reserviour of infection. The relative importance of rodent-to-man transmission has not been established (*Lancet*, 1974). The incubation period is about one week.

Diagnosis

Lassa fever should be suspected in patients with fever, pharyngitis, intestinal upset, a bleeding tendency and albuminuria with casts in the urine. The clinical aspects have been described by White (1972). A leucopenia may be present but the white cell count is variable. Liver function tests may indicate parenchymal cell damage and disturbance of normal coagulation mechanisms occurs. Renal failure has been described. Definitive diagnosis is made by virus isolation from the blood and is positive early in the disease. The virus can also be isolated from tissue at necropsy. The complement fixation test does not become positive until the fifteenth day and is negative in patients dying of the disease (Carey *et al.* 1972). Strict isolation and nursing precautions must be taken in suspected cases and post-mortem examinations should be performed with caution. Virological studies must be undertaken in a maximum security laboratory.

Pathology

The post-mortem findings would appear to bear a certain relationship to those described in the dengue group of viruses, Omsk haemorrhagic fever and Argentinian, Bolivian and Thai haemorrhagic fever (Child *et al.* 1967; Bhamarapravati *et al.* 1964). Death usually occurs about the tenth day of the disease. The most striking pathological findings were in the *liver* and *spleen*. In the liver there were focal areas of eosinophilic necrosis of parenchymal cells without an inflammatory exudate (Fig. 4.3). Eosinophilic and brownish bodies were seen in the sinusoids, the latter resembling the ochre bodies described by Villela (1941) in patients dying in the late stages of

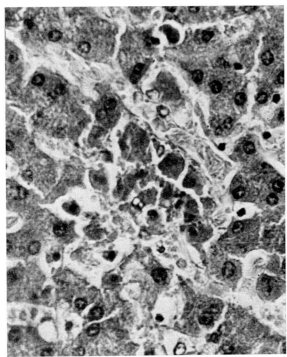

FIG. 4.3. Liver showing a focal area of eosinophilic necrosis (phloxine-tartrazine × 500). (From Edington and White, 1972, *Trans roy. Soc. trop. Med. Hyg.*, **66**, Fig. 7.)

yellow fever. Much lipochrome pigment was present in the hepatocytes. Small haemorrhages were present. The eosinophilic necrosis in the absence of bile retention, cellular infiltration, and the ochre bodies must raise the suspicion of yellow fever to a pathologist working in West Africa. However, cells in all parts of the lobule were randomly affected and there was no fatty change—nor were inclusion bodies noted. Apart from a mild cellular infiltration the portal tracts were normal. Ductular proliferation was not seen and the efferent veins were within normal limits.

The lesions in the spleen were striking and consisted of an eosinophilic necrosis surrounding depleted malpighian corpuscles associated with pavementing and a sub-endothelial lymphocytic infiltration of the splenic veins. The pulp was thickened and acellular and the sinusoids dilated. There is thus depletion of the reticulo-endothelial elements at the periphery of the malpighian corpuscles and in the pulp cords. On the other hand there was lymphocytic infiltration of the subintimal lymphatics and 'pavementing' in the trabecular veins (Fig. 4.4). These changes combined with the cellular

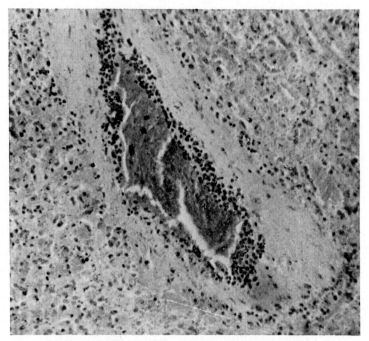

FIG. 4.4. Spleen showing pavementing and sub-endothelial lymphocytic venous infiltration (H and E × 180). (From Edington and White, 1972, *Trans roy. Soc. trop. Med. Hyg.*, **66**, Fig. 3).

infiltrate in the portal tracts of the liver would suggest that terminally the fixed structures of the lymphoid system are affected and not the mobile or recirculating pool of lymphocytes. Infiltration of the subintimal lymphatics has been noted in infectious mononucleosis, lymphatic leukaemia, myeloid leukaemia, follicular lipidosis (Goldberg and Saphir, 1959; Goldberg, 1962) and Thai haemorrhagic fever (Bhamarapravati *et al.* 1964).

In the lungs a focal pneumonitis with megakaryocytes prominent was usual. The intestine was grossly oedematous with small haemorrhages and a mild submucosal lymphocytic infiltration present. Oedema and petechial haemorrhages were present in the myocardium. The kidneys were congested. Small haemorrhages may be present and an occasional glomerulus may show an area of focal necrosis.

Haemorrhages may be present in the other organs and effusions in the serous cavities. Thrombocytopenia and prothrombin deficiency may account for the haemorrhages. On the other hand circulating antigen–antibody complexes may damage the capillaries leading to increased permeability and haemorrhage.

RABIES

Rabies is an encephalitis caused by a virus which exists in nature as a salivary gland infection of carnivorous animals, and is transmitted in the saliva by biting. All mammals are susceptible. The condition is invariably fatal in man.

Epidemiology

There are two epidemiological types of rabies: (a) Wild—the disease is maintained in animal reservoirs; many animals can act as a reservoir of infection, such as wild dogs, wolves, skunks, jackals, bats, etc. (Editorial, 1973), (b) Urban—the dog is the usual source of infection, and is particularly liable to spread the disease to man. Rabies is common throughout South West Asia, and also occurs in East and West Africa and in parts of South Africa. Rabies occurs also in India, America and Canada. In Central and South America and the Caribbean, the main vectors of the infection are bats, especially vampire bats, and the animals infected are chiefly cattle, with the dog of no importance in maintaining or spreading the disease. Though equally fatal to man its clinical course takes the form of an ascending paralysis and is more protracted (Editorial, 1965). In the Southern United States fructivorous and insectivorous bats are being increasingly incriminated as vectors. A rabies epizootic in foxes is spreading across France having previously invaded a number of other European countries. Any patient with unusual cerebral symptoms should be questioned regarding possible animal bites or contacts (Editorial, 1971; Vella, 1974; Mason-Browne, 1974).

The domestic dog is the chief source of human infection. If a normal dog, however, is bitten by a rabid animal, there is a variable incubation period of from 10 days to 8 months, but it is usually from 21 to 60 days. Once symptoms develop, the dog will die within 10 days; if it is healthy by the end of this period, it was not suffering from rabies.

There are two main forms of the disease in the dog:

(i) Dumb rabies; common in West Africa.
(ii) Furious rabies; common in the Far East.

The 'dumb' form leads to paralysis and coma, while the 'furious' type leads to extreme mania when the dog will rush around and bite indiscriminately. It is thus much the more dangerous form from the point of view of spread of infection. Not every rabid dog is infectious: the virus may not be present in the salivary glands. It should be noted that one of the early signs of rabies in the dog may be a change in temperament; the dog may appear increasingly apathetic and seek to be alone, or it may become increasingly nervous and may at this stage appear to be unusually friendly: in this stage it may be particularly dangerous as any lick will spread saliva which may contain virus. Inapparent rabies infection ocassionally occurs (Doege and Northrop, 1974).

The virus

The virus—an RNA virus—measures about 100 nm. It is a rhabdovirus and is bullet-shaped (Editorial 1973). It is relatively stable, and infected tissue stored in glycerol will remain infective for several weeks at room temperature, and for months in the refrigerator. It is rapidly destroyed by ultra-violet light and formalin, but is very resistant to phenols.

The properties of the virus are altered by serial intracerebral passage in an experimental animal. The wild 'street virus', such as may be isolated from dogs, is characterized by a long and very variable incubation period, a typical excitement phase in the disease, the tendency to reach the salivary glands, infectivity when given by any parenteral route, and the rather constant production of Negri bodies which are intracytoplasmic inclusions found in nerve cells.

If the virus is serially propagated by intracerebral passage in rabbits, its properties are changed. Such altered virus is termed 'fixed' virus. Rabies caused in the rabbit by 'fixed' virus has a short incubation period of 4–6 days; there are no Negri bodies formed: the virus cannot travel along nerves and so is not infective unless injected directly into the brain, and it is unable to multiply in the salivary glands. When given intracerebrally to rabbits it causes a rapidly fatal paralytic disease. 'Fixed' virus is used for the production of certain types of rabies vaccine: although the vaccine is killed virus, it is thought that as the fixed virus is in any case not infective except by intracerebral inoculation (tested in animals). This provides an additional element of safety in the preparation of a vaccine for use in man. The two vaccines for humans in common use for post-exposure treatment are the Semple-type vaccine and the DEV (duck-embryo vaccine). Flury LEP (low-egg-passage) vaccine virus is used for the immunization of dogs. The duration of immunity following a single intramuscular injection of 3 ml of the vaccine is at least 3 years. This vaccine has also been used for immunization of persons at risk, e.g. laboratory workers and veterinarians. The dose for humans is 1·0 ml intramuscularly on two occasions.

Pathology

The incubation period varies from 5 to 6 weeks, but may be much longer. Fever, headache and malaise may be followed by a change in sensation at the site of the bite. Coma and death may ensue or there may be a distressing stage of excitement, fear and anxiety. Clonic spasm of the muscles of the pharynx and larynx prevent swallowing (hydrophobia). Consciousness is usually retained until the late stages of the disease.

The main changes are seen in the central nervous system. The salivary glands may be soft and swollen and exhibit a mononuclear cell infiltration

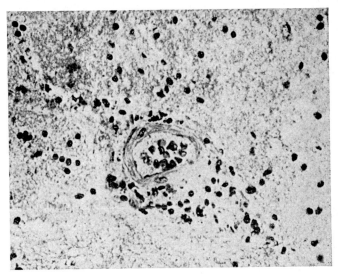

FIG. 4.5. Rabies. A small perivascular collection of leucocytes shown in the brain. (*By courtesy of Ash and Spitz.*)

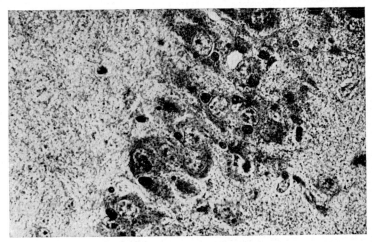

FIG. 4.6. Rabies. Dense Negri bodies are shown within the cytoplasm of nerve cells. (*By courtesy of Ash and Spitz.*)

with degeneration of acinar cells. Myocarditis may play an important role in the terminal stages of the disease—although it has not been frequently reported. The heart is macroscopically normal. Microscopically an occasional muscle cell may be necrotic and there is an interstitial infiltrate of lymphocytes, histiocytes and occasional neutrofils (Cheetham *et al.* 1970).

The findings in nervous tissue are those of neuronal degeneration especially marked in the thalamus, hypothalamus, the substantia nigra and nuclei of the cranial nerves. Perivascular and perineuronal infiltration by monocytes may be seen (Fig. 4.5). However, in 15 per cent of brains inclusions may be the sole evidence of infection without an inflammatory exudate. The characteristic changes are, however, seen in the nerve cells and a specific diagnosis can only be made if intracytoplasmic inclusions (Negri bodies) are seen (Fig. 4.6). There is a ballooning of the cytoplasm with pyknosis of the nucleus. The amount of Nissl substance is decreased. Negri bodies vary between 2–10 μm in diameter and are sharply defined, spherical, oval, or elongated eosinophilic bodies with an inner structure of basophilic granules. They are most abundant in Ammon's horn, the pyramidal layer of the cerebral cortex and in the Purkinje cell layer of the cerebellum (Earle and Dupont, 1966). Unfortunately, they are only present in about 30 per cent of human infections. They do not contain rabies virus (Matsumota, 1963) and their nature is not clear. Structureless inclusions known as Lyssa bodies are found more frequently than Negri bodies.

Diagnostic pathology

The most important aspect of diagnosis is the diagnosis of the disease in dogs, and hence the animal should be impounded and allowed to die. The head may be sent in ice to a pathologist or alternatively the dog's brain removed with strict precautions against splashing and wearing full protective clothing and goggles. One half of the brain is placed in 50 per cent glycerol saline and the other half into 10 per cent neutral formol-saline. The fixed specimen is used for examination for Negri bodies and the sample in glycerol for isolation of virus by mouse inoculation. Seller's stain★ combines simplicity with easy and rapid identification of the Negri bodies and a positive diagnosis can be made within half an hour of receipt of the specimen (WHO, 1966).

If no Negri bodies are found the mouse inoculation test must be performed. A homogenized suspension of tissue from the brain or salivary glands of the supposedly rabid animal is inoculated into the brains of mice, which are then serially killed off each day from the fifth day of inoculation onwards. The brains are examined for Negri bodies and definite identifica-

★See *Laboratory Techniques in Rabies*, 3rd Edition. WHO, 1973, No. 23.

tion of the virus depends upon demonstration of rabies antigen by the serum-virus neutralization test.

The fluorescent rabies antibody (FRA) test developed by Goldwasser and Kissling (1958) is considered the best single test currently available for the rapid diagnosis of rabies. It can be used with fresh, frozen, or glycerolated specimens and usually permits an accurate diagnosis to be established in a few hours (WHO, 1966). Several variations of the fluorescent antibody technique have been developed, including an indirect method for detection of rabies antibody in the blood serum (Thomas *et al.* 1963). Rabies virus in

TABLE 4.4. *Procedure to be adopted in case of suspected human rabies*

Nature of exposure	Biting animal:*		Treatment
	at time of exposure	during observation period of 10 days	
(1) **No lesion** Indirect contact	Rabid	—	None
(2) **Licks:**			
(i) Unabraded skin	Rabid		None
(ii) Abraded skin, scratches, un-abraded or abraded mucosa	(*a*) Healthy	Rabid	Start vaccine† at first sign of rabies in the animal
	(*b*) ? Rabid	Healthy	Start vaccine at once: stop if animal is well at fifth day
	(*c*) Rabid, escaped, killed, unknown	—	Start vaccine at once
(3) **Bites:**			
(i) Mild	(*a*) Healthy	Rabid	Start vaccine at first signs of rabies in animal
	(*b*) ? Rabid	Healthy	Start vaccine at once: stop at fifth day if animal is well
	(*c*) Rabid, escaped, killed, unknown	—	Start vaccine at once
	(*d*) Any wild animal	—	Immune serum at once, followed by course of vaccine‡
(ii) Severe (Multiple, or face, head, neck, finger)	(*a*) Healthy	Rabid	Immune serum at once: start vaccine at first signs of rabies in animal‡
	(*b*) ? Rabid	Healthy	Immune serum at once, followed by vaccine: stop if animal is healthy at fifth day
	(*c*) Rabid, escaped, killed, unknown, or any wild animal	—	Immune serum at once followed by course of vaccine‡

*Irrespective of whether the animal has itself been inoculated or not.

†Two vaccines are commonly available: (1) DEV (duck-embryo vaccine), (2) Semple type.

‡Booster doses should be given at the tenth and twentieth day following the completion of a full course of vaccine. For booster doses use vaccine of non-nervous tissue origin if available.

man has been found in the salivary glands, nasal mucosa and in the cornea as well as in other organs. Examination of a corneal impression (made by gently pressing a slide against the cornea of both eyes and then fixing in acetone for 10 minutes) by means of the direct fluorescent antibody test has demonstrated the presence of rabies antigen in corneal cells in the early stages of the disease (Cifuentes *et al.* 1971). Gel-diffusion techniques are both specific and sensitive. The recent isolation of a virus indistinguishable by complement fixation and neutralization tests from a virus isolated from shrews in Ibadan and serologically related by complement-fixation tests to the rabies virus in a child with 'aseptic meningitis' may be of interest in the field of preventive medicine (Familusi and Moore, 1972). The combined use of the serum virus neutralization test and the fluorescent antibody tests provides the quickest and most accurate way of making a definitive diagnosis. Since pathologists in the tropics are not infrequently consulted as to the procedure to be adopted in a case of suspected human rabies, we are including in Table 4.4 the recommendations of the WHO Expert Committee (1973).

SMALLPOX

Smallpox is a virus infection which was endemic in large areas of the tropical world but especially in the Indian subcontinent, South East Asia, parts of Africa and South America. The recent smallpox eradication campaign has reduced these endemic foci considerably.

Epidemiology

The most important source of infection is the person suffering from smallpox. The undetected or ambulant case is next in importance. The patient becomes infectious in the first 24 hours of the pyrexial phase and remains so until the last scabs have dropped off. Droplet spread is the mode of transmission either through direct or indirect contact, through utensils, clothing or dust infected by the patient. All ages and sexes are susceptible to smallpox. The success of the WHO global eradication campaign has resulted in foci of smallpox remaining only in India, Bangladesh and Pakistan, with sporadic cases being reported from Ethiopia (Editorial, 1973). The presence of an animal reservoir for smallpox might constitute a threat to eradication; consequently considerable attention has been focused on pox virus infections in lower primates, particularly monkey pox.

The causative virus is about 200 nm and exists in three forms which result in the severe disease *variola major* (smallpox); a mild form *variola minor* (alastrim)—a small outbreak occurred in Brazil (de Quadros *et al.* 1972); and a third variant vaccinia (cowpox) which is relatively non-pathogenic in man but very rarely can cause a fatal illness (Paradinas and Wiltshaw, 1972).

Monkey pox virus, although distinct from smallpox virus, is clearly related to it and produces in man a disease that is indistinguishable from smallpox (Editorial, 1973; Foster *et al.* 1972). Monkey-pox was first described by Von Magnus *et al.* in 1959. The condition occurs in man in West and Central Africa (Foster *et al.* 1972) and has occurred in unvaccinated individuals. No contacts have developed the disease. The virus can be distinguished from that of smallpox by the fact that it causes haemorrhagic necrotic lesions in the skin of the rabbit. The condition has recently been reviewed (Editorial, 1973).

Pathology

The changes seen after death depend upon the severity of the infection. In fulminating cases death may occur within 48 hours and there may be few abnormal findings at necropsy. The diagnosis may well be missed unless heart, blood, and skin are taken for virological studies. In these cases death has occurred from toxaemia before the smallpox eruption has appeared. The changes expected in fulminating (1–5 days), malignant (10–14 days), and benign (14–21 days) smallpox are described below (Dixon, 1962).

Fulminating smallpox

The lesions on the skin vary from a few petechiae to extensive and widespread haemorrhages. The mucous membranes are similarly affected. There may be free blood in the stomach and sometimes haemorrhages in other viscera. Virological studies are positive.

Malignant smallpox

There are gross haemorrhages in the skin with exfoliative lesions and extensive ulcerative lesions in the oral cavity, larynx, and trachea. The oesophagus may also be affected in its upper third. In the remaining organs, expecially the ovaries, testes, uterus, and kidney, there may be small focal haemorrhages. Virological studies are usually positive.

Benign smallpox

A pustular rash is present on the skin and abscesses due to secondary pyogenic infection may be present. Apart from secondary bronchopneumonia and signs of a non-specific septicaemia no other specific lesions may be noted. The central nervous system, however, may have been affected, with evidence of encephalomyelitis. Scarring is usually more pronounced in the face and this is considered to be due to the relatively larger size and greater number of sebaceous glands in this area which undergo degenerative changes leading to necrosis (Bras, 1952). Virological studies will be positive.

Complications

Pyogenic infection including osteomyelitis and empyema may cause death at a later date. A true virus-induced osteomyelitis affecting the metaphyses of growing bone—osteomyelitis variolosa—does, however, occur (Cockshott and McGregor, 1958). Alopecia may be troublesome. A serous or purulent arthritis may occur. The palpebral conjunctiva may be affected and conjunctivitis, keratitis and panophthalmitis may, rarely, cause blindness. The central nervous system may be involved and an acute psychosis may occur in the early stages of the infection with drowsiness, trismus, incontinence of urine and faeces, sensory loss, and hyperaesthesia appearing towards the end of the second week of the infection.

The clinical manifestations of smallpox are usually more severe in pregnant women, and congenital infections occur.

The *histopathological changes* in the organs in smallpox are those due to the infection itself, and those due to secondary bacterial infection (Bras, 1952).

In the epidermis in the cells of the upper layer of the rete malpighii degenerative changes with vacuolization and oedema occur. Small multilocular vesicles bordered by compressed epidermal cells are formed. Some of the trabeculae rupture forming a larger but still multiloculated vesicle. Simultaneously, the cells of the lower layers of the stratum spinosum become swollen (ballooned) and fuse, to form giant cells with two to four nuclei. Umbilication is due to active peripheral cytolysis, in contrast to the slower degenerative changes at the base and centre of the lesion. Intranuclear inclusions in the cells of the rete malpighii are striking, as, also, are variously sized intracytoplasmic eosinophilic inclusions (Guarnieri bodies). The dermis is vascular and there is a marked infiltration of lymphocytes. Histologically one cannot differentiate between variola major, and minor or vaccinia, but in varicella (chickenpox) the giant cells are more numerous, and the inclusion and the lymphocytic infiltration of the dermis are less. It requires, however, a pathologist with much experience of these lesions to differentiate them, and virological studies or electron microscopy are to be preferred.

In the pustular stage the serous and fibrinous contents of the vesicle are replaced by polymorphonuclear leucocytes, with consequent breakdown of the loculi. Congestion and inflammation occur in the dermis. Superficial ulceration occurs and the lesions heal by a process of organization with consequent scarring (pitting) and perhaps small scattered foci of leucodermia in pigmented skins.

Similar lesions may occur in the oral cavity, oesophagus, and stomach. Focal hepatitis, orchitis, oophoritis, leptomeningitis, encephalitis, and lesions in the adrenals, may be noted. Interstitial nephritis may also be an associated lesion. Proliferation of histiocytes and mononuclear cells may be found in the spleen, lymph nodes and bone marrow.

Degenerative changes in many of the organs due to the associated toxaemia may be present, and pyogenic lesions are common in various organs, especially in the subcutaneous tissues and skin.

Diagnostic pathology

The laboratory diagnosis of smallpox is based on (1) microscopic examination of smears from skin lesions, (2) culture on the chorioallantoic membrane of chicks, or tissue culture, (3) detection of antigen by agar gel diffusion or a complement-fixation test, and (4) detection of antibody in the blood during the course of the illness. Histological examination of skin lesions helps to differentiate modified variola major and alastrim from varicella. Details of the method of collecting specimens can be found in the WHO Technical Report on Smallpox, 1964 (WHO, 1964). The electron microscope can distinguish rapidly the viruses of smallpox and chicken pox.

TANAPOX

A virus of the pox group has caused epidemics in Kenya of a short febrile illness with headache and prostration. The disease was characterized by a single pock-like lesion on the upper part of the body (Downie *et al*. 1971). The virus is related to yabapox virus which produces tumours in monkeys and benign tumours in man (Editorial, 1971).

CHICKENPOX

Synonym. Varicella.

Varicella is a highly infective disease, occurring primarily, but not exclusively, in childhood. The incubation period ranges between 10–20 days. It is transmitted by the droplet route and dissemination of virus occurs up to the completion of the vesicular eruption. Patients with herpes zoster are a secondary reservoir of infection. Differentiation from smallpox in endemic areas is important. Chickenpox is rarely severe in children but some 16–33 per cent of adults develop pneumonia with a considerable mortality rate (Editorial, 1968).

Pathology

Although it is usually a benign disease, severe symptoms can result from visceral lesions (Editorial, 1966) especially in patients on steroids or immunosuppressive therapy. The lungs, liver, adrenal gland, and spleen may be affected. Glomorulonephritis, sometimes severe, may be a complication (Editorial, 1968). If the lungs are affected respiratory symptoms occur after some days and may terminate in coma and death. At autopsy papular lesions are found on the pleura, and foci of haemorrhage and consolidation a few millimetres in diameter in the lung substance. They consist of areas of focal necrosis and haemorrhage infiltrated by macrophages, lymphocytes, and polymorphs. Intranuclear and intracytoplasmic inclusions may be seen and necrosis of small blood vessels occurs.

The condition can be diagnosed radiologically in life, as extensive small shadows are seen. Calcification can occur and may be seen many years later. Virus may be isolated from the lesions post mortem.

Scrapings from the base of a vesicle stained with Giemsa will reveal multinucleate giant epithelial cells as well as cells with typical intranuclear inclusions. Patients with varicella pneumonia may show similar inclusion bodies in the sputum.

DISEASES CAUSED BY BEDSONIAE

(Trachoma, Inclusion Conjunctivitis, Lymphogranuloma Venereum, Cat Scratch Disease and Psittacosis).

The infective agents of these diseases are grouped together because of certain common characteristics. They are largely intracellular parasites 250–500 nm in diameter. The cytoplasmic colours are basophilic whereas viral inclusions are acidophilic. Both RNA and DNA are present in the particles. They are susceptible to sulphonamides and antibiotics and possess a common group antigen (Downie and MacCallum, 1967).

The agents can be isolated. The lesions in the lymphatic glands resemble those of lymphogranuloma venereum but the Frei test is negative.

TRACHOMA

Trachoma is a keratoconjunctivitis due to an agent of the psittacosis/lymphogranuloma group of atypical viruses. The agent causing inclusion conjunctivitis is closely similar, although the disease is dissimilar, and they have been referred to as TRIC agents (Gear et al. 1963). TRIC agents are now called *Bedsoniae*.

Trachoma is one of the most widespread communicable diseases, and is the greatest single cause of blindness and impaired vision. Differences in the severity of physical signs in the right and left eyes of patients have been described from Syria and Burma (Winkler et al. 1973).

Epidemiology

Trachoma occurs sporadically all over the world but the areas of greatest endemicity are North Africa, the Middle East, the northern part of the Indian sub-continent, Vietnam, China, and tropical Africa. The causal agent was first isolated with certainty in Peking by T'ang and his colleagues (1957) and confirmed in the Gambia by Collier and Sowa (1958). The aetiological role of the Gambian virus was proved by infecting blind human volunteers and inducing in them the typical lesions of trachoma (Collier *et al.* 1958).

In endemic areas the disease is acquired early in life and almost all children are infected by adolescence. Trachoma is usually spread from eye to eye by close physical contact through the fingers, fomites, or flies. In countries with a high incidence of bacterial conjunctivitis, particularly of the seasonal epidemic variety, the severity of the trachoma is enhanced and disabling complications are more frequent. In other areas, e.g. the Gambia, the disease is mild, and serious sequelae uncommon (Sowa *et al.* 1965).

Pathology

The condition is conveniently described in stages, both clinically and pathologically.

The onset is insidious and may be asymptomatic but mild irritation and watering of the eyes is usually complained of. There may be a mucopurulent discharge difficult to distinguish from bacterial conjunctivitis. This phase is usually not diagnosed in endemic areas.

In *Stage I* the conjunctivae especially of the upper lid are hyperaemic and slightly roughened due to subepithelial lymphatic hyperplasia. Pin-head greyish follicles may be noted in the upper tarsus. Spontaneous cure may occur at this stage.

Stage II is established trachoma and there are two main clinical types, one showing predominantly follicular and the other papillary hypertrophy of the tarsal conjunctiva. The follicles resemble sago grains, are soft with marginal blood vessels and are easily expressible. They are most frequent in the upper fornix. In the absence of secondary infection exudate is minimal and symptoms are mild.

The papillary type is more active and superimposed bacterial infection is present. Follicles are also present. The conjunctival vessels are dilated and there is an infiltrate of plasma cells and collections of numerous lymphocytes with prominent germinal centres. Subepithelial infiltration of the cornea by proliferating capillaries from the limbus is seen as a greyish-red lesion at the cornea-scleral junction. This is known as 'pannus'. It appears first at the upper limbus and tends to progress downwards. Necrotic changes may occur in the conjunctival and corneal stroma and in the follicles. Repair with fibroblastic proliferation occurs, leading to the next stage.

Stage III is characterized by scar formation in addition to the conjunctival changes, and the scars may be grossly visible on the conjunctival surface.

Pannus is marked. As a result of scarring, the lid margin may become irregular and inverted (entropion). Isolated eyelashes turn in against the cornea (trichiasis). Repeated attacks of conjunctivitis exaggerated by entropion and trichiasis may lead to ulceration and destruction of the cornea, with blindness a terminal event.

Stage IV is healed trachoma. The tarsal conjunctiva is fibrosed and smooth. The condition is symptomless if there are no complications. In addition to trichiasis and entropion, obliteration of the tear ducts may cause a deficiency of tears. Pannus may have affected the pupillary area, with variable effects on vision.

Diagnostic pathology

Clinically, the association of follicular conjunctivitis and pannus is diagnostic. Intracytoplasmic inclusion bodies $0 \cdot 25$–$0 \cdot 4$ μm in diameter, staining purple with Giemsa or reddish-brown by iodine, may be seen in conjunctival scrapings. These elementary particles have been termed Halberstaedter–Prowazek bodies and are the principal microscopic diagnostic feature in trachoma but are also seen in inclusion conjunctivitis of the newborn. The number of inclusions tends to be proportional to the intensity of the infection and are most numerous in scrapings from the upper lid.

In early lesions neutrophils may be abundant. In later lesions plasma cells, lymphoblasts and macrophages containing necrotic debris (Leber cells) may be seen.

The agent may be cultured in the yolk sac of the embryonated egg.

Neither serological nor skin tests are of practical value as yet but fluorescein-labelled antibody can be utilized in searching for the intracytoplasmic inclusions (Nichols *et al.* 1963).

Inclusion Conjunctivitis

In this condition even minimal eye sepsis can lead to permanent scarring of the conjunctiva and cornea with or without pannus (Watson and Gairdner, 1968). The agent resides in the genital tract, the cervix, and urethra of adults and is transmitted as a venereal infection. The eye of the newborn is affected between the fifth and fourteenth day of life. Eye-to-eye transmission is, however, rare. Typical inclusions similar to those described for trachoma are seen in conjunctival scrapings particularly from the lower lid. The exudate contains many neutrophils. The chronic type of exudate seen in trachoma does not occur.

LYMPHOGRANULOMA VENEREUM

Synonyms. Climatic bubo; paradenitis nostras; lymphogranuloma inguinale; Durand–Nicolas–Favre disease; esthiomene; venereal bubo.

Lymphogranuloma venereum is the sixth venereal disease, characterized by a transient insignificant local primary lesion followed by a lymphangitis, lymphadenitis, and minor systemic disturbances. It is caused by a member of the *Chlamydia* (*Bedsonia*) group of infective agents (Nicol, 1971).

Epidemiology

The disease has a world-wide distribution. It is common in tropical countries and has been reported from the Caribbean, Central and South America, West Africa, East and Central Africa, South India, and Indonesia. It is more common in Negroes in the U.S.A. than in the whites (Lawson, 1963). The causal agent is related to the psittacosis group of viruses. The infection is mainly transmitted by sexual contact and therefore the age incidence is that of sexual activity. The disease has occasionally been contracted by contact from infected clothing, from bathing patients and by the surgeon in removing infected lymph nodes. There are no sex or racial differences, but the disease is much more commonly detected in males than in females.

Pathology

The primary lesion may occur in any part of the external genitalia of the female or on the prepuce, glans penis, or urethra of the male. A painless vesicle, papule, or ulcer forms, and is followed in a week or so by a secondary, localized adenitis. At this stage constitutional symptoms may be marked and typhoid fever may be simulated. Pathological changes in the spleen, liver, heart, and central nervous system have been described and generalized lymphadenopathy may occur. Severe constitutional symptoms are not common in our experience.

The primary lesion consists of an ulcer surrounded by plasma cells and histiocytes containing the cone or dumbell-shaped basophilic inclusion bodies or clusters and chains of smaller azurophil elementary bodies which can be detected on Giemsa-stained smears of pus from the lesion. Occasionally eosinophils are prominent.

The secondary lesions in the lymphatics are most important from the clinical point of view. In the lymph nodes there is proliferation of monocytes, plasma cells with a few neutrophil polymorphonuclear leucocytes and eosinophils present. There is proliferation of macrophages with epithelioid cell transformation. Central necrosis and giant-cell transformation may simulate tuberculosis. The abscesses are, however, usually 'stellate' in configuration and the presence of eosinophils and plasma cells usually suggests the diagnosis. A Giemsa stain may show the presence of intracytoplasmic inclusion bodies. There is an associated marked proliferation of fibrous tissue. In the late stages a central area of necrosis may be surrounded by a palisade of scanty epithelioid cells merging with a wall of acellular hyaline material (Fig. 4.7).

In the male in the tropics bilateral involvement of the inguinal glands is usual. The individual glands may coalesce to form large, tender, inflammatory masses which may resolve or suppurate. Elephantiasis of the penis or scrotum may result. Both in the male, but more commonly in the female, the anorectal region and pelvic lymphatic glands may be affected. Proctitis arising from the perirectal tissues causes rectal stricture. In the male, homosexuality has been considered a factor. Elephantiasis of the genitalia, vaginorectal and vesicovaginal fistulae and fibrosis of the vagina are complications in the female.

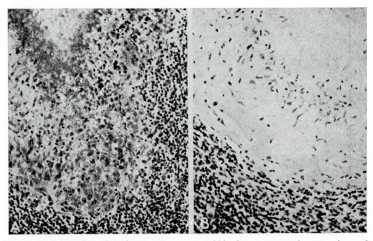

FIG. 4.7. Lymphogranuloma venereum. (A) shows central necrosis at the top of the photograph surrounded by epitheloid and rudimentary giant cells with a peripheral zone of lymphocytes and histiocytes. (B) shows a late lesion with some central necrosis with a wide area of hyalinization containing a palisade of scattered epithelioid cells. (*By courtesy of Ash and Spitz.*)

Diagnostic pathology

A smear of the lesion stained by Giemsa may reveal the presence of intracytoplasmic inclusion bodies. The histopathological features seen in biopsy material have already been described.

Diagnosis of *lymphogranuloma venereum* can also be made by (i) isolation of the virus, (ii) the Frei skin test, and (iii) the complement-fixation test. Inoculation of pus, aspirated from the buboes and inoculated intracerebrally into mice or monkeys results in a characteristic meningoencephalitis; alternatively inoculation on to the yolk sac of a developing embryonated hen's egg also results in growth of the virus. The intradermal test of Frei (see below), becomes positive 7–40 days after the onset of the adenitis and probably remains so throughout the life of the patients (Palmer *et al.* 1942). False-positive reactions do occur. Of possibly greater value in diagnosis is the complement-fixation test, when a titre of over 1:40 in a patient with clinical manifestations of the disease can be taken as confirmatory of the diagnosis, especially if acute and convalescent sera are also available (Annamunthodo, 1962). The lymphogranuloma virus is also present in the blood, cerebrospinal fluid, and faeces, as well as in buboes.

Frei skin test

The Frei skin test is an allergic test of some value in the diagnosis of lymphogranuloma venereum. It is performed by injecting into the patient intradermally an antigen containing heat-killed virus. An antigen may be made from pus aspirated from the unopened stellate abscesses in the inguinal glands of a case of the disease. The antigen most free from impurities is that made from cultures of the virus on the yolk sac of the chick embryo; it is available commercially (Lygranum S.T. Antigen, Squibb). The test is read at 48 hours and 96 hours after the injection of 0·1 ml of the antigen into the skin of the patient, and preferably also into a normal uninfected control. If positive, there is an infiltrated inflammatory dome-shaped swelling at least half a centimetre in diameter, which can both be seen and felt. In the centre of the swelling there may be a small area of necrosis surrounded by a red zone. The nodule often persists for 2 to 3 weeks.

CAT-SCRATCH DISEASE

The causal agent has not yet been isolated. The lesions in the lymphatics resemble those of lymphogranuloma venereum but the Frei test is negative.

MUMPS

Mumps is common in children in the tropics. It causes an acute inflammatory swelling of the salivary glands, mainly of the parotids with oedema and interstitial mononuclear cell infiltration. The virus is spread by droplet infection and can be demonstrated in the saliva. The incubation period is 14–21 days.

Inflammation of the testes (orchitis) occasionally occurs and rare complications are acute pancreatitis and meningo-encephalitis. A possible association of congenital infections with fibroelastisis of the endocardium of the heart has been suggested (p. 356) and also of pancreatic calcification. The diagnosis is usually clinical but the virus can be isolated from saliva, throat washings, blood, and urine. Antibodies to the virus can be demonstrated by the haemagglutination inhibition test.

Mumps is caused by an RNA myxovirus transmitted by droplet infection. The incubation period is about three weeks.

Necrosis and infiltration of 'round cells'—monocytes, plasma cells and histiocytes—occurs in the interglandular stoma of the parotid glands. The epithelium can also be affected. Other glandular structures may also be involved, including the salivary glands, pancreas, ovaries, and testes. Meningo-encephalitis, pancreatitis and cardiac and renal involvement have also been described (Mohamad and Carlisle, 1971). The condition has been reviewed by Gray (1973).

MEASLES (RUBEOLA)

Measles is a severe disease affecting young children in the tropics (Morley *et al.* 1963), and neutralizing antibodies are present in the sera of nearly 100 per cent by the age of 5 years (Hendrickse *et al.* 1964). Newborn infants are protected for about 6 months by transplacentally-acquired antibody. The mode of transmission is by droplet infection. Clinically, diarrhoea is common and a severe necrotizing gastroenteritis has been described at autopsy (Williams and Osotimehin, 1970). Mortality in some epidemics in the tropics has varied from 20 to 50 per cent (Senecal *et al.* 1962; Editorial, 1968). It should be noticed that severe atypical measles may result from exposure to natural measles infection several years after immunization by the killed or inactivated vaccine (Editorial, 1971). The symptoms are fever, cough, headache, myalgia and abdominal pain. A peripheral maculopapular rash first on the limbs spreading centripetally in contrast to measles appears about the third day. A lobar pneumonia and pleural effusion are usual (Editorial, 1971). Pereira and Benjamin (1972) described the pattern of measles in a South Indian community while a symposium on measles and its vaccination was held in Central America (Beghin, 1973). The pathogenesis of measles and the differences between the disease as seen in Africa and Europe were highlighted recently (Editorial, 1973).

Pathology

About 11 days after infection, fever and catarrh are complained of and the rash usually appears on the thirteenth or fourteenth day.

In children dying in the prodromal phase the striking feature at necropsy is the presence of syncytial giant-cells in (i) the epithelium lining the upper respiratory tract, trachea, bronchi, and bronchioles (Warthin–Finkeldey cells), and (ii) in the tissues of the reticulo-endothelial system. There may be 100 nuclei in these syncytial giant cells. In the respiratory epithelium they contain eosinophilic intranuclear and intracytoplasmic inclusions; they become separated from the basal cells and are found in the lumina of the bronchi and bronchioles in association with macrophages and cellular debris (Sherman and Ruckle, 1958). An associated interstitial pneumonitis is present. A conjunctivitis is usual. Peripheral gangrene may occur, possibly due to disseminated intravascular coagulation factors II, V, VIII and fibrinogen and the presence of fibrinolytic degradation products in the serum. This 'consumption coagulopathy' can occur in other viral diseases (Chaudhuri and McKenzie, 1970).

In the lymph nodes, tonsils, thymus, Peyer's patches, and lymphatic tissue of the appendix, giant cells with scanty cytoplasm and clumped nuclei occur. Inclusions are not usually seen. It is of interest that Osunkoya *et al.* (1973) have described multinucleated giant cells in 3-day phytohaemagglutinin-stimulated leucocyte cultures from some children with measles. Phytohaemagglutinin (PHA) normally transforms about 70 per cent of normal human peripheral lymphocytes to blast cells. These cells have a single nucleus, undergo normal mitotic cell division and have a relatively narrow range of cell size. Abnormal PHA stimulation has usually been concerned with a reduction or delay in blast formation such as occurs in some malignant lymphomas.

The giant cells seen in these cultures in measles were thought to be related to the giant cells characteristic of the histopathology of measles which are seen in lymphoid tissue, respiratory tract mucosa, skin, and kidney.

Measles viral antigen was detected on the perinuclear cytoplasm of the multinucleated giant cells and also on the cell surface of blast cells in giant-cell-positive PHA cultures.

As the virus is intimately connected with cell replication it was thought that the severity of measles might be related to the relative activity of the reticulo-endothelial system, being more severe in children in whom this system was hyperplastic.

In the brain, an encephalitis due to a hypersensitivity response with acute neuronal degeneration and occasional neuronophagia is a rare complication. Virus has not been isolated from the brain in human cases of encephalitis. Subacute sclerosing panencephalitis is a rare condition characterized by chronic mental changes, dementia, paralysis, and extra-pyramidal signs with myoclonic or athetoid movements. Gross softening and sclerosis of the cortex occurs. Characteristic intranuclear and cytoplasmic inclusions in both neurones and glial cells are seen. The condition can occur years after measles infection. It may follow measles vaccination and a second virus may be involved. It is, however, accepted that the disease is a chronic virus infection of the brain. Similar examples are cytomegalovirus infection of neonates and slow viruses such as those causing scrapie in sheep and Aleutian mink disease (Stuart Harris, 1971).

In addition to encephalitis, subacute sclerosing panencephalitis and, possibly multiple sclerosis, polyradiculoneuritis (Guillain–Barre syndrome) has also been associated with measles in a few cases (Lidin-Janson and Strannegard, 1972).

Myocarditis has also been described (Cohen, 1963) but it is a rare complication. The histopathological findings in the heart are those of minute foci of necrosis with an infiltrate of histiocytes, lymphocytes, and scanty neutrophils. Degen (1937) considered that it was doubtful if changes in the heart occurred in measles, although abnormal ECG tracings may be found in 30 per cent of patients in some series and Giustra (1954) described a condition which closely resembles idiopathic cardiomegaly following an attack of measles $5\frac{1}{2}$ years previously. This is perhaps worthy of further thought in tropical areas where the clinical manifestations of measles are so florid. Foci of necrosis may be seen in the liver. Giant-cell transformation has been noted in the epithelium of the bladder but changes in the renal tract have not otherwise been described, although they must occur as cells containing intranuclear and intracytoplasmic inclusions have been seen in the urine (Boyd and Nedelkoska, 1964).

Following the appearance of the rash the specific pathological findings usually disappear and the changes found are those of bronchopneumonia and secondary bacterial infection. In the skin there is lymphocytic infiltration around blood vessels, hair follicles, and sweat glands. The basal layer of the epidermis undergoes a fibrinoid necrosis with an associated leucocytic infiltration. Koplik's spots in the mucous membrane of the mouth are pathognomonic clinically and have similar histological features as the skin lesions. Multinucleate giant cells occur both in the epidermis and oral epithelium. Viral microtubular aggregates are present on electron microscopy both within the nuclei and cytoplasm of the syncytial giant cells (Suringa et al. 1970). In the skin focal parakeratosis and spongiosis with a few lymphocytes and syncytial giant cells are present in the epidermis.

Immediate complications are otitis media and keratitis. Kwashiorkor may be precipitated, as may tuberculosis. It has been considered until recently that the characteristic pathological changes specific for the diagnosis of measles are only seen in patients dying prior to the onset of the rash and that when death occurs in the later stages of the disease the findings are non-specific and are due to bronchopneumonia and secondary bacterial infection as described above.

Hecht, however, in 1910 described a form of giant-cell pneumonia in which there was an interstitial pneumonitis with giant cells containing intranuclear and intracytoplasmic inclusions in the bronchioles and alveoli, and Pinkerton et al. (1945) considered that this might be due to infection by the measles virus without the usual clinical manifestations. The condition is not uncommon in children in our experience but inclusion bodies have not been a noticeable feature.

McCarthy et al. (1958) isolated the virus of measles from three children dying of giant-cell pneumonia in which the giant cells showed intranuclear and intracytoplasmic includions. It is perhaps significant that the children from whom the virus was isolated were suffering from mucoviscidosis, leukaemia, and Letterer–Siwe disease. No evidence of a skin rash or any other signs of measles were noted although they had all been in contact with the infection. Koffler (1964) also demonstrated the presence of giant-cell pneumonia associated with the presence of measles virus in a 28-year-old female thought to be suffering from an immunological deficiency.

We therefore conclude that the pathology of measles in the prodromal stage is characterized by giant-cell transformation of the epithelium lining the respiratory tract and of the tissues of the reticulo-endothelial system. Following the appearance of the rash the pathological changes are usually those of secondary infection. In a proportion of patients the clinical and pathological findings may be those of a giant-cell penumonia (Hecht) in the absence of other signs of measles.

Diagnostic pathology

Leucopenia is usual. Multinucleated cells may be detected in nasal secretions and the virus can be isolated from throat washings, lachrymal secretions, or blood early in the disease by inoculation into human kidney, monkey kidney, or amnion cell cultures (Enders, 1962). Inclusion-bearing cells may be seen in the urine. A rise in antibody titre by serum neutralization, complement-fixation, or haemagglutination-inhibition tests may be demonstrated. At autopsy virus can usually be isolated from the lungs in the early stages of the infection and in the later stages only if giant-cell pneumonia is present.

RUBELLA

Rubella has a world-wide distribution. Epidemics in northern hemispheres occur irregularly at 5–7 year intervals—usually in older children and adolescents. In Britain and the U.S.A. approximately 80 per cent of pregnant women have rubella antibody. In Hawaii about 40 per cent, in Japan 65 per cent, in Uganda 76 per cent (Dudgeon, 1968).

German measles is a mild disease but its importance lies in the fact that if women are infected in the first trimester of pregnancy—especially the first month—congenital transmission can cause low birth weight, congenital heart disease, bone lesions, hepatosplenomegaly, thrombocytopenic purpura, microcephaly, cataract, deafness, and cerebral palsy in the infant (Cooper et al. 1969). The infection can be spread to susceptible contacts.

The laboratory diagnosis has been discussed in an Editorial (1970). Two serological tests are widely used—the haemagglutination—inhibition test and the complement-fixation test. The first test is reliably specific.

MARGBURG VIRUS DISEASE

In 1967 medical personnel in Margburg, Frankfurt and Belgrade in direct contact with the blood, organs or cell cultures of African green monkeys (*Cercopithecus aethiops*) from Uganda developed a serious, unknown and frequently fatal illness. The infection could spread from the patient to an auxiliary and was even spread by sexual intercourse—the semen of the husband proving infective. The disease has been extensively reviewed (Martini and Siegert, 1971; Monath, 1974). Clinically there was prostration, headache, myalgia, vomiting, watery diarrhoea, conjunctivitis, a characteristic rash, restlessness, and in severe cases, confusion, haemorrhages, haematemesis, coma and death. The incubation period varied from 3 to 9 days.

Macroscopically at post mortem the brain was congested and oedematous. Haemorrhages were present in the skin and mucous membranes. The stomach and sections of the intestines contained blood without any obvious source of bleeding. The liver was not remarkable and jaundice was not noted. Histopathological examination revealed focal necrosis in many organs without an inflammatory infiltrate (striated muscle, lung and bone excepted). The most striking lesions were in the liver and lymphatic system. In the spleen there was necrosis of follicles with loss of cells in the pulp which appeared to be replaced by finely granulated eosinophilic material. Areas of focal necrosis occurred in the liver and to a lesser extent in the testes and ovaries. Basophilic bodies 1–4 nm in diameter were noted in the vicinity of the necrotic areas, intracellularly in phagocytes and also extracellularly. A tubular necrosis was noted in the kidney and, in the brain, there was a diffuse encephalitis. In the heart only an interstitial oedema was present. There would appear to be some similarity to Lassa Fever in the pathological findings.

Diagnosis

A leucopenia is usual and peculiar forms of lymphocytes are seen in the peripheral blood in addition to plasma cells as well as pyrinophilic blast cells (immunoblasts). There is a thrombocytopenia. The plasma coagulation factors are relatively normal. The liver enzymes are markedly raised although the serum bilirubin values are normal.

Margburg virus can be transmitted to guinea pigs intra-peritoneally by blood inoculation at the height of the fever, and has been identified by electron microscopy. Immunofluorescence on liver biopsies can demonstrate the antigen. A complement-fixation test is being developed. In addition to the symposium referred to above the condition was previously reviewed by Siegert (1970).

HERPES VIRUSES

These are relatively large DNA viruses and a number of the members of the group have been associated with malignant conditions both in man, mammals, and birds. The important members of the group are shown in Table 4.5. The Epstein–Barr virus is discussed when infectious mononucleosis is considered. *H. simiae* can occasionally infect man—a fatal encephalitis ensuing.

H. saimiri and *H. ateles* can produce lymphoma-like tumours in primates and laboratory animals (Hunt and Melendez, 1972). Marek's disease virus causes neurolymphomatosis in chickens. It is of interest that the inoculation of a cell line of Burkitt's lymphoma carrying the Epstein–Barr virus caused no symptoms or signs of Marek's disease in chickens observed for 4–7 months (Ngu and Osunkoya, 1973).

TABLE 4.5. *Important members of the herpes group of viruses*

Name	Host	Disease
Herpes virus hominus	Man	*Herpes simplex*
Herpes virus varicellae	Man	Varicella-zoster
Cytomegalovirus	Man	Cytomegalic inclusion disease
Herpesvirus simiae	*Rhesus and Cynomolgus monkeys*	B. virus occasionally in man
Herpesvirus saimiri	Squirrel monkey	Malignant tumours in owl monkey and marmoset
Herpes virus suis	Pig	Pseudorabies
Epstein–Barr virus	Man, mammals	Infectious mononucleosis and associated with various malignancies
Herpesvirus ateles	Black spider monkeys	Lymphoblastic lymphomas in marmosets
Marek's disease virus	Poultry	Neurolymphomatosis

HERPES SIMPLEX

Herpes simplex is caused by *Herpesvirus hominus*. There are two antigenic strains—1 and 2. Type 2 strains are probably more virulent and are related to genital herpes—and may be related to cervical carcinoma in women (Goodheart, 1970; Editorial, 1970).

It is an acute infectious disease. The infection may be primary or recurrent. Primary infection occurs in individuals without pre-existing antibody whereas antibody is present in those with recurrent infection. Primary infection may be latent. Recurrent infection occurs from a disturbance of the host–parasite relationship and is usually mild and localized but severe and sometimes lethal infections may occur in patients with malignant lymphomas or on immuno-suppressive drugs (Juel-Jensen, 1973). Primary infections rarely can be severe and generalized. The condition has been reviewed by Dudgeon (1970).

The antibody is present in the majority of newborn infants and at one year in about 5 per cent of children. At 5 years the frequency depends on socio-economic factors—in Bantu children aged 2–3 years in Cape Town 90 per cent showed evidence of previous infection (Becker, 1966). Spread is by direct contact and droplet infection. The incubation period is 2–7 days and the infection may be subclinical in 99 per cent of patients. Antibodies are formed and remain constant throughout life. As stated above, placental passage of antibodies occur and primary infection in the neonate is uncommon.

In general the infection is usually mild with gingivostomatitis, malaise, fever and cervical lymphadenopathy being the most severe manifestations of infection. Blisters on the tongue, buccal mucosa and palate may be troublesome. There is no doubt that in the tropics herpes infection is common in children suffering from measles and kwashiorkor and a severe stomatitis may occur. It may also be an aetiological agent in cancrum oris (p. 515). Dudgeon (1970) has classified the clinical manifestations as:

(1) Cutaneous;   (2) Mucosal;   (3) Eye;
(4) Generalized; and   (5) Central nervous system.

Pathology

The characteristic lesions are vesicles 3–5 mm in diameter containing clear fluid at first which rapidly becomes pustular. Scarring is rare.

Acute kerato-conjunctivitis may be a local extension from a herpetic eruption on the face. Usually only one eye is affected and healing is the rule.

Generalized *herpes simplex* may occur as eczema herpeticum which is similar to the eruption seen in vaccinia. Vesicles appear in crops and rapidly ulcerate. The mortality may be high. Hepato-adrenal necrosis may occur especially in infants (Templeton, 1970).

Herpes hepatitis is an entity and we have seen two cases in Caucasian adults in West Africa with areas of necrosis and intranuclear inclusions in the liver similar to the histopathological picture which is seen in the neonate. The virus can be isolated from the liver at post mortem.

Herpetic infection of the central nervous system may manifest itself as:

(1) aseptic meningitis;
(2) acute encephalomyelitis with or without visceral necrosis; and
(3) acute necrotizing encephalomyelitis.

They may be primary or reactivated infections. The C.S.F. may be normal in the last condition and a space-occupying lesion may be simulated. The characteristic lesion, whether in skin or viscera, is cell necrosis associated with intranuclear changes consisting of margination of nuclear chromaton and the development of intranuclear inclusions.

Diagnosis

In cutaneous lesions multinucleated giant cells can be seen in smears stained with Giemsa. Gardner *et al.* (1968) used a specific herpetic antiserum and an indirect immunofluorescent technique on cell scrapings from skin and ocular lesions to make a rapid diagnosis. Electron microscopy on brain biopsy material makes a specific diagnosis of encephalomyelitis possible within hours (Campbell, 1969) which is most important in view of the possible therapy with idoxuridine or cytarabine. Swabs may be taken and cultured from obvious lesions. Serum may be tested for rising antibody titres, and neutralization and complement-fixation tests are of value.

INFECTIOUS MONONUCLEOSIS (GLANDULAR FEVER)

Clinically infectious mononucleosis (IM) in developed countries is a disease of children and adolescents especially of University students and similar population groups. It is characterized by fever, sore throat and lymphadenopathy. It is usually a mild disease. Splenomegaly and hepatic involvement, rarely with jaundice, are common. Skin rashes can occur.

A viral aetiology for IM has long been suspected. Recent observations have shown that the Epstein–Barr or EB virus (EBV) is intimately related to IM (Henle *et al.* 1968; Niederman *et al.* 1968; Gerber *et al.* 1968). This virus was first detected in lines of cultured Burkitt tumour cells (Epstein *et al.* 1964) and in view of its importance in this malignancy the part that it plays in infectious mononucleosis is considered in some detail. The EB virus is a herpes-type virus and grows only in cultured human cells of the haemopoietic system. It does not cause cell lysis and cells once infected remain so and pass on the infection when they divide. Antibodies to the virus are found 'normally' in a considerable percentage of most populations. The evidence which indicates that the EBV is related to IM is as follows:

1. The virus propagates only in cells of the lymphoreticular system.
2. The virus stimulates growth of lymphocytes in culture.
3. The leucocytes from IM patients in culture readily grow and develop into blastoid cell lines which all harbour EBV.
4. All patients with classical IM have shown high titres of antibodies to EBV.

5. Antibody conversion has been noted in students contracting IM—although it has also been seen in individuals in the absence of an illness recognized as IM (McCollum, 1970). However, no students with EBV antibodies developed symptoms of IM.

6. Throat washings from patients with IM have converted an indicator lymphoid cell from negative to positive for antigen of EBV as determined by the indirect immunofluorescence test (Golden *et al.* 1971).

7. Accidental transmission of the virus by blood transfusion has been shown by serological tests.

It would appear that the EBV plays an essential part in the aetiology of IM but that IM is by no means the only response to EBV infection. In spite of the above evidence, because of the lack of direct isolation of the virus, there are still some who are reluctant to accept the EBV as the aetiologic agent of IM but all evidence to date would prove that, at least, if it is not the causal agent it will be closely linked to any other agent discovered.

The relationship of the EB virus with the Burkitt tumour and other malignancies is discussed on p. 502. A prospective study of 2437 U.S. veterans with IM during service in World War II was compared with controls as to frequencies of death in the period 1946–65. No significant difference in leukaemia–lymphoma deaths were noted (Miller and Beebe, 1973).

Epidemiology

The incubation period is reported as variable—from a few days to many weeks. In Sweden it was shown that 90 per cent of neonates had antibody to the EBV at birth, presumably of maternal origin. At the age of 2 years only 12 per cent had antibodies rising to 90 per cent at 20 years of age (Demissie and Svedmyr, 1969). In developing countries IM is a disease rarely diagnosed. Diehl *et al.* (1969) identified a number of cases of glandular fever in East Africa but mostly in Caucasian children and adults, with two cases only in African students. This has been our experience in West Africa. Utilizing only standard haematological techniques, including the Paul–Bunnell test, a few cases have been diagnosed in children and Caucasian students but none in West African adults.

It seems likely therefore that in developing countries infection may occur while maternal antibodies are still present, allowing the development of immunity in some children showing no or mild symptoms of the disease, with relatively no adults exhibiting signs of the infection.

Obviously, in developed countries, as the prevalence of antibody is high, silent or mild infections must also occur.

The antibody persists for long periods after infection—probably for life as the prevalence is over 80 per cent in the elderly. It is probable that the virus persists in the lymphoreticular system which would explain the above finding and the frequent finding of the virus in cultures of leucocytes from healthy donors or patients with various diseases including leukaemia and various forms of cancer (Henle and Henle, 1970).

The mode of transmission of EBV remains obscure but their association with lymphoid tissue suggests tonsils and adenoids might contribute, and epidemics in populations of young people might be associated with kissing or through mouth-to-mouth contact or fomites.

Pathology

The lymphoreticular tissue is affected and haematological changes are marked mainly in the lymphocytic series of cells. Anaemia is unusual but rarely an autoimmune type of haemolytic anaemia with a positive Coombs test occurs.

Dodsworth and Burns (1971) have reported disseminated intravascular coagulation with hypofibrinogenaemia responding to heparin therapy as an uncommon complication.

The leucocytes may be increased, normal in number, or decreased. The striking feature, however, is the presence of variable numbers of abnormal lymphocytes in the blood smears. They are polymorphic. Some may be plasmacytoid with densely clumped nuclear chromatin and basophilic cytoplasm. Some nuclei may contain nucleoli. Larger cells are seen somewhat resembling monocytes with an oval reniform or lobulated nucleus with no nucleoli and abundant pale cytoplasm often foamy or finely vacuolated. They are peroxidase negative. These are the so called 'glandular fever cells'. They are, however, not specific and may be seen in other childhood infections. Electron microscopy studies have shown the abnormal lymphocytes to be similar to transformed lymphocytes (Carter, 1969). Leucocyte alkaline phosphatase is low early in the illness. There may be granulomatous lesions in the bone marrow and there is an increase of abnormal lymphocytes. The granulocytes show a shift to the left. A mild thrombocytopenia occurs in a number of patients and rarely may be severe.

There are striking serological changes, one of the most important being the presence of heterophile antibodies as shown by the Paul–Bunnell and other tests (see diagnosis). Antibody to the EBV can be demonstrated. The presence of a cold antibody anti-i is common. Rheumatoid and antinuclear factors have been reported and the Wasserman test may be positive. Antiplatelet and antileucocytic antibodies may develop. IgM is always present and IgG sometimes increases.

Histological examination may reveal perivascular infiltration by normal and abnormal lymphocytes in almost every organ in the body. But the lymphoreticular tissue is most severely affected. Lesions occur predominantly in lymph nodes which exhibit follicular hyperplasia and a diffuse proliferation of atypical lymphoid cells. Occasionally the follicular pattern may be destroyed, normal mitotic figures may be present and even Reed–Sternberg cells as seen in Hodgkin's disease have been described (McMahon *et al.* 1970). The danger of misdiagnosing a malignant lymphoma in these cases is considerable if clinical information is not available to the pathologist.

In the spleen there is proliferation of atypical lymphocytes and they invade the trabeculae and capsule rendering the spleen more liable to rupture. An interesting finding is lymphocytic infiltration of the subintimal lymphatics with 'pavementing' in the trabecular veins—a subject which was more fully discussed when lassa fever was considered (p. 229).

In the liver there is periportal lymphocytic infiltration and the parenchymal changes may resemble those of viral hepatitis. The liver function tests therefore may be abnormal.

A myocarditis has been described (Das and Seidelin, 1972) and pulmonary involvement has rarely been reported. Focal cellular collections may be seen in the kidney.

Nervous involvement occasionally occurs and the symptomatology is protean. Focal encephalomyelitis has been reported presenting as an expanding lesion in the occipital lobe. The pathology was that of an inflammatory demyelinating lesion consistent with allergic or post-infectious encephalomyelitis. Penman (1970), in a critical review of the literature, concluded that neurological complications were the major cause of death followed by deaths from splenic rupture and secondary infection. Rarely liver failure may occur. The nervous deaths were due to peripheral neuropathy of the Landry–Guillain–Barré type or cerebral changes secondary to encephalopathy. A terminal hyperpyrexia was not uncommon in both groups.

Diagnosis

The diagnosis depends upon:
(1) Clinical examination and a high index of suspicion.
(2) The characteristic blood smear.
(3) The positive differential heterophile agglutination test.
(4) The presence of EBV antibodies in the serum.

The Paul–Bunnell and differential heterophile agglutination tests are described in textbooks of haematology and will not be described in detail. Briefly in IM there is a heterophile antibody which is capable of agglutinating sheep's red cells in high titre. A rather similar antibody is found in low titre in normal people (Forssman antibody) but can be absorbed by guinea pig kidney and not by ox red cells. The glandular fever antibody is absorbed by ox red cells but not by the Forssman antigen in guinea pig kidney. A new commercial slide screening test utilizing horse erythrocytes (Monospot: Ortho-Pharmaceuticals Ltd.) to detect heterophile antibodies with the differential absorption characteristics of IM has been developed, which appears to be at least as sensitive and specific as the Paul–Bunnell test (Mott, 1969). False positives have been noted in a few patients with malignant lymphoma (Carter *et al.* 1970). It may be negative in a very small percentage of cases of IM but EBV antibody will be present or will develop late in convalescence (see below).

EBV antibodies may be detected in serum by immunofluoresence tests using a Burkitt cell line as antigen (Henle and Henle, 1966). The direct membrane immunofluorescence test (MIF) has been used extensively to detect membrane antigens on cultured EBV carrying lymphoblastoid cell lines of the Burkitt tumour. Hewetson *et al.* (1972) have utilized radioiodine in place of fluorescein to label the antibody to detect the membrane antigens, and claim that it is a much more sensitive test and can detect low concentrations of antimembrane antibodies in certain sera which were negative by the MIF test. Lastly a culture of leucocytes may yield a continuous line of lymphoblastoid cells. As previously stated liver function tests may be abnormal with high transaminases and positive flocculation tests.

The C.S.F. may contain an increased number of lymphocytes and protein and the pressure may be increased even in the absence of clinical C.N.S. involvement. Albumin and red blood cells may be found in the urine and urobilinogen and bile if the liver is affected.

Cytomegalic inclusion disease and toxoplasmosis can be differentiated by complement-fixation tests. Other conditions which may confuse with IM are adenovirus infections, brucellosis, trypanosomiasis, leishmaniasis, typhoid fever, and even tuberculosis.

POLIOMYELITIS AND OTHER ENTEROVIRUSES

The enteroviruses, in addition to poliovirus, include the *Coxsackie*, *Echo* (enteric cytopathogenic human orphan), and *Reo* (respiratory and enteric orphan) virus. These viruses were first isolated from the faeces of patients during poliomyelitis investigations. Healthy persons may excrete enteroviruses for short periods, and in areas where standards of environmental sanitation are low, they are prevalent among infants and young children. *Coxsackie viruses* are classified into two groups, A and B, and although frequently isolated from healthy persons they may cause a variety of human illnesses, e.g. herpangina; summer grippe; vesicular stomatitis; virus meningitis, etc. The presence of Coxsackie Group-B virus can interfere with poliomyelitis virus multiplication while a mixed Coxsackie Group A and poliomyelitis virus infection might result in a more severe paralysis (Dalldorf, 1951). Coxsackie B viruses cause pleurodynia, myalgia, aseptic meningitis, and pericarditis. It is the cause of Bornholm disease. Numerous cases of pericarditis or myocarditis have been described (Helin *et al.* 1968). Massive pulmonary haemorrhage has been reported in the newborn; there was an acute myocarditis and meningoencephalitis. The incubation period is 2–5 days, but may be longer. Illness, in this case, began on the 8th day of life.

Echo viruses are also excreted by healthy persons, particularly children, but may cause illnesses such as diarrhoea and virus meningitis. Echo virus type 5, affecting 56 newborn children and eight adults, has been reported from Singapore. No serious maternal or neonatal complications occurred (German *et al.* 1968). *Reo viruses* were first isolated from the faeces of healthy children but have been also found in children with diarrhoea and steatorrhoeic enteritis. By far the most important enterovirus in the tropics is poliomyelitis and this will be described in some detail. It should be noted that the enteroviruses (*Coxsackie, Echo, Reo*) may interfere with oral poliomyelitis vaccination campaigns in the tropics (Sabin, 1962; Montefiore *et al.* 1963). A global 4-year study of enteroviruses other than poliovirus was carried out by Assaad and Cockburn (1972).

POLIOMYELITIS

Poliomyelitis is widespread in the tropics and subtropics. In many areas infection is hyperendemic and all of the known types of poliomyelitis virus (I, II, and III) are prevalent. Within such communities the disease smoulders but epidemic outbreaks undoubtedly occur (Kaur and Metselaar, 1967). The virus strains responsible for paralytic illness in any area may vary, and at different periods in the same area one type or other may predominate (Charles and Grant, 1962; Poliomyelitis Commission, 1966).

Epidemiology

Poliomyelitis is a highly infectious disease and the alimentary tract is of prime importance as a portal of entry and exit of the virus, as it is with other enteroviruses. The factor of greatest importance in determining the incidence of paralytic poliomyelitis is the state of immunity of the affected population. In many tropical countries where sanitation is primitive and living conditions are crowded and poor, facilities for the spread of poliovirus are good; consequently infants have the opportunity of coming into contact with all three types of poliomyelitis virus early in life, and few of them reach pre-school age without having been infected with at least one strain, although, clinically, the infection is in most cases inapparent. Immunity is acquired early. In countries where the sanitary arrangements are good, the risk of contact with the virus at an early age is diminished and older persons are affected (Paul, 1955). Thus the most significant difference between the occurrence of poliomyelitis in the well-developed countries of the temperate zone and the less-developed areas of the tropics is in the distribution of cases in the various age-groups. Serum antibody surveys carried out among children in many parts of the tropics have shown that by the time they are 3 years old 90 per cent have developed antibodies against at least one type of poliomyelitis (Paul et al. 1952; WHO, 1962; Montefiore et al. 1963). Passive immunity is transmitted from mother to offspring and lasts for about 3–6 months.

Pathology

During the incubation period of 7 days the virus multiplies in the lymphoid tissue of the intestinal tract and mesenteric lymph nodes prior to the viraemia occurring. The virus eventually affects the motor neurones of the spinal cord. In the bulbar form the lesions involve the medulla and pons and may extend to the midbrain, basal ganglia, and the motor area of the cerebral cortex. In the cord the lesions are generally in the ventral horns and in the bases of the dorsal horns of the grey matter. These areas are swollen and congested and histologically the neurones show marked degenerative changes with an associated inflammatory infiltrate consisting mainly of lymphocytes. Polymorphs are present in rapidly fatal cases. Eosinophilic inclusions may be present in the nuclei of a number of the neurones. The adjacent vessels are congested and thrombosis may occur. Atrophy of the paralysed muscles occurs, and if the respiratory muscles have been affected pulmonary oedema and bronchopneumonia are usual findings. Myocarditis is a frequent complication in fatal cases, with areas of focal necrosis infiltrated by lymphocytes and macrophages the usual lesion.

Diagnostic pathology

Changes in the cerebrospinal fluid constitute one of the best aids to diagnosis. Pleocytosis is the rule in the acute period; it reaches a maximum during the first 2 days of the disease, rapidly decreases from the third day, but persists to a reduced extent during the second week of the disease. An initial polymorphonuclear leucocytosis is replaced by a lymphocytosis. The protein content of the fluid is also high.

CYTOMEGALOVIRUS INFECTION

The cytomegaloviruses previously known as salivary gland viruses induce in man a cellular response characterized by cytomegaly with prominent intranuclear inclusion bodies. Cytomegalic inclusion disease is a relatively common infection in the neonate and inclusion bodies were present in the submandibular salivary gland in 7 per cent of our necropsies performed on stillbirths and neonates (Mainwaring and Tompkins, 1963; Editorial, 1968). The disease is rare in older children and adults, but may be precipitated by the use of cytotoxic drugs, steroids, etc. (Symmers, 1960). The infant may show hepatosplenomegaly, thrombocytopenia, purpura, hepatitis, jaundice, microcephaly, and mental retardation (Weller and Hanshaw, 1962). Chorioretinitis, optic atrophy, and cerebral calcification may also be seen. Focal necroses may be seen in almost any organ—those most frequently affected are the lungs, liver, pancreas, kidney, salivary glands, and brain. An interstitial pneumonitis is usual. The pathognomonic finding is the presence of giant cells (20–40 μm) with an enlarged nucleus containing a prominent inclusion body that may be eosinophilic or basophilic. The cytoplasm may also contain small basophilic inclusions. Cytomegalic cells may be seen in sputum or urine. Specimens should be examined fresh. Liver biopsy may be diagnostic if hepatitis is present. The virus may be recovered from urine, saliva, and tissue. In neonatal infections cytomegalic cells may be present in the chorionic villi of the placenta and virus may be isolated from the mother.

SLOW VIRUS INFECTIONS

Viruses may cause subacute, chronic degenerative or even neoplastic conditions. They may be true viruses with nucleic acid cores or slow viruses which appear to be without nucleic acid and whose mode of self-replication remains uncertain. The arena viruses have been extensively reviewed by Hotchin (1971).

KURU

Kuru is a fatal neurological disease which occurs in the geographically isolated eastern highlands of New Guinea among the Fore tribe (Zigas and Gajdusek, 1957). The epidemiology of the disease seems to have altered in the last 10 years. When first described it was found to affect commonly children of either sex, and young adults of the female sex only, being rare in adult males. Today, children—especially the younger ones—are rarely affected and there has been a decline in the overall incidence and mortality of the disease. Gajdusek *et al.* (1963) suggested that predisposition to kuru might depend on a single gene, dominant in the females only, which produces fatal disease in homozygotes of both sexes in childhood and in heterozygote females in adult life. Material from brains of eight patients who had died from kuru produced, on cerebral inoculation, after long incubation a similar disease—clinically and pathologically—in chimpanzees. The possibility of a 'slow virus' being responsible was entertained

(Gajdusek *et al.* 1966) and has since been proved (Gajdusek *et al.* 1972). Gibbs and Gajdusek (1970) have extended these investigations and fourth passage kuru has now been noted in chimpanzees. The virus remains viable in human brain tissue stored at -70 °C for more than five years and is transmitted experimentally by intracerebral or peripheral inoculation. The possibility of infection by the oral route is being studied. Alpers (1970) put forward the hypothesis that the dramatic nature of the epidemiological changes may be associated with the fact that cannibalism has been abandoned among the Fore tribe with the arrival of Western civilization and the disease should soon be extinct (Editorial, 1974).

Pathology

Kuru is primarily a disease of motor-coordination with ataxia, emotional instability, and easily provoked, inordinate laughter. As the disease progresses muscular movements of all kinds cease and the patient dies about 1 year after the beginning of symptoms.

Apart from some atrophy of the cerebellar vermis the brain is macroscopically normal. It is the only organ primarily affected. Histologically the striking feature is degeneration of the neurones in the cerebellar cortex, dentate nucleus, thalamus, corpus striatum, globus pallidus, and focal areas in the cerebral cortex. The degenerative changes are most marked in the cerebellum, particularly the vermis and its afferent and efferent connections. There is a slow progressive degeneration of the spinocerebellar and lateral corticospinal tracts. Most of the cranial nuclei are spared. The cytoplasm of the affected cell becomes basophilic and vacuolated and the Nissl substance is reduced. Astroglial and microglial proliferation occur but neuronophagia is never seen (Fowler and Robertson, 1959). PAS-positive plaques (about the size of ganglion cells) are seen in the cerebellum in about half of the subjects (Klatzo *et al.* 1959). Very occasionally a blood vessel will show perivascular cuffing. A similar pathology is seen in the disease 'scrapie' in sheep and goats. A kuru-like syndrome has been produced in seven out of eight chimpanzees, 18–30 months after intracerebral inoculation of brain suspension from patients who died of kuru. The pathology was similar to that described in human kuru but the cerebral cortex was more severely affected in the apes (Beck *et al.* 1966). The pathology of both scrapie in sheep and kuru in chimpanzees has been reviewed by Daniel (1971).

In addition to kuru a similar condition has been described in the west highlands of New Guinea with much more cerebral damage and a severe ascending myelo-encephalitis has been noted. The effects of kuru on pregnancy have been described by Zigas (1973). It appears that the disease does not interfere with normal pregnancy and that the rapidly progressive deteriorating nature of kuru is slowed down by pregnancy.

5

Diseases Caused by Fungi

There is increasing evidence that fungal infections may be an important cause of chronic disease in many parts of the tropics. Their study in the tropics has been much neglected—not only due to the lack of pathological services but also probably because of the complex classification utilized by the mycologists and the specialized techniques required in the isolation and culture of fungi. In this chapter we have considered diseases caused by fungi from two broad points of view—the superficial and the systemic mycoses. The latter include those fungal diseases affecting the subcutaneous tissues. Before considering these conditions, however, some slight knowledge of mycology is required and this is dealt with very briefly. Students interested in studying the subject further are referred to the works of Alexopoulos (1962), Emmons *et al.* (1963), and Baker (1971).

Fungi are nucleated spore-bearing* organisms which do not contain chlorophyll and which generally reproduce sexually and asexually. The fungi imperfecti reproduce only by the latter method. They may obtain their nutritional requirements by attacking dead organic matter (as saprophytes) or by infecting living organisms (as parasites).

The fungi which cause disease in man include yeasts, yeast-like organisms, and the filamentous and dimorphic fungi.

Yeasts are spherical or oval unicellular organisms which reproduce asexually by budding or sexually by the production of ascospores. It is thought that the yeasts which only reproduce by budding are responsible for infection in man; *Cryptococcus neoformans* is an example.

Yeast-like organisms can produce hyphae and budding-yeast cells simultaneously; *Candida albicans* is the best example.

The filamentous fungi consist of a body, called the hypha, which consists of protoplasm containing a variable number of small nuclei and a cell wall composed of cellulose or chitin. The hypha may be unicellular (aseptate) or divided into individual cells (septate). The hyphae elongate by apical growth and branching is a feature. Masses of entangled hyphae constitute the mycelium. The mycelium tends to enlarge uniformly from the centre with the formation of a spherical colony. Sexual reproduction which implies the

*A spore is a reproductive structure which may be uni or multicellular.

fusion of two individual nuclei is not considered in this text. Asexual reproduction may occur following fragmentation of the hypha, by budding, or by division of the hypha cell to form daughter cells. Various types of spores may be formed and these are utilized in identifying and classifying fungi. Arthrospores are formed by the breaking up of a hypha into separate cells. Chlamydospores are thick-walled resistant spores formed by the enlargement of the terminal or individual cells in the hypha and vary in size and shape within a culture. Conidium is the term used for any asexual spore, but it is frequently employed to describe spores formed on hypha buds. Sporangiospores (endospores) are produced in a sac-like structure (the sporangium) which develops in buds from the hypha. Spores under favourable conditions may reproduce by budding or by the extension of a germ tube and the formation of hyphae.

The dimorphic fungi have two forms, a yeast or spore form and a mycelial form. Both these forms may be parasitic in man but the mycelial form is frequently a saprophyte in soil, etc. and the spores are the infective agent in man. Medical mycology is hampered by the multiplicity of names that have been given to fungi of medical importance. In this section the nomenclature used is that recommended by the Medical Mycology Committee of the Medical Research Council (1967).

THE SUPERFICIAL MYCOSES

Clinically, many types of superficial fungal infections can be recognized and the common name for the majority of these infections is tinea, or ringworm.

The fungi invade only the superficial skin, hair, and nails and differ from most other fungal infections in that they are contagious; towels, hair brushes, shower boards and other fomites contaminated with infected hair, epidermal scales, or contact with infected animals being responsible for the infection.

The superficial mycoses have a world-wide distribution but are more common in tropical climates. No attempt is made here to describe individual species which are identified on colonial appearance, pigment production, morphology, and biochemical and growth requirements but it must be emphasized that any lesion of the skin, hair, or nails should raise the suspicion of fungal infection and a preliminary diagnosis can usually easily be made by examining microscopically scrapings of the lesion, after treatment with 10 per cent KOH.

Hyphae and/or spores are usually readily detected. Culture is, of course, required to identify the species. The following conditions are briefly described: tinea nigra palmaris; erythrasma; tinea versicolor; black piedra;

white piedra; trichomycosis axillaris; tinea capitis, barbae, and other forms.

TINEA NIGRA

Synonyms. Keratomycosis nigricans palmaris; cladosporiosis epidermica; pityriasis nigra; microsporosis nigra.

Tinea nigra is a superficial brown or black fungal infection of the epidermis usually seen on the palm of the hands. The usual causative organism is *Cladosporium werneckii* Horta.

Epidemiology

It is most common in tropical climates and different species of fungi may be the causative organism. We have seen the plantar surface of the foot affected.

Pathology

There is marked keratosis of the epidermis with septate fungal hyphae 1–5 μm in diameter in the superficial keratotic layer. The hyphae are branched and budding cells may be noted. The brownish colour of the fungus may be seen in unstained sections. Methenamine silver stains the fungal elements well.

ERYTHRASMA

In this condition there are reddish-brown slightly scaling patches in the axillae and groins. The infection is thought to be caused by *Nocardia minutissima*, which is now thought to be a corynebacterium.

PITYRIASIS VERSICOLOR

Synonyms. Tinea versicolor; tinea flava; dermatomycosis furfuracea; liver spots.

Malassezia furfur causes a branny, scaling, sharply marginated, pale-brownish lesion of the skin. The distribution is world-wide but it is more common in tropical areas. Short hyphae and spherical cells (8 μm in diameter) are found only in the stratum corneum (Fig. 5.1).

BLACK PIEDRA

In this condition black, hard, gritty nodules (up to 1 mm in diameter) are firmly attached to the hairs of the scalp, beard, or moustache. They are composed of a mass of fungal cells and hyphae are apparent at the periphery. Growth also occurs within the hair itself. Black piedra is caused by *Piedraia*

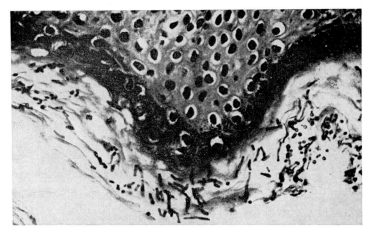

FIG. 5.1. Pityriasis versicolor. *Malassezia furfur* is shown in the stratum and corneum. Note the short blunt-edged hyphae intermingled with spores. (*By courtesy of Ash and Spitz.*)

hortae and occurs in humid tropical countries in the Americas and in Indonesia.

WHITE PIEDRA

Trichosporon beigelii grows within or on the hair of the beard or scalp, as white to light-brown nodules. It is more common in temperate regions than in the tropics.

TRICHOMYCOSIS AXILLARIS

In this condition there is a superficial infection of the axillary or pubic hair and fine nodules can be seen macroscopically. It is not uncommon in tropical climates. The aetiology is debatable. Red, yellow, and black forms have been described.

TINEA

Tinea capitis is usually caused by *Microsporum audouini* or to species of trichophyta (*T. violaceum*, *T. schoenleini*, *T. verrucosum*, or *T. mentagrophytes*). *M. audouini* is common in tropical areas but in general species of *Trichophyta* are the more common. Children are most frequently infected, boys being more commonly affected than girls. Favus, due usually to *T. schoenleini*, is confined to areas with a long, hot, dry season.

Fungae are present not only in the horny layer of the epidermis but also in the hair follicle within and around the hair. No hyphae are present in the dermis but there may be a perifollicular chronic inflammatory reaction.

Tinea corporis is caused by species of *Trichophyta*. *T. rubrum* is a common cause of superficial mycosis in India (Desai, 1963). Ringworm of the feet and hands is usually caused by *T. mentagrophytes* or *T. aubrum*, and less commonly by *T. floccosum*.

The hyphae are found in the horny layers of the skin and only two species of *Trichophyta* invade the hair follicles, namely *T. faviforme* and *T. rubrum*. A subacute inflammatory reaction is usually present in the dermis.

THE SYSTEMIC MYCOSES

The systemic mycoses have been classified in Table 5.1 according to the characteristic pathological changes they induce in the tissues. During 1972, 122 cases were reported in Great Britain, most of the infections were cases of aspergilloma (Editorial, 1974).

A number of fungi produce an acute inflammatory reaction and are usually easily seen in routine tissue sections, the infection, however, may be missed if special stains are not employed—especially in nocardiosis.

Others cause pseudoepitheliomatous hyperplasia in the epidermis with a mixed acute and chronic granulomatous inflammation in the dermis and can usually be identified from their morphology in routine sections, an exception being sporotrichosis which may only be detectable on culture.

A third group cause histiocytic proliferation with or without giant cells predominating.

Lastly there are subcutaneous phycomycosis and rhinophycomycosis in which the characteristic lesion is an eosinophilic (fibrinoid) necrosis surrounding the fungal elements.

Culture is always required for definitive species identification but the experienced pathologist can usually indicate the genus from tissue sections and indicate to the clinician the necessary form of therapy.

Any acute or granulomatous inflammatory lesion seen in biopsy material in the tropics should raise the suspicion of a mycotic infection and a PAS or methenamine silver stain will be of diagnostic help in most cases. As already stated sporotrichosis is an exception as culture is usually required to detect the organism. Staining by Gram's method is helpful if mycetoma is diagnosed. Mycobacteria may also cause necrotic inflammatory lesions and it is our practice in inflammatory lesions of unknown aetiology to request a battery of special staining methods, namely, PAS, methenamine silver, Gram, Ziehl-Neelsen, and Giemsa. A Meyer's mucicarmine stain may also be helpful. Immunofluorescent techniques are being developed and, in the future, may allow of easy identification of pathogenic fungi in surgical and autopsy specimens (Metzger *et al.* 1962).

TABLE 5.1. *Histopathological changes and the morphology of fungi seen in the tissues in the systemic mycoses*

Tissue changes	Disease	Organism	Size of fungus (μm)	Appearance of fungus
1. Acute inflammation	Candidiasis	*Candida albicans* and other species	3–4	Budding hyphae and yeasts
	Nocardiosis 'Mycetoma'	*Nocardia asteroides* See p. 271	(0·5–1) Grains	(Branched filaments). Special stains required
2. Acute inflammation with blood vessel invasion	Aspergillosis	Species of *Aspergillus*	3–4	Septate hyphae with characteristic branching
	Phycomycosis	Species of *Absidia, Mucor,* or *Rhizopus*	3–20	Haphazardly branched, rarely septate hyphae
3. Acute inflammation surrounded by a granulomatous reaction	Actinomycosis	*Actinomyces israeli*	Grain up to 300	Branching filaments with club-shaped formation at periphery
	Coccidioidomycosis	*Coccidioides immitis*	30–60	Thick-walled spores. Some containing endospores
4. Pseudoepitheliomatous hyperplasia. Mixed acute and granulomatous inflammation	North American blastomycosis	*Blastomyces dermatitidis*	8–15	Thick-walled spores. Budding forms with broad base
	South American blastomycosis	*Paracoccidioides brasiliensis*	5–30	Spores show multiple peripheral budding
	Chromomycosis	Species of *Phialophora* and *Cladosporium*	5–8	Thick-walled, dark brown, sometimes septate spores
	Sporotrichosis	*Sporothrix schenckii*	(5)	Usually no fungi seen. Asteroid body occasionally present
5. Histiocytic proliferation Necrosis	Histoplasmosis	*Histoplasma capsulatum*	3	Spores in histiocytes
6. Histiocytic proliferation Giant cells. Necrosis	African histoplasmosis	*Histoplasma duboisii*	8–15	Thick-walled spores. Budding with narrow base
	Cryptococcosis	*Cryptococcus neoformans*	4–7	Spores which stain with mucicarmine
	Cheloidal blastomycosis	*Loboa loboi* blastomycosis	8	Double spores joined by band
7. Chronic inflammation Giant cells	Rhinosporidiosis	*Rhinosporidium seeberi*	10–200	Large sporangia containing numerous endospores
8. Fibrinoid reaction round fungus. Eosinophils Granulomatous reaction	Subcutaneous phycomycosis	Species of *Basidiobolus*	5–15	Clear, thin-walled hyphae. Rarely septate
	Rhinophycomycosis	*Entomophthora coronata*	5–15	Clear, thin-walled hyphae. Rarely septate

We have made no attempt to describe the methods utilized in the culture of the pathogenic fungi or their morphology therein. Interested readers are referred to the textbook by Emmons *et al.* (1963).

CANDIDIASIS

Candidiasis is a condition caused by many species of *Candida*, the most common being *C. albicans*. They are commensals in the oral cavity, upper respiratory passages and intestinal tract.

It occurs so frequently that it is rarely reported. It causes oral (thrush), cutaneous, vaginal, pulmonary and gastro-intestinal lesions. Endocarditis may be a complication, especially after open-heart surgery.

It occurs especially in debilitated patients, premature infants, and after treatment with certain drugs (antibiotics, steroids, cytotoxic agents).

The fungus may be seen in the internal organs, in the mucous membranes and in areas of suppuration and can be detected on routine haemtoxylin and eosin or methenamine silver stains.

The yeast forms are egg-shaped, budding cells (3–4 μm in size) which stain densely as do the hyphae and enable a confident diagnosis of candidiasis to be given on tissue sections but the species cannot be differentiated.

NOCARDIOSIS

The term nocardiosis refers to a generalized mycotic infection in man caused by *Nocardia asteroides*. *N. braziliensis* and *N. caviae* are aetiological agents in the conditions known as mycetoma (see below) and are not included in the term nocardiosis. Very occasionally *N. asteroides* may cause mycetoma.

Pathology

Infection by *N. asteroides* affects primarily the lungs, and haematogenous spread to other organs occurs, a predilection for the brain and meninges being usual. It is an anaerobic, partially acid-fast branching actinomycete with hyphae which rarely exceed 1 μm in diameter. It is not found in high incidence in the tropics. It presents as a disease of the lung with secondary cerebral, renal or cardiac lesions.

It causes an acute suppurative lesion in the tissues in which branched (Gram-positive) filaments (0·5–1 μm in diameter) may be seen by Gram's or methenamine silver stains (Fig. 5.2). Granules and peripheral clubbing are excessively rare.

It cannot be detected on routine haematoxylin and eosin staining and it is possible that infection by this fungus is being missed in tropical areas.

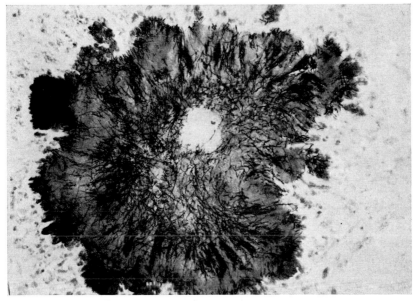

FIG. 5.2. Nocardiosis: (Mycetoma). A colony of *N. brasiliensis* is shown. Narrow, branching, Gram-positive filaments can be seen (Gram × 800). (*By courtesy of Dr. I. G. Murray.*)

THE MYCETOMAS

Synonyms. Madura foot; Madura mycosis; maduromycosis.

It must be realized that the term mycetoma does not refer to a specific condition but to a group of conditions which clinically, in the late stages, present as a chronic localized swelling involving subcutaneous tissue, fascia and bone. The lesions are usually single but may be multiple and occur most frequently on the foot but can occur anywhere on the body, the hand being the second most common site. The infecting organism can be a fungus, an actinomycete, or various types of bacteria. The most usual organisms are listed in Table 5.2. The typical lesion contains granulomata and abscesses which suppurate and drain through sinus tracts. The pus contains granules (colonies of the infecting agent) which vary in size from microscopic to more than 2 mm in diameter.

The size, colour, shape, and texture of the granules vary with the infecting organism. The subject has been extensively reviewed by Winslow (1971).

Epidemiology

The disease is of world-wide distribution but is more common in dry, tropical regions, especially in rural areas. The organism gains access to the

TABLE 5.2. *Organisms causing mycetomas*

Organisms	Colour of granules	Geographical distribution
Bacteria		
Nocardia brasiliensis	White to yellow	Nigeria, Congo, S. Africa, America
N. caviae		
Bacterium-like		
Streptomyces madurae	White or yellowish	W. Africa
S. pelletieri	Red to pink	W. Africa, Sudan, Central and South America
S. somaliensis	Yellow to brown	W. Africa, Sudan
Fungi		
Madurella mycetomi	Black to brown	W. Africa, Sudan, Algeria, Somaliland, North and South America, Europe
M. grisea	Black to brown	S. America
Allescheria boydii (*Monosporium apiospernum*)	White to pale yellow	N. America
Leptosphaeria senegalensis	Black	W. Africa
Phialophora jeanselmei	Brown to black	Martinique, U.S.A., Congo
Cephalosporium species	White to yellow	Senegal, Brazil, Puerto Rica, Japan
Pyrenochaeta romeroi	Black	W. Africa, S. America

tissues through trauma. Contaminated thorns or splinters are the usual mode of infection. No age or racial group is exempt but males in farming groups are more frequently affected because of occupational hazard.

Pathology

Irrespective of the aetiological agent the gross and microscopic tissue changes are similar. The organisms cause an acute inflammatory reaction and burrowing abscesses and sinuses are formed. Destruction of underlying bone occurs. The grains consist of colonies of organisms or hyphae with or without spores surrounded by a shell which may be rough, smooth, or spiny. The shell is an eosinophilic somewhat hyaline material and may form ray-like extensions from the periphery of a colony. It probably represents part of the host reaction. The colour of the grain depends upon the infecting organism (see Table 5.2).

On microscopy a colony of organisms is usually seen in the centre of a neutrophil polymorphonuclear exudate which is in turn surrounded by a chronic inflammatory reaction containing histiocytes and giant cells. The presence of a foreign body (thorn) may be noted. There is much fibrous tissue overgrowth with a variable cellular infiltrate. Staining by Gram's method may reveal that the grain is composed of bacteria (cocci or bacilli) and is not a true mycetoma. If Gram-positive, branching-filamentous organisms 0·5–1 μm in diameter are present, the lesion is an actinomycotic, nocardial or streptomycetal mycetoma. Anaerobic and aerobic cultures are required to make a specific diagnosis. If broad hyphae are seen with special fungal stains the lesion is a true mycetoma.

With experience the pathologist may be able to suggest the specific fungus responsible for the lesion in a high percentage of cases.

Clinically, the presence of swelling, sinuses and grains in the discharge are diagnostic of mycetoma. A knowledge of the geographical distribution of the mycetomas may allow a tentative macroscopic diagnosis to be made. Direct examination of the grain in 10 per cent NaOH may be made. The colour of the grain in routine H and E sections can be helpful (see Table 5.2) and the examination of unstained sections is frequently of value. Tissue sections differentiate the true mycetomas due to fungal infection from the actinomycetes (Gram-positive filaments) and bacterial infections (botryo-mycosis).

Radiological examination reveals the extent of bony damage and skin testing and serological investigations may be helpful in certain infections. Culture is always indicated.

ASPERGILLOSIS

A number of species of *Aspergillus* can cause disease in man, animals and birds. *A. fumigatus* and *A. niger* are the usual pathogens in man and cause chronic pulmonary lesions often with haematogenous spread to other organs. A nasopharyngeal form with unilateral proptosis has been described in the Sudan. The condition has been reviewed (Editorial 1971).

Epidemiology

The disease is world-wide in its distribution. Cases occur sporadically usually as an 'opportunistic' infection. No differences in age, race, or sex have been noted. Species of *Aspergillus* grow as saprophytes on decaying vegetation and man is exposed to the inhalation of conidia. Farmers and gardeners may become hypersensitive to the spores, with an asthmatic condition resulting. With lowered resistance in the host the inhaled spores may germinate and the fungus may invade the tissues of the lung (Seabury and Samuel, 1963). Infection has been transmitted to the neonate by exchange transfusion via the umbilical vein.

Pathology

A single, healed, calcified lesion ('coin') may be noted as an incidental finding on X-ray of the chest. Pulmonary aspergillosis may resemble tuberculosis with later signs and symptoms of cerebral, renal or cardiac involvement. Lesions of the skin or bone are not common. The aural passages and nasal sinuses may be infected (*A. niger*) with resulting otomycosis and sinusitis. Cellulitis of the face and conjunctivitis have been noted.

In the lungs of patients dying of other chronic diseases colonies of *Aspergillus* may be found in bronchi or in bronchiectatic or tuberculous cavities with little surrounding inflammatory reaction. Masses of *Aspergillus* mycelia (fungus balls) may be present in these cavities. Most

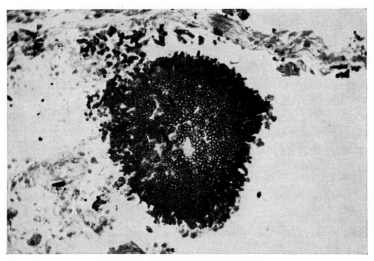

FIG. 5.3. Aspergillosis. Pulmonary aspergilloma (H and E × 200).
(*By courtesy of Dr. I. G. Murray.*)

commonly, however, the mycelia penetrate the parenchymal tissue and cause an acute necrotizing pyogenic pneumonitis (Fig. 5.3). The fungus tends to invade blood vessels, with a resulting thrombotic angiitis which is a factor in haematogenous spread. Small, acute, necrotizing abscesses with mycelia present may be found in the other viscera. The intestine is infrequently affected. Endocarditis may occur (Luke *et al.* 1963). In the nasal sinuses and orbital regions a chronic fibrotic lesion with numerous giant cells has been described.

In tissue sections the fungi may not be seen on routine H and E staining, and methenamine silver stains are preferred. The septate hyphae are

3–4 μm in diameter and characteristically demonstrate dichotomous branching. The branches arise at an angle of approximately 45 degrees. Small colonies may resemble a granule but the terminal dichotomous branching can usually be seen at the periphery. Ordinarily spores cannot be identified and the characteristic fruiting body (conidiospore) is rarely seen. If the latter is present, however, it allows a definite diagnosis of aspergillosis to be made. The hyphae of mucormycosis, which may be confused with those of *Aspergillus*, are non-septate, are two or three times greater in diameter, and do not exhibit the characteristic branching. *A. flavus* has been shown to produce a toxin with marked effects on the liver in laboratory animals (p. 559) but there is no record of aspergillosis in man producing similar lesions.

Hypha fragments and typical conidiospores may be seen in the sputum but may only indicate a saprophytic infection and repeated examinations are required to establish a diagnosis. Histological diagnosis may be made on surgically removed pulmonary lesions. The condition is most frequently diagnosed in the lungs at post mortem.

Agar gel precipitin tests are of value and may even allow of species differentiation (Longbottom *et al.* 1964).

MUCORMYCOSIS

Synonym. Opportunistic phycomycosis.

Mucormycosis is an opportunistic fungal infection caused by species of the fungal genera *Rhizopus*, *Absidia*, or *Mucor*.

It is an acute, frequently fatal, disease characterized by the occurrence of broad non-septate hyphae which tend to invade arteries and produce thrombosis and infarction (Baker, 1971).

Epidemiology

The distribution is world-wide. All age groups are affected. The fungi are common saprophytes found in soil, dying and decaying vegetable matter. Infection would appear to occur in patients whose immunological status has been altered by the presence of disease (especially diabetic ketosis, malignant disease of the reticulo-endothelial system, and malnutritional states) or by the taking of drugs (antibiotics, corticosteroids, and cytotoxic drugs) or following irradiation.

Pathology

Lesions may occur in any part of the body (Landau and Newcomer, 1962). The central nervous system is frequently affected following primary infection in the para-nasal sinuses with spread to the orbit and thence to the brain. Gastro-intestinal ulceration (oesophagus, stomach, colon) is common in the malnourished, especially children. Pulmonary, disseminated and cutaneous forms also occur.

The hyphae are abundant and cause acute inflammation and necrosis. They are highly invasive and infiltrate the walls of blood vessels causing thrombosis, mycotic emboli and infarction.

The hyphae are broad (3–20 μm), rarely septate and haphazardly branched in contrast to the regular branching of *Aspergillus*. The walls vary in thickness and some hyphae may be collapsed and twisted. They may be empty or contain strands of protoplasm—and are said to be best stained by routine H and E stains.

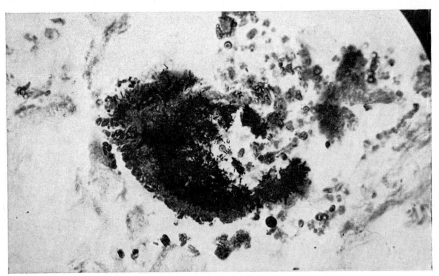

FIG. 5.4. Actinomycosis. Granule of *Actinomyces israelii* (H and E × 200). (*By courtesy of Dr. I. G. Murray.*)

The diagnosis of phycomycosis may be made on histological sections but culture is necessary to identify the species.

ACTINOMYCOSIS

Actinomycosis is caused by *Actinomyces israelii* and *A. bovis*, which produce lesions in man and cattle respectively (Fig. 5.4).

Epidemiology

The organisms are anaerobic and are commensals in the oral cavity. The mode of infection is usually endogenous in origin, infection occurring through lesions in the mouth, intestine, or skin, or by aspiration into the lungs.

Pathology

The condition presents as a chronic suppurative process in the cervico-facial region (lumpy jaw), ileocaecal region, lung, or, rarely, in the skin, nasopharynx, or lachrymal gland.

The lesions usually spread locally, and rarely haematogenous spread to the liver, brain, heart, and other viscera has been described.

Histologically pus-filled tracts and abscesses are constant findings in representative biopsies. A careful search has to be made for the character-istic 'sulphur granules'. They are round or oval bodies 100–300 μm in diameter. At the periphery there are eosinophilic, short, radiating, club-like structures which stain positively for fibrin. The granule is shown by Gram's method of staining to be a tangled mass of filaments, some of which are occasionally branched. Contaminating cocci or bacteria are usually present. Methenamine silver stains also demonstrate the fungal elements.

Nocardia asteroides may be confused with *A. israelii* but in the former con-dition granules are infrequent and filaments in the inflammatory exudate itself are common, whereas they are rare in *A. israelii* infections.

Sulphur granules, oval, rounded, yellowish structures can be recognized in pus from an actinomycotic lesion but the only certain method of diagnosis (to differentiate species of *Nocardia* or *Actinomyces*) is by culture. Serological methods are not recommended for diagnostic purposes.

COCCIDIOIDOMYCOSIS

Synonyms. Coccidioidal granuloma; valley fever; desert rheumatism.

Coccidioidomycosis is caused by the fungus *Coccidioides immitis*. The course may be benign, severe or fatal. The primary lesion is in the lung but the infection may extend to other viscera, including the bones, joints, lymph nodes, skin, and subcutaneous tissues (Figs. 5.5 and 5.6).

Epidemiology

The condition is endemic in the desert southern areas of the United States and Northern States of South America. The fungus grows in soil and spores may be airborne. Asymptomatic infections occur. The mortality is high in Filipinos and Negroes (Emmons *et al.* 1963).

Pathology

Clinically severe exposure may be followed by a short incubation period and pneumonic lesions. Symptoms of generalized aches, myalgia, fever, and

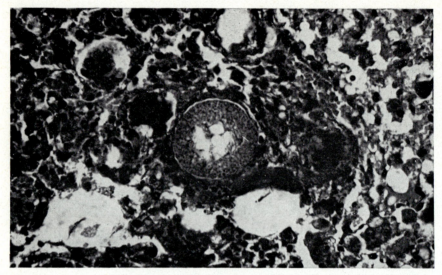

FIG. 5.5. Coccidioidomycosis. *Coccidioides immitis* in lung (H and E × 600). (*By courtesy of Dr. I. G. Murray.*)

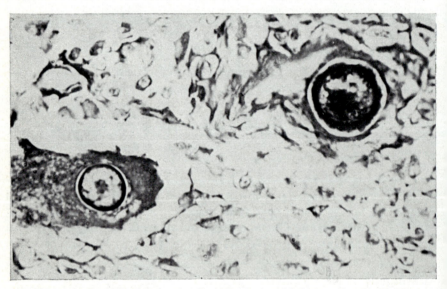

FIG. 5.6. Coccidioidomycosis. *Coccidioides immitis* in lymph node (PAS × 600). (*By courtesy of Dr. I. G. Murray.*)

anorexia may occur. Dermal lesions resembling erythema nodosum are common. Chronic pulmonary lesions occur in probably 5 per cent of infections. Dissemination may occur in many organs, and meningitis is invariably fatal.

The early lesions of coccidioidomycosis in man are those of a pyogenic pneumonitis, but sporangia (30–60 μm) with sporangiospores may be observed. Later a granulomatous lesion develops with histiocytes and giant cells which may contain sporangia. Hyphae may be seen in the lung lesions.

Large spherical thick-walled sporangia containing numerous endospores may be seen in wet films of pus or sputum in 10 per cent NaOH or in histological sections, in which they can be recognized in routine H and E preparations. The PAS technique and methenamine silver stains may be helpful.

Mice are susceptible laboratory animals.

Precipitin and complement-fixation tests give satisfactory results in coccidioidomycosis.

NORTH AMERICAN BLASTOMYCOSIS

Synonym. Gilchrist's disease.

North American blastomycosis is caused by *Blastomyces dermatitidis*. It is a chronic granulomatous and suppurative disease which originates as a respiratory infection and disseminates, usually with pulmonary, caseous, and cutaneous involvement predominating (Figs. 5.7 and 5.8).

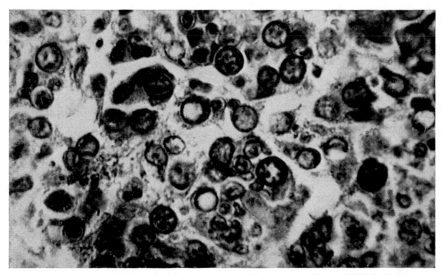

FIG. 5.7. North American blastomycosis. *Blastomyces dermatitidis* in lung (PAS × 800). (*By courtesy of Dr. I. G. Murray.*)

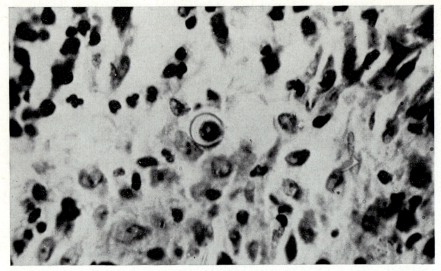

FIG. 5.8. North American blastomycosis. *Blastomyces dermatitidis* in skin
(PAS × 800). (*By courtesy of Dr. I. G. Murray.*)

Epidemiology

The condition occurs in North America and cases have been seen in
Africa. All age groups are affected, the male to female ratio being in the
region of 9 to 1. Sporadic infection is usual. The infection has been described
in dogs. Transmission is not proven but is thought to be by the inhalation
of spores from contaminated soil (Blastomycosis, 1964).

Pathology

Pulmonary symptoms suggestive of tuberculosis may be the predominating presentation. The skin, osseous, urogenital and central nervous system
may become involved. Rarely, direct infection of the subcutaneous tissues
may occur and cutaneous lesions may be the presenting symptom. The
histopathological changes may vary from acute inflammatory to chronic
granulomatous lesions with or without caseation. Pseudo-epitheliomatous
hyperplasia may be mistaken for carcinoma. The presence of the fungal cells
is the only possible method of diagnosis in tissue sections. In sections
B. dermatitidis is a cell 8–15 μm in diameter with a sharply defined wall. Larger
forms are seen. The protoplasm stains well and there may be a clear space
between the shrunken protoplasm and the cell wall. Several nuclei may be
present in the cell. Budding occurs and there is a broad basal attachment.
Hyphae are not seen. If budding is not present the resemblance to *Histoplasma duboisii* is close.

Small forms of *B. dermatitidis* have been described which resemble closely *H. capsulatum* but in the latter only one nucleus is present. Other fungi which may present a problem in the differential diagnosis in sections in the absence of budding are *Coccidioides immitis*, *Paracoccidioides brasiliensis*, and *Cryptococcus neoformans*, the last staining brilliantly with Mayer's mucicarmine.

In pus or sputum digested with 10 per cent NaOH the thick-walled spherical cells, some with wide-based buds, should be seen. The appearance in biopsy material has already been described.

Complement-fixation tests may be helpful if a rising titre is demonstrated.

Culture is necessary for accurate diagnosis. Mice are susceptible to the infection.

SOUTH AMERICAN BLASTOMYCOSIS

Synonyms. Paracoccidioidal granuloma; Brazilian blastomycosis; Lutz–Splendore–Almeida's disease.

Paracoccidioides brasiliensis causes a chronic, usually fatal, condition characterized by ulcerative granulomatous lesions of the buccal and nasal mucosa. Extension to the skin with regional and generalized lymph node involvement and haematogenous spread to the lungs, spleen, intestines, and other organs occurs (Fig. 5.9).

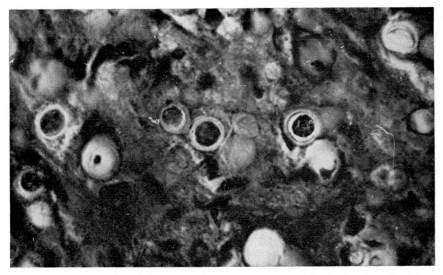

FIG. 5.9. South American blastomycosis. *Paracoccidioides brasiliensis* in skin (H and E × 800). (*By courtesy of Dr. I. G. Murray.*)

Epidemiology

The disease occurs frequently in Brazil and has been seen in most South American countries, except Chile, and in parts of Central America. It affects all age groups but its highest incidence is in the 30- to 50-year-old age group. In general, males are more frequently affected than females and rural populations more than urban. In Brazil, Japanese immigrants are very susceptible to the disease. The use of twigs contaminated with the fungus in dental hygiene may be an important source of infection. In endemic areas the organism has been isolated from dust. Dogs may be a reservoir of infection. Paracoccidiomycosis has been extensively reviewed in a Pan-American Symposium held in Colombia in 1971 (WHO, 1972).

Pathology

Lesions are seen in the nasal or oral mucosa, the conjunctiva, or anorectal mucosa. Granulomatous ulcers spread slowly but extensively. They may extend to the skin of the face, usually with regional lymphadenopathy. Haematogenous or lymphatic spread to the skin also occurs.

The entire lymphatic system is involved and lesions occur in the spleen, intestines, larynx, lungs, adrenals, and, occasionally, in bone and the central nervous system.

Histologically there is a granulomatous reaction associated with an acute inflammatory exudate. Giant cells of the Langhans or foreign-body type are conspicuous and may contain the fungus. Neutrophils may be present at the centre of epithelioid follicles. Pseudo-epitheliomatous hyperplasia with intra-epidermal abscesses are usually prominent. The fungus cells vary in size from 5 to 30 μm and are spherical structures containing a shrunken protoplasmic body.

Typical peripheral budding, if present, allows a diagnosis to be made. The entire surface of the spherule may be studded with small buds 2–5 μm in diameter. Although the yeast cells are seen on H and E preparations, the methenamine silver stain is to be preferred. They may also be seen in pus and crusts from the superficial lesions. A clinico-pathological study of deep mycotic infections during an 11-year period in Colombia has been published (Pena, 1967).

Serology is not considered very useful in diagnosis. Bilateral basal lung lesions can be seen on radiology in 80 per cent of patients.

CHROMOMYCOSIS

Synonym. Chromoblastomycosis.

Chromomycosis is caused by several fungi of the genera *Phialophora* and *Cladosporium*. Warty ulcerated lesions occur in the skin and subcutaneous tissues. Local spread by the lymphatics may occur and, rarely, cerebral lesions due to haematogenous dissemination are seen.

Epidemiology

The condition is widespread in tropical and subtropical areas and occasionally occurs in temperate climates. It is rare in children and adult males are more frequently affected, rural populations being more affected than urban. The fungus has been isolated from soil and wood, and thorn or splinter wounds are thought to be important causative factors.

Pathology

The lesions are most commonly seen in the lower limbs and usually follow minor trauma. Indolent ulcers or cauliflower-like lesions with a relatively narrow pedicle may result.

The striking feature is pseudo-epitheliomatous hyperplasia with micro-abscesses in the epidermis. Granulomatous lesions are present in the dermis consisting of epithelioid cells, foreign-body giant cells surrounded by lymphocytes, and plasma cells. Eosinophils may be present. The intervening connective tissue is infiltrated by chronic inflammatory cells. The round, thick-walled, chestnut-brown fungus cells, 5–8 μm in diameter, may be scanty, but can usually be detected in the dermis (Fig. 5.10). The pseudo-

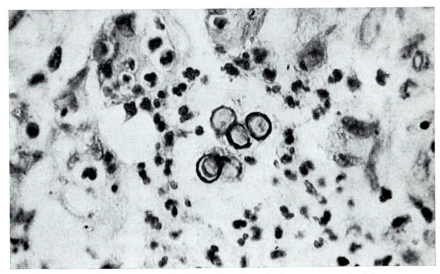

FIG. 5.10. Chromomycosis. Fungal cells of chromomycosis (chromo-blastomycosis) (H and E × 800). (*By courtesy of Dr. I. G. Murray.*)

epitheliomatous hyperplasia should raise the suspicion of chromoblasto-mycosis. The fungal bodies may be septate and can be detected on cleared unstained section. They are chestnut-brown on routine H and E stains and may be seen in giant cells. Occasionally, brown hyphae 2–5 μm wide may be seen in the superficial epithelial layers.

Long, brown, branching hyphae 2–5 μm wide may be seen in superficial crusts digested in 10 per cent NaOH. The rounded, thick-walled brown cells (6–10 μm in diameter) may be seen in pus from the lesion. The biopsy appearances have been described above. Serology is of little value as the antigens have not been standardized. Culture is essential for the accurate diagnosis of the species.

SPOROTRICHOSIS

The causative organism is *Sporothrix schenckii* and it causes chronic lesions in the skin with associated lymphatic involvement. It may become generalized involving bone joints and other organs.

Epidemiology

Sporotrichosis occurs in temperate and tropical climates. It has been described in North, South and Central America, France, and South Africa (Lurie, 1963). The fungus grows in mine timbers and the infection assumed almost epidemic proportions in miners in South Africa due to splinters infecting the skin. In other areas contaminated thorns or even metal particles penetrating the skin may cause infection.

Pathology

A small ulcerated lesion or subcutaneous nodule occurs at the site of the wound and may be the only sign of infection. The associated lymphatic channels may, however, become cord-like and the lymphatic glands enlarge and even suppurate. The syndrome of an ulcerated lesion with progressive chronic lymphatic involvement is characteristic of the infection. Haemato-genous spread may occur with involvement of bones, joints, muscles, and other viscera. On histological examination pseudo-epitheliomatous hyper-plasia of the epidermis and a mixed acute and granulomatous inflammatory response should raise the suspicion of sporotrichosis. Fungus cells may not be seen and culture is the most satisfactory method of diagnosis.

The 'asteroid body' may rarely be seen and suggests the diagnosis. It is an oval, yeast-like, basophilic structure 3–5 μm in diameter surrounded by fibrinoid material. Gram-positive, cigar-shaped, round or oval spores may rarely be noted in discharges from the cutaneous lesions. *S. schenckii* grows well in culture on glucose-neo-peptone agar at 25–35 °C. The mouse and rat are susceptible laboratory animals.

HISTOPLASMOSIS

Synonyms. Darling's disease; reticulo-endothelial cytomycosis.

Histoplasma capsulatum grows within the reticulo-endothelial cells of man involving the lymphatic tissues, lung, spleen, liver, kidneys, skin, bone marrow, central nervous system and other organs in the body.

Epidemiology

The distribution is probably world-wide and all races are susceptible. A small outbreak was recently described from Brazil (Schmidt *et al.* 1973). Children of both sexes are more frequently affected than adults in whom males predominate due most probably to occupational hazards. The disease tends to affect families or villagers in rural areas. The fungus has been isolated from soil in caves and from the interior of huts contaminated with bats' droppings (guano) (Gans and Karbaat, 1967). The soil of chicken-runs in rural areas and starlings' droppings in urban areas have been shown to be reservoirs of infection. Dogs and cats may be naturally infected. The infection has been noted not infrequently in association with malignant disease of lymphoreticular tissue.

Infection occurs by the inhalation of spores and the lungs are primarily affected. Dermal sensitivity to histoplasmin has been used in epidemiological surveys. Cross-reaction with other mycoses do however occur.

Pathology

The primary pulmonary infection may be symptomless, acute and benign, chronic, or widely disseminated and fatal. Primary lesions may also occur on the lips and mucous membranes of the mouth, pharynx, larynx or in the intestine (Fig. 5.11).

In the lungs variegated pathological changes are seen. There may be a solitary calcified nodule just beneath the pleura which on X-ray shows the 'coin' lesion. The size varies from 0·5 cm to several centimetres. *Histoplasma* cells may be found within the centre of the lesion by silver methenamine stains. Calcific bodies may be stained by the PAS technique and simulate fungi. Epithelioid-cell granulomata with or without Langhans cells and/or necrotic caseating lesions may be seen. The yeast cells are described below.

Fatal disseminated histoplasmosis is not a common condition but in addition to the lungs almost any organ in the body can be affected. The invasion of histiocytes or macrophages by yeast cells is the characteristic lesion. In the skin, however, in our experience, extracellular yeast forms are seen. Caseous necrosis can develop. In addition to the organs previously mentioned necrosis in the adrenal may cause symptoms of Addison's disease.

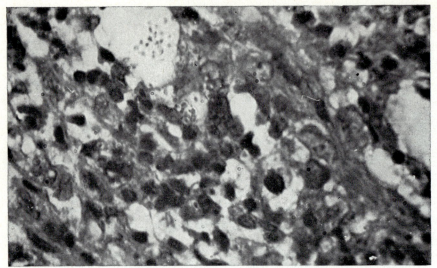

FIG. 5.11. Histoplasmosis. *Histoplasma capsulatum* in vocal cord (H and E
× 1000). (*By courtesy of Dr. I. G. Murray.*)

Endocarditis (Palmer *et al.* 1962) and pericarditis have been described
(Webb and Herring, 1962).

H. capsulatum in the histiocyte is a small spherical or oval body 1–5 μm in
diameter well demonstrated by silver methenamine stains which do not
stain *Leishmania* or *Toxoplasma*, both of which may rarely on H and E
sections be confused with *H. capsulatum*.

Examination of sputum, urine, bone marrow, excised lymph nodes, or
peripheral blood may reveal the presence of the organisms. Smears may be
stained by Wright or Giemsa stains and the yeasts appear as oval cells 2–4 μm
in size containing a vacuole and a cup-shaped mass of red-stained protoplasm
at the broad end. Budding occurs at the smaller end. Complement fixation
may show a rising titre. Culture is essential for accurate diagnosis. The
mouse is a susceptible laboratory animal.

AFRICAN HISTOPLASMOSIS

African histoplasmosis is caused by infection with *Histoplasma duboisii*
(Dubois *et al.* 1952) and occurs in a localized or disseminated form.
The literature has been reviewed by Edington (1971) and Schwarz
(1971). In the localized form lesions are confined to the skin and regional
lymph nodes, or a solitary localized osseous lesion may be seen. In the
disseminated there are multiple cutaneous lesions and the abdominal
viscera, especially the liver and spleen, are involved (Fig. 5.12). Isolated

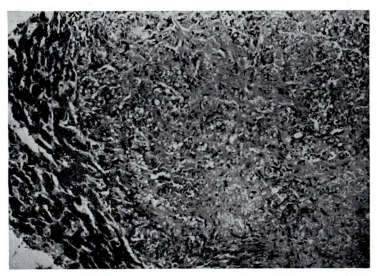

FIG. 5.12. African histoplasmosis. *Histoplasma duboisii*. Relatively acellular lesion in the liver containing numerous thick-walled yeast forms (H and E × 180).

lesions have, however, been reported in the intestine and other viscera (Cole *et al*. 1965). The lungs, in contrast to *H. capsulatum* infection, are not commonly affected. Clark and Greenwood (1968) have, however, recently discussed twelve cases with some evidence of pulmonary disease. In one Nigerian woman there were widespread lesions in the lung at necropsy. It is perhaps of interest to note that this patient was in the last trimester of pregnancy at the time of death. The central nervous system is rarely, if ever, involved but paraplegia due to vertebral involvement may occur.

Epidemiology

The condition so far has been reported in Africa south of the Sahara and north of Rhodesia. All age groups are affected, with the maximum incidence in the second decade. Males are more frequently affected than females Cockshott and Lucas, 1964; Docquier *et al*. 1974). The mode of infection is not known. Natural infection has been described in the baboon (Walker and Spooner, 1960).

Pathology

The condition varies in severity, death occasionally resulting from a disseminated infection. Various types of skin lesions have been described, the papulonodular being most common. The organs affected are enumerated above.

The yeast phase is seen in man. They are round or oval bodies 8–15 μm in their long axis. The cell wall is about 1 μm in thickness. The contained proto-plasm is irregularly dispersed and occasionally a nucleus is apparent. Budding forms usually with narrow bases occur, the bud staying attached until it reaches the size of its parent. This feature is not seen in *B. dermatitidis* infections, the yeast phase of which closely resembles that of *H. duboisii*. The ultrastructure of *H. duboisii* has been described by Williams *et al.* (1971).

The presence of the fungus cell appears in the great majority of instances to stimulate the production of histiocytes and giant cells of the foreign body or Langhan's type (Fig. 5.13). In many lesions there may be no other cellular reaction. The giant cells may contain up to thirty fungal cells and budding and growth appear to take place within them. Extracellular yeast cells may be seen, usually centrally placed in the lesion, with palisading of histiocytes, giant cells and a few lymphocytes at the periphery. Other types of lesions, however, do occur and micro-abscesses surrounding the yeasts are not uncommon, the predominant cell being the neutrophil polymorph, although an eosinophil response can occur. Extensive areas of necrosis with or without yeasts are also common and evoke a histiocytic and lymphocytic infiltration at the periphery. Epithelioid follicles in the absence of spores, resembling the tuberculous follicle, we have also seen. All these types of lesions may be

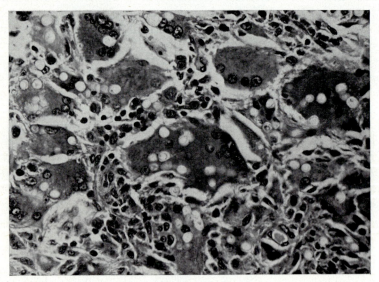

FIG. 5.13. African histoplasmosis. *H. duboisii*. Numerous giant cells containing yeast forms (H and E × 450).

seen in the one patient and the mechanisms involved in this differing response of the tissues are unclear. In the healing stage fibrosis is marked. The fungal cells are well seen on routine H and E stains but a PAS technique or a methenamine silver stain are preferred. Examination of the wet film of pus or from aspirates of lesions may be diagnostic and is a most useful laboratory procedure in our experience. It is simple to perform and frequently obviates the need for biopsy. As the mode of infection is not known the lungs should be routinely X-rayed and the sputum examined for spores in all cases.

CRYPTOCOCCOSIS

Synonyms. Torulosis; European blastomycosis; Burse–Buschke's disease.

Cryptococcus neoformans causes an acute, subacute, or chronic pulmonary, systemic, or meningeal mycosis.

Epidemiology

The distribution is world-wide and no differences in age, sex or occupation have been noted. The organism has been found frequently in pigeon's droppings and in barnyard soil and it is presumed that man must be infected frequently. The disease is probably caused by the inhalation of spores and is primarily a pulmonary infection with haematogenous spread to the skin, bones, abdominal viscera, eye, and especially the central nervous system.

Pathology

Cryptococcus cells may be found incidentally in solitary nodules in the lungs at autopsy or may be associated with the meningeal form. Active lesions in the lung are characterized by masses of cells with a surrounding low-grade inflammatory reaction. Fungus cells may be detected in the sputum.

In the central nervous system there is an insidious onset of chronic meningitis and the course may vary from a few months to 20 years. The organism may be seen in the C.S.F. and is best demonstrated in fresh preparations by the India ink method. It can be cultured and mice are susceptible laboratory animals.

Histologically the lesion is usually a pure histiocytic granuloma, and, on routine H and E sections, pale-blue, thin-walled spherical or oval bodies 4–7 μm in diameter are usually seen. In histiocytes the fungus cell usually has a clear halo 3–5 μm in width surrounding it. It has a radiate appearance with mucicarmine stains (Fig. 5.14). Budding cells may be seen but hyphae are absent. The histiocytes may be multinucleated. The fungal cells may also be shown by PAS or methenamine silver stains. Small intracellular *C.*

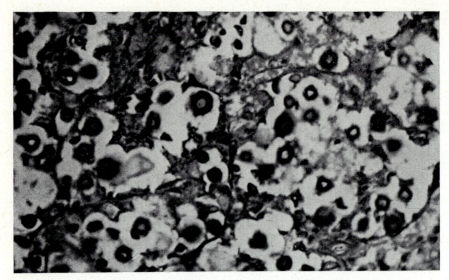

FIG. 5.14. Cryptococcosis. *Cryptococcus neoformans* in brain (H and M.C. × 600). (*By courtesy of Dr. I. G. Murray.*)

neoformans without capsules may resemble *H. capsulatum* or the small forms of *B. dermatitidis*. Mayer's mucicarmine stain, however, only stains *C. neoformans* intensely.

Serological methods are, at present, of no value in diagnosis.

CHELOIDAL BLASTOMYCOSIS

Synonym. Lobo's disease.

Loboa loboi causes keloidal warty skin lesions and occurs in the Amazon Valley, Surinam and Costa Rica.

The lesion consists mainly of giant cells which contain the fungus cells. On H and E staining, they are rounded structures 8 μm in diameter with a thick, poorly-stained wall and a central protoplasmic mass containing one or more dot-like nuclei. Double cells may be joined by a short rod-like structure. Pear-shaped buds and small chains of cells have been noted. Special fungal stains are to be preferred.

RHINOSPORIDIOSIS

Rhinosporidium seeberi causes granulomatous, hyperplastic and polypoid lesions on mucosal surfaces. The primary lesion occurs most frequently in the nasal cavity (Fig. 5.15).

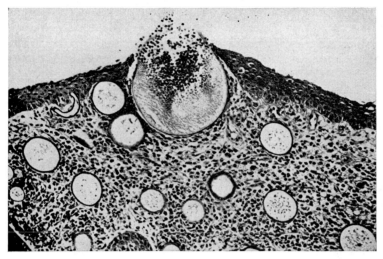

FIG. 5.15. Rhinosporidiosis. The section shows rupture of a mature sporangium with release of endospores. Numerous sporangia are present in the subepithelial tissues which are infiltrated with chronic inflammatory cells (H and E × 300). (*By courtesy of Ash and Spitz.*)

Epidemiology

The condition occurs most frequently in India and Sri Lanka but sporadic cases have been described in many parts of the world, including Africa. It occurs at any age but children and young adults are most frequently affected. Some association with water has been noted and water insects or fish may be natural hosts.

Pathology

Friable, highly vascular, sessile or pedunculated polyps may appear on any mucosal surface, and, rarely, secondary lesions are found in the skin. Lesions have been noted in the nasal mucosa, nasopharynx, soft palate, conjunctivae, lachrymal gland, larynx, bronchi, penis, vagina, rectum, and skin.

In the polypoid lesion numerous globular cysts (sporangia 10–200 μm in size) are present in the stroma which exhibits a chronic inflammatory reaction with neutrophils, plasma cells, and lymphocytes. Eosinophils are said to be inconspicuous. The cysts have a sharply-defined wall which may be up to 5 μm in thickness and contain numerous spores which when mature are about 7 μm in diameter with a well-defined wall and contain a basophilic karyosome and ten or more globular, slightly eosinophilic bodies. The sporangium may rupture with release of the spores and cause a corresponding chronic granulomatous reaction with giant cells present. The epithelium covering the lesion may also contain cysts. Special stains are not usually required but do stain the wall of the sporangium and contained spores.

Spores may be seen in the nasal secretions or sputum but examination of tissue sections is the usual method of diagnosis. Culture has not been successfully achieved nor has the condition been successfully transmitted to laboratory animals, although it is found in natural infections in horses and cattle.

SUBCUTANEOUS PHYCOMYCOSIS

Subcutaneous phycomycosis is caused by a species of *Basidiobolus*. It is characterized by a chronic progressive firm swelling of the subcutaneous tissues. Any part of the body may be affected.

Epidemiology

It was first described in Indonesia in 1956 (Lie Kain Joe *et al.*) and has now been reported in many tropical and subtropical regions.

It is predominantly a disease of childhood but is occasionally seen in adults.

Basidiobolus is a common saprophyte of soil and decaying vegetation and has been found in the gastro-intestinal tract of reptiles. Trauma is probably the portal of entry of the fungus and this is borne out by the common sites of the subcutaneous swellings, which are the limbs and buttocks. The literature has recently been reviewed by Clark and Edington (1971).

Pathology

Clinically, the condition usually presents as a firm, movable, well-defined subcutaneous swelling. Small nodules may be palpable at the advancing edge of the lesion. There is usually no pain or tenderness or constitutional upset. We have, however, seen lesions which were tender, hot and painful with accompanying pyrexia. The condition is usually benign and self-limiting but very rarely it may end fatally (Edington, 1964).

The inflammatory process affects the subcutaneous fatty tissue which becomes firm, creamy in colour and tough on section. Areas of yellowish focal necrosis may be present from which may be expressed ribbons of caseous material containing the fungal elements.

A wide variety of histopathological lesions may be seen in the one patient probably depending upon the duration of the infection and the immunological response of the host (Burkitt *et al.* 1964).

The characteristic lesion is the micro-abscess containing fungal elements at its centre and is best seen at the advancing edge of the lesion. The predominant cell in the abscess is the eosinophil polymorphonuclear leucocyte. The fungi are surrounded by a cuff of granular, intensely eosinophilic, material, which gives the staining reactions of fibrin and is thought to indicate an immunological reaction in the tissues. The fungi themselves stain poorly with H and E and, as the cytoplasm is often absent, the fungus may appear as circular, oval, or longitudinal spaces surrounded by a slight refractile envelope at the centre of the eosinophilic lesion (Fig. 5.16). The fungi stain well with methenamine silver. The hyphae vary from 5 to 15 μm

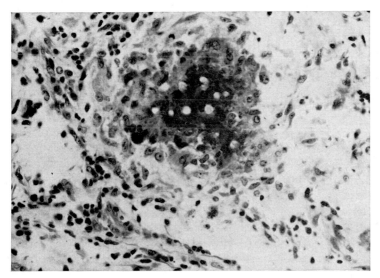

FIG. 5.16. Subcutaneous phycomycosis. Sections of the 'hyphae' can be seen as clear spaces lying in dense eosinophilic material. Palisading of epithelioid cells can be seen (H and E × 220).

in width, are thin-walled, rarely are seen branching and only occasionally are septa noted. They are discrete in the tissues.

In other areas there may be palisading of epithelioid cells round the hyphae, with plasma cells, lymphocytes, and giant cells of the foreign body or Langhans type at the periphery. Masses of disintegrating 'fibrinoid' material may be seen with a variable infiltration of eosinophils, histiocytes, lymphocytes, plasma, and giant cells. The eosinophilic material may be seen within giant cells, frequently accompanied by hyphal remnants. Areas of necrosis with micro-abscesses devoid of fungal elements may be present and extensive fibrosis with a variable cellular infiltrate occurs.

Heavy plasma-cell and lymphocytic infiltration with prominent Russell bodies are inconstant findings. Obliterative endarteritis occurs in the more chronic cases. The vessel wall is very rarely invaded by hyphae.

The histopathology is characteristic. The ultrastructure of the *Basidiobolus* species and *D. coronata* and the precipitate around the fungi have been described by Williams *et al.* (1969). Much of the precipitate consists of probably antigen–antibody complexes and has been described as the 'Splendore–Hoeppli' phenomenon. It resembles the precipitate seen around a number of parasites and fungi—notably Schistosome ova. Culture, however, is necessary to identify the fungus specifically.

RHINO-ENTOMOPHTHOROMYCOSIS

Rhino-entomophthoromycosis is caused by the fungus *Delacroixia coronata* and is characterized by nasal obstruction and swelling of the tissues of the nose, cheek and upper lip.

Epidemiology

The condition has only recently been recognized (Martinson, 1963). A few cases have been described in Nigeria, Jamaica, Kinshasa, Colombia, and Brazil. In contrast to subcutaneous phycomycosis it is predominantly a disease of adults.

D. coronata is a common saprophyte in soil and decaying vegetation and is an insect pathogen. It causes a disease in horses similar to that seen in man. The mode of infection may be by inhalation of the spores or by implantation through an accidentally self-infected wound, or by an insect bite (Martinson and Clark, 1967).

Pathology

The nasal mucosa becomes swollen and causes nasal obstruction. The lesion spreads to involve the paranasal sinuses, pharynx, palate, dorsum of the nose, cheek and upper lip. The lower lip and tissues over the mandible are never involved. The lesions in the face are similar to those of sub-cutaneous phycomycosis but differ in that they are not movable over deeper structures and the skin is movable over them. The histopathology of the lesion is identical to that seen in subcutaneous phycomycosis caused by *Basidiobolus*.

Tissue sections show the characteristic eosinophilic cuffing round the fungal hyphae. Culture is required to differentiate species of *Basidiobolus* from *D. coronata*.

MYOSPHERULOSIS

This condition has been described from Kenya and Uganda (Hutt *et al.* 1971). The cause is unknown. It presents as a subcutaneous swelling; histologically the lesion consists of cystic spaces filled with pus-like material in the subcutaneous fat. The cysts are lined by fibrous tissue and small spherules are present about 10 nm in diameter which stain positively with trichrome.

TORULOPSIS GLABRATA

T. glabrata is an opportunistic fungus which reproduces by budding. It is being found in increasing frequency in patients on immunosuppressive therapy (Marks *et al.* 1970). It causes abscesses with yeast-like cells in macrophages.

6

Bacterial Diseases

These are extremely common in the tropics, frequently with severe and florid manifestations. In this chapter the more important bacterial diseases in tropical areas have been described with certain important exceptions. *Mycobacterium tuberculosis*, for instance, is discussed in the chapter on Respiratory Diseases, as also is *Diplococcus pneumoniae*. Other equally important organisms are considered when the pathology of the organs affected by them is considered.

In the tropics the frequency of wound sepsis following surgical operations may be high, and unfortunately antibiotic- and drug-resistant bacteria are also now being found in high prevalence due to the indiscriminate and uncontrolled use of drugs in many areas. Defaulting patients are also common which aggravates the situation. In Ibadan post-operative wound sepsis has been found to be common and in 67 per cent of patients the organism was *Staphylococcus pyogenes*, of which a high proportion were resistant to penicillin, streptomycin and tetracycline. Other organisms detected were coliforms, *Proteus* spp., *Pseudomonas pyocyanea* and non-beta-haemolytic streptococci (Scott-Emuakpor, 1970). Similarly, drug-resistant strains of tubercle bacilli are being reported in high prevalence from many tropical areas.

In recent years Gram-negative organisms have emerged as causative agents of life-threatening infections and also anaemia. Apart from *Salmonella*, *Shigella* and *Proteus* organisms, coliforms and other members of the *Enterobacteriaceae* may be involved, particularly *Esch. coli*. Peripheral circulatory failure may occur. They may also cause a haemolytic anaemia which may have an immunological basis (Assoku, 1972).

THE MYCOBACTERIOSES

The organisms are slender rods occurring mostly in pairs or small clumps. Once stained they resist decolourization with acid (acid-fast). They are non-motile, non-capsulated and non-sporing. Their growth is usually slow and aerobic. All forms of animal life may be affected by various species of these bacteria. The most important are

Mycobacterium tuberculosis and Mycobacterium leprae. The former is discussed in the chapter on the respiratory system and the latter is discussed below.

Myco. johnei causes a chronic enteritis in cattle and sheep (Cruickshank, 1965).

Mycobacteria, however, also cause ulcerative skin lesions.

Myco. ulcerans was reported from Australia in 1948 (McCallum *et al.* 1948) and *Myco. balnei* from Sweden in 1954 (Linell and Norden). Various other species may cause ulcers and all biopsies or smears from non-specific ulcers in the tropics should always be routinely stained by Ziehl-Neelsen. These however may be negative if due to *Myco. balnei* and culture on Löwenstein-Jensen's medium at 31 °C is necessary for diagnosis. There is a group of acid-fast bacilli which does not produce disease in guinea pigs and which may be associated with human disease and has been named anonymous or atypical mycobacteria. Over 400 strains have been identified and have been classified into seven groups (Marks and Richards, 1962). Little is known about their importance as pathogens in the tropics but their prevalence is high.

LEPROSY

Leprosy is a widespread contagious disease which is particularly common in Africa and the Indian subcontinent, where it is estimated that 4 million and 3 million people respectively are affected. The disease is also common in S.E. Asia (Bechelli *et al.* 1973). Chile is one tropical country which is said to be exempt from the disease, although it is common in other countries in South America. Although of recent years several million people from countries where leprosy is prevalent have migrated to the industrialized west, bringing leprosy with them, secondary cases in the receiving lands are extremely rare or practically unknown, even among the immigrant population (Browne, 1973).

Epidemiology

The reputed cause of leprosy is *Mycobacterium leprae*, which is a slender rod 5 μm long and 0·5 μm in breadth. The organism has never been grown in pure culture, and has only recently been successfully inoculated into animals (Shepard, 1960). Rees *et al.* (1969) have succeeded in reproducing in mice a picture very similar to the human disease. Armadillos seem to be particularly susceptible to *M. leprae* and can be experimentally infected relatively easily. The dissemination of the bacilli in mice has been studied by Widdell *et al.* (1970). Characteristically, *Myco. leprae* are found grouped together in tightly packed formations (globi) consisting of thirty or more bacilli, enclosed perhaps within the cellular confines of a reticulo-endothelial cell, surrounded by a glial membrane, or lying free in the tissues. *Myco. leprae* is alcohol- and acid-fast. The viable organism stains deeply and uniformly; irregular staining or beading indicates non-viability. In leprosy, there are two pathological extremes, characterized on the one hand by unrestrained multiplication of *Myco. leprae* (lepromatous leprosy) and on the other by very scanty multiplication of the organism (tuberculoid leprosy). The infectiousness of leprosy is not high, and repeated skin to skin contact would ordinarily seem to be necessary. The mechanism of contagion probably consists of the transfer of living *Myco. leprae* from skin to skin, and the introduction of the bacilli into the corium by some slight and unremembered trauma (Doull, 1962). There is no positive evidence for the existence of an extrahuman reservoir of leprosy bacilli; nor, having regard to the fact that *Myco. leprae* cannot be cultured, for different strains. It is possible that fomites contaminated by skin squames or by nasal secretion may serve as a vehicle for the dissemination of bacilli. Conjugal infections are usually 5 per cent or less.

While prolonged and intimate contact is classically considered to be necessary for infection to develop, there are well-authenticated cases of patients acquiring the infection after a brief or passing contact with a person suffering from leprosy. It is quite rare for workers in leprosaria to contract leprosy. Although leprosy is commonest in hot and humid lands, climatic factors *per se* are probably not important. Children and adolescents are commonly held to be more susceptible than adults, as are males more than females, but these generalizations are not as definite as they are sometimes made out to be (Newell, 1966). Hormonal influences may play a part, since there seems to be an increased incidence at puberty in both sexes, and clinical exacerbation of the disease may occur during pregnancy and particularly after parturition. Racial and genetic susceptibility affect the spread of the disease from Central Africa, eastwards or westwards (Browne, 1962), the ratio of lepromatous to tuberculoid patients increasing. It is possible that genetic factors may play an important role in deciding susceptibility to lepromatous leprosy (Thomas and Job, 1972). A comparison of the modes of spread and the incidence of tuberculosis and leprosy was made by Rees and Meade (1974). The status of BCG in leprosy seems uncertain.

The natural history of leprosy can conveniently be represented as follows:

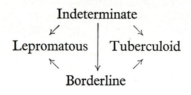

Immunology

All persons exposed to repeated contact with open cases of leprosy do not contract the disease, and, moreover, a variable proportion of those who do develop leprosy, suffer from a self-healing form. Many persons infected with leprosy manifest a vigorous response to the organism, while a variable proportion develop the severe progressive form of the disease characterized by minimal response. In spite of the deficiency of cell mediated immunity in lepromatous leprosy, there is no increase in cancer mortality in leprosy patients (Olernick, 1969).

Thus, the pathological and clinical characteristics of leprosy form a spectrum from LL to TT. What mainly determines the place of an individual patient's disease on this spectrum is the extent to which cellular immunity is expressed. In tuberculoid leprosy cellular immunity and hypersensitivity are well developed while in lepromatous leprosy they are absent (Bryceson and Pfaltzgraff, 1973; Goodall et al. 1971; Turk and Bryceson, 1971). Godal et al. (1971) have studied lymphocytic transformation with Myco. leprae in tuberculoid and lepromatous patients. In the former the average lymphocyte transformation was $11 \cdot 1$ per cent whereas in the latter there was a complete lack of response. This lack of response was found to be specific for Myco. leprae in lepromatous patients and was thought to indicate immunological tolerance.

Increased autoantibodies are found in leprosy; they include rheumatoid factor, antithyroglobulin antibody, cryoglobulins, c reactive protein and false positive biological tests for syphilis such as the Wassermann reaction. Titre levels are variable (Bonomo et al. 1965; Petchelai et al. 1973; Wright, 1973).

The lepromin test

The antigens used for the lepromin test are prepared by the maceration of tissue containing great numbers of bacilli, such as a nodule obtained from a patient suffering from active lepromatous leprosy. The organisms are killed by heat or by other means. A refined lepromin is obtained by treating the tissue with chloroform and ether, and then centrifuging at high speed. The deposit is suspended in carbol-saline. The test is performed by injecting $0 \cdot 1$ ml of antigen intradermally; the site of injection is inspected after 24 hours, and daily thereafter. There are other methods of preparing a suitable antigen from bacillus-containing material and sundry modifications of the test.

There are two types of cutaneous response to the lepromin test. The early reaction of Fernandez consists of an erythematous infiltrated area which appears 24–72 hours after injection. The Mitsuda reaction is nodular in form and most intense 21–30 days after injection. The early reaction is now interpreted as a response to soluble substances of the bacillus, and the late reaction as resistance to the bacillus excited by insoluble substances. Variation of the intensity of the lepromin test occurs among leprosy patients as well as among contacts. The best site for the inoculation is the anterior aspect of the forearm.

Neither an early nor a late lepromin reaction proves immunity. The lepromin test is essentially an allergic reaction, though many leprologists believe that the reaction tests both allergy and immunity to leprosy bacilli (Dharmendra, 1966). The proportion of persons in endemic areas giving positive Mitsuda reactions increases with age from nil at birth up to 80 per cent in adults (Guinto *et al.* 1954; Davey *et al.* 1958). Rotberg (1957) speculated that an intrinsic natural factor exists—which he calls factor N (N for natural)—that gives an individual the capacity to react specifically to *Myco. leprae*. He points out that about 20 per cent of the population, for no apparent reason, will not become lepromin-positive however strong the natural or artificial extrinsic stimuli may be, and that this minor group lacks intrinsic factor N. The Mitsuda reaction is negative in pure lepromatous leprosy and strongly positive in major tuberculoid leprosy; variably positive in intermediate forms (borderline or dimorphous; atypical lepromatous; atypical and minor tuberculoid). B.C.G. vaccination may result in conversion of a negative lepromin reaction to positive, this conversion occurring in a variable proportion of subjects to a variable degree, and for a variable period (Rosemberg *et al.* 1960; Mukerjee and Kundu, 1961). Miranda (1963) has shown that an extract of normal skin, obtained according to the technique for the preparation of the Mitsuda antigen, produces a late skin reaction of tuberculoid structure similar to the Mitsuda in at least half the patients who have tuberculoid leprosy. This is known as the *Faria reaction* and has been repeated and confirmed by numerous investigators. It is therefore difficult to assert that the Mitsuda reaction specifically implies the existence of a heightened resistance to clinical infection with *Myco. leprae*.

Antibodies to certain fractions of old tuberculin are present in the sera of many leprosy patients, as demonstrated by the Middlebrook–Dubos haemagglutination reaction, but the presence of these antibodies is of problematical relation to defence mechanisms in leprosy. Cottenot (1965), using the fluorescent antibody technique, reported that sera from leprosy patients showed fluorescence against the bacillus and the highest titres were in patients with severe lepromatous leprosy, while Lim and Fusaro (1963) have reported a small increase of IgA in tuberculoid and lepromatous leprosy, while IgM was markedly increased in five out of six lepromatous sera with no rise in tuberculoid patients. Associated with these findings, is the occurrence of positive tests for syphilis especially in patients with long-standing lepromatous leprosy (Daguet and Languillon, 1961).

Pathology

The latent or silent period (sometimes known as the incubation period) varies from a few weeks to possibly 20 years, the usual period being 2–4 years.

There may or may not be an early indeterminate phase, which is difficult to recognize. Healing may occur at this stage, or the disease may progress to other forms. In considering the pathology the following forms of leprosy will be described.

(1) Indeterminate leprosy.
(2) Lepromatous leprosy.
(3) Tuberculoid leprosy.
(4) Borderline (dimorphous) leprosy.
(5) Pure polyneuritic leprosy.
(6) Masked leprosy.
(7) The Lucio phenomenon.
(8) Reactional states in leprosy:

   (a) Erythema nodosum leprosum and acute exacerbation.
   (b) Progressive lepra reaction.

Following the description of these differing forms of leprosy the changes that occur in the different organs are described and the association of leprosy with amyloidosis discussed.

The two most common types are the lepromatous and the tuberculoid. In the lepromatous the resistance of the host to *Myco. leprae* is minimal or absent. Numerous bacilli are found in the lesions with little cellular reaction, and the Mitsuda reaction is negative. In the tuberculoid type, on the other hand, small numbers of bacilli excite a vigorous granulomatous reaction similar to that seen in sarcoidosis or proliferative tuberculosis. This reaction is thought to indicate a degree of 'allergy' or immunity to the infection. The Mitsuda reaction is strongly positive.

Indeterminate leprosy

Patients in an endemic area of leprosy may present with complaints of paraesthesiae and one or more ill-defined slightly hypopigmented macules in the skin in which sensory loss is minimal or absent. Thermal sensation may be slightly impaired. Smears of the lesion are usually negative for *Myco. leprae*.

Skin biopsy reveals a non-specific mild mononuclear and lymphocytic infiltration of the dermis. Acid-fast bacilli are not usually detected by routine staining or by fluorescent techniques. The aggregation of the cellular infiltrate around the finest nerve fibres and in association with adnexal structures in the dermis may indicate the aetiology of the lesion. The

Mitsuda reaction is negative. The condition may heal or progress to any of the other three types of leprosy, and diagnosis may be possible only in retrospect.

Lepromatous leprosy

The first sign is usually an ill-defined and slightly hypopigmented macule, which appears on the extensor surface of the body or buttocks. The lobes of the ears, forehead, lips, and nose are involved later. The prelepromatous and lepromatous macules coalesce while the areas affected become raised and nodular and the characteristic 'leonine facies' may result. The nodules may break down and ulcerate. The serosanguineous fluid contains large numbers of *Myco. leprae*. Multiple, ill-defined, erythematous, raised and soft lesions may be present. In the early stages nervous disturbance is minimal, in contrast to the tuberculoid type. Later, however, there is enlargement and hardness of nerves, with increasing loss of function. Thermal sensation usually is impaired first, to be followed by light touch; sensation to pain remains longest. The nerves most commonly affected are: the ulnar, external popliteal, posterior tibial, the great auricular, radial, and supraorbital. Destruction of the autonomic nervous pathways leads to loss of sweating (anhidrosis) and lack of tone in the blood vessels with cyanosis and oedema, most marked in the hands and feet. Wasting and paralyses in the regions affected occur, resulting in 'trophic' changes, ulceration, and even gangrene. Facial paralyses, claw hand, and foot drop are common. Many of these late neurological signs are common to both lepromatous and tuberculoid leprosy. The remarkably stereotyped distribution of motor and sensory deficits in lepromatous leprosy may be conditioned by temperature, the cooler areas of the skin being most frequently affected as *Myco. leprae* is thermo-sensitive in the mouse footpad (Sabin, 1970). Lymphadenopathy is usual, and *Myco. leprae* can usually be seen in material obtained by a puncture of the lymphatic nodes of the extremities. The mucosa of the nasal cavity, epiglottis, larynx, and trachea is frequently involved, and scrapings from the mucosa covering the nasal septum usually contain many bacilli, often in globi; bacilli may persist in the nasal mucosa after they have disappeared from the skin and may reappear on relapse before becoming apparent in the skin. The Mitsuda reaction is negative.

When the bacilli gain entrance to the skin they rapidly multiply within the histiocytes and cells of the reticulo-endothelial system. They pass along lymphatics to the regional lymph nodes, and enter the blood stream to affect the liver, eyes, bone marrow, spleen, and testes. They penetrate the Schwann cells and peripheral nerves. An unusual feature in leprosy is this marked affinity of *Myco. leprae* for peripheral nerve tissue. The nerves may be affected throughout their length, but the most marked lesions are seen where the nerves are in close apposition to bone. The central nervous system is almost never affected.

In the dermis the histiocytes become large with vacuolated cytoplasm of foamy appearance containing large numbers of *Myco. leprae*. These are the lepra, Virchow, or foamy cells characteristic of lepromatous leprosy (Fig. 6.1). The foamy appearance is due to lipid material and metabolic products of the bacilli which form clear zones in the cells giving the 'soap-bubble' appearance. The nuclei are pale with a delicate chromatin network and contain one or two distinct nucleoli. *Myco. leprae* frequently occur in rounded masses, termed globi, which have the appearance of tightly-packed

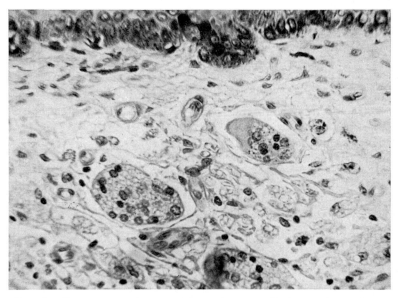

FIG. 6.1. Lepromatous leprosy. Foamy lepra or Virchow cells are shown in the dermis (H and E × 400). (*By courtesy of Dr. S. G. Browne.*)

bundles of cigars. The clumps of bacilli appear to be bound together by a lipid-like substance, the glia, and the masses may be intra- or extracellular (Cochrane and Davey, 1964). Globi may also be formed by the coalescence of Virchow cells (Khanolkar, 1964). A granuloma is formed in the dermis, composed mainly of histiocytes with a few lymphocytes and plasma cells. Aggregations of histiocytes are present round the adnexal structures in the immediate vicinity of the granuloma, but the nerve fibrils themselves are remarkably free from cellular infiltration, despite the presence of *Myco. leprae* lying between the neurofibrils. Characteristically, there is a narrow, clear, hyalinized subepidermal zone free from infiltrate. The epidermis is thinned, there is loss of rete pegs, and pigment in the malpighian layer is reduced.

Later, lepra cells, lymphocytes, and plasma cells appear in the nerve bundles. Degeneration of myelin sheaths and axis cylinders occur with consequent sensory, motor, and trophic changes. Job (1970) has studied the ultrastructure of radial cutaneous nerve biopsies. *Myco. leprae* were present in large numbers in Schwann cells, macrophages, endothelial cells and occasionally in perineural cells. The lesions in the skin or mucous membrane may ulcerate, with consequent scarring. Loss of the nasal septum or stricture of the larynx may occur.

The lymph nodes most frequently affected are the femoral, inguinal, and axillary. They are soft, discrete and moderately enlarged. There is proliferation of the histiocytic sinusoidal lining cells, many of which contain *Myco. leprae* and lymphocytes and plasma cells. There is replacement of the lymphocytes in the paracortical area (thymus-dependent region) by histiocytes. The germinal centres and plasma cell populations do not appear to be greatly altered indicating that humoral antibody production is not greatly affected (Turk and Waters, 1968). The nodes rarely break down and ulcerate.

The liver is invariably affected (p. 309).

Miliary lepromata are also found in the spleen, bone marrow, and testes. Eventual healing by scarring produces few clinical symptoms, except in the testes, which are concerned with the occurrence of gynaecomastia—a not uncommon complication (p. 311).

Lepromatous infiltration of the cornea and iris can occur with blindness resulting, and iridocyclitis is a common complication of the reactional states (p. 308).

Amyloidosis is frequently found in the late stages of the disease, and is discussed on p. 723.

Tuberculoid leprosy

Clinically the main presenting feature is a hypopigmented anaesthetic lesion in the skin which is firm and in which healing tends to occur from the centre. Minute papules (tubercles) can often be seen at the periphery. Anhidrosis, loss of thermal sense, touch and pain occur early (in contrast to lepromatous leprosy, in which they occur, typically, late). The peripheral nerves may become thickened and hard in the early stages: the nerves involved may be cutaneous twigs in the vicinity of the lesion, or the corresponding nerve trunk; later all the main peripheral nerves may be enlarged, hard and tender. In the late stages, muscular wasting, extensive anaesthesia, and trophic changes occur.

Histopathological examination of the lesion reveals a marked cellular reaction around the skin appendages and nerve elements. Langhan's giant cells, epithelioid cells, monocytes, lymphocytes, and plasma cells in a follicular arrangement are found in the dermis at all levels (Fig. 6.2). The subepidermal zone does not escape. The neurovascular plexus, sweat glands, and hair follicles are invaded at an early stage. Acid-fast remnants of *Myco. leprae* or even the bacillus itself may be found in the giant-cell systems, but this is rare. Nerve fibrils, in addition to perineuritic cuffing, are invaded by chronic inflammatory cells at an early stage. Adnexal structures are eventually destroyed by the chronic granulomatous process (Fig. 6.3).

The epidermis is thinned, the rete pegs completely flattened and the function of the melanocytes is destroyed, with consequent loss of pigment in the malpighian layer. The histological picture resembles closely that of tuberculosis or sarcoidosis, the distinguishing feature being the marked adnexal and neural involvement. Caseation does not occur except in nerves: granulomatous follicles in nerves may undergo necrosis and, in our experience, are indistinguishable from a caseating tuberculous focus—the so-called nerve abscess. This condition is said to be relatively common in India but rare in Africa and other parts of the world. The abscess may rupture through the sheath and discharge a fluid containing flakes of fibrin;

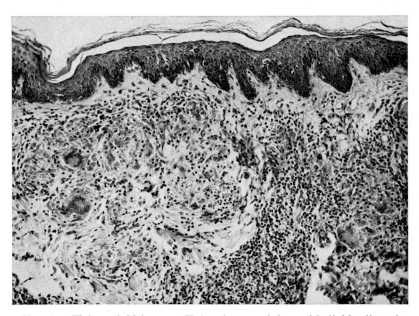

FIG. 6.2. Tuberculoid leprosy. Tubercles containing epithelioid cells and giant cells are surrounded by a dense collection of lymphocytes. The epidermis is still relatively unaffected (H and E × 200).

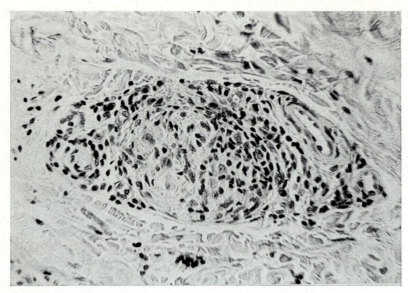

FIG. 6.3. Tuberculoid leprosy. Infiltration of a nerve bundle by lympho-cytes and epithelioid cells (H and E × 400). (*By courtesy of Dr. S. G. Browne.*)

it is usually sterile on culture. *Myco. leprae*, however, may be present, but are scanty.

Tuberculoid follicles are frequently seen in the liver, subserously or in the portal tracts, but cause no symptoms.

The nasal mucosa is only affected by direct encroachment of a neigh-bouring lesion and skin smears are negative to standard methods of examination. The Mitsuda reaction is often strongly positive. In the reactional phase (see p. 308) mild generalized symptoms occur, skin smears may become positive and the Mitsuda reaction temporarily negative.

Borderline leprosy (dimorphous)

In this type of leprosy, clinical and pathological features of both lepro-matous and tuberculoid leprosy are present. It occupies an intermediate position between both, and may develop towards one of the polar types.

Skin biopsies may reveal a purely histiocytic reaction in areas with a monocytic and lymphocytic infiltration around the skin appendages and terminal nerve endings. Lepra cells may be deep in the dermis. Function impairment of the dermal adnexae is usually minimal. The nerve trunks may be early involved.

Skin smears are usually positive for *Myco. leprae*; the Mitsuda reaction is variable: it is usually slightly positive and the degree of positivity may change in the course of the disease.

In the reactional phase the skin smears become more highly positive.

Pure polyneuritic leprosy

Polyneuritic or pure anaesthetic leprosy is a relatively common clinical entity, signs of neural involvement occurring without skin manifestations. This form of leprosy is to be differentiated from the secondary polyneuritic form which may complicate the tuberculoid, lepromatous, or borderline types. Clinically it is manifest by peripheral anaesthesia, nerve enlargements, muscular paralyses, and trophic changes.

The nerves most frequently involved are the ulnar, peroneal, and the 5th and 7th cranial. Glove and stocking anaesthesia may occur—thermal tactile, pain and pressure sense are lost in that order. Claw hand, drop foot, facial paralyses, and corneal insensitivity may occur. Anaesthesia and injury cause mutilating lesions of the hands and feet.

Diagnosis can only be achieved by nerve biopsy, which may reveal granulomatous lesions with *Myco. leprae* present. Scanty bacilli may, however, also be present in the skin of anaesthetic areas. A spastic paralysis has been described as a complication among New Caledonian leprosy patients and may be nutritional or toxic in origin (Brody *et al.* 1969).

Masked leprosy

In this concealed type of leprosy, *Myco. leprae* may be present in the skin in the absence of overt disease.

The Lucio phenomenon

This is a form of lepromatous leprosy described by Lucio and Alvarado in 1852. The skin is smooth, but a generalized thickening can be felt on palpation. The eyebrows are lost early. Erythematous macules appear which become haemorrhagic and necrotic centrally, with ulceration.

Histologically there is proliferation of histiocytes in the dermis and numerous leprosy bacilli. Polymorphonuclear leucocytes may be present. There is also a marked vascular inflammatory reaction associated with thrombosis and occlusion affecting the smaller dermal blood vessels. In the ulcerated areas there is a chronic inflammatory reaction with a superficial layer of fibrin and acute inflammatory cells. *Myco. leprae* may be present in the reticulo-endothelial cells of the viscera, with little cellular reaction. The Mitsuda reaction is negative.

Reactional states

In all types of leprosy certain patients may clinically exhibit a sudden exacerbation of their symptoms or, in the case of lepromatous leprosy, present with certain well-recognized acute skin lesions. These reactional states are thought to be an immunological reaction to the products of mycobacterial breakdown, and have many of the features of an autoimmune disease. In tuberculoid leprosy there is an exacerbation of the lesions with tenderness and local oedema prominent. Borderline leprosy reacts similarly but more violently. Histologically, bacilli can usually be demonstrated and there is evidence of a superimposed acute inflammatory reaction.

In lepromatous leprosy the reactional states are usually classified as (*a*) erythema nodosum leprosum, and (*b*) progressive lepra reaction.

Browne (1966), however, has described papilliform skin lesions containing numerous normal *Myco. leprae* appearing suddenly in patients who had had several years treatment for lepromatous leprosy and who were clinically quiescent. The bacilli were not dapsone-resistant and the majority of patients responded to long-term therapy.

(*a*) Erythema nodosum leprosum

This occurs in lepromatous leprosy and rarely in lepromatous leprosy with borderline features. The patient may be febrile and complain of malaise, neuralgia, arthralgia (perhaps with effusion), and the sudden appearance of crops of 'red spots' or bluish-scarlet macules on the face and limbs. An acute diffuse iridocyclitis may occur, and acute painful polyneuritis. The sudden onset of this condition is usually associated with certain precipitating factors such as chemotherapy, an associated pyrexial illness, smallpox vaccination, or an emotional upset. Changes may occur in the peripheral blood (which are described when the progressive reaction is being considered).

The pathological changes are those of lepromatous leprosy with a superimposed acute inflammatory reaction and a fibrinoid vasculitis. Wemambu *et al.* (1969) have noted granular deposits of immunoglobin, complement and soluble mycobacterial antigen in the acute inflammatory lesions in some patients. It was considered that these findings were consistent with the lesions being a manifestation of the Arthus phenomenon. In a few patients the level of the third component of complement in the serum was raised.

(*b*) Progressive lepra reaction

An attack of erythema nodosum leprosum may be of short duration, but it may recur or persist and merge into a more severe and lengthy reaction.

Fever, nerve tenderness, hepatosplenomegaly, arthralgia and severe irido-cyclitis may occur. In addition to the lesions of erythema nodosum other skin eruptions may be noted. Multiple subepidermal nodules 2–4mm in diameter coalesce to form a hard, firm, dermal infiltrate attached to the subcutaneous tissues, which tends to break down and ulcerate.

Hypoalbuminaemia and a raised γ-globulin are found in the serum and serum antinuclear factor, L.E. cells, rheumatoid factor, thyroglobulin antibodies, and significantly high levels of cryoproteins, in addition to false-positive biological tests for syphilis, may also be present. A number of these findings may be positive in lepromatous and borderline leprosy in the non-reactional phase.

Histologically, lepromatous lesions are present with a marked infiltration of lymphocytes and plasma cells. *Myco. leprae* are present in large numbers. The Mitsuda reaction is negative.

Changes in individual organs

(a) The liver

The liver is affected in all types of leprosy, but more especially in the lepromatous. Clinical evidence of liver damage is most unusual, but liver-function tests may show abnormalities, especially in patients with *Myco. leprae* and leprous granulomatous lesions on biopsy (Karat *et al.* 1971), e.g. the thymol turbidity and flocculation tests may be positive, the serum bilirubin may be raised and bromsulphthalein retention may be marked. A reversed albumin/globulin ratio is the rule. C-reactive protein may also be increased (Ross, 1964). A high frequency of the Australian antigen has been noted in some areas in patients with lepromatous leprosy but not in others (Shivi and Zuckerman, 1972).

Drugs used in therapy may also damage the liver either by direct toxic action or due to an idiosyncracy. Hepatitis or subacute hepatic necrosis in association with an exfoliative dermatitis (Browne, 1964) may occur.

Histologically, there is proliferation of the Kupffer cells, which contain *Myco. leprae*. Miliary lepromata consisting of lepra cells and varying numbers of lymphocytes and plasma cells are found in the sinusoids, portal tracts, and parenchyma. The bacilli may persist in the Kupffer cells when they have disappeared from the skin and nasal mucosa following therapy, and perhaps furnish a reservoir of viable bacteria of epidemiological import-ance. In tuberculoid leprosy follicles may be present. Secondary amyloidosis may also affect the liver.

(b) The skeletal system

The bone changes in leprosy are of three main types (Paterson and Job, 1964).

   (i) Specific—due to the action of *Myco. leprae* in bone.
  (ii) Non-specific inflammatory or degenerative—due to sensory loss.
 (iii) Osteoporotic—due to disuse.

Approximately 20–25 per cent of patients will exhibit bone damage of one or more of the types listed above, the most common being the non-specific.

(*i*) *Specific bone changes.* This is not a common condition and occurs with by far the greatest frequency in lepromatous patients. The lesions are most commonly found in the small bones of the hands and feet. The nasal septum may also be involved. *Myco. leprae* is found frequently in the bone marrow in lepromatous leprosy and infection is thought to spread from that site in the majority of cases (Job, 1963). Clear-cut areas of bone destruction are seen radiologically.

Histologically the bony trabeculae are invaded by inflammatory granulation tissue consisting mostly of histiocytes. Scattered lymphocytes and occasional plasma cells are also present. *Myco. leprae* are seen in histiocytes. Fragments of dead bone and proliferating osteoid tissue are present in the lesion.

(*ii*) *Non-specific inflammatory or degenerative lesions.* The loss of sensation in the hands and feet render them much more liable to unnoticed trauma and to infection, since the normal mechanisms of tissue protection and repair are grossly interfered with. Vascular lesions may cause degenerative changes or aseptic necrosis of the tissues, which are liable to secondary infection. Septic lesions and penetrating ulcers, especially of the foot, are common. Chronic osteitis and periostitis cause slow absorption of bone. The shafts of long bones may taper off to points or become absorbed.

Acute arthritis may occur and may be unnoticed due to loss of sensation, and effusion into the joint may occur in the course of acute exacerbation in lepromatous disease. The ligaments may be affected with consequent subluxation of the joint.

(*iii*) *Osteoporosis.* With disuse, osteoblastic activity is depressed and osteoclastic activity predominates. Rarefaction of bone occurs and liability to fracture is increased.

(c) *The eye*

The eye may be affected in leprosy in a number of ways.

  1. Direct spread may occur from lepromatous involvement of the eyelids, face or nose.

  2. In lepromatous leprosy *Myco. leprae* may be found in the tissues of the eye. The infection is usually considered to be blood-borne but neural spread cannot be eliminated.

3. In reactional states ocular tissues may become sensitized by leprous processes elsewhere in the body.

4. Involvement of the 5th and 7th nerves can cause corneal anaesthesia and lagophthalmos, with consequent liability to secondary infection and perforating corneal ulcers.

The most common cause of blindness in leprosy is involvement of the iris and ciliary body by *Myco. leprae* (Choyce, 1964), but cranial nerve involvement may also result in blindness though the following sequence of events (facial nerve → lagophthalmos → exposure keratitis → corneal ulcer → panophthalmitis). Posterior segment lesions are unusual (Weerekoon, 1972).

It should be remembered that other conditions, such as trachoma and onchocerciasis, may be common in certain endemic leprosy areas and complicate the ocular findings.

(d) The testes

Orchitis, with or without *gynaecomastia*, is a well known complication of leprosy, almost always occurring in the lepromatous type but very occasionally in the borderline (Job, 1961). Gynaecomastia is usually bilateral but occasionally may be unilateral and asymmetric; the nipple, areola, and breast tissue may be involved separately.

A number of factors may be concerned in the production of gynaecomastia —testicular atrophy, hepatic disease, hormonal disturbances, and nutritional deficiencies (see p. 595). Testicular atrophy may be present without gynaecomastia necessarily developing. The ovaries in the female are rarely affected.

Both the seminiferous tubules and the connective tissue are affected. *Myco. leprae* and even globi may be present in the epithelial lining cells. Lepromatous granulomatous tissue is present in the connective tissue and eventually leads to fibrosis and hyalinization of the tubules. Hypertrophy and hyperplasia of the interstitial (Leydig) cells occurs, and occasional bacilli may be found in their cytoplasm. As would be expected from the pathology, permanent sterility may result. Pulmonary tuberculosis is a frequent complication.

(e) The kidney

Renal failure is a frequent cause of death. Proteinuria is common. Renal biopsy and autopsy studies have revealed that proliferative glomerulonephritis, chronic glomerulonephritis, amyloidosis, chronic interstitial nephritis and hypertensive nephropathy are associated with leprosy. Especially in lepromatous leprosy it has been considered that the deposit of immune complexes in the glomeruli may be the cause of glomerulonephritis. No association with the Australian antigen or antibody, malaria or beta-haemolytic streptococci have been noted in the leprosy patients with renal disease studied.

(f) Other organs

The endocrine glands, excluding the testis, are rarely involved in leprosy. Lepromata have been described in the cortex of the adrenal and lepra cells noted in the parathyroids. Amyloid change can occur in any organ, including the thyroid and pituitary glands. Nodular lepromatous lesions have been noted in striated muscle (Convit *et al.* 1960) and may become more noticeable and painful in reactional states.

In lepromatous leprosy granulomatous lesions with cellular infiltration occur in muscular tissue. *Myco. leprae* are numerous (Mansour *et al.* 1970). Segmental atrophy of muscle fibre with sarcolemmal proliferation may occur (Slotwiner *et al.* 1969).

Leprosy and amyloidosis

Secondary amyloidosis is found in approximately 50 per cent of post mortems performed on patients dying of lepromatous leprosy in the United States. It is very much less common in India, Africa, Mexico, and Japan (Williams *et al.* 1965). The reason for this difference in incidence is obscure, and the lowered intake of animal fat in the areas of low incidence has been suggested as a possible factor. A form of primary renal amyloidosis and secondary amyloidosis in tuberculous subjects are, however, not uncommon findings in tropical Africa (Edington and Mainwaring, 1964)—so it is unlikely that this will be found to be the sole explanation.

Contributory factors in the production of amyloidosis are: frequent erythema nodosum reactions, the concomitant presence of tuberculosis or extensive ulceration from neurotrophic disease.

Diagnostic pathology

The cardinal points in diagnosis are the presence of anaesthesia in a chronic skin condition and the demonstration of *Myco. leprae* in a smear of the lesion stained by the Ziehl–Neelson method (Ridley and Ridley, 1971). The best sites for taking smears are the following:

(1) the active edge of the most active lesion,
(2) the ear lobes,
(3) the mucosa of the nasal septum.

Biopsy of typical macules, nodules, infiltrations or enlarged nerves is often used. A decrease in total serum lipids, cholesterol, and phospholipids (Misra and Ventetrasubramamian, 1964), and a raised level of 5-hydroxytryptamine in the C.S.F. of patients with leprosy, have been reported (Singh *et al.* 1965). Cave *et al.* (1963) have advocated arteriography of hands and feet as a routine particularly in osseous leprosy lesions, since an authentic arteritis has been found in some patients. Bacterial assessment of patients with leprosy is made by counts on skin smears or biopsy specimens, from which two indices can be derived—(a) the *Morphological Index* (M.I.), and (b) the *Bacteriological Index* (B.I.). In the former, an assessment of viability of bacilli is made by counting the percentage of solid-staining acid-fast rods; in the latter, an assessment is obtained of the numbers of bacilli in the smears (Ridley, 1967).

GRANULOMA MULTIFORME

This condition was described by Leiker *et al.* (1964) in Northern Nigeria where it was known as Mkar disease. It is a chronic skin granuloma with polymorphic appearance and has been seen in large numbers of patients attending leprosy clinics in Northern Nigeria. Browne (1966) has reported a high prevalence of the condition in three groups of villages in Eastern Nigeria where it is known as Nkanu. It may be a similar condition to that reported by Clarke (1959) as erythema annulare centrifugum and it was referred to as granuloma annulare by Dr. H. N. Gray from Mkar in a private letter to one of us (G.M.E.) in 1961.

The early lesions are usually papulo-nodular and develop into plaques or circinate lesions. They may be moderately hypopigmented. The diameter varies between 1 and 15 cm. Some lesions may subside and new lesions appear. The course may extend over 10 years. The lesions are usually on the upper part of the body and affect the older age groups. It is more common in females. Histologically the epidermis is normal or slightly atrophic with some loss of pigment. The dermis shows a tuberculoid infiltrate. There may be a clear sub-epidermal zone. The infiltrate consists of histiocytes, lymphocytes, epithelioid cells and giant cells of foreign body or Langhans type. Eosinophils and plasma cells may be present. Central collagenous degeneration is common. Appendages and nerves are not affected. The condition has been frequently mistaken for leprosy. It can be distinguished clinically by the presence of itching, lack of sensory impairment and anhidrosis. Hypopigmentation is less marked. Nerves are never affected.

The aetiology is unknown.

DIPHTHERIA

Coryne bacterium diphtheriae is the causative organism of diphtheria in which there is an inflammatory lesion in the throat with the formation of a false membrane. In addition, a highly potent exotoxin is produced which may cause myocardial damage (p. 372) and toxic fatty changes in the viscera in addition to a degenerative demyelination of nerve roots and proximal portion of the nerves leading to paralyses. Diphtheria is a disappearing disease in developed countries owing to the success of preventive immunization. It is thought to be uncommon in tropical areas—indeed it was thought to be rare in West Africa until recently (Wyatt, 1974). Deaths from faucial diphtheria do occur in children in Ibadan and Ghana but not in anything like the number which would be expected in a population which is not actively immunized. Immunity has, however, been shown to be high by Schick testing. In this test a weak solution of diphtheritic toxin is injected into the skin. If there is antitoxin in the blood no reaction takes place—indicating immunity.

Obviously children in West Africa are being immunized at an early age —perhaps by cutaneous infections (see Veld Sore, p. 728). The pathology of diphtheria is not further dealt with here as it is well described in most standard textbooks.

Erysipelothrix and *Listeria*, which are closely related members of the *Corynebacteriaceae* family, are primary pathogens in animals but sometimes cause infection in man.

CHOLERA

This is a disease of rapid onset caused by *Vibrio cholerae* and characterized by vomiting; profuse dehydrating diarrhoea with 'rice water stools' and marked toxaemia. Muscular cramps, suppression of urine and shock occur later. The *incubation period* is 1 to 7 days.

Classical cholera, caused by *Vibrio cholerae*, classical biotype is now virtually limited to the Indo-Pakistan subcontinent and notably in the deltas of the Ganges and Brahmaputra rivers. Cholera El Tor, caused by *Vibrio cholerae*, El Tor biotype was originally confined to a limited geographical area in the Celebes in Indonesia but has been spreading in a pandemic form since 1961 to Indonesia, Sarawak, the Philippines, Sabah, Taiwan, Korea, Hong Kong, the Chinese mainland, West New Guinea, Malaysia, Singapore, Burma, Thailand, India, Pakistan, Afghanistan, Iran, Bahrein, Nepal, Turkey and Iraq. Recently it has been reported from Egypt, Libya, Tunisia, the Southern U.S.S.R., Czechoslovakia and now, for the first time, has entered Africa south of the Sahara, with cases in Guinea, Ghana, Nigeria and East Africa. It has also occurred in Ethiopia, Sudan and Spain and has recently been imported to Australia and New Zealand (Editorial, 1972; Editorial, 1973).

Epidemiology

The reservoir of infection is a sick person, a convalescent patient or a carrier through the faeces or vomit. For every typical case of the disease there may be 10–100 other symptomless persons excreting the vibrio.

Cholera may begin suddenly as a water-borne disease. In Calcutta, where cholera is endemic, the supply of filtered water falls short in summer and the people are found to use both unfiltered and tank water. Cholera also spreads by close personal contact, by contaminated food (e.g. dates in the Egyptian epidemic of 1947), infected inanimate objects and by flies. Intra-familial spread also occurs. In order to flourish, cholera requires a combination of dense population and poor sanitation. For many years there was a tendency to overlook the role of symptomless carriers in the transmission of cholera, until it was shown that the carrier state in cholera El Tor may last for more than 7 years ('Cholera Dolores' in the Philippines) and that the vibrio can establish itself in the gall bladder.

Cholera El Tor has been proved capable of speedy and extensive spread over much wider areas than classical cholera, and in several such areas cases due to cholera El Tor have displaced those of classical cholera. In Calcutta, for instance, by the end of 1964 there was only one case of classical cholera for every ten or more cases of cholera El Tor. This epidemiological phenomenon is explained by the demonstration that the El Tor biotype eliminates the classical biotype in a few hours both *in vitro* and *in vivo*. Cholera has a seasonal pattern but the season varies from locality to locality—thus in Dacca, Bangladesh, the cholera season follows the monsoon rains and slowly disappears during the hot, dry months; while in Calcutta, India, the disease rises to a peak during the hot, dry season and ends with the onset of the rains.

The major changes in the epidemiology of cholera have been (i) recognition of the increasing importance of carriers, (ii) the frequency of personal contact infection (case to case spread) rather than water-borne epidemics and (iii) the predominance and alarming spread of the El Tor biotype. Wollf (1971) has formulated a quantitative approach to the cholera problem.

V. cholerae was discovered by Koch in 1883 and is a delicate Gram-negative organism. There are two biotypes, classical and El Tor. Each biotype contains three serotypes—Inaba, Ogawa and Hikojima. The El Tor biotype is named after the El Tor quarantine station in Egypt, where it was first isolated in 1920; it is distinguished from the other three strains by being able to produce a soluble haemolysin which is active against sheep and goat erythrocytes and by other characteristics.

Pathogenesis and pathology

Cholera usually manifests itself by the sudden onset of effortless vomiting, diarrhoea, thirst, muscle cramps (abdominal and in the extremities), oliguria, hoarseness proceeding to aphonia, lethargy and collapse. In children there may be mental confusion and convulsions (perhaps due to hypoglycaemia). The stools rapidly become colourless (rice water) and as much as 24 l a day may be passed. Death results from severe dehydration, loss of electrolytes, acidosis, and, in some patients, renal failure. In the past, mortality was, in certain epidemics, as high as 80 per cent, but with modern replacement therapy it can now be almost nil. Wallace *et al.* (1966) have shown that there is no significant difference in the clinical and biochemical manifestations of infection with *V. cholerae* and with *V. El Tor*, and the disease is similar in most respects in children and adults (Lindenbaum *et al.* 1966).

The stools are isotonic, with a low concentration of protein of about 0·1 G per cent. The pH is about 7·5, and the electrolyte content in mEq/l is: sodium, 139; potassium, up to 24; chloride, 106; and bicarbonate, 48 (Pollitzer, 1959; Phillips, 1963; Greenhough, 1965). The average daily stool volume is 24·0 l, compared with 6·1 l in non-choleraic diarrhoea (Carpenter *et al.* 1965). A suitable replacement fluid is '5:4:1 solution' (Greenhough *et al.* 1964) which contains 5 G sodium chloride, 4 G sodium bicarbonate and 1 G potassium chloride per litre. The solution is prepared and sterilized with the appropriate amounts of sodium and potassium chloride, the sodium bicarbonate being added just before the infusion is set up, as autoclaving causes decomposition of sodium bicarbonate. The differential serum proteins show a general marked increase (Rahman, 1965), and sera of cholera patients also exhibit a rise in immunoglobulins, especially in IgA and IgM, the IgA values being particularly elevated in patients with *El Tor* cholera (Goldstein, 1966; Felsenfeld *et al.* 1966).

Formerly it was considered that a massive outpouring of fluid occurred through denuded and desquamated areas of intestinal epithelium, but this opinion is no longer tenable in view of the low protein content of the stools. In addition, it has been shown that ^{131}I-labelled polyvinylpyrrolidone given intravenously in cholera patients is excreted at a normal rate into the intestinal lumen, which suggests that the mucosa is intact. Also, the intestinal mucosa has been found to be intact in biopsy specimens taken from twenty-three patients, though the villi were blunted and there was an infiltration of lymphocytes and monocytes in the lamina propria; alkaline phosphatase was diminished and subepithelial bullae were noted. (Fresh *et al.* 1964).

The mechanism of the fluid and electrolyte loss is still not certain. Dutta *et al.* (1959, 1963) demonstrated that a condition resembling cholera could be produced in suckling rabbits by administering orally sterile filtrates of lysates of suspensions of cholera vibrios, and Benyajati (1966) has confirmed these findings in human volunteers. Finkelstein *et al.* (1966) have shown that, in certain liquid media, *V. cholerae* produces a factor, which they called cholergan, that results in a cholera-like disease in the infant rabbit and human volunteers. Cholergan can be separated into two components: Procholergan A, which is the active principle, and Procholergan B, which protects A against the action of the acid gastric juice when given orally. It is suggested that the A substance causes an increase of villus capillary permeability in the small intestine and may be a major factor in the pathogenesis of cholera. Phillips (1963) has described an inhibitory factor in cholera stools and cholera culture filtrates which inhibited sodium absorption by frog skin membranes and which, it was thought, might inhibit the active transport of the sodium ion from the gut lumen to the plasma and cause retention of fluid in the intestinal lumen. This inhibition of the 'sodium-pump' has, however, been noted in other conditions and does not explain the high concentration of bicarbonate in the cholera stool. It has been shown that aspiration of duodenal and upper jejunal contents reduces the stool output in cholera and that the common bile duct is patent when liquid colourless stools are passed (Greenough, 1965). It has been suggested that the cholera vibrios in the upper gut stimulate the hypersecretion of secretin or secretin-like hormones, and that the fluid and electrolyte losses are the combination of an outpouring of fluid into the duodenum and of non-specific defective absorption by the intestine. From the foregoing it will be realized that the exact mechanism of fluid loss is still undecided; although recent work indicates that it is mainly due to excessive secretion. Thus, it has been shown that exotoxin from *Ch. vibrio* increases the activity of an enzyme adenylcyclase which stimulates intestinal secretion (Editorial, 1972). In the later stages of the disease haemoconcentration, hypovolaemia, hypotension and shock may cause ischaemic necrotic lesions in the intestine and an acute tubular necrosis in the kidney.

Diagnostic pathology

A definite diagnosis of cholera can be made only after isolation of *V. cholerae* from the faeces of patients. The faeces should be transported to the laboratory as rapidly as possible in alkaline peptone water (pH 9·0). Three methods are available for the rapid recognition of cholera vibrios: (i) the selective enrichment/fluorescent-antibody technique, (ii) the oblique-light technique and (iii) the gelatin-agar method (Finkelstein and Gomez, 1963). Microscopic examination of a stool specimen may show large numbers of vibrios.

Serological identification is an essential step; thus to-day we recognize the following schema of antigenic structure:

1. H flagellar antigens—common to many species of vibrios and hence of very little use in identification.

2. O somatic antigens—there are three antigens of which antigen A is common to all *V. cholerae*; antigen B and antigen C are specific to Ogawa and Inaba types respectively, while the presence of all the three antigens ABC characterizes the Hikojima serotype. El Tor has the same antigens as the classical types (Inaba, Ogawa, or Hikojima) but can be distinguished from these vibrios by the tests listed below (Vella, 1972).

(*a*) Mukerjee's phage typing (Mukerjee, 1963).
(*b*) Haemolysin production.
(*c*) Fowl cell agglutination.
(*d*) Voges–Proskauer reaction: production of acetyl methylcarbinol.
(*e*) Antibiotic sensitivity: polymyxin B.

CLOSTRIDIAL INFECTIONS

The clostridia are Gram-positive anaerobic rod-like organisms and produce endospores. Several species form exotoxins and are pathogenic. The most important of these are *Clostridium botulinum, Cl. tetani,* and *Cl. welchii.*

BOTULISM

There are a number of types of *Cl. botulinum.* They produce a powerful exotoxin in food which, when ingested, is absorbed from the upper part of the intestine and causes vomiting, constipation, ocular pareses, and pharyngeal paralysis, ending in coma and delirium. Mortality may be high. Diagnosis may be made by injecting food into unprotected and antitoxin-treated mice. The food itself may be cultured. Cultures from liver and spleen may be positive at post mortem and toxin may occasionally be recovered from the liver (Topley and Wilson, 1964).

GAS GANGRENE

A number of Clostridia cause gas gangrene, the more common being *Cl. welchii, Cl. sporogenes, Cl. oedematiens,* and *Cl. septicum.* Mixed infections are usual.

The condition follows tissue injury and is a rapidly spreading necrotizing inflammation. The production of gas causes crepitus in tissues. The presence of large, Gram-positive bacilli in fluid aspirated from the affected site is diagnostic. Culture of the organism can be undertaken anaerobically but the diagnosis is essentially clinical as isolation of the organism is too time consuming and, indeed, the demonstration of *Cl. welchii* in a wound is by itself of little diagnostic significance as it may be a simple contaminant. Gas gangrene is common in the tropics but as its pathology is similar to that seen in temperate climates it is not considered further.

CL. WELCHII AND INTESTINAL DISEASE

The exotoxins of *Cl. welchii* have been considered by some to play a part in the 'toxaemia' seen in acute intestinal obstruction. Infection with *Cl. welchii* may be responsible for outbreaks of food poisoning. Reheated or cold cooked meats are the usual source of infection. A diffuse sloughing enteritis of the jejunum, ileum, and colon (enteritis necroticans, 'pigbel') has been described in Germany and New Guinea (Murrel *et al.* 1966). It is the commonest acute abdominal condition requiring laparotomy in hospital practice in the highlands of New Guinea. The disease in this area, in both epidemic and sporadic forms, is related to pig feasting, which is an integral and complex part of the indigenous cultures of all highland tribes. Males are affected more than females. Clinically, the disease follows the ingestion of a large pork meal and is characterized by anorexia, severe upper abdominal pain, bloody diarrhoea, and vomiting. The fatality rates vary from nil to 85 per cent. There is also a necrotizing enteritis affecting mainly premature infants which has a high fatality rate and has been reported from Singapore (Tan *et al.* 1972). van Enk (1971, personal communication) has reported an increasing incidence of necrotizing jejunitis of variable severity in children, young adults and adults in his hospital in Ashanti, Ghana. The aetiology has been obscure.

Cl. perfringens (*Cl. welchii*) type C has been isolated from a significant proportion of resected bowel segments but it has not yet been conclusively established that a direct aetiological relationship exists between *Cl. perfringens* type C and enteritis necroticans. In the tropics a necrotizing colitis has also been thought to be due to *Cl. welchii* infection. This condition occurs in West Africa but the role that *Cl. welchii* plays in its aetiology is unknown. Extensive sloughing and necrosis of almost the entire large bowel occurs. Infection in the liver and spleen with the production of gas-filled cysts have been described in patients with debilitating disease on rare occasions (Ashley, 1965).

TETANUS

Tetanus is one of the commonest causes of death found in post-mortem material in Ibadan, West Africa and occurs in high incidence in many areas (Adams *et al.* 1959; Brown *et al.* 1960; Vakel *et al.* 1964). The exotoxin of *Cl. tetani* causes tonic spasms of the voluntary muscles which may be localized or generalized. The mortality may be high and involvement of the muscles of respiration is the most frequent cause of death.

Epidemiology

Cl. tetani is a Gram-positive, slender, motile rod up to 5 μm in length. Large terminal endospores, giving the appearance of a tennis racquet, are often present. The spores are resistant and will only germinate with growth and multiplication of vegetative forms if the surrounding oxygen tension is low. They are, therefore, harmless in clean wounds with no tissue necrosis present. Factors which favour the germination of spores are trauma with haemorrhage and tissue necrosis, the presence of foreign bodies, the presence of toxins of, and infection by, other bacteria. Experimentally the presence of certain chemicals such as lactic acid, saponin, and ionized calcium salts favour growth. Spores may remain dormant in healed wounds for many years and growth may occur following trauma or operative interference or no exciting cause may be noted—the so-called idiopathic tetanus.

Tetanus occurs most commonly after perforating or puncture wounds. Such lesions are usually contaminated with *Cl. tetani* spores from contaminated soil or street dust or from gunshot, nails, and splinters. Bites or scratches from carrion-eating animals are dangerous. Neonatal tetanus is common in the tropics, occurring in the first 10 days of life. The methods of dividing the cord vary in different areas. Bamboo is used in some and the cord tied with hemp and other vegetable material. Dressings of leaves are frequently applied and the possibility of infection entering through the cord is great (Tompkins, 1958; Schofield *et al.* 1961; Barten 1973). Puerperal tetanus is also common and may be due to primitive midwifery, e.g. the use of cow dung as a topical application in the vagina (Suri *et al.* 1964). Tropical ulcers, middle-ear disease in children and other causes of chronic ulcers (fungal, etc.) are common portals of entry. Infection may follow vaccination or the injection of antitoxic sera, bacterial vaccines and other medicaments. Tetanus has also occurred following surgical operations, tooth extractions, and burns. The incubation period of tetanus varies from 2 to 30 days, with an average of 7–10 days. A notational system for the classification of tetanus giving a severity index which should be comparable for all areas, as well as a concise method of recording the progress of the disease and the response to treatment, has recently been produced by Phillips (1967). A mathematical model of tetanus based on the natural history and dynamics of the infection was constructed by Cvjetanovic *et al.* (1972).

Pathology

The bacilli produce a powerful exotoxin at the site of the lesion. The absorption and mode of action of this toxin is controversial (Wright, 1955). Spasm may occur in the muscles adjacent to the injury and this is considered to be due to the toxin being absorbed by the motor nerve endings and passing up the nerve to affect the anterior horn cells of the spinal cord. Following this local spasticity, generalized symptoms may or may not appear. Tetanus, however, usually presents as a generalized condition with the muscles of the jaw (trismus, lock jaw), face (the sardonic smile, risus sardonicus), fore limb, trunk (opisthotonos), and lower limbs affected in that order. It is thought that the toxin is carried by the lymph from the local wound to the blood stream and then to the brain. Hyperpyrexia is a not infrequent complication and myositis ossificans has also been described (Femi-Pearse and Olowu, 1971).

At autopsy the changes are frequently minimal and non-specific. Many deaths are due to respiratory difficulty either to spasm of the respiratory muscles or involvement of the respiratory centre (apnoeic crisis). Cardiac arrest also occurs. Many factors are involved, including age, severity of the infection, the presence of intercurrent infection (tracheobronchitis, infection from a tracheostomy wound), and associated disease. The lungs may show only congestion or be haemorrhagic and oedematous, with areas of consolidation or collapse present. Swelling of the nerve cells in the motor ganglia of the spinal cord and medulla with chromatolysis and neuronal lesions in the dorsal vagal nuclei have been described (Montgomery, 1961). Crush fractures of the vertebrae, usually T4–8, especially in sickle-cell disease, due to spasm of the back muscles with opisthotonos occur, and actual rupture of muscles has been described (Davies and Rowland, 1965). A local source of infection should be sought for. The presence of sickle-cell haemoglobin may have an adverse effect on mortality from tetanus, and pulmonary embolism, following thrombosis of the veins of the leg, occasionally occurs.

Diagnostic pathology

Diagnosis is frequently difficult and may depend solely on the clinical findings. The typical bacilli may be seen on Gram-stained smears of the pus from an obvious wound. The organism may be cultured in Robertson's cooked-meat medium or in anaerobic cultures in 4–12 days. Mice or guinea-pigs may be inoculated subcutaneously.

THE TYPHOID FEVERS

These infections are caused by members of the *Salmonella* group, *Salmonella typhi* and *S. paratyphi A, B,* or *C*. There are many phage types of *S. typhi*.

Epidemiology

Typhoid fever presents one of the classical examples of a water-borne infection, it has a world-wide distribution although it is endemic only in communities where the standards of sanitation and personal hygiene are low (Kanhemeva and Isebaert, 1973). All ages and both sexes are susceptible.

Contamination of water—the cause of major outbreaks—can occur through cross-connection of a main with a polluted water supply, faecal contamination of wells, or faulty purification. An outbreak of water-borne transmission of chloramphenicol-resistant *S. typhi* occurred in Mexico (Gonzalez-Cortes *et al.* 1973). Typhoid can also be spread by shell-fish. particularly oysters which mature in tidal estuaries and are thus exposed to contaminated waters. Milk-borne outbreaks occur either by direct contamination from a carrier or indirectly from utensils. Ice-cream, other milk products, ice, vegetables, duck eggs, and salads may be infected directly or indirectly. Flies and infected dust may be sources of infection. Person-to-person spread can occur through an intermediary common vehicle (McGregor and Reinhart, 1973). The *paratyphoid fevers* are food-borne rather than water-borne infections. It must be borne in mind, however, that food (e.g. corned beef), as in the Aberdeen outbreak of 1964, can also cause epidemics of typhoid fever. In Rhodesia the case incidence begins to rise as water supplies contract to their minimum just before the hot, wet season starting in October, and reaches a peak when the early rains have resulted in the transfer downstream of contaminated water from one pool to another (Weeks *et al.* 1971).

About 2–4 per cent of typhoid patients become chronic carriers of the infection. The majority are faecal carriers. Urinary carriers also occur and seem more common in association with some abnormality of the urinary tract and in patients with *Schistosoma haematobium* infection (Farid *et al.* 1972). In some patients the focus of persistent typhoid infection in carriers may be not only in the gall bladder but in the deep biliary passages of the liver (Erlick and Reitler, 1960). An equal sex incidence of typhoid carriers occurs among the Chinese in Hong Kong, and the carrier state there, unlike in Europe and the U.S.A., is maintained by a focus of infection within the liver rather than in the gall bladder. In view of a higher incidence in typhoid carriers of infection of the bile ducts with the liver fluke, *Clonchorchis sinensis*, McFadzean and Ong (1966) conclude that this infection may be a factor responsible for the persistence of *S. typhi* within the liver. *Salmonella septicaemia* has been described in association with *S. mansoni* infection in Brazil and Egypt (Rocha *et al.* 1971). Chloramphenicol resistant typhoid fever has become a global problem (Editorial, 1973; Butler *et al.* 1973).

Phage typing has proved of value in dealing with the carrier problem and in tracing the source of outbreaks. Symptomless infections also occur. Cvjetanovic *et al.* (1972) have constructed an epidemiological model of typhoid fever.

Pathology

Clinically, headache, abdominal discomfort, joint pains, constipation (or, less commonly, diarrhoea), vomiting, cough, and backache are the most

frequent symptoms. Constantopoulos *et al.* (1973) has described fulminant diarrhoea associated with acute haemolysis in G-6-PD deficient
patients. The patient is apathetic and mentally dull. There may be grave
toxaemia and the typhoid state with delirium and coma.

Following ingestion the bacilli multiply in the second part of the
duodenum, the bile present forming an excellent culture medium. During
the incubation period jejunal biopsy studies have shown an inflammatory
reaction in the jejunum which may be diffuse or granulomatous, the exudate
consisting of histiocytes, plasma cells, lymphocytes and a few polymorphonuclear cells. Eosinophils and mast cells are also slightly increased
(Sprinz *et al.* 1966). The bacilli multiply in the lymphoid tissue of the
Peyer's patches and mesenteric lymph nodes and eventually pass into the
blood stream, probably via the thoracic duct, with general dissemination,
particularly to the liver, spleen and reticulo-endothelial system.

They pass into the bile and multiply rapidly, and enter the intestinal tract
for the second time. This heavy reinfection of the lymphoid tissue is probably
responsible for the major pathological changes in the bowel. Death of the
organism releases an endotoxin so, in addition to the local changes initiated
by the bacteria, generalized signs of toxaemia are present in the organs—
cloudy swelling and necrosis of the heart and voluntary muscle respectively
being examples. In addition the toxaemia leads to a general lowering of
resistance, and laryngitis, bronchitis, and pneumonia may be caused by
invasion of secondary organisms as well as by the typhoid bacillus itself.
Sudden fatal hypothermia following treatment with chloramphenicol can
occur (Mulligan, 1971), and one of us (G.M.E.) has seen a Jarisch–Herxheimer reaction simulating perforation occurring following therapy.

The gastro-intestinal tract

The typhoid bacillus affects the lymphoid tissue of the small and large
intestine. The Peyer's patches at the lower end of the ileum are most
frequently affected but lesions may be seen proximally as high as the
jejunum and the large intestine may also exhibit lesions usually in the
ascending colon. In *paratyphoid B infection* there may be, in addition, ulcers
in the stomach and large intestine, including the rectum.

The pathology can be described in four stages—hyperaemia, necrosis,
ulceration, and healing—which crudely approximate to the weeks of the
disease. In the hyperaemic stage the lymphoid tissue becomes congested
and projects from the surface of the bowel wall. There is an infiltration of
large monocytes (phagocytes) derived from the reticulo-endothelial system.
They are palely eosinophilic with a well demarcated eccentric nucleus and
are the predominant cell seen in typhoid fever ('typhoid cells'). They are
phagocytic and may contain erythrocytes, bacilli, lymphocytes, and cellular

debris. Monocytes, lymphocytes, and plasma cells are usually also present but polymorphonuclear leucocytes are rarely seen. Necrosis occurs in the lymphoid tissue in the areas of histiocytic infiltration due to the toxin released from the dead bacilli and extends in the mucosa and submucosa. Thrombosis and blockage of small blood vessels also play a part in the process. Sloughing and ulceration occur in the third week. The cellular exudate still consists of the typhoid macrophage with variable numbers of plasma cells and lymphocytes. Polymorphonuclear leucocytes are scanty. Typically, the ulcers are oval and lie in the long axis of the intestine on the antimesenteric border. The edges are soft, raised, and undermined, and the floor may contain necrotic greenish-black slough or the muscularis may be visible. They are usually separate, up to 3–4 cm in length, but may be confluent in the iliocaecal region. The intervening mucosa usually shows a catarrhal hyperaemia.

The stage of healing commences in the fourth week. Fibrosis and scarring are minimal and strictures never occur.

A fibrinous exudate may be found on the peritoneal surface in the absence of macroscopic perforation and ileus is a complication (Bohrer, 1966). Perforation is a not uncommon complication and occurs about the end of the third week. It is especially common in Ghana and this may be due to: (1) many cases of typhoid fever not coming to hospital—only those severely ill; (2) an extremely virulent local *Salmonella* strain; (3) a lowered host resistance. Many perforations occur in the first week of the disease—a finding which has also been noted in Southern India where perforation is not so frequent. Investigations are required on host resistance factors (Archampong, 1969). The perforation may be single or multiple and occurs in the distal ileal region. Haemorrhage is a further complication and neither the occurrence of perforation nor of haemorrhage is related to the clinical severity of the disease—nor indeed are the number and size of the ulcers in all instances. Intussusception is a very rare complication (Leech and Wright, 1944).

Liver and gall bladder

Toxaemia causes cloudy swelling of the hepatic cells and small globules of fat may be present. The striking feature, however, is the presence of typhoid nodules, which are small lesions usually situated in the parenchyma in the outer third of the hepatic lobule, and consist of collections of macrophages and lymphocytes with or without central necrosis (Fig. 6.4). Bacilli may or may not be detected. Typhoid abscesses have been described. Cholangitis is rare.

Typhoid bacilli multiply readily in bile, and the gall bladder is the usual seat of infection in the carrier. Acute cholecystitis is unusual but chronic

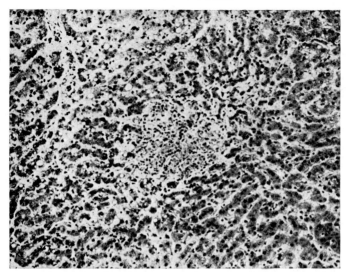

FIG. 6.4. Typhoid fever. A 'typhoid nodule' consisting of necrotic cells and macrophages is demonstrated. Bacteria may or may not be demonstrable (H and E × 125). (*By courtesy of Ash and Spitz.*)

cholecystitis occurs in the carrier state and there is a superficial infiltrate of mononuclear cells with secondary lymphoid follicles in the mucosa and submucosa. Chronic cholecystitis is, however, not common in most tropical areas in which typhoid occurs and McFadzean and Ong (1966) have shown that the gall bladder carrier is rare in the Chinese in Hong Kong. Further information on the pathology of the gall bladder in the typhoid carrier state in other parts of the tropics is required. Gall stones are said to be a relatively common secondary complication in Europe but are rarely seen in tropical Africa, possibly due to altered cholesterol metabolism.

The reticulo-endothelial system

The spleen is enlarged, hyperaemic, and cherry-red in colour, but in areas of stable malaria the macroscopic picture is complicated by the presence of pigment in children and it may appear greyish-red. There is marked proliferation of the reticulo-endothelial histiocytes in the sinusoids and pulp and the typhoid nodules described in the liver may be present. Erythrophagocytosis may be noted and there is a predominance of histiocytes in the germinal centres.

The mesenteric lymph nodes are swollen and hyperaemic or haemorrhagic and the sinusoids are packed with histiocytes and monocytes from the blood. Pyogenic infection and suppuration may occur but are rare.

Typhoid nodules may be seen in the bone marrow and there is variable myeloid hypoplasia. Haemoglobinuria has been described in typhoid on rare occasions (Smith, 1951; Gelfand, 1972). A leucopenia with a relative lymphocytosis usually occurs in the peripheral blood. Haemolytic anaemia has been described as a not infrequent complication of *S. typhi* infections (McFadzean and Choa, 1953). In addition to the usual signs of a haemolytic anaemia the Coombs test has been positive when performed. The mechanism is obscure. Chloramphenicol does not immediately affect the haemolytic process and its response to A.C.T.H. is suggestive of an immunological basis, alternatively G-6-PD deficiency may be implicated (Meyer, 1973). Acute haemolysis complicating co-trimoxazole therapy for typhoid fever in patients with G-6-PD deficiency has been reported (Owusu, 1972; Chan and McFadzean, 1974).

Genito-urinary system

Prior to chloramphenicol therapy 20–30 per cent of patients excreted bacilli in the urine in the third week of the illness and the lesions described were a toxic nephrosis and/or 'typhoid nodules' in the kidney. Clinically, a condition resembling acute nephritis has been described but the pathology is unknown (Huckstep, 1962). Massive intravascular haemolysis due to G-6-PD deficiency with acute tubular necrosis has been reported as a complication (Lwanga and Wing, 1970). Chronic infections can, however, occur in the kidney in *Salmonella* infections. Perinephric abscesses, pyelonephritis, and pyelitis have been described but usually occur in patients with pre-existing structural damage (Belzer *et al.* 1965). Infection with *S. paratyphi A* complicated by schistosomiasis with hepatic fibrosis has a characteristic clinical picture, which is different from that of classic enteric infection in patients without schistosomiasis (Hathout *et al.* 1967). Other aspects of the relationship between salmonellosis and schistosomiasis are discussed on p. 176.

Orchitis is a rare complication and is presumably due to the presence of 'typhoid nodules' in the interstitial tissue of the testes.

Respiratory system

Ulceration and oedema of the larynx have been described but are rare. Mild bronchitis and pneumonitis occur in many patients and lung abscesses have been described (Hanne, 1964). Secondary infection is common and bronchopneumonia in children and lobar pneumonia and occasionally empyema in adults are not unusual complications.

Cardiovascular system

Pericarditis has been described but is very rare. Fatty degeneration of the myofibrils of the heart due to toxaemia is said to be common and clinically the heart would appear to be affected. Sudden death due to heart failure can occur. This has not been common in our experience. Anaesthesia has been considered dangerous due to the heart lesions.

Venous thrombosis in the lower limbs (in some instances spreading to the inferior vena cava) with subsequent pulmonary embolism was a not uncommon complication in Europe but would appear to be much less of a hazard in tropical areas.

The central nervous system

Meningism is a not infrequent finding in typhoid with normal findings in the cerebrospinal fluid and is presumably due to the toxaemia. A pyogenic type of meningitis does, however, occur (Vaizey, 1959) although it is not common. Clinically, peripheral neuritis has been described but there is little information on the pathology. Chanmugam and Waniganetti (1969) have described the Guillaine–Barré syndrome (distal paraesthesia, muscle pain and weakness spreading proximally with increased C.S.F. protein and a normal cell count) associated with typhoid fever.

Skeletal system

Osteomyelitis is not common in the acute stage of typhoid fever but usually occurs in convalescence or even years after infection (Huckstep, 1962). It occurs in the long bones. The vertebrae may also be affected with the development of typhoid spine. Osteomyelitis is a common occurrence in children with blood dyscrasias associated with the presence of sickle-cell haemoglobin—the infecting organism is usually a *Salmonella* (see p. 446). Typhoid osteitis, usually affecting the long bones and running a chronic course, is very occasionally seen (Groll and Smith, 1965).

In addition to the bony lesions typhoid nodules may also be present in the marrow.

Other organs

Otitis media and parotitis may be complications due to secondary infection. Alopecia may be troublesome. Zenkers degeneration in voluntary muscle (the rectus abdominus, diaphragm, and thighs) is a focal hyaline degeneration with fragmentation of the muscle fibres caused by the toxaemia. Very occasionally a true typhoid arthritis may occur, and deep-seated abscesses in the back and buttocks have been reported in addition to the breast (Barrett and McDermott, 1972). *Rose spots* are macules about 1–2 mm in size which appear usually on the abdomen and chest about the seventh to tenth day of the illness. Histologically there is hyperaemia of the dermis with an associated monocytic infiltration. Typhoid bacilli may be present in clumps.

Diagnostic pathology

Blood culture in bile-salt broth during the first 2 weeks of the disease usually yields *S. typhi*. It has been suggested that 'clot' culture is even more efficient (Editorial, 1966). After about the tenth day the Widal test (O and H agglutinins) becomes positive and rises progressively—a rising titre rather than absolute values is necessary for a positive diagnosis. A leucopenia with relative lymphocytosis is often seen. The diazo test is a red coloration given by the froth of the urine of typhoid patients when mixed with the diazo reagents, despite its definite limitations it is a simple and useful diagnostic aid which becomes positive after the fifth day of clinical illness. Culture of the faeces and urine may have to be repeated at frequent intervals before a positive result is obtained. The Vi reaction is of no value either in the diagnosis of the acute attack or in the forecasting of clinical relapse; it is, however, of help in the detection of the carrier state (Forrest *et al.* 1967).

BACILLARY DYSENTERY

Bacillary dysentery is caused by one of the pathogenic species of bacteria belonging to the genus *Shigella*. Species and varieties of the genus *Shigella* are numerous and they can be conveniently classified into four main subgroups (Topley and Wilson, 1964).

Subgroup A: Ten antigenically distinct serotypes, including Shiga's bacillus, Schmitz's bacillus, and the Large-Sachs organisms.

Subgroup B: *Sh. flexneri.* Six main serotypes and a number of sub-serotypes, all antigenically interrelated.

Subgroup C: *Sh. boydii.* Fifteen antigenically distinct serotypes.

Subgroup D: *Sh. sonnei.*

The proportion of infections due to individual serotypes varies considerably from country to country, and in the same country at different times, but the organisms of greatest clinical importance are *Sh. shigae*, various types of *Sh. flexneri* and *Sh. boydii*, *Sh. schmitzii* and *Sh. sonnei*. The disease caused by Shiga's bacillus tends to be the most and that by Sonne's bacillus the least severe. The dysentery bacilli are non-motile, Gram-negative organisms.

Epidemiology

Bacillary dysentery has a world-wide distribution but is commoner in tropical than in temperate climates, lack of adequate sanitation and personal hygiene being mainly responsible. Infection is derived from ambulant cases of the disease, from healthy convalescents, and from symptomless carriers. The organisms, which are excreted in the faeces, may gain access to food through the imperfectly cleansed fingers of the patient or carrier; or they may pass from one person to another by contact with inanimate articles. Fly-borne infection is important in the tropics. Epidemic infection may result from the contamination of milk or of ice-cream. Occasionally dysentery is water-borne. Young children are more liable than older persons to acquire *Shigella* infections and when infected to suffer from clinical disease.

During a period of 5 years (1960–1965) diarrhoeal diseases surveys were carried out by the WHO Diarrhoeal Advisory Team in Mauritius, Sudan, United Arab Republic, Ceylon, Iran, East Pakistan, and Venezuela. The studies mainly concentrated on the pre-school population showed that morbidity and mortality was highest among children under the age of 3. An increase of the diarrhoea rate could be noticed during the period of weaning and the difference in diarrhoea incidence between breast-fed children and those receiving bottle milk or other types of food was statistically significant. Shigellae were isolated both from children suffering from diarrhoea and from those having no diarrhoea. In West Pakistan *Shigella* was the commonest bacterial pathogen found in children under 2 years of age (Ingram *et al.* 1966).

Bacillary dysentery has a short incubation period, about 48 hours as a rule. It is essentially a local disease; the bacilli remain confined to the intestine and to the mesenteric nodes and they do not invade the blood stream. The disease may run a chronic course.

Pathology

The lower end of the ileum and colon are affected. The mucosa is hyperaemic and oedematous and there is lymphoid hyperplasia. A superficial infiltration of polymorphs, macrophages, and plasma cells with ulceration and fibrinous exudation occurs. The ulcers remain superficial unless secondary pyogenic infection occurs. The intervening mucosa may become hypertrophic and polypoid in appearance. Perforation is rare. It is said that secondary infection may lead to a form of ulcerative colitis or simulate pseudo-malignant lesions. It is doubtful if these changes occur frequently in the tropics. Subepithelial cysts may arise from submucosal nests of epithelium isolated during the inflammatory process. Cerebral oedema and extensive acute changes in the nerve cells of the cerebral cortex with destruction of the glial processes have been described in children in Japan and haemorrhagic lesions may also be present in the stomach and duodenum (Suwa, 1966). Convulsions in children, pneumonitis, conjunctivitis, iritis, corneal ulcers, parotitis pyelonephritis and arthritis, have also been noted (Barrett-Connor, 1970). The arthritis usually follows 2–5 weeks after the acute illness. Cultures of joint fluid are usually sterile and bacteraemia is not present. There may be an associated conjunctivitis and urethritis. The arthritis is thought to be a hypersensitivity phenomenon. Rarely, myocarditis and polyneuritis are further complications.

Diagnostic pathology

The isolation of the specific organism from the faeces cultured as early as possible in the disease provides the best means of diagnosis. In the early stages macroscopical examination of the mucus shows a striking number of red blood cells and polymorphonuclear leucocytes. Tillett and Thomas (1974) have provided a statistical method for estimating the true isolation rate from culture of the faeces.

BRUCELLOSIS

Brucellosis is one of the most important zoonoses. Human disease is attributed to *Brucella abortus*, *Br. suis*, and *Br. melitensis* from cattle, swine, and goat exposure especially. Brucella are small, non-motile, non-sporing, Gram-negative coccobacilli. Apart from their different CO_2 requirements, the members of this group resemble each other closely in their cultural characters. Table 6.1 summarizes the chief differential features of members of this group.

TABLE 6.1. *The differential features of brucella organisms*

Species	CO_2 Requirement	H_2S Production	Growth		Agglutination in non-specific sera	
			Thionin	Basic fuchsin	*abortus*	*melitensis*
Br. abortus	+	+ 4 days	−	+	+	−
Br. melitensis	−	−	+	+	−	+
Br. suis	−	+ 5 days	+	−	+	−

Epidemiology

Brucellosis is more prevalent in the tropics than is generally supposed and has been widely reported from Africa, South America, and India (Polding, 1956; Cox, 1966; Collard, 1962). In these days of wide travel, 'holiday brucellosis' should always be borne in mind (Vella and Goode, 1973).

Many animals can serve as sources of infection for man, among which the most important are cattle, swine, goats, and sheep (Spink, 1956). The modes of transmission are ingestion, contact, inhalation, and inoculation from animals which are discharging brucella. Infection by ingestion may occur by the gastro-intestinal route, and by penetration of the mucous membrane of the oral cavity and throat. The transmission of brucella by ingestion of contaminated milk, milk products, especially cheese, meat and meat products is well recorded. Viable brucella may be present in the viscera and muscles of infected carcasses for periods of over 1 month. Camel meat and water are also vehicles of infection. Contact with infected material, e.g. placentae, urine, carcasses, etc., is a common source of infection in some countries. It is an occupational disease of veterinarians, farmers, etc. (Williams, 1974; Rogus et al. 1974). Air-borne infection through the mucous membranes of the eye and respiratory tract can occur, while accidental inoculation has been recorded among veterinarians and laboratory workers (WHO, 1964). Chronic brucellosis is frequently missed and the prevalence is unknown (Editorial, 1974).

Immunoglobins have been studied in both acute and chronic cases of brucellosis; in the latter the serum reactivity is mainly confined to the IgG and IgA fractions while in the acute cases IgM globulins are also involved (Coghlan and Weir, 1967).

Pathology

Following an incubation period of 1–3 weeks brucellosis may present as an acute, severe, non-specific febrile illness, as an undulant type of fever or as an atypical intermittent chronic type. The course of the disease is lengthy but usually patients recover within a year. The mortality is low. Lymphadenopathy and splenomegaly are usual and occasionally hepatomegaly occurs. The severity of the pathological lesions depends upon the species of Brucella. The least severe are produced by Br. abortus, complications are greater with Br. melitensis, and Br. suis causes chronic lesions with suppuration.

The organisms are found intracellularly in the reticulo-endothelial system, and small miliary granulomas resembling sarcoid or tuberculosis are formed in the lymph nodes, spleen, liver, and bone marrow. They consist of epithelioid cells surrounded by lymphocytes, monocytes, and fibroblasts. Giant cells are inconstantly present. Necrosis and suppuration can occur but caseation is not seen. Complications occur and almost any organ in the body can be the seat of lesions. Orchitis, epididymitis, arthritis, osteomyelitis of long bones and vertebrae, mastitis, oöpheritis, and meningoencephalitis have all been recorded. Although the granuloma may be seen in liver-biopsy material, hepatitis is not a feature of the condition clinically. Centrilobular necrosis and extensive destruction of liver parenchyma has been described and rarely cirrhosis may be a sequel. Acute pyelonephritis and subacute bacterial endocarditis may be found at necropsy. Ocular lesions, iritis, choroiditis, and uveitis may occur. Hypersplenism is a complication and, with associated lesions in the marrow, thrombocytopenia and purpuric manifestations in conjunction with a leukaemoid reaction in the peripheral blood may be superimposed and complicate the haematological picture. An association with Hodgkins' disease and lymphosarcoma has been noted.

Diagnostic pathology

The laboratory diagnosis of brucellosis includes bacteriological and serological methods as well as allergic tests. The various methods have been described in detail by Alton and Jones (1967) and Kerr *et al.* (1968). *Brucella* organisms can be most easily cultured from the blood and bone marrow but brucellae can be isolated from other sources, e.g. synovial fluid, lymph nodes, etc. A progressive rise of antibody titre occurs in acute brucellosis and the serum agglutination test nearly always gives significantly positive results in the presence of active infection. The interpretation of the agglutination test is not always easy since, owing to the occurrence of latent and past infections, a certain proportion of the population of any country is found to contain serum antibodies capable of reacting to a variable titre (Henderson and Hill, 1972). The complement-fixation test can also be used in the diagnosis of chronic brucellosis. The intradermal test when positive only indicates a state of specific allergy and must be interpreted with great caution. It is a useful adjunct to other methods of diagnosis and is particularly useful in epidemiological surveys. Detection of IgG has been found to be of particular help in clinically doubtful cases (Macdonald and Elmslie, 1967).

ANTHRAX

Anthrax is enzootic in many areas of the world and can be conveniently divided into its agricultural and industrial aspects. It is caused by *Bacillus anthracis*, a Gram-positive, aerobic, spore-bearing, rod-shaped organism.

Epidemiology

The disease occurs in the economically important domestic animals—cattle, sheep, goats, etc. and it is largely from contact with these animals, or with industrial raw materials derived from such animals (hair, hides, etc.), that man becomes infected. In the tropics human anthrax is prevalent in many parts of Africa, South America, the Near and Middle East, and in the Indian subcontinent.

In agricultural areas concomitant contamination of the soil with the spore forms of *B. anthracis* occurs. The spores are very resistant to chemical and environmental influence and can survive for years in certain types of soils and animal products, e.g. hides and wool. Anthrax spores have been found in samples of bone meal carried from India and Pakistan (Levy Committee, 1959). The main sources of infection in agricultural workers are contact with contaminated carcasses, wool, hides, and hair. The ingestion of insufficiently cooked meat derived from infected animals is another source of infection; thus intestinal anthrax is the commonest form of anthrax encountered in Kenya (Fendall and Grounds, 1965).

Cutaneous anthrax is the most frequent form of the disease among industrial workers. Hair, wool, bones, hides, and skins are the usual sources of infection. Inhalation anthrax occurs but is rare.

Pathology

In animals suspected of having died of anthrax, a post-mortem examination should not be made; otherwise blood will be spilt on the neighbouring ground and will provide a source of infection for the other beasts. The pathology of cutaneous anthrax is that of a haemorrhagic necrosis. The malignant pustule commences as a red, painful papule which becomes necrotic, with the formation of a central black eschar. The regional lymph nodes are enlarged. Septicaemia with a haemorrhagic meningitis may occur and in our experience this may be found in the absence of skin lesions. A small pustule surrounded by brawny oedema should raise suspicion of anthrax.

In those working with the skins of animals (wool sorters' disease) lesions may occur in the lungs due to the inhalation of the spores. In the pulmonary form haemorrhagic ulcerative lesions occur in the lower trachea and bronchi associated with haemorrhagic necrotic lesions in the hilar lymph nodes. Necrosis and haemorrhage in the lungs associated with haemorrhagic pleural and pericardial effusions are usual. In all these lesions the paucity of neutrophils and cellular infiltration is remarkable. There are many bacilli in the lesions and they can be demonstrated by Gram's stain. The intestinal form occurs in our experience in West Africa and should be suspected at post mortem if the duodenum and upper jejunum are oedematous with haemorrhagic necrotising lesions in the mucosa. Associated lesions in the lymph nodes may be noted. It has to be differentiated from enteritis necroticans (p. 319). Dutz *et al.* (1970) have reported primary anthrax of the stomach with massive ascites in an Iranian woman.

Diagnostic pathology

Microscopical examination of fresh material derived from lesions shows the typical *B. anthracis* organisms. Culture and animal inoculation are usually used for confirmation of the diagnosis.

PLAGUE

Plague is a rapidly fatal disease due to *Yersinia pestis* which can manifest itself in a variety of ways—bubonic, pneumonic, and septicaemic forms. The organisms are small, Gram-negative, ovoid bacilli, showing bipolar staining.

Epidemiology

Although the number of cases of plague have gradually declined, foci of the disease still exist in South East Asia, South America, the Indian sub-continent, and parts of Africa. A noteworthy feature is the continuing importance of the disease in Vietnam where 1203 cases were reported in 1972. Recent outbreaks have occurred in Africa in Lesotho, The Libyan Arab Republic, The Malagasy Republic, the United Republic of Tanzania and Zaire (WHO, 1973).

The bubonic disease—which is the commonest—is transmitted by the bite of an infected rat flea *Xenopsylla cheopis*. Meteorological conditions exert an important role upon the epidemiology of plague, both in deter-mining the survival of plague bacilli and the life of the vector fleas. The natural reservoir of plague is in wild rodents—sylvatic plague—and epizoo-tics affect many different species throughout the world. The infection is transferred to rats living in urban areas from wild rodents and thence to man. In rural areas, man can be infected in the fields, bring the disease home, infect his own rats and fleas and thereby his family. Pneumonic plague is transmitted from person to person by contact with patients suffering from primary pneumonic plague or from patients with bubonic plague who develop terminal plague pneumonia. A mixed pneumonic bubonic plague outbreak occurred recently in Vietnam (Pham Trong *et al.* 1967) and *P. pestis* was recovered from the throats of asymptomatic healthy carriers (Marshall *et al.* 1967). Ray and Kadull (1965) have developed an agar-gel precipitation inhibition test for determining plague antibody.

Pathology

The incubation period is 2–4 days. The septicaemic form presents with meningitis and pneumonia. The pneumonic form may be primary or secondary to the septicaemic or bubonic types. Bubonic plague presents suddenly with chills, fever, nausea, vomiting, and oliguria. Mental anxiety is marked. A leucocytosis of about 40,000 is usual and blood culture may be positive in about 50 per cent of patients. The buboes are painful tender swellings of the lymphatic glands and may be single or multiple. They appear on the second to fifth day of the illness. The inguinal, axillary, and cervical lymph nodes are affected in that order of frequency.

The whole vascular system is often seriously involved. The endotoxin affects the vascular endothelium of all organs and haemorrhages and necroses with many bacilli present are the characteristic lesions. In the vessels in the region of the bubo these lesions may be especially prominent.

The liver is often enlarged and congested. Fatty degeneration commonly occurs and there may be minute, greyish nodules containing degenerate and necrotic parenchymal cells, polymorphs, and many bacilli. The heart is dilated and flabby with fatty changes in the muscle fibres. Severe lesions in the lungs may be found, with bronchopneumonia and sometimes pus formation. Congestion, oedema, petechial haemorrhages of the brain, and a frank *Yersinia* meningitis have been described.

Diagnostic pathology

Y. pestis may be detected in smears of material aspirated from buboes, from sputum, or even from the blood stained by Gram's method. Culture and animal inoculation should be performed. Smears from the spleen are positive at necropsy. Fluorescent antibody, complement fixation, and haemagglutination techniques have also been used (Chen and Meyer, 1966).

PASTEURELLA PSEUDOTUBERCULOSIS

P. pseudotuberculosis causes acute mesenteric lymphadenitis mainly in young males between 5 and 15 years of age (Mair, 1968). The diagnosis is established by isolation of the organism, by the demonstration of specific antibodies in the serum, by histological examination of the lymph nodes and by the response to a specific skin-test antigen. If death occurs the organism can be cultured from the numerous abscesses found in the liver and spleen. Histologically the lesions in lymph glands consist of small abscesses and palisading of histiocytes may be seen reminiscent of cat scratch fever and lymphogranuloma venereum.

TULARAEMIA

Tularaemia is a disease of animals caused by infection with *Pasteurella tularensis*. It is mainly a disease of temperate climates (Editorial, 1971) and causes fever, chills, headache associated with respiratory symptoms contracted from direct contact with sick or dead animals, eating under cooked infected meat or drinking infected water. It can also be transmitted by arthropods. There are focal necroses in many of the viscera. The diagnosis is usually made by a positive agglutination reaction or culture of blood or the lesion at site of location.

DONOVANOSIS

Synonyms. Granuloma venereum; ulcerating granuloma of the pudenda; Donovaniasis.

Donovanosis is a chronic granulomatous condition usually affecting the genital organs and is caused by *Donovania granulomatosis*.

The organism is an encapsulated, Gram-negative coccobacillus which in lesions in man is seen within phagocytes—the Donovan bodies. It can be cultured in the yolk sac of the developing chick embryo. An ultrastructural study has been undertaken by Davis (1970). It occurs in the Caribbean, East Indies, and in parts of South America, Africa, and India. It is generally but not invariably a venereal disease, and occurs in both sexes between the ages of 20–40 years.

Pathology

The incubation period varies from days to several months. It commences as a papule which ulcerates. The edges are indurated, sharp and deep and the floor is covered by a thick, yellow, offensive, purulent exudate. It extends peripherally and may reach a very large size. A characteristic feature of the condition is the scarring which occurs. The scars may be nodular and keloidal. The perineal, perianal region, anus, vagina, cervix, and penis are the more usual sites. Extragenital lesions occur on the lips, oral cavity, oesophagus, and larynx and may be caused by autoinoculation or by haematogenous spread. Bone involvement occurs, the clavicle, skull, and ribs being most frequently affected (Siebes, 1965). Satellite papules may occur along the line of lymphatic drainage and lymph nodes may suppurate. Mutilating ulceration of the genitalia occurs and deformity and elephantiasis are common complications.

There is pseudoepitheliomatous hyperplasia of the epidermis at the edge of the ulcer. The dermis and subcutaneous tissues are infiltrated by chronic inflammatory cells, mainly plasma cells and lymphocytes. In the superficial portion, clusters of polymorphonuclear leucocytes are conspicuous and they may also be present in the deeper layers. Large, vacuolated hysticocytes are prominent and contain the pathogenic Donovan bodies (Fig. 6.5). In tissue sections the presence of these histiocytes in association with clusters of polymorphs are highly suggestive of the diagnosis. The Donovan bodies can be demonstrated by a Giemsa stain or by silver impregnation methods. The latter method stains the capsule. Intracellular Donovan bodies may be demonstrated in biopsy material, in tissue smears, or on examination of the exudate from the lesions (Fig. 6.5).

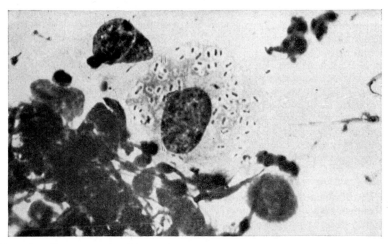

FIG. 6.5. Donovanosis. Photomicrograph of Donovan bodies in a large mononuclear cell in a tissue smear (H and E × 800). (*By courtesy of C. P. Douglas.*)

BARTONELLOSIS

Bartonellosis appears in two distinct forms: (*a*) Oroya fever, and (*b*) verruga peruana.

Oroya fever is an acute, febrile illness associated with a rapidly developing anaemia and a high mortality. Verruga peruana is a non-fatal disease exemplified by generalized cutaneous lesions. It usually occurs following recovery from the Oroya fever stage although it occasionally arises apparently spontaneously. The infection is limited to Peru, Colombia, and Ecuador. The causative organism is *Bartonella bacilliformis*. Although known since 1905 it was first cultured in 1928 by Noguchi from an acute case of Oroya fever and the culture produced the nodules of verruga in monkeys. Oroya fever is also known as Carrion's disease since Carrion, a medical student, inoculated himself with material from a verruga lesion and died from Oroya fever 39 days later. The disease is transmitted from man to man by the bites of various species of sandflies which live at altitudes of 2000–8000 feet and bite only at night.

The organisms are pleomorphic Gram-negative coccobacilli and are found in blood smears, either free in the plasma or within red cells, in Oroya fever. They are sparse in the nodules in verruga and culture of material on serum agar is the most reliable method of isolation.

Pathology of Oroya fever

The incubation period is 3 weeks and the patient presents with pyrexia, bone and joint pains, and signs of a rapidly increasing anaemia of a haemolytic type. Normal transfused erythrocytes are also destroyed, but erythrocytes from patients with verruga peruana are said to survive normally. The organisms stain well with Giemsa and are easily detectable in blood smears. There is a polymorphonuclear leucocytosis. The spleen and liver are enlarged.

At autopsy the organisms are found widely distributed in the reticulo-endothelial cells of the bone marrow, liver, spleen, and lymphatic glands. In addition to the signs of a haemolytic anaemia (hyperplastic marrow, siderosis, etc.) areas of necrosis are present in the bone marrow and probably account for the bone pains. Centrilobular necrosis occurs in the liver and there is marked erythrophagocytosis by Kupffer cells. Areas of infarction and necrosis are common in the spleen. The pulp cords are congested and erythrophagocytosis and hypertrophy of the sinusoidal lining cells containing organism are seen.

There is proliferation of the sinusoidal histiocytes which in lymph glands contain red blood cells and organisms. The principal cause of mortality is a particular susceptibility of patients with Oroya fever to septicaemic infection with *Salmonella* organisms, commonly *Salm. typhimurium* (Cuadra, 1956).

Pathology of verruga peruana

Verruga peruana usually is seen 5–6 weeks after an attack of Oroya fever but it may occur spontaneously with an incubation period of about 2–3 months. The skin lesions may be miliary or nodular. The miliary lesions are small nodules and papules which appear in crops and are widely distributed. The mucous membranes may be affected. The lesions bleed easily and often are ulcerated and covered with crusts. Dysphagia, haematemesis, melaena, and vaginal haemorrhage may occur.

The nodular lesions are sparse and may reach considerable size. They are present in the subcutaneous tissues and are prone to occur in the region of joints. Mortality is virtually nil.

The striking feature of the histopathology is the marked proliferation of capillaries and it is said that the lesions may resemble Kaposi's disease. *Bartonella* may be seen within the endothelial cells of the blood vessels. The organisms, however, are far less numerous than in the visceral form and culture is the most certain method of diagnosis. The superficial portions become oedematous and haemorrhage and ulceration occur. With infiltration of leucocytes and plasma cells, the lesion may resemble a pyogenic granuloma.

CHANCROID

Synonyms. *Hæmophilus ducreyi* infections; soft chancre.

Chancroid is an acute venereal disease caused by *Haemophilus ducreyi*. The incubation period is about 2 weeks. A necrotic ulcer develops on the genitalia, usually the penis in males and the labia minora and majora in females. Autoinoculation frequently leads to multiple chancres. The ulcer may be up to 3 cm in diameter. The base is not indurated in contrast to the syphilitic chancre. In 1 or 2 weeks the lymph nodes become enlarged and painful and may suppurate (buboes). Constitutional symptoms are mild. The condition is usually self-limiting.

Histologically the surface of the ulcer consists of fibrin and necrotic debris lying on a layer of vascular granulation tissue. Capillaries and endothelial cells are prominent. Vasculitis may lead to thrombosis or necrosis of the vessel wall. Deep to the granulation tissue there is a third zone of chronic inflammatory cells and fibrous tissue. The lymphatic glands show a similar reaction surrounding the necrotic tissue at the centre of the abscess.

Diagnosis can be suggested on tissue biopsy material but isolation of the organism is preferable. *H. ducreyi* is a short, plump, Gram-negative coccobacillus about 1–2 μm in length and 0·6 μm in breadth which can be isolated in media containing mammalian blood (Topley and Wilson, 1964).

MELIOIDOSIS

Melioidosis is a disease of man and animals caused by a slender, motile, Gram-negative bacillus variously named *Bacillus whitmori, Loefflerella whitmori,* and *Pseudomonas pseudomallei.* It may be bipolar or filamentous.

The disease is almost entirely confined to South East Asia and a considerable proportion of healthy adults in Thailand have been shown to have complement-fixing antibodies in their serum to *L. whitmori* (Nigg, 1963). Rodents are frequently infected and the organism has been found widely distributed in soil and water. It has been postulated that the ingestion of water contaminated by the urine or faeces of infected rodents is the method of transmission, but recently traumatic damage to the skin has been thought to be the portal of entry (Editorial, 1970). Melioidosis has been recognized as a military problem in South East Asia (Fournier, 1965). Some cases may simulate tuberculosis or disseminated fungus infections (Duong-Hong-Mo and Tran-Hiep-Cuong, 1967). Neonatal melioidosis has been described (Osteraas *et al.* 1971).

Pathology

The disease is usually recognized in non-immunes and the course is usually brief, death occurring within 3–4 weeks. More chronic forms, however, occur. A stellate abscess surrounded by epitheloid and giant cells may be misinterpreted as cat scratch disease, tularaemia, lymphogranuloma venereum, sporotrichosis or *Pasteurella pseudotuberculosis* (especially if in mesenteric glands). Diarrhoea, mild abscesses, chronic lung disease, or a rapidly septicaemia may occur.

At autopsy the common findings are focal areas of consolidation in the lung with multiple minute abscesses in the lungs, spleen, liver, kidneys, heart, eye, and bones, which tend to coalesce and contain bright green pus. Microscopically, polymorphonuclear leucocytes and giant cells are found.

The organism can be cultivated on glycerol agar from the blood, abscesses, and the urine. Rarely it may be found in the cerebrospinal fluid. Inoculation of guinea-pigs or hamsters should be undertaken. Agglutination tests are not of much value.

MYCOPLASMAS

Mycoplasmas are the smallest free-living organisms known. They were formerly known as pleuro-pneumonia-like organisms. They possess both ribonucleic and deoxyribonucleic acids. They cause respiratory disease and polyarthritis in animals. *Mycoplasma pneumoniae* causes cold-agglutmin-positive primary atypical pneumonia in man (Editorial, 1965).

The subject has been reviewed by Taylor-Robinson (1971) and Thomas (1971).

Little is known about their importance in pathology in the tropics. By examining urine and urethral and cervical swabs Osoba (1972) found *M. hominus* and T-strain mycoplasma in 1–42 per cent and 24–60 per cent of blood donors, gynaecology outpatients and female consorts of males with sexually transmitted diseases in Nigeria. It was concluded that both organisms could not be pathogenic in the genito-urinary tract and that there was no racial factor governing their frequency.

7

Spirochaetal Disease

THE TREPONEMATOSES

The human treponematoses can be subdivided into two main groups: (i) the non-venereal treponematoses, which are transmitted mostly among children, and (ii) venereal treponematosis, which occurs mostly among adolescents and adults and is caused by *Treponema pallidum*. The epidemiological pattern of venereal disease and endemic treponematoses has undergone important changes in recent years in both developing and developed countries. Idsoe *et al.* (1973) have reviewed the situation.

Syphilis is uncommon in many parts of the tropics where yaws is endemic. There is nothing remarkable in its pathology in the tropics, apart from the fact that tabes dorsalis is said to be rare, and it is not considered further. There is, however, a condition termed *endemic syphilis* which is caused by the organism of syphilis (*T. pallidum*), attacks children, and is not transmitted venereally. A classification of the non-venereal treponematoses is given in Table 7.1.

TABLE 7.1. *Classification of non-venereal treponematoses*

Non-venereal treponematoses (endemic treponematoses of childhood)	Causative organisms
(1) Pinta (mal del pinto; carate)	*T. carateum*
(2) Yaws (pian, framboesia, bouba)	*T. pertenue*
(3) Endemic syphilis (Bejel)	*T. pallidum*

Epidemiology of non-venereal treponematoses

About 20 years ago it was estimated that approximately 50 million people suffered from the endemic treponematoses of childhood, but the vigorous mass-treatment campaigns carried out by the World Health Organization have caused a rapid regression of the prevalence of these infections.

The natural histories of the three endemic treponematoses of childhood (Pinta, yaws, and endemic syphilis) are very similar and have been described in detail by Hackett (1963). The treponeme enters the body through the mucosa or through a break in the epidermis. While the initial lesion is developing treponemes reach the neighbouring lymph glands, which become enlarged; at a later date treponemes enter the blood stream and are carried throughout the body. They then multiply in the skin to produce the papillomata. The initial lesions of yaws and pinta appear on any exposed part of the skin but in yaws they are most frequent below the knee (Hackett, 1957); in endemic syphilis the initial lesions are infrequent. The early skin lesions of *yaws* are discrete, proliferative moist papillomata, containing numerous treponemes; in *endemic syphilis* they are moist and circinate papules and condylomata. The initial and early lesions of *pinta* are spreading, scaly plaques, and later bluish pigmentary skin changes occur. Years later these dyspigmented areas become depigmented.

Pinta extends from Mexico down to the upper Amazon basin and the number of positive serological tests in the population accurately reflects the prevalence of the disease in childhood (Marquez *et al.* 1955).

Yaws was endemic throughout large parts of the tropics and was by far the most important endemic treponematosis (Hackett and Loewenthal, 1960). It extended from the Caribbean Islands and South America, through the equatorial belt of Africa extending to South East Asia and the Pacific islands. The disease is transmitted by contact among children living in warm, humid climates, where the standards of personal hygiene are low (Hackett, 1967).

Endemic syphilis occurs in Africa north and south of the equatorial belt and in Asia in the rural areas of Syria, Saudi Arabia, Iraq, and Iran. It is a disease of warm, dry climates. In Senegal, Senecal *et al.* (1962) have reported prevalences of seroreactors of 92 per cent and of clinically active cases of 4 per cent. Luger and Schmid (1961) have remarked on the rarity and mildness of late neurosyphilis and cardiovascular lesions in rural populations in whom endemic syphilis is prevalent.

Pathology of pinta, yaws, and endemic syphilis

Hudson (1965) has suggested that all the treponemal infections are one disease caused by one treponeme and their differing clinical and epidemiological patterns are due to differing climatic and sociological conditions.

The pathology of these three conditions is similar. Congenital forms do not occur. Visceral lesions and changes in the C.N.S. are uncommon in endemic syphilis and do not occur in yaws (excluding bones) and pinta. The striking feature of the pathology is the infiltration of lymphocytes and plasma cells in the more acute lesions. Perivascular infiltration is not as severe as that seen in syphilis and endarteritis of blood vessels is unusual. In the late stages fibrosis and endarteritis or chronic ulcerative lesions with epithelioid cells predominating may be seen. Spirochaetes may be demonstrable by Levaditi's stain.

Diagnosis by histopathological means is rarely required in these conditions with the exception of the isolated ulcer or juxta-articular node and serological and clinical tests are the most common methods employed.

Diagnostic pathology

Serological findings reveal no differences between the human treponemes and diagnostic tests fall into two categories.

A. Non-treponemal tests

These include precipitation, flocculation, and those complement-fixation methods which utilize antigens derived from animal tissue extracts. The two most commonly employed are the Kahn precipitation test (the antigen is lipids from beef heart) and the Venereal Disease Research Laboratories (V.D.R.L.) flocculation test (the antigen is cardiolipin, cholesterol, and lecithin). These tests are highly specific but occasionally biologically false-positive reactions occur in normal individuals. Other conditions such as smallpox vaccination, leprosy, tuberculosis, malaria, and kala azar may also cause false-positive reactions. The serology of yaws has been reviewed by Fischman and Skorepova (1973).

B. Treponemal tests

The *Treponema pallidum* immobilization (TPI) test involves the principle that treponema antibodies have the property of immobilizing *T. pallidum*. The percentage of spirochaetes immobilized over a 48-hour period by the test serum is estimated. The test distinguishes individuals with biologically false-positive non-treponemal test but does not distinguish yaws and syphilis.

An antigen has also been produced from *T. pallidum* which gives results similar to the TPI test by complement-fixation methods (TPCF). A fluorescent treponemal antibody test has also been evolved and also distinguishes between treponemal and non-treponemal positive reactions in standard tests. The most satisfactory serological method for testing for venereal syphilis may involve three tests (Carpenter *et al.* 1960) and refined techniques are required (Editorial, 1965).

THE RELAPSING FEVERS

Relapsing fever is due to infection of the blood by morphologically indistinguishable strains of spirochaetes which are transmitted by ticks resulting in endemic disease, and by body lice resulting in epidemic disease.

TICK-BORNE RELAPSING FEVER

Non-epidemic relapsing fever is due to infection with *Borrelia duttoni* and is transmitted by a number of ticks, of which the African *Ornithodorus moubata* is one of the most important.

Epidemiology

The disease occurs in Central, East and South Africa as well as in North Africa, North, Central and South America, the Middle East and northern India. In most areas *B. duttoni* normally affects rodents and occurs only accidentally in man, while in central Africa it primarily affects man, in whom it is endemic.

The tick lives in the soil of the floor, or the mud plaster walls of African huts; they are also found in caves and in the soil of bush or scrub country. The female lays batches of eggs each of which hatches to produce a larval tick with three pairs of legs. The larval forms pass through about five moults at intervals of 2 weeks. Larval forms and adults feed by sucking blood. A proportion of the offspring of infected female ticks are infected transovarially; thus the infection may persist through several generations. During feeding a saline fluid, called coxal fluid, is excreted from glands near the attachment of the legs.

It is generally believed that the infected fluid exuded by the coxal glands, saliva, and bowel contaminates the wound made by the bite of the tick and spirochaetes enter the blood stream.

Humans entering caves, working in bush country, living in infected African huts, or sleeping in rest houses in the vicinity of infected villages are liable to acquire the infection. The incubation period is usually about a week (5–10 days). It seems that babies and little children are very susceptible to the disease and it appears that immunity is acquired with increasing age by those living in endemic areas (Bell, 1956). There are several reports in the literature of new-born infants developing relapsing fever within the first 10 days after birth (Geigy and Mosser, 1955), but no case of congenital infection has been recorded. Garnham (1936) suggested that infection was transmitted after birth during the process of suckling, possibly from cracks in the nipples, to abrasions in the child's mouth. Heisch (1950) has shown experimentally that *B. duttoni* will infect lice. But no large-scale change in vector has been proved to occur under natural conditions.

LOUSE-BORNE RELAPSING FEVER

This disease is more common in temperate than tropical climates, but outbreaks of epidemic louse-borne relapsing fever have occurred in parts of

Africa, India, and South America. The only definite endemic focus of louse-borne relapsing fever in the world is in Ethiopia (Rijkels, 1971). Bryceson et al. (1970) carried out a meticulous clinical and laboratory study and reviewed the literature. Like epidemic typhus fever, which it may accompany, it is associated with poor sanitation and personal hygiene, particularly overcrowding, undernutrition, and lice-infested clothing. It is conveyed from one man to another by the human body louse, *Pediculus humanus*, and the spirochaete responsible is *Borrelia recurrentis*. The blood of a patient suffering from relapsing fever contains spirochaetes only during the febrile periods and lice become infected at this time. In contrast to ticks, no transovarial transmission in lice occurs. Infection is conveyed to human beings not by the bite of the louse, but by contamination of the wounds (made by biting or by scratching) with the body fluids of the louse. The incubation period is usually from 2 to 10 days.

Pathology

The pathology of tick-borne and louse-borne relapsing fever is similar. The mortality is usually low but was reported to be high in one epidemic in West Africa. When spirochaetes are disappearing from the blood of patients with louse-borne relapsing fever there occurs an abrupt rise of body-temperature, arterial pressure, heart rate, respiratory rate, and worsening of the lesions—a series of events reminiscent of the Jarisch–Herxheimer reaction. The leucocyte-count falls suddenly when these changes begin, suggesting that the reaction may be due to the liberation of leucocyte or endogenous pyrogen (Schofield et al. 1968). The most consistent haematological abnormality is thrombocytopaenia, with platelet counts below 150,000/cm. This was attributed to increased consumption due to intravascular clotting and to pooling in the enlarged spleen. Treatment of louse-borne relapsing fever is followed by a sudden increase in fibrin-degradation productions (FDP) (Perine et al. 1971a and b; Perine et al. 1974).

Jaundice and haemorrhages into the skin, stomach, intestine and kidneys are usual findings at necropsy. The spleen is enlarged and miliary lesions may be obvious in the gross specimen. They consist of mononuculear cell infiltrates and congestion with numerous organisms usually present. Infarctive lesions are common. The liver is enlarged and congested and areas of focal necrosis may be present. Lesions may also be present in the heart, kidneys, lymphatic glands, and bone marrow, and the spirochaetes may be demonstrated by silver stains. Intracranial haemorrhage and, rarely, meningitis may occur. Bronchopneumonia is a frequent complication.

Diagnostic pathology

Blood should be taken during the pyrexial period and examined either by dark-ground illumination or after staining with a Romanovsky stain. *B. duttoni* is about 15 μm long and made up of spiral turns occupying 2–3 μm. The numbers present in a blood film vary from case to case; at the height of the first pyrexial attack they arc often numerous. Blood infection is less heavy in the tick-borne than in the louse-borne disease. The organisms may be recovered by culture or by intraperitoneal inoculation of blood into laboratory animals (e.g. mouse or rat). The Wasserman reaction may be positive. Ginger and Katz (1970) separated *B. duttoni* from blood by DEAE cellulose anion exchanger.

B. recurrentis is morphologically similar to *B. duttoni* and similar diagnostic methods as described above are used. Animal inoculation into small animals is only possible, however, after passage through monkeys. The Weil-Felix test may be positive for Proteus OXK (Robinson, 1942).

LEPTOSPIROSIS

Synonyms. Weil's disease; spirochaetal jaundice; mud, field, or swamp fever; Japanese seven-day fever.

Leptospirosis is caused by infection with spirochaetal organisms, belonging to the genus *Leptospira*. A large and increasing number of leptospiral serotypes have been recognized in various countries and a list of their global distribution has been recently compiled (Leptospiral serotype distribution lists, 1966).

Epidemiology

Leptospirosis has a world-wide incidence and the disease varies in its symptomatology, depending to some extent on the nature of the causative organism; *L. icterohaemorrhagiae* is widely distributed in man while *L. canicola* is mainly found in dogs. *L. bataviae* is very common in South East Asia while *L. grippotyphosa* is the commonest serotype in man in Thailand (Sundharagiati *et al.* 1966). The leptospiral organisms are slender, closely wound spirochaetes which vary in length from 8 to 24 μm. The spirals are shallow and regular, each being about $\frac{1}{4}$ μm in length.

Leptospirosis occurs chiefly in damp, badly drained, rat-infected situations, and infection probably occurs directly or indirectly by contamination of the abraded skin or of a mucous membrane such as that of the eye, nose, or mouth, with rat's urine. It has been established by numerous workers that the rat—particularly *Rattus norvegicus*—is a very frequent carrier of pathogenic leptospirae. *L. canicola* is excreted in the urine of dogs and pigs and the disease has occurred in persons who have been in close contact with a sick dog and have cleaned up its dejecta, as well as in workers in piggeries. Water and sewage exposed to frequent and heavy contamination by rats are common sources of infection. It has been suggested that in certain circumstances human excreters of leptospirae in the urine may be the source of spread of the disease (Spinu *et al.* 1963). Leptospirosis was thoroughly discussed in Antwerp in 1966 (International Colloquium on Leptospirosis. 1966a, b), and recently reviewed by Turner (1973).

Pathology

The leptospiroses are acute febrile diseases, variable in their severity and symptomatology. They can be grouped as those presenting with classical leptospiral jaundice (Weil's disease) and the 'benign' or anicteric leptospiroses. Only the pathology of the former type will be described. The incubation period is about 10 days and three stages of the infection are usually recognized:

(1) Septicaemic lasting about 1 week with myalgia, especially of the calf muscles, jaundice, and purpuric manifestations the most prominent symptoms.

(2) A combined icteric and uraemic phase in the second week with haemorrhage and symptoms of renal failure common.

(3) The stage of convalescence.

At post mortem there are haemorrhages in many tissues and these are considered to be due to damage to the capillary walls rather than to hepatic insufficiency. In the liver there are subcapsular and parenchymal haemorrhages. The parenchymal cells may be relatively unaffected and the mechanism of the jaundice is unclear. Central or areas of focal necrosis with an infiltrate of mononuclear cells, bile stasis, and fatty degeneration may be present. Spirochaetes may be demonstrable by Levaditi's stain.

Subcapsular haemorrhages are present in the kidneys, which are swollen and tense. Necrosis of the proximal tubular epithelium with large numbers of leptospirae lying between the necrotic cells and hyaline and bile casts in the distal convoluted tubules are the usual findings microscopically. The interstitial tissue is oedematous and is infiltrated by plasma cells and lymphocytes either in a diffuse or focal fashion.

In the voluntary muscles there are areas which show vacuolation, loss of striation, hyalinization, and infiltration, with histiocytes, polymorphs, and plasma cells present. Large clumps of hyaline material with surrounding proliferation of sarcolemmal cells are suggestive of the diagnosis.

A vegetative endocarditis and fibrinous pericarditis may be present and occasionally a mononuclear-cell meningitis may be a complication or even the presenting feature of the disease.

Diagnostic pathology

A polymorphonuclear leucocytosis is usually present. The organism can be demonstrated in the blood during the first week of the disease and in the urine during the subsequent weeks, while serological examination confirms the diagnosis. Leptospiruria may persist for as long as 11 months (Johnson, 1960). Renal biopsy demonstrates infiltration of the interstitial tissue with lymphocytes and histiocytes, tubular damage, and focal thickening of the glomerular basement membrane (Penna et al. 1963; De Brito et al. 1965). The long-term prognosis of patients who recover from an attack of lepto-spirosis is good and renal function returns to normal in the majority of the cases (Simpson et al. 1967). The organisms can readily be cultured on a variety of simple media, and inoculation of infected blood into guinea-pigs is also used. For ease and rapidity of diagnosis serological methods are mainly relied upon (Galton et al. 1962). Agglutinins, lysins, and comple-ment-fixing bodies appear towards the end of the first week of the disease and increase to reach their maximum after 4–7 weeks. Dried blood on filter paper is a practical alternative to serum samples for the agglutination test (Sundharagrati et al. 1967).

8

The Circulatory System

For many years accurate information on the frequency of cardiovascular disease in the tropics was lacking and misconceptions arose from clinical impressions, the supposed rarity of essential hypertension and rheumatic heart disease being examples. The opening of new medical schools in developing countries with consequent improvement in diagnostic techniques and, not least, more time being available to the clinician to give to his patients, have greatly enhanced our knowledge of the frequency and type of heart disease in various areas of the tropical world (Trowell, 1960; Gelfand, 1961; Imperial and Felarca, 1963; Parry, 1966, Harling et al. 1965. Kallichurum 1969; Brockington and Edington, 1972; Kallichurum, 1972).

THE HEART

There is little information available regarding the anatomy of the normal heart in tropical areas. What little there is would suggest that, although the heart weight is less, its percentage weight to body weight is as would be expected in Europe (Coles and Davies, 1959; Hayes and Lovell, 1966). Surveys carried out by various investigators in rural and urban Jamaica and in a village in Guyana have shown cardiac enlargement and left ventricular hypertrophy to be common by the criteria applied in normotensive subjects (Ashcroft, 1972). One of the reasons is an average smaller thoracic diameter with a similar cardiac diameter to Caucasians. There is some evidence to suggest that the coronary anastomotic pattern may differ in various parts of the world—whether due to inherited or environmental factors has still to be defined—and this is discussed more fully when the geographical pathology of coronary artery disease is considered.

With the exception of coronary artery disease—and, in many areas, thyrotoxic heart disease and those conditions affecting the aged in the population, such as senile amyloid disease—it should be remembered that the well-described conditions occurring in temperate climates occur probably just as frequently in the tropics and often with more florid manifestations —acute bacterial endocarditis being a case in point, and diphtheritic myocarditis should not be forgotten. Brown atrophy and the thrush-breast heart of anaemia are not just textbook descriptions as they now are in the

Western world. Dietary deficiencies, toxins, viruses, and parasitic and bacterial infections are important agents in heart disease in the tropics and these are dealt with in appropriate chapters.

Excluding parasitic and nutritional disease, there are a number of conditions affecting the myocardium seen in the tropical areas of the world which would appear to be rare or much less common in temperate climates. These are idiopathic cardiomegaly (IC) and endomyocardial fibrosis (EMF) which are dealt with in some detail in the following pages. The occurrence of cardiac aneurysms in Africa is also of interest. El-Hassan and Wasfi (1972) have described the pattern of cardiovascular disease in Khartoum while Miall *et al.* (1972*a*, *b*, *c*) have carried out longitudinal studies of heart disease in a Jamaican rural population.

The conditions mentioned above are, however, only a relatively small proportion of the diseases affecting primarily the myocardium, and a classification of these conditions modified after Fowler (1964) is given in Table 8.1. Shaper (1972*a*, *b*, *c*, *d*), has reviewed the whole subject of cardiovascular disease in the tropics while WHO (1974*a*, *b*, *c*) is engaged in an intensive effort to stimulate international cooperation in cardiovascular problems.

I. PRIMARY MYOCARDIAL DISEASE

(a) Idiopathic familial heart disease

If the hereditary ataxias and metabolic diseases are excluded at least two forms of idiopathic heart disease occur. The first resembles idiopathic cardiomegaly but glycogen may be present in the myofibrils. The second type is known as obstructive cardiomyopathy (asymmetrical hypertrophy) and may cause sudden death in young adults. Both sexes are affected and it may be inherited as a Mendelian dominant. The lesion is a localized hypertrophy of cardiac muscle, usually in the septum, causing subaortic narrowing of the outflow path. Histologically there is hypertrophy and atrophy of the myofibrils with fibrosis. Glycogen is absent. The condition has been well described by Teare (1958) and the literature reviewed by Hudson (1965).

TABLE 8.1. *Classification of the myocardiopathies*

I. Primary myocardial disease
  (*a*) Familial
  (*b*) Idiopathic cardiomegaly and intracardiac postoperative thrombosis
  (*c*) Idiopathic cardiomegaly occurring in late pregnancy and the puerperium
  (*d*) Endocardial fibroelastosis
  (*e*) Endomyocardial fibrosis
  (*f*) Congenital heart disease
  (*g*) Annular subvalvular left-ventricular aneurysms

TABLE 8.1.—*continued*

II. Secondary myocardial disease

A. Myocarditis

   (i) Viral (poliomyelitis, Coxsackie B, and rickettsial etc.)
   (ii) Giant cell
 (iii) Rheumatic
 (iv) Bacterial endocarditis
  (v) Diphtheritic
 (vi) Syphilitic and tuberculous
 (vii) Parasitic and mycotic
(viii) Loeffler's disease
 (ix) Toxic
  (x) Acute Suppurative myocarditis

B. Cor pulmonale

C. Hypertensive heart disease

D. Atherosclerosis and coronary artery disease

E. Degenerative conditions

   (i) Thrush-breast heart
  (ii) Cloudy swelling
 (iii) Fatty change
 (iv) Calcification
  (v) Ischaemic atrophy

F. Metabolic disorders

   (i) Glycogen-storage disease
  (ii) Thyrotoxicosis
 (iii) Myxoedema
 (iv) Haemochromatosis
  (v) Nutritional deficiency
      (*a*) Brown atrophy
      (*b*) Kwashiorkor
      (*c*) The heart in anaemia
      (*d*) Beriberi and alcoholic heart disease

G. Collagen disease

H. Sarcoidosis

I. Amyloid disease

J. Neuromuscular and neurologic disorders

   (i) Progressive muscular dystrophy
  (ii) Friedreich's ataxia
 (iii) Myotonic muscular dystrophy

K. Primary and metastatic tumours including the carcinoid syndrome

(b) Idiopathic cardiomegaly (ICM)

Synonyms. Primary myocardial disease; myocardosis; idiopathic cardiac hypertrophy; idiopathic cardiomyopathy; cardiopathy.

The condition has received much attention in Africa and the various synonyms used in that continent in contrast to those used on a global scale are given in the footnote below.* At a recent symposium in London the International Society of Cardiology reviewed the present state of knowledge of the cardiomyopathies and drew attention to issues which remain contentious (Shaper, 1972; Editorial, 1973).

Idiopathic cardiomegaly can be defined as an acute, subacute, or chronic disorder of heart muscle of unknown aetiology often with associated endocardial or sometimes with pericardial involvement but not atherosclerotic in origin (Goodwin, 1964). Intracardiac thrombosis and embolic episodes are common.

It is common in West Africa and is one of the most common heart conditions seen in the Bantu in South Africa. It has been described in southern Rhodesia (Gelfand, 1952) and probably occurs in East Africa. Cases have been seen in the West Indies (Stuart and Hayes, 1963; Fodor et al. 1964), Colombia (Correa et al. 1963), in children in Africa (Altman and Stein, 1956; Antia et al. 1969), and the United States (Bloomfield and Liebman, 1963). The condition has been reported in whites and non-whites (probably being more frequent in this group), Italians and Chinese in the United States, Europeans and Coloureds in South Africa, Indians, Malays, Australians and, occasionally, in Britain. It is our opinion that idiopathic cardiomegaly will probably be found in most tropical areas as facilities for cardiological investigations improve. Idiopathic cardiomegaly occurs in all age groups but the majority of the patients are over 30 years of age. Both sexes are affected. No familial tendency has been noted and a study of veterans in the United States has shown that the condition is acquired (Muehsam et al. 1964). No race would appear to be exempt. The lower socio-economic groups are more likely to be affected. The multiplicity of synonyms testifies to the ignorance surrounding the aetiology of this condition or perhaps it would be wiser to say group of conditions as, in different areas, different pathological processes are most probably involved as causative factors. Numerous factors have been considered in the aetiology of the condition, viral infections, alcoholism, malnutrition, an immune mechanism, and dietary deficiencies being most frequently mentioned. The

---

*Nutritional heart disease (Gillanders, 1951); the heart in chronic malnutrition (Higginson et al. 1952); cardiovascular collagenosis with parietal endocardial thrombosis (Becker et al. 1953); obscure cardiopathy, dilated ventricle type (Nwokolo, 1955); idiopathic hypertrophy of the heart in African children (Altman and Stein, 1956); cryptogenic heart disease (Higginson et al. 1960); heart muscle disease (Edington and Jackson, 1963).

possibility of an infective agent being responsible for cases in Britain has recently been discussed (Braimbridge *et al.* 1967). Vitamin E, copper, and selenium deficiency are known to cause heart disease in animals, but there is no evidence that they are aetiological agents in man. Before a pathological diagnosis of ICM can be made it is necessary to exclude the following conditions:

1. Significant systemic hypertension.
2. Organic valvular disease.
3. Coronary artery disease.
4. Intra- or extra-cardiac shunt.
5. Obstructive cardiomyopathy.
6. Histological evidence of myocarditis or systemic disease.
7. Cor pulmonale with right ventricular dilatation and hypertrophy (Fejfar, 1968).

Pathogenesis

The onset of cardiac failure may be acute, subacute, or chronic. Spontaneous remissions and transient hypertension in the absence of fundal or renal changes may occur. Bouts of pyrexia have been described in the South African cases (Becker, 1963). Cardiac enlargement with breathlessness, nocturnal dyspnoea, cough, haemoptysis and cardiac pain are usual. The pulse is of small volume. Although a pericardial effusion is frequently seen at necropsy, clinical signs of pericardial involvement are not usual. Embolic phenomena may be frequent. Eosinophilia and anaemia are unusual and the response to treatment is usually poor.

Macroscopically at necropsy a straw-coloured pericardial effusion of varying severity is usual. Although all chambers of the heart are usually dilated and hypertrophied (weights as great as 850 g have been recorded) occasionally right or left ventricular enlargement may predominate and hypertrophy of the pulmonary outflow path may be a marked feature and may be related to pulmonary thrombo-embolism. The heart tends to be globular and the muscle of soft consistency, with small focal patches of fibrosis scattered throughout the myocardium of one or both ventricles in a few instances. The trabeculae carneal at the apices of the ventricles and the papillary muscles are flattened. There may be an increase of white fibrous bands running between the trabeculae, even, rarely, spanning the ventricular cavity, and this, with the flattening of the trabeculae and sometimes deepening of the inter-trabecular spaces, gives a 'lacework' appearance in the lower third of the ventricles. Thrombi are present in decreasing frequency in the right and left atrial appendages and the apices of the left and right ventricles in about 70 per cent of hearts but it should be noted that

Becker *et al.* (1953) found thrombi in the left ventricle in all hearts examined. The thrombi may be pale and firm or red and friable, the latter being considered an agonal phenomenon. In the ventricles they are found at the apex between the trabeculae carneae. Plaques of white fibrous tissue may be found at the apices or in the endocardial surfaces of the inflow tracts of the ventricles. Occasionally the myocardium at the apex of the left ventricle may be thin and is somewhat reminiscent of the lesion commonly seen in Chagas' disease. From these plaques fibrosis may extend into the underlying myocardium. The valves are unaffected and mild atherosclerosis of the coronary arteries may be present in the older age groups. The great vessels are usually macroscopically normal.

Histological examination

Excluding the presence of a terminal pericarditis, lesions in the pericardium are not usual. A mild lymphocytic infiltration of the epicardium may be present.

The endocardium may be normal but there are usually localized and patchy areas of fibroelastosis, superimposed on a mucinous oedema of the connective tissue—these lesions being most frequently noted in the endocardium of the papillary muscles and inflow tract. Small foci of lymphocytes, macrophages, and plasma cells have been described in the endocardium but are unusual in our experience. The valves are normal.

Thrombi in various stages of organization, most often between the interstices of the trabeculae carneae, may be present. The thrombi are frequently formed of fused platelets and fibrin. In others, varying numbers of red cells and leucocytes are present. Endocardial necrosis subjacent to the thrombus has been described. At the base of the thrombus, vascular granulation tissue with a variable number of chronic inflammatory cells and haemosiderin deposits are present, superimposed on which is a layer of collagen of varying degrees of vascularity, on the surface of which there may be a layer of fibrin. The late stage of such a lesion is represented by a fibrous plaque lying on a disrupted elastica, variable in extent, and fibrous tissue may penetrate for a few cells thicknesses into the myocardium. In the collaginous areas enclosing the trabeculae carneae, thin-walled vascular spaces are present. Fibrin thrombi in the Thebesian and luminal veins have been noted.

In the myocardium there are diffuse changes in the muscle cells. They are enlarged with bizarre vacuolated nuclei, many of the 'staghorn' type being present. The cytoplasm is granular and vacuolated. Loss of striation is a variable feature. An increase of perinuclear lipochrome pigment is not unusual. Areas of myocytolysis may be present. This is a non-specific lesion and has been well described by Schlesinger and Reiner (1955). The cytoplasm of the affected group of myofibrils disappears—the term 'falling out necrosis' has been used. The sarcolemma is preserved. There is no cellular reaction and fibrous repair commences at the periphery of the lesion— (Fig. 8.3, p. 363), eventually a fibrous scar is formed containing pigment, which is PAS positive, resembling the perinuclear pigment found in the myofibrils. These lesions are most frequently found in the central portion of the papillary muscle and trabeculae carneae of the left ventricle. They are situated at the periphery of the pure coronary vascular circulation.

Basophilic (mucinous) degeneration of the muscle fibres has been described but is rare in our material. It is, however, worthy of description as it may simulate a parasitic condition. The fibres are granular and stain blue on routine H and E staining. There is no surrounding cellular infiltration. The changes are non-specific and are present in a variety of cardiovascular, renal and malignant conditions (Scotti, 1955). A deficiency of the enzyme succinic dehydrogenase has been noted in one case (Kobernick et al. 1963).

The interstitial tissue shows mucinous oedema with occasionally a scanty lymphocytic infiltrate. Patchy fibrous scars most marked in the inner third of the ventricular muscle, independent of thrombus formation, with surviving muscle cells between the scarred areas and the endocardial surface are usual. The most marked scarring is, however, seen in the papillary muscles and trabeculae carneae. Perivascular fibrosis is an inconstant finding. Aschoff nodes are never seen.

Atheromatous change in the larger coronary arteries may be present in mild degree in the older age groups but injection studies have excluded coronary artery disease as a causal agent. Very rarely an embolus may cause occlusion. Changes in the smaller blood vessels have been described (notably by South African workers); these include necrotizing arteriolitis and areas of fibrinoid necrosis in the heart itself, intimal focal nodular swellings, giant-cell intimitis of the pulmonary vessels, and increased metachromasia of the aorta. Occasionally we have noted organized thrombi in the smaller pulmonary vessels.*

---

*It should be noted that Becker (1963) in South Africa has reported an acute form of 'mural endocardial disease' characterized by the presence of large thrombi in the cardiac cavities, almost invariably the left ventricle, with associated thrombi in the pulmonary artery in six of twenty-four patients. The endocardium of the ventricle was swollen and thickened, with focal inflammatory cells and haemorrhages present. Degenerative changes were noted in the myocardium—most marked in the inner third. In the chronic form the condition resembled ICM. The similarity to EMF was noted and the author considered that the two conditions might represent modified manifestations of essentially the same disease process. Edington and Jackson (1963) could not separate pathologically the 'early' case of EMF from 'heart muscle disease'. However, in view of the geographical differences in the distribution of the two conditions and the uncertain state of our knowledge they have in this text been considered entirely separate entities.

Changes in the other organs

These are essentially those of chronic venous congestion with over half the patients, in contrast to the findings in EMF, exhibiting infarctive lesions. Peripheral oedema, ascites, pleural effusion, and changes of chronic venous congestion in the lungs, liver, spleen, kidney, and brain are usual. The most frequent sites of infarction are the lungs, kidneys, spleen, and brain, and minute embolization of the glomerular capillaries has been described. Occasionally we have noted changes suggestive of multiple emboli in the vasculature of the lung. Although Gillanders (1951) noted cirrhosis of the liver in all his South African patients subsequent investigations have not confirmed this finding and moderate to severe siderosis of the liver has only been described in the expected incidence in cases from South Africa. Liver disease has not been a feature in other parts of the world.

Diagnostic pathology

Radiologically there is generalized enlargement of the heart, the ventricular chambers, the left being predominantly affected (WHO, 1965). The lungs often show peculiar clouding, enlargement of pulmonary veins, pulmonary oedema, and pleural effusions. Electrocardiographic features include: sinus rhythm with or without ventricular ectopic beats; various degrees of left bundle branch block; and left axis deviation. Angiocardiography generally reveals a dilated left ventricular cavity and atrioventricular incompetence. Blood culture is negative, while the transaminases and erythrocyte sedimentation rate are normal. Cardiac biopsy is being increasingly used in the diagnosis of obscure cardiomyopathies (Editorial, 1972).

Intracardiac post-operative thrombosis

This is an unusual condition which has been described by Letac *et al.* (1953) in Senegal. Massive recent mural thrombi are found more frequently in the right ventricle but also in the left, usually as a complication of surgical procedures. Organized lesions are described in the endocardium. The aetiology is unknown but is probably multifactorial. The writers state that this form of thrombosis may replace the venous thrombosis (which is rare in Senegal) of temperate climates as a postoperative complication.

(c) Idiopathic cardiomegaly occurring in late pregnancy and the puerperium

The term peri-partum cardiomyopathy has been suggested by Brigden (quoted by Hughes *et al.* 1970). Congestive cardiac failure may occur suddenly in the last few weeks of pregnancy or in the puerperium. Transitory hypertension is a not uncommon finding in the initial stages. Recovery is usual but the condition tends to recur in succeeding pregnancies. It is probably more common in the coloured races (Walsh *et al.* 1965) and it is not uncommon in Africa (Payet *et al.* 1961), and in Saudi Arabia (Perrine, 1967). The cause is unknown. Malnutrition, vitamin deficiencies, a form of toxaemia, hypersensitivity to drugs or trophoblastic tissue and viral infections have all been considered. Embolic phenomena are not unusual (Middleton, 1964).

The pathology of the heart is similar to that described in ICM but a pericardial effusion is unusual and focal areas of necrosis are found in the myocardium and may be associated with a cellular infiltrate of lymphocytes, histiocytes, and occasionally neutrophils and eosinophils—findings which are unusual in our experience in ICM. Ultrastructural studies have been reported by Sakakibara *et al.* (1970).

(d) Endocardial fibroelastosis

The endocardium consists of a number of layers. Beneath the endothelial cells is a layer of delicate collagen fibres superimposed on somewhat thicker collagen fibres strengthened by elastica and carrying lymphatic channels and blood vessels. Lastly there is a layer of smooth muscle. Patchy areas of fibroelastosis on the ventricular walls are found in many conditions and probably represent a reaction to stress. Fibrin is probably deposited from the blood stream with subsequent development of elastic fibrils (Dyson and Decker, 1958). There are, however, two well-recognized forms of endocardial fibroelastosis which occur in newborn and older children. The first is associated with congenital defects of the heart, especially those causing obstruction to the aortic outflow path, and appears to be secondary to them or to have occurred simultaneously during their development, as the condition has been seen in children dying shortly after birth (Forfar *et al.* 1964) and in stillbirths.

The second group shows well-marked endocardial thickening with no anatomical abnormality to account for it—so-called primary endocardial fibroelastosis. The aetiology is unknown but the mumps antigen skin test is positive in 100 per cent of cases.

Any chamber may be affected but the left ventricle is most frequently involved. The endocardium is covered with white fibrous tissue giving the 'sugar icing' effect. The valves may be involved in the process. The ventricles are usually enlarged but may be small. Histologically the endocardial thickening is composed of fibroelastic tissue.

The condition can be diagnosed clinically by (*a*) the appearance of congestive failure in the first 8 months of life (in the great majority of cases), (*b*) the absence of organic heart murmurs, (*c*) an abnormal increase in voltage of R in V6 and S in V1 or both together, and (*d*) a flat or inverted T wave in V6 (Sellers *et al.* 1964). Angiography shows an enlarged thick-walled left ventricle with absent or minimal changes in contour in systole or diastole and delay in emptying.

(e) Endomyocardial fibrosis

Endomyocardial fibrosis is a progressive heart disease characterized in the established condition by fibrosis in the inflow tract and the apex of one or both ventricles.

The disease has been seen in Uganda, Nigeria, Ghana, Tanzania, Kenya, and the Congo territories. It has also been reported from India, Sri Lanka, Malaya, and Colombia but is rare or absent within the hot and dry tropical areas of the Sudan and Mali, and the more temperate climate of Rhodesia. The disease has occasionally been observed in the United States, Britain (Brockington *et al.* 1967), and other countries. It is uncommon in Dakar (Payet *et al.* 1967). Workers at Kampala, found that in Uganda EMF was three times as common among the migrant Ruandra tribespeople as among the indigenous Baganda. The sexes are equally affected and the disease is most common in patients under 30 years of age.

Epidemiology

Although the clinical and pathological manifestations of the disease have been fully described, the natural history is little understood and the aetiology completely unknown. In fact, the concept of active disease in EMF has only recently been introduced (Parry and Abrahams, 1965) to complement the earlier classical descriptions of a static fibrotic process. Several hypotheses have been put forward to explain the aetiology of EMF. Farrer-Brown and Tarbit (1972) have found it difficult at times to delineate the spectrum of endomyocardial fibrosis.

Environmental factors

The striking geographical distribution of EMF has led to the belief that, like Burkitt's lymphoma, this disease is climatically determined—but whether this is due to humidity, rainfall, temperature, altitude, or other environmental factors is not clear.

Socio-economic factors

Most of the patients that have been studied belonged to the lower socio-economic groups. Such persons are prone to undernutrition as well as to increased exposure and susceptibility to bacterial and other infections. It is interesting to note in this respect however, that the disease has been met in sophisticated and well-fed expatriates resident in the tropics (Gray, 1951).

Filariasis

French workers (Gerbaux *et al.* 1957) have considered filarial heart disease an entity and the similarity in geographical distribution between *Loa loa* infection and EMF has led some workers to postulate an aetiological relationship between the two conditions (Ive *et al.* 1967). It is of interest that in European patients a considerable eosinophilia has usually been found (Brockington *et al.* 1967) and that EMF occurs in Kerala, India, where filariasis is present (WHO, 1967). It may be that EMF is a variant of the cardiopathy which occasionally complicates long-standing eosinophil leucocytosis including eosinophilic leukaemia (Brockington *et al.* 1970). Roberts *et al.* (1969) have reported extensive endomyocardial fibrosis with superimposed thrombi similar to that described in Löeffler's fibroblastic parietal endocarditis in two patients with eosinophilic hyperplasia of the bone marrow and spleen. Occasional thrombosed small arteries in the heart, spleen, kidneys and lungs were noted. It was thought that this might be a manifestation of a 'collagen disease' and its similarity to EMF was noted.

Dietetic factors

It has been noted in Uganda that the disease is commonly found in areas where plantains (*Musa* spp.) or root crops are used as a staple foodstuff, but does not occur with the same high frequency where cereals or relatively high protein diets are used. It has therefore been suggested that EMF may be analogous to carcinoid heart disease since plantain is the richest natural source of 5-hydroxytryptamine, and lesions similar to those of EMF have been experimentally produced in guinea-pigs fed on a plantain diet (McKinney and Crawford, 1965). It has recently been demonstrated from West Africa that in patients with EMF as well as other miscellaneous cardiopathies, 5-H.T. derived from a plantain meal, as well as endogenous 5-H.T., are not detoxicated or excreted as effectively as in normal, healthy subjects (Ojo and Parratt, 1966). It should be noted, however, that the pathology of EMF in no way resembles that described in the heart in the 'carcinoid' syndrome. It is also surprising that in Jamaica, where bananas are liberally consumed, EMF does not occur. On the existing evidence therefore, there seems little reason to associate EMF with increased dietary intake of 5-H.T.

Immunological factors

It has been suggested that EMF may be an unusual expression of the rheumatic process (Abrahams, 1959; Shaper, 1967). In Uganda, a high frequency of circulating heart antibodies is present in African patients with and without known cardiac disease, and there is some suggestion that the frequency of these antibodies is higher in patients with EMF. Moreover, presence of fibrin deposits shown by immunofluorescent techniques and high incidence of pericarditis in patients with endomyocardial fibrosis suggests a propensity to auto-immune reactivity (van der Geld *et al.* 1966; Shaper *et al.* 1967).

Other considerations

Adi (1963) reported from Nigeria right-sided EMF occurring in two brothers. Patel *et al.* (1971) have also described nine cases occurring in four families in Uganda—five of which had also the tropical splenomegaly syndrome. Although the authors state that genetic factors may be operative in the aetiology the writers consider that environmental factors and an altered immunological status of the host are by far the most important factors in the majority of patients. Experiments on rats have shown that a comparatively brief period of treatment with certain corticoids plus sodium salts produced myocardial necroses which tended to heal by the formation of thick scar tissue, producing a condition resembling EMF. In rats in which these subendocardial necroses were prevented by the prophylactic administration of magnesium chloride, the secondary fibrosis did not develop (Selye, 1958); Miller *et al.* (1963) produced significant endomyocardial pathology in dogs following chronic impairment of cardiac lymphatic drainage.

It is difficult to draw any single conclusion on the aetiology of EMF; present evidence, however, favours an infective and/or immunological basis for the disease.

Pathology

Macroscopic

The condition, often of severe degree, may be found as an incidental feature at necropsy in patients dying from some unrelated cause and not exhibiting, or perhaps it would be more accurate to say not complaining of, symptoms related to cardiac disease.

A pericardial effusion, frequently large, may be present. Cardiac enlargement is found in 50 per cent of subjects, in the remaining 40 per cent the heart is normal or small and contracted, and heart weights varying from 120 g to over 600 g have been recorded.

Any or all chambers of the heart may exhibit endocardial lesions but the most marked changes are found in one or both ventricles, usually said to be more extensive in the left, but in our experience being equally frequent in the right. In right-sided EMF a characteristic external malformation of the heart is produced. The right atrium is enormously dilated and hypertrophied, with a marked sulcus between the apices of the ventricles and, in addition, there is dilatation of the conus and infundibulum. These findings have been well described by Davies in East Africa (1948, 1956). Internally in the heart there is no valvulitis and the pulmonary and aortic valves are in all instances normal, unless a superimposed bacterial endocarditis or rheumatic carditis is present.

There is gross fibrous thickening of the endocardium of the inflow tract in either or both ventricles usually most marked at the apex and frequently extending up the posterior wall behind the posterior cusps of the atrioventricular valves. The papillary muscles are embedded in the fibrous tissue, which extends to the chordae tendinae causing shortening with distortion of the valvular cusps which in themselves usually appear normal (Figs. 8.1 and 8.2).

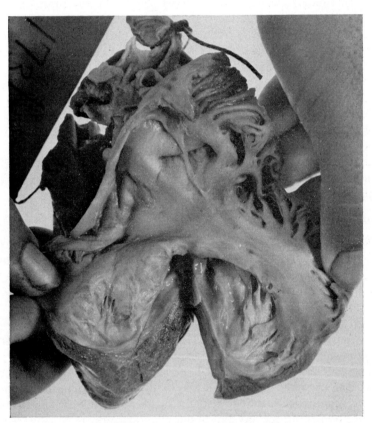

FIG. 8.1. Right-sided endomyocardial fibrosis, showing gross hypertrophy and dilatation of the right atrium. The ventricular cavity is reduced to about one-third of its normal size and the cusps of the grossly dilated tricuspid valve are bound down to the endocardial fibrotic process.

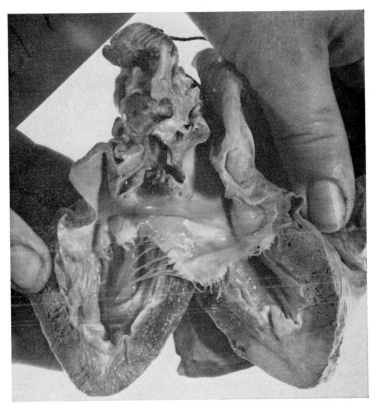

FIG. 8.2. Left-sided endomyocardial fibrosis. Note the fibrous tissue penetrating into the apical myocardium. The mitral valve is normal.

We have seen, in a few instances, a fibrous plaque in the endocardium posteriorly to, and to which may be adherent, the posterior cusp of the mitral and the inferior cusp of the tricuspid valve in the absence of or presence of minimal fibrosis of the endocardium at the apex of the left or right ventricles. Even in advanced cases in the left ventricle the endocardial fibrosis extends for only a short distance up the septal wall and terminates in a thick, rolled edge—the inferior surface often being roughened, concave, and greenish in colour, suggestive of recent thrombus formation. This lesion we have never seen in the right ventricle.

The most severe lesions are seen in the right ventricle and two-thirds of its cavity may be obliterated by fusion of the opposing walls due to fibrosis extending from the apex, leaving only a saucer-shaped depression lined by pearly-white fibrous tissue from which the affected papillary muscles stand out rigidly, as Davies states, as 'marble pillars'. The chordae tendineae are grossly shortened and the tricuspid valve is finally represented as a dilated, rigid, non-functioning ring. Occasionally in the right ventricle fusion of the opposing walls may take place some distance above the apex, leaving a small endocardial lined crypt at the apex.

Lesions are present in the atria in about 60 per cent of cases and depend upon the severity of the ventricular lesions, the most usual being patchy sclerosis associated with ante-mortem thrombi in the appendages.

When the right ventricle is severely affected the right atrium is enormously dilated and hypertrophied, showing prominent trabeculation and patchy endocardial sclerosis frequently associated with a massive 'ball thrombus' —indeed the thrombotic process may extend into the superior vena cava and large tributary veins of the head and neck.

From the thickened endocardium of the apex and inflow tract, tongues of white fibrous tissue may be seen penetrating the inner third of the myocardium of the ventricles and, in some instances, thinning of the myocardium at the apex of the left ventricle is a noticeable feature. Ante-mortem thrombi are not uncommonly seen superimposed on the ventricular as well as on the atrial lesions.

Although the lesions of EMF are predominantly those of the inflow tract, it is not unusual to find the endocardium of the outflow tract slightly thickened and in these cases a mild fibroelastosis is noted on histological examination—the changes in the outflow path being thought to be due to a compensatory mechanism.

Histological findings

The pericardium may or may not show evidence of a recent pericarditis, and a mild lymphocytic infiltration of the epicardium is not unusual.

On the luminal surface of the ventricles there is usually a layer of fibrin or an ante-mortem thrombus superimposed on dense hyalinized avascular tissue in which areas of calcification are inconstantly present. This layer merges with a layer of granulation tissue containing loose collagen fibres, dilated blood vessels and a mild infiltrate of chronic inflammatory cells. Granules of haemosiderin may be present. In other areas the hyalinized collagen merges with the subendocardial myofibrils.

Elastic tissue may be present in the superficial layers of the collagen and in its depths at the site of the obliterated endocardium, but it never resembles in extent or uniformity the picture of fibroelastosis.

Tongues of fibrous tissue extend within the inner third of the myocardium. The papillary muscles and trabeculae carneae are embedded in avascular fibrous tissue. The central vessel of the papillary muscle is usually thickened, the muscle fibres are degenerate, areas of myocytolysis may be present and there is elastosis in the area of the obliterated endocardium. In the fibrous tissue between the trabeculae and papillary muscles thin-walled blood vessels suggestive of recanalization are present and, rarely show small mural fibrin thrombi. In the depths of the lesion large, thin-walled vascular channels, presumably Thebesian veins, are also seen, and may contain fibrin or ante-mortem thrombi.

Associated with the endocardial sclerosis is subendocardial fibrosis and degeneration and necrosis of the muscle fibres of the inner third of the myocardium.

The endocardium of the outflow tract usually shows a mild fibroelastosis.

The most marked changes in the myocardium occur in the inner third of the ventricular wall, but, in our experience, may be diffuse and extensive. The myofibrils vary in size, are granular and vacuolated giving a 'moth-eaten' appearance. Cross-striations persist. An excess of perinuclear lipochrome pigment is not unusual. The nuclei are enlarged, exhibit bizarre forms, and are frequently vacuolated. Areas of myocytolysis may be present (Fig. 8.3). Patchy fibrosis in the myocardium may occur—the fibrous scars containing a scanty cellular infiltrate with muscle pigment lying free or within macrophages. The yellow brown pigment can be readily differentiated from haemosiderin in that it is negative with Perl's stain and stains

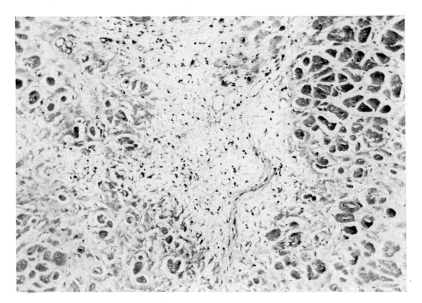

FIG. 8.3. Endomyocardial fibrosis. Myocytolysis. Note the acellular central 'falling out' necrosis. The sarcolemmal sheaths of the myofibrils can still be distinguished (H and E × 180).

positively with a periodic acid Schiff technique. The fibrosis is not usually perivascular in situation.

The interstitial tissue is oedematous. There is no valvulitis unless a concomitant rheumatic carditis is present. Isolated lesions of the tricuspid and mitral valves do, however, occur but the posterior cusp of the mitral valve is most frequently affected. A pad of loose areolar fibrous tissue is present on the inferior surface of the cusp and the subjacent endocardium is thickened and fibrous. Lesions with central fibrinoid change have been noted in the endocardium with this type of valvular involvement. The cusp may be completely bound down to the endocardium by dense fibrous tissue. These valvular lesions may occur with minimal endocardial involvement elsewhere in the ventricles. Myocardial changes are, however, present.

The larger coronary vessels are normal but medial hypertrophy and endarteritis may be seen in smaller vessels in the affected subendocardial regions and papillary muscles.

There is an absence of cellular infiltration, haemorrhage, or frank necrosis, unless there is an associated terminal illness. Aschoff nodes are not seen unless there is a concomitant rheumatic carditis. Neither amyloid, fatty, nor glycogen infiltration has been reported. Microfilariae have been noted very occasionally in the myocardium in Nigeria (Fig. 8.4).

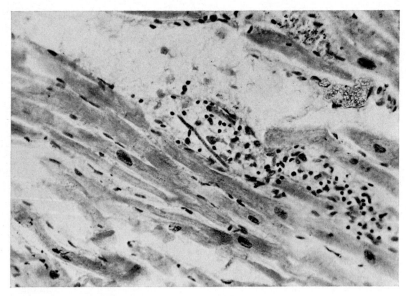

FIG. 8.4. Endomyocardial fibrosis. A microfilaria in heart muscle with surrounding cellular reaction in endomyocardial fibrosis (H and E × 180).

Other organs

Embolic phenomena are not common but do occur. We have seen one young woman with unsuspected EMF (which is a not unusual finding at necropsy) who was admitted *in extremis* and on post-mortem examination was found to have a saddle embolus at the bifurcation of the aorta. There was the roughened, concave, greenish-brown lesion present on the lower third of the septal left ventricular wall suggestive of a recent thrombus, which has already been described. Rarely, cardiac emboli may affect other branches of the aorta.

Splenic and rarely renal infarcts can occur but pulmonary emboli are not uncommon.

If the heart lesion is the cause of death (excluding embolism) chronic venous congestion is invariably present in the other organs. In right-sided EMF the liver is severely affected and clinically the patient may present with massive ascites in the absence of peripheral oedema, high venous pressure, stunting of growth, and early finger-clubbing. Arterial oxygen desaturation is sometimes present. Liver biopsies in these patients have revealed severe central congestion leading to central fibrosis and even cardiac cirrhosis. The reason for the oxygen desaturation is not clear, but is related to the post-sinusoidal portal hypertension. A shunt between the azygos and pulmonary veins has been suggested (Abrahams and Parry, 1963). Similar oxygen desaturation of the arterial blood occurs in cirrhosis of the liver and in the pipe-stem fibrosis seen in schistosomiasis. Osunkoya *et al.* (1972) have described small granulomata in the liver in a high proportion of patients dying at EMF and also noted that cirrhosis was more frequent than in rheumatic heart disease subjects similarly studied.

Diagnostic pathology

Electrocardiographic abnormalities are present but have no constant or specific features. Extrasystoles are not uncommon, but other arrhythmias are rare. Cardiac catheterization in advanced or moderately severe disease reveals, as expected, disordered function, and the presence of pulmonary hypertension. Angiography is useful, especially in patients with left-sided EMF (Cockshott, 1965). Antistreptolysin-O titres are raised in many of the patients. Serum transaminase is normal in the established case.

(f) Congenital heart disease

The incidence and distribution of congenital heart disease in the tropics are, in general, no different from those of the temperate zones (Muir, 1960; Watler, 1960; Schrire, 1964). Wallooppillai and Jaysinghe (1970), however, have analysed 555 cases of congenital heart disease in Sri Lanka.

Coarctation of the aorta and aortic stenosis were rare when compared with figures from other parts of the world.

(g) Annular subvalvular left-ventricular aneurysm

Annular subvalvular left ventricular aneurysms are aneurysms of unknown aetiology which occur almost exclusively in the Negro race. They may be single or multiple and communicate with the ventricular cavity below the fibrous ring of the aortic or mitral valves. They extend into the ventricular wall including the septum usually in a circular fashion and may track superiorly within the wall of the left atrium producing an aneurysmal dilatation within the cavity. There is an absence of coronary artery disease.

Epidemiology

These aneurysms have been reported most frequently in Africa but have also been noted in France, the United States, the West Indies, and the British Isles. Where the race has been stated the patients have, with two exceptions (Pocock *et al.* 1965), been Negro. The sex incidence is probably equal (Abrahams *et al.* 1962) and the age range is from 6 to 45 years.

The usual cause of cardiac aneurysms in temperate climates is coronary artery disease but this has been excluded as an aetiological agent in these patients by post-mortem and coronary artery injection studies (Edington and Williams, 1968). In addition it would be most unusual for coronary artery disease to cause aneurysms at the base of the heart. Rheumatism, dyscollaginosis, syphilis, and trauma can be dismissed on clinical and pathological grounds as possible causative agents. Tuberculosis has been an associated finding in a number of patients and amyloidosis has been described in only one subject. These findings are considered fortuitous and there is no valid pathological evidence to incriminate tuberculosis in the aetiology of these aneurysms. In the Congo, however, tuberculous left-ventricular aneurysms with characteristic histopathological changes have been described and would appear to be a separate entity (Beheyt and Vandepitte, 1958). No evidence suggestive of a systemic disease process has been found in other organs nor have parasites been incriminated.

It is more difficult to exclude the possibility of a low-grade localized infective process in the heart being responsible for the lesions. Blood cultures have, however, been consistently negative in all patients so far investigated and such lesions have not been described in other races in the pre-antibiotic era. It has been suggested that these aneurysms originate as 'herniae' through a congenital weakness in the ventricular wall in the region of the atrio-ventricular groove (Robertson and Jackson, 1960). In the light of present knowledge this would appear to be the most acceptable explanation of the racial factor and constant site of these aneurysms. Macleod *et al.* (1970) have reported an aneurysm arising from the posterior wall of the left atrium just above the mitral valve in an American Negro female aged 10 years. It was successfully operated upon and was thought to be congenital in origin.

Pathogenesis

The aneurysms may be unsuspected and be found incidentally at necropsy, or patients may present with aortic or mitral incompetence. There are no diagnostic auscultatory sounds but systolic clicks and late systolic murmurs at the mitral area in the presence of electrocardiographic abnormalities are suspicious findings. The presence of a subaortic aneurysms should be suspected in a patient with aortic incompetence and negative serological tests for syphilis (Pocock *et al.* 1965). The macroscopic appearances of the heart depend upon the site and size of the aneurysm or aneurysms. Aneurysms occurring below the aortic valve and posterior cusp of the mitral are usually small with relatively little anatomical distortion, whereas those below the anterior cusp of the mitral may enlarge laterally, anteriorly, and superiorly, distorting the surface of the left ventricle and compressing the left atrium (Fig. 8.5). A chronic pericarditis is usual over the surface of the aneurysm. Occasionally the aneurysms may track upwards between the endocardium and left atrial muscle, producing a cystic swelling in the atrial cavity (Edington and Williams, 1968). A fistulous opening between a ventricular aneurysm and the left atrium has been described (Chisler *et al.* 1965). The orifices vary in size from a few millimetres to 2 cm and are surrounded by dense, white, fibrous tissue on the endocardial surface of the left ventricle and are situated a little below the atrio-ventricular fibrous ring. The valve cusp adjacent to the orifice may be thickened and fibrous but the unassociated valves are normal. There is usually associated hypertrophy of the left atrium and ventricle due to either mitral or aortic incompetence. The right side of the heart is usually normal although some obstruction to the pulmonary outflow path by a septal aneurysm is theoretically possible (Figs. 8.6 and 8.7).

Associated rheumatic carditis, EMF, tuberculosis, subacute bacterial endocarditis, and chronic interstitial myocarditis have been noted in a few patients and have been considered fortuitous findings.

Angiographic and autopsy injection studies have shown that the coronary arteries are normal. Large submitral aneurysms may stretch and thin the circumflex branch of the left coronary artery. Thrombosis of this branch has been reported in only one instance.

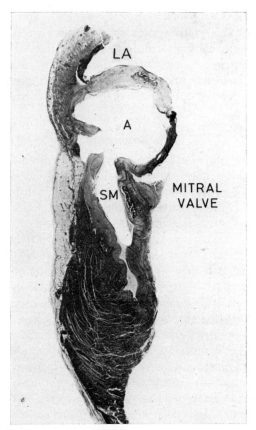

FIG. 8.5. Subvalvular left ventricular aneurysms. A section of the left atrium and ventricle, showing a submitral aneurysm (SM) with extension into the left atrium (LA). Note the atrial aneurysm lies between the endocardium and the myocardium.

Histological examination

The findings are non-specific. The endocardium around the orifice shows fibrous thickening with some thickening of the original elastic layer, which continues for a short distance into the lining of the aneurysmal cavity where it merges with the fibrous tissue of the wall of the aneurysm. Calcification and even heterotopic bone containing marrow elements may be found in this area or in the wall of this aneurysm. The wall itself consists of laminated thrombus or fibrin deposits superimposed on avascular fibrous tissue containing a variable number of chronic inflammatory cells and haemosiderin deposits, dense collagen, and compressed muscle fibres. In areas vascular granulation tissue and lymphocytic and plasma-cell infiltrates may

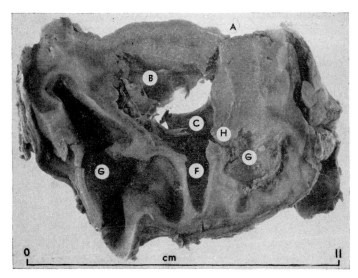

FIG. 8.6. Sub left ventricular aneurysms. Transverse section of the left ventricle viewed from below, showing how the loculated aneurysms circumscribe the mitral valve. A: original section of left ventricular wall made at necropsy; B: anterior cusp of mitral valve; C: posterior cusp of mitral valve; F: ostium below posterior cusp of mitral valve; G: aneurysm; H: ostium below posterior cusp of initial valve closed surgically. (*By courtesy of the Quarterly Journal of Medicine.*)

be noted. Obliterative endarteritis of the smaller vessels in the wall is usual. The fibrosis and muscle changes may be present for some distance from the aneurysm and, in areas, the wall of the myocardium may be replaced by the fibrotic aneurysmal wall. An overlying chronic pericarditis is usual in these cases.

The findings in the myocardium remote from the aneurysm are those of hypertrophy and there may be non-specific ischaemic changes. A chronic interstitial myocarditis has occasionally been noted but stigmata of rheumatic heart disease or other specific conditions have not been seen.

Other organs

If congestive cardiac failure has been precipitated the changes of chronic venous congestion will be present in the other organs. No specific changes have been noted in any organ but embolic lesions occur. Infarctive cortical scarring is not unusual in the kidney and care must be taken to distinguish these lesions from chronic pyelonephritis, which has been not uncommonly reported in these patients.

Diagnostic pathology

Radiologically a submitral aneurysm may give a characteristic bulge on the left border of the heart and angiography may show paradoxical systolic expansion of the aneurysm.

The electrocardiographic findings are non-specific but will differentiate an aneurysm due to coronary artery disease.

The changes in the blood are not helpful and blood culture is negative.

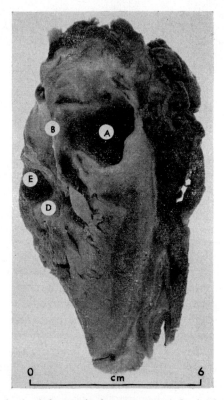

FIG. 8.7. Subvalvular left ventricular aneurysms. Sagittal section through the left ventricle, showing two aneurysms. A: anterior submitral aneurysm; B: anterior mitral cusp; D: thickened endocardium; E: posterior submitral aneurysm. (*By courtesy of the Quarterly Journal of Medicine.*)

II. SECONDARY MYOCARDIAL DISEASE

Only those conditions which are specially applicable to students in the tropics are considered in any detail below.

A. MYOCARDITIS

(i) Viral myocarditis

The term myocarditis is used when active inflammation is proven in the heart which is not due to the so-called 'collagen' diseases or other well-known entities. It may occur in viral, bacterial, or parasitic infections or be caused by toxins and drugs (Gore and Saphir, 1947). In many instances no detectable cause may be found and these have been termed 'isolated' or Fiedler-type myocarditis. In the last-named type, however, giant cells may be found.

Many of these cases of isolated myocarditis are no doubt due to viral infections and, with improving laboratory facilities, the aetiologic agent should be recovered in more and more patients. Viral disease is common in the tropics and our knowledge is constantly expanding. Not long ago poliomyelitis was considered rare in West Africa whereas it is now known to be extremely common and, until prophylactic inoculation was introduced, was the greatest cause of death in unprotected immigrants once the dangers of malaria and yellow fever had been overcome. The Coxsackie-B virus is common and may affect the heart of the neonate (Javett et al. 1956). Bornholm disease (epidemic pleurodynia) is also seen. Outbreaks of influenza can occur. The subject has recently been reviewed by Burch and Giles (1972).

The heart resembles macroscopically that seen in idiopathic cardiomegaly but histologically there is widespread interstitial infiltration by eosinophils, monocytes, histiocytes, and plasma cells.

(ii) Giant-cell myocarditis

This is probably a distinct form of heart disease (Hudson, 1965) but other conditions causing giant-cell granulomatous lesions must be excluded (tuberculosis, sarcoid, syphilis, and fungal diseases). It occurs in young and middle-aged adults and the sexes are equally affected. It has been noted in association with tuberculosis and syphilis and a viral or allergic aetiology has been suggested.

The heart is enlarged and yellowish streaking may be noted in the myocardium of the ventricles. Histologically the lesion consists of Langhans or foreign-body-type giant cells in an infiltrate of lymphocytes, plasma cells, and eosinophils. The giant cells may resemble multinucleated myocardial cells and transition forms may be seen.

(iii) Rheumatic heart disease

Until recently, rheumatic heart disease was thought to be rare in the tropics. It is now a well-recognized entity and an important cause of illness in many tropical areas, and in India it is the main cardiac problem (Garcia-Palmieri, 1962; Beet, 1956; Muir, 1958; Rosenblatt and Stokes, 1963; Back and de Pass, 1957; Payet and Pene, 1955; Rahman et al. 1953; Sujoy et al.

1963). It is of interest that a high prevalence of elevated antistreptolysin-O titres has been found in most tropical and subtropical countries (Strasser and Ratta, 1973).

It has been stated, however, that it may differ somewhat in its clinical presentation, chorea and severe acute rheumatic fever being infrequently seen. There is no doubt that classical rheumatic endocarditis with mitral stenosis occurs, the fibrotic manifestations in the valves extending down the chordae tendineae being in marked contrast to the apical fibrosis with extension up the inflow tract seen in endomyocardial fibrosis. The relationship between the two conditions is discussed on p. 358.

(iv) Bacterial endocarditis

Both the acute and subacute varieties occur and do not differ in their pathology from the well-described forms in the Western hemisphere.

(v) Diphtheritic myocarditis

Contrary to some reports, diphtheria as shown by Schick testing is common in many tropical areas although clinically it is thought to be rare. Diphtheritic lesions of the skin (veldt sore, p. 728) are known to occur and may be aetiological agents in the Schick reaction and diphtheritic myocarditis. If the heart is affected it is dilated, pale, and flabby, and yellow streaking may be present in the myocardium. The myofibrils show hyaline, granular and perhaps fatty change. An infiltrate of histiocytes, plasma cells, and lymphocytes may be present in the stroma, and polymorphonuclear leucocytes and eosinophils have also been described. Scarring may result and probably accounts for the conduction defects seen clinically. The SGOT activity is raised in patients with evidence of myocarditis.

(vi) Tuberculous and syphilitic myocarditis

The heart may be involved in miliary tuberculosis and occasionally a tuberculoma occurs. In syphilis a gumma is occasionally seen but the heart is most frequently affected secondarily to aortic disease with valvular involvement.

(vii) Parasitic myocarditis

There are numerous parasites which affect the heart in the tropics, by far the most important being *Trypanosoma cruzi*. In our experience, however, in West Africa, where Chagas' disease does not occur, parasitic myocarditis has not presented itself directly as a problem of any magnitude. The part that parasites may play indirectly, however, in such conditions as idiopathic cardiomegaly or EMF has still to be assessed. The effect of individual parasites on the heart is considered when their pathology is described elsewhere in the text.

(viii) **Loeffler's disease**

(**Synonym.** Fibroblastic parietal endocarditis).

Loeffler's disease is a condition which causes progressive congestive heart failure. There is an associated eosinophilia and embolic episodes are common. The endocardium is fibrotic in areas and mural thrombosis is usual.

Epidemiology

Loeffler's disease occurs predominantly in middle-aged males. It has been described most frequently in Europe and occasional cases have been seen in Africa. The cause of the disease is unknown and, although parasites have not been excluded, there is little evidence that they may be incriminated in the aetiology (Weiss-Carmine, 1957). Lennox (1948) has suggested that it is a disease of altered sensitivity due to some as yet unidentified allergen.

Pathology

In the acute stage no macroscopic abnormalities are present in the heart. Microscopically there may be an eosinophilic arteritis with an associated eosinophilic interstitial myocarditis. There may also be evidence of a generalized vascular condition affecting many organs, including the central nervous system, in a number of patients (Davies and Coles, 1960). In the more chronic stages the heart is enlarged and hypertrophied. There is greyish-white fibrosis and scarring of the endocardium of the inflow and occasionally the outflow tracts of one or both ventricles, the left being almost always involved. The papillary muscles and chordae tendineae may be affected, with mitral incompetence the usual complication. Vegetations may occasionally be present on the valves themselves. Mural thrombi are usual. In the myocardium the inner third is maximally involved. Histologically there is fibrous thickening of the affected endocardium with variable amounts of elastic tissue present, and superimposed thrombi may be attached. Vascular granulation tissue underlies the thrombi and haemosiderin may be present. The fibrosis may affect the inner third or even more of the myocardium. Patchy fibrous scars may be present. The myofibrils are hypertrophied and may undergo basophilic degeneration. The Thebesian veins are dilated and their walls thickened. The smaller coronary arteries show endarteritis and degenerative changes. Focal collections of inflammatory cells (lymphocytes, plasma cells, and eosinophils) are usually present in the endocardium and interstitial tissue.

Other organs

Infarctive lesions are common in the lungs, spleen, and kidney. Vascular changes may be found in any of the viscera. An eosinophilic pneumonia has been described in the lung (Brink and Webber, 1963) and eosinophils may be prominent in the spleen and lymph nodes.

(ix) **Toxic myocarditis**

Clinically unexplained cardiac failure is not uncommon in the tropics and toxic substances must always be considered in their aetiology. The difficulty experienced in obtaining an accurate history, the peripatetic habits of many of the patients and the frequent use of native medicines often render an accurate diagnosis impossible. Possible toxic agents can be classified as follows:

(1) Drugs, including native medicines.
(2) Dietary.
(3) Poisons.
(4) Venoms. These are considered when the poisonous snakes are described (p. 725).

Drugs

Many drugs used in the therapy of tropical diseases have serious effects on the heart and we have experience of death occurring especially in patients undergoing emetine (Brem and Konwaler, 1955) and antimony (Chien Ten and Liu, 1957) therapy. Arsenic (Edge, 1946), the sulphonamides (More et al. 1946), antibiotics (Haden and Langsjoen, 1961), and smallpox vaccine (Finlay Jones, 1964) can also cause adverse cardiac complications. Native medicines are usually considered hepatotoxic agents and have not been, as yet, implicated as causative agents in cardiac disease.

Dietary

The contamination of wheat in South Africa by the seeds of *Argemone mexicana* caused a small outbreak of a cardiomyopathy syndrome. These poppy seeds contain a toxic principle which affects the heart and has been responsible for epidemic dropsy in India (Brink et al. 1965). A number of plants in South Africa may affect primarily the heart of sheep and cattle, with myocytolysis and fibrosis occurring (Watt and Breyer-Brandewijk, 1962).

Poisons

Carbon monoxide poisoning may occur in huts heated by braziers in the cold season in areas of the tropics, and cardiac damage may be one of the complications. Poison on arrows may contain toxic saponins but strophanthus is the main ingredient in West Africa (Degroote, 1960).

B. COR PULMONALE

The term implies hypertrophy of the right ventricle with or without associated cardiac failure, and pulmonary hypertension is the common factor in its aetiology. Many factors are, however, concerned in the production of pulmonary hypertension and the term cor pulmonale is usually reserved for pulmonary hypertension caused by disorders originating in the lung. If at post mortem both ventricles are hypertrophied and there is no evidence of cardiac disease (mitral stenosis, congenital defect, or pulmonic stenosis) cor pulmonale is usually considered to be present if the weight of the right ventricle is greater than 50 per cent that of the left.

The factors that are concerned in pulmonary hypertension are complex and are listed below:

(1) Chronic lung disease (emphysema, chronic bronchitis, bronchiectasis, fibrocystic disease, tuberculosis, pneumoconiosis, sarcoidosis, idiopathic pulmonary fibrosis (Hamman–Rich), 'the collagen diseases' pulmonary carcinomatosis and berylliosis) causes hypoventilation and a rise in the alveolar carbon dioxide content. This is considered to produce the additional factor of vascular spasm of the pulmonary arterioles.

(2) Reduction in the pulmonary vascular bed by obliteration of the pulmonary arterioles by micro-emboli or other disease processes (sickle-cell disease, schistosomiasis, scleroderma, amyloidosis, arteritis (including syphilis), or tumour emboli). Atherosclerosis of the larger pulmonary arteries is common after the age of 40 years in Western communities. Its degree is independent of coronary or aortic atherosclerosis. Pulmonary hypertension accelerates the process and, in our experience in tropical areas, severe pulmonary atherosclerosis is secondary to pulmonary hypertension and is not an aetiological factor in the condition.

(3) An increased blood flow in the pulmonary arterial circulation due to vascular shunts between the left and right side of the heart which is especially common in congenital defects. With increasing pulmonary hypertension the flow may be reversed from right to left and, with resulting cyanosis, is regarded as a grave prognostic sign. Such conditions are ventricular septal defect, patent ductus arteriosus, aortic septal defect and atrial septal defect.

(4) Increased pulmonary capillary resistance with associated chronic venous congestion and haemosiderosis in the lungs, such as is seen in left heart failure due to mitral stenosis, pulmonary venous obstruction due to various causes and myxoma of the left atrium.

(5) Restriction of respiratory movements and compression of vessels which may occur in kyphoscolosis.

(6) Increased blood viscosity which occurs with polycythaemia vera or from O_2 unsaturation of the arterial blood as is seen, *par excellence*, in mountain sickness.

(7) Idiopathic pulmonary hypertension. This occurs most commonly in young adults with females being more frequently affected (Wade and Ball, 1957; Sleeper *et al.* 1962). The aetiology is unknown but genetic factors, spasm of the pulmonary arterioles and amniotic fluid embolism in pregnancy have been considered possible aetiological agents by various authors. The smaller pulmonary arterioles (less than 100 μm) are thin-walled structures consisting of an endothelial lining and a thin elastic lamina. In idiopathic pulmonary hypertension, muscular hypertrophy, damage to the elastica, necrosis, and thrombosis in these smaller arterioles occur. Fibrinoid necrosis

and arteriolitis may also be seen. Plexiform and angiomatoid lesions described in the lungs in schistosomiasis may also be present and also occur in secondary pulmonary hypertension from other causes.

Statistics regarding the incidence of cor pulmonale and pulmonary hypertension are difficult to compile in temperate climates and are almost non-existent in developing countries. A high incidence of cor pulmonale has been noted in Delhi in an entirely non-industrial population (Padmavati and Pathank, 1959). Men were only slightly more affected than women and there was a preponderance of rural over urban cases. The patients were comparatively young. Untreated chronic respiratory infections owing to poverty and lack of medical care were considered the underlying factors. Mitral stenosis is also a potent cause of pulmonary hypertension in India. Emphysema has been reported to be probably as common in Thailand and the West Indies as in Europe (Hayes and Summerell, 1963) and cor pulmonale is not uncommon. Diffuse fibrosis of the lung, the Hamann–Rich syndrome, also accounted for cor pulmonale in the West Indies (Hayes and Richards, 1964).

It is our impression that pulmonary hypertension is common in post-mortem material in West Africa and is not uncommon in East Africa (Turner, 1962). Recently a condition termed pulmonary veno-occlusive disease has been described with internal thickening and fibrosis of the pulmonary veins. The evidence suggests that the venous obstruction is thrombotic in origin. Virus infections may be important in the aetiology (Editorial, 1972).

Asthma is certainly common but little is known about its aetiology. Parasites in childhood and fungal spores in humid climates are possible aetiological agents in the adult. Bronchiectasis and tuberculosis are common. The part that sickle-cell disease and schistosomiasis play in the aetiology of cor pulmonale is discussed on pp. 441 and 175.

C. HYPERTENSIVE HEART DISEASE

It has been stated that essential hypertension is rare in developing countries, and that in some populations, e.g. Melanesians and Polynesians in Oceania, there is no increase of mean blood pressure with age during adult life (Lowenstein, 1961; Maddocks and Vines, 1966). There is no doubt, however, that in many parts of the tropics essential hypertension is common and often severe (Colbourne et al. 1950; Abrahams et al. 1960, Miall et al. 1962; Padmatavi, 1962; Imperial and Felarca 1963; Fodor et al. 1964; Sacks, 1959). Shue (1964) showed that hypertension was more common in the South African Bantu than in Coloureds or whites in Cape Town in spite of the fact that aortic and coronary atherosclerosis was much less common. Moreover, although coronary artery disease mortality was lower in the Bantu than in the white population, mortality from cerebral catastrophies was as high, if not higher, in the former group. It is our experience in West Africa that essential hypertension is common and, in necropsy material, is associated with cerebral atherosclerosis in relatively young age groups, the relative absence of coronary and aortic atherosclerosis being remarkable. Sterling (1960) has shown that there is evidence of hypertension in 31 per cent of adult Jamaicans coming to necropsy and that essential hypertension is more common than renal. It is unlikely that these findings will be uniform throughout all areas of the tropics and further geographical studies are indicated. Secondary hypertension due to renal disease is also common in the tropics.

D. ATHEROSCLEROSIS AND CORONARY ARTERY DISEASE

In contrast to the findings in hypertensive heart disease, necropsy studies (Florentin *et al.* 1963; Goodale *et al.* 1964; Lee *et al.* 1964) have shown a low incidence of atherosclerosis in East and West Africans and Koreans when compared with U.S. white and non-white populations. Coronary artery disease has also been shown to be low in many parts of Africa (Payet *et al.* 1960; Wainwright, 1961; Shee, 1963; Walker, 1963) and there is a virtual absence of acute clinical episodes. Coronary artery disease is also found in low incidence in Japan, Thailand, and China. Japanese living in America show a higher incidence than that recorded in the population of Japan. The situation in India is variable, a relatively high incidence being reported from the Punjab (Wig *et al.* 1962) and Madras (Subramanian and Kulangra, 1967) and a low incidence in Agra. Indeed, in the Pubjab the prevalence rates in men and women were similar to the rates found in Michigan, U.S.A. (Sarvotham and Berry, 1968). It is of interest that in northern India the intake of animal fat is much greater than that found in southern India (Malhotra, 1967). Muslims and Parsees are said to be more affected than Hindus. The incidence of coronary artery disease is high in Indians living in South Africa. In Israel it is more common in Jews born in Europe and America than in those born in Asia and North Africa.

South African workers (Anderson *et al.* 1959) have compared the degree and chemical content of atherosclerosis of the aorta in the South African Bantu and white populations. Atherosclerosis was significantly less in the Bantu and there were differences in the ash, calcium, and cholesterol concentrations. It would appear, therefore, that environmental factors rather than racial or genetic are concerned in this differing incidence and that probably a low intake of animal fat might be important in the low incidence of atherosclerosis and coronary artery disease. This, however, is not borne out by the studies of Mann *et al.* (1965) in the Masai of Tanzania whose diet is rich in animal products and dairy fat and who are almost free from coronary artery disease. They are, however, an exceptionally fit and athletic people. It has also been suggested that the gall bladder bile of the Masai has an enormous reserve capacity to dissolve cholesterol and that this system protects them from cholesterol gallstone formation (Editorial, 1971). Similarly the Somalis, whose diet consists largely of camel's milk containing an excess of saturated fatty acids, also rarely suffer from myocardial infarction. Essential hypertension is not rare in these populations and it should be noted that their serum cholesterol values are low. This is, however, probably the one parameter that is most often directly proportional to the incidence of atherosclerosis and coronary artery disease in population groups. The pattern of atherosclerosis in the African living in Nigeria has been described by Williams (1969).

Trace elements in soil are now receiving considerable attention (WHO, 1972). Lower tissue chromium has been reported in coronary-prone populations which may be due to an excessive consumption of refined foodstuffs, especially sugars, which lack chromium and enhance its urinary excretion. Raw sugars contain chromium. There may be a positive correlation between cadmium content of the kidney and hypertension. Nickel and manganese have been found to be raised in the serum in ischaemic heart disease. Zinc, manganese and vanadium may have beneficial effects on lipid metabolism and atherosclerosis, whereas copper may have an atherogenic effect as it is a lipid peroxidation catalyst and serum levels may be high in patients with infarction. Intensive international studies are being undertaken at present on these and related possible aetiological factors.

Other factors, rather than dietary, may, however, be involved in the rarity of coronary artery disease in tropical populations. There is some evidence to show that there may be increased fibrinolytic activity in the blood of Africans which might inhibit thrombus formation in coronary arteries (Merskey et al. 1960). There may be more frequent anastomoses between left and right coronary arteries which might militate against sudden infarctive lesions (Pepler and Meyer, 1960; Ferguson et al. 1970). Lagundoye et al. (1973), however, in 147 unselected necropsies in Ibadan noted that the frequency of the so-called third primary division of the coronary artery was very much less than that reported in the South African Bantu and that in only 8 subjects was atherosclerotic disease noted by post-mortem angiography and this was of the mildest degree. The part that multiple infestations play, with parasites constantly present in the peripheral blood, on thrombus formation has never been assessed. There is little information available on platelet function in tropical areas and in view of their importance in thrombosis and serotonin metabolism they are worthy of further study. Essien (1973) has shown that the normal platelet count in the lower socio-economic groups in Nigeria is very much lower than that regarded as normal in temperate zones. The platelets present may also have a different functional ability as has been noted by Retief and Vandenplas (1970) in the healthy Bantu when compared with the white South African—notably decreased early *in vivo* adhesion. Platelet function has recently been reviewed by Hirsh and Doery (1971).

The factors concerned in the aetiology of atherosclerosis are numerous and the reasons why atherosclerosis is less severe and coronary artery disease less common in parts of the tropics have still to be elucidated. No single hypothesis—diet, hypocholesterolaemia, exercise, stress, genetic, hormonal, coagulation, or anatomical factors—can satisfactorily explain the differences in prevalence that have been recorded but, in our opinion, parasitic load and coagulation factors are worthy of further study.

E. METABOLIC DISORDERS

Glycogen-storage disease occurs in the tropics but its presentation is not remarkable nor its incidence high. Thyrotoxicosis is rare in many areas of the tropics and myxoedema is not common. Haemochromatosis is discussed on p. 569. Brown atrophy is seen in wasting diseases and lipofuscin in the myofibrils of the heart is commonly seen in idiopathic cardiomegaly and heart conditions in the tropics. The changes in the heart in kwashiorkor are discussed on p. 678. Anaemia is a common cause of heart disease in the tropics and with beriberi and alcoholic heart disease are described in some detail.

The heart and anaemia

A remarkable feature of medicine in the tropics is the extremely low levels of haemoglobin which can be tolerated in patients without heart failure supervening (3g/100ml or less). It is uncommon to see a patient dying of congestive cardiac failure due to anaemia without some secondary contributory factor or factors being present. Exceptions must be made, of course, in cases of acute anaemia due to trauma, haemolysis, or malaria in young children. Anaemia in pregnancy is also an important cause of mortality. Deficiency of folic acid or vitamin B_{12} may also precipitate a fatal crisis in patients suffering from various forms of chronic anaemia, and fatal crises in sickle-cell disease due to these deficiencies or to marrow embolism are not uncommon, the last mentioned being especially frequent in the last trimester of pregnancy.

In acute anaemia there is a sudden decrease in the blood volume and a rapid reduction in the circulatory red cell mass with consequent anoxia. If fatal, changes in the heart and other viscera at necropsy are usually non-specific. Pulmonary oedema is usually a noticeable feature and if haemolysis and/or malaria has been responsible changes in the spleen and reticulo-endothelial system will be prominent. If recovery ensues renal changes with anuria are not infrequent complications.

The changes induced in the heart and other viscera by chronic anaemia are ill understood. Acute coronary insufficiency may rarely be precipitated. The lack of oxygen may cause nutritional degenerative changes in the myocardium. The anaemia causes a decreased blood viscosity and there is possibly a decreased resistance in the peripheral vessels, resulting in an increased cardiac output, tachycardia, and increase of the jugular venous pressure. The heart consequently undergoes dilatation and hypertrophy and congestive cardiac failure may result. The oedema is multifactorial—a weakened myocardium, venous congestion, changes in the osmotic pressure of the plasma, and altered cellular metabolism due to anoxia all playing a part.

In temperate climates anaemia may precipitate clinical evidence of underlying cardiac pathology—atherosclerosis, etc.—but, in our experience this is not common in the tropics. Efficient therapy usually restores cardiac function to normal. The presence of anaemia in childhood has been considered as a possible aetiological factor in a number of cardiac conditions occurring in tropical areas but as yet it has not been conclusively shown that these hypotheses have any factual basis.

Beriberi and alcoholic heart disease

In the literature there are frequent references to Oriental and Occidental beriberi. The former is caused by dietary deficiency of vitamin B_1 (thiamine) and the latter is commonly found in chronic alcoholics. Both types are seen in the tropics.

Beriberi heart disease should not be diagnosed unless there is an absence of other aetiological agents, a history of inadequate dietary intake suggestive of thiamine deficiency, and an adequate response to thiamine therapy or necropsy proof of diagnosis. Clinically there may be evidence of peripheral neuritis, cardiomegaly, oedema, anaemia, hypoproteinaemia, minor non-specific electrocardiographic changes, and increased venous pressure.

This definition would appear to exclude the Occidental type occurring in alcoholism but the role of alcohol is not clear and dietary deficiencies or imbalance are thought to be important in the aetiology of the condition.

Beriberi is characterized clinically usually by a relatively sudden onset precipitated by sudden increase in calorie intake without corresponding increase in aneurin intake. There is gross oedema without evidence of severe myocardial disease and the venous pressure is high. The symptoms respond rapidly to aneurin therapy but syncope, shock, and sudden death can occur.

Heart disease can present in this fashion in alcoholics and a form known as 'palm wine-tappers heart' has been described in the Gambia (Walters and Smith, 1952; Harling *et al.* 1965). The sap of the palm tree if allowed to ferment for 24 hours is a pleasant and mildly alcoholic beverage. The tappers work is arduous and involves climbing probably thirty to forty palm trees 30 feet or so in height twice a day—it is not surprising that large quantities of the product are imbibed with, unfortunately, the development of oedematous heart disease which, fortunately, responds rapidly to vitamin B_1 if medical help is available. Usually in alcoholics in the West, however, the onset is insidious with phases of spontaneous remission.

A certain number of alcoholics present with severe heart failure and signs of marked myocardial disease, a low cardiac output, a small pulse pressure and evidence of peripheral vasoconstriction. Transient hypertension may occur, the cause of which is obscure. They do not respond to aneurin therapy and should not be included as cases of Occidental beriberi (Brigden and Robinson, 1964).

There is little evidence to suggest that the Oriental form progresses to this low-output type seen in the West (Griffith, 1952) but the possibility should not be dismissed. Hepatomegaly is a common finding in both groups of patients but signs of severe liver damage or cirrhosis are unusual. Neurological symptoms are not usually severe but psychopathological changes, paraesthesia, tenderness in the calf muscles and/or absent deep reflexes may be present.

The cause of the high output is obscure. In addition to myocardial lesions there is thought to be both increased blood volume and decreased peripheral resistance (Akbarian *et al.* 1966).

Many factors are probably concerned in the non-beriberi type of alcoholic heart disease, socio-economic, poor diet, and gastro-intestinal disease associated with long-standing excessive alcohol intake contributing to the pathological changes. There is an increased excretion of magnesium in the urine, leading to hypomagnesaemia (Heaton *et al.* 1962) and it is known that deficiencies of potassium, magnesium, and chloride aggravate induced cardiac lesions in laboratory animals.

Magnesium is the fourth most abundant cation in the body. Roughly one half is present in bone and the remaining half inside the body cells. Only about 1 per cent is in the extra-cellular fluid and the plasma concentration is maintained at a remarkably constant level ($1 \cdot 5 – 1 \cdot 8$ mEq per litre) (Macintyre, 1967). The parathyroid glands may be responsible for the control of magnesium metabolism. Experimental magnesium deficiency causes hypercalcaemia and a reduction in muscle potassium content in the presence of a normal plasma potassium. Calcification of the kidney has been described. Magnesium deficiency in man occurs in the malabsorption syndrome, parathyroid disease, chronic alcoholism, vomiting and diarrhoea, diuretic therapy, hypercalcaemia, renal tubular acidosis, portal cirrhosis, kwashiorkor and primary aldosteronism. Oral magnesium therapy would also appear to be life-saving in the very rare, severe form of Bartter's syndrome in the infant where there is failure to thrive with hypokalaemic and hypochloraemic alkalosis (Mace *et al.* 1973).

A deficiency of aneurin, riboflavin, nicotinic acid, pantothenic acid, biotin, pyridoxine, vitamin B_{12}, and folic acid has been noted in the peripheral blood of alcoholics with and without peripheral neuropathies (Fennelly *et al.* 1964) and mitochondrial damage has been shown in the heart by histochemical techniques (Ferrans *et al.* 1965).

Pathology

The pathology of the heart is non-specific. It is invariably enlarged and all chambers are dilated; hypertrophy of the left ventricle being usual. In Oriental beriberi there is oedema of the interstitial tissues and hydropic degeneration of the myofibrils and of the conducting tissue. Mural thrombi may be present.

The non-beriberi type of alcoholic heart resembles macroscopically the heart described in ICM. Histologically, however, fatty change and loss of cross-striations may be seen. Small focal areas of necrosis accompanied by a mild cellular reaction may be present in addition to areas of myocytolysis.

A form of beriberi heart disease has been described in infants in South East Asia breast fed by thiamine-deficient mothers where polished rice was the staple diet (see p. 684).

Other conditions

None of the remaining conditions listed in Table 8.1 (collagen disease, sarcoidosis, amyloidosis, or neuromuscular and neurological disorders) are considered to be common causes of heart disease in the tropics. Metastatic tumours are, however, not uncommon and because of the possible importance of 5-hydroxytryptamine in heart disease in the tropics (Crawford, 1963) the carcinoid syndrome is dealt with in some detail on p. 541.

J. PRIMARY AND METASTATIC TUMOURS OF THE HEART

Primary tumours of the heart are rare but secondary tumours are common in areas in which there is a high incidence of lymphoreticular tumours and/or the Burkitt tumour. Cardiac involvement is not infrequently seen also in patients suffering from liver-cell carcinoma, Kaposi's sarcoma, malignant melanoma and chorioncarcinoma.

THE PERICARDIUM

The conditions affecting the pericardium can be classified as follows:

(1) Rheumatic.
(2) Acute idiopathic including viral.
(3) Pyogenic or bacterial.
(4) Uraemic.
(5) Amoebic.
(6) Tuberculous, including chronic constrictive pericarditis.
(7) The 'collagen diseases'.
(8) Myocardial infarction.
(9) Malignant conditions.

Rheumatic and acute idiopathic pericarditis due probably to Coxsackie or Echo virus infections are rarely seen by the pathologist. Pyogenic and pneumococcal pericarditis are common complications of localized infections elsewhere in the body. In persons dying of uraemia a fibrinous pericarditis is not unusual. Amoebic pericarditis is an entity (p. 73). Hydropericardium is common in patients dying of anaemia, ICM, or EMF. A localized pericarditis is usual with left ventricular aneurysm (p. 369).

Tuberculosis is one of the most important conditions affecting the pericardium (Somers, 1967). It is usually of the caseating type with much caseous material lying between the thickened layers of the pericardium, in which numerous tuberculous follicles can be seen histologically. Associated tuberculomas are usually present in the myocardium. The acute pericardial effusion associated with pulmonary tuberculosis also occurs and the fluid is straw-coloured with flakes of fibrin present. In spite of the high incidence of tuberculosis in our post-mortem material, constrictive pericarditis is not common and severe cardiac fibrosis in the liver is much more frequently due to right-sided endomyocardial fibrosis than to constrictive pericarditis— at least in areas where EMF occurs. In India, however, constrictive pericarditis due to tuberculosis is not uncommon (Basu, 1965). Adhesive pericarditis with no symptoms is common. The importance of the collagen diseases in the pathogenesis of pericarditis in the tropics is unknown. A haemorrhagic pericarditis may result from metastatic spread of primary tumour of the breast or kidney. Lymphoreticular tumours (including the Burkitt), Kaposi's disease, and chorioncarcinoma may also affect the pericardium.

THE ARTERIES

There are few comparative studies of the histology of arteries in the neonate in the tropics. It has been shown, however, that the coronary arteries in the newborn African child resemble histologically those of their European counterpart (Robertson, 1960). Evidence is accruing from geographical studies that the pattern of atherosclerosis may differ considerably from that found in temperate climates. An unusual form of diffuse intimal thickening of the aorta possibly associated with atherosclerosis has been noted in India (Duggal *et al.* 1966) and in Africa the aortic circumference has been thought to be less, the media thinner and degeneration of elastic tissue very common (Dick, 1947; Pepler, 1955).

Apart from atherosclerosis, arterial disease in the tropics, with one exception, would not appear to differ greatly from that seen in temperate climates, diseases associated with the aged, however, such as temporal or giant-cell arteritis and Mönckeberg sclerosis, being much less commonly seen, probably due to the differing age structure of the populations at risk. The arterial lesions in diabetes are less severe. The exception is a form of arteritis affecting mainly the aorta and its larger branches which has been described in children and young adults in Japan, Africa, India, Singapore, and China. It is discussed below under the term arteritis of obscure aetiology.

ARTERITIS OF OBSCURE AETIOLOGY

Synonyms. Takayasu's disease; pulseless disease; young female arteritis type of aortic arch syndrome; idiopathic arteritis in young Africans; primary arteritis of the abdominal aorta in children; anomalous or abdominal coarctation.

There are at least two conditions affecting the aorta and its larger branches which have a similar pathology and whose aetiology and interrelationship with each other are obscure. These are Takayasu's disease and an idiopathic aortitis described in African, Indian, and Chinese children and adults (Isaacson and Wayburne, 1957; Danaraj *et al.* 1959 and 1963; Abrahams and Cockshott, 1962; Sen *et al.* 1962; Hwang and Liv, 1962). Cases have been reported from Colombia (Munoz and Correa, 1970) in which there has been coagulative necrosis surrounded by fibroblasts, monocytes and occasional giant cells in the aorta.

Reddy *et al.* (1970) in South India have described extensive densely adherent periaortic lymphadenopathy. The lymph nodes showed the changes described in toxoplasmosis. In three patients the sera were strongly positive.

At one time Takayasu's disease was thought to affect only young females and the pathological lesions to be restricted to the aortic arch and its major branches—it has been referred to as the young female arteritis type of aortic arch syndrome. It has, however, now been reported in childhood (Zerpa *et al.* 1966; Warshaw and Spachs, 1965) and not infrequently in males. The thoracic and abdominal aorta or lower-limbs arteries may be involved (Strachan, 1966) and even the endocardium (Chhetri *et al.* 1970). The findings in many cases are similar to those reported in idiopathic aortitis in the tropics, in which the arch of the aorta and its branches may also be affected (Isaacson, 1961) and the pulse may be absent in the upper extremities as well as the lower. We have been unable to satisfy ourselves from the available pathological information that these conditions are separate entities, and they are consequently described as 'arteritis of obscure aetiology'. Included in this syndrome is the panarteritis causing aorto-iliac thrombosis in three South African Bantu (Pepler and Simson, 1959). Temporal or giant-cell arteritis is, however, excluded as it would appear to be a separate entity—affecting a much older age group and differing in its pathology, and being as far as we know uncommon in tropical areas (Kinmont and McCallum, 1965; Garrett, 1961). Cystic myxomatous degeneration of the arteries is also rare (Bliss *et al.* 1963).

Epidemiology

The condition has been described in all parts of the world but would appear to be more common in Africa, India, and the Orient, and probably more common in non-whites in the United States.

It occurs in childhood and in relatively young adults. It is uncommon in the middle-aged and elderly. Females are more frequently affected than males. The aetiology is unknown and many factors have been considered, including rheumatic fever and streptococcal sensitivity, tuberculosis, syphilis, toxins, and the collagen diseases. None has as yet proved acceptable. An auto-immune reaction to vascular elastic tissue has been proposed without convincing supporting evidence. The fact that steroids have been considered helpful in preventing the progress of the disease in a few cases is perhaps suggestive of an immunological basis (Strachan, 1966).

Pathogenesis

There may be general symptoms prior to the onset of localizing arterial disease or the prodromal phase may be symptomless. Fever, pleurisy, haemoptysis, muscle pains, polyarteritis, skin lesions, fatigue, and weight loss may be complained of. These symptoms have rarely been described in tropical areas. Anaemia and an elevated sedimentation rate are usual. The tuberculin test is usually positive and γ-globulin is raised in the blood.

If the aortic arch is involved there are absent or diminished pulses in the upper extremities. The head may be held in a flexed position and cerebral and ocular symptoms with loss of hair occur.

If the abdominal aorta is involved renal artery occlusion is usual, with consequent hypertension. Hypertension, encephalopathy, or congestive cardiac failure have been the most common presenting symptoms in children in the tropics. Abdominal pain and weakness and claudication in the lower limbs may be noted. The larger peripheral arteries may be solely involved and popliteal and femoral aneurysms in Africans have been described.

Necropsy findings

Obliteration of the larger branches of the aortic arch may be found, with associated ischaemic changes in the brain, eye, and muscles supplied. The aorta shows wrinkling of the intima with segmental areas of stenosis and aneurysmal dilatation. In the stenotic areas the wall is thickened and there are thick white plaques on the intima. It should be noted that multiple aneurysmal dilatations of the aorta would appear to be more common in Africa (Jackson and Brew, 1961; Abrahams and Cockshott, 1962; Penn, 1963; Joffe, 1965) and have been noted in Negroes in America (Henry, 1963; Austen and Blennerhassett, 1965) and genetic factors have been considered by some authors in their aetiology. They are uncommon in Japan (Nasu, 1963). Thrombosis of the lower abdominal aorta and iliac vessels may occur and dissecting aneurysms have been described in Sri Lanka (Thenabadu et al. 1970). If the renal arteries are affected the kidneys may be unilaterally or bilaterally contracted and granular and generalized uraemic manifestations may be present. Cardiac hypertrophy, with signs of chronic venous congestion in the other organs, is usual. Encephalomalacia and splenic infarcts may be noted.

Histologically, in the early stages a segmental periarteritis is present with an infiltration of lymphocytes, histiocytes, and plasma cells, with associated perivascular cuffing and endarteritis of the vessels in the vasa vasorum. Polymorphonuclear leucocytes may be present but eosinophils or fibrinoid degeneration have not been reported. A similar inflammatory infiltrate occurs in the media, with disruption of the elastica and subsequent fibrosis. Occasionally, giant-cell systems may be present and these are thought to be a non-specific reaction to degenerate elastic tissue (Isaacson, 1961). The giant cells may be of the Langhans or foreign-body type. Degeneration and fibrosis of the intima with superimposed intra-arterial thrombosis with consequent organization and, in some instances, recanalization, occur. Calcification, in these lesions is said to be rare but has been observed. Eventually the arterial wall is represented by a collagenous cord, the end result of a panarteritis. Stenosis and/or aneurysmal formation is the eventual outcome.

CAROTID ARTERITIS

A form of arteritis has been described in children in the United States causing thrombosis of the internal carotid artery (Shillito, 1964).

Upper respiratory infections, fevers, sepsis, and trauma have been considered as aetiological agents.

The main lesions would appear to occur in the region of the base of the skull. The pathology is indeterminate but might possibly be initiated by a periarterial inflammatory process.

SYMMETRICAL GANGRENE

Synonym. Idiopathic peripheral gangrene of the tropics.

This condition has been seen in Africa (Gelfand, 1947; Turpie *et al.* 1967; Barr *et al.* 1972; Steiner and Hutt, 1972), and India (Subramanian, 1949). Clinically, the tips of the digits, nose, and ears may be effected or the lesions may be confined to the lower legs or hands. It may present as symmetrical painful oedema of the lower leg with gangrene ensuing in a few days. It has been associated with anaemia, syphilis, vitamin-B deficiency, acute infections including typhoid, typhus fever, and malaria. It is not related to diabetes, arteriosclerosis thromboangitiitis obliterans, or ergotism. It occurs in children and young adults of both sexes. It has been associated with tropical thrombophlebitis (Gelfand, 1949), arteriolar spasm being considered responsible for the gangrene. The pathology has not been satisfactorily described and the aetiology is unknown. Barr *et al.* (1972), however, have described coagulation abnormalities which cause shortening of the clotting and thrombin time. Thrombotic vascular occlusion is therefore not surprising. Herbal preparations containing stimulants to uterine and smooth muscle have now been considered in the aetiology of the condition.

We have seen occasionally young children suffering from symmetrical gangrene in Africa. The condition has recently been reviewed by Lloyd *et al.* (1967) who considered polyarteritis nodosa to be the causative lesion in temperate climates. Absence of pulses in the peripheral arteries has occasionally been a feature in Africa and the aetiology may differ from those cases reported in the Western world. Peripheral gangrene associated with polyarthritis has been reported in a child aged 8 years in Zambia (Lowenthal, 1967).

THE VEINS

Apart from tropical phlebitis or thrombophlebitic diseases of veins these would not appear to pose any special problems in the tropics. In the previous edition we stated that it was our impression that varicose veins and varicose ulcers of the lower extremities were uncommon and this has been confirmed by Burkitt (1972). Varicose veins are rare in all developing countries and in the rural African in contrast to the American Negro in whom the prevalence is high. It was considered that the aetiological agent was faecal arrest associated with a low residue diet as defined by Cleave *et al.* (1969).

Constipation causes increased intraluminal pressure in the colon and intra-abdominal pressure when straining at stool with consequent pressure transmitted to the veins of the lower limbs. The relative rarity of haemorrhoids and deep vein thrombosis (see below) can be explained in a similar fashion.

PHLEBOTHROMBOSIS AND PULMONARY EMBOLISM

Pulmonary embolism following thrombosis of the internal iliac, femoral, or deep calf veins in the leg is thought to be rare in areas in the tropics (Davies, 1948; Elmes, 1958). Phleboliths in the pelvic veins have rarely been seen radiologically in East Africa (Brown, 1943). Postoperative pulmonary embolism and phlegmasia alba dolens are also uncommon. In addition, thrombo-embolic episodes in the lungs were noted to be far less common at necropsy in East Africans when compared with a series in North Americans (Thomas *et al.* 1960). The incidence of postoperative deep vein thrombosis diagnosed by radioisotope scanning in 100 Sudanese patients aged 40 or over was 12 per cent—this compares with a prevalence of 30 per cent in patients in British hospitals (Hassan *et al.* 1973).

In Nigeria, however, venous thrombosis does occur in malnourished subjects—cerebral sinus thrombosis in kwashiorkor and of the leg veins in malignant disease and tuberculosis being entities. A series of fifty-four patients dying of pulmonary embolism in a 5-year period in Ibadan has recently been described by Nwokolo and Ikoku (1967). The majority of incidents occurred in medical patients but eleven followed surgery. There was suggestive evidence that pulmonary embolism was more frequent in carriers of the sickle-cell gene; the incidence of the S trait is 24 per cent and that of the C trait 6 per cent in the population at risk. Three patients in the series were suffering from SC disease. Kallichurum (1969) has shown deep vein thrombosis to be common in the Bantu in Natal and pulmonary embolism occurred.

The reasons for the apparent rarity of venous thrombosis in some areas are complex. Bronte-Stewart (1965) suggested that a low intake of animal fat in the diet might be responsible as it inhibits fibrinolysis. Vegetable fats do not have this effect. A fall in the incidence of postoperative thrombo-embolic accidents was noted in Europe during World War II and dietary factors were considered important in the aetiology. It should be noted, however, that an increase in circulating fibrinolysins has been suggested in certain tropical populations, and the habit of many patients in the tropics of refusing to remain inactive in bed even on the first postoperative day must also be considered in the presumed lowered incidence of postoperative complications of venous thrombosis. The possible effects of a high residue diet with frequent bulky stools preventing increased intracolonic and intra-abdominal pressure and thus preventing increased venous pressure in the lower limbs is mentioned above.

MULTIPLE (IDIOPATHIC) THROMBOPHLEBITIS

Synonym. Tropical phlebitis.

Venous thrombosis can occur as a complication of any acute infectious illness but there is a form of idiopathic thrombophlebitis which has been described in Africa (Fisher, 1941) and has been referred to as tropical phlebitis. An outbreak has been recorded in East African troops where over 600 were affected (Charters and Manson-Bahr, 1946). It bears a close resemblance to thrombophlebitis migrans but relapses are not as common. The aetiology is unknown but in one outbreak it was described as common in troops undergoing antisyphilitic treatment and a possible viral infection has been postulated.

Young adults are commonly affected and the onset is abrupt, with pyrexia and pain and tenderness over the affected segment of the vein. Local oedema follows and is thought to be due to arteriolar spasm. This may be severe enough to cause gangrene of the digits (Gelfand, 1949). The femoral vein is most frequently affected but the subclavian, jugular, mesenteric portal, splenic, and even the cerebral sinuses may be involved. Death occasionally occurs. There is a relative lymphocytosis in the peripheral blood. Blood cultures are negative.

The media and intima of the veins are infiltrated by neutrophils and proliferating capillaries. Histiocytes are present and may contain eosinophilic inclusions shown by the phloxine-tartrazine stain (Fisher *et al.* 1946). Thrombosis occurs secondarily to the mural lesion.

9

The Respiratory System

Respiratory conditions are common in the neonate, the most common conditions being, in our experience, the respiratory distress syndrome, pulmonary haemorrhage, and bronchopneumonia.

In the respiratory distress syndrome either simple atelectasis or hyaline membrane atelectasis may be seen on histological examination of the lungs. At post mortem the lungs are heavy and congested and associated cerebral haemorrhage may be present. Microscopical examination may reveal widespread collapse of terminal air spaces with oedema of the interstitial tissues and distended lymphatics. An acidophilic membrane (hyaline) may replace the lung epithelium of the respiratory bronchioles and alveolar ducts. Congestion is marked and intra-alveolar haemorrhages and an inflammatory infiltrate are usually present.

Pulmonary haemorrhage is usually unexplained but may be associated with dysmaturity, cerebral haemorrhage due to birth injuries, infection, or haemorrhagic disease.

Bronchopneumonia and alveolar haemorrhage are also common findings in the neonate. In infants *Pneumocystis carinii* infection has been reported (Ariztia *et al.* 1957; Abioye, 1967), as has also cytomegalic inclusion disease (Mainwaring and Tompkins, 1963). Kerosene poisoning in children is not uncommon in certain parts of the tropics and 100 cases have been reported from Baghdad (Nouri and Al-Rahim, 1970). There is cough, cyanosis, vomiting and constipation or diarrhoea. There are also signs of central nervous system involvement. A chemical pneumonitis occurs and bronchopneumonia is a usual complication.

Whooping cough, measles and other viral infections, and bronchopneumonia associated with nutritional, bacterial, and parasitic diseases (especially malaria) and giant-cell pneumonia are all common conditions. The migratory stages of many parasitic infections may cause respiratory symptoms, and these are mentioned in their appropriate context. Special attention is given to tropical eosinophilia.

Asthma, bronchitis, bronchiectasis, and lung abscess are common. Excluding the parasitic infections (paragonimiasis, amoebiasis, etc.) their pathology is not remarkable. It should be remembered, however, that direct microscopic examination of the sputum is a valuable diagnostic procedure in the tropics. Rhinitis and coryza and true bronchial asthma have been reported in those working with African hardwoods. Allergic contact dermatitis is, however, the most serious hazard. The smoking of 'black fat tobacco' may cause interstitial pulmonary fibrosis in middle-aged and elderly individuals in Guyana (Editorial, 1972). Primary pulmonary hypertension with eosinophilia is not uncommon in Sri Lanka and has been considered to be associated with filariasis (Obeysekere and De Soysa, 1970).

Pulmonary fibrosis, emphysema and other conditions concerned in the aetiology of cor pulmonale are discussed on p. 374.

The pneumokonioses are problems which are directly related to the presence of a mining industry. Asbestosis is found in a limited area of South Africa and is associated with a high incidence of mesothelioma of the pleura (Working Group, 1965) and less often of the peritoneum (Enticknap and Smither, 1964; Bolio-Cicero et al. 1961).

Lobar pneumonia is still a common and serious disease, with jaundice, toxaemia, pericarditis, and empyema common complications. Jaundice is a particularly common complication and is considered to be due to liver-cell damage (Hall and Parry, 1963). Tugwell (1973) has shown that in Northern Nigeria the liability to jaundice in this infection is associated with glucose-6-phosphate dehydrogenase deficiency. Theron et al. (1971) in an electron microscopy study in Bantu patients considered that toxic injury to the liver cells and cholestasis were precipitated by lobar pneumonia.

Pulmonary embolism and infarction have been discussed on p. 388.

The pleura

Pleural effusion and empyema are common in the tropics. An eosinophilic pleural effusion may be seen in a wide variety of diseases (Campbell and Webb, 1964). The occurrence of mesothelioma in association with asbestosis has been mentioned. Widespread deposits of lymphosarcoma are occasionally seen. Chylothorax is not common. It occasionally follows chest trauma or is found in association with malignant disease involving the thoracic duct—or following surgery of the heart and great vessels (McFarlane and Holman, 1972).

In this section only tropical eosinophilia (eosinophilic lung) and tuberculosis are considered in detail; sarcoidosis and malignant disease are briefly described.

TUBERCULOSIS

Pulmonary tuberculosis is prevalent throughout the tropics, being particularly common in the Indian subcontinent, parts of Africa, and the

Far East. Extrapulmonary tuberculosis, although less common, is neverthe-less an important public health problem in many tropical countries.

Epidemiology

The observed prevalence of pulmonary tuberculosis in the tropics depends very much on the methods of examination used—the three techniques most commonly employed, either singly or in combination, are: (i) bacteriological examination and culture of sputum, (ii) radiology of the chest, and (iii) the tuberculin test. A person once infected is likely to harbour live tubercle for the rest of his life, and these can cause the development of disease at any time if suitable circumstances exist. The natural history of tuberculosis in the human body has been studied in detail by Myers (1959a, b, 1961, 1962, 1963).

Tuberculosis is to some extent a household infection and it was found in Kenya that household contacts, especially of the younger age groups, were infected five to ten times more frequently than the general population from which they derived (WHO tuberculosis Chemotherapy Centre, 1961). Similarly, in Madras, a high prevalence of tuberculous lesions was found in household contacts. It appeared, however, that the main risk to relatives and others living, cooking, and feeding with tuberculous patients arose from exposure before the diagnosis was made. After diagnosis and with well-managed chemotherapy the risk was small and much the same whether the patient was treated at home or in a sanatorium. Moreover, tuberculous patients in Madras and elsewhere in the tropics have been treated effectively by chemotherapy even when they continued hard manual work and remained undernourished (Editorial, 1961; Fox, 1963). In Africa there is more tuberculous infection in the male than in the female population while, as one would expect, the level of infection is consistently higher in urban than in rural areas (Albert *et al.* 1972; Poffenbarger, 1972). The prevalence of bacillary excretors is low (< 1 per cent), (Roelsgaard *et al.* 1964). Detailed bacteriological investigations have shown that isoniazid-sensitive tubercle bacilli isolated from patients in South India are on average less virulent than bacilli from British patients (Mitchison, 1963). This risk to the community from patients who are excreting isoniazid-resistant tubercle bacilli, either because they were primarily infected with such organisms, or after un-successful treatment, lies mainly in the fact that isoniazid-resistant infec-tions militate against successful treatment with isoniazid-containing combinations (Fox, 1962).

Until recently the tuberculin test was universally accepted as an almost infallible means of determining whether or not an individual had been infected with tubercle bacilli. Edwards and Palmer (1953) showed, however, that tuberculin sensitivity is not invariably related to tuberculous infection and suggested that this allergy can be due to infection with a microorganism, that is similar to, but not identical with, *Myco. tuberculosis*. The geographical extent of this 'non-specific' tuberculin sensitivity has been reviewed by Nyboe (1960), who emphasized that this phenomenon is particularly prevalent in the tropics and subtropics. Although it is not known what causes this non-specific sensitivity, it has been shown in India (Bates *et al.* 1951) that the causative agent is associated with low more than with high altitudes; similar findings have been reported from tropical Africa. It appears that persons giving weak reactions to low doses of tuberculin and strong reactions to high doses have a non-specific type of allergy and are not likely to be infected with tubercle bacilli (Palmer, 1953). A dynamic model for the study of the epidemiology of tuberculosis capable of rapid solutions by a computer has recently been constructed by Waaler and Oecon (1967).

Pathology

In many areas of the tropics the primary or childhood form of tuberculosis which was rare in adults in temperate climates until the advent of chemotherapy, is considered the most common form in all age groups. Histologically it is exemplified by acute caseating necrosis with a peripheral infiltration of histiocytes, epithelioid cells, lymphocytes, and occasional eosinophils. The Langhans giant cells and fibroblastic proliferation which are features of the secondary or adult type are absent or minimal.

Tuberculosis of the respiratory tract

The primary infection consists of the Ghon focus, which is situated subpleurally in any part of the lungs. It consists of, at first, an infiltration of acute inflammatory cells, to be followed in a few days by the appearance of histiocytes, epithelioid cells and, later, typical tuberculous follicles if resistance is acquired. Healing or lymphatic spread to the hilar mediastinal glands may occur. In the childhood type of tuberculosis which is considered common in the tropics, thin-walled abscesses filled with caseous pus are present in the lungs and there is massive involvement of the hilar and mediastinal glands. Pressure of the glands on the bronchi may cause collapse of lobes. Calcification is unusual and miliary tuberculosis, bronchopneumonia, pericarditis, and extensive extrapulmonary dissemination is frequent from the glandular focus. In our experience in West Africa this type is seen in children, many under the age of 1 year, and frequently in older children associated with protein-calorie deficiency disease. Many children, however, exhibiting the primary complex recover, and calcification of the foci in the parenchyma and hilar lymph nodes is seen. Calcified nodes become smaller with treatment and are not common in adolescents or adults in Ibadan, which suggests that calcium may be absorbed from the healed lesions in a certain proportion of cases (Bohrer, S., personal communication). The adult type of tuberculosis with fibrocavitary or fibrocaseous lesions in the apical regions of the lungs and minimal lymph node involvement is occasionally seen in children (Brew, 1962). Tuberculous bronchiectasis and empyema with pulmonary collapse are common complications and the destroyed lung is not uncommonly seen in India (Basu, 1965).

Although in other areas of the tropics the childhood type may be common in adults (Large, 1964), in West Africa the secondary or 'adult' type is usual (Henshaw, 1959). This is to be expected, as 80 per cent of the population are tuberculin-positive by the age of 24 years. The childhood type is, however, seen in adults, usually in the presence of some other condition which has interfered with the immunological status of the patient—leukaemia, Hodgkin's disease, steroid therapy, etc. The danger of the occurrence of miliary tuberculosis in patients undergoing steroid therapy cannot be too strongly emphasized and we have seen a number of undiagnosed deaths from this cause. Radiological findings may be indeterminate and the Heaf test negative.

Associated tuberculosis of the larynx and trachea occur. Isolated nasopharyngeal tuberculosis is uncommon but a few cases have been described (Martinson, 1967). Pleural effusion is common in all age groups. Pleural punch biopsy has been found a most useful diagnostic procedure in patients in whom there has been no bacteriological or radiological evidence of tuberculosis (Lucas and Mainwaring, 1962).

Amyloidosis is a complication which usually occurs in adults, but we have seen the condition in a child of 6 years (p. 723).

Tuberculosis of lymphatic glands

In many areas of the tropics the milk of cattle is not consumed and consequently infection due to the bovine strain of *Myco. tuberculosis* is not seen. Instead of the localized tonsillar gland complex previously seen in temperate areas cervical-gland involvement in these areas tends to be diffuse. Tuberculous lymphadenopathy is extremely common in the tropics and forms a relatively large part of our surgical biopsy material. It is due to the human strain of *Myco. tuberculosis*. It may be generalized, discrete, and painless, and be seen in relatively well-nourished children with hepatomegaly and splenomegaly (Trowell, 1960), or can occur in cachectic patients with widely disseminated tuberculosis. Mesenteric adenopathy is discussed when intestinal tuberculosis is described.

The lesions, especially in children, are frequently of the acute necrotizing type with few giant cells present. Lymphoedema of the extremities or breast are not uncommon complications and phlyctenular keratitis is frequently associated with cervical adenitis. The histopathological diagnosis in the great majority of instances has to be presumptive, as the acid-fast bacilli are rarely demonstrable in tissues. In addition to histological examination, a smear of fresh tissue should be examined for the presence of tubercle bacilli, and culture and animal inoculation should be undertaken when feasible.

Tuberculosis of bone

Even in the absence of bovine strains tuberculosis of bone is common in the tropics, the spine being most frequently affected. The larger joints are also affected (Basu, 1965), but less commonly, and extensive lesions of the vault of the skull have been described (Barton, 1961). Dactylitis is uncommon.

The thoracic, lumbar, and cervical spine are affected in that order and 'spindle' thoracic, psoas, and cervical and retropharyngeal abscesses occur (Konstam, 1963).

Children under 15 years are mainly affected but the condition is not infrequent in adults.

The lesion commences in the body of the vertebra, and collapse may follow caseous necrosis. In addition to paravertebral abscesses, kyphosis and paraplegia are complications. In the latter condition toxic and vascular reactive changes have been described in the cord. Compression by tuberculous granulation tissue or pus in the epidural space are added factors. The paravertebral abscess may track along muscle and discharge with the formation of fistulous sinuses. Calcification of the psoas tendon has been described as causing flexion deformity of the hip. Phlyctenular keratitis may also occur.

In West Africa bony repair can occur with anterior bridging along the anterior and lateral spinal ligaments (Konstam, 1963), unlike the lesions in Central Asia where rarefaction and destruction are the most important features (Serafino et al. 1960). De Tavera and De Leon (1967) studied spinal tuberculosis in children in the Philippines. Gross lymphatic tuberculosis was present in all cases and all were positive tuberculin reactors. Children with gross lymphatic involvement were therefore examined carefully and clinically unsuspected spinal involvement was noted in 7 of 39 children examined. Spinal tuberculosis may be a direct extension of tuberculous infection of the vertebral bodies resulting from thrombotic localization in prevertebral lymphatic tissues.

Tuberculosis of the central nervous system

Tuberculous meningitis is common in children in the tropics especially under the age of 1 year. It also occurs in adults but is very much less common (Lauckner, 1959). It is usually considered to be secondary to a lesion elsewhere in the body, although very occasionally such a lesion may not be detectable. The meninges may be affected by miliary spread, by rupture of a small isolated tuberculoma, or occasionally by direct extension of a tuberculous focus in bone. The inflammatory process is of a more acute type, with a predominantly monocytic and lymphocytic infiltrate accompanying necrosis of tissue with few giant cells present. The base of the brain is most frequently affected. The cerebrospinal fluid is clear but it may have an opalescent appearance and give a fine web of fibrin on standing. The number of cells is raised, often being 200 per mm³ or even higher; the majority are lymphocytes. The protein is increased and the glucose and chlorides are diminished. Tubercle bacilli can usually be found on microscopic examination of the centrifuged deposit or in the fibrin web which forms in the fluid. Choroidal tubercles are present at the onset in about half the cases and provide an immediate diagnostic clue. They are easily found in a well-sedated child whose pupils are fully dilated (Editorial, 1971).

Tuberculomas of the brain are not uncommon. Tuberculosis of the spinal epidural space is a complication of tuberculosis of the spine.

Tuberculosis of the alimentary tract

Tuberculosis of the oral cavity would not appear to be common and the great majority of lesions of the alimentary tract are limited to the small intestine. Very rarely ulceration of the tongue and buccal mucosa occurs secondarily to pulmonary tuberculosis and a tuberculoma of the tongue may occur. Occasionally lesions of the stomach have been recorded. Abdominal tuberculosis with ascites is common in many parts of the tropics in all age and sex groups. In Ibadan it accounts for 24 per cent of all adult patients presenting with ascites (Nwokolo, 1967). It may be a primary condition or secondary to tuberculosis of the lungs (Francis, 1972).

In the secondary type it may be part of a miliary spread or ulceration of the intestine may occur following ingestion of infected sputum. The Peyer's patches are affected and transverse ulcers with undermined edges and nodular margins are formed. There is fibrosis of the muscular coat and stenosis, but perforation is not usual. However, loops of intestine become adherent and perforation between loops occurs. Hypertrophic ileocaecal tuberculosis occurs and may simulate carcinoma (Anand, 1956). The appendix may be affected. Tuberculous peritonitis and the malabsorption syndrome are complications of intestinal tuberculosis. Subtotal villous atrophy may be seen on jejunal biopsy.

The most frequent type of abdominal tuberculosis is, however, in our experience the glandular—often without a demonstrable primary lesion in the intestine—and it may be associated with enlargement of glands in the neck, groin, or axilla. The mesenteric, para-aortic, and upper abdominal glands are enlarged and present a variable appearance on section. They may be firm and white with yellowish areas of caseation present or be almost entirely replaced by yellow creamy pus. With rupture of a gland, the whole of the mesenteric and peritoneal surface may be studded with tubercles. The ascitic fluid is yellow and contains flakes of fibrin. It occasionally may be haemorrhagic. The protein content is usually high (over $2 \cdot 5 \, G/100 \, ml$) with numerous lymphocytes present, and bacilli may be seen on stained smears or isolated on culture and/or by animal inoculation. Hypoprotein-aemia and anaemia due to a malabsorption defect are common complications.

Peritoneal tuberculosis may occasionally be secondary to infection of the Fallopian tube in females.

Tuberculosis of the blood-forming organs

In tuberculosis almost every type of anaemia has been described. In uncomplicated cases a mild iron-deficient anaemia is usual. The monocyte is an important cell in the pathology of the condition as it transforms in the presence of products of the bacillus to the epithelioid cell. A monocytosis is said to be an unfavourable sign, whereas a lymphocytosis is suggestive of resistance developing (Wintrobe, 1961). A polymorphonuclear leucocytosis is rarely seen. A haemolytic type of anaemia has been described and purpura may also occur (Dalgleish and Ansell, 1950).

Miliary tubercles may be present in the marrow and can cause pancyto-penia and macrocytosis with a hyperplatic or aplastic picture on marrow puncture (Evans *et al.* 1952; Fountain, 1954).

Leukaemoid reactions are common and may be of the lymphocytic, monocytic, or myeloid type. The most frequent form is probably the acute myeloblastic with a white cell count which may be as high as 100,000 cells per mm³ in the peripheral blood and 50 per cent may be myeloblastic (Hughes *et al.* 1959). The additional signs of severe anaemia, lymphadeno-pathy and splenomegaly, renders the diagnosis difficult. The leucocyte alkaline phosphatase reaction in the peripheral blood, and splenic puncture, may be helpful in diagnosis.

Tuberculous strictures and fistulae in the small intestine may cause a macrocytic anaemia due to vitamin B_{12} or folic-acid deficiency with a corresponding leucopenia. The marrow is hyperplastic and megaloblastic. The haematological findings may be indistinguishable from pernicious anaemia, but free HCl is usually present in the gastric juice.

In a certain number of younger patients caseating tuberculosis may be responsible for myelofibrosis with mild splenomegaly and lymph node enlargement (Fountain, 1954; Crail *et al.* 1948).

Tuberculosis of the genito-urinary system

In our experience caseating renal tuberculosis is rare and if the kidney is affected it is usually part of a miliary spread; in consequence the ureters and bladder are also infrequently affected. In contrast is the relatively frequent infection of the genital tract. However, in China and India caseating renal tuberculosis is common and would appear to be not uncommon in Britain (Editorial, 1971).

In males the epididymis is affected from a focus elsewhere, or occasionally as an isolated lesion. Spread to the vas, seminal vesicles, and prostate occurs. The testicle is affected in the late stages.

In the female, infection in the Fallopian tube may remain localized or spread to the ovary, uterus, and cervix. Pyosalpinx and tubo-ovarian abscesses may lead to extensive pelvic tuberculosis and acute tuberculous peritonitis. The endometrium may be affected by miliary or local spread. Typical follicles may be seen on histological examination of material obtained by curettage. In the absence of follicles, tuberculous endometritis should be suspected if lymphocytic aggregates are present in the stroma, or if pus and inflammatory debris are present in the glands. The occasional gland may be cystic (Govan, 1962). Guinea-pig inoculation is, however, the most reliable method of detecting tuberculous endometritis and is more sensitive than histological or cultural methods.

Other organs

Miliary tubercles are commonly found in the liver with dissemination of the disease, and occasionally a tuberculoma may be found. Similar lesions are seen in the spleen. Tuberculosis of the breast is an entity.

Primary lesions have been reported on the scalp, face, knee, elbow, hand, or forearm, but are rare in our experience. Lupus vulgaris occurs, as also does erythema nodosum. A primary tuberculous ulcer of the skin occasionally occurs, and scrofuloderma seems more common in India than Africa. Localized subcutaneous tuberculous abscesses can occur (Editorial, 1971). Phlyctenular keratitis has already been mentioned.

The blood vessels may be affected on the adventitial or intimal surface. In addition to miliary tuberculosis of the intima, lesions involving all layers of the vessel wall and mycotic aneurysms of the aorta or peripheral vessels may occur. The possible association of tuberculosis and idiopathic arteritis of unknown origin is discussed on p. 385.

Tuberculosis of the heart and pericardium are discussed on pp. 374 and

383. Tuberculous constrictive pericarditis is not uncommon in India (Basu, 1965). The adrenal gland is discussed on p. 661.

Tuberculosis and pregnancy

Tuberculosis is more frequently seen in emergency obstetric admissions than in patients regularly attending ante-natal clinics. Pregnancy does not affect the disease adversely with adequate therapy (Lawson, 1962). Congenital transmission is rare.

Diagnostic pathology

The laboratory diagnosis of tuberculosis is bacteriological, radiological, and histological. The use of fluorescent microscopy for the detection of tubercle bacilli has been described by many authors, who almost unanimously came to the conclusion that it has pertinent advantages over the time-honoured Ziehl–Neelsen technique. Strains of 'anonymous' mycobacteria (atypical acid-fast bacilli) are sometimes isolated from sputum specimens submitted for examination for *Myco. tuberculosis*; their possible pathogenic role in tropical countries where tuberculosis is prevalent is difficult to determine (Snijder, 1965; Wong, 1964).

TROPICAL EOSINOPHILIA

Synonyms. Eosinophilic lung; tropical pulmonary eosinophilia.

This is the name given to a clinical syndrome characterized by paroxysms of coughing with marked eosinophilia, which usually responds favourably to treatment with diethylcarbamazine. A similar symptomatology with eosinophilia can occur, however, in the course of known parasitic infections such as strongyloidiasis, loiasis, schistosomiasis, ascariasis, toxocariasis, and pulmonary gnathostomiasis, as well as in more cosmopolitan allergic conditions such as Loeffler's syndrome and asthma (Beaver and Danaraj, 1958; de Langen, 1928; Mainzer, 1938; Beaver *et al.* 1962; Prijyanonda *et al.* 1955; Crofton *et al.* 1952).

Epidemiology

It is generally accepted that tropical eosinophilia is caused by occult filarial infections. The evidence in favour of this hypothesis has been accumulating over the years and comprises (i) the demonstration of a consistently high titre of filarial complement-fixing antibodies in the absence of evidence of microfilaria in the blood (Danaraj *et al.* 1959); (ii) clinical, haematological, and serological response to therapy with diethylcarbamazine (Danaraj, 1958); (iii) the experimental production of a syndrome very similar to tropical eosinophilia in a volunteer inoculated with infective larvae of two species of animal filaria (Buckley, 1958); and (iv) the demonstration of microfilariae in the lungs of individuals showing the typical signs of eosinophilic lung (Webb *et al.* 1960). It was noted in Singapore that Indians who constituted only 7 per cent of the general population provided 80 per cent of tropical eosinophilia cases there (Danaraj, 1958), yet in India, Chaudhuri (1956) reported that evidence of pulmonary disease was merely frequent and not invariable in his patients with tropical eosinophilia and that the response to antifilarial treatment was not constant. Other series of cases reported in India have likewise shown wide variations in symptoms and clinical findings (Ball and Treu, 1950). On the other hand a series of cases such as that described in Singapore has also been reported from India (Viswanathan, 1948).

Wong (1964) has shown that whereas microfilariae introduced intravenously into the non-immune dog circulate for periods of up to several weeks, in the immune dog similarly introduced microfilariae promptly disappear from the circulation. It is possible therefore that eosinophilic lung results from an alteration of host immunity to a filarial parasite, giving rise to allergic phenomena manifested by persistent hypereosinophilia and pulmonary symptoms (Danaraj *et al.* 1966).

Pathology

Clinically the patient usually presents with respiratory symptoms and radiological evidence of pulmonary involvement. Hepatomegaly and lymphadenopathy are variable findings.

The pathological changes depend upon the host's reaction to the microfilariae in the lungs, liver, spleen, and lymph nodes. The microfilariae are found in the tissues and not in the blood.

Macroscopically small white nodules may be scattered throughout the lung tissue and be present in lesser numbers in the liver and less commonly the spleen. Lymphatic glands may be enlarged soft and fleshy with small brownish-grey areas evident on the cut surface. Sheathed microfilariae resembling *W. bancrofti* have been noted in wet-drop preparations (Webb *et al.* 1960).

In the lungs groups of alveoli may be packed with eosinophils and fibrin. Eosinophilic abscesses with portions of microfilariae at the centre may be seen. In other areas there may be a central zone of eosinophilic necrosis containing microfilariae surrounded by histiocytes of epithelioid type, fibroblasts, giant cells, lymphocytes, plasma cells, and eosinophils, in varying proportions (Danaraj *et al.* 1966). Others may have a centre of acidophilic hyaline material containing inconstant fragments of microfilariae—the so-called Meyers–Kouwenaar bodies—surrounded by epithelioid cells. The microfilariae measure about 3–7 μm in width and, on serial sectioning, about 200 μm in length. Positive identification is difficult, if not impossible, in sections.

The lesions do not appear to be related to blood vessels or bronchi, and surrounding them may be focal areas of compensatory emphysema and collapse. Bronchiectasis has been recorded as a complication.

Similar lesions, ranging from the acute eosinophilic to the granulomatous, with microfilariae inconstantly present, are seen in the liver parenchyma. The lobular pattern is preserved but the portal tracts may be focally infiltrated with eosinophils.

The architecture of the lymph node or spleen is preserved. Aggregates of eosinophils are formed in the sinuses or cords and microfilariae may be present. Central eosinophilic necrosis, granulomatous lesions, and the hyaline change already described, may all be noted. The capsule is thickened and infiltrated with lymphocytes and eosinophils.

Diagnosis is confirmed by the presence of an eosinophilia, radiological changes in the lungs, and a positive filarial complement-fixation test (Donohugh, 1963).

SARCOIDOSIS

Although there is a predominance of sarcoidosis in Negroes in the United States compared to the white population, it would appear to be rare in Africa and the tropics as a whole (Wade, 1962). It is rare in Venezuela, parts of India, Singapore, Hawaii, the Philippines, Vietnam, Taiwan, and China (Present and Siltzbach, 1967). It is also rare in California, in American Indians, and Canadian Eskimos. We have seen the occasional case in West Africa, and sarcoidosis has been reported from the Zambia (Fletcher, 1966). The condition was once thought to be rare in Japan but is now known to occur. Perhaps with increasing awareness it may be found to be more common in areas where it is at present considered a rarity.

Sarcoidosis is a systemic disease in which characteristic granulomatous follicles are present in various organs. The sarcoid follicle resembles that of the tuberculous follicle without central caseation. The giant cells may contain curious star-shaped bodies (asteroid or Schaumann bodies). No organ of the body is exempt from attack. Pulmonary infiltration, enlargement of lymph nodes, spleen, liver and lesions in bone as well as in the skin, eyes, salivary, lachrimal and pituitary glands and central nervous system have been described. Primary myocardial disease may also occur (Editorial, 1972). Intradermal injection of a sterile suspension prepared from a sarcoid lesion (Kviem Test) causes a similar lesion to appear in about six weeks in patients with sarcoidosis. Positive Kviem tests, however, have also been found in patients with Crohn's disease (Editorial, 1971).

CARCINOMA OF THE NASOPHARYNX

The incidence of carcinoma of the nasopharynx is high in the Chinese and in the emigrant Chinese in Malaya, Singapore, Indonesia, Australia, and America. A lower incidence, but still greater than that in the Western world, is found in Malays, Filipinos, and Indonesians (Shanmugaratnam, 1966). It is common in Formosa and Kazakhstan (the U.S.S.R.), and is the most common cancer in males in Taiwan and the third most common in females (Yeh, 1966). Small foci of relatively high incidence are seen in Kenya (Clifford, 1965). It is uncommon in other parts of Africa, America, Sri Lanka, India, and Japan.

The cause of the high incidence is unknown. Heredity, smoke from the burning of incense in China and from wood fires in Africa, and the taking of snuff, have been considered factors (Sturton et al. 1966). No association has been noted in the Chinese in the U.S.A. with incense burning, tea drinking, or cigarette smoking (Zippin et al. 1966). Snuff is associated with a raised incidence of carcinoma of the maxillary sinus in the Bantu (Harrison, 1964). An interesting development is the discovery of a close association between high anti-EB virus titres and this tumour in patients in Africa, Sweden, France, China and America (Klein, 1971). It is possible that this tumour arising in close association with lymphoid tissue becomes thus infected. The higher titres could be accounted for by the large number of cells infected and prolonged stimulation. The association of the EB virus with infectious mononucleosis and the Burkitt tumour are discussed on pp. 255 and 502. The part that the EB virus plays in the aetiology of nasopharyngeal cancer is obscure, as areas of high frequencies of this tumour do not correspond with those of the Burkitt tumour, and the EB virus is implicated in both. Obviously some other factor or factors must be concerned. Sturton et al. (1970) have suggested that a chemical carcinogen (possibly a nitrosamine) associated with a virus infection might be the possible aetiological agents.

Clifford and Bulbrook (1966) noted that patients with nasopharyngeal carcinoma had a high excretion of oestrogen metabolites in the urine. The possibility of oestrogenization altering the columnar ciliated epithelium of the nose to squamous, and/or producing a vasomotor rhinitis, was discussed. It was suggested that the high oestrogen/androgen ratios in these patients might act as promoters in the development of nasopharyngeal carcinoma. The male preponderance (4·5:1) has, however, to be explained, and it was thought that the cyclical oestrogen excretion in women in contrast to the constant in males might mitigate the cancer-promoting effects on the nasal epithelium.

The pathology of the tumour is that of a squamous-cell or undifferentiated carcinoma. All gradations of differentiation are seen and a transitional cell type occurs. Lymphocytic infiltration may be a marked feature in the so-called lympho-epithelioma. Most neoplasms are unilateral and arise in the lateral or superoposterior walls. Occasionally the anterior wall is affected or there may be widespread dissemination in the nasopharynx. Metastases to cervical glands, bones, lung, and liver and local intracranial spread occur. An adenocarcinoma of the nasal cavity and sinuses has been described in workers exposed to wood dust possibly from hard woods such as beech and oak (Editorial, 1968).

Other malignant conditions

Sarcomas (including rhabdomyosarcoma) occasionally affect the upper respiratory tract.

Carcinoma of the larynx is not a common tumour but does occur, the recorded incidence being somewhat higher in Cali, Colombia, than in other areas of the tropics.

Carcinoma of the lung would appear to be uncommon in most areas of the tropics, with Jamaica showing an intermediate incidence between the low figures in the tropics and the high incidences found in temperate zones. It is our impression that the sex incidence tends towards equality and that histologically the adenocarcinoma is not uncommonly seen.

Malignant lymphomas not infrequently affect the mediastinum and lung, but the rarity of deposits of the Burkitt tumour in the lung is remarkable.

IO

The Haemopoietic System

ANAEMIA IN THE TROPICS

In certain rural areas of the tropics as many as 90 per cent of the population may be anaemic by the accepted normal haematological values of the Western world. In spite of the widespread anaemia, however, studies of selected population groups (soldiers, nurses, etc.) have tended to show that the optimum haematological values in tropical and temperate zones are similar (WHO, 1959). These optimum values are, however, rarely seen in hospital and outpatient practice and anaemia is one of the greatest medical problems in the tropics. This should be remembered in the planning of comprehensive health services, medical schools, etc., as more personnel and space are required for the haematological services than would be necessary in Europe.

The aetiology of anaemia in the tropics is multifactorial and the agents will vary in incidence and degree in different parts of the tropics and even in similar geographical areas. The most important factors are malaria, dietary deficiencies (iron, folic acid and, in certain areas, vitamin B_{12}), hookworm infection, other parasitic and bacterial infections, malnutrition, and pregnancy. Anaemia associated with a number of these conditions has been described in its appropriate context. In addition, in many areas abnormal haemoglobin diseases and thalassaemia may be present in high incidence.

It should be remembered that most of the anaemias that are seen in temperate climates, with the possible exception of Addisonian pernicious anaemia (which is uncommon), are present in the tropics; they are only briefly mentioned. Standard haematological techniques are not described but certain technological procedures necessary for the diagnosis of the abnormal haemoglobin diseases are given in the appendix. The conditions discussed in detail in this section are listed below. Malnutrition and anaemia is discussed on p. 674.

A. Iron-deficiency anaemia.

B. Megaloblastic anaemia.

C. Dimorphic anaemia.

D. Anaemia in pregnancy.

E. Haemolytic anaemia:

(i) The abnormal haemoglobin diseases.
(ii) The thalassaemia syndromes.
(iii) G-6-PD deficiency.
(iv) Blackwater fever.

F. The purpuras and other haemorrhagic disorders.

G. Leukaemia.

H. Blood transfusion in the tropics.

I. The spleen and the idiopathic tropical splenomegaly syndrome.

J. Tumours of lymphoreticular tissue and the Burkitt tumour.

Target cells

Excluding films obtained from persons homozygous or heterozygous for haemoglobin C, a high percentage of target cells in normal blood films has been observed in Ghana, Nigeria, and from East Africa. Thus Edington (1953) found that 61 out of 156 healthy boys aged 8–19 years had increased numbers of target cells, for which no cause could be found. Blackman (1962) noted similar findings in healthy village children in Uganda. It has been suggested by various authors that changes in serum proteins or lipids may be possible factors in the origin of these target cells, but the question is far from settled.

Eosinophils

A high eosinophil count is a classical finding in parasitic disease and occurs throughout the tropics, especially in association with helminthic infections. Ezeilo (1972) showed that eosinophil values in Zambia were higher in Africans than in Europeans and that neutropenia was common in the African and was related to diet.

Erythrocyte sedimentation rate

High erythrocyte sedimentation rates in 'healthy' individuals have been recorded from various parts of Africa, with mean values of 25–31 mm (Lassman, 1939; Courdurier and Brygoo, 1947). The reason for the increased E.S.R. is to be found in the different serum protein pattern of Africans (Deegan *et al.* 1956). The diagnostic value of a raised erythrocyte sedimentation in these circumstances requires reassessment.

IRON-DEFICIENCY ANAEMIA

The main basic causes of iron deficiency in the tropics are:
  (i) an inadequate dietary iron content;
  (ii) excessive losses of iron from the body;
  (iii) disturbance of iron metabolism by bacterial and other infections;
  (iv) interference with absorption of iron from the intestine;
  (v) increased demand—pregnancy.

There is a lack of availability of iron-containing foods (meat, eggs, and green vegetables) in some parts of the tropics, and many of the vegetable staples commonly used, such as cassava, rice, and plantain, have a low iron content. Although true dietary deficiency of iron exists in the tropics (Mitra, 1953; Stott, 1961), in many areas the daily dietary iron intake is adequate (Ramalingaswami and Patwardham, 1949; Nicol, 1952) and in most cases in which iron deficiency develops other factors, e.g. increased requirements, excessive loss, or deficient absorption or utilization, are mainly responsible (Chatterjea, 1964).

The most important cause of excessive loss of iron from the body in the tropics is undoubtedly heavy hookworm infection, the role played by excessive sweating, although invariably mentioned, is probably minimal. Bacterial and other infections are extremely common in the tropics and are an important cause of anaemia—tuberculosis being a case in point, p. 397. It seems most likely that the anaemia of infection is the result of impaired erythropoiesis and shortened survival of the red cells; it can be either microcytic and hypochromic or normocytic and normochromic. There may be toxic granules and Dohle bodies in the polymorphonuclears which show a shift to the left. Finally, some tropical diets have a high phytate and phosphate content and these substances may play some part in the aetiology of iron-deficiency anaemia as they form insoluble complexes with iron salts, thus hindering absorption (Foy and Kondi, 1956). The absorption of iron is also impaired in the malabsorption syndrome. Anaemia in pregnancy is discussed on p. 412.

The haematological findings are usually those described in temperate climates with a mean corpuscular haemoglobin concentration of less than 30 per cent and microcytosis and hypochromia evident in the peripheral blood film (Fig. 10.1). The fasting serum iron is less than 50 μg/100 ml and the plasma unsaturated iron-binding capacity is high being between 300 and 400 μg/100 ml. In the presence of other conditions, however (malnutrition, etc.), the iron-binding capacity may be low.

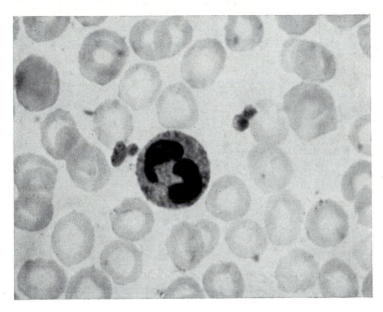

Fig. 10.1. Anaemia due to iron deficiency. The red cells show marked central pallor, and slight anisocytosis and poikilocytosis ($\times$ 1575). (*By courtesy of Dr. John Watson Williams.*)

Stainable iron is not detectable on marrow smears or sections and differentiates a true iron-deficiency anaemia from one in which there is failure to utilize iron, as occurs with infection. Recently it has become possible to detect ferritin in serum by immuno-radiometric assay and it is considered that its concentration in serum may quantatively measure the amount of storage iron available (Jacobs *et al.* 1972).

Despite a high incidence of severe chronic iron-deficiency anaemia in Africa, glossitis, stomatitis, dysphagia, and koilonychia are rare (Jacobs, 1963). In northern Nigeria, however, koilonychia occurs (Fleming, A. F., pers. corr.)

MEGALOBLASTIC ANAEMIA

Although reports of Addisonian pernicious anaemia can be found in the literature (Jayaratnam *et al.* 1967) it is rare in tropical countries where megaloblastic anaemia is much more frequently due to nutritional deficiency of folic acid or vitamin B_{12} in association with other factors (Chatterjea, 1967). Its aetiology is therefore often complex and is best exemplified by the classification given in Table 10.1

TABLE 10.1. *Aetiological classification of the megaloblastic anaemia*
(modified from Girdwood, 1963)

I. Folic-acid depletion

  1. Dietary lack:
    Nutritional megaloblastic anaemia
  2. Increased demand:
    Infancy—pregnancy—haemolytic anaemia—leukaemia—chronic infections
  3. Impaired absorption:
    Malabsorption syndromes
  4. Impaired storage:
    Possibly liver disease
  5. Interference with metabolism:
    Administration of folic-acid antagonists
    Primidone—aminopterin—Daraprim in large doses

II. Vitamin-B_{12} depletion

  1. Dietary lack:
    Nutritional megaloblastic anaemia
  2. Deviation of vitamin B_{12} by bacteria or parasites in the small intestine:
    Diphyllobothrium latum
    Bacteria in diverticula or blind loops of the small intestine
  3. Impaired absorption:
    Malabsorption syndromes
  4. Lack of intrinsic factor:
    Addisonian pernicious anaemia
    Gastrectomy

III. Others

  1. Folic-acid deficiency in association with ascorbic-acid deficiency
  2. Pyridoxine responsive megaloblastic anaemia

I. FOLIC-ACID DEPLETION

The main source of folic acid is green vegetables, but it is also present in liver and kidney. Up to 10 per cent of the folic-acid content of the diet may be lost in cooking, so in addition to diet, local cooking habits are important in influencing the incidence of folic-acid deficiency in a community. Milk is deficient in folic acid, so that any condition causing an increased demand in infants, e.g. infection, haemolytic anaemia, etc., is liable to precipitate a megaloblastic anaemia. Similarly in pregnancy the increased demands of the fetus in the last trimester may precipitate a folic-acid-deficient megaloblastic anaemia in women on a marginal intake. There is no doubt that an increased demand for folic acid occurs in haemolytic anaemias and megaloblastic change is a frequent complication—often precipitating a sudden and rapid fall in the circulating red cell mass. Chronic infection especially tuberculosis may also induce a megaloblastic anaemia. Folic-acid deficiency is common in the malabsorption syndromes. The megaloblastic anaemia associated with liver disease is discussed on p. 549. The increasing use of chemotherapeutic agents in malignant diseases in the tropics may precipitate folic-acid disease in some patients.

II. VITAMIN-B_{12} DEFICIENCY

Vitamin B_{12} is contained only in foodstuffs of animal origin and its consumption is generally low in most tropical countries. Dietary intake, however, and available body stores, are more critical in the case of folic acid than with regard to vitamin B_{12}, and this may be one reason why megaloblastic anaemia due to B_{12} deficiency is not as common as would be expected. Dietetic vitamin B_{12} deficiency has, however, been observed in patients with megaloblastic anaemia in Singapore (Wells, 1958) and in Vegans in India who exclude from their diet all foods of animal origin, including not only meat but milk, cheese, and eggs (Wokes *et al.* 1955).

Disturbances of the bacterial flora in the gut and competition by bacteria for vitamin B_{12} have been shown to be other probable causes of megaloblastic anaemia in the tropics (Foy and Kondi, 1956). The anaemia of *D. latum* infection is discussed on p. 208. Failure to absorb vitamin B_{12} is very occasionally the cause of a megaloblastic anaemia in Africa (Watson Williams and Fleming, 1966). Inadequate intrinsic factor may be congenital or related to gastric atrophy, gastric resection or neutralization by antibody. This is rare in most parts of the tropics. Other causes of vitamin B_{12} deficiency are chronic pancreatitis, the Zollinger–Ellison syndrome, drugs, coeliac disease, and tropical sprue. Intestinal diverticula are rare as is the blind loop syndrome. Lymphoreticular tumours may occasionally be a factor in the latter condition.

III. OTHERS

Occasionally a megaloblastic anaemia is seen which does not respond to either folic acid or vitamin B_{12} and responds to pyridoxine.

The diagnosis of the megaloblastic anaemias

In the tropics there is frequently a mixed picture of iron deficiency, haemolytic, and megaloblastic anaemia. Excluding Addisonian anaemia and anaemia due to gastric causes, the incidence of achlorhydria should be similar to that found in the general population. The M.C.V. may be normal or increased and the M.C.H.C. is frequently low. Leucopenia and a degree of thrombocytopenia are usual. The thrombocytopenia does not usually produce symptoms but may do so in the acute anaemia, which may occasionally result in pregnancy from folic-acid deficiency. The presence of macrocytes, especially macro-ovalocytes, anisocytosis, poikilocytosis, and large hypersegmented polymorphs in the peripheral blood film is diagnostic (Fig. 10.2), and the examination of the buffy coat may be helpful. If more than 3 per cent of the polymorphs are five-lobed a deficiency of folic acid or vitamin B_{12} should be suspected. It should be remembered, however, that the presence of hypersegmented neutrophils is by no means a substitute for serum vitamin assays if available (Johnson *et al.* 1969). Unconjugated serum bilirubin may be moderately elevated and urobilinogen increased in the urine and faeces.

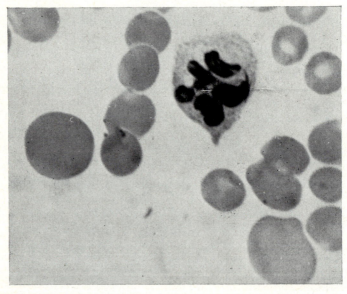

FIG. 10.2. Anaemia due to folic-acid deficiency. The red cells are filled with haemoglobin and some are very large. Anisocytosis and poikilocytosis are marked. The polymorphonuclear neutrophil has at least six lobes in its nucleus ($\times$ 1575). (*By courtesy of Dr. John Watson Williams.*)

Megaloblastic erythropoiesis will be present in marrow aspirates and is characterized by haemoglobinization of the red cell series proceeding at a faster rate than nuclear maturation. The chromatin network of the promegaloblasts and megaloblasts is more open and finer, and in more mature forms gives a finely stippled appearance. In severe cases maturation arrest may occur and many of the cells are promegaloblasts and basophilic megaloblasts. Abnormalities are present in the granulocytic series and 'giant stab' cells (metamyelocytes) are seen. This cell is large (30 μm) and has a U-shaped irregular nucleus with usually pale-blue cytoplasm with a few granules present. The megakaryocytes may be decreased and abnormally formed.

The differentiation between B_{12} and folic-acid deficiency in the absence of first-class laboratory facilities is difficult. Folic-acid therapy in B_{12} deficiency may be dangerous and precipitate the development of nervous manifestations. This is unlikely to occur in megaloblastic anaemia in the tropics, where folic-acid deficiency is usual. A therapeutic trial of $0 \cdot 4$ mg folic acid daily for 10 days will induce a haematological response in folate deficiency but not in B_{12} deficiency (Marshall and Jandl, 1960). If laboratory facilities are available B_{12} deficiency can be shown by:

(i) the assay of serum B_{12} concentration utilizing the growth requirements of *Euglena gracilis* or *Lactobacillus leichmanii*,

(ii) the use of radioactive vitamin B_{12} absorption or urinary excretion methods.

(iii) The injection of two micrograms of vitamin B_{12} and noting a maximum reticulocyte count of the 5th, 6th or 7th day. The response is directly related to the degree of anaemia. There is an increased excretion of methylmalonic acid in the urine. Intrinsic factor can be assayed in the gastric juice and an antibody may be demonstrable in the serum (Broadsheet, 1973).

Folic-acid deficiency can be confirmed by (1) assaying its activity in the serum by utilizing the growth requirements of *L. casei*, (2) utilizing folic-acid clearance tests, or (3) the histidine-loading test or the formiminoglutamic acid (FIGLU) excretion test. Folic acid is required for the conversion of histidine to glutamic acid. In its absence histidine is metabolized to FIGLU and no further catabolism occurs. FIGLU is excreted in the urine and can be estimated quantitatively by spectrophotometry. The test may give anomalous results with cirrhosis of the liver, in some cases of B_{12} deficiency, and in pregnancy (de Gruchy, 1966).

DIMORPHIC ANAEMIA

In this condition, deficiencies of iron and folic acid operate together to produce a mixed haematological picture. This type of anaemia occurs commonly throughout the tropics. The blood picture may be macrocytic or normocytic and the cells are usually, but not uniformly, hypochromic. A number of the nuclei of the polymorphonuclear leucocytes may be hypersegmented in the peripheral film (Fig. 10.3. Giant metamyelocytes may be detected in the marrow, and the nuclei of erythrocyte precursors have the finely stippled reticulin of the megaloblast (Trowell, 1943).

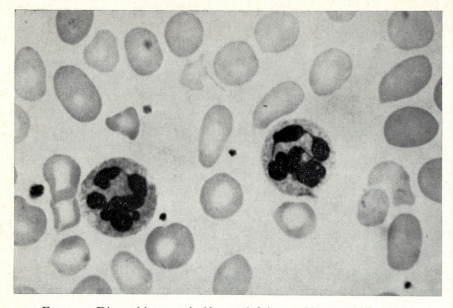

FIG. 10.3. Dimorphic anaemia (due to deficiency of iron and folic acid). Some of the red cells are hypochromic and microcytic, whilst others are normochromic and macrocytic. There is marked anisocytosis and poikilocytosis. The leucocytes have multilobed nuclei ($\times$ 1575). (*By courtesy of Dr. John Watson Williams.*)

ANAEMIA IN PREGNANCY

During pregnancy increased requirements of iron, folic acid, and vitamin B_{12} are needed to meet the demands of the foetus. The additional monthly requirements of iron, for example, rise from about 30 mg in the first trimester to 115 mg in the last. Moreover, anorexia in early pregnancy, and the hypochlorhydria commonly found, further affect the intake and absorption of the essential haemopoietic factors.

In the tropics a complex haematological pattern may be found, as in addition to the factors mentioned above, protein deficiency, parasitic, and bacterial infections are common. Chronic hepatic and renal disease may also complicate the picture. Obstetric haemorrhage is also common and the presence of a preceding anaemia greatly increases the risk of peripheral circulatory shock.

Anaemia in pregnancy is extremely common and accounts for 20–40 per cent of maternal deaths in India, lack of folic acid or vitamin B_{12}, or both, being important factors in its aetiology; dimorphic anaemia also occurs (Devi, 1966). In Hong Kong, on the other hand, iron-deficiency anaemia is by far the most common type seen and megaloblastic anaemia is rare (Todd and Kau, 1965). Anaemia in pregnancy is also a common cause of mortality in West Africa (Lawson and Stewart, 1967) and presents features of interest. Megaloblastic change is present in the marrow of over 90 per cent of patients and folic-acid deficiency has been confirmed by folic-acid assays. There is no deficiency of vitamin B_{12}. Iron deficiency is not a factor of importance as stainable intracellular deposits of iron pigment can be demonstrated in marrow smears (Harrison, 1967). In over 75 per cent of severely anaemic patients a haemolytic process with a raised reticulocyte index is found. Hepatomegaly and splenomegaly are common. It is considered in Ibadan that this haemolytic process is indirectly related to *P. falciparum* infection. It usually responds well to antimalarial and folic-acid therapy. A small number of patients may not respond and prednisolone has been found helpful in therapy (Fleming and Allan, 1969). Thus in parts of West and East Africa a megaloblastic anaemia due to folic-acid deficiency with evidence of a haemolytic process is the common type of severe anaemia seen in pregnancy. The glomerular filtration rate is increased in pregnancy and renal tubular function is altered. The mean folate clearance is also much raised in normal pregnant women (Fleming, 1972). Iron deficiency would not appear to be an important aetiological agent. Folic-acid deficiency usually manifests itself in the third trimester or in the puerperium and it may cause an acute and sudden drop in the haemoglobin in a patient who has been relatively well. Blood transfusion may be necessary as a life-saving measure (Fullerton and Turner, 1962). The effect of folic-acid deficiency in the abnormal haemoglobin diseases in pregnancy is discussed on p. 436. The cause of the folic-acid deficiency is most probably a combination of increased demands of the fetus, low dietary intake and, in malarious areas, increased haemolysis due to *P. falciparum*. Very occasionally there is evidence of impaired absorption (Fleming, A., personal communication) and further investigations are required on the metabolism of folic acid in pregnancy. In certain parts of the tropics anaemia in pregnancy may be seasonal depending upon the availability of local foodstuff (Fleming, 1970). Haemoglobin A_2 has been reported as raised in pregnancy by some authors but not by others (Benster and Cauchi, 1970). With severe folic-acid deficiency thrombocytopenia and a haemorrhagic diathesis may occur. Although vitamin-B_{12} deficiency has been described in pregnancy in India it is rare in Africa.

The necropsy findings in the megaloblastic type of anaemia are those of severe anaemia with pulmonary oedema. The spleen is usually enlarged and meaty-red on section. Histologically the splenic pulp is congested and megaloblasts may be distinguishable. Erythrophagocytosis may be noted in the histiocytes of the reticulo-endothelial system. In our experience, granules of iron pigment are usually present in the periportal parenchymal cells of the liver, with small amounts in the marrow and spleen.

HAEMOLYTIC ANAEMIA

Haemolytic anaemia is extremely common in the tropics, and a classification is given in Table 10.2. Only the conditions shown in heavy print are discussed in any detail in this section. Dacie (1974) has reviewed the subject of the hereditary haemolytic anaemias.

TABLE 10.2. *Classification of the haemolytic anaemias of importance in the tropics*

1. Hereditary intracorpuscular defects:
   Abnormal haemoglobins—thalassaemia—glucose-6-phosphate dehydrogenase deficiency—hereditary spherocytosis—hereditary elliptocytosis
2. Infectious agents:
   Malaria—kala-azar—toxoplasmosis—Bartonellosis—clostridial infections—cholera—typhoid—tuberculosis—relapsing fever—viral infections—pyaemia
3. **Tropical splenomegaly syndrome:**
   Hypersplenism
4. **Blackwater fever**
5. Secondary haemolytic anaemia:
   Tumours of lymphoreticular tissue—disseminated carcinomatosis—hepatic and renal disease
6. **Transfusion reactions including haemolytic disease of the newborn**
7. Vegetable and animal poisons
8. Physical agents
9. Chemical agents:
   Many drugs
10. Vitamin deficiencies:
    Vitamin B_{12}—folic acid—vitamin C
11. Idiopathic acquired haemolytic anaemia
12. Paroxysmal cold haemoglobinuria
13. Puruvate kinase (PK) deficiency
14. Autoimmune haemolytic anaemia (Dacie, 1970)

Haptoglobins

Haptoglobins are a family of plasma-proteins which bind haemoglobin, they constitute a major portion of the α_2-globulins. The most striking property of haptoglobins is their ability to combine with haemoglobin liberated into the plasma. When intravascular release of haemoglobin is continuous, as in many haemolytic anaemias, e.g. sickle-cell anaemia and thalassaemia major, the haptoglobin levels in the plasma fall considerably and may even be undetectable. Smithies (1955) found that three haptoglobin patterns could be distinguished in human populations. They are designated Hp 1-1, Hp 2-1 and Hp 2-2 as shown on starch gel electrophoresis. Several variations in the usual Hp 2-1 and Hp 2-2 electrophoretic patterns have been described. The molecule consists of two dissimilar polypeptide chains, the alpha and beta linked by disulphide bonds. The beta chains appear to be identical in all three phenotypes whereas amino acid substitutions may occur in the alpha chains. Normal values of haptoglobin per 100 ml of plasma have been reported to be between 65 and 200 mg. As the hapto-globin-haemoglobin complex is readily removed from the circulation, the levels of haptoglobin will depend on the presence or absence of haemolysis as the presence of free haemoglobin in serum rapidly leads to its (hapo-globin) disappearance. Haemoglobin cannot be demonstrated in the urine until the serum haptoglobin has been saturated. A fall in the haptoglobin content of the serum may indicate increased red cell destruction. The human haptoglobins have recently been reviewed by Ofosu (1972). A surprising finding in the tropics has been the extremely low levels of haptoglobins in some persons with no apparent disease (Allison *et al.* 1958; Arends and Gallango, 1962; Bennett, 1961).

THE ABNORMAL HAEMOGLOBINS AND THE ABNORMAL HAEMOGLOBIN DISEASES

In few subjects in medicine have such rapid advances been made in knowledge in the last two decades as in the field of abnormal haemoglobins. The subject has been extensively reviewed by WHO (1972), Stoller, (1974), Lehman, (1974). Although sickle-cell anaemia was described in 1910 it was not until 1949 that the inheritance of the S gene was understood. In the same year sickle-cell anaemia was shown to be a 'molecular disease', the electric charge on the molecule differing from that of normal haemoglobin. The chemical structure of the haemoglobin molecule was defined in 1957 and the chemical structure of many of the abnormal haemoglobins is now known. It should be realized that not all abnormal haemoglobins produce disease, and the abnormal haemoglobin diseases can be defined as conditions in which there is an inherited abnormality of the haemoglobin, part or all of the normal haemoglobulin in the erythrocyte being replaced by an abnormal variant with the clinical manifestations of a disease process. The most important abnormal haemoglobins in the tropics are haemoglobin S, C, D, and E. Haemoglobin H and Barts are also important but as they are asso-ciated with thalassaemia (p. 453) they are described when that condition is considered. It should be noted that the heterozygous inheritance of thalas-saemia with other abnormal haemoglobins is also common. Fetal haemo-globin and haemoglobin A_2 may be affected in the abnormal haemoglobin diseases so they are described in some detail. The laboratory techniques required in the diagnosis of these conditions are described in the Appendix. For postgraduate students interested in the subject brief notes are given on the less common haemoglobin variants, including the 'unstable' haemo-globin diseases.

The structure of normal haemoglobin

In 1957 the haemoglobin molecule was described as an ellipsoid structure made up of two identical half molecules each containing two haem groups and two coiled, chemically-different polypeptide chains, the alpha (α) and beta (β) chains (Rhinesmith et al. 1958). These chains were shown to be made up of sequences of amino acids, the α chain containing 141 and the β chain 146 (Fig. 10.4). Normal adult haemoglobin can thus be represented as $\alpha_2\beta_2$.

A second minor fraction of normal haemoglobin which usually comprises about 2·5 per cent of the total was later discovered and named A_2. In this fraction the α chain was similar to that found in normal adult haemoglobin (A) but the β chain differed in its amino-acid composition and was named delta (δ) so A_2 could be represented as $\alpha_2\delta_2$ (p. 425). Another fraction, A_3, has been described but is now thought to be senescent molecules of normal haemoglobin.

In addition to A and A_2 a third haemoglobin is normally found in the new-born child in high concentration (50–80 per cent) and is known as fetal (F). It differs from haemoglobin A and A_2 in the β and δ chains respectively and can be represented as $\alpha_2\gamma_2$. The γ chain contains 146 amino-acid residues and is closely similar to the β chain of haemoglobin A. These three normal haemoglobins can be represented as:

Normal adult haemoglobin (A) $\alpha_2\beta_2$
Normal adult haemoglobin (A_2) $\alpha_2\delta_2$
Normal fetal haemoglobin (F) $\alpha_2\gamma_2$

The nomenclature of the abnormal haemoglobins

Sickle-cell anaemia was first described in 1910 by Herrick in a West Indian youth. In 1949 Pauling and his associates demonstrated that sickle-cell haemoglobin differed in its electrophoretic behaviour from normal haemoglobin. Shortly afterwards Itano and Neel (1950) described a second abnormal haemoglobin (C) which differed in its electrophoretic behaviour from both normal (A) and S haemoglobin. Many other haemoglobin variants

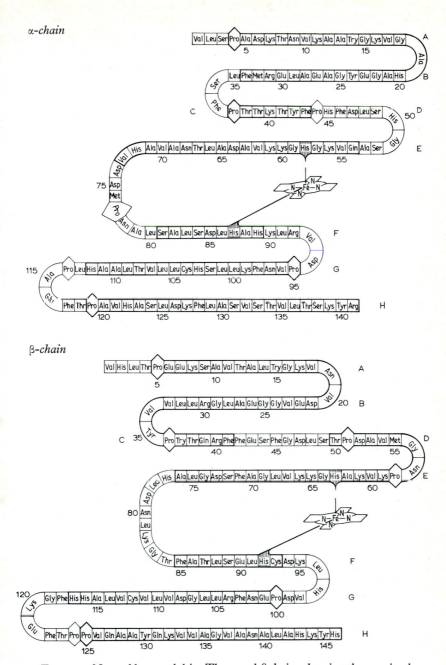

α-*chain*

β-*chain*

Fig. 10.4. Normal haemoglobin. The α and β chains showing the proximal and distal histidine residues and the turns in the chains. Helical portions are thickly boxed. (*By courtesy of North Holland Publishing Co.*)

were described in the next few years and the alphabet down to Q has now been utilized. Ingram (1957, 1959) illustrated by 'finger printing' techniques* that in the abnormal haemoglobins S and C there were specific amino-acid substitutions in the β chain of normal haemoglobin; valine and lysine being substituted respectively for glutamic acid in the sixth position, and these haemoglobins can be represented thus:

Haemoglobin S: $\alpha_2^A\beta_2^S$ or $\alpha_2\beta_2^S$ or $\alpha_2\beta_2^{6VAL}$ or $\alpha_2\beta_2^{6GLU\text{-}VAL}$

Haemoglobin C: $\alpha_2^A\beta_2^C$ or $\alpha_2\beta_2^C$ or $\alpha_2\beta_2^{6LYS}$ or $\alpha_2\beta_2^{6GLU\text{-}LYS}$

Glutamic acid is negatively charged, valine is neutral, and lysine is positive. In an electric field, therefore, in an alkaline buffer solution (usually at pH 8·6), normal adult haemoglobin (A) having a greater negative charge (glutamic acid) moves more rapidly towards the positive pole (anode), haemoglobin S (neutral valine) less rapidly, and haemoglobin C (positive lysine) least rapidly. Other haemoglobins have been found which move more rapidly than A and haemoglobins are termed 'slow' or 'fast' depending on whether they have a greater or lesser positive charge respectively than A. The substitution of different amino acids of similar charge in either the α or β chains of haemoglobin may thus give a similar pattern on paper electrophoresis. Haemoglobin D, for instance, has a similar mobility to S and a number of haemoglobins which move as D have been found to have a differing amino-acid composition.

A recommended nomenclature was agreed at the Tenth International congress of Haematology in Stockholm in 1964. The alphabetical nomenclature already in use was retained. Haemoglobins have been named from A to Q (excluding B, for which S is used). The remaining letters of the alphabet should not be used and new haemoglobins should be named after localities.

Some letters describe a group of haemoglobins with similar electrophoretic patterns. If the abnormal polypeptide chain has been identified it can be indicated thus: Hb Dα or Hb Dβ. The place of origin should also be noted, for example Hb Gα Philadelphia; Hb Gα Norfolk; Jb Gβ San Jose; Hb Gβ Accra.

Haemoglobin A_2 ($\alpha_2\delta_2$) and F ($\alpha_2\gamma_2$) have also abnormal forms and the nomenclature follows a similar pattern, e.g. Hb $A_2\delta$ Flatbush, showing that the abnormality is in the delta chain, and Hb Fα Norfolk, showing that the abnormality is in the α chain.

---

*'Finger printing' consists essentially of tryptic digestion of the globin moiety of haemoglobin followed by electrophoretic and chromatographic analyses on paper. Characteristic peptide patterns are produced for individual haemoglobins and are compared with the peptide pattern of normal haemoglobin. The abnormal peptide can then be eluted and the amino-acid composition determined.

The chemical structure of many abnormal haemoglobins is now known and, if so desired, haemoglobin C could be designated thus: $\alpha_2\beta_2^{6\text{GLU-LYS}}$, showing that lysine has replaced glutamic acid in the sixth position in the β chain, or more simply: $\alpha_2\beta_2^{6\text{LYS}}$.

A haemoglobin may have both abnormal α and β chains and these 'hybrids' should be designated by the names of the abnormal haemoglobins with which they share their abnormality. A haemoglobin may have an abnormal α chain identical with the α chain found in haemoglobin I and a β chain identical with that found in haemoglobin C, and would be represented thus: Hb $\alpha_2^I\beta_2^C$ or Hb I/C.

The inheritance of the abnormal haemoglobins

In 1949 it was shown by Neel that the S gene, i.e., the gene responsible for the production of sickle-cell haemoglobin (S), was inherited in the autosomal Mendelian pattern and in its homozygous expression (SS), in which no normal adult haemoglobin (A) is found, was responsible for a severe congenital haemolytic anaemia, sickle-cell anaemia; whereas in the heterozygote (AS) it resulted in the relatively harmless sickle-cell trait in which both normal and sickle-cell haemoglobin are present in the erythrocyte.

The mode of inheritance can be shown as follows:

FATHER		MOTHER	
A S		A S	
AA	AS	AS	SS
Normal	S Trait	S Trait	S Anaemia

Later, the dissociation–reassociation studies of Itano and Singer (1958) and Itano and Robinson (1959) were of the greatest importance. Haemoglobin in mild acid solution dissociates into sub-units which reassociate on neutralization.

If two abnormal haemoglobins are mixed and treated in this way the result of the interaction depends upon the polypeptide chains affected. If a haemoglobin with an abnormal α chain (I) and one with an abnormal β chain (S) are so treated, two new molecular species are formed:

$$\alpha_2^A\beta_2^S + \alpha_2^I\beta_2^A = \alpha_2^A\beta_2^A \text{ Normal} + \alpha_2^I\beta_2^S \text{ Hybrid}$$

If, however, two haemoglobins with abnormalities in the same chain are treated (e.g. S and C) no doubly abnormal haemoglobin is formed:

$$\alpha_2^A\beta_2^S + \alpha_2^A\beta_2^C, \text{ no change}$$

This is a relatively simple method of determining which polypeptide chain in an unknown variant is abnormal.

Itano and his collaborators (1959) postulated that the alpha and beta chains were synthesized under independent genetic control so that double heterozygosity at the α and β loci should result in four different haemoglobins in the same individual.

Subsequently patients have been described with four different haemoglobins present in the peripheral blood (Atwater *et al.* 1960). We have ourselves seen examples in Nigeria.

The rather complicated inheritance which occurs is best exemplified in Table 10.3. If the father's gene constitution is $\alpha^A \alpha^G / \beta^A \beta^A$ and the mother's $\alpha^A \alpha^A / \beta^A \beta^C$ the possible offspring are shown in Table 10.3.

TABLE 10.3

Genotype*	Phenotype*	Haemoglobin
$\alpha^A \alpha^A / \beta^A \beta^A$	$\alpha_2^A \beta_2^A$	A
$\alpha^A \alpha^A / \beta^A \beta^C$	$\alpha_2^A \beta_2^A : \alpha_2^A \beta_2^C$	A+C
$\alpha^A \alpha^G / \beta^A \beta^A$	$\alpha_2^A \beta_2^A : \alpha_2^G \alpha_2^A$	A+G
$\alpha^A \alpha^G / \beta^A \beta^C$	$\alpha_2^A \beta_2^A : \alpha_2^A \beta_2^C : \ \alpha_2^G \beta_2^A \ \ \alpha_2^G \beta_2^C$	A+C+G+hybrid GC

Genotype = total genetic make-up of an individual. *Phenotype* = the information derived from the examination of a single individual without reference to family data.

Combinations of abnormal α and β chains are, however, not common and in West Africa where there is a high incidence of haemoglobins S and C and where G, K, H, P, and possibly E, occur in low incidence, patients with this type of inheritance do not present a clinical problem of practical importance —although such patients are occasionally seen.

It should be noted that the γ and δ chains are also under separate genetic control, so there are four separate structural loci on the chromosomes responsible for the synthesis of the α, β, γ and δ chains respectively and forming normal haemoglobin (A) $\alpha_2 \beta_2$, haemoglobin (A$_2$) $\alpha_2 \delta_2$, and fetal haemoglobin (F) $\alpha_2 \gamma_2$.

The α and β loci would appear to be widely separated but the δ and β loci are closely linked and this has genetic implications which are discussed when Hb Lepore is considered.

The classification of the abnormal haemoglobins

The abnormal haemoglobins have been classified in the past according to their mobility on paper electrophoresis at pH 8·6. This is an unsatisfactory method of classification as there are many haemoglobins with a similar mobility, for instance ten types of haemoglobin G have been described and haemoglobins with abnormalities in either the α, β, or γ chains have been noted.

As the chemical structure of the polypeptide chains of many of the abnormal haemoglobins is now known, an accurate chemical classification is evolving and they are probably best classified as α-, β-, δ-, or γ-chain variants of the normal haemoglobins with their specific amino-acid abnormality designated (Finch and Perutz, 1974).

It should be noted that if the abnormality is in the α chain all three normal haemoglobins, A ($\alpha_2\beta_2$), A$_2$ ($\alpha_2\delta_2$), and F ($\alpha_2\gamma_2$), will be affected. For example in the heterozygous inheritance of haemoglobin I the following haemoglobins will be present

$$A \text{ and } AI: \alpha_2\beta_2, \alpha_2^I\beta_2$$
$$A_2 \text{ and } A_2I: \alpha_2\delta_2, \alpha_2^I\delta_2$$
$$F \text{ and } FI: \alpha_2\gamma_2, \alpha_2^I\gamma_2$$

If the abnormality is in the β, δ, or γ chain only haemoglobin A, A$_2$, or F will be respectively affected.

α-chain variants are not common and do not present a problem of any importance in the tropics.

As it is unlikely that facilities for determining the chemical composition of the polypeptide chains will be available in the great majority of laboratories in the tropics and as, in our experience, paper electrophoresis of the haemoglobin in combination with routine haematological investigations and family studies are adequate for most practical diagnostic purposes in areas where abnormal haemoglobins are found in high incidence, no attempt is made to include a chemical classification as outlined above.

The electrophoretic mobility of the more important haemoglobins in alkaline buffer is shown in Table 10.4.

TABLE 10.4. *The mobility of haemoglobins on paper electrophoresis in alkaline buffer (pH 8·6)*

	'Slow'		'Fast'	
Cathode −	CE:O:DS:LPH:G:FA$_2$:	AM:	K:JN Barts:HI	Anode +

The diagnosis of the abnormal haemoglobins and the abnormal haemoglobin diseases

From a consideration of the electrophoretic mobility of the abnormal haemoglobins shown in Table 10.4 above, it will be seen that haemoglobins C and E, D and S, and L, P, and H, move closely together. In addition, F, H, and Bart's are not easily detected and variants of A$_2$ cannot be detected, on paper electrophoresis. Further laboratory procedures are therefore required for their diagnosis and, as the diagnosis of the individual haemoglobin is discussed when their pathology is described in the following pages, it was considered that some understanding of these more involved techniques was necessary prior to a consideration of the pathology. This is the reason why, contrary to our usual procedure, the general methods advised in the diagnosis of the abnormal haemoglobin diseases are described in this portion of the text.

In general, heterozygotes inheriting an abnormal haemoglobin and haemoglobin A are usually symptomless, haemoglobin S and the 'unstable' haemoglobin diseases being exceptions. Not all abnormal haemoglobins cause disease. The homozygote for haemoglobin G Accra is symptomless and was discovered on follow up of a routine survey in which paper electrophoresis was employed and the presence of a 'slow' haemoglobin noted. These symptomless bearers of an abnormal haemoglobin are usually detected on field surveys or as an incidental finding on routine laboratory examination. The methods of diagnosing a 'symptomless' abnormal haemoglobin are given in paragraph 3 of Table 10.5.

An abnormal haemoglobin disease may occur in an individual homozygous for an abnormal haemoglobin gene, e.g. SS or CC, or in a doubly heterozygous individual, e.g. SC or SD, or in one who has inherited the gene

TABLE 10.5. *Methods employed in the diagnosis of an abnormal haemoglobin disease*

1. History and clinical examination

2. Evidence of a haemolytic anaemia:
   (i) Reticulocyte count
   (ii) Serum bilirubin estimation (unconjugated raised)
   (iii) Urinary and faecal urobilinogen (increased)
   (iv) Serum iron (raised)
   (v) Coombs' test (negative)
   (vi) Osmotic fragility (decreased)
   (vii) Red-cell survival studies (shortened life span)
   (viii) Peripheral blood film (presence of target cells, inclusion bodies, or intra-erythrocytic crystals and abnormal forms (sickled, etc.) suggest the presence of an abnormal haemoglobin)
   (ix) Incubation with brilliant cresyl blue

3. Haemoglobin analyses:
   (i) Sickling test (Appendix)
   (ii) Estimation of fetal haemoglobin (slide test and alkali denaturation)
   (iii) Solubility studies (to differentiate S and D)
   (iv) Electrophoretic, chromatographic and 'finger printing' techniques

4. Family studies

responsible for an abnormal haemoglobin from one parent and a gene responsible for a haematological disorder from the other, e.g. E-thalassaemia, S and congenital spherocytic anaemia.

A patient suffering from an abnormal haemoglobin disease exhibits primarily the signs and symptoms of a haemolytic anaemia which will be diagnosed on routine laboratory investigations. The general methods advised in the diagnosis of the abnormal haemoglobin diseases are outlined in Table 10.5.

History and clinical examination

In areas of high S incidence the history is most important. A history of 'joint pains' associated perhaps with 'yellow eyes' and dark urine and an examination of the blood smear may be presumptive evidence of sickle-cell anaemia or sickle-cell disease (p. 432). We have had patients referred to us with the correct diagnosis based only on the history and clinical examination prior to haematological investigation.

An examination of the peripheral blood film, a sickling test and electrophoresis of the haemoglobin are usually sufficient to allow of a diagnosis being made. Details of the sickling test are given in the Appendix and electrophoresis is discussed below, with brief comments on additional tests which may be required. Screening for sickle-cell disease was reviewed in *British Medical Journal* (1974).

Incubation with brilliant cresyl blue

If haemoglobin H is suspected (p. 458) the erythrocytes should be incubated with brilliant cresyl blue to detect the presence or absence of inclusions (Appendix, p. 768).

Estimation of fetal haemoglobin

The staining of a peripheral blood film for the presence of fetal haemoglobin reveals whether fetal haemoglobin, if present, is distributed uniformly or at random in the red blood cells. The former distribution is found in the condition 'hereditary persistence of fetal haemoglobin' (p. 426). In other conditions with raised F the distribution is random.

The amount of F present can also be determined by estimating the alkali resistant haemoglobin in the blood (Appendix, p. 766).

Solubility studies

S is much less soluble than other haemoglobins and this allows differentiation from haemoglobin D, which has the same electrophoretic mobility.

Electrophoresis

When an electric potential difference is passed across a solution of haemoglobin, the molecules move toward the attracting electrode. Since the iso-electric point of haemoglobin (pH 6·8) is below pH 8·6, in a buffer of this alkalinity they will move towards the positive pole (anode) and in acid buffer (pH 6) towards the negative (cathode). A supporting medium to carry the haemoglobin is utilized and this may be paper, cellulose acetate, starch gels, or starch blocks. There are many variables in this technique, especially in the tropics, one of the most difficult requirements to obtain being a constant voltage, and resort may have to be made to dry batteries in series. Known controls are necessary with every processing.

Paper electrophoresis

This technique had already been discussed when the classification was considered. Although starch-gel electrophoresis at pH 8·6 is now the method of choice, paper electrophoresis is still a useful rapid screening procedure in areas where abnormal haemoglobins are found in high incidence.

Paper electrophoresis in acid buffer (pH 6·0) may separate haemoglobins which move closely together in alkaline buffer.

Starch-gel electrophoresis

This is particularly valuable in separating haemoglobin A from F and for detecting A_2. It is becoming the electrophoretic method of choice.

Starch-block electrophoresis

In contrast to the gel, whole grains of starch are present to which little of the haemoglobin adsorbs. Consequently a large proportion of the haemoglobin in a particular band can be recovered for further chemical investigations if required.

Chromatography and 'finger printing'

Column chromatography using various resins has been employed to obtain fractions of haemoglobin variants. As a diagnostic procedure it has largely been superseded by the 'finger printing' technique, details of which are given by Lehmann and Huntsman (1966). Antibodies have also been produced to the various polypeptide chains and have been utilized in immuno-electrophoretic techniques (Boerma and Huisman, 1964). These procedures are unlikely to be available in many laboratories in the tropics and are not discussed further.

Family studies

Ideally, a patient should never be diagnosed as homozygous for a gene responsible for an abnormal haemoglobin disease unless the electrophoretic diagnosis has been confirmed by a family study.

Haemoglobin A_2 and abnormalities in the δ chain

Haemoglobin A_2 is a normal constituent of human haemoglobin and constitutes about $2 \cdot 5$ per cent of the total. The molecule consists of four haem groups and two pairs of polypeptide chains the α and δ chains and is represented as $\alpha_2\delta_2$. The δ chain, containing 146 amino-acid residues, is very similar to the β, differing in only ten amino acids, and the β and δ loci are closely linked. Small amounts are normally seen in cord blood by starch-block electrophoresis and by immuno-electrophoretic techniques. Abnormal A_2 haemoglobin occurs in the α-chain abnormal haemoglobin diseases. A_2 may be split up into two fractions in the Negro, A_2 and A_2^1 (B_2), with an abnormality in the δ chain in the latter (Huisman *et al.* 1961). An abnormal A_2 haemoglobin has been described, haemoglobin A_2 Flatbush (Ranney *et al.* 1963) and two abnormal δ chains have been seen in one individual, (Huisman and Lee, 1965).

In the hereditary persistence of fetal haemoglobin, A_2 is reduced in the heterozygote and absent in the homozygote. In β thalassaemia the A_2 levels are variable, on occasion being increased and in others depressed.

In α thalassaemia small amounts of haemoglobin δ_4 may be present at birth and it is occasionally seen in the adult.

On paper or starch-gel electrophoresis in alkaline pH A_2 and E run together. A_2, however, rarely exceeds 5 per cent of the total haemoglobin, whereas E in the heterozygote usually forms 30–40 per cent. Ultimately the only satisfactory method of differentiation is 'finger printing'.

A_2 is not usually seen if a barbitone buffer is used and Tris buffer is to be preferred (Lehmann and Huntsman, 1966). If A_2^1 is present the A_2 band on starch-gel electrophoresis is duplicated.

Fetal haemoglobin and abnormalities in the γ chain

In young embryos in the first few months of fetal life, two haemoglobins are present which differ from A, A_2, and F.

At about the third month, these haemoglobins disappear and fetal haemoglobin is formed ($\alpha_2\gamma_2$). The α chain is identical to that found in normal adult A ($A_2\gamma_2$) and A_2 ($\alpha_2\delta_2$) haemoglobin. The γ chain contains 146 amino-acid residues and resembles the β chain of haemoglobin A. Before birth the rate of γ-chain production decreases and β- and δ-chain production is initiated. At birth, fetal haemoglobin forms 50–80 per cent of the total, being higher in prematures. Three minor components are also present (Karaklis and Fessas, 1963). It gradually decreases during the first 3 months of life, reaching about 1 per cent by the end of 1 year, and about 0·4 per cent is present in the normal adult, amounts of 1 per cent or over being considered abnormal.

It is increased in conditions in which there is impairment of normal adult haemoglobin synthesis such as is seen in the congenital haemolytic anaemias including the abnormal haemoglobin diseases. It may also be increased in leukaemia, aplastic anaemia and in pregnancy. There is also a hereditary condition in which F is increased: 'hereditary persistence of high fetal haemoglobin' (see below).

Abnormal fetal haemoglobins are found in α-chain variants and abnormalities may also occur in the γ chain. Abnormal F haemoglobins are Alexandra (Fessas *et al.* 1959), Aegina (Fessas *et al.* 1961), haemoglobin Roma (Silvestroni and Bianco, 1963), Texas (Schnieder *et al.* 1964), and F γ Galveston.

The detection of fetal haemoglobin

Fetal haemoglobin is denatured more slowly by alkali than other haemoglobins, and Singer *et al.* (1951) have described a useful and rapid test for its detection (Appendix, p. 766). It is, however, only accurate when there is more than 2 per cent fetal haemoglobin present. On paper electrophoresis A and F are not easily separated but on starch-gel electrophoresis F travels well ahead of A, with haemoglobin S behind.

The intracellular distribution of F can be studied on blood smears by the acid dilution technique of Kleihauer *et al.* (1957).

Ultraviolet spectroscopy can also be used.

The hereditary persistence of fetal haemoglobin

This condition was first described in Ghana by Edington and Lehmann (1955) in a patient whose haemoglobin on paper electrophoresis appeared to be predominantly S but who exhibited no haematological abnormalities. Subsequent family studies revealed that one parent was heterozygous for haemoglobin S and that the other had a high level of fetal haemoglobin in the peripheral blood but S was absent. It was thought that this might be due to the presence of an unusual thalassaemia-like gene.

Similar cases have been described and are now thought to be due to the double heterozygous inheritance of the S gene and of a gene responsible for the production of high fetal haemoglobin.

The 'High F' gene is inherited as a Mendelian dominant and is thought to be closely linked, or allelic, to the haemoglobin β-chain locus. It impairs the switch over of the production of γ to β and δ chains in the fetus and thus inhibits synthesis of Hb A and A_2, with the consequent persistence of haemoglobin F ($\alpha_2\gamma_2$) into adult life. F may form up to 40 per cent of the haemoglobin in the heterozygote, the remainder being normal adult haemoglobin (A and A_2).

Hereditary persistance of fetal haemoglobin occurs in about $0 \cdot 1$ per cent of American Negroes and the incidence is probably the same in parts of West Africa, and has also been seen in Mediterranean areas, Greece, Switzerland, Jamaica, and East Africa.

Heterozygotes and homozygotes are asymptomatic. The homozygotes show only fetal haemoglobin (Baglioni, 1963).

Individuals doubly heterozygous for the high F and S, C, or thalassaemia genes, have been reported.

The high F gene suppresses the production of β and δ chains, so with S and F there may be little A or A_2 present. The amount of S is enhanced (presumably because its abnormal β chain is unaffected and has a greater avidity for α chains than the γ of F) and may form 80 per cent of the total haemoglobin. On paper electrophoresis the pattern resembles SS. Clinically, however, the patient is little affected. Haemoglobin F is also present in a uniform pattern in the erythrocytes in a peripheral blood smear, in contrast to its random distribution in sickle-cell anaemia (SS) and other haemoglobinopathies, and starch-gel electrophoresis reveals the presence of F. This illustrates again that homozygosity should never be accepted from laboratory tests and that family studies are essential. The presence of F haemoglobin in the erythrocyte is considered to inhibit the sickling properties of S, as it does not interact when S precipitates *in vitro* and accounts for the mild symptomatology (Brown *et al.* 1972). Similarly, FC may resemble on electrophoresis CC, and haemoglobin F-β-thalassaemia is a relatively mild condition.

The relationship between haemoglobin F and malaria is discussed on p. 468.

Haemoglobin S

The S gene is inherited as a Mendelian dominant characteristic and, as are the other abnormal haemoglobins, is an allele of the gene responsible for the production of normal haemoglobin (A). The abnormality is in the β chain and glutamic acid in the sixth position is replaced by valine ($\alpha_2\beta_2^{6VAL}$).

The red blood cells containing S, when deprived of oxygen assume filamentous, sickle, holly, or oat-leaf shapes, and sludging of blood with blockage of vessels may occur. In the heterozygote (AS) the usually harmless sickle-cell trait is present, but in the homozygote (SS) a severe form of congenital haemolytic anaemia complicated by infarctive lesions—sickle-cell anaemia—occurs.

Numerous individuals have been seen doubly heterozygous for S and other abnormal haemoglobins, and S has been described in combination with 'high fetal' haemoglobin and thalassaemia. The clinical and pathological effects of these doubly abnormal heterozygotes are described when sickle-cell anaemia is considered on p. 431.

The sickling mechanism

It should be noted that sickling of the erythrocytes has been reported by at least two groups of workers in the presence of haemoglobin I and Barts with no haemoglobin S present (Thompson *et al.* 1965). Sickling also occurs in haemoglobin C. This, however, is rare. In the presence of S haemoglobin, sickling of the red blood cell occurs when the oxygen tension is lowered, the protein of the haemoglobin precipitating to form 'tactoids' or paracrystalline aggregates of low solubility. With reoxygenation the majority of erythrocytes resume their normal shape. This physicochemical change is utilized in the 'sickling test' when chemical-reducing agents are mixed with a drop of peripheral blood under a sealed coverslip to reduce the oxygen tension and thus induce sickling. Bacterial cultures can be used in a similar manner (Robinson, 1945).

The degree of oxygen desaturation necessary to produce sickling depends not only upon the proportion of S haemoglobin in the erythrocyte but also upon the type of inherited haemoglobin in the heterozygote. In the sickle-cell trait (AS), in which the proportion of S varies from 20 to 40 per cent, sickling does not occur until the oxygen tension falls to 10 mm Hg, in the double heterozygote for S and F (SF), where S may represent 70 per cent or more of the haemoglobin, at 30 mm Hg, but in sickle-cell haemoglobin C disease (SC), where S represents only 50 per cent of the haemoglobin, sickling may occur at a tension of 50 mm Hg.

It has also been observed that with lowered oxygen tension the viscosity of the blood, if sickle-cell haemoglobin is present, decreases and the rate of change has been noted during deoxygenation (Charache and Conley, 1964). In sickle-cell anaemia (SS) there is a rapid increase in viscosity, SF shows a slower increase and AS slower still. SJ has been shown to behave as AS. This is important when the pathology of sickle-cell disease is considered, as blockage of blood vessels and infarctive lesions most commonly occur in these conditions in which there is a rapid increase in the viscosity of the blood. As stress may precipitate *in vivo* sickling, Djabanor (1972) studied the effects of adrenalin, noradrenalin and hydrocortisone on the sickling process *in vitro* and found that they did not have any significant effect. On the other hand sickling may be prevented by urea, cyanate and carbamyl phosphate and trials of oral urea as a prophylactic are being undertaken. It can be stated therefore that the pathological effects of the sickling phenomenon in the erythrocyte depends upon the presence, and to a certain extent the concentration, of S haemoglobin, the duration of exposure of the red cell to reduced oxygen pressure, the type of the associated haemoglobin, and also upon the pH of the surrounding medium, as sickling is enhanced in an acid medium. Stasis will lead to acidosis and therefore favour the formation of sickle cells. It should be noted that sickle-cell haemoglobin is distributed fairly uniformly throughout the red-cell population.

The sickle-cell trait (AS)

The S gene is widely distributed but its highest incidence is found in tropical Africa, where the incidence of the trait in different tribes may vary from 12 to 40 per cent. The reason for this high incidence is discussed on p. 466.

It is present in the descendants of West Africans in the United States, the incidence being about 7 per cent, the West Indies, and South America. Isolated pockets of relatively high incidence are found in Sicily, Greece, South Turkey, South Arabia and in the Indian peninsula.

The proportion of S haemoglobin present in the erythrocyte varies from 20–45 per cent but is usually constant in the individual. It has, however, been reported to vary with the occurrence of anaemia, and a similar phenomenon has been noted with haemoglobin E (Grode and Laszlo, 1966).

Pathology

Excluding the 'unstable haemoglobin diseases' the heterozygous inheritance of an abnormal haemoglobin disease is usually considered to be a harmless anomaly. Bearers of the sickle-cell trait show no haematological abnormalities apart from a possible decrease in osmotic fragility. Clinically, however, the trait has been associated with hyposthenuria, haematuria, splenic infarction, and sudden unexplained deaths. Bearers of the trait have also been reported as showing an increased susceptibility to splenic abscess, *Salmonella* infection of bone, and pyelonephritis in pregnancy (Whalley *et al.* 1964), and to react more severely to typhoid fever, pneumonia, tetanus, and anaesthesia. A decreased susceptibility to leprosy and hookworm anaemia has been suggested, the latter being unproven in surveys.

In populations, however, in which the incidence of the trait is high and in which there are many other possible inherited anomalies of the red blood cell, caution should be exercised in attributing pathological changes to the presence of the sickle-cell trait alone, and detailed and comprehensive studies of the haemoglobin and enzyme content of the erythrocyte in these patients as well as family studies should be undertaken before accepting that the disease process is due solely to the presence of the trait.

In an extensive post-mortem study we could produce no evidence that the incidence of the trait was greater in patients dying of pneumonia, typhoid fever, or pyelonephritis. There was suggestive evidence that its presence might adversely affect the prognosis in tetanus, which is perhaps not surprising when the degree of anoxia produced is considered. We have seen sudden unexplained deaths in subjects whose haemoglobin at post mortem on electrophoresis showed the AS pattern but who were otherwise inadequately investigated. The findings in the organs at post mortem resembled those of the sequestration crisis of SC disease, which is described later. This has also been described in Negroes in the United States (Jones et al. 1970). Extensive infarction of the liver has been described (Mengel et al. 1963).

There is no doubt that splenic infarction can occur in trait carriers when the oxygen content of the air is lowered, and the majority of these episodes have occurred in individuals flying in unpressurized aircraft (Rotter et al. 1956), but may also occur in pressurized aircraft (Green et al. 1971). Splenic abscess has been reported in the Congo and Nigeria. Hyposthenuria and haematuria would also appear to be entities. Migraine is generally regarded as uncommon in Africa. 'Complicated' migraine consisting of amaurosis, ptosis, opthalmoplegia, localized weakness, sensory loss, disturbance of speech and equilibrium or loss of consciousness and lasting more than one hour associated with the headache of migraine has been found to be more common in bearers of the sickle cell trait (Osuntokun and Osuntokun, 1972).

Impairment of the concentrating power of the kidney (hyposthenuria) has been noted in the sickle-cell trait, and in sickle-cell anaemia in the United States (Cochrane, 1963), and has been confirmed in Africa by Vandepitte (1959). The degree is mild in trait carriers but increases with age. It is associated with the high osmotic pressure which occurs in the interstitial fluid in the region of the renal papillae, causing increased viscosity, anoxia, and restricted blood flow to the cortex. The sodium/potassium excretion ratio is also lowered in patients with SS anaemia (Addae and Konotey-Ahulu, 1971). Vascular occlusions may occur in the region of the papillae and pelvis and be responsible for the unilateral or bilateral haematuria which is seen clinically in trait carriers (Bennett et al. 1967; Akinkugbe, 1966). Renal papillary necrosis has been described and demonstrated radiologically (Harrow et al. 1963; McNulty, 1966). It is essential in patients suffering from haematuria to exclude the possibility of S haemoglobin being an aetiological agent, as nephrectomy, which we have seen performed unnecessarily, is usually contraindicated.

Sickle-cell trait blood survives normally when transfused and, in an area where the incidence is 24 per cent, is utilized for storage and transfusion without untoward effect in the great majority of patients. It should not, however, be utilized for exchange transfusion in severe anaemia in pregnancy (Edington, 1963) or in the newborn (Veiga and Vaithianathan, 1963). It can be used as a marker in transfusion studies, and we have followed its appearance in the peripheral blood following intraperitoneal infusion with interest.

Diagnosis

Routine haematological investigation reveals no abnormality. Small numbers of target cells in the peripheral blood smear and a decreased fragility have occasionally been reported. The sickling test is positive and the red cells assume 'holly leaf' or oat shapes. Filamentous forms (the common form in sickle-cell anaemia) are rarely seen. On paper electrophoresis in alkaline buffer the characteristic AS pattern is seen. In the solubility test almost 70 per cent of the haemoglobin may precipitate, whereas 80–90 per cent precipitates in SS. It must be emphasized once again that if an individual thought to be a trait carrier shows evidence of possible sickle-cell disease associated factors should be searched for, and the haemoglobin fully investigated and family studies undertaken.

Sickle-cell anaemia (SS) and sickle-cell disease

Sickle-cell anaemia is due to the homozygous inheritance of the S gene. It produces a severe congenital haemolytic anaemia with infarctive lesions in the viscera especially marked in bone. Haemoglobin S may be found in association with other abnormal haemoglobins and clinically the double heterozygote may suffer from classical sickle-cell anaemia, from a mild haemolytic anaemia with infarctive lesions, or be symptomless depending upon the physicochemical characteristics of the second inherited abnormal haemoglobin. Any condition in which sickle-cell haemoglobin is concerned in the production of a disease state is termed 'sickle-cell disease'. Apart from sickle-cell anaemia, the most common forms are sickle-cell haemoglobin-C disease (SC), and sickle-cell thalassaemia (STh), both of which produce milder forms of sickle-cell anaemia. Approximately 3 per cent of children born in West Africa suffer from sickle-cell disease (SS or SC) and there are probably 1,000,000 sufferers in tropical Africa so the problem is enormous and, to date, there is little prospect of its solution. Rare forms of sickle-cell disease are S Stanleyville II, which produces the symptoms of sickle-cell anaemia; SD Punjab may also produce severe symptoms but other SD forms may be mild, as are those of SKβ Woolwich and SE disease. SKβ Cameroon, SG, SJ, SF, S Hopkins II, and SP are harmless conditions, and should not properly be included in the term sickle-cell disease.

Apart from SS and SC disease the pathology has not been well described. As the clinical aspects of sickle-cell anaemia differ somewhat in the States and Africa and also from those of SC disease they are described separately. The pathology of both conditions, however, is similar and is described on p. 437, and differences in the two conditions are commented upon when the pathology of the individual organs is considered.

Sickle-cell anaemia (SS)

Sickle-cell anaemia does not usually manifest itself until the third or fourth month of life, as the presence of F haemoglobin protects against the pathological effects of the sickling phenomenon. Sickle cell disease and haemoglobin C disease can, however, be diagnosed in cord blood samples by agar-gel electrophoresis (Yawson et al. 1970).

In the United States a number of patients reach adult life and survival to the age of 66 years has been reported, the diagnoses having been confirmed by 'finger printing' techniques (Charache and Richardson, 1964). This has also been noted in the West Indies (Sergeant et al. 1968) where incidentally duodenal ulceration was a not uncommon complication after puberty. Although in Africa death still occurs frequently before the age of puberty, with increasing medical care and urbanization a pattern similar to that reported in America and the West Indies is emerging. It has been noted in tropical Africa that the 'crises' are most frequently seen during or just after the rainy season when malaria transmission is most intense, and that suppressive antimalarial therapy diminishes their number and intensity. Although, therefore, the presence of S haemoglobin in the heterozygote protects the bearer from the lethal effects of P. falciparum malaria, in the homozygote (SS) the malarial infection may be a 'trigger' mechanism in inducing increased haemolysis and vascular stasis, with consequent severe pathological effects on the homozygote and early mortality. (Adeloye et al. 1971). Infection is also known to precipitate crises, especially respiratory, and urinary tract infection (Konotey-Ahulu, 1971; Lambotte, 1974).

Sickle-cell anaemia should be suspected in young children presenting with swelling of the hands or feet (dactylitis), joint pains, and fever. Vascular stasis may rarely cause peripheral arterial or venous gangrene. The signs and symptoms of a haemolytic anaemia are present. Hepatomegaly and altered liver-function tests are not unusual and hepatitis may be simulated. Cholelithiasis is common in America but rare in Africa. Splenomegaly is common in young children but in America disappears as the child grows older, due to multiple infarctions with subsequent fibrosis and scarring. Splenic abscesses occasionally are seen. Splenomegaly, however, tends to persist in Africa, due to the effects of stable malaria (Hendrickse, 1965). Crises occur with pain, prostration, and shock, and either the muscles and joints of the limbs or the abdomen may be affected, at times simulating acute osteomyelitis or an acute abdominal catastrophe. The crises have been reviewed by Biggs (1965). Lactic acid dehydrogenase is elevated in patients in crises (Neely *et al.* 1969).

In these crises there is usually no evidence of excessive haemolysis (Naumann *et al.* 1971) and the symptoms and signs are due to stasis and sludging of blood in smaller vessels, with consequent anoxia. Fibrinolytic activity is reduced during episodes of clinical crisis (Mahmood *et al.* 1967). Ho Ping, Kong and Alleyne (1969) have noted no evidence of metabolic acidosis in ten adult Jamaican patients with sickle cell anaemia in crisis.

A sudden rapid sequestration can, however, occur with folic-acid deficiency or with infection suppressing erythropoiesis (aplastic crisis), p. 436.

It cannot be too strongly emphasized that sickle-cell anaemia has been well named 'the great masquerader' and in areas where S haemoglobin occurs no operative interference, especially in children, should be undertaken without a rapid sickling test being performed and a peripheral blood smear examined. A straight X-ray of the abdomen in an abdominal crisis may reveal dilated loops of gut with fluid levels. Anaesthesia is a hazard in sickle-cell anaemia patients (Gilbertson, 1965) and, if necessary, exchange transfusion with normal blood should be considered prior to the anaesthetic being given. Indeed transfusion is considered desirable prior to anaesthesia and surgery in all patients with sickle cell disease as it reduces the viscosity by dilution of the abnormal cells (Celle and Weed, 1971). Oduro and Searle (1972) have described their methods of anaesthesia in 505 patients with various haemoglobinopathies in Ghana. We have seen a number of fatalities occur from unnecessary laparotomies in children in an abdominal SS crisis. Limbs have also been lost due to the injudicious use of the tourniquet in orthopaedic procedures, the anoxia induced causing sickling and thrombosis with subsequent gangrene.

The heart is usually enlarged in sickle-cell anaemia and cor pulmonale due to thrombi in the pulmonary arteries occurs after the age of 10 years in a proportion of patients.

Renal lesions may cause haematuria and papillary necrosis. An increased liability to pyelonephritis has been suggested. Priapism may be a complication and may even be the initial clinical complaint (Campbell and Cummins, 1951). Cerebral accidents may occur and vascular changes in the retina are described.

Chronic ulcers of the leg are common in the United States but would not appear to be a striking feature of the disease in Africa, the higher and more uniform temperature perhaps militating against stasis and thrombosis in the superficial vessels. The most marked changes are seen in the skeletal system and are discussed when the pathology is considered. Patients with sickle-cell anaemia tend to have a certain type of habitus, with tower skull, parietal bossing, and long, slender limbs. Intelligence is not impaired. If pregnancy eventuates, the course may be hazardous and intensive ante-natal care is essential.

In West Africa we have occasionally seen pregnancy in SS disease, and the spleen in those patients has invariably been much enlarged. Van Enk *et al.* (1972) have described in Ghana two patients with SS associated with alpha-thalaasaemia who had 6 and 7 children successfully. Electrophoresis in those patients showed haemoglobins S, F, A, and a trace of fast-moving haemoglobin in the position of Hb Barts. Hendrickse *et al.* (1972) have described thirty-eight pregnant women with sickle-cell anaemia in Nigeria. Complications occurred in all patients and included bacterial infections, severe anaemia, bone pain and acute sequestration crises and pre-eclampsia.

Diagnosis

On haematological investigation there is evidence of a haemolytic anaemia, the haemoglobin usually varying from 5 to 9 G/100 ml. The peripheral blood smear shows marked poikilocytosis, anisocytosis, target and sickled cells. In crisis, normoblasts and a leucocytosis will be present. The rapid sickling test is positive and filamentous forms are present. The majority of the haemoglobin present will be shown to be S on paper electrophoresis. Fetal haemoglobin is usually present and may be detected by starch-block electrophoresis and by the alkali denaturation test. It is distributed in a random fashion in the cells. SF, STh, and SD may give a similar pattern to SS on paper electrophoresis. Family studies should differentiate these various conditions.

SF is symptomless and fetal haemoglobin is distributed uniformly in the red cells.

Clinically, STh is a milder condition and small amounts of A may be noted on agar-gel electrophoresis at pH6, but occasionally family studies may be the only method of differentiating the conditions (Lehmann and Huntsman, 1966). SD may be distinguished from SS by the solubility test, the amounts of insoluble haemoglobin detected being 60 and 80–90 per cent respectively.

Haemoglobin C

Haemoglobin C was first described by Itano and Neel (1950). The abnormality is in the β chain ($\alpha_2\beta_2^{6LYS}$).

It is found in its highest incidence in Northern Ghana and the neighbouring Volta territory (18 per cent) and falls in incidence to the south, where it is not found east or south of the River Niger, and west and north where it is rare in Liberia and Sierra Leone. The incidence in Southern Ghana is about 12 per cent and in Western Nigeria 6 per cent. It is absent in East Africa. It has been described frequently in the American Negro, where its incidence is approximately 2·5 per cent, and occasionally in North Africa and Italy. The geographical distribution of this gene is interesting and suggests that it arose in the region of Northern Ghana and spread as outlined above.

The C trait and pure haemoglobin-C disease

In the C trait, C forms about 30–40 per cent of the haemoglobin and the condition is harmless. Target cells may be present in the peripheral blood film and the osmotic fragility may be increased. Gangrene of both legs following exposure to cold in a West Indian male with haemoglobin-C trait has been described (Smith and Wright, 1963). In the homozygote (pure haemoglobin-C disease, CC) no A is present and the percentage of F may be increased. Patients may suffer from a mild haemolytic anaemia with splenomegaly and are frequently unaware of the condition. It would not appear to be a hazard in pregnancy providing ante-natal care is adequate (Hendrickse et al. 1972). The condition has mostly been detected accidentally, in surveys or in prospective blood donors. Target cells are numerous in the peripheral blood and intracellular crystal-like structures have been seen in the red blood cell and are best demonstrated in 3 per cent sodium chloride solution (Conley, 1974). Areas of osteoporosis have been decribed in the mandible and have proved to be diagnostic (Halstead, 1970). The pathology is that of a chronic haemolytic anaemia and is exemplified by hyperplasia of the reticulo-endothelial system, siderosis, and bone changes due to marrow hyperplasia.

Diagnosis

On electrophoresis in barbitone buffer at alkaline pH, C moves slowly behind E or A_2 and in Tris buffer slightly in front. On agar electrophoresis E runs with A, as does D Punjab, and C runs behind, as does S. F is found in front of A.

Haemoglobin C and other abnormal haemoglobin disease

The heterozygous inheritance of C has been noted with J Baltimore, thalassaemia, the high fetal gene and, of course, frequently with S. It has also been seen with Gα Baltimore in an individual with four major haemoglobins in the peripheral blood. CJ and CF are symptomless but the electrophoretic pattern of the latter may resemble CC (see p. 427). C thalassaemia causes a mild haemolytic anaemia with target cells and fragmented erythrocytes in the peripheral film. The severity of sickle-cell haemoglobin-C disease varies and the pathology is described below.

SC disease occurs in high frequency in West Africa, where there is a high incidence of haemoglobins S and C in the population. It is due to the inheritance of the S gene from one parent and the C gene from the other. It does not occur in the neonate as the great percentage of the haemoglobin is F. Clinically it produces a milder haemolytic anaemia than is found in SS disease, and the condition may even be symptomless. We have seen SC disease diagnosed by electrophoresis in volunteer blood donors and SC blood has been used once for transfusion, with disastrous effects on the recipient. The usual history given is that of joint pains and fever, improving with age. Cerebral and renal lesions can occur. Cardiomegaly is unusual. Bone lesions, especially in the hip joint, are common, and ocular complications would appear to be more common than in SS disease, although they are not common in Africa. Micro-aneurysms of the retinal vessels, retinitis proliferans, obliteration of vessels, and retinal and vitreous haemorrhages have been described (Edington and Sarkies, 1952; Goodman *et al.* 1967; Goldberg, 1972).

It is in pregnancy, however, that the most severe effects of SC disease are seen. Once again its effects are variable, as we have seen death occur in a female in her eighth pregnancy, the previous seven having been unremarkable. Severe manifestations usually occur in the last few weeks of pregnancy or during or shortly after labour and take two forms—the sequestration crisis, or bone-marrow infarction with embolic phenomena in the lungs.

In the sequestration crisis the haemoglobin may drop 4–5 G in 24 hours and is usually due to folic-acid deficiency (Fullerton and Watson-Williams, 1962). The splenic pulp and hepatic sinusoids are packed with sickled erythrocytes, the patient literally having bled to death into the spleen, p. 438.

The rapid and sudden fall in the haemoglobin can be satisfactorily managed by exchange transfusion with packed normal cells. Management of bone-marrow embolism is more difficult and, in our experience, deaths are still occurring from this cause. Normoblastaemia and thrombocytopenia occur in the peripheral blood. Fat globules may be seen in the sputum. Bone marrow infarction can also be detected by isotope scanning and with successful therapy, marrow regeneration takes place (Hutchinson *et al.* 1973). Post-delivery heparinization in patients with bone or joint pains is considered a valuable preventive measure. Curzen (1964) has described sclerosis of the uterus in sickle cell disease with a low-grade necrosis of the inner myometrium due to blockage of capillaries by sickle red blood cells.

Anaesthesia in patients with SC disease is hazardous and the application of a tourniquet in bone surgery may result in thrombosis and gangrene of the limb involved.

Diagnosis

The characteristic pattern of the haemoglobin on electrophoresis (SC) associated with the presence of numerous target cells in the peripheral blood and evidence of a mild haemolytic anaemia usually presents no difficulty in diagnosis (Figs. 10.5 and 10.15).

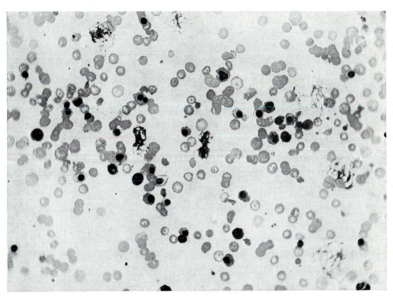

FIG. 10.5. Peripheral blood film in SC disease in pregnancy, illustrating a normoblastic crisis. Note the target cells. (Jenner-Giemsa × 400)

Pathology of sickle-cell anaemia and sickle-cell haemoglobin-C disease

The pathology of sickle-cell disease depends upon the presence of a haemolytic anaemia, infarctive changes in the organs, and the presence or absence of associated conditions (Edington 1955). Bacterial infections are extremely common in the younger age groups, including pyogenic hepatic abscess (Schulman and Beem, 1971).

The haemolytic anaemia causes the non-specific changes of hypertrophy of the reticulo-endothelial system, siderosis in the spleen, liver, and bone marrow, and perhaps anoxic fatty changes in the viscera and cardiomegaly. Siderosis is more marked in SS than SC disease and the degree would appear to vary in different areas, being much less pronounced in Western Nigeria than in Southern Ghana. It is frequently severe in the United States where therapy probably is important in this connection. Various infections frequently cause death in younger patients with sickle-cell anaemia but the most common cause of death in sickle-cell disease is either the sequestration crisis or catastrophes following thrombosis and embolism. Anaesthesia may also cause fatalities. The mechanism of the sequestration crisis has already been discussed (see p. 436) and the infarctive lesions are described when the individual organs are considered.

In the sequestration crisis at post mortem there is gross pallor of all the organs, with the exception of the liver and spleen. The spleen is, in our experience, pathognomonic, being enlarged, firm, elastic, and slaty-blue in colour (see below). Mild icterus and a mild degree of peripheral oedema may be present. The macroscopic findings when death has been due to infarctive lesions are not specific, but the spleen may once again point to the cause of death. If sickle-cell disease is suspected it is essential that as much of the marrow should be examined for infarctive lesions as is feasible, and a radiological survey of the skeletal system may be helpful. A rapid sickling test may be done at post mortem and electrophoresis of the haemoglobin is done routinely in all necropsies performed in our department and is advisable if an abnormal haemoglobin disease is suspected.

The spleen

In sickle-cell anaemia the spleen weight may vary from a few to 2600 g. The enlarged spleen is dark blue in colour, of rubbery consistency and the cut surface is dark red and dry. Histologically the splenic pulp is packed with sickled erythrocytes and the sinusoids are compressed and empty. Erythrophagocytosis and haemosiderin deposits may be seen in the sinusoidal lining cells and in the pulp histiocytes. Haemorrhages round the malpighian corpuscles may be prominent and perivascular haemosiderin deposits are usually present in the trabeculae. This is the usual pathology of SS disease in the young child and SC disease in all age groups and is characteristic of the sequestration crisis. Megaloblasts may be distinguishable in the sinusoids (Fig 10.6).

In older children in SS disease areas of fibrosis with deposition of iron and calcium salts occur—the so-called Gandy-Gamna bodies or siderofibrotic nodules. Yellowish bamboo-like crystals surrounded by fibrosis and foreign-body giant cells are commonly seen (Fig. 10.7). Eventually the spleen may be represented by a greyish-brown, gritty, fibrous remnant weighing only a few grams. This type of spleen is not commonly seen in areas of stable malaria although it does occur. Malarial pigment in these areas is a constant concomitant finding in both conditions.

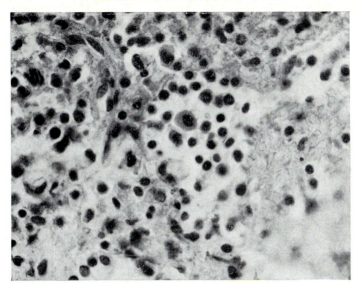

FIG. 10.6. Megaloblasts in the splenic sinusoids (28-year-old pregnant woman) (H and E × 488). (*By courtesy of Blackwell Scientific Publications Ltd.*)

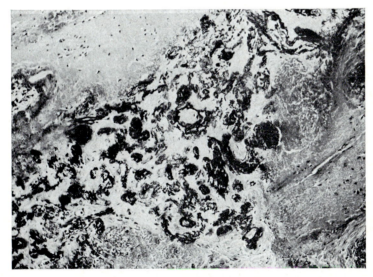

FIG. 10.7. Spleen in sickle-cell anaemia. There is complete destruction of the splenic architecture. There is extensive fibrosis with massive deposition of iron and calcium salts. The occasional bamboo crystal can be distinguished (H and E × 130).

As previously stated, splenic infarction and abscesses may be complications. The areas of calcification may be noted radiologically in life on a straight X-ray of the abdomen.

The liver

The liver is usually enlarged, and pathological changes due to anaemia, sickling of the red cells in the sinusoids with fibrin deposition and hyaline thrombi, and obstruction to the flow of blood by engorged Kupffer cells are common. Areas of focal necrosis and fibrosis are commonly seen and cirrhosis is a not uncommon complication in the United States in SS disease, and is now seen not infrequently in West Africa (Alli and Lewis, 1969) although previously described as uncommon (Brew and Edington, 1965). Clinically there is evidence of hepatic dysfunction in most patients suffering from sickle-cell anaemia (Helkovitz and Jacobson, 1961). Haemosiderosis is more marked in sickle-cell anaemia than in other forms of sickle-cell disease and the part that multiple transfusions may play in the pathology of the liver, including serum-transmitted jaundice, must be borne in mind. In our experience areas of extra-medullary erythropoiesis are unusual. Erythrophagocytosis of sickled cells by the Kupffer cells is a marked feature (Fig. 10.8). Ultrastructural studies of the hepatocytes have revealed changes suggestive of hypoxia (Rosenblate *et al.* 1970).

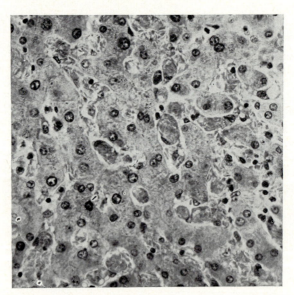

FIG. 10.8. Section of the liver, showing marked erythrophagocytosis (25-year-old pregnant female, SC) (H and E × 400). (*By courtesy of Blackwell Scientific Publications Ltd.*)

Gall stones are infrequently seen in West Africa in sickle-cell disease, in contrast to the American findings where it has been stated that cholelithiasis occurs in approximately one-third of patients suffering from sickle-cell anaemia (Margolies, 1951; Cameron *et al.* 1971).

The kidney

The possible pathogenesis of hyposthenuria has already been discussed. The most constant findings are dilatation and congestion of the capillaries of the glomerular tuft with sickled cells, and the presence of atrophied and digitate glomeruli. In the medulla, congestion of the intertubular capillaries occurs and the vessels beneath the epithelium of the renal papillae may be dilated and congested, with focal haemorrhages present. Venous thrombosis has been reported but is rare in our experience—nor have we found an increased incidence of pyelonephritis in our material. Papillary necrosis and scarring have been reported. Haemosiderin is inconstantly present in the tubular epithelium. Fat emboli may be seen in the glomerular capillaries, with associated marrow infarction. The nephrotic syndrome has been associated with sickle cell disease in a few patients. The light and electron microscopic alterations observed were similar to those reported in the nephrotic syndrome induced by saccharated iron oxide in laboratory animals, viz: atrophy and collapse of renal parenchyma, iron-containing pigment in the glomeruli and tubular epithelium, loss of epithelial foot processes, proliferations of mesangial matrix and duplication of the glomerular basement membrane (McCoy, 1969). Sickle cell disease may be associated with the nephrotic syndrome but in a large series of renal biopsies in children with the nephrotic syndrome in West Africa, where the frequency is about 3 per cent, no such association was noted.

The lungs

In the sequestration crises the predominant feature is pulmonary oedema. In SS disease pulmonary venous thrombosis with organization and recanalization may be seen and be the causal factor in the pulmonary hypertension which occurs in that condition (Figs. 10.9 and 10.10).

Marrow and fat embolism occur in both SS and SC disease but is more common in the latter in pregnancy (Fig. 10.11). Large marrow fragments are present in the pulmonary arteries and fat globules are scattered widely in the alveolar septal capillaries. Infarctive necrotic areas can be detected in the marrow (Fig. 10.13). Pulmonary bone marrow embolism may also occur following fractures of bone and is a not unusual complication of external cardiac massage. It has very rarely been reported as a complication of sternal marrow puncture (Carstens, 1969).

Massive pulmonary embolism from thrombosed internal iliac or femoral

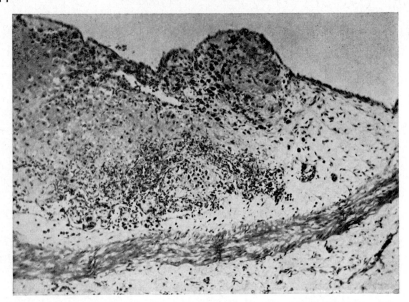

FIG. 10.9. Thrombus being incorporated in the wall of a pulmonary artery (5-year-old boy, SS) (H and E × 117). (*By courtesy of Blackwell Scientific Publications Ltd.*)

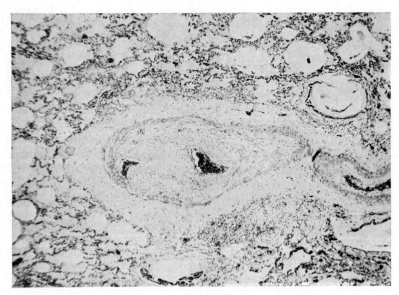

FIG. 10.10. Recanalization of a pulmonary artery (40-year-old female, SC) (H and E × 52). (*By courtesy of Blackwell Scientific Publications Ltd.*)

veins is relatively rare in West Africa but is a not uncommon complication of sickle-cell disease, and this complication should be considered in all patients with sickle-cell disease undergoing prolonged bed rest or operative procedures.

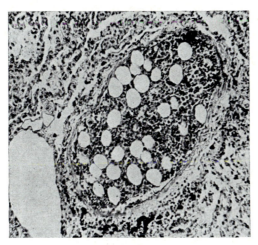

FIG. 10.11. Bone-marrow embolus in a pulmonary artery (23-year-old pregnant woman, SC) (H and E × 59). (*By courtesy of Blackwell Scientific Publications Ltd.*)

The heart

The heart is usually enlarged and hypertrophied in SS disease and is less affected in SC disease. Cardiovascular abnormalities are usually more common in children with low haemoglobin levels. Cor pulmonale is a common finding in SS disease in the United States. There is no evidence that the presence of sickle-cell haemoglobin predisposes to other forms of heart disease.

The central nervous system

Subarachnoid haemorrhage and multiple thromboses may occur. Extensive haemorrhage in the cerebral haemospheres or in the Virchow–Robin spaces have been described. Focal necroses in the anterior lobe of the pituitary gland have been seen. All these complications are more common in sickle-cell anaemia, and we have found pneumococcal meningitis to be a not uncommon complication. Adeloye and Odeku (1970) have recently reviewed the literature.

The skeletal system

The bony changes are caused by two mechanisms (1) marrow hyperplasia, and (2) marrow infarction (Cockshott, 1965).

The changes caused by marrow hyperplasia are non-specific and are seen in their most advanced forms in sickle-cell anaemia and thalassaemia major. Marrow hyperplasia causes absorption of bone, osteoporosis, and softening. Later, sclerosis may occur.

In the skull there is widening of the diploe, clinically exemplified by bossing in the parietal region. The outer table becomes thin and is partially absorbed, trabecular definition is lost and perpendicular striations from the inner table give the 'hair-on-end' appearance rarely seen in sickle-cell haemoglobin-C disease. Patches of localized osteoporosis later becoming sclerotic also occur. Osteoporotic changes are also seen in the ribs and, in the spine, thinning of the trabeculae of the vertebrae may cause flattening of the bodies and bulging of the disks into their substance, with consequent 'cupping'. Massive infarction with complete collapse of vertebral bodies may rarely occur. Back pain is common in both conditions (Figs. 10.12, 10.13, and 10.14).

In the long bones vascular red marrow with little fat is found throughout their length, with subsequent thinning of the cortex and frequent multiple pathological fracture in sickle-cell anaemia. In some instances the destruction of cortical bone by marrow hyperplasia may be followed by irregular thickening due to new bone formation. Acute diaphyseal cortical infarcts are common in SS disease. Infarction of almost the entire shaft may occur in young infants whereas localized infarctions are more common in older infants. The distal femora and proximal tibiae are most commonly involved (Bohrer, 1970).

In young children sickle-cell anaemia infarctive lesions would appear to be especially common in the small bones of the hands and feet. Infarctive lesions in the phalanges are followed by local osteoblastic activity and soft tissue swelling, giving the picture of an aseptic dactylitis. Shortening of digits due to these lesions can occur.

In the larger joints (especially the hip and shoulder) the circulation in the vascular loops that supply the cartilage is sluggish and the oxygen tension is reduced and would appear to favour intravascular sickling and thrombosis, as lesions in these joints are common in SC disease. Avascular necrosis of the head of the femur has been described in SS disease, but in general, lesions of the hip joint are more common in sickle-cell haemoglobin-C disease and can be distinguished from Perthes' disease in that they occur in a later age group and the epiphyseal line is fused.

Permanent damage to joints may also occur from focal haemorrhages causing a chronic synovitis.

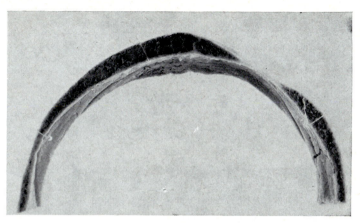

FIG. 10.12. Section of the skull, showing hyperplasia of marrow and an area of collapse due to infarction and fibrosis (37-year-old male, SS). (*By courtesy of Blackwell Scientific Publications Ltd.*)

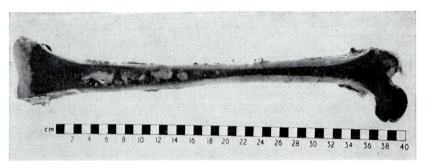

FIG. 10.13. Infarctive areas in the bone marrow of the femur (24-year-old pregnant woman, SC). (*By courtesy of Blackwell Scientific Publications Ltd.*)

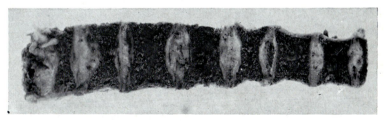

FIG. 10.14. Hyperplasia of the vertebral marrow with flattening and collapse of the bodies (37-year-old male, SS). (*By courtesy of Blackwell Scientific Publications Ltd.*)

Infarctive lesions in the marrow are not infrequently seen at necropsy in SC disease (p. 444) and are the cause of the embolic lesions in the lungs already described (Fig. 10.11).

Salmonella infection of bone in the early years of life is common. The organisms most frequently encountered are *Salm. dublin, Salm. typhimurium, Salm. enteritidis, Salm. kisangani,* and *Salm. oranienburg. Salm. typhi*; staphyloccocal, and *Esch. coli* infections also occur but are rare. There is possibly a diminished resistance of the gastro-intestinal tract to invasion by *Salmonella* organisms and small necrotic foci in the marrow presumably form a favourable medium for their growth. Osteitis and osteomyelitis are seen in SS and SC disease and have also been described in trait carriers. The long and small bones of the limbs are most frequently affected.

Delay in skeletal maturity due to folic-acid deficiency has also been described (Fig. 10.15).

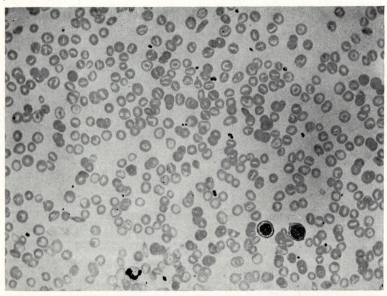

FIG. 10.15. Peripheral blood film in sickle-cell haemoglobin-C disease in pregnancy. Note the numerous target cells, occasional sickled cell, and presence of megaloblasts (Jenner–Giemsa × 500).

Haemoglobin D

This was first described by Itano in 1951. Both α- and β-chain variants have been described. The α-chain type was seen in a Turkish Cypriot and is rare. Dβ Ibadan is also rare. The common form is Dβ Los Angeles or Punjab. It is found in 3 per cent of Sikhs in the Punjab and in lower incidence in Bombay in India, in American Negroes, in the Mediterranean area, and rarely in Britons, Turks, Persians, Nigerians, Congolese, and Indonesians.

The heterozygotes (AD) are completely symptomless.

The homozygotes (DD) show a mild haemolytic anaemia and spleno-megaly, with target cells in the peripheral blood. Virus or other infections may precipitate severe symptoms. It has been found in association with thalassaemia and haemoglobin S when a haemolytic anaemia results. Patients suffering from sickle-cell haemoglobin-D disease may exhibit mild or severe symptoms of sickle-cell disease—or be symptomless.

On electrophoresis, D moves as S, and SD may be mistaken for SS. It can be distinguished by its higher solubility and by the fact that on agar-gel at pH 6 it moves as A and not as S, which travels behind A.

Other abnormal haemoglobins

Approximately 150 abnormal haemoglobins have been described and it is obviously impossible to describe them in this text. Short comments are given on a few below and the amino acid substitutions of these and others are shown in Table 10.6 (Rucknagel and Laros, 1969).

Haemoglobin E

Haemoglobin E was first described by Itano et al. (1954). The abnormality is in the β chain. It is found in high incidence in the Burmese and in adjacent Thais and Eastern Malayans, incidences of 19 to 35 per cent being quoted. The highest incidence recorded from India was 3·9 per cent in Bengalees. A focus has been noted in the Veddas of Ceylon, and isolated instances in Turkey, Egypt, and Holland. It has recently been described in the Vietna-mese (Blackwell et al. 1965). The heterozygote (AE) is symptomless and the homozygote exhibits a mild haemolytic anaemia with target cells in the peripheral blood. Haemoglobin E is found frequently in association with thalassaemia, and the symptomatology is variable and at times severe. With β thalassaemia, as E has an abnormal β chain, its production is not suppressed and high E and F values may be found in the absence of A. The electrophoretic pattern may be mistaken for EE and family studies are always required to prove homozygosity. E has also been noted in association with ovalocytosis (Lie Injo Luan Eng, 1965). Pregnancy aggravates the condition and infant mortality may be high. The E homozygote is only at a slight disadvantage compared with his normal brother but in countries with a high incidence of thalassaemia there is a considerable loss of genes. It has been suggested that increased iron absorption in the E trait carrier

TABLE 10.6. *Amino acid substitutions of abnormal human hemoglobins* (From Rucknagel and Laros, 1969. *Clin. Obstet. Gynec.* **12**, pp. 54–55)

Abnormal Hb	Position	Amino acid substitution HbA → Abnormal Hb	
Alpha chain variants			
J-Toronto	5	Ala	Asp
J-Paris	12	Ala	Asp
J-Oxford	15	Gly	Asp
I	16	Lys	Glu
J-Medellin	22	Gly	Asp
Memphis	23	Glu	Gln
G-Honolulu, G-Hongkong, G-Singapore	30	Glu	Gln
L-Ferrara, Umi, Kokura, Michigan-1, Tagawa II, Yukuhashi II, Beilinson	47	Asp	Gly
Mexico	54	Gln	Glu
Shimonoseki, Hikoshima	54	Gln	Arg
Norfolk, Kagoshima, Nishiki I, II, III	57	Gly	Asp
M-Boston, Leipzig-2, M-Osaka, M-Koln	58	His	Tyr
N-Seattle	61	Lys	Glu
G-Philadelphia, G-Bristol, G-Azuokoli, D-St. Louis, D-Washington	68	Asn	Lys
Ube II	68	Asn	Asp
M-Iwate, M-Kankakee, M-Oldenberg	87	His	Tyr
Chesapeake	92	Arg	Leu
J-Cape Town	92	Arg	Gln
Chiapas	114	Pro	Arg
J-Tongariki	115	Ala	Asp
O-Indonesia	116	Glu	Lys
Beta chain variants			
Tokuchi	2	His	Tyr
S	6	Glu	Val
C	6	Glu	Lys
C-Harlem	{ 6 { 73	{ Glu { Asp	{ Val { Asn
G-San Jose	7	Glu	Gly
Siriraj	7	Glu	Lys
Porto Alegre	9	Ser	Cys
N-New Haven, J-Baltimore	16	Gly	Asp
E-Saskatoon	22	Glu	Lys
Freiburg	23	Val	Deletion
E-Nagasaki	26	Glu	Lys
Hammersmith	42	Phe	Ser
G-Galveston, G-Port Arthur, G-Texas	43	Glu	Ala
K-Ibadan	46	Gly	Glu
G-Copenhagen	47	Asp	Asn

TABLE 10.6 (*Continued*)

Abnormal Hb	Position	Amino acid substitution HbA → Abnormal Hb	
J-Bangkok	56	Gly	Asp
Hikari, Ube-3	61	Lys	Asn
M-Saskatoon, M-Kurume, M-Chicago, M-Emory, M-Radon, M-Hita, M-Arhus	63	His	Tyr
Zurich	63	His	Arg
M-Milwaukee-1	67	Val	Glu
Sydney	67	Val	Ala
J-Cambridge	69	Gly	Asp
J-Iran	77	His	Asp
G-Accra	79	Asp	Asn
D-Ibadan	87	Thr	Lys
Gunn-Hill	91–95 or 93–97		Deletion
M-Hyde Park	92	His	Tyr
N-Baltimore, N-Memphis	95	Lys	Glu
Köln	98	Val	Met
Yakima	99	Asp	His
D-Punjab, -Cyprus, -Chicago, -Los Angeles, -Portugal, -N. Carolina	121	Glu	Gln
O-Arabia, -Bulgaria, -New York	121	Glu	Lys
K-Woolwich	132	Lys	Gln
Hope	136	Gly	Asp
Kenwood	143	His	Asp
Ranier	145	Tyr	His
Gamma chain variants			
F-Texas	5	Glu	Lys
F-Galveston	6	Glu	Lys
Delta chain variants			
Sphakia	2	His	Arg
B₂	16	Gly	Arg
Flatbush	22	Ala	Glu

might confer an advantage, but there is no evidence that the trait carrier does absorb more iron. The possible protection HbE confers against malaria is discussed on p. 468.

On paper electrophoresis with barbiturate buffer E moves in front of C and with Tris buffer behind C. At acid pH it migrates with S. On agar-gel electrophoresis E does not separate from A, whereas C separates widely (Lehmann and Huntsman, 1966).

Haemoglobin G

Haemoglobin G was first described in Accra by Edington and Lehmann (1954). α- and β-chain variants are as follows: Gα Bristol, Gα Baltimore, Gα Chinese, Gα Hong Kong, Gα Honolulu, Gα Ibadan, Gα Norfolk, Gα Philadelphia, Gβ Accra, and Gβ San Jose.

No clinical or haematological abnormality has been attributed to the presence of haemoglobin G and the Gβ Accra homozygote was perfectly normal. Haemoglobin Gα Baltimore has been noted with C—in the peripheral blood of an individual with four haemoglobins present (Rieder and Naughton, 1965).

On paper electrophoresis at alkaline pH, G lies between A and S. Starch gel, starch block at alkaline pH, and agar-gel electrophoresis at acid pH are used in differentiation.

Haemoglobin I

Haemoglobin I was first described by Page et al. (1955) and reviewed by Thompson et al. 1963). Isolated cases have been seen in Algerian, French Canadian, Indonesian, and Indian families. It is an α-chain variant and the abnormal A_2 and F forms have been seen. In the heterozygote I Interlaken a mild anaemia is present and occasional inclusion bodies may be noted in red cells.

Haemoglobin Iα thalassaemia has been described and, as the abnormality is in the α chain, I is found with Barts (γ_4) in the infant and with haemoglobin H (β_4) in the adult.

On electrophoresis in alkaline pH Hb I is a 'fast' haemoglobin and moves as haemoglobin H. In acid pH it moves towards the negative pole and H remains stationary nor does I show inclusion bodies on incubation with cresyl blue.

Haemoglobin J

Haemoglobin J was first described by Thorup et al. (1956) and has been seen in isolated families of different ethnic groups. Both α- and β-chain variants have been reported, as follows: Jα Oxford, Jα Toronto, Jβ Trinidad, Jβ Jamaica, Jβ Baltimore, and Jβ Ireland. Jβ Korat is not uncommon in Thais (Blackwell et al. 1965). It has been diagnosed in combination with S, C, and thalassaemia. Both SJ and CJ resemble the harmless sickle-cell trait (Weatherall, 1964). HbJ Tongariki (α 115 Ala → Asp) has been reported in high frequency in New Britain (Abramson et al. 1970). In the heterozygote (AJ) J comprises more than 50 per cent of the haemoglobin, so its rate of synthesis must be greater than A. On alkaline electrophoresis it moves more rapidly than A and slightly more rapidly than K and Hopkins 2, but slower than haemoglobin Bart's and Mexico.

No pathological abnormalities are ascribed to its presence.

Haemoglobin K

This was first described by Cabannes in Algeria (Cabannes and Buhr, 1955). It was also described later in Liberia as Liberia II. Hopkins II may be a similar haemoglobin. It has been seen in India, Northern Ghana, St. Thomas Island, Guinea, Nigeria, and the West Indies. Both α- and β-chain variants have been described (O'Gorman et al. 1963). Heterozygous inheritance of S and K haemoglobins have been diagnosed in two individuals, one with a mild haemoglobinopathy (SKβ Woolwich) and the other with no clinical or haematological disability (SKβ Cameroon) (Allan et al. 1965). It moves slightly further towards the anode than A on electrophoresis at alkaline pH, and behind J. At acid pH it is slightly faster than J. It causes no disability.

Haemoglobin L

Haemoglobin L was first described in a Hindu in 1957 by Ager and Lehmann. The abnormality is in the β chain. An α-chain variant has also been reported from Italy (Bianco *et al.* 1963). On alkaline electrophoresis L moves closely with D but is easily distinguished on ion-exchange chromatography. No anomalies have been reported due to its presence.

Haemoglobin M

This was first described by Horlein and Weber (1948) and the subject has recently been reviewed by Jaffe and Heller (1964) and Lehmann and Huntsman (1966). The condition probably occurs in most parts of the world. Cyanosis can be caused in two ways: either (1) due to a deficiency of the methaemoglobin reductase enzyme system which is transmitted as an autosomal recessive trait, or (2) due to the presence of the abnormal haemoglobin M. Various types of the latter have been described, haemoglobin Mα Iwate, Mβ Milwaukee, Mβ Saskatoon, and others (Hayashi *et al.* 1966). If the abnormality is in the α chain, cyanosis is evident at birth, as A, A$_2$, and F are affected, but if in the β it does not appear until F is replaced to a great extent by A. M does not show normally on electrophoresis. The haemoglobin has to be converted to methaemoglobin first when it will then separate from A. The absorption spectrum also differs. Both these tests will also differentiate the enzyme deficiency as in this abnormality the methaemoglobin behaves as normal adult haemoglobin. Apart from cyanosis the patients are little affected.

Haemoglobin N

This 'fast-moving' haemoglobin was first described as Liberia I by Robinson *et al.* (1956). It has been reported in Liberia, North West Africa, the United States, and Italy (Silvestroni *et al.* 1963). The abnormality is in the β chain and no clinical anomalies have been reported.

Haemoglobin O

This was first described as haemoglobin X in a Buginese by Lie Injo Luan Eng (1958) and is now known as Oα Indonesia. A β variant has been described in an Arab family (Oβ Arab). The former is present in 2 per cent of Buginese and 3 per cent of Makassars. Oβ Arab has been seen in the Middle East in combination with S. There is increased resistance to hypotonic saline in trait carriers but otherwise no abnormalities have been reported.

On alkaline electrophoresis it moves between E and S and on chromatography is slower than S. Lehmann and Huntsman (1966) have pointed out that it may be difficult to differentiate O Arab and C and E on paper electrophoresis, and that some examples of C and E reported from the Middle East and Africa may be O.

Haemoglobin P

This haemoglobin was first called haemoglobin G Galveston, and described by Schnieder and Haggard (1958). It has been found in an American family and in the Congo and Italy (Silvestroni *et al.* 1963). The abnormality is in the β chain.

Haemoglobin Q

Haemoglobin Q was described in 1958 by Vella *et al.* in a Chinese who was also a carrier of haemoglobin H. It is an α-chain variant and has been described in association with α thalassaemia. It moves more slowly than A and slightly faster than G.

Haemoglobin Lepore

This abnormal haemoglobin was described by Gerald and Diamond (1958). It has been seen in Italian Americans (Lepore Washington) and in New Guinea (Lepore Hollandia). Isolated cases have been reported in Portugal, Italy, and Greece, and in Italians in Britain (Barkham et al. 1964).

It is close to haemoglobin A on paper electrophoresis if Tris alkaline buffer is used and moves as haemoglobin S on starch-gel or starch-block electrophoresis (Lehmann and Huntsman, 1966). At least two forms have been described with abnormalities in the β chain. The abnormal chain contains portion of normal β and normal δ chains. Baglioni (1963) has suggested that the abnormality arises as the result of non-homologous crossing over of the β and δ chains. In the heterozygote only small amounts of Lepore haemoglobin are present (10–16 per cent). Homozygotes have been described and, as would be expected, no A ($\alpha_2\beta_2$) or A$_2$ ($\alpha_2\delta_2$) is present, but there are large amounts of F ($\alpha_2\gamma_2$) and Lepore itself ($\alpha_2\beta_2$ Lepore).

Haemoglobins Stanleyville I and II

Stanleyville II has been described in association with haemoglobin S, and the S/Hb Sta patient presented as classical sickle-cell anaemia. It has the mobility of S on paper electrophoresis at pH 8·6 but can be separated from it by resin chromatography. It is an α-chain variant (Hall-Craggs et al. 1964).

Both haemoglobins might be placed in the haemoglobin-D group.

Hopkins 1 and 2

Hopkins 1 is a β-chain variant and moves as haemoglobin I. Hopkins 2 is an α-chain variant and has about the same electrophoretic mobility as J. They were described by Smith and Torbert (1958).

Haemoglobin Norfolk

This is a 'fast-moving' haemoglobin described by Ager et al. (1958).

There is an α-chain anomaly and no clinical symptoms have been reported. On electrophoresis it moves as N.

Haemoglobin Beilinson

This was described by O'Gorman et al. (1963). It is an α-chain abnormality and moves behind haemoglobin A in the L position.

Haemoglobin Caserta

This was described by Ventrouto et al. (1965).

Haemoglobin Porto Alegre

This was described by Tondo et al. (1963). The homozygote is symptomless.

Haemoglobin Shimonoseki

This was described by Miyrji et al. (1963). It shows an α-chain abnormality and moves slightly faster than S ($\alpha_2^{54arg}\beta_2$).

Haemoglobin Mexico

This is a 'fast-moving' haemoglobin described by Lisker *et al.* (1963). The abnormality is in the α chain and it moves between J and K.

The 'unstable haemoglobin' diseases

These have recently been reviewed by White and Dacie (1971). Clinically their presence results in so-called congenital Heinz-body haemolytic anaemia. At least 30 different molecular variants have so far been described. In these conditions an amino-acid substitution produces a haemoglobin molecule which is less stable than normal and haemolysis can occur, with the proportion of the abnormal haemoglobin being less than 50 per cent. Haemoglobin Zurich disease was described by Frick *et al.* (1962). It is a β-chain abnormality. On electrophoresis in alkaline pH it migrates between A and S. The haemoglobin molecule is abnormally sensitive to methaemoglobin-forming drugs and a severe haemolytic crisis can be precipitated by sulphonamides. Haemoglobin Zurich usually forms only 40 per cent of the total haemoglobin. Fragmentation of erythrocytes is marked and inclusion bodies (Heinz) in the erythrocytes due to deposition of denatured haemoglobin is usual. A mild haemolysis may be present in the quiescent stage and the red cell survival time is shortened.

Haemoglobin UBE-1 disease was described by Shibata *et al.* (1963). No abnormality was noted in the parents and the abnormal haemoglobin migrated between S and C, with the same mobility as O.

Haemoglobin Seattle disease was described by Huehns *et al.* quoted from Huehns (1965). The abnormality is in the β chain and Seattle usually forms 40 per cent of the total haemoglobin. It does not separate from A on paper electrophoresis and requires a special buffer system when it migrates as J. A mild haemolytic anaemia is present and the red-cell survival time is shortened.

Haemoglobin St. Mary's disease was described by Buchanan *et al.* quoted from Huehns (1965). It moves as A on paper electrophoresis but can be separated by starch-gel electrophoresis. A haemolytic anaemia with occasional crises occurs.

Haemoglobin Koln disease was described by Pribilla (1962). It moves close to S and the abnormality is in the β chain. A second family has been described in Scotland. A mild haemolytic anaemia with Heinz-body formation in the erythrocytes is present.

Heat-unstable haemoglobin disease was described by Grimes and Meisler (1962). No abnormal haemoglobin is seen by the usual techniques but a proportion of the haemoglobin is readily denatured on heating to 50°C. Heinz bodies are present.

THE THALASSAEMIAS

In these conditions there is no inherited abnormality of the structure of haemoglobin as such, but there is genetic interference with the rate of production of adult haemoglobin.

There are two principal varieties of thalassaemia—β *thalassaemia,* where the defect of synthesis is in the β chains of haemoglobin; and α *thalassaemia,* in which the α chains are involved. Serum-immunoglobulin levels (Ig) G, A and M are higher than normal in thalassaemia of both α and β varieties (Wasi *et al.* 1971).

β Thalassaemia major

Synonyms. Cooley's anaemia; thalassaemia major.

'β *thalassaemia*' implies that the condition results from defective synthesis of the β chain of haemoglobin A ($\alpha_2\beta_2$). This reduction in β chains is associated with the continued synthesis of the γ chains of haemoglobin F ($\alpha_2\gamma_2$), beyond the normal period, and a relative or absolute increase in δ-chain synthesis—haemoglobin A$_2$ ($\alpha_2\delta_2$).

Thalassaemia major is the name given to the severe clinical form of the disease and is usually the result of inheritance of the abnormal gene from both parents. The haemoglobin pattern of the homozygous state is characterized by a 10 to 40 per cent increase in haemoglobin F and low, normal, or increased levels of A$_2$. The parents of such a patient both usually have increased levels of haemoglobin A$_2$.

β *thalassaemia* has a world-wide distribution, with high incidence areas in the Mediterranean region and the Middle and Far East, and it occurs sporadically in nearly every ethnic group. (Malamos *et al.* 1962; Aksoy, 1959; Chatterjea, 1959; Na-Nakorn, 1959; Vella and Ibrahim, 1961). It seems likely that the β thalassaemia gene has a relatively low incidence in tropical Africa (Vandepitte, 1959; Watson-Williams, 1965), excluding Liberia where the incidence may be as high as 10 per cent (Olesen *et al.* 1959). It has been described in the British (Knox-Macauley *et al.* 1973; Vella, 1973).

Anaemia is always severe, there is marked hypochromia and aniso-poikilocytosis. Target cells are usually present, there is marked basophilic stippling of the red cells, and nucleated red cells appear in the peripheral blood. A slight reticulocytosis and leucocytosis occur. The red cell osmotic fragility is markedly decreased while the red cell life span is shortened (Fessas, 1967). Fessas (1963) has described inclusion bodies in the cytoplasm of both nucleated red cells and reticulocytes; they stain with methyl violet, are well seen on phase contrast microscopy, and commonly occur in splenecto-mized patients. These inclusion bodies almost certainly represent denatured haemoglobin consisting of an excess of α chains which is produced in the presence of a gross deficit of β chains. The serum bilirubin and plasma haemoglobin levels are raised, with an absence of haptoglobins. Seitanidis (1973) studied complement levels in β-thalassaemia major.

The radiological manifestations of Cooley's anaemia have been reviewed by Baker (1964), and they are basically the result of marrow overstimulation occurring early in life. The medullary portion of the cranial bones is thickened and there is a striking vertical striation 'hair-on-end' appearance. The cortex of the long bones is thin, the bone is unusually transparent, and the medulla reticulated. The iliac and scapular bones show a marked fan-like striation. The small tubular bones of the hands show coarsened trabeculae in the metacarpals and phalanges as well as retardation of maturation. Tubulation of the femurs and the 'rib-within-rib' pattern of the chest are other characteristic radiological findings. There is deformity of the maxilla and dental arch with a resultant protuberance of the front teeth (Asbell, 1964). Papavassiliou (1965) has described erythropoietic tissue masses located along the spine which protrude into the posterior mediastinum. Though usually symptomless they occasionally produce dull, girdle pains and rarely paraplegia; they occur in older patients.

Recurrent pericarditis with gross pericardial effusion and concomitant pleural effusion occurs. Cardiac involvement with congestive cardiac failure, often with arrhythmias and heart block, is the main cause of death (Engle, 1964).

The autopsy findings are those of a chronic severe haemolytic anaemia with marked siderosis in all the organs. The heart is hypertrophied, dilated, and rusty-brown in colour. Myocardial cell destruction is pronounced and marked interstitial fibrosis is present. Erythrophagocytosis by the reticulo-endothelial system, gross congestion of the pulp of the spleen with haemorrhages and infarctive lesions and associated bone changes as described in the pathology of sickle-cell disease, are noted. A mild form of β-thalassaemia major has been described from Singapore (Boon and Wong Hock, 1973).

β Thalassaemia minor

β thalassaemia minor is the heterozygous state of Cooley's anaemia and it shows great variability. At one end of the scale there may be no symptoms and the blood picture merely shows minor morphological changes of the red cells with diminished saline fragility—*thalassaemia minima* (Silvestroni and Bianco, 1946). At the other end, the symptomatology and clinical signs may be so severe as to resemble the homozygous state. An intermediate form with mild anaemia, moderate splenomegaly, gall stones, bone pains, leg ulcers, and chronic jaundice—*thalassaemia minor*—also occurs. In the Negro populations, heterozygous thalassaemia is always mild, while the severe 'intermediate' forms are commonly seen in Greece and Italy (Weatherall, 1964). Thalassaemia minor may cause severe anaemia in pregnancy with secondary folic acid deficiency (Meital *et al.* 1961; Goldberg and Schwartz, 1954).

Haematologically, the M.C.H. and the M.C.V. are low, there may be microcytosis, poikilocytosis, and hypochromia. The distinction between β-thalassaemia minor and iron-deficiency anaemia of mild to moderate degree has been improved by England and Fraser (1973) and Raper (1973). Target cells are usually present. Basophilic stippling is common in Italian and Greek heterozygotes. The saline fragility is invariably reduced, while the main diagnostic feature of heterozygous β thalassaemia minor is the elevation of haemoglobin A_2. Haemoglobin F, if detectable at all, is present in only small amounts (1–5 per cent). It has recently been claimed that a rise in haemoglobin A_2 occurs in acute falciparum malaria, the implication of this finding in population studies in malarious areas is obvious (Arends, 1967).

Other rarer forms of heterozygous β thalassaemia have been described, these are: (i) β thalassaemia associated with normal levels of haemoglobin A_2 and high levels of fetal haemoglobin, (ii) δ-chain thalassaemia. For details the student is referred to the excellent monograph by Weatherall and Clegg (1974).

Interaction between β thalassaemia and the abnormal haemoglobins

Heterozygotes for both β thalassaemia and β-chain abnormal haemoglobins have been extensively studied. Various combinations have been described: (1) sickle-cell thalassaemia, (2) haemoglobin C-thalassaemia, (3) haemoglobin E-thalassaemia, (4) haemoglobin D-thalassaemia, (5) haemoglobin J-thalassaemia, (6) haemoglobin N-thalassaemia, (7) haemoglobin G-thalassaemia.

The most striking feature of these β thalassaemia–abnormal haemoglobin combinations is the great variation in the clinical and haematological findings which occurs in affected individuals. On the whole a good correlation is found between the clinical manifestations of the disorders and the presence or absence of haemoglobin A. Thus in sickle-cell thalassaemia the individuals with little or no haemoglobin A detectable on electrophoresis behave like sickle-cell anaemia patients, while the presence of 15–30 per cent haemoglobin A usually, but not invariably, results in a milder syndrome.

Sickle-cell thalassaemia in pregnancy

Pregnant women with sickle-cell thalassaemia are occasionally liable to crises, abortion, premature delivery, and bacterial infection. Dunn and Haynes (1967) reported upon two Negro patients with sickle-cell thalassaemia who developed pulmonary infarction, a haemolytic crisis, and post-partum bleeding secondary to faulty involution. Both were delivered of a viable infant. Hendrickse et al. (1972) have reported anaemia, bone pain crises and an increased risk of post-partum haemorrhage in pregnancy in West Africa.

Pathology of β thalassaemia haemoglobin-E disease

The clinical picture of β thalassaemia haemoglobin-E disease resembles that of thalassaemia major in many aspects. Hepatosplenomegaly is present in almost all cases. Invariably present are hypochromia, microcytosis, anisocytosis, poikilocytosis, polychromasia, basophilic stippling, and reticulocytosis. Serum iron is normal or elevated. The significant pathological findings are anaemia and parenchymal and reticulo-endothelial haemosiderosis; hyperplasia of haematopoietic tissue and cirrhosis may be a complication. There are in some cases proliferative lesions in the glomeruli and an increase in lipochrome pigment in the visceral organs and smooth muscle (Bhamarapravati *et al.* 1967).

α Thalassaemia

In α-chain thalassaemia there is a depression of α-chain production, thus affecting haemoglobin A $(\alpha_2\beta_2)$, A_2 $(\alpha_2\delta_2)$, and F $(\alpha_2\gamma_2)$. This results in *infancy* in excess production of γ chains which then aggregate to form the tetramer-γ_4 $(\gamma_4 = $haemoglobin Bart's); and in *adult life* it results in excess of β chain production to form β_4 $(\beta_4 = $haemoglobin H). There are two important clinical forms of α thalassaemia. (1) A severe form of α thalassaemia associated with almost 100 per cent haemoglobin Bart's (γ_4), which is incompatible with life and results in hydrops fetalis (Poortrakul *et al.* 1967). This probably represents homozygosity for an α-thalassaemia gene. (2) A milder form of α thalassaemia associated with excess β production and presenting in adult life as *haemoglobin-H disease* (β_4). This probably results from the interaction of two milder α thalassaemia genes.

1. Severe homozygous α thalassaemia

The homozygous inheritance of the gene is incompatible with life, and hydrops fetalis results, with stillbirth occurring between the twenty-eighth and thirty-fourth week (Lie Injo Luan Eng *et al.* 1962). The placenta is large and friable and there is much extra-medullary erythropoiesis in the spleen, liver, and other organs. Peripheral blood smears reveal severe erythroblastosis, reticulocytosis, and many target cells. In the parents of the hydropic babies there is no increase in fetal or A_2 haemoglobin; the morphology of the red cells is, however, slightly abnormal. There are no simple tests for the detection of α thalassaemia trait (heterozygotes). The main characteristics of severe α thalassaemia are given in Table 10.7 and are contrasted with the heterozygous condition.

2. Haemoglobin-H disease

Haemoglobin H, the first of the 'fast-moving' haemoglobins to be discovered, was described by Rigas *et al.* in 1955. It was later shown to consist of four β chains (Jones *et al.* 1959).

TABLE 10.7. *Characteristics of α thalassaemia* (modified from
Weatherall, 1965)

	Homozygote	Heterozygote
Haemoglobin electro-phoresis in infancy	Mainly Hb Bart's. Traces of A and H	5–15% Hb Bart's.* Traces of Hb, H, F, and A
Haemoglobin electro-phoresis in adult life	—	Normal or traces of Hb Bart's or H
Haemoglobin A, and F	—	Normal
Clinical severity	Incompatible with fetal survival. Stillbirths	Very mild. May be completely 'silent'
Red-cell inclusion bodies	Present	Occasional
Red-cell morphology	Marked hypochromia. Many target cells. Erythroblastosis	Varies from normal to moderate hypo-chromia with target cells
Red-cell osmotic fragility	Not reported	Slightly decreased
Other haematological findings	Tendency for red cells to sickle on wet pre-parations	Low M.C.H. with normal serum iron. High red cell count
Distribution	Far East. No cases found elsewhere to date	Far East; Mediterranean littoral; Africa

Haemoglobin Bart's has been reported from several parts of the world (Tuchinda *et al.* 1959; Hendrickse *et al.* 1960; Fessas, 1961; Weatherall and Boyer, 1962). It is found in variable amounts. It is alkali resistant but less so than F. It has a characteristic ultraviolet spectrum and moves slightly faster than J at pH 8·6, and at pH 6·5 separates from A.

It is common in Chinese, Greeks, Italians, Indians, Indonesians, Burmese, and Thais (Rigas *et al.* 1955; Ceppellini, 1959; Gouttas, 1955). It has been described in Sweden, Britain, and American Negroes (Hendenberg, 1958; Woodrow *et al.* 1964).

Clinically, the manifestations of haemoglobin-H disease are very variable. They include easy fatiguability due to long-standing anaemia, recurrent attacks of jaundice and fever, generalized joint pains, pain in the right upper quadrant, and splenomegaly (Fessas, 1959; Lie Injo Luan Eng *et al.* 1961). Haemoglobin H can cause severe refractory anaemia in pregnancy (Brain and Vella, 1959) and the haemoglobinopathy may be masked by severe iron deficiency. Keng and Khoo (1970) have described the changes in the liver. Portal fibrosis was an inconstant finding but haemosiderosis in the periportal parenchymal cells was usual—sometimes severe.

On paper electrophoresis haemoglobin H is a 'fast-moving' haemoglobin which moves ahead of Bart's and has a similar mobility to I. The abnormal haemoglobin forms about 5–30 per cent of the total haemoglobin, the remainder being A with perhaps small amounts of A_2 and δ_4 present. Occasionally, Bart's may be seen. H and Bart's can be further differentiated on normal starch-gel electrophoresis or in a phosphate buffer system at pH 7·7. Inclusion bodies are present in the majority of all of red cells in haemoglobin H and can be demonstrated by incubation with brilliant cresyl blue; they are also visible after splenectomy, and are precipitated by sulphonamides and other drugs causing haemolysis in G-6-PD-deficient persons, p. 460. Similar inclusion bodies are occasionally seen with Bart's.

On electrophoresis in acid pH haemoglobin H remains stationary and I moves towards the negative pole. Inclusion bodies are not seen in erythrocytes containing haemoglobin I.

The main differences between α and β thalassaemia are given in Table 10.8.

TABLE 10.8. *Summary of the main differences between α and β thalassaemia* (modified from Weatherall, 1965)

Thalassaemia type	Hb F	Hb A_2	Hb Bart's and H	Known combinations with abnormal haemoglobins
α thalassaemia	No increase	No increase	May be present	I; Q; S; C; F; E
β thalassaemia	Usually increased	Usually increased	Absent	S; C; E; D; J; N; G; H

α Thalassaemia$_1$/α thalassaemia$_2$/haemoglobin-E disease

The inheritance of three abnormal genes—namely the severe type of α thalassaemia gene, the milder α thalassaemia gene, and haemoglobin-E, has been described from Thailand and results in a disease clinically similar to thalassaemia major (β thalassaemia). The haemoglobin phenotype is A + E + Bart's and in contrast to haemoglobin-H disease only a few of the red cells show inclusion bodies (Wasi *et al.* 1967).

Hereditary spherocytosis and elliptocytosis

Hereditary spherocytosis and elliptocytosis are said to be rare in Negroes, but have been reported in the South African Bantu (Metz, 1959) and have been seen in West Africa (Charles and Smithers, 1959). Ringelhann *et al.* (1970) have reported hereditary persistence of fetal haemoglobin and heterozygous elliptocytosis in a Ghanaian adult male. Malaria has been thought to precipitate a haemolytic anaemia in elliptocytosis (Nkrumah, 1972).

GLUCOSE-6-PHOSPHATE DEHYDROGENASE DEFICIENCY

Glucose-6-phosphate dehydrogenase (G-6-PD) deficiency of the red cells has been demonstrated in many parts of the world. It is particularly common among Mediterranean, Middle Eastern, Far Eastern, and African populations (Siniscalco *et al.* 1966; Szeinberg, 1963; Omer *et al.* 1972; Flatz and Sringam, 1963; Chan *et al.* 1964; Gilles *et al.* 1960; Luzzatto *et al.* 1965). This red cell enzyme defect is apparently harmless unless the red cells are challenged in some way, most usually by the administration of one of a large group of drugs. G-6-PD deficiency is inherited as a sex-linked trait, with full expression in male hemizygotes and female homozygotes, and with variable expression in female heterozygotes (Childs and Zinkham, 1959). This means that the male hemizygote and the female homozygote are always deficient, whereas the female heterozygote is only partially deficient. Many variants of G-6-PD deficiency have been distinguished (WHO, 1967). The two clinically most important are the 'Negro' type of G-6-PD deficiency, which is characterized by a rapid (A) band in starch-gel electrophoresis; and the 'Mediterranean' type, which has more severe clinical effects and is characterized by a slow (B) band. Chan *et al.* (1972) reported for the first time the existence of G-6-PD B(—) Chinese. A third group of G-6-PD-deficient persons have congenital non-spherocytic haemolytic disease (CNSHD), characterized by chronic reticulocytosis and anaemia which may occur spontaneously as well as in response to infection and drugs. Beutler (1970) has emphasized that a surprising number of G-6-PD deficiencies exist, of varying severity. Juvenile cataracts occasionally occur. Oni *et al.* (1970) have noted that in a Nigerian woman, some of whose red cells contained the A variant of the enzyme and some the B, who was also suffering from paroxysmal nocturnal haemoglobinuria, the cells bearing the PNH abnormality were confined to those bearing the B variant. This was considered to be evidence that the PNH abnormality consists of a clone of cells which arises by somatic mutation.

G-6-PD deficiency plays an important role in the pathogenesis of a variety of haemolytic anaemias in the tropics. A fall with age in the frequency of G-6-PD deficiency occurs (Editorial, 1970).

Drug-induced haemolysis with or without haemoglobinuria

Primaquine was the first drug to be shown to produce haemolytic anaemia in enzyme-deficient individuals (Beutler, 1960), and since then many drugs in common clinical use have been implicated.

A list of some of these potentially haemolytic substances is given in Table 10.9.

Although chloroquine appears on the list of haemolytic drugs, this substance has been used widely and rarely causes clinically significant

TABLE 10.9. *Some potentially haemolytic substances in G-6-PD-deficient subjects*

1. *Antimalarials*
   Primaquine
   Pamaquine
   Quinocide
   Pentaquine
   Mepacrine
   Chloroquine

2. *Sulphonamides*

3. Sulphones

4. *Antipyretics and analgesics*
   Acetylsalicylic acid
   Acetanilide
   Acetophenetidin (Phenacetin)
   Phenazone
   Aminophenazone

5. *Nitrofurans*
   Nitrofurantoin (Furadantin)
   Furazolidone (Furoxone)
   Nitrofurazone (Furacin)

6. *Other drugs*
   Dimercaprol (BAL)
   Methylene blue
   Naphthalene (moth balls)
   Ascorbic acid
   Phenylhydrazine
   Probenecid (Benemid)
   Vitamin K
   Trinitrotoluene
   Neosalvarsan
   Quinidine (C)*
   Chloramphenicol
   Niridazole
   Co-trimoxazole

7. *Peas, beans, other vegetables*

*(C): Haemolysis so far only observed in Caucasians.

haemolysis. Co-trimoxazole and niridazole have also been incriminated (Chan, 1972; Chan and McFadzean, 1974).

The haemolysis is self-limiting if the initial dose is not excessive, even when the same dose of drug is continued, because the older and most susceptible erythrocytes are destroyed and the remaining younger erythrocytes are relatively resistant to haemolysis (Dern *et al.* 1954). The severity of haemolysis is sometimes dosage-dependent, and it usually begins on the third day after drug administration. In Negro hemizygotes the enzyme deficiency is less severe (usually activities are around 15 per cent of normal), occasionally, however, complete absence of G-6-PD activity may occur in the African Negro (Owusu, 1972). Acute reversible renal failure precipitated by anaemia and urinary tract infection has been described in G-6-PD deficient patients (Owusu *et al.* 1972.)

Haemolysis during infection

Bacterial, parasitic, and viral infections can all act as an exogenic trigger mechanism in G-6-PD-deficient individuals. Thus *typhoid fever* has been incriminated in Malaysia, Israel, South Africa, and elsewhere (Charmot *et al.* 1966; Hersko and Vardy 1967; Levin, 1967; Chan *et al.* 1971). A high frequency of G-6-PD deficiency in patients with typhoid fever has been reported from Accra, Ghana (Owusu *et al.* 1972). Devakul *et al.* (1966) in Thailand, noted a greater degree of haemolysis in G-6-PD-deficient patients with malaria, despite a lower parasitaemia, than in malarial patients with normal enzyme levels. Thus, G-6-PD-deficiency seems to predispose to malarial anaemia. A finding, also noted by Lewis and Jilly (1966). Acute haemolytic anaemia caused by viral infections, e.g. infective hepatitis, has also been reported (Choremis *et al.* 1966). Morrow *et al.* (1968) reported a high frequency of G-6-PD deficiency in patients with viral hepatitis. The relationship between jaundice, lobar pneumonia and G-6-PD deficiency has already been mentioned p. 391 (Tugwell, 1973; Parent, 1973).

Favism

Fava beans can produce haemolytic anaemia in G-6-PD-deficient individuals (Sansone *et al.* 1958). Favism is common among the inhabitants of Sardinia, Southern Italy, and other parts of the Mediterranean littoral. Other plants will produce a similar syndrome, e.g. peas and male fern. Not all G-6-PD-deficient persons experience haemolysis after ingestion of fava beans and additional factors may be involved. The onset of haemolysis occurs much more rapidly than it does with drugs, appearing within 24 hours, and in the case of fava pollen inhalation it occurs immediately and is severe (Larizza *et al.* 1961).

Neonatal jaundice

Neonatal jaundice in infants whose red cells are deficient in G-6-PD has been widely reported (Doxiades *et al.* 1961; Gilles and Taylor, 1961). Recently, a case of kernicterus has been described from Nigeria; this is of interest because it is commonly said that in Negroes neonatal jaundice caused by this enzyme defect is mild (Ifekwungwe and Luzzatto, 1966). It has been suggested on the basis of family studies that an unknown additional inborn defect might be responsible for severe jaundice in babies with G-6-PD-deficiency (Fessas *et al.* 1962).

The determination of G-6-PD-deficiency can be made by qualitative as well as quantitative tests. The most commonly used qualitative tests for screening populations are (1) the brilliant cresyl blue dye test,* (2) the methaemoglobin reduction test, and (3) the MTT-linked spot test. Quantitative assay of G-6-PD activity is an essentially research procedure. There is usually no difficulty in the detection of enzyme-deficient males and homozygous females of any racial group. The detection of heterozygotes is more difficult and special methods have been devised (Gall *et al.* 1965).

*See Appendix.

BLACKWATER FEVER

Blackwater fever is an acute haemolytic condition associated with fever, anaemia, jaundice, and haemoglobinuria. It is generally considered as of malarial origin and is only found in regions where *P. falciparum* infection occurs. It can occur in either sex and at any age.

The pathogenesis is unknown but certain factors seem to be essential: (i) it occurs only in *non-immune* individuals living in, or having returned from, an area of *P. falciparum* malaria. Therefore, only children in areas of *stable* malaria are usually affected (Jelliffe, 1951). (ii) It used to be closely associated with repeated infections inadequately treated with quinine. Since the introduction of the synthetic antimalarial drugs blackwater fever has become relatively rare. However, the reintroduction of quinine as a method of therapy in non-immune patients infected with chloroquine-resistant strains of *P. falciparum* has increased its incidence. It has been encountered, however, during the course of a severe attack of falciparum malaria unrelated to quinine therapy in comparatively new arrivals in endemic areas of malaria.

Caution must be evinced in accepting all patients presenting with haemoglobinuria in areas of malaria as cases of blackwater fever. It has been shown that the enzyme G-6-PD may be deficient in up to 20 per cent of the population of some of these malarious areas and a drug-induced haemolytic anaemia due to this enzyme deficiency must be excluded before a diagnosis of blackwater fever can be accepted (Gilles and Ikeme, 1960).

The condition develops suddenly and is, in effect, a severe exacerbation of the intravascular haemolysis seen in malaria, although parasites may be scanty or even absent in the peripheral blood. The haematological findings are those of a severe haemolytic anaemia as described in malaria (p. 23), but a direct positive Coombs test has been noted in a number of non-immune patients associated with the administration of quinine. In addition severe renal lesions occur and renal failure is a common complication.

Pathology

The pathology is similar to that seen in malaria. Haemozoin may be, however, less marked in the reticulo-endothelial system, and lesions in the central nervous system are variable. A heavy parasitaemia is rarely seen in the vessels. Kruatrachue and Harinasuta (1970) have recorded a reduction in red cell thickness accompanied by reduced osmotic fragility during the period of haemolysis. The liver is yellow-brown in colour, with centrilobular changes and evidence of biliary stasis present.

The mechanism of the massive intravascular haemolysis is ill understood and was fully discussed when malarial anaemia was considered (p. 23). The most attractive theory is that of an antigen–antibody reaction precipitated by the administration of quinine, or by some other factors. In normal subjects haemoglobin is present in the plasma in small amounts (5 mg/100 ml) and amounts up to about 110 mg/100 ml can be bound by haptoglobins (see p. 414). Over this amount other mechanisms come into play and some haemoglobin unites with albumin to form methaemalbumin (a haematin/albumin complex) which is constantly found in the serum in blackwater fever and can be detected by Schumm's test. The remainder of the haemoglobin in unbound and free in the plasma. The bound haemoglobin does not appear in the urine, but unbound haemoglobin (mol. wt. 68,000) can pass across the normal glomerular basement membrane, with consequent haemoglobinuria which is characteristic of the disease. This occurs when the release of large amounts of haemoglobin into the blood stream overcomes the maximum binding capacity of the haptoglobins. Small amounts of haemoglobin in the glomerular filtrate are reabsorbed by the proximal tubules of the kidney, the remainder appearing in the urine. In the proximal tubules some of the haemoglobin is broken down and haemosiderin is formed and re-excreted and can be detected in the urinary sediment by the Prussian blue reaction and can occur in the absence of frank haemoglobinuria. Unconjugated bilirubin is invariably, and conjugated bilirubin usually, raised in the blood.

At one time the *renal lesions* were thought to be due to tubular blockage by haemoglobin precipitated by acidosis and increased salt concentration. This formed the basis of alkali therapy. However, anuria in malaria is not invariably related to haemoglobinuria and evidence of tubular dysfunction may precede, or occur, without haemoglobinuria, so this theory is untenable. In addition large amounts of haemoglobin have been given to man and animals without adverse effects. Neither parasites nor haemozoin are considered to be direct factors in the renal pathology. The lesions are now considered to be most probably due to ischemia of the renal cortex arising from reduced renal blood flow, the fundamental lesion being renal vasoconstriction with a juxtaglomerular shunt at the junction of the cortex and medulla, rendering the cortex and peripheral glomeruli ischaemic and causing marked changes in the tubules.

The initial renal vasoconstriction should theoretically result in an increase of antidiuretic hormone in the blood, later accentuated by further renal ischaemia, and causing maximal reabsorption of water from the glomerular filtrate, finally leading to stasis and formation of haem casts in the tubules and, possibly, obstruction to the nephron. A combination of reduced glomerular filtration rate, excessive tubular reabsorption, and, possibly, nephron blockage, finally results in anuria. The part that parasite metabolism and catabolism play is at present unknown, but it is not thought to be great. Macroscopically, the kidneys are enlarged and swollen. The cortex is pale with perhaps small haemorrhages present, and the medulla is congested. Microscopically, the glomeruli are usually little affected and are avascular. Amorphous hyaline material is usually present in the capsular space and gives a variable reaction to haemoglobin and free-iron stains. The capsular epithelium may be cuboidal.

The most marked changes are in the epithelium of the ascending limb of Henle's loop and in the distal convoluted tubules, and are patchy in distribution. The epithelium of the proximal and collecting tubules is not usually severely affected. The affected cells in the loops of Henle and distal convoluted tubules show all degrees of degenerative change up to complete necrosis. The tubules are dilated and contain epithelial, hyaline, or granular casts and other casts giving the staining reaction of haemoglobin. In some instances the casts give a positive Prussian blue reaction for iron. Regeneration of tubular epithelium, tubulo-venous anastomoses, and interstitial casts, with a corresponding lymphocytic infiltration, may be present. Malarial parasites and haemozoin are rarely seen.

In short, the changes are those of a non-specific tubular necrosis as described in many conditions, including the 'crush syndrome' (Maegraith and Findlay, 1944); haemoglobin casts are evidence of the sudden severe haemolysis which has occurred. As would be expected from the renal changes, urea retention and acidosis are marked. Hyperkalaemia is an added hazard.

The *urinary changes* vary with the severity of the condition. In the milder forms, albuminuria, casts, haemosiderinuria, some methaemoglobin, and increased urobilinogen, all of slight degree, may be found. The amount of urine decreases with advancing severity until complete suppression may occur. Increasing amounts of albumin in the urine, oxy- and methaemoglobin, casts, urobilinogen, scanty red blood cells, and bile are found with increasing severity. A corresponding increasing retention of urea is present in the blood, with a fall in the urinary content of urea and chloride. The urine is light red when first passed but rapidly changes colour to dark red and brown as the oxyhaemoglobin is reduced to methaemoglobin.

If recovery ensues, the urinary signs rapidly regress, but the blood urea falls more slowly. The excessive loss of electrolytes in the diuretic phase may be a danger in the later stages.

GENETIC ASPECTS OF MALARIA IMMUNITY

Haemoglobin S, haemoglobin C, haemoglobin E, the thalassaemia gene, haemoglobin F, G-6-PD, and the Rh factor, have all been implicated as possibly playing a part in malaria immunity.

Haemoglobin S and malaria

The high incidence of a gene lethal in its homozygous expression (SS) in many parts of tropical Africa (very few homozygotes reproduce) was difficult to explain until Beet (1946) and Allison (1954) independently suggested that this might be due to the selective advantage the heterozygote enjoyed against the lethal effects of *P. falciparum* malaria, the loss of normal genes due to this cause outweighing the loss of the S gene in sickle-cell anaemia patients. This hypothesis is now accepted and various facts confirm its veracity.

(1) The sickle-cell gene is found in its highest incidence in areas where *P. falciparum* malaria is, or was until recently, endemic.

(2) In areas of stable malaria, high *P. falciparum* densities are significantly less commonly found in children with the sickle-cell trait (AS) than in normal children (AA).

(3) Post-mortem studies have revealed that death from cerebral malaria does not occur in the S heterozygote (AS).

(4) There is evidence that the incidence of the sickle-cell trait in a population increases with advancing years, which is suggestive of differential survival with a greater loss of normal genes (Fig. 10.16).

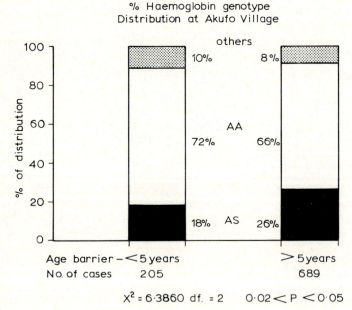

Fig. 10.16. Percentage haemoglobin genotype distribution in a West African village (Akufo).

that malaria is involved. The evidence to date is inconclusive (Kidson and Gorman, 1962; Stammatoyannopoulos and Fessas, 1964).

G-6-PD and malaria

Confirmation of the malaria-protection hypothesis has been sought in various ways: gene-frequency-distribution studies in populations living in areas of different malarial endemicity; malaria-parasite-density surveys in G-6-PD normal and deficient children; induced-falciparum malaria in human volunteers; and G-6-PD deficiency among patients with severe clinical falciparum malaria. Except for gene-frequency-distribution studies, the results have always been conflicting. The results of recent studies, however, have provided evidence that G-6-PD deficiency offers a selective advantage to the carrier against potentially lethal malaria infection, although the results are not as conclusive as for haemoglobin S (Gilles *et al.* 1967). In blood from female children with acute *P. falciparum* malaria the parasite rate was 2 to 80 times higher in normal than in deficient erythrocytes (Luzzatto *et al.* 1969; Luzzatto *et al.* 1972).

Rh-negative gene and malaria

Gorman (1964) has put forward a most interesting hypothesis about the possible selection against the Rh-negative gene by malaria. The incidence of the Rh gene is generally low in areas in which malaria is or was endemic. It was suggested that a population subject to a heavily malarious environment might be superior antibody producers owing to selection by elimination of poor antibody producers. If this were so, erythroblastosis fetalis should be more intense in malarious areas, and Rh-negative genes should be selectively eliminated if the frequency of the gene is or was below 0.50 (Wiener, 1942). Hence Rh-negative mothers in a malarious area should show a higher incidence of sensitization to an Rh-positive fetus than their counterparts in northern areas. In Ibadan, Nigeria, over 400 Rh-negative pregnant multiparae were studied and, apart from some who had had previous transfusions of Rh-positive blood, the evidence of those sensitized by pregnancy was only 2.5 per cent—a lower incidence than the figures recorded from Europe and elsewhere. This evidence does not, therefore, substantiate Gorman's hypothesis.

THE PURPURAS AND OTHER HAEMORRHAGIC DISORDERS

Bleeding due to coagulation defects is comparatively rare in the tropics, whereas haemorrhage from larger vessels due to erosion in malignant disease or rupture is common. Purpura is difficult to detect in many of the darker-skinned people in the tropics and can be most satisfactorily diagnosed by carefully examining the mucous membranes. A brief standard classification is given in Table 10.10.

TABLE 10.10. *Classification of the purpuras and other haemorrhagic disorders*

A. Due to capillary defects
    (i) Allergy: Henoch–Schonlein purpura
    (ii) Vitamin-E deficiency. Scurvy.
    (iii) Toxic: acute infections, drugs, snake-bite poisons
    (iv) Metabolic: senile purpura, malignant disease, uraemia

B. Due to platelet deficiency
    (i) Primary or essential thrombocytopenia
    (ii) Secondary:
        Aplastic anaemia due to drugs and poisons (chemotherapy)
        Malignant disease of bone marrow
        Occasional megaloblastic anaemia
        Acute leukaemia
        Infections

C. Defects of coagulation
    (i) Fibrinogen deficiency
        Congenital (rare)
        Defibrination syndrome
    (ii) Hypoprothrombinaemia
        Congenital: haemorrhagic disease of the newborn
        Malabsorption of vitamin K: steatorrhoea, biliary obstruction, hepato-cellular damage
        Anticoagulant drugs

D. Haemophilia and related disorders

The haemorrhagic manifestations of *scurvy* are not associated with thrombocytopenia but are considered to be due to increased capillary permeability. *Henoch–Schonlein purpura* is considered to be due to a similar defect and is rare in our experience. Non-thrombocytopenic purpura can occur following the administration of many drugs, iodides, quinine, mercury, procaine penicillin, and phenacetin being the most likely agents in the tropics. It can also occur as a complication of viperine and crotaline snake bites. Drug-induced purpura has, however, in our experience been of the thromocytopenic type. The purpuras of meningococcal septicaemia and uraemia are relatively common.

Essential thrombocytopenia is uncommon in the American Negroes (Wintrobe, 1961) and is not common in West Africa.

There is a condition called *onyalai* which occurs in East and South Africa which is a form of thrombocytopenic purpura. Haemorrhagic bullae in the mucosa of the oral cavity are, however, a striking clinical feature. It occurs in young adults and children. Megakaryocytes are present in the bone marrow in normal or increased numbers but the platelet life span is reduced (Lurie *et al.* 1969). Attempts to demonstrate a thrombocytopenia-inducing factor, as has been done in idiopathic thrombocytopenic purpura, were unsuccessful by the technique employed. Splenic sequestration of platelets is variable but if present splenectomy will cause remission. It was considered by these authors that the retention of the term *onyalai* as indicative of a separate disease entity was unwarranted. *Thrombocytopenic purpura* is not uncommon following the use of certain drugs. The most important are the chemotherapeutic agents used in malignant disease, and quinine and pamaquine in children may also be causal. Drugs should be suspected if unexplained thrombocytopenia occurs in an adult. The condition may occur as the result of snake or insect bites and is a complication of heat stroke. It is commonly seen with malignant invasion of the bone marrow and is a constant feature of acute leukaemia. Thrombocytopenic purpura is a very real complication of the acute megaloblastic anaemia occasionally seen with folic-acid deficiency.

Hypoprothrombinaemia due to a deficiency of vitamin K, which is a precursor of Factor VII, is a not uncommon cause of haemorrhagic disease of the newborn. Secondary hypoprothrombinaemia is common, especially as the result of liver disease, and the prothrombin time of the blood should be estimated prior to liver biopsy being performed.

Haemophilia is a constitutional anomaly of blood coagulation which depends on the hereditary transmission of a sex-linked recessive Mendelian trait and is characterized by a life-long tendency to prolonged haemorrhage, as well as markedly delayed coagulation time in affected males (Wintrobe, 1961). The bleeding is known to be due to the absence of a clotting factor— antihaemophilic globulin or factor VIII. The absence of other clotting factors can cause a similar condition clinically. It is not intended to discuss these further. The condition is rare in the American Negro (Boyles and Currie, 1958) and is thought to be rare in Africa. However, we have seen a few cases in Ibadan and the possibility of haemorrhage following circumcision causing some deaths in infancy must be considered. Forbes *et al.* (1966) have described five patients with haemophilia and five with Christmas disease in Kenya, and cases have been described in South and West Africa and the Congo so the condition may not be so rare in Africans as previously thought (Essien and Adeloye, 1972). The condition is said to be rare in the Chinese but occurs in Japan. Von Willebrand's disease, an autosomal-dominant inherited bleeding disorder characterized by a prolonged bleeding time and a low antihaemophilic factor (factor VIII level) is rare in Asiatic and Negro races. It has, however, been reported in a Bantu family in South Africa (Gomperts *et al.* 1969).

LEUKAEMIA

There are marked geographical and racial variations in the incidence of leukaemia both in tropical and temperate climates. The incidence is very much less in the U.S. non-white than in the white but in the latter group mortality statistics show a downturn for all ages from 1 to 74 years. In South Africa the incidence in whites is higher than that seen in Europe and the U.S.A. and is very much less in the Bantu. In Western Nigeria and Jamaica the incidence is similar to that found in Western populations. The incidences are low in Mozambique, Uganda, and in the Bantu in South Africa. The lowest incidence is recorded in the Chinese in Singapore (Doll *et al.* 1966).

The pattern of leukaemia is also variable. Acute leukaemia is rare in children in the Chinese in Singapore, the Japanese in Hawaii, Western Nigerians, and in the peoples of Mozambique and Uganda, whereas the maximum mortality for acute lymphatic leukaemia in England is 3 years and there is a peak of acute myeloid leukaemia at 2–4 years (Court-Brown and Doll, 1961).

Why acute leukaemia in the 0–4-year-old age group is not seen in certain tropical areas is not known but it is known that there is a low mortality from leukaemia in countries in which death rates from communicable diseases are still high (WHO, 1962). Court-Brown and Doll (1961) showed that the mortality peak in children only occurred after 1920 in England and has become more pronounced since 1940. This peak is also apparent in U.S. white children and is beginning to emerge in the U.S. Japanese and non-white children (Rucknagel, 1966; Fraumeni and Miller, 1967). In Ohio, U.S.A., there is a lower incidence in children of low-income families regardless of race (Browning and Gross, 1968). In South Africa it is rare in the Bantu but the peak is evident in children of higher-income white parents (Utian and Heymann, 1963).

Leukaemia mortality is less in Israel in populations of African and Asian origin than it is in those of Israeli or European origin but mortality in children of African and Asian origin in the 1950–58 period has more than tripled whereas those of the latter have doubled. The childhood peak is also absent in South American countries.

In Africa, in children, lymphomas may exceed leukaemia by a ratio of 10:1. In Jamaica the frequencies in children of leukaemia and lymphomas were 30·5 and 12·6 per cent, resembling the Western pattern, and there was a high incidence of acute leukaemia in young children (Watler *et al.* 1961). It should be noted that over 90 per cent of the Jamaican population is either pure Negro or of predominantly Negro descent (Bras *et al.* 1969). It is of interest to note that malaria has been eradicated from Jamaica (Ashcroft *et al.* 1969) and that the Burkitt tumour is rare. Environment is obviously therefore important in acute leukaemia in childhood and we would agree with Davies (1965) that in some areas of the tropics young children may possess some factor of resistance to leukaemia. It would appear that the peak incidence at the age 2–4 is associated with improved standards of living and it is tempting to speculate that the absence may be related to the multiple infestations and infections so commonly found, the raised gamma-globulin values in the neonate in Africa (Michaux *et al.* 1966) exerting a transient protective action against some oncogenic factor in early childhood thus explaining the absence of acute leukaemia in the 0–4-year-old age group and its emergence in the 5–9. On the other hand, improved methods of therapy in the higher income groups may save the leukaemia-prone neonate. These theories are, of course, speculative but there is some evidence that infective factors may be concerned in the aetiology of leukaemia, viz: possibly clustering, greater mortality in town dwellers and the occurrence of complete remissions especially in childhood. The possible introduction of a carcinogen with improved standards of living and the early death of the leukaemia-prone child in poor social surroundings from infectious causes are other factors to be considered. Davies and Owor (1965) noticed chloromatous deposits in 8 of 13 children suffering from myeloid leukaemia in Uganda. Lothe (1967) noticed a much lower incidence. Essien (1972) recorded three instances in his large series of leukaemic patients in Ibadan. The reason for the apparent greater tendency of African children to exhibit this lesion is unknown.

Children born to mothers who had an influenza infection in pregnancy may be more likely to develop leukaemia or Hodgkin's disease (Editorial, 1972). Chicken pox in pregnancy may also be a factor in leukaemia developing in children (Aldestein and Donovan, 1972). Children who have a history of viral infection, bacterial infection or allergy are also more prone to develop leukaemia after exposure to low doses of ante-natal irradiation.

It should be noted that in Mozambique, Uganda, and Western Nigeria the Burkitt tumour is found in high incidence and it was suggested at one time that this lymphoma might be the expression of the acute leukaemia of childhood seen in temperate climates. The Burkitt tumour, however, has its peak incidence in an older age group and very, very rarely terminates with a leukaemic blood picture. The possibility that cases are being missed must be considered (Lothe, 1967). It has been suggested that the heritable disorders associated with cytogenic defects predispose to leukaemia whereas disorders associated with immunological deficiencies are related to the lymphomas (Fraumeni and Miller, 1967). It is most unlikely that leukaemia associated with recognizable cytogenetic defects accounts for the differing incidence of acute leukaemia in childhood in England and Africa.

In 78 adult patients suffering from leukaemia in Ibadan the following types were seen: acute leukaemia 21; acute monocytic 7; subacute myeloid 1;

chronic myeloid 24; chronic lymphatic 25. The findings in East Africa in a smaller series were similar and the overall incidence of the various types is the same as that reported in the United States (Wintrobe, 1961). Poly-cythaemia vera is rare in the tropics. Although the pattern is similar in Western countries and in Africa, there is some evidence that the clinical presentation in chronic lymphatic leukaemia may differ. In Africa the spleen is usually markedly enlarged with absent or minimal lymphadenopathy (Haddock, 1967). A lymphocytosis is present in the peripheral blood and the majority of the cells are mature lymphocytes. The marrow is infiltrated with lymphocytes, and liver biopsy shows a marked lymphocytic infiltration of the portal tracts and sinusoids. A few patients presenting with this clinical and haematological picture have temporarily responded to long-term anti-malarial therapy only to finally succumb to a malignant lymphoma of the acute lymphoblastic or reticulum-cell type. The differential diagnosis between this type of chronic lymphatic leukaemia and the tropical spleno-megaly syndrome is discussed on p. 497. Chronic lymphatic leukaemia is said to be rare in the West Pacific Region, especially in Japan.

Chronic myeloid leukaemia would not appear to differ in its clinical presentation in Africa but information on the incidence of the Philadelphia 1 chromosome in the tropics as a whole is lacking (Editorial, 1966). It has been detected in a few patients in Ibadan. Acute erythraemic myelosis is generally considered a rare type of leukaemia and even more rare in the African. Luzzatto and Lewis (1972), however, have recently noted three cases in Nigeria. It should be remembered that leukaemoid reactions are relatively common in the tropics and may present diagnostic difficulties. Alkaline phosphatase is said to be diminished in the granulocytes in chronic myeloid leukaemia but increased in the leukaemoid reaction (Editorial, 1968).

BLOOD TRANSFUSION IN THE TROPICS

The high incidence of all types of anaemia including the abnormal haemoglobin diseases, the severe complications of childbirth, acute surgical emergencies in anaemic patients, and, lastly, the mounting toll of road accidents frequently involving large numbers of people, emphasize the tremendous need for transfusion services in the tropics. Unfortunately in many areas these are not available and it falls upon the hard-worked medical officer working in isolation to provide his own. With enthusiasm this can be done and we have seen efficient small blood banks being run by the single doctor in charge of a hospital which may be serving a population of 100,000 or more. In certain areas, due to ignorance or prejudice it may be difficult to obtain donors, but slowly, as the dramatic effects of transfusion are seen by patients and their relatives, it becomes more and more simple to persuade relatives to donate blood. The method of blood-donor recruitment in Ibadan has been well described by Maclean (1958) and the blood bank in the University College Hospital (500 beds) now processes over 8000 units per year. The following discussion on blood transfusion techniques is aimed at assisting the inexperienced practitioner to understand the problems which he may be confronted with in the tropics, more sophisticated readers are referred to standard textbooks on the subject. Blood-grouping techniques have been described in a Medical Research Council Memorandum (1958) and are not described in detail in this chapter.

The subject is dealt with under the following headings:

(a) Blood groups and transfusion
    (i) Blood-group antigens
    (ii) Blood-group antibodies
    (iii) The ABO system
    (iv) The Rh system
    (v) Other blood-group systems
    (vi) Compatability tests (cross-matching tests)

(b) Transmission of disease by blood transfusion

(c) Selection of donors
    (i) Technique of venesection
    (ii) Storage of blood

(d) Methods of blood transfusion
    (i) Intraperitoneal blood transfusion
    (ii) Autotransfusion

(e) Incidence of complications and reactions
    (i) Simple febrile and allergic reactions
    (ii) Haemolytic transfusion reactions
    (iii) Infected blood
    (iv) Transfusion and severe anaemia
    (v) Citrate toxicity
    (vi) Thrombophlebitis
    (vii) Air embolism
    (viii) Transfusional siderosis

(f) Haemolytic disease of the newborn

(a) Blood groups and transfusion

(i) Blood-group antigens

There are at least fourteen human blood groups systems: ABO, P, MNSs, Rhesus, Lutheran, Kell, Lewis, Duffy, Kidd, I, Auberger, Xg, Diego, and

Cartwright (Mollison, 1967). The most important in blood transfusion are the ABO and Rh blood-group systems. The groups are genetically controlled and their incidence varies in different races in various parts of the world. The world-wide variations have been described by Mourant (1954), Boyd (1958), and Race and Sanger (1962) and are not discussed in any detail in this text, our remarks being mainly confined to West Africa where most of our experience has been gained. The part that selection plays in the incidence of the various blood groups should, however, be of interest to workers in the tropics. Haemolytic disease of the newborn must have a selective disadvantage against certain blood-group antigens and the possible association of malaria and the incidence of the Rh negative individuals is discussed on p. 469. In addition there is an association between blood groups and certain diseases (Reed, 1961). It is possible that susceptibility to diseases such as diphtheria, typhoid, influenza, and pneumonia might be influenced by the ABO genotype and affect their incidence in population groups. Similarities between the blood-group O antigen and the plague bacillus, and the A antigen and the smallpox virus, have been noted. It is now too late in the Western world to investigate possible associations between these diseases and blood groups but such investigations are still possible in areas of the tropics. In population groups a comparison of gene frequencies in the elderly and young children might reveal interesting selective advantages of various blood group systems. Blood groups and malignant disease are dealt with in their appropriate context.

(ii) Blood-group antibodies

Blood-group antibodies can be classified by the way they are produced into *naturally-occurring*, that is antibodies that occur without any obvious antigenic stimulus, and *immune*, that is antibodies that are produced in response to the parental administration of foreign red-cell antigens. The naturally-occurring antibodies are usually large molecular weight (mol. wt. = 1,000,000) antibodies of the immunoglobulin class, IgM. They are frequently 'cold' antibodies, that is they agglutinate the appropriate red cells more strongly at temperatures below 37 °C. They have probably been produced in response to antigens on bacteria and other organisms, some of these antigens having chemical structures in common with red-cell antigens. Immune antibodies, on the other hand, while they may be of the immunoglobulin class IgM when first produced often rapidly become smaller molecular weight (mol. wt. = 150,000) antibodies of the immunoglobulin class, IgG. They are warm antibodies, that is they agglutinate the appropriate red cells more strongly at 37 °C and in contradistinction to the IgM antibodies they pass readily through the placental barrier and can give rise to haemolytic disease of the newborn.

Blood-group antibodies can also be classified according to the way they react with the appropriate red cells in the laboratory into *complete*, that is antibodies which agglutinate the red cells when they are suspended in saline, and *incomplete*, that is antibodies that will not agglutinate the appropriate cells suspended in saline but will agglutinate them when a suitable medium such as bovine albumin is used. The reason for their two different types of reaction is probably largely based on the size of the immunoglobulin molecule involved. IgM antibodies are mainly *complete* and IgG antibodies *incomplete*, although there are some exceptions. Thus it will be seen that naturally-occurring antibodies are usually complete antibodies and immune antibodies though they may at first be complete, normally rapidly become incomplete in type.

(iii) The ABO system

There are six common groups in the ABO system A_1, A_2, B, A_1B, A_2B, and O. The H antigen present in saliva is also present in red cells but varies in quantity according to the ABO group. The greatest activity with anti-H serum is seen in group O cells and the least with group A_1B. To determine the ABO group on blood donors tile grouping is not recommended, as weak A antigens of subgroup A_2 may be missed. Standard tube methods should be employed. However, if speed is essential a slide method may be used and is described in the Appendix.

TABLE 10.11. *The ABO blood-group system*

Group	Antigen on the red cells	Antibody in the serum (or plasma)
A A_1	$A + A_1$	Anti-B
A_2	A	Anti-B (2% Anti-A)
B	B	Anti-A + A_1
AB A_1B	Both (i.e. $A + A_1 + B$)	None (i.e. not anti-A or anti-B)
A_2B	Both (i.e. $A + B$)	None (i.e. not Anti-A or Anti-B) (25% Anti-A_1)
O	None (i.e. not A or B)	Both (i.e. anti, $A + A_1 + B$)

'Immune' anti-A and anti-B as opposed to naturally-occurring antibodies have been described and are important factors in ABO haemolytic disease of the newborn, the incidence of which is high in West Africa. Three per cent of infants born in Ibadan have been found to be jaundiced, possibly due to this cause. Haemolytic disease of the newborn occurs in group A or group B children born of group O mothers. However, it is very difficult to predict the occurrence of ABO haemolytic disease by examination of the mother's blood as almost all the sera of group O adults give a positive indirect antiglobulin (Coombs) test with adult A or B cells indicating the presence of immune antibodies. Lytic anti-A and/or anti-B antibodies occur in 56 per cent of group O bloods tested within 24 hours of taking. The diagnosis of the disease itself may also be difficult as the direct antiglobulin test on the baby's blood is often negative or only weakly positive. Evidence of increased red-cell production in cord-blood films with spherocytosis of the red cells and an increased osmotic fragility of the baby's blood is helpful as the last two findings do not occur in Rh incompatibility. Lysis of a 4 per cent suspension of the baby's cells by fresh maternal serum is probably a more significant test of ABO haemolytic disease but this test may also be positive in unaffected infants. The possibility of an associated G-6-PD deficiency must always be considered and appropriate tests undertaken. The reason for the high incidence of ABO haemolytic disease of the newborn in West Africa is unknown. In this connection, the findings of Oliver-Gonzalez and Torregrosa (1944) that anti-A and to a less extent anti-B titres in Group O subjects exposed to *P. falciparum* malaria were far greater than in control Group O subjects might be relevant.

(iv) The Rh system

In 1940 Landsteiner and Wiener prepared in laboratory animals an anti-rhesus monkey erythrocyte serum. It was found that this serum would agglutinate the red cells of about 85 per cent of white persons tested. These cells were referred to as Rh positive and the cells of the remaining 15 per cent as Rh negative. Subsequently many human examples of what is now called anti-D were discovered and for a long time it was considered that human anti-D and the anti-Rh monkey serum were identical, and the whole system was called the rhesus system. It is now known, however, that the anti-Rh monkey serum does not identify the same determinant as anti-D and, because the whole system cannot be renamed, the anti-Rh monkey serum is called anti-LW. The system is now extremely complex. It is simplest to consider that three genes are responsible for the Rh antigens and that each gene is responsible for at least two alternate forms Cc, Dd, Ee. Each chromosome carries three genes which may be a combination of these forms, and numerous genotypes exist, e.g. CDe/cde, cde/cde, etc. The terms Rh positive and Rh negative refer to the presence or absence of the D antigen. Rh negatives are most common in Europe, the highest incidence being found in the Basque peoples. In all areas of the tropics the incidence among the aboriginal populations is low. In Asia and the Pacific the closely linked chromosomic combinations CDe and cDE are the principal ones found, whereas Africans are mainly cDe. Among Asians east of Burma this incidence of Rh negative becomes 1 in 3000, or less. In the American Indians similarly the rhesus negative is very low or absent. Only in Africa (4–6 per cent), Western Asia, India, and Pakistan (7–10 per cent) is the Rh negative appreciable. There is, consequently, a low incidence of haemolytic disease of the newborn due to rhesus incompatibility in most areas of the tropics.

In West Africa the incidence of rhesus negative individuals is in the region of 4–6 per cent and haemolytic disease of the newborn due to rhesus immunization does occasionally occur. An interesting finding has been that, although the frequency of immunization in rhesus-negative women transfused with rhesus-positive blood is as expected elsewhere, the frequency of immunization by pregnancy is low, being only 2·5 per cent (Worrledge *et al.* 1968). The reason for this is obscure. Although the incidence of the rhesus-negative individuals is low in the tropics rhesus grouping should not be ignored, especially in girls and women of child-bearing age, as 50 per cent of rhesus-negative patients transfused with rhesus-positive blood will develop antibodies. Rh haemolytic disease, however, can now be prevented. Sensitization of the mother occurs most frequently in the first pregnancy at the time of delivery by transplacental haemorrhage of fetal red cells into the maternal circulation. The injection of Rh antibody into the mother following delivery blocks the antigen on the surface of the fetal red cells and prevents maternal sensitization. Anti-D serum may, however, transmit serum hepatitis, therefore an Rh immunoglobulin (7S) has been isolated from plasma which obviates this danger. This treatment has no place in a woman who is already sensitized but should be given to all unsensitized Rh negative women following delivery if the child is Rh positive. Similar preventive measures should be used in the case of abortion.

All rhesus-negative results in blood donors should be confirmed by the use of antiglobulin serum, as the Du antigen may react weakly with anti-D serum. A test for emergency slide-test rhesus grouping is given in the Appendix (b).

(v) Other blood-group systems

The remaining blood-group systems also differ in their incidence. There is, for instance, a U group of the MNss system which is peculiar to the Negro, and anti-M, anti-N, and anti-S antibodies are found in about 2 per cent of all blood samples in Ibadan. There is also a high incidence of Le (A-b-) individuals in West Africa and naturally-occurring Lewis antibodies are found in 10 per cent of samples received. Negroes have a high incidence of the Fy (a-b-) which has not been seen in Europeans (Sanger *et al.* 1955).

The Diego system is not found in Europeans or Negroes but is present in South American Indians, Japanese, and Chinese. The Sutter (Js^a) is an antigen which is part of the Kell system and is not present in Caucasians or Mongoloids (Giblett and Chase, 1959). The Kell antigen is almost unknown in all tropical areas except perhaps the Australian aboriginal. The association of an anti-P antibody and hydatid disease is discussed on p. 205.

Almost all these remaining blood-group systems may occasionally cause transfusion reactions and some may cause haemolytic disease of the newborn. Special tests may be required to detect the antibody. Lewis antibodies are best detected in fresh serum. Other antibodies are more active at 4 °C or 20 °C and difficult to detect at 37 °C. Others may only be detected by the indirect antiglobulin test.

(vi) Compatability tests (cross-matching tests)

The ABO and rhesus groups of the recipient and donor should be determined and blood of the same group utilized for transfusion. Cross-matching tests of the donor red cells against the recipient's serum should never be omitted. These tests must be capable of detecting agglutinating antibodies and a wide range of incomplete antibodies. A saline agglutination, an in-albumin test at 37 °C and an indirect antiglobulin test should be performed, and these tests are described in the Appendix (c).

About 10 per cent of group O individuals in temperate climates have haemolysins or high-titre anti-A agglutinins in their serum sufficient to cause a transfusion reaction in group A or B patients, and the figure is higher in the tropics (56 per cent in Nigeria); these should be tested for in all group O donors [see Appendix (d)]. This, however, will usually be impracticable in most areas of the tropics. 'Universal donor' group O blood should not therefore be employed for transfusing A or B recipients without prior investigation, except in unavoidable emergencies.

(b) Transmission of disease by blood transfusion

The most frequent and serious disorder likely to be transmitted by blood transfusion is, just as in temperate climates, *hepatitis*. The incidence is considered to be in the region of 1 per cent in Ibadan and, of course, the risk to the recipient is increased the greater the number of units transfused. In an exchange transfusion 10 pints may be utilized. A further complication in the tropics is the difficulty in obtaining a clear-cut history of jaundice from donors, thus probably increasing the risk of hepatitis. In few areas will it be possible to screen the donors for the presence of the Australia antigen (p.

578). Even if this were possible, however, it is doubtful if, in the present stage of our knowledge, large numbers of donors should be rejected in areas of high frequency. Care, however, should be taken in transfusing immigrants from populations who have a low frequency of the antigen. There is little information available on the severity of transfusion-transmitted hepatitis in the tropics.

Where *malaria* is endemic it has not been an hazard in our experience if the patient is indigenous. The neonate is passively protected and adults are immune. Theoretically, infants and young children may develop a severe infection and it is justifiable to prescribe a course of antimalarial therapy in these patients. The peripheral blood of donors in Ibadan is not examined for the presence of malarial parasites as it is known that approximately 10 per cent will be positive for *P. falciparum* malaria. If non-immunes are transfused the risk of transmitting malaria is very great and can be obviated by administrating chloroquine diphosphate (600 mg) to the recipient either before or following the transfusion. Malarial parasites survive for at least 14 days in blood stored at 4 °C and all blood transfused in an area of stable malaria should be regarded as infected. In Europe, *P. malariae* has occasionally been transmitted by blood transfusion.

The spirochaetes of *syphilis* and *yaws* probably do not survive for more than 72 hours in stored citrated blood. If fresh blood is transfused in an endemic yaws area, or from a donor in whom the possibility of a syphilitic infection cannot be excluded by serological tests, it is probably wise to prescribe suitable antibiotic cover for the recipient.

Brucellosis has been transmitted by blood transfusion in very rare instances.

The presence of *microfilariae* in the peripheral blood of a donor is of little importance as passage in the insect vector is necessary before infection can be established. Allergic reactions in the recipient may, however, occur (Bird and Menon, 1961). The *microfiliariae* survive for 14–21 days in stored blood at 4 °C. The question of *Chagas' disease* poses a much more difficult problem as it may be transmitted by apparently healthy people. In Sao Paulo, Brazil, 2 per cent of donors may be infected by *T. cruzi*. All potential donors in areas in which Chagas' disease is endemic must be screened for the presence of this infection and rejected if infected. Attempts are being made to ensure sterility of the blood by the addition of anti-parasitic agents.

The African form of *trypanosomiasis* has similarly been transmitted by blood transfusion. Extensive attempts are being made to eradicate this infection and it might be wise to reject donors from areas where the parasites are still endemic.

The transmission of *leishmaniasis* has been reported but must be very rare. The estimation of the haemoglobin should lead to the rejection of the donor. The whole subject of blood transfusion and tropical disease was reviewed (*Lancet*, 1973).

(c) Selection of donors

Shortage of staff and the high incidence of endemic diseases makes the screening of donors a difficult problem. In addition where there is a scarcity of volunteer donors a large percentage cannot be lightly discarded as unsuitable.

The hazards of transfusion-transmitted disease have already been discussed. Donors should be between the ages of 18 and 65 years. The haemoglobin level of the prospective donor should be estimated and a minimal level of 12·5 g/100 ml is a realistic acceptable figure in both sexes and can be rapidly and easily estimated by the use of a copper-sulphate solution of specific gravity 1053. A drop of blood taken into a capillary tube is allowed to fall a distance of 1 cm into the solution and will sink if the haemoglobin content is 12·5 g or more per 100 ml. If it floats the haemoglobin content is less than required. The blood pressure should be taken and, if high, the donor should be carefully supervised during venesection or rejected.

In areas where there is a high incidence of the abnormal haemoglobin diseases or thalassaemia, ideally the electrophoretic pattern of the haemoglobin should be analysed and a peripheral blood film examined. Trait blood can be used for transfusion purposes but sickle-cell trait blood should *not* be utilized in packed cells for exchange transfusion purposes as we have seen anaemic patients with normal haemoglobin in their erythrocytes dying during, or following, transfusion in whom at necropsy the spleen and liver have resembled those seen in the sequestration crisis described on p. 438. If electrophoresis is not available a rapid sickling test should be performed and, if positive, SC disease should be excluded by the examination of a peripheral blood film—the presence of numerous target cells and the occasional sickled cell being diagnostic. In other areas the haemoglobin level should exclude the possibility of donors having homozygous abnormal haemoglobin disease or thalassaemia. An abnormal haemoglobin-trait (other than S) or thalassaemia-trait blood is quite suitable for transfusion. Hazards have been ascribed to the deficiency of G-6-PD in the red cell. In our experience, in an area where the incidence is over 20 per cent, no apparent danger results from transfusing G-6-PD-deficient blood; this is probably due to the fact that in the Negro form of G-6-PD deficiency only the older cells are susceptible to oxidant drugs, while in the Caucasian form all the red cells are susceptible.

A husband's blood should not be transfused to his wife of the childbearing age in view of the danger of stimulating antibody formation with the future occurrence of haemolytic disease of the newborn.

(i) Technique of venesection

The veins of the antecubital region are most suitable. The skin should be treated with 0·5 per cent chlorhexidine (Hibitane, ICI Laboratories) in 70 per cent alcohol. A sphygmomanometric cuff at a pressure of 60mm Hg should be placed round the upper arm. An intradermal injection of 1 per cent procaine should be given adjacent to the vein, and the needle inserted into the vein. 420ml of blood is taken into 120ml of the acid–citrate–dextrose anticoagulant mixture with frequent agitation to ensure adequate mixing. A few millilitres of blood are then taken into two pilot bottles, one containing anticoagulant for cross-matching purposes and the other containing no anticoagulant for grouping and other serological tests. The pressure on the cuff is then released and a sterile dressing firmly applied to the puncture wound.

Following venesection the donor should rest for 15 minutes and be given suitable fluid. Ferrous sulphate tablets may be prescribed and blood should not be further donated for a period of 3–6 months.

(ii) Storage of blood

The blood should be stored at 2–6 °C. It should be discarded at the end of 21 days. Freezing or infection may cause haemolysis or clotting of blood and if haemolysis is detected in the supernatant plasma the blood should be discarded. A domestic refrigerator is not really suitable and small, thermostatically-controlled refrigerators are available commercially.

(d) Methods of blood transfusion

The usual method of giving blood is via a simple venepuncture or by cutting down on a vein. Blood can also be given via the tibial marrow in infants, by the intraperitoneal route, or a patient's own blood may be utilized in cases of intraperitoneal haemorrhage. Only the last two methods are described in detail. Following transfusion, every bottle should be retained for 24 hours in the refrigerator with the recipient's pretransfusion sample. This enables a transfusion reaction if it occurs to be adequately investigated. The temperature should be taken half-hourly during the transfusion and for at least 2 hours after its cessation.

(i) Intraperitoneal blood transfusion

Blood can be given intraperitoneally to the fetus, infant, or adult following adequate cross-matching tests. Our experience is limited to children suffering from protein-calorie deficiency disease in whom the presence of hypoproteinaemia, oedema, and anaemia not only raised technical difficulties in the giving of blood intravenously but made the danger of 'overloading' a real problem (Ofori Atta, 1958). The blood is slowly absorbed from the peritoneal cavity. In one child with normal haemoglobin who was given sickle-cell trait blood intraperitoneally, sickle cells slowly appeared in the peripheral blood, reaching their maximum concentration in 9–21 days. The method is therefore not of value in patients requiring urgent blood replacement but is a simple and safe procedure in slowly making effective whole blood (including its protein content) to anaemic and malnourished patients.

(ii) Autotransfusion

In areas of the tropics where blood banks are unknown and donors difficult to obtain, it should be remembered that blood recently shed within the peritoneal cavity can be utilized for transfusion. This method is particularly applicable to patients suffering from traumatic rupture of a viscus or a recently ruptured tubal pregnancy. The apparatus required is simple: a sterile ladle or container to remove the blood and sterile gauze to filter it into a standard sterile transfusion bottle containing 120 ml of acid–citrate–dextrose mixture. The bottle can then be connected to a standard giving set and the blood given intravenously in the usual fashion. Autotransfusion has the advantage of being rapidly carried out without the necessity of grouping and cross-matching tests and complications have rarely been reported. It should be noted, however, that the blood removed from the abdominal cavity should be transfused immediately and storage for even a few hours is not permissible as the risk of infection is great. The procedure has been described in 530 patients by Pathak and Stewart (1970).

(iii) Intra-uterine transfusion

This is a special technique used in the treatment of haemolytic disease of the newborn and has been well described by Walker and Ellis (1970).

(e) Incidence of complications and reactions

In Accra, Ghana, the incidence of transfusion reactions was in the region of 6 per cent (Edington, 1956) and the major factor was lack of care in cleaning equipment. The major hazard was over-enthusiastic transfusion therapy in the anaemic patient. The first can be overcome by paying scrupulous attention to the cleaning and rinsing of apparatus in pyrogen-free distilled water and sterilization procedures. Better still, in inadequately staffed laboratories, disposable plastic giving and taking sets and containers containing anticoagulant should be used. These are available commercially. Blood transfusion in the severely anaemic patient is described separately on p. 487.

The complications and reactions are described below.

(i) Simple febrile and allergic reactions, including those due to sensitivity to plasma and white cells

A mild febrile reaction may be due to the presence of pyrogens which are polysaccharide products of bacterial metabolism. The incidence of this type of reaction can be reduced to a minimum by scrupulous care in the preparation of the ACD solution (p. 769) and equipment used in transfusion work. Pyrogen-free chemicals and distilled water should always be used.

A few patients may have developed isoagglutinins to leucocytes in the donor's blood and others may be sensitive to the plasma.

Allergic reactions may occur in patients with a history of allergy. Either an antigen or antibody may be present in the donor's blood which reacts with the corresponding antibody or antigen in the patient. Allergic skin lesions, pyrexia, and generalized symptoms may occur. Severe reactions are uncommon but do occur. They can be prevented by the administration of antihistamine drugs. Corticosteroids may have to be employed in severe reactions.

(ii) Haemolytic transfusion reactions

The symptoms and signs of haemolytic transfusion reactions are very variable. At their most severe they may occur within 2–3 minutes of injecting a few millilitres of blood; at their least severe, they may be delayed 1–2 hours after the start of the transfusion. The classical symptoms are a feeling of heat along the vein, pain in the back, flushing of the face, and a constricting feeling in the chest. These, however, are symptoms of a severe reaction and they should not be ignored for collapse and circulatory failure may follow. More usually, however, the only sign is a fever, often accompanied by a rigor. When morphine and/or an anaesthetic have been given these initial signs and symptoms may not occur. In this case, the first signs that grossly incompatible blood has been given may be bleeding at a previously dry operation site or, if less incompatible blood has been given, there may only be jaundice or a failure of haemoglobin to rise satisfactorily. After the initial signs and symptoms are over the danger of incompatible blood transfusions lies in the development of renal damage and anuria.

If the classical symptoms occur the transfusion should, of course, be stopped at once. If, however, the patient only gets a mild fever the transfusion should be slowed and a sample of blood taken from the other arm. The serum of this is compared by eye with the pre-transfusion sample; if there is any suggestion of haemolysis or jaundice the transfusion should be stopped, if not it can be continued cautiously.

Severe haemorrhage following incompatible blood transfusion is due to a defibrination syndrome. This can also occur in amniotic fluid embolism, following major surgical procedures or the bite of certain venomous snakes.

This is thought to be due to the release of thromboplastin-like substances from the agglutinated red cells. This results in widespread intravascular clotting with the subsequent removal of the clots by the fibrinolytic system. The diagnosis can be established by showing there is a low concentration of fibrinogen in the blood. Rapid screening tests have been described (Hardisty *et al.* 1964). The treatment must be directed toward preventing further clotting and the patient should be given heparin in sufficient doses to render the blood incoagulable (4–5000 units at once and repeated as necessary). Fibrinogen (3–6 g is the usual dose) or triple strength plasma may also be necessary. Fresh blood as a source of platelets is often given.

Renal damage probably only occurs when the renal blood flow has been impaired and dextran, plasma or compatible blood should be given until the blood volume is normal. The urine should be collected and measured over the next 24 hours. If oliguria develops the patient should be treated as a case of acute renal failure (Chapter 13).

To investigate a suspected haemolytic transfusion reaction the following samples are needed: the pre-transfusion sample of blood from the patient; all the bottles given and the post-transfusion sample of blood from the patient taken from the other arm as soon as possible after the reaction. The pre- and post-transfusion sera should be compared and any change in colour suggestive of an increase in bilirubin and/or haemoglobin noted. The pre- and post-transfusion samples and all the blood bottles should be regrouped by a tube method and the cross-matching tests repeated using the indirect anti-globulin test and allowing a maximum incubation time. Any atypical antibodies should be identified against a large panel of red cells of known blood groups. The blood bottles given should be spun and the plasma inspected for haemolysis. If O blood has been given to an A or B patient, immune anti-A or anti-B should be looked for in plasma of the bottles. Finally, blood films should be made of the blood remaining in the bottles and these should be stained by Gram's stain and examined for bacteria.

Haemolytic transfusion reactions usually could have been prevented. They are more often the result of administrative errors than of errors in technique. Every suspected transfusion reaction should be thoroughly investigated and if a mistake is found the whole administrative and technical process reviewed so that it may not occur in the future.

(iii) Infected blood

The transfusion of infected blood may mimic the signs of an incompatible transfusion reaction. Contamination of blood on venesection is not uncommon but as blood is bactericidal harmful effects are unusual. Cold-growing contaminants are a danger and may be present in the absence of overt haemolysis in the stored blood. To detect contaminants, culture at 4 °C, 20 °C, and 37 °C should be performed. Microscopical examination of the blood itself is not completely dependable. To prevent contamination, bottles should not be opened until the transfusion is about to commence. Pilot bottles should be used for cross-matching purposes. Packed cells should be prepared immediately prior to the transfusion, utilizing every care in the removal of the plasma, and only with blood which has been stored for less than 2 weeks.

(iv) Transfusion and severe anaemia (overloading)

The haemodynamics of the circulation in severe anaemia have been described on p. 379. Such patients tolerate transfusion badly, as instead of the usual response of increased cardiac output to an increase in pressure in the right auricle, the cardiac output may fall and pulmonary oedema follow (overloading).

Transfusion is virtually never required in non-pregnant patients suffering from severe megaloblastic anaemia (Editorial, 1965). It is life saving, however, in the severe anaemias of pregnancy and iron-deficiency anaemias seen in the tropics and is required in the anaemia of renal failure and the hypoplastic anaemias. An exchange transfusion of packed cells is the treatment of choice in the severe anaemias of pregnancy admitted as emergencies in the tropics (Fullerton and Turner, 1962). In many areas, however, this may not be technically feasible and then 500 ml of packed cells may be given and the rate of transfusion should not exceed 1·0 ml/kg of body weight per hour. If symptoms of overloading (shortness of breath, tightness in chest) ensue, the transfusion should be stopped and the patient propped up if not already in that position. Pulmonary oedema, however, may develop insiduously within 12 hours of the transfusion and evidence of overload should be treated by withdrawal of blood. Ledingham (1964) and Harrison and Lawson (1966) have added a rapidly acting diuretic (ethacrynic acid 0·7 mg/kg body weight) to the packed cells and claim that the prompt diuresis produced mitigates against the possibility of 'overloading'.

Packed red cells may be prepared by removing the supernatant plasma citrate from blood in which the red cells have been allowed to settle. A certain amount of plasma (about 30 per cent of volume of blood) should be left to enable the blood to flow. The risk of contamination is great unless plastic containers are used, when the plasma can be expressed aseptically. The packed cells prepared from standard transfusion bottles should be utilized within a few hours to minimize the risk of bacterial contamination.

(v) Citrate toxicity

In exchange transfusions (especially in the newborn or in patients with impaired hepatic functions) muscular tremors, hypotension and cardiac abnormalities—even arrest—may occur due to citrate toxicity, which causes a fall in ionized calcium. They can be abolished by the use of 2–10 ml of 10 per cent solution of calcium gluconate, depending upon the age of the patient. Associated potassium toxicity may also be a factor.

(vi) Thrombophlebitis

This occurs most frequently following cannulation of the vein and is related to the length of the transfusion, the risk increasing the longer the transfusion lasts.

(vii) Air embolism

This is a rare complication. It may occur at the commencement of a transfusion or when air is introduced with the transfusion bottle under pressure and the bottle becomes empty unnoticed. It may also occur when bottles are being changed. It causes pain in the chest, severe dyspnoea, and cyanosis.

(viii) Transfusional siderosis

This is unlikely to be a problem of any magnitude in the tropics for some time to come. It is seen most commonly in patients with aplastic anaemia or chronic haemolytic anaemia who require repeated transfusions over a long period. Rarely, a condition indistinguishable from haemochromatosis results (p. 574).

(f) Haemolytic disease of the newborn

In this condition the life span of the infant's red cells is shortened by the action of specific IgG antibodies derived from the mother by placental transfer. The haemolytic process lessens in severity as the concentration of maternal antibody diminishes, and is therefore maximal at the time of birth. Jaundice, however, may increase after birth as the infant can excrete bilirubin via the placenta *in utero*. The rarity of haemolytic disease of the newborn in most areas of the tropics due to rhesus incompatibility and the diagnostic signs of ABO incompatibility have already been mentioned. It is possible for ABO incompatibility to cause intrauterine death but if hydrops fetalis occurs the more likely possibility of α-chain thalassaemia should be considered (p. 457). The majority of the causes of neonatal jaundice are discussed in the section on the liver (p. 568) but the possibility of over-dosage of synthetic vitamin-K analogues or the presence of a hereditary anaemia (spherocytosis) are not mentioned. The part that the deficiency of G-6-PD may play in neonatal jaundice has been discussed on p. 478.

The severity of haemolytic disease of the newborn is best assessed by estimating the haemoglobin and bilirubin concentration of the cord blood. If the infant's red cells give a positive antiglobulin test and the cord haemo-globin is less than 14 g/100 ml and the bilirubin value greater than 4 mg/100 ml the possibility of exchange transfusion should be considered. Sixty to 90 ml/kg body weight of a concentrated suspension of compatible red cells (preferably washed group O cells in ABO incompatibility) should be given by intermittent withdrawal and reinjection of blood into a plastic catheter in the umbilical vein. Septic thrombophlebitis and perforation of the umbilical vein are additional possible complications to those trans-fusional hazards already described.

Exchange transfusion may also be necessary in the other conditions causing jaundice—especially prematurity—in order to prevent the occur-rence of kernicterus.

Pyruvate kinase (PK) deficiency

Pyruvate kinase (PK) deficiency haemolytic anaemia is inherited as an autosomal recessive trait and has been reviewed by de Gruchy and Grimes (1968). It causes a non-spherocytic congenital haemolytic anaemia. Other enzymatic deficiencies may be involved.

Autoimmune haemolytic anaemia

Autoimmune haemolytic anaemia can only be diagnosed when drugs, iso-antibodies and other causes have been excluded. The direct antiglobulin test is usually strongly positive with the red cells and evidence of increased red cell destruction is present. It can be classified into six groups depending upon the proteins found on the red cell surface: IgG only; IgG plus complement; IgM only; IgM plus complement; IgA plus complement and complement only (Editorial, 1969).

THE SPLEEN

The weight of the normal spleen in adults in Europe varies between 150 and 200 g. In the tropics, however, in areas of stable malaria the spleen weight is proportionately and absolutely much heavier in all age groups, the average in African adults being twice that of normal (Bruce Chwatt, 1967). The pattern of splenomegaly in malaria is discussed on p. 14.

Splenomegaly is common throughout the tropics and the various causes are listed in Table 10.12 (Trowell, 1960). The tropical and other specific conditions causing splenomegaly are discussed elsewhere in the text and are not considered in this chapter. In many instances, however, no apparent cause for the splenomegaly can be found and this is discussed under the heading of tropical splenomegaly syndrome (T.S.S.). The syndrome of hypersplenism is also common in tropical areas and is described in the following pages.

TABLE 10.12. *Causes of splenomegaly*

I. Inflammatory and parasitic
   1. *Acute*: blood-stream infections, bacterial endocarditis, malaria, infectious mononucleosis and allied states, splenic abscess
   2. *Chronic*: malaria, kala azar, trypanosomiasis, schistosomiasis, brucellosis, histoplasmosis, tuberculosis, syphilis (especially congenital), Felty's syndrome, sarcoidosis

II. Portal splenic hypertension
Cirrhosis and liver disease, portal thrombosis, diseases of splenic vein and other causes

III. Diseases of blood and reticulo-endothelial system
   1. Haemolytic anaemia, haemoglobinopathies, thalassaemia, myelosclerosis, and infarction
   2. Other anaemias—pernicious and megaloblastic anaemia, iron-deficiency, etc.
   3. Thrombocytopenic purpura
   4. Leukaemia, reticuloses, polycythaemia vera
   5. 'Hypersplenism'

IV. Tropical splenomegaly syndrome, Banti's syndrome

V. Abnormal storage
In Gaucher's Niemann–Pick, Hand–Schueller–Christian disease, amyloidosis, etc.

VI. Cysts, neoplasms

VII. Spontaneous haemorrhage and rupture of spleen

Hypersplenism

The term hypersplenism denotes splenic enlargement with marked diminution in the circulating blood of erythrocytes, platelets (thrombocytopenia) or granulocytes (splenic neutropenia) or of all three (pancytopenia). The reticulo-endothelial cells of the spleen may selectively destroy any one of the three cells with the other two only slightly affected, or all three may be affected. Three explanations have been proposed to explain the splenic mechanism.

   (i) Some splenic factor causes marrow inhibition.
   (ii) The spleen may form antibodies which destroy the formed blood elements.
   (iii) Hypersequestration of blood may occur in the spleen.

In our experience the last explanation is the most likely in the tropics, possibly combined with abnormal immunological reactions. Hypersplenism is usually described as primary or secondary. In primary hypersplenism no cause is detected for the increase in spleen size or functional activity. Secondary hypersplenism occurs in association with other conditions such as leukaemia, lymphosarcoma, and infectious conditions including parasitic diseases (schistosomiasis, kala azar, malaria, etc.). It is a common finding in T.S.S. The bone marrow is hyperplastic. Anaemia is marked and infection and haemorrhages may be present if the leucopenia and thrombocytopenia are severe. The changes in the spleen are described below.

Pathology

In our experience the following description of the spleen (Prankerd, 1963) would appear to satisfy the clinicopathological and morbid anatomical findings in those patients in whom splenomegaly and anaemia have been the important presenting clinical signs.

Arterial blood is conveyed into the splenic cords of Billroth, which consist of lymphatic tissue and cells of the reticulo-endothelial system. The blood then filters through this system into the splenic venous sinusoids thence to the splenic vein and liver via the portal circulation. The circulation in the spleen is best considered as intrasinusoidal (referring only to blood in the venous sinusoids) and extrasinusoidal (referring to blood outside the sinusoids).

Normally, blood passes rapidly through the spleen and little is present in the extrasinusoidal spaces. Under certain conditions the 'lymphatic filter' is impeded and gross congestion in the extrasinusoidal tissue results. A vicious circle is initiated, with more and more erythrocytes packing the extrasinusoidal tissue. This stasis of blood is known as 'pooling' and can be caused by:

(1) Changes on the surface charge of the red cell (as occurs in malaria).
(2) Alteration in the size and shape of the red cell (sickle-cell disease, hereditary spherocytosis, thalassaemia, etc.)
(3) Lymphatic and reticulo-endothelial hyperplasia in the extrasinusoidal tissue.
(4) Abnormal conditions affecting the reticulo-endothelial cells, lymphosarcoma, leukaemia, and Gaucher's disease.

The most dramatic effects of 'pooling' are seen in the sequestration crisis of sickle-cell disease where up to 40 per cent of the total circulatory red cells may be trapped in the extrasinusoidal tissue, the patient literally having bled to death into the spleen.

In contrast to these findings, in anaemia due to hereditary non-spherocytic anaemia where the morphology of the red cell appears normal both extra- and intrasinusoidal congestion are usual. In chronic venous congestion there is intrasinusoidal congestion and the changes in the erythrocyte, which occur with pooling and are described below, are absent.

The effects of pooling (extrasinusoidal congestion)

Pooling does not always imply intrasplenic destruction of red cells and the time factor in the intrasplenic circulation is considered important—the longer the delay, the greater the likelihood of destruction. Irrespective of the cause erythrocytes in the splenic vein show an increased osmotic and mechanical fragility. There is also an alteration in the potassium/sodium ratio in the red cell. Stasis in the spleen may also cause metabolic damage to the cell from glucose deprivation and the membrane may be injured by lysolecithins. The possible absorption of antigen/antibody complexes leading to opsonization or even outright lysis must be considered in malaria and other infections. The packing of red cells into the extrasinusoidal tissue causes an increase in the plasma volume with a 'dilution' anaemia superimposed upon the haemolytic.

If pooling is present normal transfused cells have been shown to be sequestered in the spleen.

The role of splenectomy

The justification for the term 'hypersplenism' is due largely to the fact that in many instances splenectomy abolishes or relieves the existing cytopenia. Splenectomy, however, should not be lightly undertaken in the tropics and, ideally, evidence of a shortened red-cell survival, an increased plasma volume, and the presence of intrasplenic pooling, should be demonstrated prior to operation. In addition, in areas of stable malaria, splenomegaly with evidence of hypersplenism has been shown to respond favourably to long-term suppressive antimalarial therapy. The role of splenectomy in T.S.S. has been discussed by Cook *et al.* (1963).

Tropical splenomegaly syndrome (T.S.S.)

Synonyms. Cryptogenic splenomegaly; gross splenomegaly of obscure origin; postinfective malarial splenomegaly; idiopathic splenomegaly; tropical splenomegaly; big spleen disease, splenomegalie algerienne; Bengal splenomegaly (Tropical cryptogenic splenomegaly).

Tropical splenomegaly syndrome can be defined as a syndrome with no recognizable cause in which there is splenomegaly and anaemia, and sometimes thrombocytopenia, a relative or absolute lymphocytosis in the peripheral blood, and lymphocytic infiltration in the bone marrow. Hepatic sinusoidal lymphocytosis usually occurs. It has been encountered in Algeria (Cattoir and Marell, 1950); South Arabia (Fawdry, 1955); India

(Chaudhuri *et al.* 1956); Hong Kong (Cook *et al.* 1963); Uganda (Mardsen *et al.* 1965); the Sudan (Mustafa, 1965); Ghana (Ratnesar *et al.* 1966); and New Guinea (Pryor, 1967a). The subject of chronic splenomegaly in the tropics was reviewed by Hutt and Lowenthal (1974).

Epidemiology

Chronic malaria has been considered a possible factor in Aden, parts of India, and in East and West Africa. The syndrome is thought to represent an abnormal immunological reaction to malarial antigen. On the other hand, the racial distribution of the syndrome in Uganda (Shaper, 1969) and its familial distribution in the Upper Watut Valley of New Guinea suggests that a genetic predisposition may be involved (Crane, 1972). Dacie *et al.* (1969) have reported a similar syndrome in Britain in individuals who have not been exposed to malaria, possibly due to cellular proliferation in the spleen and liver in response to an autoantigen in contrast to the malarial antigen responsible for the condition in endemic malarial areas. Lowenthal and Hutt (1970) reported a case of T.S.S. in a Caucasian resident in Zambia who had taken antimalarials regularly for 17 years.

In areas of stable malaria, splenomegaly is a constant finding in a certain proportion of adults, the incidence in females being higher than in males (Colbourne *et al.* 1950; Butler *et al.* 1973). The relationship of this 'normal splenomegaly' to T.S.S. has not yet been satisfactorily investigated. In some patients a history of repeated attacks of mild fever suggestive of malaria is given. In East Africa patients with T.S.S. have shown a high level of malarial antibody titres and *P. malariae* has been noted in the peripheral blood in a significant number of patients (Marsden *et al.* 1965). Perhaps of greater significance is the observation that, in Ibadan, a number of patients with T.S.S. respond to long-term antimalarial suppressive therapy. A further factor in favour of the malarial hypothesis for the condition in Africa is the rarity of T.S.S. in the South African Bantu (Trowell, 1960), in whom malaria is rare. Nevertheless, from a consideration of the clinical and pathological aspects of T.S.S. described in various parts of the tropics, we are not convinced that the condition is a single disease entity. There would appear to be two types of presentation. In one group of patients the presenting symptoms are those of splenomegaly with portal hypertension and its complications, in the second splenomegaly and the associated haematological findings of hypersplenism predominate. Perhaps the concept of a 'postinfective splenomegaly' with disturbance of the immunological mechanisms is the most sensible attitude to adopt regarding the aetiology of T.S.S. until more widespread and detailed geographical studies are undertaken. Charmot and Vargues (1963) suggested a possible malarial cause with some immunological disorder, as reflected by the high globulin level and the presence of macroglobulins encountered in their African patients.

In this connection it is interesting to note that McFadzean and Tsang (1956) showed that, providing the liver was not cirrhotic, a satisfactory haemolytic response was elicited to the intravenous injection of washed sheep erythrocytes in patients with T.S.S. On the other hand the response to the injection of a subcutaneous antigen (*S. typhi*) was lower than in controls and was corrected by splenectomy. Humoral immune response in T.S.S. were also studied in New Guinea. Crane *et al.* (1973) showed that for flagellin and influenza vaccine immune response was lower in New Guineans with T.S.S. than in other groups. The effect of the spleen on plasma cells was considered a possible factor in this phenomenon.

In New Guinea Marsden *et al.* (1967) could find no association between parasitaemia, malaria antibody titre, and hepatic sinusoidal infiltration, in malarious villages.

Pathology

The condition is more common in relatively young adults and both sexes are affected. The patient may have been aware of the enlarged spleen or have suffered from repeated attacks of mild fever and abdominal pain and discomfort for 1 to 30 years. The liver is enlarged in about 20 per cent of patients. Clinical evidence of portal hypertension is common in Hong Kong and India but less common in Africa although the intrasplenic pressure is raised and portal venograms are suggestive of portal hypertension (Leather, 1961; Williams *et al.* 1966). Chronic leg ulcers, infantilism, dwarfism, failure of the secondary sex characteristics, and amenorrhoea have been noted in Hong Kong and have responded dramatically to splenectomy (Cook *et al.* 1963). Vascular fragility has also been reported as increased in Hong Kong, and haemorrhagic episodes are not uncommon in Hong Kong and India (Basu, 1965).

The blood-forming organs

The marrow may be normal or show erythroid hyperplasia. Myeloid maturation arrest has been described. Megaloblastic change, especially in pregnancy, has been noted. In the peripheral blood a normocytic or slightly macrocytic anaemia is usual. The reticulocytes are variable but are usually between 2 and 5 per cent. Neutropenia and thrombocytopenia may occur and there may be a relative or absolute lymphocytosis. There is increased mechanical and osmotic fragility. Signs of active haemolysis may be slight except in pregnancy (Marsden *et al.* 1965) but faecal stercobilin is increased. The Coombs' test is negative and there is no evidence of any haemolytic factor, apart from hypersplenism. The plasma volume is invariably increased. An excessive uptake of chromium-tagged red cells has been noted in the spleen and/or liver.

The spleen is enlarged and may weigh up to 5000 g. It is of firm consistency and the cut surface is dark red. Perisplenitis is usual. Infarcts may be prominent. Histologically there is periarterial and trabecular fibrosis and siderofibrotic nodules (Gandy-Gamna bodies) may be prominent (Basu and Aikat, 1963). The reticulo-endothelial cells in the extrasinusodial tissue show marked proliferation and multinucleated giant cells have been described (Chaudhuri *et al.* 1956). Lymphocytes and plasma cells are conspicuous. Erythrophagocytosis and haemosiderin deposits are usual. Malarial pigment is not usually seen. The sinusoids may be congested and dilated but the greatest degree of congestion is extrasinusoidal. Endophlebitis of the portal vein is present.

In New Guinea positive tests for rheumatoid factor and a high incidence of cold haemagglutinins with anti-i specificity have been found in the serum (Pitney, 1968). Haemolytic anaemia and erythrophagocytosis in liver and spleen which occur in New Guinea may be related to the presence of cold agglutinins of high thermal range.

The liver

Liver biopsies in Hong Kong, Aden, India, East and West Africa, and New Guinea (Pryor, 1967a) have shown a variable infiltration of lymphocytes in dilated sinusoids, with hyperplasia and hypertrophy of the Kupffer cells (Fig. 10.17). The lymphocytes may be single, in rows, or clustered, and

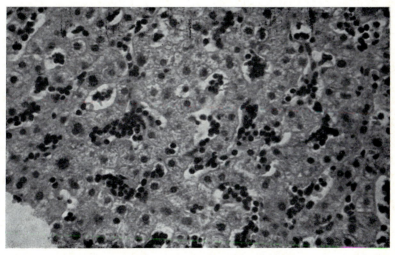

FIG. 10.17. 'Tropical Splenomegaly Syndrome'. Severe hepatic sinusoidal lymphocytosis (H and E × 400).

may be so increased as to resemble lymphatic leukaemia. Variability of sinusoidal lymphocytosis is usual and no correlation between HSL gradings in the liver sinusoids and the absolute lymphocyte count in the peripheral blood has been noted. Hepatic sinusoidal lymphocytosis is not pathognomonic of T.S.S. (Sagoe, 1971). Occasional histiocytes, eosinophils, mast cells, or immature cells may be seen. In Africa very occasionally malarial pigment may be seen in the Kupffer cells or in histiocytes in portal tracts. The Kupffer cells contain large amounts of IgM (Bryceson, personal communication). There is no cholestasis or evidence of liver-cell necrosis. Sinusoidal reticulum is normal. Portal-tract fibrosis is inconstant in African material but is more common in India and Hong Kong, where post-necrotic cirrhosis is also common. Portal tracts may be infiltrated with lymphocytes, plasma cells, and some eosinophils, and may be present in the absence of sinusoidal changes. Fluck et al. (1973) studied the ultrastructure of the hepatic sinusoids in T.S.S. and concluded that the general appearance is consistent with a complex immunological reaction occurring in the liver sinusoids.

The large percentage of patients with cirrhosis in Hong Kong and India contrasts with the finding in Africa and this may well be a different condition. In some series in Africa patients with splenomegaly and cirrhosis have not been considered as suffering from T.S.S. and have been excluded from the series. Portal hypertension has been found in all areas either by demonstrating a raised intrasplenic pressure or abnormal portal venograms, often with abnormal collaterals. The venogram may resemble that seen in clay pipe-stem fibrosis or idiopathic portal hypertension (p. 550). Portal hypertension in East Africa could not be correlated with the presence of an increase of lymphocytes in the sinusoids not with constant changes in the portal tracts (Leather, 1961; Williams et al. 1966). Indeed, Leather (1961) emphasized the common occurrence of portal hypertension in the absence of hepatic fibrosis. The presence of this portal hypertension in T.S.S. is interesting. Boyer et al. (1967) for instance, in India, have discussed idiopathic portal hypertension. In their patients splenomegaly was the predominating abnormality but portal-tract fibrosis was considered an important aetiological agent and possibly concerned with the multiple infestations and infections present in childhood. Hypersplenism was not a feature of the condition. The association between this condition and T.S.S. must remain conjectural. Bilirubin is occasionally raised. Liver-function tests are usually normal. Gamma globulin and β macroglobulins are raised and higher titres of malaria antibodies have been noted in East Africa by fluorescent antibody techniques (Gebbie et al. 1964). P. malariae has been noted in the peripheral blood of some patients.

Evidence from New Guinea suggests that the natural history of T.S.S. is that of a progressive disease with a high mortality in the fully developed case (Crane *et al.* 1972). Whether the increased portal blood flow and portal hypertension leads to cirrhosis is debatable. In our experience it does not (Sagoe, 1971). Complications of portal hypertension may cause death. Splenectomy has been shown to reduce the liver blood flow in one patient— not in another (Williams *et al.* 1966).

Splenectomy corrects the excessive haemolysis and the expanded plasma volume and leucopenia and thrombocytopenia if present (Hamilton *et al.* 1967; Pryor, 1967b; Crane *et al.* 1972). In the tropics this procedure should not be lightly undertaken (p. 492) and it is not justified until long-term antimalarial therapy has been tried (Watson-Williams and Allan, 1968; Stuiver *et al.* 1971; Crane *et al.* 1973; David-West, 1974). The role of plasma proteins in chronic expansion of plasma-volume in T.S.S. has been defined by Crane *et al.* (1974). Chronic leg ulcers, dwarfism, failure in development of secondary sex characteristics, and amenorrhoea are also improved. It may reduce portal blood flow and perhaps prevent the development of cirrhosis. Excessive fibrinolysis is a hazard of the operation, and following splenectomy malaria, piroplasmosis, pneumococcal and streptococcal infections may occur. Tropical splenomegaly syndrome may in some patients end up in lymphosarcoma (Anand and Davey, 1965).

Diagnostic pathology

The diagnosis of T.S.S. is arrived at by a process of exclusion, and standard haematological and radiological investigations are required. Isotope studies, estimation of plasma volume, barium swallow, splenic smears, intrasplenic venous pressure, splenic and portal venography, post-sinusoidal wedge pressures, and immunological studies have all been carried out by various investigators at some time or other. Liver biopsy is an important diagnostic procedure. Dilatation of the sinusoids together with lymphocytosis may be seen. Alterations of the immunoglobins IgG and IgM have been reported (*Brit. med. J.*, 1967; Ziegler and Stuiver, 1972). Sagoe (1970) has shown that high IgM values and normal lymphocyte transformation scores when stimulated by phytohaemagglutinin distinguish T.S.S. from atypical forms of chronic lymphatic leukaemia or other malignant lymphomas.

Banti's syndrome

In 1894 Banti described a syndrome in which there was anaemia with hypersplenism; later this was followed by a transitional stage with jaundice and disturbance of gastro-intestinal function. Latterly there was the ascitic stage with cirrhosis. In the transitional stage there was endophlebitis of the portal and splenic veins with minimal increase in liver fibrosis (Banti, 1937). These observations were made in an area where malaria was holoendemic and although much doubt has been expressed about Banti's observations they would appear to us to describe a syndrome very similar to T.S.S.

Other conditions

Primary splenic abscess of unknown aetiology is an entity (Islam, 1967). Splenic abscesses have also been noted in sickle-cell disease and in bearers of the sickle-cell trait. Gas-forming organisms may be present (Jelliffe, 1949). Other conditions which have been implicated as causal factors in splenic abscesses are amoebiasis, pyaemia, relapsing fever, tropical phlebitis, typhoid fever and infarction in malarial infection.

Splenic cysts and neoplasms are uncommon, excluding tumours of the reticulo-endothelial system and chorion cancer which are common in many areas of the tropics.

TUMOURS OF LYMPHORETICULAR TISSUE

Based on the relative proportions of all tumours, malignant disease of this system would appear to be high in Nigeria, Francophone West Africa, Egypt, Iran (Arnim, 1966), and Saudi Arabia (Taylor, 1963). In South Africa the mortality of the white population is twice that of the coloured or Bantu.

In Great Britain and the United States Hodgkin's disease is the most prevalent form of malignant lymphoma, whereas reticulum cell sarcoma is the most prevalent in Japan (Anderson *et al.* 1970). It is possible that the undifferentiated histological types may be more common and the follicular or nodular types of lymphoma uncommon in certain parts of the tropics. There are therefore differences in the incidence and pattern of lymphoreticular tumours in differing geographic areas. The reasons for this are obscure. As long ago as 1954 Camain suggested that the presence of multiple parasites in the population of Francophone West Africa might play a part in the high frequency of RE tumours recorded in that part of the world. The possibility of stable malaria, which causes intense hyperplasia with perhaps blockade of the reticulo-endothelial system, conditioning this system to a greater liability to malignant proliferation or altering the immunological surveillance of the host, is now considered a factor in the high incidence of the Burkitt tumour found in tropical Africa and New Guinea (Editorial, 1970). Multiple infections and infestations therefore may play a part in influencing the incidence and pattern of tumours in which immunological factors are thought to be particularly important and this would apply to tumours of lymphoreticular tissue. It is of interest that it has been shown in an autopsy study that RE tumours were more frequent in subjects suffering from schistosomiasis when compared with controls (Edington *et al.* 1970). Apart from differing incidences and perhaps pattern, the histopathology of these tumours in the tropics (excluding the Burkitt tumour) would appear to conform to the well-described types in the Western world. The only condition therefore that is dealt with in any detail in this section is the Burkitt tumour.

Lymphosarcoma and reticulum-cell sarcoma are found in high incidence until the age of 65 years in Nigeria, until the age of 39 in Laurenco Marques and in Uganda until the age of 49 years. In contrast they are relatively rare in the Johannesburg Bantu. Modan *et al.* (1969) have found a highly significant difference in incidence in three ethnic groups is Israel and Haenzel and Kurihara (1968) noted that the mortality rates of lymphomas in immigrant Japanese in the U.S.A. were much closer to the U.S.A. figures than to the low incidence recorded in Japan. Environmental factors are therefore important in the aetiology of these tumours.

The incidence of Hodgkin's disease is lowest in Japan and the Chinese in Singapore, otherwise it does not differ markedly throughout the world. There is, however, some evidence that it may be more common in children in Africa and South America and that the more aggressive histological types (mixed cellularity and lymphocyte depleted) are more common than in temperate climates where the nodular sclerosing type is more frequently seen in children (Edington *et al.* 1973). Recently a significant increase in EB virus antibodies has been noted in patients with Hodgkin's disease (Levine *et al.* 1971) and impairment of cell-mediated immunity has been demonstrated (Kaplan, 1971). Prior appendicectomy and tonsillectomy enhances the liability to Hodgkin's disease and its occurrence may be seasonal. Vianna *et al.* (1972) have described a striking series of cases of Hodgkin's disease in a group of persons who attended or were connected with a certain high school in Albany, New York. The findings were thought possibly to suggest that Hodgkin's disease was due to an infective condition with a carrier state and a long incubation period. Lymphoid tissue might act as a barrier to infection. If these conclusions are valid the possibility of a breakdown in immunological surveillance being associated with Hodgkin's disease is indeed a possibility.

Myelomatosis would appear to be more common in the West Indies, the American Negro, the white American and in Western Europe than in tropical Africa, Asia or South America (Talerman, 1969). Environment would once again appear to be important in the aetiology of this condition. It would appear that the environmental factors concerned must differ from those of lymphosarcoma, reticulosarcoma and the Burkitt tumour in view of its differing geographical incidence from these tumours. Leukaemia is discussed on p. 472.

The tumours of lymphoreticular tissue can be classified as follows:

1. Reticulum cell sarcoma (diffuse or nodular)
    (a) Undifferentiated (Stem cell)
    (b) Histiocytic
2. Lymphosarcoma (diffuse or nodular)
    (a) Poorly differentiated (lymphoblastic)
    (b) Well differentiated (lymphocytic)
3. Mixed lymphocytic—histiocytic malignant lymphoma (diffuse or nodular)
4. Hodgkin's disease (Lukes *et al.* 1966)
    (a) Mixed cellularity (granuloma)
    (b) Lymphocyte depleted (sarcoma)
    (c) Lymphocyte predominant (paragranuloma)
    (d) Nodular sclerosing
5. The Burkitt tumour
6. Mastocytoma
7. Proliferative diseases with dysproteinaemia
    Multiple myeloma
    Primary macroglobulinaemia of Waldenstrom
    Heavy chain disease
8. Histiocytosis
    (a) Malignant histiocytosis
    (b) Acute differentiated histiocytosis (Letterer–Siwe disease; histiocytosis X)
    (c) Chronic differentiated histiocytosis (Hand–Schuller–Christian disease; chronic disseminated histiocytosis X; eosinophilic granuloma of bone)
9. Myelosclerosis with myeloid metaplasia
10. Unclassified
    Mycosis fungoides
    Sezary's disease

THE BURKITT TUMOUR

Synonyms. African lymphoma; lymphosarcoma; small, round-celled sarcoma; multicentric sarcoma; malignant lymphoma, undifferentiated lymphocyte type.

The Burkitt tumour is a malignant neoplasm of lymphoreticular tissue which occurs most commonly in children, frequently involving the facial bones and periorbital region. Abdominal viscera may however be primarily affected. Involvement of the central nervous system is also not uncommon.

The tumour possesses distinctive morphological (Wright, 1963) and growth characteristics in short-term cultures (Pulvertaft, 1964) which are considered diagnostic. Fialkow *et al.* (1970) have studied the glucose-6-phosphate dehydrogenase types of normal and malignant tissues in seven patients heterozygous for the enzyme suffering from the tumour. Two enzyme types were present in normal tissues but only one type was found in the malignant cells which was thought to be suggestive that the tumour has a clonal origin.

It was Burkitt in 1958 who first gave a concise clinical description of the tumour in Uganda children, and O'Conor and Davies in 1960 described the pathology.

Epidemiology

The Burkitt tumour is the commonest tumour of childhood in Uganda and in Ibadan, accounting in these areas for 50 per cent and 70 per cent respectively of all childhood malignancies (Edington and Maclean, 1965). In addition to the high incidence in tropical Africa (Burkitt, 1964; Camain and Lambert, 1965) it is common in New-Guinea (Ten Seldam *et al.* 1966) and isolated cases have been reported from the United States (O'Conor *et al.* 1965), England (Wright *et al.* 1967), Brazil, Colombia (Beltram *et al.* 1966), Cuba, Puerto Rico, Canada, India, and Vietnam.

The geographical distribution of the tumour in high incidence is mainly controlled by two climatic parameters—temperature and humidity. Thus it is most common in those areas of tropical Africa where the mean monthly temperature is over 60 °F ($15 \cdot 5$ °C) and the relative humidity is high (Burkitt, 1962). A careful survey in Uganda showed that in lowland areas along the Nile the tumour was twenty times as common as in the mountainous regions (Burkitt and Wright, 1966).

The tumour is rarely seen under the age of 2 years and in endemic areas it is uncommon over the age of 15 years. It is most frequently seen in the 5- to 9-year age groups with a median of approximately 7 years both in Africa and in the relatively few cases reported in the United States, whereas in the mountainous areas of Uganda where the tumour is not common, the average age of onset is said to be $16 \cdot 2$ years (Burkitt and Wright, 1966). The tumour is not uncommon among adult immigrants to Uganda coming from the mountainous districts of Rwanda and Burundi, where the disease is almost unknown. Boys are affected about twice as frequently as girls and no race would appear to be exempt. It seems to be relatively rare among the higher socio-economic group of Africans living in endemic areas.

The apparent climatic influence on the incidence of Burkitt's tumour and its striking age distribution has led to a variety of hypotheses relating to the aetiology of the disease. However, it would now appear that the presence of the tumour in high incidence in a population is associated with two factors: (1) the presence of stable malaria due to *P. falciparum* infection and (2) the presence of the Epstein–Barr virus (EB virus). Before discussing these two factors, however, previous hypotheses are described.

One suggestion—now discarded by most—was that it might be an African biological variant of lymphatic leukaemia (O'Conor and Davies, 1960). Pulvertaft (1964) considered that the lymphocytes transformed by the bean extract, phytohaemagglutinin, resembled closely the Burkitt cell. It is known that a similar transformation can occur if lymphocytes are exposed to toxoid, tuberculin, and viruses to which the patient has been previously exposed, and the transformation is considered to be the result of an antigen–antibody reaction. Beans are widely consumed in Africa and presumably the phytohaemagglutin could produce the reaction described above. It was thought, however, that beans by themselves were unlikely to be causative but that an infective agent might cause this transformation. It was also suggested that the widespread incidence of periodontal disease with lymphocytic infiltration in children might explain the predilection of this tumour for the jaw region, the lymphocytes perhaps being transformed by an antigenic stimulus. With regard to the EB virus Burkitt (1962) suggested that an arthropod-borne virus might be causal. Haddow (1964) has argued that if the hypothesis of a virus aetiology were correct the distribution would indicate a very high rate of infection early in life; the great majority of persons infected would develop immunity, and only a small minority would develop malignant tumours. The rarity of the disease above the age of 15 years in endemic areas, except possibly in non-immune immigrants, would fit the hypothesis. Moreover, the cumulative age incidence of Burkitt's tumour closely parallels the changes in yellow fever immunity rates in Uganda.

Raised titres of antibody to the EB virus have been found in patients with the Burkitt tumour, nasopharyngeal carcinoma and Hodgkin's disease when compared with controls in the population. The virus is closely associated with infectious mononucleosis (p. 255) and Cohen *et al.* (1970) have reported the occurrence of a Burkitt tumour in a 17-year-old American girl 16 months after the infection and in whom antibody was present and viral antigen was detected in buffy coat material after long-term culture. Four separate antigenic complexes have been defined in cultured Burkitt tumour cells and four corresponding antibodies detected in patients' sera (Editorial, 1971).

These are:
(1) E.B.-virus capsid antigen.
(2) The E.B.-virus associated membrane antigen.
(3) The 'early' EB-virus antigen.
(4) The soluble antigen which evokes precipitins.

(1) and (2) are the best documented. The capsid antigen is demonstrated by indirect immunofluorescence on fixed target cells. It is the conventional system for titrating EB-virus antibodies. The membrane antigen is detected by immunofluorescence on living target cells—but the more reliable 'blocking' test is now used (Klein et al. 1969). Other factors in favour of an infective agent being involved in the aetiology of the Burkitt tumour are the time–space clustering reported by Morrow et al. (1971) and the findings of McFarlane et al. (1967) who noted that the acute-phase proteins, C-reactive protein, ceruloplasmin and haptoglobin were markedly elevated in children with acute manifestations of the tumour. It is of interest that antibodies to the EBV have been detected in monkeys in Africa but not in the Americas (Dunkel et al. 1972) and that mosquitoes have been implicated in its possible transmission (Editorial, 1967). Species of herpes viruses have produced malignant lymphomas in monkeys. However, the distribution of the EB virus is world-wide and the only evidence to date that it is causal is the raised antibody titres found in Burkitt tumour patients. There must be some other factor which accounts for the increased incidence of this tumour in certain tropical areas. This has been considered to be to an altered immunological surveillance of the host due to parasitic infection—especially the presence of stable P. falciparum malaria. The immunosuppressive effects of malarial parasites have been demonstrated in mice infected with P. berghei (Greenwood et al. 1971) and mice repeatedly infected with the same parasite have developed a malignant lymphoma morphologically similar to the Burkitt tumour (Jerusalem, 1968). Wedderburn (1970) has shown experimentally the synergic action of a plasmodium and a potentially oncogenic virus in the same animal. No one who has examined sections of the liver in children in areas of stable malaria could fail to notice the tremendous hypertrophy and phagocytosed pigment in the cells of the reticuloendothelial system. Williams (1966) and later Pike et al. (1970) showed that the frequency of the sickle-cell trait was less than expected in Burkitt tumour patients—perhaps indicating that those protected from heavy infections of P. falciparum malaria were less likely to develop the tumour. Low IgM values and spontaneous remissions have been noted. Fulminating tumours of the breast have been seen in pregnancy in Ibadan and also reported by Shepherd and Wright (1967)—one of whose patients underwent spontaneous regression following delivery. Fass et al. (1970) reported that delayed hypersensitivity reactions to autologous tumour extracts in twelve Burkitt's lymphoma patients showed that only one patient reacted before treatment and that that patient was the only one with localized disease. Seven responded when tested after treatment and were all in remission and have remained well. By contrast 4 of the 5 patients in whom positive skin tests did not develop have relapsed. The correlation between positive skin tests and the

clinical state of the disease is impressive and would imply that cell-mediated immunity is important in the prognosis of the tumour. Deficiency of cell-mediated immunity appears to be correlated with poor prognosis and may be related to dysplastic changes observed in the thymuses of patients dying of the disease (Osunkoya, 1971). Furthermore, the degree of lymphocytic infiltration at the tumour site during treatment appears to influence prognosis (Osunkoya *et al.* 1970). An Editorial (1970) stated that the epidemiological evidence incriminating malaria in the aetiology of the Burkitt tumour was now beyond dispute. To sum up it would appear possible that in children or even adults with altered immunological surveillance due to intense parasitic infection or even pregnancy the EB virus may become oncogenic and cause transformation of lymphocytes into the 'Burkitt cell'.

Chromosomal abnormalities have been noted in tumour cells in over 80 per cent of untreated cases but they have been inconstant and variable, while the chromosomes in the cells in the peripheral blood and marrow were normal (Jacobs *et al.* 1963). Dorfman (1965) believes that there is a distinct overlap between what is defined as Burkitt's lymphoma in Africa and conventional childhood lymphosarcoma of the lymphoblastic type.

Pathology

The clinical presentation and organ distribution of the Burkitt tumour do not resemble any of the more common malignant lymphomas described in temperate climates.

One of the most common forms of clinical presentation is that of facial swelling. The jaws, one or more quadrants, are most frequently affected. Periorbital tumour deposits also occur but are less common. As many as 70 per cent of children have been said to present with jaw lesions but the actual percentage probably depends upon the age of the patient and the duration of the disease when first seen. Primary jaw tumours (if the term primary may be used in this condition) are said to be more common in the younger age groups, less common in older children, and rare over the age of 15 years. Deposits in the jaw can also occur in children who have presented at first with deposits elsewhere in the body.

Abdominal swelling is the next most common presentation, especially in girls in whom bilateral ovarian deposits are common. Any of the abdominal organs may be involved, however, including lymph nodes. Paravertebral and retoperitoneal masses are not uncommon.

Sudden flaccid paraplegia may occur due to pressure of a tumour on the cord and a number of areas in the cord may be affected.

Almost any organ in the body, however, with the usual exception of the lung, may be affected, and in children in Ibadan the diagnosis of the Burkitt tumour should always be considered in the differential diagnosis of a possibly malignant condition. In spite of frequent deposits in the intestine, intussusception has not been common in our experience and the rarity of superficial lymph-node involvement is remarkable.

Generally, the tumour is considered to be multicentric in origin, although the frequent occurrence of deposits in ovaries, abdominal lymphatic glands, kidneys, and mediastinal glands and heart are suggestive of lymphatic spread. Grossly, the tumour is of fairly soft consistency yellowish-white in colour with bright yellow areas of necrosis and small haemorrhages. It usually appears fairly well demarcated from the surrounding tissue—an observation not borne out microscopically.

The most common sites of tumour deposit are in the skeletal system, namely the mandible and maxilla, where it commences in the marrow space and extends into the soft tissues, the antra, base of the skull, or orbit, depending upon the original site. Multiple foci may be present. Other bones are less frequently affected but none are exempt and in one case the presenting tumour was in the diaphysis of the femur.

Lymphoreticular tissue. Excluding the cervical glands peripheral lymphatic glands are not commonly affected. Involvement of mediastinal and abdominal lymph nodes is, however, common and deposits may be present in the spleen.

Bone-marrow deposits are not uncommon—especially in the ilium, and marrow puncture can be a useful diagnostic procedure. In spite of bone-marrow involvement leukaemic manifestations are rare, although malignant cells may occasionally be seen on buffy coat examination.

Cardiovascular system. Tumour deposits in the pericardium or heart are not uncommon and associated mediastinal involvement is usually found in these cases.

Respiratory system. The lungs are very rarely the seat of macroscopic deposits but microscopic involvement may be evident in a low percentage of cases.

Central nervous system. This system is involved in approximately 30 per cent of patients. The brain and its coverings are more frequently involved than the spinal cord. The neurological complications have been well described by Odeku *et al.* (1973), Singh *et al.* (1973) and Nkrumah and Perkins (1973). The meninges may be affected primarily or by extension of an existing tumour in the bones of the skull. In the case of the cord it is most frequently affected by extension of intra-abdominal para-vertebral tumour masses, and plaques of tumour tissue are found in the extradural space. Isolated tumour deposits in the brain have been described but are not common. Perineural involvement of the cranial and other nerves is, however, common with extension to the meninges, Virchow–Robin spaces, and adjacent parenchymal tissue (Fig. 10.18). Burkitt cells can be

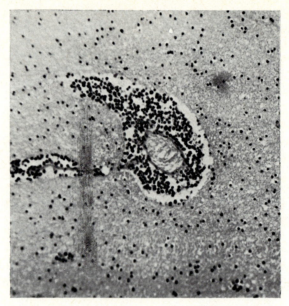

FIG. 10.18. Burkitt tumour. Perivascular cuffing in Burkitt meningo-encephalitis (H and E × 80).

found in the cerebrospinal fluid and this form of Burkitt 'meningo-encephalitis' would appear to be becoming more common terminally when chemotherapy has failed (Janota, 1966).

Alimentary system. The salivary glands and palate are not infrequently affected, and, occasionally, tonsillar deposits are seen. Umbilicated deposits frequently occur in the stomach, small intestine, appendix, and large intestine. Intestinal haemorrhage is a complication but intussusception is not common. Multiple deposits may be found in the liver and pancreas. Retroperitoneal and paravertebral masses are common. Gross ascites is unusual but fluid usually can be recovered on aspiration if the abdominal organs are involved, and typical Burkitt cells can be seen in cytological preparations or by phase contrast examination.

Endocrine glands. Direct extension to the pituitary occurs and deposits are frequently seen in the thyroid and adrenals. The thymus is rarely involved.

Genito-urinary system. The ovaries are frequently involved, the testes very much less so. The tumour masses in the pelvis and retroperitoneal tissues may cause hydronephrosis and renal impairment. The kidneys themselves are frequently the seat of multiple tumour deposits. Deposits have been noted in the breasts in both sexes, and may grow rapidly and reach a large size in pregnancy in rare instances.

Other organs. The subcutaneous tissues may be affected but usually as a late manifestation of the disease.

The microscopic appearances are distinctive in satisfactory paraffin-embedded sections. The tumour consists of sheets of 'blast' cells scattered among which are large histiocytes which have an eccentric nucleus and a large amount of pale-staining cytoplasm containing pyknotic nuclear remnants and cell debris (Figs. 10.19 and 10.20). On processing, some of these histiocytes may be lost, leaving clear spaces. These clear spaces and the pale histiocytes interspersed at intervals on the background of the sheets of darkly-staining tumour cells give the 'starry sky' appearance (Fig. 10.21). The histiocytic cells are not thought to be malignant but to represent a host reaction. The 'starry sky' appearance is not specific for the Burkitt tumour and can be seen in other tumours. The striking cellular uniformity is a useful diagnostic feature and is mimicked by few other tumours.

The 'blast' cell consists of a large round, oval, or reniform nucleus surrounded by a rim of cytoplasm which is indistinct in paraffin sections. The nuclear membrane is well defined, the chromatin material is in small clumps or short strands and one or more small eosinophilic or dark nucleoli are present. There is frequently a background of pale, bluish, granular material which represents cytoplasmic remnants. Mitotic figures are variable in number. Extensive areas of necrosis may be present and there may be

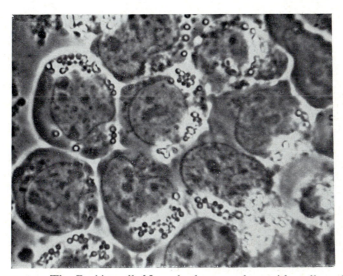

FIG. 10.19. The Burkitt cell. Note the large nucleus with well-marked nucleoli. Lipid granules in the cytoplasm are obvious (phase contrast × 1200). (*By courtesy of Dr. B. O. Osunkoya.*)

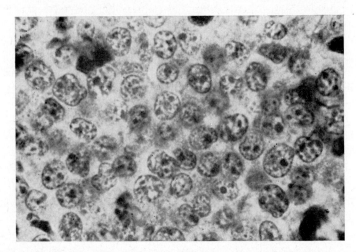

FIG. 10.20. The Burkitt cell. Sheets of Burkitt cells which appear to consist of nucleus only. Nucleoli are well marked and there is a background of granular material. Compare with the appearance on phase contrast (H and E × 500).

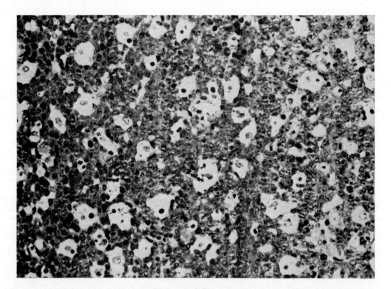

FIG. 10.21. Burkitt tumour. Sheets of Burkitt tumour cells with numerous histiocytes present. The small pyknotic nuclei can be seen and debris is present in a number of the histiocytes. An exaggerated 'starry sky' pattern (H and E × 180).

numerous small, darkly-staining cells representing the pyknotic nuclei of the blast cells. Lymphocytes are not usually present in any numbers. Vascularity is not a feature. The reticulin framework is scanty and encloses sheets of tumour cells.

Press preparations of fresh tissue stained by Jenner–Giemsa confirm the large nucleus with a rather coarser and more clumped chromatin pattern than is present in the lymphoblast. Up to five small, dark nucleoli may be present. There is a rim of basophilic cytoplasm containing usually a variable number of vacuoles which represent lipid granules and are probably a sign of early degenerative change. These vacuoles are non-specific and are seen in marrow preparations in various haematological conditions.

In the press preparations there may be some variations in cell size, coarseness of the nuclear chromatin pattern, and basophilia of the cytoplasm suggestive of different stages of maturity. However, in only a few instances have we noted possible 'differentiation' of the primitive cells to the lymphocytic series in jaw tumours in older children which were clinically characteristic of the Burkitt tumour, but which on histological, cytological, phase contrast, and tissue culture examination were in fact lymphosarcomas. Wright in Uganda, who has examined many hundreds of these tumours, has not reported this 'differentiation' so its significance must remain conjectural.

The histiocyte contains a pale, basophilic, finely-stippled nucleus usually containing one or two nucleoli with a large amount of faintly basophilic cytoplasm and engulfed nuclear remnants and cell debris present. The histochemistry of the tumour has been studied by Wright (1963) in Uganda. In the blast cell there was no evidence of alkaline or acid phosphatase or 5-nucleotidase activity, but there was slight non-specific esterase activity. It was PAS-negative. These findings, excluding the slight non-specific esterase activity, are similar to those expected in the poorly differentiated type of lymphosarcoma, but differ from the pattern expected in the histiocytic reticulum cell which exhibits acid phosphatase and non-specific esterase activity. The cells are pyronin positive.

Phase contrast and tissue culture

Pulvertaft (1965), and later Osunkoya working in Ibadan, have shown that phase contrast examination of cells from the tumour itself, from ascitic, pleural, and cerebrospinal fluid, or from marrow or splenic aspirates, is a most valuable and accurate diagnostic aid. On phase contrast, the cells are twice the diameter of lymphocytes, non-coherent, spherical, dark, opaque, and non-motile, with a few superficial lipid granules situated at one pole or in a broad band round the equator. The nucleus occupies most of the cell and is pale and indented with large bizarre nucleoli (Fig. 10.19). This cell is readily and rapidly distinguished from those of neuroblastoma, retinoblastoma, and Wilm's tumour, all of which can be confused, in poor biopsies, with the Burkitt tumour.

On tissue culture the Burkitt cell is said to be quite distinctive and has not been seen in many hundreds of malignant lymphomas cultured in London, although it was stated that in this series not many childhood malignancies were examined (Pulvertaft, 1965). In contrast to other lymphoreticular tumours the Burkitt tumour is not difficult to maintain in continuous culture. Minor culture differences have been noted in a few of the nine strains maintained in Ibadan and these are mainly in mobility, size, and lipid granular content, and probably correspond to the slight variations noted on press preparations (Osunkoya, 1966). The cells are sluggishly motile, do not adhere to glass but may or may not adhere to each other. They survive well on thyroid feeder layers, do not lyse collagen and autolyse rapidly in T.C.199 medium at 3 °C. The tumour cells are frequently seen within histiocytes—a phenomenon which Pulvertaft has termed 'emperipolesis'. This is non-specific and thought to be concerned with immune reactions in the host.

Diagnostic pathology

Consideration of the clinical history and a satisfactory biopsy usually establish the diagnosis. However, in a number of instances the biopsy may be small, a necrotic area may have been excised, or the tissue may have been compressed on removal. In these circumstances the greatest difficulty may be experienced in differentiating the tumour from retinoblastoma, neuroblastoma and Wilm's tumour. It is therefore, our practice in Ibadan to attempt to obtain, in addition to tissue for processing for histological examination, (1) a press or imprint preparation of the tumour on slides, which are then fixed in methyl alcohol and stained by May–Gruenwald or Jenner–Giemsa, (2) a suspension of cells in T.C. 199 medium to be examined by phase contrast, and (3) culture (for details see Pulvertaft, 1965). The combination of histological, cytological, and phase-contrast examination will almost certainly allow accurate diagnosis in all cases. The electron microscope reveals numerous ribosomes in the cytoplasm of Burkitt's tumour cells and a high cytoplasmic content of R.N.A. by pyronin and acridine orange staining. Wright et al. (1967) consider this pyroninophlia to be a useful histological feature which aids the separation of Burkitt's tumour from other malignant lymphomas and with this we would agree.

Rosettes, pseudo-rosettes, and neurofibrils are never seen in the Burkitt tumour; and histologically the presence of these may be of help in differentiating the tumour from a neuroblastoma, which on phase contrast shows faceted cells adherent to each other and which on culture tend to adhere to glass.

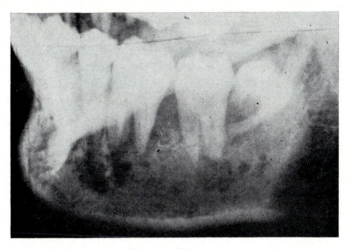

FIG. 10.22. Burkitt tumour. The mandible, showing osteolytic deposits and loss of the lamina dura. (*By courtesy of Dr. W. P. Cockshott.*)

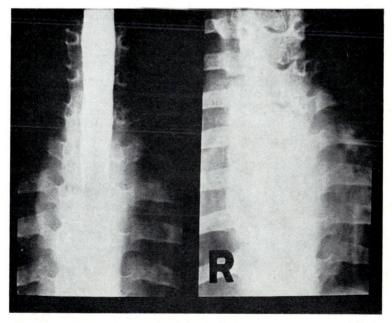

FIG 10.23. Burkitt tumour. The paravertebral soft tissue mass can be seen on the right and a complete spinal block is shown by myelography. (*By courtesy of Dr. W. P. Cockshott.*)

The retinoblastoma occurs in a somewhat younger age group but in Africa is usually undifferentiated. On culture it shows branching chains of cells adherent to each other. The presence of epithelial cells on press preparation allows easy differentiation from Wilm's tumour.

The radiological findings have been well described by Cockshott (1965). The tumour deposits show as osteolytic lesions in bone and any bone may be affected. In the mandible and maxilla patchy, minute areas of trabecular bony destruction occur and a striking feature is the erosion of the trabeculae of the lamina dura of the teeth. With extension of the process, teeth are lost (Fig. 10.22). Extension within the surrounding soft tissues occurs and maxillary deposits extend into the antra and nasal passages. Deposits may arise primarily in the ethnoid or sphenoidal sinuses and diploe of the skull. The radiological appearances in the maxilla or mandible are not specific and can be simulated by neuroblastoma or leukaemia. Paravertebral masses may be seen, the vertebral bodies may be affected, and myelography may show a complete spinal block (Fig. 10.23). The iliac bones are more frequently and extensively involved than is the sternum. The long bones are occasionally involved and the tumour may erode the cortex with elevation of the periosteum, simulating a Ewing's tumour, a reticulum-cell sarcoma, or secondary neuroblastoma.

11

The Alimentary System

INTRODUCTION

The diseases of the alimentary tract which affect the neonate would not appear to differ greatly in temperate and tropical climates. Congenital malformations occur. Congenital umbilical hernia is more common, while pyloric stenosis, cystic fibrosis of the pancreas and meconium ileus are probably less common than would be expected in temperate climates. Umbilical herniae may be present in 66 per cent of pre-school children in Western Nigeria, which is a figure considerably higher than those quoted for East and South Africa. There is a striking fall in prevalence with age in Western Nigeria but this is not noticeable in South Africa (Wyatt and Matthew, 1972). It is more common in children of the lower socio-economic group but does occur in the elite society. Factors in the aetiology of the condition may be heredity, malnutrition, splenomegaly, bulky carbohydrate diet and heavy intestinal parasitic infections. A world-wide survey of congenital malformations has recently been completed to which interested readers are referred (Editorial, 1967). Necrotizing enterocolitis in premature infants occurs.

Bacterial, viral, and parasitic infections are extremely common (typhoid, amoebiasis, etc.) and are discussed in their appropriate chapters.

The variable incidence of volvulus and intussusception as causes of intestinal obstruction is interesting, as is the recent report of lactase deficiency in the intestinal epithelium of the U.S. Negro and the Baganda and Bantu tribes of East Africa. These are briefly discussed. Diverticulitis is rare in most parts of the tropics. Hirschprung's disease is not uncommon, the common symptoms being vomiting, abdominal distension, abnormal stools and constipation or diarrhoea. It usually presents in the first week of life and a ganglionosis has been present in our material. Caecal perforations have been reported (Ajayi *et al.* 1969). Malignant disease of the alimentary tract is considered as a whole, the high incidence of oral cancer and cancer of the oesophagus in areas of the tropics being noteworthy.

THE ORAL CAVITY

Generalized stomatitis, cheilosis, and angular stomatitis are common conditions and are associated with malnutrition and vitamin deficiencies, especially ariboflavinosis. We have occasionally seen an acute epiglottitis causing sudden death in the young child. Smoothness and pallor of the tongue are common in anaemia. Thrush is common in young children. Scurvy, metallic poisons, tuberculosis, and syphilis may affect the oral cavity. Epulides occur in adults, more commonly in females. In about 26 per cent of children in East Africa pigmentation of the fungiform papillae of the tongue unassociated with signs of malnutrition was noted by Beet (1948). A similar finding was recorded by Raper (1948) in about 50 per cent of adult Africans. The pigmentation is due to melanin deposition and increases in amount with age. In contrast to periodontal disease dental caries is not common in most areas of the tropics. Investigations in Papua–New Guinea, however, have shown an association with a varying content of elements in soil and vegetables and caries prevalence (Barnes *et al.* 1970). In many areas up to 80 per cent of children may be affected. Inflammation of the gingiva leads to bony destruction, with consequent loss of teeth. Leprosy, rhinoscleroma, the traponematoses, the leishmaniases and the mycoses may affect the oropharynx, and haemorrhagic bullae are seen in onyalai.

Dental fluorosis occurs in isolated areas in the tropics but is prevalent in Thailand (Leatherwood *et al.* 1965) and in India (Jolly *et al.* 1968; Teotia *et al.* 1971). The subject has been reviewed in a WHO monograph (1970). A distressing feature in parts of West Africa is the frequency with which uvulectomy is practised by the native barber surgeons. Haemorrhage, sepsis, and gross scarring may result. Oral submucous fibrosis, parotid gland enlargement, and cancrum oris are common in the tropics and are discussed below. Tumours of the oral cavity are considered later.

ORAL SUBMUCOUS FIBROSIS

Synonyms. Atrophia idiopathica (trophica) mucosae oris (Schwartz, 1952); submucous fibrosis of the palate and pillars (Joshi, 1953), diffuse oral submucous fibrosis (Lal, 1953); sclerosing stomatitis (Behl, 1962).

Submucous fibrosis is an insidious, chronic disease affecting any part of the oral cavity and sometimes the pharynx, exemplified by a fibro-elastosis in the submucosal tissues and epithelial atrophy, causing loss of elasticity in the oral mucosa with resulting trismus. It may be preceded by, or associated with, vesicle formation into the mucosa, and a juxta-epithelial inflammatory reaction is constant (Pindborg, 1965).

Epidemiology

Oral submucous fibrosis has been reported mainly in India but has been seen in Indians living in East Africa, and in the occasional European in India, as well as in Nepal, Sri Lanka, Malaysia, Thailand, and South Vietnam. It has been estimated that there may be 2,000,000 cases in India. The majority of patients are in the 20- to 40-year-old age group and the sexes are equally affected, as are all social classes. The aetiology is unknown but the prolonged action of a mild irritant has been suggested. The chewing of betel nut is considered an unlikely factor but the irritant principle of chillies (*Capsicum annum*), especially if associated with low levels of vitamins A, B, or C in the diet, may be important in the aetiology of the condition (Wahi *et al.* 1966).

The incidence of oral cancer is high in India and oral submucous fibrosis may be a precancerous condition (Pindborg *et al.* 1968). Oral leukoplakia is frequently an associated condition.

Pathology

Patients may present with painful vesicles in the oral mucosa. The mucosa later becomes blanched and opaque. The distribution is symmetrical and white fibrous bands run in a vertical direction. The soft palate, uvula, and anterior pillars of the fauces, and even the pharynx, may be involved. Marked changes in the lower lip and the floor of the mouth may occur.

Hyalinized collagen in the submucosa with atrophy of the mucosa are constant findings. In the early stages, eosinophils are seen but later an inflammatory exudation of lymphocytes and plasma cells occurs. Obliteration of blood vessels is seen in the late stages.

CANCRUM ORIS

In this condition there is gangrene of the gingival tissues and soft tissues of the cheek. The bone of the mandible and/or the maxilla is exposed, with usually sequestrum formation. It is a growing problem in many parts of the tropics, as many children, who in the past would have died, survive on antibiotic therapy. The resulting facial defects present an insoluble problem in areas where plastic surgery is not available.

Epidemiology

Children aged between 2 and 5 years are mainly affected. However, it has been reported in adults in concentration camps (Dawson, 1945) and affects young adults in Western countries. The well-fed, healthy child is not affected. Systemic diseases such as measles, anaemia, and smallpox are predisposing factors, especially in malnourished children. The condition is not, however, a common complication of kwashiorkor. It most probably commences as a herpes simplex infection of the gingiva. Invasion by *Borrelia vincenti* and *Fusiformis fusiformis* follow, and spreading gangrene occurs. In Nigeria no discrepancies in the ABO blood groups or secretor status of the patients have been noted. The incidence of the sickle-cell trait was as expected and acatalasaemia was not found (Emslie, 1963). The last condition has been implicated as a factor in oral gangrene in Japan (Takahara, 1952).

Pathology

There is usually ulceration of the gingiva, with exposure of bone. The lesion extends to the facial tissues and a dark spot shows on the outer surface. Sloughing follows with perforation and loss of facial tissue. The edges of the ulcerated area are usually fairly sharply defined in the late stages but a rapidly spreading cellulitis may be present. Extensive necrosis of bone may occur.

Histologically the striking feature is necrosis of tissue with the organisms present at the advancing edge of the lesion, where there is an infiltrate of chronic inflammatory cells. In the healing stage granulation tissue and, later, extensive fibrosis occurs. The resulting deformity may be great.

Lung abscesses and bronchopneumonia are complications.

Diagnostic pathology

Fusiformis fusiformis is a cigar-shaped, Gram-positive organism 5–12 μm in length with a straight or slightly curved axis. It is easily decolourized on Gram's stain and is non-motile. It can be cultured anaerobically on serum agar or serum broth. The culture is pleomorphic and the organism has little effect on laboratory animals.

Borrelia vincenti is a delicate organism 5–10 μm in length with three to eight irregular spirals present. It is actively motile, Gram-negative and stains poorly. It can be demonstrated in fresh material by dark-ground examination. It can be cultured anaerobically on serum agar or serum broth. It has no effect on the guinea-pig. However, if both organisms from lesions are inoculated infection occurs.

Both these organisms can be demonstrated on smears from ulcerated lesions by Gram's stain. Dark-ground examination is also useful. Culture and animal inoculation are further diagnostic procedures.

The parotid gland

Bilateral enlargement of the parotid glands may be classified as inflammatory or non-inflammatory. Examples of the former are: acute pyogenic or viral parotitis (mumps is common in the tropics), bilateral salivary duct calculi, acute post-operative parotitis, sarcoidosis, tuberculosis, fungal infections and Sjorgen's syndrome.

Non-inflammatory bilateral parotid gland enlargement occurs in a variety of conditions including bilateral lymphomas, diabetes mellitus, pregnancy and lactation, malnutrition, obesity, alcoholism with liver disease, and following starch, heavy metal and some drug ingestions (Kaltreider and Talal, 1969).

Bilateral painless enlargement of the parotid gland is, however, not uncommon in many areas of the tropics. The other salivary glands are not usually affected. The condition has been observed in prison camps and pellagrins in Europe and is associated with a low-protein, high-carbohydrate diet in the tropics. It has also been noted in patients suffering from cirrhosis of the liver.

The aetiology is obscure. Biopsy has shown hyperplasia of the gland and a large number of secretory granules in the cells (Salamon, 1958). The hypertrophy of the ductular and glandular systems has been confirmed by sialograms (Farago, 1964). Various theories have been advanced to explain the hyperplasia. It may be functional in response to a high carbohydrate intake or to a nutritional surplus after a prolonged period of malnutrition. The condition is not associated with severe malnutrition in which atrophy of the gland is found. It has also been suggested that depression of the cholinesterases which occurs in undernourished individuals may favour increased parasympathetic action and hyperfunction of the parotids. Endocrine factors have also been considered in the aetiology of the condition. No entirely satisfactory explanation, however, fits the varying incidence in different geographical areas. The most important factor, however, would appear to be dietary. It has been produced experimentally in laboratory animals by reducing the food intake. Histologically the glands showed hyperplasia (Buchner and Sreebny, 1970).

Children over the age of 5 years and young adults are most frequently affected.

THE OESOPHAGUS AND STOMACH

OESOPHAGUS

Inflammatory lesions of the oesophagus are relatively rare and oesophageal varices secondary to portal hypertension is probably the most common pathological condition affecting the oesophagus in the tropics. In spite of widespread anaemia the Paterson–Brown–Kelly syndrome of dysphagia, spasm, inflammation, and stenosis of the lower pharynx (Editorial, 1967), would appear to be uncommon as is postcricoid carcinoma. Mega-oeso-phagus is common where Chagas' disease is endemic (p. 43).

Corrosive oesophagitis due to chemical burns is not uncommon (Martinson, 1967) and may follow attempted suicide by the ingestion of lysol. Caustic soda, widely used for the making of soap in homes, sulphuric acid for car batteries, and nitric acid in the goldsmith's trade are frequently stored in bottles in the home. Young children and adults may be affected. The caustics may be imbibed accidentally, for suicidal purposes, or utilized as medicine by traditional healers.

Burns are produced in the mouth, pharynx, oesophagus, stomach, and larynx, and shock may be marked in the acute phase. Ulceration ensues and heals by granulation tissue with fibrosis and scarring. Strictures are almost always multiple and occur most commonly at the level of the bifurcation of the trachea and lower third of the oesophagus.

Complications of the acute stage are perforation of the oesophagus or stomach and tracheo-oesophageal fistulae. Bronchiectatis or lung abscess may ensue. In the chronic stage bouginage may cause rupture, and gastric ulceration and even pyloric stenosis may occur.

Dilatation and ulceration of the oesophagus above the stricture are common.

Cancer of the oesophagus is discussed separately.

PEPTIC ULCER

Gastric ulcer is rare in most parts of the tropics. When it occurs it is usually prepyloric in position and occurs in the lower socio-economic groups (Nwokolo, 1966). The male/female ratio would appear to be similar to that reported in England, being about $2 \cdot 4 : 1$. The greatest numbers of patients are seen in the fifth and sixth decades. It is of interest that we have occasionally seen a perforated acute gastric ulcer in the neonate and a benign giant gastric ulcer has been seen in a young female at necropsy. Gastric ulcer is much more common in Negroes in the U.S.A. than it is in Africans (Joly, 1956). The reason for this relative rarity of gastric ulcer in Africa and India (Dogra, 1940) is not known. No difference has been found in acid curves of normal Nigerians and Englishmen (Rose, 1935). Perforation and obstruction are more common complications than haemorrhage.

Duodenal ulcer, on the other hand, is common in southern India and parts of Africa and the duodenal/gastric ulcer ratio may be as much as $30:1$, whereas in Britain it is $2 \cdot 1 : 1$ (Dogra, 1940; Davey and Dickson, 1964). All social classes tend to be affected and the male/female ratio is $3:1$. The free hydrochloric acid level is high (Konstam, 1955).

In southern India and Nigeria the diet is generally low in protein and high in carbohydrate, and is consequently bulky. The staples are rice and tapioca, and yam and cassava respectively. Spices are consumed but are also consumed in areas where the ulcer incidence is low (northern India).

Deficiencies of thiamine and riboflavin are possible factors. Ascariasis and hookworm are endemic but are unlikely to be causal agents (Chuttani *et al.* 1967). Tovey (1974) reviewed the geographical distribution of peptic ulcer.

Pathology

The ulcer is usually situated in the posterior wall of the upper part of the duodenum. It may be deep and penetrate into the head of the pancreas. Fibrous overgrowth is marked and perforation is not common in West Africa but does occur in Kampala. Stenosis and haemorrhage are complications and stomal ulcers following gastro-enterostomy occur. A fistulous communication between the duodenum and the biliary system may also be a complication (Lewis and Bohrer, 1969).

APPENDICITIS

Appendicitis occurs in most areas of the tropics, and seems to be more common in urban than rural communities (Janssens and Muynck, 1966). It is responsible for about 14 per cent of abdominal emergencies in Ibadan (Joly and Thomas, 1954; Badoe, 1967) but would appear to be less common in East Africa (Trowell, 1960). The part that intestinal parasites play, therefore, in the aetiology of the condition cannot be great and is mentioned when the individual parasites are described. In our experience schistosomiasis is the only condition occurring with any frequency in surgically-removed appendices and the infection probably renders the appendix more liable to secondary infection in a minority of patients (p. 163). A carcinoid tumour of the appendix is occasionally seen.

INFLAMMATORY CONDITIONS OF THE GASTRO-INTESTINAL TRACT

Apart from the specific infections which are discussed elsewhere, salmonella and staphylococcal food poisoning commonly occur in the tropics but their manifestations do not differ from those described in standard textbooks.

S. typhimurium is the most common of the many salmonella serotypes which cause acute food poisoning. The incubation period is 6 to 24 hours. The onset is sudden with fever, vomiting and diarrhoea. The infection is usually confined to the intestinal tract and recovery is the rule unless the patient is debilitated. A carrier state may persist for some months.

Staphylococcus aureus

Certain phage types produce an enterotoxin which can cause acute diarrhoea and vomiting. Cold meat dishes are the usual source of infection. The toxin is heat stable. The incubation period is short—usually less than four hours. The illness is generally brief with complete recovery the rule but we have seen a choleraic-like epidemic in Burma with a considerable mortality. Bacteriological examination may be negative if the organisms have been killed by cooking.

Clostridium welchii

Severe outbreaks may occur in hostels, etc. in the tropics. Spores may resist boiling for a number of hours and may germinate as food cools. A rapid recovery is usual. The organism can be easily isolated from suspected food and from the patient's stools in which it usually persists for a number of days after the attack.

Enteritis necroticans is discussed on p. 319. We have seen haemorrhagic necrosis of the small intestine in a few children in West Africa but were unable to determine its cause. Cases of enteritis necroticans have been described in East Africa (Wright and Stanfield, 1967) and Headington et al. (1967), have described segmental infarcts of the small intestine and mesenteric adenitis in Thai children, the cause of which was obscure. Segmental vasospasm of the mesenteric vascular bed was thought the most likely explanation although the initiating factor could not be determined. These children present with acute febrile watery diarrhoea with faeces strongly positive for occult blood. Ileus and shock then occur with X-ray evidence of a segmental lesion of the small intestine. This condition may be more widespread than the literature would suggest so it should be considered in any child with the above-mentioned symptoms as surgical intervention is life-saving. It is of interest that 'ischaemic' colitis in young adults has been recently reported in the Western world (Clark et al. 1972). The role of HL-A antigens in inflammatory bowel disease is reviewed by Russell and Schlaut (1974).

An interesting condition brought about by movement to a new place, not necessarily but commonly in the tropics, is a non-specific enteritis referred to as a traveller's diarrhoea.

TRAVELLER'S DIARRHOEA

Diarrhoeal attacks of varying severity are a common consequence of persons travelling from one area of the world to another and are one of the hazards of travel to the tropics and subtropics. It affects the newcomer but not the inhabitant; most attacks are mild and of short duration, some are more severe, interfere with a programme of activities, or may even necessitate treatment in bed. Their causation is indeterminate (Turner, 1967).

ULCERATIVE COLITIS

Most reports would suggest that ulcerative colitis is uncommon in most parts of the tropics (Zuidema, 1959; Trowell, 1960). It is virtually non-existent in south-east Asia (Tinkler, 1966) and it is our impression that it is rare in Ibadan. Billinghurst and Welchman (1966) have reported four cases in Africans in East Africa. Ulcerative colitis is, however, not rare in India, where it seems to be a milder disease than in Europe since it remains limited to the rectum, sigmoid colon, and descending colon (Chuttani *et al.* 1967). Coincident salmonella infections and ulcerative colitis occur (Dronfield *et al.* 1974).

The cause of the condition is unknown. Many factors have been considered in its aetiology. Recently, antibodies to colonic mucosa have been demonstrated in the serum of patients with ulcerative colitis and the possibility of auto-immunization being an aetiological factor was considered, McGiven *et al.* (1967), however, found that the auto-antibodies were not specific for colonic mucosa and suggested they were not the cause of mucosal damage but reflected cellular activity by auto-immune lymphoid cells. If the view of Acheson and Truelove (1961) that artificial feeding in the first few weeks of life is an aetiological agent in ulcerative colitis is correct, it would suscribe to the present body of opinion that ulcerative colitis is rare in the tropics.

The pathology of the condition is that of a chronic ulcerative process affecting mainly the mucosa and submucosa of the colon. The infiltrate is mainly lymphocytes, plasma cells, and histiocytes, but occasionally eosinophils are prominent. Crypt abscesses, consisting of neutrophils, eosinophils, red cells and mucus within crypt lumina are conspicuous and the coalescence of these ruptured abscesses causes the ulcerative lesion which seldom extends more deeply than the submucosa. Polypoid hyperplasia of the mucosa between the ulcers is a notable feature. Carcinomatous change is common in long-standing cases. Ulcerative post-dysenteric colitis and regional ileitis have to be considered in the differential diagnosis. In the former the amoebic gel diffusion test is positive and in the latter a 'sarcoid' reaction is seen histologically.

REGIONAL ILEITIS (CROHN'S DISEASE)

This would appear to be an uncommon condition in the tropics but the diagnosis may well be being missed as the pathology is that of a chronic granulomatous condition, affecting usually the lower end of the ileum. A changing epidemiological pattern of the disease is taking place (Hiller *et al.*

1974). Giraud *et al.* (1969) has reported five cases in the Transvaal Bantu. The stomach and large bowel can, however, be involved. Thickening of the bowel wall and narrowing of the lumen is usual and the term 'hose pipe' has been used.

The most useful diagnostic feature is the presence of a sarcoid reaction in the tissues of the bowel wall, and regional lymph nodes. Schaumann bodies may occasionally be present in the giant cells. Occasionally this reaction may not be seen and fissures from the ulcerated mucosal surface penetrating deeply in the muscular coat or even the serosa are suggestive of the diagnosis. Superficially there is necrosis with an infiltrate of polymorphs, lymphocytes, and plasma cells. In the later stages histiocytes replace the polymorphs. Mast cells as shown by staining with polychrome methylene blue and the periodic acid–Schiff method are also numerous (Rao, 1973). It differs from ulcerative colitis, which is essentially a superficial lesion. The aetiology has recently been discussed in an Editorial (1970) and genetic, infective and immunological factors have been considered.

EOSINOPHILIC GRANULOMA OF THE INTESTINE

The aetiology of this condition has been the subject of much discussion. It was suggested that the cause might be an allergic reaction to ingested foodstuffs or other substances (Smith, 1956; Leinbach and Rubin, 1970). One of the most likely causative agents of the condition is undoubtedly *Eustoma rotundatum*, a nematode parasite commonly occurring in the peritoneum of the North Sea herring (Ashby *et al.* 1964). Kuipers and his colleagues investigated the parasite extensively, and found that it occurred in large numbers in the peritoneal cavity of the herring, the numbers varying directly with the length of the herring.

The pathology is that of a diffuse or focal eosinophilic infiltration of the gastro-intestinal tract. Macroscopically there may be diffuse or localized lesions, the gut being thickened and yellowish to red-blue in colour. Polypoid lesions may be present. Ulceration is not common. The pyloric antrum is most frequently affected. Lesions are common in the small intestine and less common in the caecum and colon.

Histologically there is a massive infiltration of eosinophils in the submucosa splitting the muscularis. The muscle coats may be invaded but the serosa is intact. The mucosa is also usually intact but ulceration can occur. There is accompanying oedema and congestion of blood vessels and dilatation of lymphatics. Villous atrophy and abnormalities of the surface epithelium have been described and a malabsorption syndrome may result. Fragments of larvae may or may not be identified in the lesion.

Eosinophilic granulomas of the gut have been described from many parts of the world. *Eustoma rotundatum* cannot be implicated in all cases and other parasitic infections may be implicated (Ashby *et al.* 1964). A macro-cytic anaemia has been described in a few patients prior to the onset of symptoms. A peripheral blood eosinophilia may or may not be present. Cortico-steroids may be of value in therapy.

INTESTINAL OBSTRUCTION

The most common cause of intestinal obstruction is strangulated inguinal hernia. Femoral and internal herniae are not commonly seen. Occasionally an acquired adult umbilical hernia may strangulate but this is rare in the infantile type which is common in Africa (Jelliffe, 1954).

There is, however, a remarkable variation in the incidence of volvulus and intussusception in different parts of the tropics and these are discussed when they are considered below. Tuberculosis may cause intestinal obstruc-tion either by stenosis of the lumen or, less commonly, by pressure of enlarged lymph nodes on the third part of the duodenum or jejunum (Anand and Pathak, 1961; Davey and Pearson, 1965).

Pyloric stenosis is a frequent complication of carcinoma of the stomach but less frequently is carcinoma a cause of large-bowel obstruction.

The presence of bands and adhesions, and mesenteric thrombosis are not frequent causes of obstruction in the tropics although they do occur. Acute colonic obstruction due to *S. japonica* infection is not uncommon in China (Nai-Kuang and Pen-Ching, 1957)

Ileus associated with peritonitis is a not infrequent condition. The role of *ascariasis* is mentioned on p. 101.

Volvulus

Volvulus of the small intestine is rare in temperate climates but not uncommon in parts of India and East and South Africa. In Ibadan, Nigeria, it is more common than volvulus of the large intestine (Cole, 1965) but the incidence is not high. Young adult males are usually affected. The whole of the root of the mesentery usually acts as the pedicle. No specific cause has been noted but frequent intestinal infections with mesenteric glandular enlargement and dietary factors may play a part in the aetiology.

Volvulus of the sigmoid colon is common in many parts of the world. The incidence varies markedly. It accounts for 2·5 per cent of all causes of intestinal obstruction in Great Britain and between 1 and 4 per cent in the U.S.A. (excluding mental institutions, where the incidence is higher), whereas the figures from Germany and Russia are 31 per cent and 50 per cent respectively. The figures in Ibadan, Nigeria, and Accra, Ghana, are 1–2 per cent (Joly and Thomas, 1954; Cole, 1965) and 2·7 per cent (Badoe, 1965) respectively. Much higher figures are found in South Africa, 15·3 per cent (Skapinker, 1953); Uganda, 20 per cent (Shepherd, 1967);

Rhodesia, 33 per cent (Gelfand, 1957); Brazil, 25 per cent (Oliveira *et al.*
1963); Western India, 24 per cent (Anderson, 1956); and Peshawar,
30 per cent (Ahsan and Rahman, 1967). In America, volvulus of the sigmoid
colon is much commoner in Negroes than in whites (Pool and Dunavent,
1951).

In Brazil, sigmoid volvulus is considered most probably to be a complication of Chagas' disease (see p. 47). In megacolon in East Africa vacuolization
and chromatolysis of neurones has been noted, although their numbers are
not reduced (Bohm and Smith, 1966).

The condition is much more common in males than females, and adults
of any age may be affected.

The reasons for these differing incidences are not clear. It has been postulated that in these patients there is a long loop with a short mesenteric base
holding the two limbs of the sigmoid colon in approximation. Whether this
is racial or induced is not known. Teubes (1963) considered that dietary
distension of the colon with high-residue diets and periods of starvation
followed by an enormous meal were the most important aetiological factors.
The low incidence of the condition in areas of West Africa is, however,
difficult to explain as a high-residue diet is consumed and Mohammedan
fasts are religiously observed.

A history of attacks of abdominal pain, constipation, and distension
followed by sudden relief and the passage of a bulky stool may be given, and
suggests previous attacks of partial obstruction and that self-correction can
occur. The pathology depends upon the duration of the symptoms. The
colon is dilated and twisted, usually in an anti-clockwise direction, through
an angle of 180°. All grades of congestion of the wall up to death of tissue and
gangrene may occur. Scarring and adhesions around the base of the mesentery may be present. Double volvulus of small bowel and sigmoid colon
may occur, being not uncommon in Uganda (Trowell, 1960). There is
an anti-clockwise twist of the sigmoid colon and the small intestine follows
to make a loop about the sigmoid and passes down to be trapped beneath its
own mesentery. If this occurs the symptoms are much more acute, gangrene
occurs more rapidly, and the mortality rate is high. Radiological examination in the supine position shows the distribution of gas in the grossly
distended sigmoid colon. The erect film shows fluid levels in the sigmoid
loop.

Intussusception

In temperate climates intussusception usually occurs in children, and
precipitating factors are rarely found (Peck *et al.* 1963). A virus infection
affecting the mesenteric lymph nodes has been considered a possible cause
(Potter, 1964).

Secondary intussusception is a rare disease which may occur in children or adults and is due to a localized lesion in the intestine.

In Ibadan, Nigeria, the most common condition presenting as an abdominal emergency after a strangulated hernia is intussusception (Joly and Thomas, 1954). It occurs in adults and is relatively rare in children. It is also common in Korea in adults (Dietrick and Moon Ho Lee, 1965), in Kampala (Burkitt, 1952), and in the Congo, South Africa, and Egypt. It is usually the caput caeci type and the ileocaecal valve lies alongside the apex of the intussusception—obstruction is therefore not always complete. The aetiology is unknown but it has been suggested that there may be greater mobility of the caecum and ascending colon and a long retrocaecal appendix may be factors in the condition. Dietary factors are also probably involved.

The condition occurs slightly more frequently in males in the 20- to 40-year-old age group. Intermittent griping abdominal pain alternating with constipation and diarrhoea is usual. A mass is usually palpable but there is absence of tenderness or rigidity. Radiographs may show an empty right iliac fossa. The pathological changes are those typical of necrosis and haemorrhage at the apex of the intussusception if resection is performed.

DIVERTICULAR DISEASE OF THE COLON

This condition is rare in many of the developing countries of Africa and Asia (exceptions, however, occur—Ethiopia for example) whereas it is the commonest pathological process involving the large bowel in temperate climates. It is a frequent source of morbidity and a not uncommon cause of death (Editorial, 1969). The sigmoid colon is most frequently affected. Muscle thickening is usually associated with the presence of diverticula. The cause is unknown but increased pressure within the colon with hypertrophy of the circular muscle or with the development of diverticula or usually with both are thought to be factors in the aetiology. Dietary factors are considered important (Cleave et al. 1967). The American negro develops diverticula with an equal frequency to his white compatriot. The low bulk diet may fail to provide adequate dilatation of the colon with progressive contraction of the circular muscle in contrast to the high-residue diet of so many areas of the tropics. The condition has recently been reviewed by Painter and Burkitt (1971).

PERFORATION

Although in Europe the most common types of intestinal perforation are of the stomach and duodenum, this is not necessarily so in the tropics. Gastric ulcer is not common and perforation is said to occur less commonly in duodenal ulcers because of their site and the overgrowth of fibrous tissue which occurs at the base of the ulcer. Probably the most common type of perforation seen is the typhoid ulcer. This usually occurs in the lower ileum. Perforation may also occur through a solitary small, punched-out ulcer with indurated edges in the lower ileum and has been attributed by some to *Ascaris* infection. On other occasions *Ascaris* worms may not be detectable and the condition has been called 'idiopathic'. The role of *Ascaris* in this condition is debatable (Evans Amfon, 1963). Primary non-specific ileal ulcers in children who present with anaemia and acute and chronic rectal bleeding have been reported by Grosfeld *et al.* (1970). These differed in their aetiology from the ulcers seen in adults due to the ingestion of enteric-coated potassium containing medications. The cause is unknown. Typhoid fever should always be considered and appropriate laboratory tests undertaken. Amoebiasis may cause perforation of the large intestine but a localized peritonitis in the absence of perforation is more usual. Rarely, a tuberculous ulcer may perforate.

ANORECTAL DISEASE

Lymphogranuloma venereum is a common cause of rectal stricture and an amoeboma may simulate carcinoma. Rectovaginal fistulae may be due to lymphogranuloma venereum, obstructed labour, or, less commonly, rectal tuberculosis. Enemata are widely used in the tropics and irritant and caustic preparations may cause severe proctitis and stricture. Schistosomiasis may cause polypoid lesions which are otherwise not common. Prolapse of the rectum is common in malnourished children, with associated intestinal parasites present, and is also seen in the elderly, with urinary obstruction at times a precipitating factor. Haemorrhoids and their complications occur, and condyloma acuminata, fistula in ano, and anal fissure are common conditions.

THE MALABSORPTION SYNDROME

Intestinal malabsorption, in a broad sense, may be defined as any state in which there is a disturbance of the net absorption of any constituent across the intestinal mucosa (Jeffries *et al.* 1964). Although malabsorption may affect one or a variety of different substances, malabsorption of fat is the most commonly encountered defect. Excessive loss of fat in the stool (steatorrhea), may be a clinical manifestation in a variety of disorders. Sleisenger's classification (1967), based on etiologic mechanisms, lists the following:
 1. Inadequate digestion
     Gastric resection
     Pancreatic insufficiency
     Biliary obstruction
     Biliary cirrhosis

2. Biochemical abnormality
   Coeliac disease, adult and childhood
   Tropical sprue
   Deficiency of sugar-splitting enzymes
   A-beta-lipoproteinaemia

3. Inadequate absorptive surface
   Jejunal exclusion
   Gastro-ileostomy
   Large fistulas
   Massive bowel resection

4. Disease of the intestinal wall
   Ileo-jejunitis
   Amyloidosis
   Radiation injury
   Acute bacterial and viral enteritis

5. Lymphatic obstruction
   Lymphoma*
   Whipple's disease*
   Tuberculosis (tabes mesenterica)*

6. Altered bacterial flora
   Blind loop syndrome
   Multiple jejunal diverticula
   Multiple strictures
   Scleroderma*
   Small fistulas
   Neomycin therapy

7. Miscellaneous
   Carcinoid syndrome
   Diabetes mellitus
   Islet cell tumour of the pancreas
   Hypoparathyroidism
   Hypothyroidism
   Hypogammaglobulinaemia
   Mesenteric artery insufficiency

Clinical manifestations of the malabsorptive syndromes are protean and highly variable. From Volwiler's diagram (1957, Fig. 11.6), it will be noted that at least twelve different problems may present themselves.

Steatorrhea is always present during exacerbations. Diarrhoea is not an

---

* These disorders also involve the intestinal wall.

essential feature of the syndrome, but is ordinarily present during its acute phase. General malnutrition with protein deficiency is probably the most serious single feature and often results secondarily in additional malfunction of the small intestine and of pancreatic acinar cells. The metabolic bone disorder resulting from prolonged steatorrhea is probably due to combined deficiencies of protein (osteoporosis) and calcium (osteomalacia) (see discussion in following section).

In recent years a more accurate and thorough understanding of the pathologic lesions involved in the various malabsorptive disorders has been achieved through the peroral procurement of intestinal biopsy specimens. This technique has made available non-autolysed small intestine mucosa for study and has led to recognition of pertinent histologic alterations (Shapiro, 1971). Post-infective temporary malabsorption has recently been described (Montgomery *et al.* 1973).

The chief causes of the malabsorption syndrome in the tropics are given in Table 11.1.

TABLE 11.1 *Main causes of malabsorption in the tropics*

Primary	Secondary
Tropical sprue	1. Tuberculosis, p. 396
	2. Pancreatic disease, p. 665
	3. Intestinal parasites:
	(*a*) Strongyloidiasis, p. 107
	(*b*) Giardiasis, p. 80
	(*c*) Hookworm, p. 97

The subject of intestinal absorption has recently been comprehensively reviewed (*Brit. med. Bull.*, 1967). Standard textbooks will provide the reader with a formidable list of the many conditions that can give rise to steatorrhoea, all of which may be seen in the tropics but are relatively uncommon compared to the above. Thus coeliac disease and its adult counterpart idiopathic steatorrhoea are responsible for only a few cases of primary malabsorption in India (Walia *et al.* 1966; Misra *et al.* 1966; Desai and Jeejeebhoy, 1967). Both coeliac disease and, to a lesser extent, idiopathic steatorrhoea, respond favourably to a gluten-free diet and are often referred to as 'gluten-induced enteropathies'; in contrast, tropical sprue is not influenced by a gluten-free diet.

Tropical sprue

Tropical sprue has been defined as a primary malabsorption syndrome occurring in people resident in, or previously resident in, the tropics, usually associated with defective absorption of fat, carbohydrates, vitamins and other nutrients and with radiological changes in the small intestine (Baker *et al.* 1962). The disease has a peculiar geographical distribution and even in sprue-endemic areas the distribution is irregular. It has been reported most frequently from India, south-east Asia, Indonesia, and Puerto Rico. It seems extremely rare in Africa (Harries, 1964). The natural history of the disease is influenced by the age of the patient (Stefanini, 1948), climatic conditions (Webb and Simpson, 1966), previous nutritional deficiency (Ayrey, 1948), and by the duration of the illness (Gardner, 1958). Although cases of sprue are usually sporadic, epidemics sometimes occur (Mathan *et al.* 1966). The aetiology of the disease is unknown and various factors—none conclusively proved—have been incriminated, e.g. folic-acid deficiency; dietary deficiency; allergy; bacterial, viral, and fungal infections. Tomkins' *et al.* (1975) have suggested that *enterobacteria* may be responsible for persisting jejunal abnormalities in tropical sprue.

Pathogenesis

The pathogenesis of tropical sprue is best explained by a consideration of the absorptive functions of the proximal and distal small intestine in man. Figure 11.1 represents the small intestine as a simple tube and illustrates the sites of absorption of the various substances which largely determine the type of nutritional deficiency that occurs in tropical sprue.

Thus, glucose, xylose, iron, water-soluble vitamins, and divalent cations are absorbed in the jejunum. Fat, protein, and certain fat-soluble vitamins are also absorbed to a large extent proximally but, because they are absorbed more slowly, the peristaltic movements of the jejunum propel them to the ileum, where absorption is complete. The ileum is a reserve area for absorption of the above substances and also absorbs vitamin B_{12} (Booth, 1965). In most series of patients studied a reasonably good correlation has been found between the degree of malabsorption and the duration of symptoms.

Thus in the early stages intestinal malabsorption of fat, glucose, xylose, vitamin B_{12}, and folate deficiency are found, suggesting that both the jejunum and ileum are affected. After 4 months the intestinal mucosa, both jejunal and ileal, has the appearance of partial villous atrophy, megaloblastic anaemia due to folate deficiency occurs, and there is a considerable fall in the serum vitamin B_{12} concentration (O'Brien and England, 1966). Folate deficiency and megaloblastic anaemia do not, however, invariably occur (Sheehy *et al.* 1963; 1965), nor is it clear why discrepancies in the absorption of one substance or another sometimes occur in patients with tropical sprue. Booth and Mollin (1964) recorded subacute combined degeneration of the cord in patients with chronic tropical sprue and Kalro and Stewart (1974)

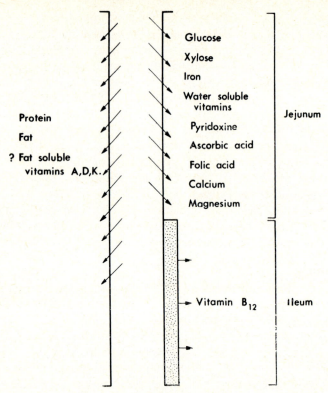

FIG. 11.1. Sites of absorption in the small intestine. (*After Booth*, 1965.)

pernicious anaemia. The level of ionic plasma calcium and magnesium may be low. In severe cases the prothrombin index is low, as are the serum concentrations of the fat-soluble vitamins. Intestinal loss of 'albumin' occurs in sprue patients but no correlation is found between this loss from the gut and the degree of hypo-albuminaemia (Vaish *et al.* 1965). It seems likely that the hypoproteinaemia and hypoalbuminaemia found in tropical sprue (Garcia Lopez *et al.* 1949; Baker, 1957) are due to a combination of four factors—diminished protein intake, defective absorption of dietary protein, protein loss from the gut, and diminished albumin production by the liver.

The main differential features between adult coeliac disease and tropical sprue are given in Table 11.2.

In the malabsorption associated with early intestinal parasitic infections the xylose absorption curve is frequently normal and may help to differentiate this type of malabsorption from tropical sprue. In tropical sprue the fat is split, as pancreatic enzymes are present. Changes are present in the

TABLE 11.2. *Differential features between adult coeliac disease and tropical sprue*

Adult coeliac disease	Tropical sprue
Proximal small bowel disease	Generalized small bowel disease
Related to dietary gluten	Unrelated to dietary gluten
Rare in tropics	History of sojourn in tropics
Osteomalacia common	Osteomalacia rare
Vitamin B_{12} deficiency rare	Vitamin B_{12} absorption commonly subnormal
Intestinal mucosa severely affected	Intestinal mucosa less severely affected
Broad-spectrum antibiotics ineffective	Broad-spectrum antibiotics favourable effect
Folic acid ineffective	Folic acid favourable effect
Diarrhoea relatively uncommon	Diarrhoea very common

gastric and upper intestinal mucosa. In the stomach there is depression of gastric secretion with a varying degree of gastritis and mucosal atrophy. No relationship has been noted between the severity of the gastric and intestinal lesions (Vaish *et al.* 1965).

On examination of jejunal biopsy specimens by the dissecting microscope, the villi in the early stages are shortened, broad, and leaf-shaped. Later the surface becomes convoluted and in the most severe stages an almost flat surface with a few crevices results (Swanson and Thomasson, 1965).

The histopathological changes are non specific and have been described in many conditions (Collins, 1965). The villi are shortened and thickened but the changes are not uniform. Partial villous atrophy is usual but not the almost total type seen in coeliac disease (Fig. 11.2). Measurements of the villi are given by O'Brien and England (1966). There is a narrowing of the mucosa with a predominance of plasma cells, histiocytes, lymphocytes and eosinophils in the lamina propria. Histiocytes containing PAS-positive granules may be seen at the tips of the villi. There is an initial rise in the mitotic index of the epithelial cells lining the crypts and goblet cells are increased. Adenosine triphosphatase (A.T.P.) has been shown to be present in the surface epithelium and lipoid vacuoles are seen in the thickened basement membrane separating the surface epithelium from the lamina propria. In coeliac disease, on the other hand, A.T.P. is markedly reduced and lipid vacuoles are seen in the surface epithelium (Schenk *et al.* 1966). Paneth cells are also reduced in numbers as shown by phloxine tartrazine stains.

Deaths most commonly occur in the first 10 years of life and in the older age groups. At autopsy, the body is very emaciated, with absence of sub-cutaneous fat. The skin is dry with irregular, pigmented scattered areas and sometimes petechial haemorrhages. The heart often shows brown pig-mentation. Ceroid, a lipid pigment, may be found in the smooth muscle of the gastro-intestinal tract, blood vessels, prostate, uterus, urinary bladder and lymph nodes in certain malabsorptive states. The condition has been termed lipfuscinosis or brown bowel syndrome. It has also been described in Northern Thailand in the absence of malabsorption and Vitamin E defi-ciency and a high intake of unsaturated fat have been mentioned as possible factors in its aetiology (Troncale *et al.* 1968). Lipofuscins are a group of pigments formed by oxidation of cellular lipoids and lipoproteins and have variable but characteristic staining properties depending upon the degree of oxidation and type of lipid in the cell. Pigmentation of the alimentary tract also occurs in melanosis coli due to the ingestion of anthracene laxatives which is now a rare disease and has not been described in the tropics. The red bone-marrow may be increased diffusely as the result of megaloblastic hyperplasia or may be replaced by pale, fat-free gelatinous tissue. Changes in the bones resembling osteoporosis and osteomalacia have been rarely reported.

Diagnostic pathology

The diagnosis of tropical sprue is confirmed by biochemical, histological, and radiological examination. Faecal-fat excretion, D-xylose absorption, glucose absorption, vitamin-A absorption, vitamin-B_{12} absorption, and serum-folate activity will reveal evidence of malabsorption of some or all of these substances (Sleedem and Kumar, 1973). The findings in jejunal ileal biopsies have already been described, while radiological examination using non-flocculable barium (Raybar) will reveal in the more severe cases thickened transverse mucosal folds with or without dilatation of the jeju-num. In the tropics, these diagnostic findings are not always easy to interpret since a remarkably high incidence of malabsorption and histological evidence of chronic enteritis has been noted in asymptomatic apparently normal individuals in Thailand, South India, Puerto Rico, Haiti, and West and East Pakistan (Sprinz *et al.* 1962; Baker *et al.* 1962; Angel *et al.* 1963; Klepstein *et al.* 1966; Russell *et al.* 1966; Lindenbaum *et al.* 1966). Thus, xylose absorption was subnormal in 20–100 per cent of asymptomatic subjects in these countries, while jejunal villous architecture was also abnormal by both dissecting and light microscopy; a finding also noted in Uganda where tropical sprue is rare (Banwell *et al.* 1964). Lindenbaum (1965) has shown that in Pakistanis with acute intestinal infections with a

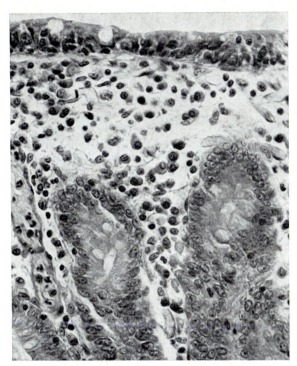

FIG. 11.2. Coeliac disease. Jejunal biopsy, illustrating damage to the surface epithelium in total villus atrophy. The crypt epithelium is relatively normal (H and E × 180). (*By courtesy of Dr. J. H. Yardley.*)

variety of organisms, widespread, moderate to severe impairment of absorptive function was the rule and some individuals showed continued malabsorption weeks or months after the acute infection. It cannot, therefore, be excluded that failure to recover absorptive function after single or repeated bouts of intestinal infection may not be responsible for the widespread abnormalities of intestinal structure and function noted above in asymptomatic individuals from several tropical countries.

Lactase deficiency

Many American Negroes suffer from milk intolerance due to a deficiency of lactase in the epithelium of the small intestine. This deficiency can be shown by the indirect evidence of a 'flat' lactose-tolerance curve following the ingestion of 50 g, or directly by histochemical methods, or assay of the intestinal mucosa obtained by jejunal biopsy (Cuatrecasas *et al.* 1965; Bayliss and Rosensweig, 1966). The incidence of this deficiency is also high in the Baganda and Bantu tribes of Uganda (Cook and Kajabi, 1966) and is probably also high in India (Jeejeebhoy *et al.* 1966). The reasons for these high incidences are unknown but it is considered most probably to be genetically determined. Deficiency of lactase can, however, also occur in disease states and has been noted in coeliac disease and acute ulcerative colitis (Lubos *et al.* 1967; Chalfin and Holt, 1967). Children allergic to milk may not necessarily exhibit this deficiency. Normal levels of disaccharidases including lactase have been found to be normal at birth in the newborn Baganda but fall with ageing—hypolactasia being present (as shown only by the lactose-tolerance test) as early as 6 months (Cook, 1967). The possible importance of the lack of this enzyme in children suffering from mild abdominal pain and diarrhoea, and the part that it might play in protein calorie deficiency disease, should be borne in mind.

TUMOURS OF THE ALIMENTARY SYSTEM

The macroscopic and microscopic pathology of the tumours of the alimentary system in the tropics is similar to that seen in temperate zones and will not therefore be described in any detail. It is possible that anaplastic tumours are more common owing to the younger population at risk. The geographical distribution and relative incidence of these tumours, is, however, of great interest and will be dealt with below.

TUMOURS OF THE ORAL CAVITY

In Africa the common tumours seen in the oral cavity, excluding such benign tumours as epulides, etc., are salivary gland tumours, ameloblastomas, and the Burkitt tumour, p. 500 (Edington and Sheiham, 1966). In Egypt, however, squamous cell carcinoma is common, the tongue being frequently affected. Salivary-gland tumours and ameloblastomas are briefly discussed below. Fibro-osseous dysplasia or ossifying fibromas and giant-cell tumours (osteoclastoma) of the jaw are not uncommon in our experience and intra-osseous fibromas and fibro-osteomas occasionally occur. Fibro-, osteo-, and chondrosarcomas occur in low incidence. Malignant lymphomas, plasmacytoma, neuroblastoma, retinoblastoma, and leukaemia have also been seen affecting the jaw.

The incidence of carcinoma of the oral cavity in Africa is much lower than that recorded in temperate climates and the sex incidence is equal. It is also recorded in low incidence in most areas of South America, Japan, Hawaii, and in the Chinese population in Singapore. On the other hand, carcinoma of the oral cavity is present in high incidence in certain parts of India, in Thais (Tansurat, 1961), and in New Guinea (Atkinson *et al.* 1964). Betel-nut chewing is common in these areas. The admixture of lime may be important. Tobacco added to the betel and lime in the quid enhances its carcinogenic effect on the buccal mucosa in Ceylon (Chin and Lee, 1970). Oral submucous fibrosis is also a precancerous lesion.

Chutta cancer occurs in India and is a squamous-celled carcinoma of the hard palate associated with the habit of smoking chutta (a coarse type of cheroot) with the burning end inside the mouth. It is more common in women. A high incidence of oral cancer has also been noted in certain areas of Colombia where the habit of smoking with the lighted end inside the mouth is also usual.

Khaini cancer occurs in Bihar and is associated with the chewing of a tobacco leaf and lime mixture. A squamous-cell carcinoma occurs between the lips and front teeth. Vitamin-A deficiency may be an important associated factor.

In areas of Russia the habit of chewing nass (a mixture of tobacco, ash, oil, and lime) may be associated with carcinoma of the anterior two-thirds of the tongue and mandibular alveolar margins. In areas where the quid is held under the tongue carcinoma of the floor of the mouth may occur.

SALIVARY-GLAND TUMOURS

Salivary-gland tumours are common. The site distribution is parotid (46–68 per cent), submandibular (5–30 per cent), and palate (3–19 per cent) (Edington and Sheiham, 1966). Occasionally the lips, cheek or buccal cavity may be affected. The sex incidence is equal, exluding the palatal tumours which may be more common in the female sex (Davies *et al.* 1964).

The histological pattern is not remarkable and the benign tumours can be classified as mainly cellular, mucinous, and mixed cellular and mucinous. Malignancy is diagnosed on the grounds of cellular pleomorphism and increased mitotic figures. The incidence of malignant change is considered to be in the region of 20–30 per cent.

AMELOBLASTOMA

Synonym. Adamantinoma.

The relative incidence of ameloblastomas in Africa has been considered by Edington and Sheiham (1966) and they form from 0·3 to 2·7 per cent of tumours in various studies. No marked sex, age, or racial differences have been noted, apart from the fact that in Ibadan the majority of the tumours affect the anterior portion of the mandible (Akinosi and Williams, 1968) and this has been considered to be related to the increased incidence of periodontal disease and of calculus deposition in Nigerian patients.

The histopathology of the tumour is not remarkable, both solid and cystic types being seen. Small amounts of melanin may be present in 10 per cent and we have seen one melanotic ameloblastoma (Williams, 1967).

CANCER OF THE HYPOPHARYNX

A high frequency of cancer of the hypopharyngeal–laryngeal region in both sexes has been reported from North Thailand. It is thought to be associated with the smoking of a local variety of the cigar called 'Keeyo'. The cigar contains approximately equal amounts of Thai tobacco and the chopped bark of the 'koi' tree (*Streblus asper*). Bronchial cancer occurs in an equal frequency in both sexes (4 per cent) and is somewhat higher than the frequency recorded in some other tropical areas (Menakanit, 1971).

CANCER OF THE OESOPHAGUS

The incidence of cancer of the oesophagus differs widely in different areas of the tropics. It is one of the commonest cancers seen in China and is common in the Chinese in Singapore but is rarely seen in the Chinese in Hawaii. In China itself the incidence varies markedly in different provinces (Li *et al.* 1962). The condition is common in Chile, Assam, Jamaica, Curaçao (Hartz, 1958), Puerto Rico, Japan, and Kazakhstan in the U.S.S.R. The late Dr. R. J. W. Burrell described the recent pronounced increase in cancer of the oesophagus in the Transkei region of South Africa where it assumed almost 'epidemic' proportions. High frequencies have been noted in many areas of South, Central, and East Africa. Its relative infrequency in West and North Africa is remarkable. In South Africa, whites and Asians are not affected. In the United States there are substantial racial and geographic variations. There is a rising non-white mortality at all ages and it is more pronounced in males. The mortality has been relatively stable in the white population (Schoenberg *et al.* 1971). All the evidence would point to circumscribed environmental factors being important in the aetiology of the condition. Burrell emphasized the soil–plant–animal relationship as possible aetiological factors (Rose, 1965). Geological differences have been noted between regions of high and low incidence. In areas of high incidence in the Transkei the 'gardens' have been poorer agriculturally. Deficiencies of molybdenum, copper, and manganese in the soil were common and it was thought might lead to the growth of plants less resistant to fungal infections (Burrell *et al.* 1962). It is known that, in the laboratory, nitrosamine compounds, irrespective of the route of administration tend to induce cancer at specific sites—especially the eosophagus (Boyland *et al.* 1964). Fungal disease of staples might well produce nitrosamines with specific carcinogenic activity in the eosophagus. It is, however, likely that in different geographic areas differing causal agents will be found. For instance, betel chewing has been implicated in Sri Lanka—an area where females are more frequently affected than males (Stephen and Uragoda, 1970). This is an unusual sex incidence as males are more commonly affected, the ratio varying from 12:1 to less than 2:1 in different areas. In Northern Iran the female frequency rate is also high and compounds of the N-nitrosamine groups have been found in the special 'pregnancy diet' which is widely used. Multiparous women aged 35–45 years are affected (McGlashan, 1970). In East Central and South Africa, McGlashan (1969) considered that there was a significant correlation between the geographical pattern of the disease and the drinking of sugar-based alcoholic spirits. Analysis of this drink in Central Africa (Kachasu) revealed a high zinc content and dimethylnitrosamine was isolated in concentrations of 1–3 parts per million which would be carcinogenic in laboratory animals as first described by Magee and Barnes (1956). This view has been supported by Cook (1971). It is also of interest that Du Plessis *et al.* (1969) have shown the presence of dimethylnitrosamine in the juice of *Solanum incanum*, a food additive in Bantu diets. Lastly it is of interest that carcinoma of the oesophagus is common in Chagasic megaoesophagus—but malignant change is rare in megacolon due to the same cause (Koberle, F. personal communication). The possibility of nitrosamines acting as environmental carcinogens has been reviewed by Lisinsky and Epstein (1970).

Iron-deficiency anaemia is not a factor as siderosis is common in areas of high and low incidence, and the absence of post-cricoid carcinoma is noteworthy.

The youngest patients are seen in the third decade and the mean ages for males and females fall within the sixth and fifth decades respectively. Although no difference in the socio-economic groups have been noted, the relative absence of carcinoma of the oesophagus in South African Asians and whites would suggest that the rural Bantu population of the poorer classes is more exposed to the carcinogenic agent.

The tumours are invariably squamous-cell carcinomas, and the thoracic portion of the oesophagus is primarily affected. The site of neoplasms of the oesophagus should be classified as follows:

(*a*) Cervical oesophagus (subcricoid but above the sternal notch).
(*b*) Thoracic oesophagus not involving the cardia.
(*c*) Distal oesophagus involving the cardia.

If substantial gastric involvement occurs the tumour should be regarded as of gastric origin unless shown to be a squamous-cell carcinoma.

CANCER OF THE STOMACH

Japan and Iceland have probably the highest incidence rates of cancer of the stomach in the world. In the Hawaiian Japanese the incidence is considerably lower than that recorded in Japan (Doll *et al.* 1966). The Scandinavian countries show the next highest incidence and are followed by the United Kingdom, Chile, Colombia, Puerto Rico, and Israel. In Israel a

higher incidence has been noted in those of European extraction as compared with those whose origins were in Africa or Asia (Modan *et al.* 1966).
The incidence in the United States is slightly lower than in the last two
countries quoted and is steadily decreasing. It has been stated that cancer
of the stomach is more common in the U.S. non-white than the white, but
the figures quoted by Dorn and Cutler (1958) show a higher incidence in
the white. The incidence in Africans in Africa is low excluding perhaps
the Kivu province in the Congo, whereas the incidence in South African
coloureds, whites, and Asians far exceeds the incidence in the United States,
being highest in the coloureds in both sexes (Oettle, 1964). In Nigeria the
incidence is similar to that seen in the United States until the age of 50 years
and is then very much less in the older age groups. A low incidence has been
found in India and in the Chinese in Singapore. Jamaica would appear to
occupy an intermediate position between the low incidence found in Africa
and the moderate incidence found in the U.S. non-white.

The evidence thus is that environmental rather than racial or genetic
factors are concerned in the aetiology of the condition. A relationship with
blood group A, however, has been noted in some areas of the world.

The carcinogenic action of hydrocarbons in grilled or smoked meat or fish
has been suggested as a possible factor. Grilled meat, is, however, probably
more widely consumed in the U.S. than in any other country and there the
incidence of stomach carcinoma is steadily decreasing. It has been suggested
that the heavy consumption of dairy produce and fresh vegetables might be
responsible for this decreasing incidence, but in Japan, where the consumption of these products is increasing, the incidence of stomach cancer is
rising. In parts of Africa, where dairy produce is seldom consumed, the
incidence is low and this was found to be so in various tribes on different
diets, of different religions and in varying sociological situations. Gastric
cancer does occur not infrequently in rural farmers in Nigeria where, it
should be noted, gastric ulcer is rare and pernicious anaemia does not occur.
Pernicious anaemia is also rare in Japan. The part that gastic ulcer plays in
the aetiology of gastric cancer is still controversial in some parts of the
world (Editorial, 1970), but the most recent evidence would suggest that
it is of little importance. Vitamin-A deficiency has also been mentioned as
a possible factor but this deficiency occurs frequently in tropical areas of
low gastric cancer incidence. Alcohol and smoking are not considered
factors. It has been suggested that a maize diet may have a protective effect.
As yet, however, no specific dietary factor or factors have been definitely
proven to be causal in gastric cancer.

It has also been suggested that the hardness of water or composition of
the soil, notably the presence of a high zinc content in north Wales may be
factors. Certain diseases have also been associated with the occurrence of

gastric cancer, namely dental caries, achlorhydria, atrophic gastritis, and pernicious anaemia.

No striking differences in the pathology have been noted in tropical areas. Kim *et al.* (1972) noted no significant differences in the histological appearances of gastric carcinoma in Korea as compared with findings from Japan and the U.S.A. Males are more usually affected than females, in a ratio of 2:1. The age-incidence has already been mentioned. The majority of tumours originate in the pyloric or prepyloric region. The ulcerative form of gastric cancer is the most common but polypoid and infiltrative types occur. Irrespective of the macroscopic appearances, the tumour is an adenocarcinoma and the histological pattern varies from the well-differentiated to the anaplastic, the latter being most usual in the infiltrative type of growth. Mucin secretion is common either intracellularly (signet ring) or extracellularly.

OTHER TUMOURS OF THE STOMACH

Benign polyps are rare in our experience. Other benign tumours do, however, occur. Sarcomatous tumours would not appear to differ in their presentation in tropical and temperate zones. Primary reticulum-cell sarcoma and lymphosarcoma have been seen. Disseminated tumours of the reticulo-endothelial system (including the Burkitt tumour) frequently affect the stomach (Edington and Easmon, 1967).

CANCER OF THE SMALL AND LARGE INTESTINE

Cancer of the small bowel is rare throughout the tropics, as it is in temperate zones. Primary lymphomatous tumours are, however, not uncommon in some areas of Africa, particularly in the United Arab Republic and French-speaking West Africa. The carcinoid tumour is described on p. 541.

Cancer of the large intestine is found in low incidence throughout the tropics. No tropical area has reported anything approaching the incidences recorded in the United Kingdom, United States, or New Zealand. This is remarkable when the multiplicity of parasites (including *S. mansoni*) affecting the intestine is considered. The reasons for this low incidence are obscure. Ulcerative colitis, diverticulitis, polyposis coli, and adenomatous polyps would appear to be uncommon in tropical areas and this rarity may partially be responsible for a low incidence of cancer. There is some evidence to suggest that the normal microflora of the intestinal tract may be concerned in converting an inactive substance into a carcinogen. It is tempting to speculate that dietary habits and multiple infections and infestations in the tropics may reduce the risk of large bowel cancer by altering the microflora. Bowel habits may also be important, frequent defaecation allowing any carcinogenic substance lesser contact with the mucosa. Walker and Walker

(1969) have shown that Bantu children and adults have more frequent stools and a shortened intestinal transit time when compared to white South Africans in whom the incidence of colonic cancer is much higher. It is, perhaps, strange however, that carcinoma rarely occurs in megacolon in Chaga's disease where stasis must be excessive.

Hill *et al.* (1971) considered that the geographical variations of colonic cancer correlated with variation in the fat content of the diet. It was thought that intestinal bacteria might be able to produce carcinogens from dietary fats and from bile steroids, and differences in diet might bring about differences in the bacterial flora of the intestine. The examination of faeces from Western countries (high incidence) and from Uganda, South India and Japan (low incidence) showed that the former had higher counts of bacterioides and lower counts of enterococci and other aerobic bacteria than the 'low incidence' populations. They also contained a higher concentration of steroids which were also more degraded than the concentrations found in Africa and Asia. It was considered that intestinal bacteria may be aetiologically related to cancer of the colon. There is, however, little information available on the physiology of the large intestine in the tropics. There is some evidence to suggest that the incidence of carcinoma of the colon varies independently in incidence from that of the rectum. Classification of the site of the large bowel cancer in tropical areas is thus important and a classification suggested by a symposium on tumours of the gastro-intestinal tract in Africa is given below.

The World Health Organization classification of tumours of the large intestine (see below) should be employed whenever possible. Squamous-cell carcinoma of the anal canal should not be included among tumours of the large intestine.

WHO classification of tumours of the large intestine

153. Malignant neoplasm of large intestine, except rectum:
    0·0. Caecum, appendix, and ascending colon.
    0·1. Transverse colon, including hepatic and splenic flexures.
    0·2. Descending colon.
    0·3. Sigmoid colon.
    0·8. Large intestine (including colon), part unspecified.
    0·9. Intestinal tract, part unspecified.

154. Malignant neoplasm of rectum and rectosigmoid junction:
    0·0. Rectosigmoid junction.
    0·1. Rectum and anal canal.

Such a detailed classification, however, may present certain difficulties in areas of the tropics where patients present late with advanced and extensive tumours. In these circumstances the site of the tumours should at least be classified into:

1. Right colon from caecum to splenic flexure inclusive.
2. Left colon and rectum.

The sex ratio varies from 1:1 to 3:1 males to females in both sites in different areas of the tropics. The mean age in both males and females is similar and tends to occur in the fifth decade. Age-specific rates show a falling-off in the incidence of colon and rectum carcinomata in the older age groups.

Protuberant, ulcerative, and infiltrative growths occur, the last being more common in Africa than in temperate zones. The tumour is an adeno-carcinoma. The incidence of mucoid and anaplastic tumours has been reported to be higher in parts of Africa than in American and British series and is probably due to the higher proportion of the younger age groups in African patients. Just as in stomach malignancies there may be a higher ratio of primary lymphomatous tumours of the large intestine in areas of the tropics, and leiomyosarcoma is not rare in our experience.

THE CARCINOID SYNDROME

Serotonin (5-hydroxytryptamine) is normally produced from the amino-acid tryptophan by specialized cells in the gastro-intestinal tract, the argentaffin cells of Kulschitsky. Serotonin is deaminated by the enzyme monoamine oxidase in the liver and lung to 5-hydroxyindolacetic acid and excreted in the urine, where it may be detected by Erlich's aldehyde reagent. The tumours termed 'carcinoids' or argentaffinomas arise from these cells and similar tumours may arise in the bronchial glands of the lung, the bronchial adenomas of 'carcinoid' type. It has been suggested that carcinoids arising in the bronchus and stomach might have a different cell of origin from those arising in the ileum and appendix (Black and Maffner, 1968).

The term kinin is a generic term for a group of polypeptides with potent biologic activities capable of influencing smooth muscle contraction, inducing hypotension, increasing blood flow, and microvascular permeability, inciting pain and perhaps causing the emigration of granulocytic leukocytes (Kellermeyer and Graham, 1968). They have been implicated in several physiological and disease processes. They have been considered to be associated with serotonin in the 'carcinoid syndrome'.

The tumours are firm and yellow and consist of masses of spheroidal or polyhedral cells with a finely granular cytoplasm rich in lipid. The granules reduce silver salts and also diazonium to an orange colour. They arise in the gastro-intestinal tract and may metastasize to the liver, when the excess serotonin formed causes the carcinoid syndrome which is exemplified by symptoms pointing to involvement of the vessels of the skin, the valves of the right side of the heart, respiratory and gastro-intestinal symptoms, and a high level of 5-hydroxytryptamine in the serum and an increased excretion of 5-hydroxy-indole acetic acid in the urine. Fibrotic thickening occurs on the pulmonary and tricuspid valves superficial to the elastica of the endocardium, at the free margins of the cusps, and at the commissures. The thickening is probably initiated by deposition of platelets and fibrin and may spread down the chordae tendineae of the tricuspid valve. As serotinin is inactivated in the lung, lesions on the left side of the heart are less common (Roberts and Sjoerdsma, 1964). Fibrotic plaques may also be found in the inferior vena cava and elastic sclerosis of the mesenteric blood vessels has been described in the presence of ileal tumours (Anthony and Drury, 1970).

There is a high content of serotonin in bananas and plantains and the urinary output of 5-hydroxy-indole acetic acid has been shown to be high in areas of Africa. It has been suggested that the high ingestion of serotinin may be a factor in endocardial lesions of the heart in Africa. This is discussed on p. 358.

DISEASES OF THE LIVER AND GALL BLADDER

Metabolic, toxic, fungal, viral, bacterial, and parasitic conditions frequently affect the liver in the tropics. Specific conditions are dealt with in their appropriate context, including the hepatomegaly found 'normally' in populations living in areas of stable malaria (p. 13).

A high incidence of primary liver-cell carcinoma, however, is one of the outstanding problems in many tropical areas and is closely associated with cirrhosis of the liver. In temperate climates 5–15 per cent of cirrhotic livers exhibit malignant change, whereas in areas of high incidence in the tropics malignant change may occur in 50–80 per cent. A common type of cirrhosis in temperate climates is considered to be 'portal' in contrast to the 'post-necrotic' type which is considered to be more common in the tropics. Considerable attention has therefore been paid to the morphological description of these two types of cirrhosis and to the factors which may be concerned in their aetiology with special emphasis on geographical studies.*

Particular attention is also paid in this section to other specific forms of cirrhosis peculiar to the tropics, veno-occlusive disease of the liver, African siderosis, and Indian childhood cirrhosis being examples.

There is some evidence that the pathology of infectious hepatitis may

---

*The terms portal and postnecrotic would probably be better expressed morphologically as micronodular and macronodular respectively.

differ in temperate and tropical areas and related conditions have been retained in this section rather than in the chapter on virology.

A classification of liver disease is given in Table 11.3. Mathematical models for the diagnosis of liver disease have been devised (Fraser and Franklin, 1974).

I. THE LIVER OF THE NEONATE

There is little information available on the normal liver in neonates in the tropics. In our experience fatty change in the parenchymal cells and areas of extensive extra-medullary erythropoiesis are not unusual findings. The amount of histochemically demonstrable iron pigment varies in different areas depending upon a number of factors including the dietary iron content of the mother.

Neonatal giant-cell hepatitis is not uncommon in the tropics and can be caused by congenital malformations of the bile ducts, erythroblastosis fetalis (rare), viral infections, and inborn errors of metabolism (Smetana et al. 1965). Toxoplasmosis, cytomegalic inclusion disease, herpes simplex (Bird et al. 1963), infective hepatitis virus A, and rubella virus (Editorial, 1966) have all been implicated as causal agents. We have seen two cases of congenital hepatic fibrosis in Ibadan and the condition has been described in Jamaican children (Thorburn et al. 1967).

Umbilical sepsis in the newborn is common and may spread along the umbilical vein, causing pyogenic infection in the liver. Tetanus may also be a complication of this condition. This is discussed on p. 319.

II. LIVER ABSCESS

Infection may reach the liver by either (1) the hepatic and portal circulation, (2) the biliary system.

The most common cause of liver abscess in the tropics is amoebiasis, and this has been considered on p. 72. Ascariasis has also been considered a factor (p. 100).

Infection may, however, also reach the liver via the portal vein from foci in the gastro-intestinal tract including gastric ulcer and appendix abscess either as emboli or as a spreading infective thrombosis (pylephlebitis). Many organisms including *Streptothrix actinomyces* may be involved. Spread by the biliary system (suppurative cholangitis) is a feature of infections caused by the liver flukes, and a condition described as oriental cholangitis of obscure aetiology is discussed on p. 600.

TABLE 11.3. *Classification of liver disease*

I. The liver of the neonate

II. Liver abscess

III. Portal and postnecrotic cirrhosis (micronodular and macronodular)
   1. The morphology of portal cirrhosis
   2. The morphology of postnecrotic cirrhosis
   3. Comparison of portal and postnecrotic cirrhosis
   4. The morphology of mixed cirrhosis
   5. Additional findings in cirrhosis
   6. Aetiology of portal and postnecrotic cirrhosis:
      (*a*) Geographical distribution
      (*b*) Age, sex, and social class
      (*c*) Alcohol
      (*d*) Malnutrition
      (*e*) Virus infections
      (*f*) Parasitic infections
      (*g*) Hypersensitivity
      (*h*) Dietary toxic factors:
         (i) Chemicals
         (ii) Drugs
         (iii) Plant alkaloids
         (iv) Mycotoxins
      (*i*) Associated conditions

IV. Biliary cirrhosis

V. Central cirrhosis:
      (i) Cardiac cirrhosis
      (ii) Veno-occlusive disease
      (iii) The Budd–Chiari syndrome

VI. Pericellular cirrhosis, including 'interstitial'

VII. Special forms of cirrhosis:
      (*a*) Hereditary and neonatal disease
      (*b*) Disturbances of iron metabolism
      (*c*) Indian childhood cirrhosis

VIII. Specific affections of the liver:
      (i) Infectious hepatitis and homologous serum jaundice
      (ii) Active chronic hepatitis
      (iii) Massive liver-cell necrosis
      (iv) Acute fatty liver of pregnancy
      (v) Congenital dilatation of the intrahepatic bile ducts

IX. Tumours of the liver

X. Diseases of the gall bladder

III. PORTAL AND POSTNECROTIC CIRRHOSIS

Our knowledge of the morphology and aetiology of cirrhosis in the tropics is not great but is expanding rapidly. Most of the evidence would suggest that the most usual type of cirrhosis seen in the tropics is post-necrotic, and that in some areas malignant change may occur in over 50 per cent of patients. This is in contrast with the findings in temperate climates where portal cirrhosis is common and malignant transformation is much less common. Comparisons of the incidence of cirrhosis and its complications in differing geographical areas demand, therefore, a morphological diagnosis. A number of experienced workers in the tropics have utilized the classification of cirrhosis described by Gall (1960), to which interested readers are referred, but we have retained a somewhat less elaborate classification which is discussed below.

When considering a satisfactory morphological definition a distinction must be made between fibrotic changes in the liver, which are especially common in tropical areas and frequently parasitic in origin, and cirrhosis—one of the most important distinguishing features between the two being evidence of widespread nodular regeneration in the latter.

The following definition is based on the findings of an International Committee which considered the nomenclature and classification of cirrhosis in 1956. Anatomically the term cirrhosis implies widespread fibrosis throughout the liver with complete or almost complete destruction of the normal lobular architecture. Cellular necrosis may or may not be present but is considered to have occurred at some stage of the disease. Fibrous linkage of central veins and portal tracts occurs and nodular regeneration is present.

The classification of cirrhosis may be made either on an aetiological or anatomical basis and neither is entirely satisfactory. The same agents may lead to differing patterns of cirrhosis (Dible, 1951). Thus alcohol can produce portal and occasionally postnecrotic cirrhosis. Moreover, there are differing patterns of cirrhosis for which the causal agent, or agents, are unknown—and by some authorities are thus termed 'cryptogenic cirrhosis'. The Australia antigen (hepatitis association antigen) has been noticed in relatively high frequency in 'cryptogenic cirrhosis' in temperate climates. The term is not used commonly in the tropics as a morphological classification is usually employed. The antigen has been noted in much higher frequency in the tropics in postnecrotic cirrhosis than in portal.

Morphologically cirrhosis is usually classified, excluding biliary and other specific types which will be discussed later, as either portal or postnecrotic. Where difficulty is experienced in differentiating between these two conditions the term 'mixed' is used.

I. THE MORPHOLOGY OF PORTAL CIRRHOSIS

A number of synonyms have been used in the literature, such as Laënnec's atrophic, diffuse septal, cryptogenic, micronodular, alcoholic, or nutritional. They confuse aetiological and morphological concepts and it is suggested that the term portal cirrhosis should be employed in those cases which conform to the description given below.

Macroscopically, the liver is usually reduced in size and varies in colour from pale yellow to brownish-green. It is tough on section and shows a uniform fine nodularity, the nodules not usually exceeding 4mm in diameter. The normal shape of the liver is retained.

Microscopically the liver is traversed by relatively fine fibrous tissue joining portal tracts and central veins and containing nodules roughly the size of lobules. The fibrous tissue contains bile ducts, pseudoductules, blood vessels, and a variable number of lymphocytes, histiocytes, and polymorpho-nuclear leucocytes. There is no evidence of thick scarring with lobular collapse. Fatty vacuoles may be present without a surrounding inflammatory reaction. Normal portal tracts are not seen. The micronodules of parenchymal tissue do not show the usual lobular structure and hepatic-vein radicles, which are rarely present, are eccentric in position.

The liver cells are relatively uniform in appearance, bizarre cells being uncommon in the late stages. They may be swollen and contain fatty vacuoles compressing the nucleus to one side. Inconstantly present is a peculiar form of cellular necrosis first described by Mallory (1911). A coarse, irregular hyaline network which stains deeply with eosin and phosphotungstic-acid haemotoxylin appears in the cytoplasm of the affected cells (Mallory's alcoholic hyaline); this is followed by leucocytic infiltration and by destruction of the affected cells or group of cells. This type of degenerative change is most frequently seen in the vicinity of the fibrous trabeculae and is best demonstrated by Mallory's phloxinemethylene blue method by which it stains intense red. It is due to swelling and degenerative changes in the mitochondria. It is not peculiar to portal cirrhosis and is found in other types of cirrhosis, including primary biliary and the Indian childhood type, Wilson's disease and primary liver cell carcinoma (Nayak et al. 1972). The combination of fatty infiltration and this type of degeneration is, however, most frequently seen in portal cirrhosis in patients with a history of chronic alcoholism (Fig. 11.3).

Intracanalicular bile thrombi are not unusual. The sinusoids are narrowed and difficult to detect. There may be an increase of haemosiderin in the Kupffer and parenchymal cells. Areas of necrosis may be seen in post-mortem specimens when there has been gross haematemesis or other vascular accidents prior to death.

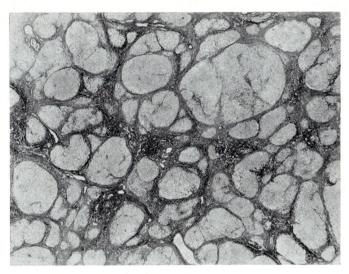

FIG. 11.3. Portal cirrhosis (from an alcoholic). The regeneration nodules are small and relatively uniform and are separated by bands of fibrous tissue of uniform thickness (Silver impregnation ×7). (*By courtesy of Churchill Ltd. In: Recent Advances in Pathology*, 1960.)

2. THE MORPHOLOGY OF POSTNECROTIC CIRRHOSIS

Once again many synonyms have been used in the literature—cryptogenic, coarsely nodular, macronodular, posthepatitic, post-toxic, nodular cirrhosis, nodular hyperplasia of the liver, or healed subacute yellow atrophy. We consider the term postnecrotic cirrhosis should be employed in those areas which conform to the description given below.

The liver is reduced in size and its normal shape may or may not be retained. Greyish-white fibrous tissue of irregular thickness divides the reddish-brown to green liver tissue into nodules, varying in size from a few millimetres to centimetres. Yellow or greenish areas of necrosis may be present and simulate malignant change.

Microscopically, the liver is traversed by bands of fibrous tissue varying greatly in width and containing nodules, in some of which lobular structures can be recognized (central veins and portal tracts). This differentiates portal from postnecrotic cirrhosis (Harrison, 1960) (Fig. 11.4). Thick scars are present representing the juxtaposition of three or more portal tracts and are evidence of lobular collapse following necrosis of parenchymal cells. The fibrous tissue contains an excess of bile ducts, pseudoductules, vascular channels, and histiocytes and lymphocytes with occasional plasma cells.

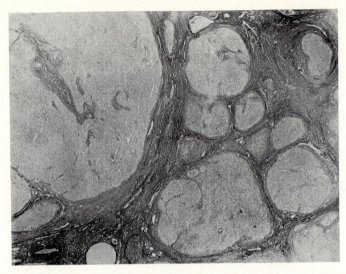

FIG. 11.4. Postnecrotic cirrhosis. The regeneration nodules vary greatly in size and are separated by fibrous bands of variable thickness. The nodule at bottom centre is 5 mm in diameter (Silver impregnation × 7). (*By courtesy of Churchill Ltd.* In: *Recent Advances in Pathology*, 1960.)

The nodules vary in size and signs of regeneration in the liver cells (variation in size, binucleated and multinucleated forms, enlarged nucleoli) may be marked. The liver-cell cords are broadened, being two or more cells in breadth. There may be bile retention in the canaliculi, Kupffer, and parenchymal cells, but this is usually focal in distribution. Fatty change is unusual and alcoholic hyaline is not commonly seen. Haemosiderin deposition is not a feature. Terminal haemorrhage from oesophageal varices with consequent anoxaemia may cause widespread nodular necrosis.

3. COMPARISON OF PORTAL AND POSTNECROTIC CIRRHOSIS

Macroscopic	*Portal cirrhosis*	*Postnecrotic cirrhosis*
Scarring	Fine	Mixed
Nodules	Uniform 4 mm	Size varies
Microscopic		
Intact lobules	Absent	Present
Fat	May be prominent	Usually absent
Central veins	Absent	Present
Haemosiderin	May be present	Usually absent
Alcoholic hyaline	May be present	Usually absent

Clinical

Alcoholism	Some association	Rare
Pancreatitis	Some association	Nil
Liver-cell carcinoma	Low incidence	Higher incidence
Gall stones	More common	Can occur
Oesophageal varices	Occurs	More common
Peripheral neuritis	Occurs	Nil
Course	Insidious	Can be rapid

4. THE MORPHOLOGY OF MIXED CIRRHOSIS

In a number of instances it may be difficult to decide into which category the macroscopic and histopathologic changes in the liver should be classified. If lobular collapse is evident the term postnecrotic should be used; otherwise the changes can be classified as 'mixed'. It should be noted that a form of 'interstitial cirrhosis' is described when pericellular cirrhosis is considered.

5. ADDITIONAL FINDINGS IN CIRRHOSIS

Clinically, the course of many patients suffering from cirrhosis in the tropics (usually postnecrotic) may be silent and rapid, and complicated by the presence of carcinoma. We have seen, for example, athletes dying from cirrhosis and carcinoma of the liver within a few months of good athletic performances.

The usual causes of death in cirrhosis of the liver are hepatic coma and haemorrhage from oesophageal varices. The coma is precipitated by impairment of blood supply causing damage to the liver cells. Haemorrhage and sudden alterations of the haemodynamics of the hepatic circulation, the cause of which is often obscure, are the important factors in liver-cell damage.

Cyanosis and hypertrophic osteoarthropathy (clubbing) may be present. The arterial blood shows a low percentage of oxygen saturation, the cause of which is obscure but may be due to venous arterial shunts, blood entering the pulmonary veins (arterial) either from the portal system (porto-pulmonary anastomoses) or from the hepatic and azygos veins. A disorder of the pulmonary microvasculature has also been postulated (Stanley *et al*. 1972). Anaemia may be prominent and numerous factors contribute to the haematological changes seen in cirrhosis. In chronic liver disease there is proliferation of the cells of the reticulo-endothelial system, erythrocyte survival is diminished, blood coagulation defects occur and gastro-intestinal bleeding is common. A haemolytic anaemia complicated by 'hypersplenism' may occur. Leucopenia, thrombocytopenia, macrocytosis, and target cells may be seen in the peripheral blood.

Prothrombin deficiency may result from defective synthesis in the liver or lack of absorption of vitamin K in obstructive jaundice. Plasma fibrinolysins are frequently increased and fibrinolysis following surgery is a hazard. The liver stores vitamin B_{12} and high levels are found in the serum in liver disease.

Portal hypertension is an invariable complication and increased pressure in the portal venous system may be due to various causes, which can be classified as follows:

A. Extrahepatic (thrombosis of portal vein)
B. Intrahepatic:
   (i) Presinusoidal   (a) Congenital
                      (b) Schistosomiasis (*mansoni: japonicum*)
   (ii) Postsinusoidal (a) Central lesions
                      (b) Cirrhosis
C. Idiopathic

Irrespective of the aetiological agent, portal hypertension causes congestion of the alimentary canal with digestive disturbances, splenomegaly, anastomoses between the portal and systemic circulations at the lower end of the oesophagus, inferior haemorrhoidal veins, the veins around the umbilicus and the vestigial vein in the ligamentum teres.

Fluid accumulates in the peritoneal cavity (ascites) and has the character of a transudate with protein not exceeding 1–2 G/100 ml. Hypoalbuminaemia and increased aldosterone secretion with reabsorption of sodium cause transudation of fluid through the capsule of the liver or serosa of the gut and mesentery into the abdominal cavity.

In the classification of portal hypertension A and B are self-explanatory. It is of interest that Miller (1967) in East Africa has reported the common occurrence of extraportal obstruction in teenage children with normal livers. The possibility of an old pyelephlebitis being responsible was considered. In a small proportion of patients, however, portal hypertension can occur without apparent pathological changes in the liver or portal vein (Polish *et al.* 1962; Siderys and Vellios, 1964). The splenic-pulp pressure is increased but the hepatic-wedge pressure is usually normal. No abnormalities are noted on liver biopsy or in the liver-function tests. The portal vein is patent and dilated and there may be sclerotic plaques on the intimal surface. The cause is not known but is considered to be related to increased portal-blood flow due to splenic and other factors. It is of interest to note that portal hypertension in 'tropical splenomegaly' has also been recorded in the absence of demonstrable hepatic pathology.

Boyer *et al.* (1967) have described a form of idiopathic portal hypertension in India in which there is portal fibrosis associated with intra-and extrahepatic portal vein sclerosis. The porto-splenogram resembles that seen in pipe-stem fibrosis caused by schistosomiasis, and sometimes tropical splenomegaly syndrome. There is no increase of lymphocytes in the sinusoids of the liver which has been described in some cases of 'tropical splenomegaly' (p. 495). Nayak and Ramalingaswami (1969) have described a condition in India in which obliterative occlusion of the portal veins in the liver occurs unassociated with cirrhosis or extrahepatic portal vein obstruction. There is marked subendothelial thickening of the larger intra-hepatic branches of the portal vein with a patchy segmental distribution leading, it is thought, to portal hypertension. These findings have been reported in other parts of India and there is reason to believe that the syndrome is widespread in that country. The aetiology is also unknown.

In addition to portal hypertension a number of other conditions may be associated with the presence of cirrhosis and should be looked for at necropsy. Spider naevi may be present in the skin. Palmar erythema is difficult to detect in coloured races. Peripheral oedema and jaundice are usual. Parotid-gland enlargement and *gynaecomastia* with loss of axillary and pubic hair and testicular atrophy may be seen in males. It is considered that the failure of the damaged liver to inactive circulating oestrogens is responsible for these changes, and an increased urinary oestrogen and diminished 17-ketosteroid excretion has been noted in life. It has been suggested, however, that increased secretion rather than impaired catabolism in the liver may be responsible for these findings (Brower *et al.* 1964). Amenorrheoa occurs in females. The severity of atherosclerosis is said to be reduced.

Chronic relapsing pancreatitis, peptic ulcer and gall stones are rarely associated factors in the tropics, also the reduced severity of atherosclerosis reported in temperate climates would be less noticeable. A 'silent' peritonitis has been described (Editorial, 1964). Evidence of haemorrhage from eosophageal varices may be present and deficiency of coagulation factors may be responsible for haemorrhages in the substance or cavities of any of the viscera. The clotting defect is complex in its aetiology. Factors V, VII, IX and prothrombin are involved. In sophisticated centres the following laboratory investigations should be performed: peripheral blood count including platelet count; bleeding time; whole blood clotting time, one stage prothrombin time; thrombo test or partial thromboplastin time; prothrombin consumption index and euglobulin lysis time (Donaldson *et al.* 1969).

It is essential to estimate coagulation factors prior to diagnostic liver biopsy as intra-abdominal haemorrhage from the punctured liver is a real danger. We have seen one or two deaths from this complication in patients suffering from primary liver cell carcinoma on whom diagnostic liver biopsy had been performed. In rural areas the bleeding time and clot retraction should be done.

The kidneys may be bile-stained, and histologically bile-pigment casts and necrosis of the proximal tubules may be found. Other renal changes have been described. Spider naevi may be seen in the pleura and arterial dilatation of the peripheral branches of the pulmonary artery with, rarely, pulmonary arteriovenous anastomoses, have been noted in the lungs (Berthelot *et al.* 1966).

Degenerative changes have been described in the basal ganglia in the brain.

6. AETIOLOGY OF PORTAL AND POSTNECROTIC CIRRHOSIS

Many factors have to be considered in the aetiology of portal and post-necrotic cirrhosis.

(a) Geographical distribution

As previously stated most investigations in developing countries would suggest that postnecrotic cirrhosis is more common than portal. Unfortunately, crude death rates as compiled by WHO (1963) do not differentiate between the various types of cirrhosis, but the highest figures are shown for Chile, Mexico, Austria, France, and West Berlin. Low figures are given for Egypt, Panama, the Philippines, Thailand and Iraq. The incidence in the U.S.A. non-whites is lower than in the whites. Post-mortem figures from South Africa have not shown great differences in the incidence of cirrhosis in the Bantu, Coloured, and white populations (Becker and Chatgidakis, 1961; Thomson, 1961). A striking feature, however, was the large proportion of cirrhotic livers in the Bantu which showed malignant change and this accounts for the increased incidence of liver-cell carcinoma in the Bantu and is also found in other areas of the tropics where liver-cell carcinoma is common.

The highest frequencies of cirrhosis probably occur in areas of Europe and America. The incidence is low in Cali, Colombia, although fatty livers secondary to protein deficiency are prevalent, (Correa and Llanos, 1966) and the incidence is probably low in Brazil (Montenegro *et al.* 1958) and Jamaica (Bras *et al.* 1961).

The present recorded geographical distribution of cirrhosis is therefore of little help in elucidating the probable aetiological agents involved excluding perhaps alcoholism in temperate climates.

(b) Age, sex, and social class

Cirrhosis of the liver occurs in younger age groups in the tropics, the condition being not uncommon under the age of 20 years in East Africa

(Gelfand, 1961). It would appear to be more common in males, ratios of 3 : 1 being quoted. The rise in incidence of carcinoma of the liver associated with cirrhosis after the menopause would perhaps suggest that sex hormones may be important factors. This is borne out by experiments on laboratory animals—male rats being more susceptible to cirrhosis-producing diets than female (Patek *et al.* 1969). There is no evidence that social class influences the incidence.

(c) Alcohol

The relationship between chronic alcoholism and cirrhosis cannot be denied (Steiner, 1964) but the mechanism of the liver damage is unknown. In addition to a high intake of ethyl alcohol other factors such as chronic gastritis with associated dietary deficiencies and/or infections may play a part. An acute alcoholic hepatitis occurs (Sherlock, 1963) and may progress to a portal type of cirrhosis with fatty change and alcoholic hyaline in the liver cells, frequently referred to as nutritional cirrhosis, a type of cirrhosis which is rare in the tropics. Thus aetiological factors cannot always be established from the morphological appearances of the liver, as a postnecrotic type of cirrhosis may occasionally be found in patients with a long history of chronic alcoholism.

(d) Malnutrition

Two facts, (*a*) that dietary deficiencies in laboratory animals produced fatty change, necrosis, cirrhosis and neoplasms in the liver, and (*b*) that there was a high incidence of carcinoma complicating cirrhosis of the liver in man in certain tropical areas where concomitant protein deficiency and fatty change in the liver in childhood were common, led to the belief that there was probably a causal relationship between protein-calorie deficiency disease (kwashiorkor) and cirrhosis and carcinoma of the liver. There is little direct evidence, however, that protein deficiency *per se* in man leads to cirrhosis of the liver, perhaps excluding, in rare instances, cirrhosis in alcoholic subjects. In Ghana and Nigeria we have been unable to trace in autopsy material a continuous progression from the stellate fibrosis, seen in kwashiorkor and other conditions (p. 677), to frank cirrhosis. In addition, followup studies in children who have suffered from kwashiorkor have not shown the subsequent development of cirrhosis (Srikantia *et al.* 1958; Bras *et al.* 1961; Camain, R. personal communication; Cook and Hutt, 1967). Also, it is not uncommon for cirrhosis in Nigeria to occur in members of relatively well-to-do families who are unlikely to have suffered from malnutrition in childhood. The sex incidence in kwashiorkor approaches unity, and stellate fibrosis is slightly more common in girls—whereas cirrhosis occurs more frequently in males.

The geographical distribution of high incidence rates of liver-cell carcinoma associated with cirrhosis does not correspond to that of high incidence of protein-calorie deficiency disease in childhood. For instance in Egypt, parts of South America and India, and the West Indies (if central cirrhosis is excluded) carcinoma of the liver and/or cirrhosis is relatively uncommon, although protein calorie deficiency disease may be abundant in childhood. In addition Correa and Llanos (1966) considered that cirrhosis of the liver was uncommon in Cali, Colombia, although the fatty liver secondary to protein deficiency is prevalent. It is of interest that Bhuyan *et al.* (1965) have shown that rats challenged by carbon tetrachlorate are less liable to the development of cirrhosis if on a low-protein diet.

Further evidence against this hypothesis is obtained from a study of the types of cirrhosis seen in the tropics where malnutrition is common, as the usual type is postnecrotic with little fat or alcoholic hyaline present. 'Nutritional' cirrhosis is considered to be portal, with small nodules and usually much fatty change in the hepatic cells and, on occasion, there is alcoholic hyaline.

From a consideration of those facts there would appear to be little justification for the theory that protein-calorie deficiency disease in childhood is responsible for cirrhosis and/or carcinoma of the liver in the tropics. Even the possibility that liver damage due to non-dietary factors with eventual cirrhosis is more likely in populations with a poor dietary intake of protein is not clearly borne out by present geographical studies.

(e) Virus infections

The part that viral infection may play in the aetiology of neonatal giant-cell hepatitis is discussed on p. 568. The common viral infections causing severe liver lesions in children and adults are infectious hepatitis (virus A), homologous serum jaundice (virus B), and yellow fever. Infectious mononucleosis may also cause liver damage but has not been considered a factor in the aetiology of cirrhosis in the tropics—nor has yellow fever, which is discussed on p. 220. We have seen two cases of herpes hepatitis both fatal in Caucasians in West Africa without the predisposing factors usually present in temperate climates (Editorial, 1973). The liver shows multiple discrete areas of necrosis of liver cells with the intranuclear inclusions characteristic of herpes-infected cells present. Similar changes may be seen in the adrenals. The virus can be isolated from the liver or may be seen on electron microscopy. Liver biopsy is the best method of diagnosis and therapy with cytosine arabinoside should be considered.

Infectious hepatitis and homologous serum jaundice have been considered causative factors in cirrhosis. Cirrhosis of the liver is rarely found as a sequel to epidemics of viral hepatitis in temperate climates and even in the tropics. However, considerable rethinking is necessary in view of the studies on the Australia hepatitis-associated antigen in the tropics which are discussed on p. 578. The antigen has been found in higher prevalence in the tropics in patients with postnecrotic cirrhosis but not with portal. Mosquitoes may be vectors and oro-faecal transmission may occur. There is no doubt that hepatitis is endemic in many areas of the tropics—certain towns in West Africa, for instance, being notorious for the occurrence of hepatitis in newly arrived immigrants. As the pathology may differ somewhat from that described in Europe, the condition is considered in some detail on p. 581. In spite of the discovery of the Australia antigen there are still discrepancies to be explained.

Viral hepatitis affects both sexes equally under the age of 15 years but there is then a greater incidence in females with more deaths (Sherman and Eichenwald, 1956). This is borne out by our own post-mortem figures in which hepatitis is more common in women, 4·4 per cent compared to 0·8 in males. Cirrhosis, in contrast, is more common in males. Moreover, as has already been said, there is a low incidence of cirrhosis in certain tropical areas in South America, Jamaica, and India, where infectious hepatitis is endemic.

It has been stated that viral hepatitis may be more severe in malnourished populations with, perhaps, a greater liability to subsequent liver pathology. The rarity of cirrhosis in the areas mentioned above would not support this statement. Many of the facts quoted would suggest that viral hepatitis is not a potent factor in causing cirrhosis but certain patients have been shown to develop postnecrotic cirrhosis following hepatitis (Sherlock, 1963; Camain, 1957), and many patients suffering from active chronic hepatitis have apparently a typical attack of infectious hepatitis at the commencement of the condition. Camain reported that in Senegal 15 per cent of patients with viral hepatitis developed cirrhosis. The evidence is thus conflicting but it would appear that, under certain conditions, viral hepatitis can proceed to cirrhosis of the liver usually of a postnecrotic type. The reason for the apparent disparity in the incidence of viral hepatitis and cirrhosis in various areas of the tropics is obscure and the possibility that there may be differing viral strains is perhaps worthy of consideration.

(f) Parasitic infections

Many parasites affect the liver including those of malaria, schistosomiasis and the liver flukes. Granulomatous lesions of the liver are common in the tropics and frequently the aetiology is obscure—the most common in our experience being tuberculosis and schistosomiasis. Sarcoidosis should be considered in some areas. Granulomatous lesions of unknown aetiology are common in temperate climates (Gibson, 1973). Certain of the liver flukes cause dilatation of the bile ducts and cholangitis, and are associated with malignant change in the lining epithelium, but are not considered to cause cirrhosis. Malaria and *S. mansoni* and *S. japonicum* have, however, been considered as possible causal factors of cirrhosis.

Regarding malaria, there is no doubt that in areas of stable malaria 100 per cent of children gaining their immunity have much pigment in the Kupffer cells and portal tracts (p. 28). Stellate fibrosis in the portal tracts has been associated with the presence of the pigment as well as with kwashiorkor, but in our experience it also occurs in the absence of both. Boys and girls show an equal incidence of malaria and, in addition, adult pregnant females are more prone to relatively heavy infections than males, the sex in which the incidence of cirrhosis is greatest. Furthermore, cirrhosis is common in areas where malaria is absent—notably in the Bantu in South Africa. We do not consider that malaria is an aetiological agent in cirrhosis of the liver.

In *S. mansoni* infection cirrhosis is not found very commonly in Brazil (Montenegro *et al.* 1958; Cheever and Andrade, 1967), or Puerto Rico, where *S. mansoni* is endemic in areas (Martinez *et al.* 1965), nor is it thought to be common in Egypt (Hashem *et al.* 1961). *S. mansoni* produces a portal fibrosis which is responsible for presinusoidal portal hypertension but a true cirrhosis rarely if ever occurs. It is more difficult to evaluate the role of *S. japonicum* but as yet there is no convincing proof that it produces true cirrhosis in man. It must be realized that, in areas where possible causal parasitic diseases are endemic, carefully planned, controlled studies are required if incidental and causal infections are to be differentiated.

(g) Hypersensitivity

The importance of autoimmune processes in the aetiology of chronic liver disease are as yet undecided but considerable evidence is accruing that they may be important in at least three conditions (Doniach, 1970; Walker, 1974).

1. Primary biliary cirrhosis.
2. Active chronic hepatitis (lupoid hepatitis; juvenile cirrhosis).
3. Certain cases of cryptogenic cirrhosis.*

Autoimmune processes have been considered important in these conditions because the patients show a high frequency in their serum of anti-nuclear factor and serum smooth muscle and mitochondrial antibodies. In addition the cell-mediated response to liver antigens using the leucocyte-migration test gives a high frequency of abnormal responses in all three

---

* Note the term cryptogenic cirrhosis is used in the aetiological classification of cirrhosis and should be reserved for patients found to have inactive cirrhosis on liver biopsy with no clinical evidence of previous active liver disease.

conditions in contrast to the findings in patients with various other liver disorders (Smith *et al.* 1972). It is possible that following an initial insult continuing damage to the liver may be perpetuated by autoimmune mechanisms. Primary biliary cirrhosis is discussed on p. 561 and active chronic hepatitis on p. 584. The pathological response of the liver to certain drugs, such as chlorpromazine, is thought to be a sensitivity type of reaction and is discussed below.

(h) Dietary toxic factors

These can be considered under four headings: chemical; drugs; plant alkaloids; mycotoxins.

(i) Chemicals. Although selenium deficiency may cause liver disease in experimental animals it has not been incriminated as a factor in man. Little information is available on the other trace elements. Zinc and cobalt have been shown to be increased and molybdenum reduced in the liver in cirrhosis and liver-cell cancer in South Africa (Butt and Higginson, 1957). Zinc deficiency has also been shown to occur in alcoholic liver disease (Sullivan and Heaney, 1970). Siderosis is discussed on p. 570.

(ii) Drugs. Many drugs are known to damage the liver and the subject has been reviewed by Sherlock (1968). Drugs should be given with caution to patients with underlying liver disease as the normal prescribed dosage may precipitate untoward reactions—this is especially important if sedation is required. Drugs may affect the liver in a number of ways and these are discussed below.

(*a*) *Interference with bilirubin metabolism.* Drugs may induce haemolysis and increase the metabolism of unconjugated bilirubin in the liver cell. Others may compete with serum bilirubin for the binding of bilirubin or may interfere with the transport of bilirubin through the liver cell. Conjugation of bilirubin in the liver may be disturbed. Excluding the newborn, however, the most important effect of drugs affecting the liver can be considered as either a hepatotoxic or a hypersensitivity reaction.

(*b*) *Hepatotoxic drugs.* The heavy metals, carbon tetrachloride, chemotherapeutic agents and antituberculous drugs are hepatotoxic and the parenchymal damage in the liver is directly related to dosage. Salicylates have also recently been incriminated (Editorial, 1973).

(*c*) *Sensitive type cholestasis.* Chlorpromazine is an example and induces a cholestatic hepatitis not directly related to dosage.

Sensitivity would appear to be an important aetiological factor, as steroids may help in therapy. Bile pigment is present in the canaliculi (most marked centrilobularly) liver and Kuppfer cells. Mild degenerative changes may be present in the parenchymal cells with an associated infiltration of monocytes and eosinophils in the portal tracts. A similar appearance may be seen

in what is possibly a form of cholestatic viral hepatitis. This is a not uncommon finding on liver biopsy in our experience in Ibadan, especially in
females, and drugs have not been directly incriminated. The possibility,
however, of 'native medicines' being causative agents cannot be discounted.
The histopathology of drug-induced liver disease has been reviewed by
Smetana (1963). It is of interest that the computer has been utilized in the
diagnosis of drug-hypersensitivity jaundice with apparently considerable
success (Stern *et al.* 1973).

(iii) **Plant alkaloids.** Many plants may damage the liver. They may be
ingested accidentally in food or in herbal remedies or may be given deliber-
ately as poisons. The study of medicinal and poisonous plants is an enormous
subject, interested readers are referred, as an example, to the textbook by
Watt and Breyer-Brandwijk (1962) which deals with the human and veter-
inary toxicology of the flora of South East Africa. The types of possible
hepatotoxic plants vary from area to area. There are over 1000 species of the
genus *Senecio* and 400 of *Crotalaria*, in addition to many other genera, and
only a few examples are given here.

The action of species of *Senecio*, *Crotalaria*, and *Heliotropium* will be
discussed when veno-occlusive disease is considered, but it should be noted
that *C. fulva*, and related species, are considered to cause cirrhosis in
Jamaican children and that this type of cirrhosis, in relatively high incidence,
is limited to that particular geographical area.

The eating of the unripe fruit (ackee) of the tree *Blighia sapida* causes
vomiting, convulsions, coma, and death in children in Jamaica (Jamaican
sickness) and West Africa. It should be noted, however, that the role of ackee
has been questioned (Fistein, 1960) and that different plants are thought to
be involved in other areas of the world where somewhat similar syndromes
occur with marked hypoglycaemia and fatty change in the liver. Polypeptides
(hypoglycin A and B) isolated from the fruit have produced fatal hypoglycaemia in laboratory animals and a high incidence of fetal abnormalities
in rats (Persuad, 1967). At post mortem in these children there may be
petechial haemorrhages in the intestine, pleura, and endocardium. Fatty
change is marked in the liver and kidneys and occasionally in the pancreas
and myocardium. Areas of necrosis may also be present in the liver and
kidneys.

Herbal medicines in South Africa have also been considered to cause
liver damage with jaundice, spontaneous hypoglycaemia, or acute tubular
necrosis (Neame and Pillay, 1964).

We have also seen on a few occasions hypoglycaemia in Nigerian children
following the ingestion of 'cow's urine' a common native medicine in use in
Western Nigeria. To the urine are added various chemicals and plant
products of which tobacco is the most usual. Acute renal failure with tubular

necrosis has been, however, the most usual presentation at post mortem in these cases.

Symptoms of hepatic disease have been reported from Northern Rhodesia in groups of villagers eating various roots and tubers in times of famine. Central necrosis in the liver with fatty degeneration were constant findings at autopsy (Steyn, 1965).

Yams (*Dioscorea rotundata*), one of the staples of the diet in areas of the tropics, has been shown to produce liver necrosis in laboratory animals (Gilbert and Gillman, 1963) and wild yam poisoning has been reported in Nyasaland (Stevenson, 1962).

In Guam, cyasin obtained from *Cycas circinalsis* L. produces hepatic and renal tumours in mice (Laqueur *et al.* 1963), but there is no evidence that it produces the same effect in man. The bark of the sasswood tree has also been implicated in liver disease (Akenlade, 1967).

(iv) Mycotoxins. The association of peripheral gangrene in man with fungal contamination of rye (ergotism) has been known for many years. The toxins of many species of mushrooms, particularly those of the genus *Amanita*, are known to be hepatotoxic, and *Fusarium sporotrichoides*, a fungus which may contaminate cereals, causes alimentary toxic aleukia in Russia. This condition is characterized by an acute gastroenteritis followed by pancytopenia, purpura, and associated secondary infection (Pomeranz, 1964; Davidson, 1963). In addition, various toxic substances have been isolated from moulds contaminating animal foodstuffs during this century, sporodesmin isolated from *Pithymyces chartarum* and causing liver necrosis and cirrhosis in sheep being an example.

Penicillium islandicum, a contaminant of rice in the Far East, has been shown to produce at least two hepatotoxic compounds which cause acute liver injury, cirrhosis and primary liver-cell carcinoma in mice and rats (Miyake *et al.* 1960). It has been considered a possible aetiological agent in cirrhosis and carcinoma of the liver in man.

The outbreak of hepatic disease in turkeys in Great Britain in 1960, was shown to be due to contamination of Brazilian groundnut meal by the fungus *Aspergillus flavus* and this focused attention on the possible importance of such fungal contamination of staples in the aetiology of liver disease, especially cirrhosis and primary liver-cell carcinoma. The hepatotoxic principle was named aflatoxin (Lancaster *et al.* 1961; Sargeant *et al.* 1961), and from it four related chemical compounds have been isolated. Two of these, named B_1 and G_1, are, in rats, by far the most active heptocarcinogens known (Editorial, 1964). Locally manufactured peanut butter in the Philippines has been shown to be highly contaminated with aflatoxin B_1 and has been shown to be excreted in the urine as aflatoxin M_1 which is the hydroxylated product of B_1 (Campbell *et al.* 1970).

With the exception of sheep, all laboratory and farm animals (pigs, calves), tested have been shown to be sensitive to the toxin. Hepatic lesions have been produced in rhesus monkeys.

Liver tumours have been produced in rats, ducks, mice, and trout. The young laboratory animal is more vulnerable than the adult and carcinoma of the liver in rats can appear, following the initial challenge, after 1 year or more on a normal diet. This fact, combined with the knowledge that aflatoxin is rapidly metabolized and excreted, renders the possibility of investigating its importance as a causal agent in chronic liver disease in man most difficult. However, Campbell *et al.* (1970) have reported the finding of aflatoxin M_1. The hydroxylated product of B_1, in the urine of children in the Philippines eating contaminated peanut butter and further studies on populations with a high incidence of primary liver cell cancer are indicated.

Large doses of the toxin cause massive necrosis of liver cells with diffuse haemorrhage in weanling ducks, smaller doses cause proliferation of bile ducts within the liver-cell cords and portal fibrosis. The extent of this bile-duct proliferation is a reliable biological indication of the relative toxicity of the material under test.

Cows fed on highly toxic meals secrete a 'milk factor', toxic to ducklings, and a similar phenomenon has been noted in rats.

Many other species of *Aspergillus* are known to produce substances which are toxic to animals.

The fungus penetrates the kernel when the shell of the groundnut is damaged during harvesting or transport. Moisture is essential for the growth of the fungus, and reduction in the moisture content of the environment is the best method of preventing contamination and/or controlling germination of the fungal spores and further growth.

The fungus may be cultured or aflatoxin may be detected by chemical techniques and either, or both methods, have detected contamination of market produce in many areas of Africa. In addition, in Addis Ababa, *P. islandicum* has been isolated (Coady, 1964). Aflatoxin is heat stable, but edible groundnuts, peanut butter, and refined groundnut oil are said to be safe from contamination.

Although conditions in many areas of the tropics favour the growth of fungi on stored food-stuffs there is, as yet, no direct evidence that mycotoxins are implicated in the aetiology of widespread liver disease in these areas. The circumstantial evidence in Africa is, however, considerable.

(i) Associated conditions

Many conditions produce granulomatous lesions in the liver—brucellosis, tuberculosis, and sarcoidosis being examples. There is no evidence that they are agents of importance in the aetiology of cirrhosis.

Ulcerative colitis may cause fatty infiltration in the liver with pericholangitis and the development of postnecrotic cirrhosis, but it is not common in the tropics. Other conditions such as diabetes mellitus, thyroid disease, leukaemia, and porphyria have been associated with cirrhosis, but once again are only of minor interest in the overall pattern of the condition.

IV. BILIARY CIRRHOSIS

Biliary cirrhosis may be primary or secondary. Primary biliary cirrhosis is a chronic non-suppurative cholangitis affecting mainly women in middle age. Cirrhosis develops at a late stage. Secondary biliary cirrhosis is due to obstruction or congenital absence of the bile ducts. The types of biliary cirrhosis noted in the tropics do not apear to differ from those described in temperate climates, with the possible exception that secondary biliary cirrhosis due to obstruction of the main bile ducts would appear to be less common. An abnormal lipo-protein (X) has been described in the serum of patients suffering from obstructive jaundice. It is detected by immunoelectrophoretic methods and has been found to be associated with cholestasis most frequently in extrahepatic obstructive jaundice (75 per cent) and primary biliary cirrhosis (48 per cent). It is less commonly present in cholestatic hepatitis. Its significance is unknown (Ross et al. 1970).

In this connection it should be noted that it has been claimed that primary biliary cirrhosis may be differentiated from extrahepatic biliary obstruction by immunological techniques (Goudie et al. 1966). Krohn et al. (1970) detected the Australia antigen (see p. 578) in 9 of 10 cases of primary biliary cirrhosis and particles were detected in the sera of 11 of 12 cases by electron microscopy identical to those described in carriers of the antigen. MacSween et al. (1973) also noted, a significantly higher incidence of the antigen (15·6 per cent) in patients with primary biliary cirrhosis when compared with controls using a radio-immunoprecipitation technique. The antibody was present in 9·4 per cent. In lymphocyte transformation studies one of twenty-four patients' lymphocytes transformed on stimulation with an AU-rich serum.

This failure to show delayed hypersensitivity to AU was considered perhaps to be due to the impairment of cellular immunity which has been reported in primary biliary cirrhosis. On the other hand lymphocytic transformation occurs in patients who have recovered from AU-associated viral hepatitis on exposure to serum-rich antigen (Yeung Laiwan, 1971) and this lack of transformation might be taken as evidence against the AU antigen being an aetiological agent in primary biliary cirrhosis. The relationship between the antigen and biliary cirrhosis is uncertain. The disease may be caused by AU/anti-AU complex formation or the increased frequency may be due to impaired immune mechanisms in these patients. It is of interest that the frequency of primary biliary cirrhosis has not been reported to be high in tropical areas where the antigen and antibody are found in high prevalence.

Although in the tropics there is a high incidence of intestinal parasites, many of which are found in the bile ducts, biliary cirrhosis has not been ascribed to their presence and the rarity of gall stones, in many areas, is also noteworthy. Biliary cirrhosis is monolobular in type and consists essentially of fibrosis emanating from the portal tracts with bile retention a notable feature. The end stages may not be distinguishable from portal cirrhosis.

V. CENTRAL CIRRHOSIS

Central cirrhosis can be brought about by cardiac causes, veno-occlusive disease, and the Budd–Chiari syndrome.

(i) CARDIAC CIRRHOSIS

With elevation of the hepatic venous pressure, centrilobular congestion occurs in the liver. The consequent anoxaemia causes atrophy and loss of liver cells so that the centrilobular regions are represented by capillaries and stroma, the peripheral cells showing perhaps fatty change and hyperplasia. With prolonged, increased venous pressure, and especially with intermittent episodes in children, centrilobular and portal fibrosis occur. Linkage of central veins to each other and to portal tracts can be seen and eventually a true cirrhosis may occur with hyperplastic nodules present. The two most common causes of cardiac cirrhosis are constrictive pericarditis and right-sided endomyocardial fibrosis. In our experience, liver bioposies in the latter condition may not exhibit congestion, (an artefact of the procedure) but centrally-dilated sinusoids and fibrosis are prominent. It should be remembered that the liver is affected in a focal fashion and the biopsy may not be representative. Fibrosis and linkage of the central veins is usually apparent in post-mortem material and, with the associated cardiac condition, differentiate this type of cirrhosis from other forms.

(ii) VENO-OCCLUSIVE DISEASE

Definition: Veno-occlusive disease of the liver is an acute, subacute, or chronic condition affecting primarily the central and sublobular hepatic veins.

Geographical distribution

It has been reported most frequently from the West Indies, but also occurs in North and South Africa, Jerusalem, and India.

Aetiology

It has been known for many years that pyrrolizidine-containing alkaloids in plants can damage the liver of cattle. Alkaloids of various genera of this group, especially *Crotalaria*, *Senecio*, and *Heliotropium*, have produced liver injury in all animal species in which they have been tested, including primates. Many factors influence their toxicity, including the condition of the soil, the state of growth of the plant, and the portion of the plant (root, seed, stem leaves) ingested. Large doses cause centrilobular liver damage, oedema of the lungs, and death in a few days. Cirrhosis may develop in survivors. Malignant transformation is unusual after one dose but does occur after repeated intermittent administration. Giant-cell transformation of hepatic cells has been described. The toxicity of the alkaloid under test is usually greater in male when compared to female, in young when compared to adult, and in protein-deficient when compared to well-fed laboratory animals. Female rats may secrete the toxic factor in their milk (Schoental, 1963; Schoental and Magee, 1959). Senecio poisoning occurs naturally in animals in many parts of the world (Hill, 1960). In South Africa *C. dura* is responsible for hepatic and pulmonary lesions in the disease 'jagsieket' in horses, and *C. retusa* and *C. crispata* are responsible for Kimberley horse disease in Australia, a marked feature of which is centrilobular cell necrosis and fibrosis in the liver with associated pulmonary emphysema (Gardener *et al.* 1965). Veno occlusive disease has also been produced in *Macaca speciosa* monkeys by injecting intraperitoneally 0·125 gm of monocrotaline per Kg of body weight (Allen *et al.* 1969).

In man the ingestion of bread from imperfectly winnowed wheat contaminated by a *Senecio* weed was known to cause centrilobular liver lesions as long ago as 1920 (Willmott and Robertson) in South Africa and a further outbreak has been reported (Selzer and Parker, 1951). It is now generally accepted that veno-occlusive disease in the West Indies is due to the ingestion of 'bush tea' containing the alkaloids of *C. fulva*, which produces a similar condition in rats (Hill *et al.* 1958; McLean *et al.* 1964). *C. retusa* may be the causal factor in Barbados. Children in the 1- to 6-year-old age group are most frequently affected and a familial incidence may be noted. The sex incidence is equal. The disease has also been described in adults in India (Gupta *et al.* 1963). A sudden outbreak of veno-occlusive disease in three Bedouin families has been described in Iraq (Al-Hasany and Mohamed, 1970).

Pathology

Clinically, the condition usually presents as acute hepatomegaly and ascites in children. About 50 per cent of those affected recover, about 20 per cent die in the acute stage and the remainder pass into the subacute or chronic stage with signs of portal hypertension (Stuart and Bras, 1957).

The primary pathological change involves the central and sublobular hepatic veins (Fig. 11.5). There is subendothelial oedema followed by intimal overgrowth of connective tissue and narrowing and occlusion of the lumina, best shown histologically by a reticulin stain. Centrizonal

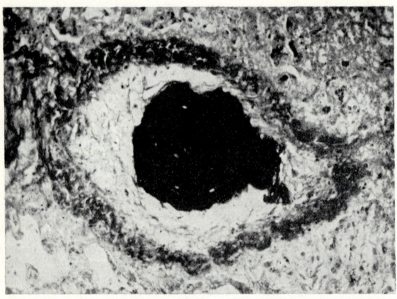

Fig. 11.5. Acute veno-occlusive disease of liver. West Indian girl aged 3 years. The hepatic venous tree was injected post-mortem with Indian-ink gelatin; the vessel has a narrowed lumen due to subintimal thickening (Mallory trichome stain) (× 190). (*From Trowell, Non-Infective Disease in Africa, 1960. Edward Arnold.*)

congestion, atrophy or necrosis of liver cells, with consequent fibrosis, leads to gross changes similar to those described in cardiac cirrhosis. There is an absence of cellular infiltration in the early stages and no generalized vascular changes. On electron microscopy endothelial damage is seen in the sinusoids, subterminal, and terminal hepatic veins with extravasation of red blood cells into Disse's space (Brooks *et al.* 1970). Thrombosis of the larger hepatic veins is said to be rare though it is a feature of the Chiari syndrome and of certain cases reported from South Africa and Egypt

(Selzer and Parker, 1951; Safouh and Shebata, 1965). Freiman *et al*. (1968) have described an acute form in fifteen children in Johannesburg, ten of whom died. Liver failure with hypoglycaemia occurred in four. *Crotalaria fulva* was thought to be concerned in the aetiology. On histological examination the centrilobular nature of the cirrhosis can be distinguished from the portal and postnecrotic varieties. In the West Indies cirrhosis due to veno-occlusive disease accounts for approximately 30 per cent of all types (Bras *et al*. 1961). Malignant transformation is most unusual. The changes in the remaining organs are those of portal hypertension with its associated complications. Liver biopsy is necessary for definitive diagnosis. Liver-function tests are variable. Flocculation tests are positive and the trans-aminases are slightly raised. Serum bilirubin may be raised although jaundice is not usual.

(III) THE BUDD-CHIARI SYNDROME

In this syndrome centrilobular lesions occur in the liver following the pattern of those caused by chronic venous congestion due to cardiac lesions and are caused by occlusion of the ostia of the hepatic veins at their union with the inferior vena cava. The occlusion was considered by Chiari to be due to a primary infection of the veins but congenital abnormalities have also been suggested (Gibson, 1960). A web or membrane in the inferior vena cava, which may be amenable to surgery and which can be diagnosed radiologically, has been described (Schaffner *et al*. 1967; Takuchi *et al*. 1971). The possibility that *Senecio* alkaloids may be implicated as causal factors in the syndrome must always be considered (Selzer and Parker, 1951). Children and young adults are affected. The use of oral contraceptives has also been implicated as a rare possible causal factor (Editorial, 1971).

Secondary thrombosis of the hepatic veins due to pressure from tumours, puerperal caval thrombosis, or sepsis may cause a similar condition. It may also occur rarely as a complication of paroxysmal nocturnal haemoglobinuria due to a thrombophlebitis of the hepatic veins.

VI. PERICELLULAR CIRRHOSIS

This is the classical lesion of congenital syphilis and frequently is not a true cirrhosis. There is fibrous tissue proliferation extending between portal tracts and throughout the lobules. Individual parenchymal cells are surrounded by cellular fibrous tissue infiltrated with histiocytes and lymphocytes. Spirochaetes are present and can be demonstrated by Levaditi's stain. Areas of hyperplasia with giant-cell transformation can simulate the so-called 'neonatal giant-cell hepatitis'.

In adults in Mexico, a diffuse interstitial cirrhosis has been described which to a certain extent is pericellular—small groups of cells being involved in the process and regenerative nodules being inconspicuous (Perez-Tamayo, 1958). Its aetiology is obscure.

Pericellular fibrosis may also be an incidental finding in liver biopsies in Indian childhood cirrhosis.

VII. SPECIAL FORMS OF CIRRHOSIS

These are discussed under the headings of hereditary and neonatal diseases, disturbances of iron metabolism, and Indian childhood cirrhosis.

(A) HEREDITARY AND NEONATAL DISEASES

The hereditary and developmental diseases associated with liver cirrhosis are listed in Table 11.4. They do not cause a high incidence of cirrhosis in the tropics.

TABLE 11.4. *Hereditary and neonatal diseases associated with cirrhosis*

   (i) Haemochromatosis (see p. 569)
  (ii) Hepatolenticular degeneration (Wilson's disease)
 (iii) Galactosaemia
 (iv) Fructose intolerance
  (v) Cystic fibrosis
 (vi) Porphyria
 (vii) Sickle-cell disease (p. 440)
(viii) Giant-cell hepatitis and causes of jaundice in the neonate
 (ix) Developmental abnormalities
  (x) Glycogen storage disease

(i) Haemochromatosis

Haemochromatosis is not common in the tropics and its relationship with siderosis is discussed on p. 572.

(ii) Wilson's disease

In this condition there is a deficiency of caeruloplasmin in the plasma which normally transports copper. The copper is loosely attached to albumin and is deposited in the tissues causing a postnecrotic type of cirrhosis of the liver and bilateral softening and degeneration of the basal ganglia in the brain. The liver cells are large with clumped glycogen in the nucleus and fatty change is usual. Lipofuscin is found round the bile canaliculi.

(iii) Galactosaemia

Galactosaemia is due to the absence of the enzyme galactose-1-phosphate uridule transferase and is transmitted as an autosomal recessive gene.

It may appear in the first few weeks of life when jaundice, diarrhoea, hepatomegaly, and weight loss occur, or the condition may not be recognized until later in life.

The liver shows pseudoglandular and fine fatty changes in the liver cells with some bile retention. Regenerative nodules and cirrhosis occur (Smetana and Olen, 1962). Diagnosis can be made by estimation of the enzyme activity in the erythrocytes or hepatic tissue (Walker *et al.* 1962). A non-glucose reducing sugar is present in the urine. The condition does occur in the tropics but its incidence is unknown.

(iv) Fructose intolerance

This condition is due to a reduction in the enzyme fructose-1-phosphate aldolase (Cornblath *et al.* 1963), and is transmitted as an autosomal recessive. Clinically, an intolerance to fruit juice is noted. The liver damage resembles that described in galactosaemia.

(v) Cystic fibrosis

This appears to be a rare condition in the tropics. The function of the exocrine glands is affected. Clinically, recurrent respiratory infections and malabsorption due to pancreatic disease occur. Cirrhosis of a biliary type may develop (di Sant Agnese and Blanc, 1956; Roberts, 1962). There is an increased chloride content in the sweat. It has been suggested that the increased salt-loss in the sweat may have a further selective disadvantage against the gene in tropical areas and account for its apparent rarity.

(vi) Porphyria

Abnormal porphyrins are manufactured in the bone marrow (porphyria erythropoietica) or in the liver (hepatic porphyria). The erythropoietic form does not develop disease of the liver although the porphyrins responsible for the photosensitivity of this disease are apparently of hepatic origin (Iber and Maddrey, 1965). These writers classified hepatic porphyria as follows:

(a) Acute intermittent porphyria (or Swedish type) which is autosomal dominant. Acute intermittent porphyria with abdominal pain, peripheral neuritis, and psychological disturbances may not be as uncommon in tropical Africa as recently thought (Greenwood, 1967).

(b) Porphyria variegata (or South African type) which is autosomal dominant.

(c) Porphyria cutanea tarda which is frequently familial.

(d) Acquired porphyria (Turkish type) which may occasionally be familial.

Fibrous changes and cirrhosis of the liver occur in all types except the acquired. Haemosiderin is commonly present. A high incidence of chronic alcoholism has been noted in patients with porphyria. Alcoholic patients with liver disease occasionally have porphyrinuria and the condition cannot be differentiated from hepatic porphyria. Acquired porphyria may also follow the ingestion of hexachlor benzene (Granick, 1964). The pathology of the subject has been reviewed by Elder *et al.* (1972).

(vii) Sickle cell disease

See p. 440.

(viii) Giant-cell hepatitis and causes of jaundice in the neonate

The causes of giant-cell hepatitis have already been mentioned at the beginning of this chapter (p. 543).

Glucuronyl transferase is necessary for the conjugation of bilirubin in the liver and thus allow its excretion as bilirubin diglucuronidase. The activity of this enzyme is deficient in premature infants and an excess of unconjugated bilirubin is present in the blood (physiological jaundice). An excess of unconjugated bilirubin is also found with excessive haemolysis in erythroblastosis fetalis which is rare in the tropics, in ABO incompatability, and in deficiency of the enzyme glucose-6-phosphate dehydrogenase. A hereditary deficiency of glucuronyl transferase occurs in the Crigler–Najjar syndrome, cases of which die of kernicterus in infancy. Gilbert's syndrome also causes raised values of unconjugated bilirubin. The nature of the defect in this disease is unknown and the clinical symptoms are usually mild (Foulk *et al.* 1959). It is an inherited condition probably in a dominant form with incomplete penetrance and variability of expression. The liver in these two diseases is normal. An additional abnormality occurs in which there is marked siderosis of the liver with excess urobilinogen in the faeces (Israels *et al.* 1963).

An increase of conjugated bilirubin is found in the Dubin-Johnson and Rotor syndromes. The conditions are essentially similar and are differentiated only by the presence of an unidentified pigment in the liver in the former. They are probably, however, a manifestation of the same defect in the excretion of bile. Bromsulphthalein excretion is impaired. A number of cases have been reported from Papua and New Guinea, and the geographical pathology described (Vaughan *et al.* 1970). Infection especially by gram-negative organisms is also a cause of neonatal jaundice.

(B) DISTURBANCES OF IRON METABOLISM

Heavy deposits of iron pigment are found in the viscera without anaemia or other evidence of blood destruction in two conditions: haemochromatosis and African siderosis. Repeated blood transfusions in patients suffering from aplastic anaemia or other blood dyscrasia may produce a similar effect. These conditions are discussed below.

(i) Haemochromatosis (synonym: bronzed-diabetes)

Haemochromatosis is due to an inherited metabolic abnormality leading to excessive iron absorption from the intestine, widespread deposits of haemosiderin in certain organs, cirrhosis, and pancreatic fibrosis with associated diabetes mellitus.

Aetiology

Some doubt has recently been cast on the theory that this disease is due to an inherited metabolic defect. It has been reported that iron pigment (haemosiderin) is present in the liver of 30–80 per cent of patients with portal cirrhosis and all grades of severity may be observed. Patients with cirrhosis may absorb more iron from the intestinal tract. The reason for this is not known but pancreatic deficiency and an increased alcoholic intake have been suggested as possible factors. Haemochromatosis may therefore represent one end of the spectrum of a common condition in which there is an increased absorption of iron and increased deposition in the liver and other viscera (MacDonald and Mallory, 1960; MacDonald and Baumslag, 1964). This view is, however, not generally accepted and haemochromatosis is usually considered a rare inherited disease (MacSween and Jackson, 1966). It may be of value to examine the first degree relatives of patients with idiopathic haemochromatosis in order to detect those affected. Serum iron and serum total iron binding capacity should be estimated, and if justified, liver biopsy performed. Those with histologically grade 3 or 4 iron pigment in the liver should be treated by venesection (Powell, 1967.)

Haemochromatosis probably has a world-wide distribution. It is more common in males and may be familial. A history of alcoholism is not unusual.

Pathology

Clinically the patient with haemochromatosis presents with an enlarged, firm liver, diabetes mellitus and, in a certain proportion of Caucasian patients, a brownish or leaden hue in the skin. The skin changes are due first to an excessive deposition of melanin pigment with later haemosiderin deposits in macrophages and adnexal structures in the dermis. Pigmentation of the oral mucosa also occurs.

Transferrin is not increased but may be fully saturated instead of the normal 35 per cent. Serum iron values are raised. The pigment is considered to be essentially parenchymal in distribution.

Heavy deposits are found in the liver, upper abdominal lymph nodes, pancreas, gastric glands, heart muscle, stomach, thyroid, etc. The deposits are less in the spleen and kidney. A specific arthropathy has been described with the radiological appearances of chondrocalcinosis. Acute attacks of inflammatory synovitis may also occur due to the liberation of calcium pyrophosphate crystals into the joint fluid (Editorial, 1969).

It has recently been suggested that a deficiency of the enzyme xanthine oxidase as shown by liver studies may be concerned in the pathogenesis (Magee and Sacklem, 1966). This enzyme assists in the reduction of ferric to ferrous iron facilitating its transfer to the plasma where it is bound to transferrin. The enzyme levels have also been noted to be low in cirrhosis of the liver.

The liver usually shows a fine cirrhosis of the portal type but post-necrotic cirrhosis has been described. It is reddish-brown in colour. Histologically, the cirrhotic process is not always quantitatively directly related to the amount of iron pigment present and it has been stated that the cirrhosis may precede the pigment deposition. Haemosiderin is present in Kupffer cells, parenchymal cells and either in histiocytes or lying apparently free in the portal tracts or scar tissue. It may also occur in the epithelium of the bile ducts. Lipofuscin may be seen in the parenchymal cells. The iron content of the liver may be as much as 5 per cent of its dry weight. Malignant transformation in the liver in haemochromatosis is more common than in non-pigmentary portal cirrhosis in both Europe and the United States—figures of about 18 per cent being quoted.

The pigment is present in the epithelial cells and connective tissue of the pancreas. The degree of pancreatic fibrosis and atrophy is not quantitatively related to the amount of iron pigment. Lipofuscin is found in the smooth muscle of blood vessels and ducts.

Jejunal biopsy studies have shown iron-containing granules in the columnar epithelium of some villi and much pigment in macrophages in the lamina propria (Astaldi et al. 1966). Lipofuscin has also been described in the non-striped muscle of the intestine. Associated findings at necropsy in haemochromatosis are those due to cirrhosis of the liver and diabetes mellitus. An arthropathy may be a complication. It is of interest that repeated venesection may benefit the patient and the fibrotic process in the liver (Crosby, 1969).

(ii) African siderosis

It has been known for over 30 years that heavy iron deposits are frequently found in the tissues of the Bantu population in southern Africa (Strachan, 1929) and a similar finding, in lesser incidence, has been described in Ghana (Edington, 1954) and in Zambia where it is associated with osteoporosis and scurvy (Lowenthal et al. 1967). It does not occur in East Africa, Western

Nigeria, Gambia, and Senegal. Various terms have been used in describing
the condition: haemochromatosis (Strachan, 1929); cytosiderosis (Gillman
and Gillman, 1951); siderosis (Wainwright, 1957); haemosiderosis; nutritional siderosis (Edington, 1959).

Males are affected more frequently than females in the 20- to 50-year-old
age group but after the menopause the sex-difference is less striking.
Various hypotheses have been elaborated to account for the condition.
Prolonged malnutrition with pancreatic damage and derangement of
intracellular metabolism has been suggested. In laboratory animals a high
iron intake and a predominantly maize diet or a diet deficient in folic acid
has produced the condition. On the other hand, the intake of iron in Ibadan
is high, malnutrition is common in childhood, maize is consumed and folic-
acid deficiency is common, but siderosis is rare. The use of iron cooking
pots increasing the intake of dietary iron has been mentioned as a possible
factor. The possibility has been considered that anaemia in childhood may
condition the mucosal mechanism to the absorption of increased amounts
of iron in the diet and that this may persist into adult life. In the adult the
absorbed iron would no longer be utilized for growth and would accumulate
to produce a gradual increase in the body's iron stores. It is of interest that
Ringelhann *et al.* (1970) have noted increased iron absorption in young
adult males in Ghana.

Numerous other factors including liver disease, alcohol, copper, cobalt,
pyridoxine, pancreatic insufficiency, phytic acid, and phosphorus have been
shown to influence iron metabolism and the cause of the condition is still
obscure. Leucocytic ascorbic acid may be reduced in African siderosis and
would appear to influence the concentrations of serum iron. No significant
correlation was noted between the serum iron levels and marrow iron
gradings until ascorbic therapy was instituted. Serum iron can only be used
therefore as an index of iron overload in the Bantu after repletion with
ascorbic acid (Wapnick *et al.* 1970). The absence of siderosis, however, in
Western Nigeria and its presence only 400 miles away in Ghana is intriguing.
It is perhaps relevant that, in the former area, the usual alcoholic drink is
fermented in calabashes, whereas in Accra illicit distilled and brewed liquors
are probably produced in metal containers.

Pathology

One school of thought maintains that the iron deposited in the organs is
mainly parenchymal, the other that it is mainly reticulo-endothelial.

In most studies the liver has been the organ primarily examined and the
deposition of iron pigment in that organ can be classified as follows:

A. Iron pigment present in Kupffer cells alone, the amount varying from
a blue haze to a heavy granular deposit.

B. Iron pigment present in the periportal parenchymal cells alone.
C. A combination of A and B.
D. Iron pigment present in large amounts in the Kupffer cells, parenchymal cells and portal tracts in the absence of cirrhosis.
E. Type-D distribution in the presence of cirrhosis.

In siderosis, pigment is thought to be deposited primarily at the biliary poles of the periportal parenchymal cells and to extend through the lobule with increasing severity. Lipofuscin may be present in the centrilobular cells. All types of iron distribution may, however, be seen and the pathology of the liver may be indistinguishable from that seen in haemochromatosis. Pigment is unusual in the stomach, choroid plexus, pancreas, thyroid, skin, adrenals, and heart, whereas deposits are heavy in the duodenum, jejunum, spleen, and bone marrow, and this distribution is said to be a differentiating feature from haemochromatosis (Fig. 11.6).

In Ghana we found that both a parenchymal and reticulo-endothelial type of pigment deposition occurred (Edington, 1959) and that in some instances siderosis could not be differentiated from haemochromatosis. Nine per cent of diabetics in Ghana (Dodu, 1958) and 25 per cent of diabetics in South Africa (Seftel et al. 1960) appeared to be suffering from haemochromatosis. In the pancreas both acinar and islet cells contain iron pigment with interstitial fibrosis present. Porphyria cutanea tarda was a frequent complication in these patients, with siderosis of the pancreas and associated diabetes in South Africa (Seftel, 1963). It must be concluded that siderosis may simulate idiopathic haemochromatosis both clinically and pathologically, and that the cirrhosis and the diabetes are most probably secondary to the iron overload or to associated factors. This is further borne out by the type of cirrhosis which occurs in the Bantu in association with siderosis as it is usually of the portal (monolobular or nutritional) type and malignant transformation is said to be unusual, whereas the usual type of cirrhosis in the Bantu is postnecrotic and malignant transformation occurs in at least 50 per cent (Higginson, 1963).

The upper abdominal lymph glands are heavily pigmented. In the spleen the pulp histiocytes and sinusoidal cells are packed with haemosiderin and the capsule and trabeculae are also encrusted. Fibrosis is not a feature. In the kidney small amounts of pigment are present in the proximal tubules distributed in a focal fashion and a little may be present in the interstitial tissue (Wainwright, 1957).

In the bone marrow, pigment is present in the histiocytes and extracellular tissue. The staining of marrow biopsies for the presence of histochemically demonstrable iron is a useful screening procedure for the presence of siderosis (Edington and Dodu, 1957).

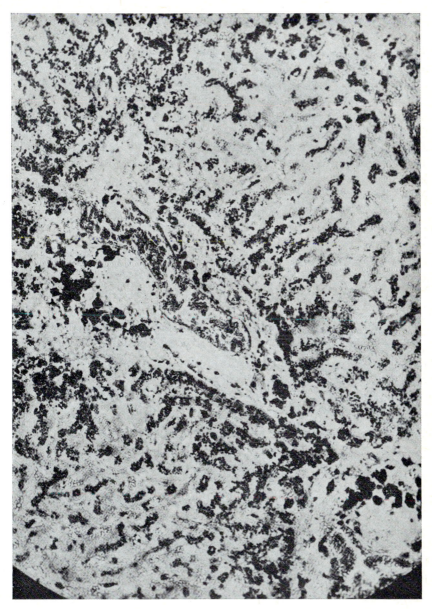

FIG. 11.6. African siderosis of the liver. Heavy deposits of iron in the liver of a Ghana male aged 38 years (Perl's stain) (× 185). (*From* Trowell, *Non-Infective Disease in Africa*, 1960. *Edward Arnold.*)

The plasma iron and iron-binding capacities may be low or normal with fairly severe siderosis, but in patients with type-E livers high values comparable with those in haemochromatosis may be found. It is of interest to note that high plasma iron values have been recorded in male Bantus, among whom iron-deficiency anaemia is uncommon (Bothwell and Bradlow, 1960). The association of siderosis and anaemia in Ghana has been discussed (Edington, 1954). Peritonitis may be a complication (Buchanan, 1970).

To summarize: siderosis would appear to be a fortuitous and common condition in the South African Bantu and southern Ghanaian and is being reported from other parts of the world. Dietary factors and perhaps alcohol are concerned in its aetiology. In a proportion of individuals a condition indistinguishable from haemochromatosis occurs.

(iii) Transfusional and haemolytic siderosis

Following repeated transfusions in the therapy of refractory anaemia, heavy deposits of haemosiderin may be found in the viscera. The distribution is first reticulo-endothelial but later the parenchymal cells of the liver, pancreas, and other organs may be involved. Rarely clinical diabetes and haemochromatosis may occur.

Heavy deposits of iron pigment may also be found in long-standing haemolytic anaemia, especially the severe forms of thalassaemia and sickle-cell anaemia.

(c) INDIAN CHILDHOOD CIRRHOSIS (ICC)

This condition was defined in India as follows: infantile cirrhosis of the liver is a disease peculiar to India affecting infants and young children and with a tendency to run in families. It is characterized in its early stages by enlargement of the liver which is felt to be hard, and usually also by enlargement of the spleen with ascites. The symptomatology is vague, the course variable but generally slow, and it usually terminates fatally. The aetiology is unknown (Sing *et al.* 1961).

Aetiology

It occurs most commonly between the age of 1 and 3 years. In some series boys have been affected much more frequently than girls and in other series the sexes have been equal. A familial incidence has been noted but whether this denotes environmental or genetic factors is not known. It is more common in middle-class communities and children in vegetarian sects are frequently affected.

It would appear to be restricted to India where it has been reported in southern India, Calcutta, and the Punjab. The only other common type of cirrhosis affecting children in considerable incidence is that caused by veno-occlusive disease, which is found in the West Indies, but from a consideration of the pathology the two conditions do not appear to be related. The limited geographical distribution also appears to exclude the usual virus of infectious hepatitis as a causal agent. However, Chandra (1970) using the double diffusion in agar technique described the presence of hepatitis associate antigen (HAA) in 6 per cent of thirty patients. More sensitive techniques would undoubtedly reveal a higher frequency.

Serum immunoglobulins G, A, and M were significantly raised and the complement component B_1C reduced. Antibody to smooth muscle was present in 82 per cent of patients. It was suggested that liver cell damage in early life, perhaps by the HAA, was perpetuated by a secondary immunological mechanism.

On the other hand Yadgiri et al. (1970) have identified a substance in the urine and liver of children with ICC, which has a close resemblance to aflatoxin B_1, by fluorescent studies on thin-layer chromatogram. However, the ultraviolet and infrared spectra of this compound and absorption spectra differed from those of aflatoxin B_1. The nature of this compound is thus in doubt. Aflatoxin M_1 which is the hydroxylated product of B_1 has been detected in the urine of children eating aflatoxin-contaminated peanut butter in the Philippines (Campbell et al. 1970). Amla et al. (1971), however, have suggested that aflatoxin may be important in the aetiology and have reported the development of cirrhosis in children eating peanut meal contaminated by aflatoxin. Nayak et al. (1972) have noted the presence of alpha-fetoprotein in the serum by the gel diffusion technique. Malnutrition is an unlikely cause of it since this type of cirrhosis is not as common in poor families and does not occur in other tropical areas where malnutrition is rife. It is difficult to exclude dietary, toxic, or even deficiency factors, and inborn metabolic errors have to be considered. Even the possibility of an, as yet, undiscovered infectious agent being responsible for the condition cannot be dismissed.

Pathology

Clinically, the condition may be fulminant, acute, or subacute. In the acute type the child presents with symptoms and signs resembling infectious hepatitis. In the subacute there is a gradual onset of signs of portal hypertension with jaundice an inconstant feature in the early stages. The clinico-pathological findings in the acute stage are those of infectious hepatitis, and in the subacute and chronic stages those of cirrhosis and portal hypertension. Caeruloplasmin levels in the plasma have been found to be normal and no L.E. cells have been detected. There is hypoalbuminaemia and the flocculation tests are positive. Bromsulphthalein is retained. Alkaline phosphatase activity is usually normal. Bilirubin and urobilin are present in the urine.

Hypersplenism and an autoimmune haemolytic anaemia may occur (Perkash *et al.* 1971).

We have been fortunate in being able to examine in consultation with Dr. Sriramachari liver biopsies from children suffering from this condition. The appearances suggest a severe progressive affection of the parenchymal cells which show ballooning and variation in size, with enlarged pale nuclei containing enlarged nucleoli. Alcoholic hyaline is inconstantly present but fatty change is rare. Nayak *et al.* (1969) have reported that the alcoholic hyaline is similar to Mallory's which is found in liver damage associated with alcohol and that it was present in the liver cells in all their patients suffering from ICC. It was considered to represent toxic injury to the hepatocytes and the prognosis was directly related to the number of cells affected. It is of interest that alcoholic hyaline is not commonly seen in our material in Ibadan where ICC does not occur and where the incidence of primary liver cell carcinoma is high. Eosinophilic degeneration with a leucocytic infiltration may affect individual cells. Lipofuscin is inconstantly present in the Kupffer cells. In the later stages giant-cell transformation and bile stasis occur. The central veins are not occluded. Reticular collapse occurs in areas and there is proliferation of fibrous tissue in the portal tracts which are infiltrated by lymphocytes, histiocytes, and occasional polymorphonuclear leucocytes. The fibrosis extends periportally and may surround individual cells focally in the lobule (Sing *et al.* 1961). Bile-duct proliferation occurs and progressive fibrosis eventually produces cirrhosis. The cirrhosis has been described as portal (Smetana *et al.* 1961) and also as postnecrotic (Achar *et al.* 1960). The occurrence of malignant transformation in Indian childhood cirrhosis has not been remarkable. Apart from the liver function tests mentioned above, liver biopsy is a valuable diagnostic procedure and haematological investigations should be undertaken.

The pathological findings would suggest that the causal agent or agents have a direct toxic affect on the hepatocytes and it is tempting to suggest that the hepatitis associated antigen associated with some unknown toxic factor is responsible. As previously stated the limited geographical distribution makes it unlikely that the HAA and aflatoxin are the only factors involved as these are found in association in many tropical areas where ICC does not occur.

VIII. SPECIFIC AFFECTIONS OF THE LIVER

(1) INFECTIOUS HEPATITIS AND HOMOLOGOUS SERUM JAUNDICE

(Viral hepatitis type A and viral hepatitis type B.)

Although many viruses may cause hepatitis there are two main types—infectious hepatitis and homologous serum jaundice. It is now recommended that these conditions be redesignated viral hepatitis type A and viral hepatitis type B respectively (WHO, 1973). Until recently, differences between the two main types were dependent on epidemiological observation. The discovery, however, of the association between hepatitis and the Australia antigen has permitted the differentiation serologically of these two types of hepatitis, as it is now generally agreed that the antigen is related to the 'serum' type of hepatitis (type B). Feinstone *et al.* (1973) using immune electron microscopy have identified a virus in the stools of patients with hepatitis A.

Viral hepatitis type A

The 'Milan antigen' was at first thought to be associated with type A hepatitis but later studies showed that it was a non-specific abnormal lipoprotein. An antigen has also been detected in faeces but as yet studies are inconclusive. Attempts to demonstrate particles in serum by electron microscopy have failed. Studies on human volunteers have demonstrated the route of transmission. The transmission of hepatitis A to marmosets and non-human primates has been reported but as yet the results are not universally accepted.

Viral hepatitis type A has a world-wide distribution (Hill and Bras, 1957). It is endemic in most areas of the tropics but occasionally epidemics take place. Like poliovirus, the virus of infectious hepatitis gains entry to the body via the alimentary tract and multiplies there with excretion of the virus in the stools. Virus is excreted not only during the acute phase of the illness but also during the long incubation period, which varies from 15 to 45 days. The main pathway of infection is the gastro-intestinal tract, but since the virus is also present in the blood the disease may—like the virus of homologous serum jaundice—occasionally be transmitted by infected blood. Spread by inhalation of droplets has been postulated but not proved (MacCallum *et al.* 1951).

Most epidemics of infectious hepatitis are spread by contact with infected patients (Editorial, 1968), though some extensive outbreaks have also been traced to the consumption of contaminated water, food, and milk. In contrast to contact-spread epidemics, water-borne and food-borne outbreaks are usually explosive and sudden in onset. One of the most dramatic water-borne epidemics occurred in Delhi in the winter of 1955–56, when about 29,000 cases of infectious hepatitis appeared in a 7-week period after the main water supply of the city had been contaminated with sewage some 6 weeks earlier (Indian Council of Medical Research, 1957). Raw shellfish and clams have also been responsible for food-borne epidemics. The mortality in pregnant females suffering from infectious hepatitis is high.

Australia antigen and viral hepatitis type B

Precipitating antibodies against a series of beta-lipo-protein antigens were discovered in some patients who had had multiple transfusions (Blumberg *et al.* 1962). An antibody was found in the serum of two American haemophiliacs which reacted with the serum of an Australian aborigine, and this antigen was therefore named Australia antigen (Blumberg *et al.* 1965). Extensive studies of this antigen have now been undertaken in many populations, and the Australia antigen, also known as AU(1), SH (Prince, 1968) and hepatitis antigen, is now usually described as the 'hepatitis-associated' antigen (HAA) or HBAg and has been shown to be closely associated with the long incubation type of viral hepatitis (serum hepatitis, Type B or MS-2 strain).

The antigen is rare in normal North American and European communities but occurs in frequencies as high as 20 per cent in some apparently healthy populations in the tropics (Blumberg *et al.* 1970; Prince, 1970; Bagshawe and Nganda, 1973). It also occurs more frequently in the serum of patients who have received multiple transfusions, institutionalized patients with Down's syndrome, in some forms of leukaemia, Hashimoto's disease and in lepromatous leprosy. It has been detected in post-transfusional hepatitis, in carriers of serum hepatitis in blood donors, in patients and staff of renal dialysis units, in patients attending VD clinics and in some patients with chronic hepatitis and cirrhosis.

The antigen is present in the serum of most patients with viral hepatitis type B in the acute phase but disappears in the first 6–12 weeks of convalescence. A few patients develop long-lasting antigenaemia and may develop chronic liver disease (Editorial, 1972).

Levene and Blumberg, however, in 1969 reported that different samples of Australia antigen were not serologically identical. Bouvier (1972) showed that all samples of Australia antigen tested shared a common antigen 'a' but differed in the possession of a second antigen which are most frequently *ad* or *ay*. Other antigens have been described (Editorial, 1973). Subtype *ay* is common in drug addicts whereas *ad* tends to be the predominant type among asymptomatic carriers. Most cases of hepatitis are due to *ay*. All cases in a single outbreak have been due to the same subtype. Iwarson *et al.* (1973) have reported a high incidence of liver disease among thirteen donors with *ay* in their blood. Only 3·3 per cent of recipients of *ay* positive blood and only 0·7 per cent of recipients of *ad* positive blood, however, developed hepatitis after transfusion. Donors incubating the disease were thought to be more dangerous sources of infection than long-time carriers with no signs of liver disease.

Characteristic particles have been described by electron microscopy in the serum and cytoplasm of hepatic cells of patients who have been shown to be carrying the hepatitis-associated antigen (Almeida, 1971; Haynes *et al.* 1972) about 20 nm in diameter and tubular forms of similar width. Larger particles about 42 nm in diameter have been described by Dane *et al.* (1970) and by Williams and Almeida (1972), who suggested that these variations might be helpful in prognosis. All the evidence would suggest that the HAA is the agent responsible for serum hepatitis in man.

The antibody to HAA is rarely found after primary exposure to the antigen and persists for only a few weeks. It is found most frequently in individuals who have been repeatedly exposed to the antigen. Its incidence in 105,724 blood donors in the West of Scotland was 0·006 per cent (Wallace *et al.* 1972) whereas in Uganda it was present in 30 per cent of the population (Anthony *et al.* 1972) and was found to be of no diagnostic significance in diseases of the liver whereas the antigen itself was present in significantly higher frequency in cirrhosis of the liver and hepato-cellular carcinoma than in controls (Vogel *et al.* 1972).

The HAA was associated with postnecrotic cirrhosis and not with portal and was also associated with liver cell dysplasia, i.e. nuclear and cytoplasmic enlargement, gross nuclear pleomorphism, double nuclei and occasional mitotic figures. These findings were thought to support the hypothesis that viral hepatitis type B infection was a factor in the ultimate development of hepatocellular carcinoma in some Ugandan patients. Alpha-fetoprotein-positive patients with hepatocellular carcinoma were HAA positive significantly more often than AFP negative patients—a finding previously noted in the United States (Prince *et al.* 1970).

Smith *et al.* (1972) have shown experimentally that mosquitoes can transmit the antigen and detected its presence in one of 300 mosquitoes caught in the wild in Nigeria. Prince *et al.* (1972) have also detected the antigen in 28 of 187 pools of mosquitoes caught in the wild in Kenya and Uganda. Similar studies have been carried out in Greece (Papaevangelore, 1974). So it is possible that an arthropod vector may transmit hepatitis in Africa. Hepatitis is a major urban disease in Accra, where it is more severe in the lower socio-economic groups. HAA has been identified in the faeces of hepatitis patients (Grob and Jemelka, 1971). So in the tropics a fecal–oral type of transmission is also possible (Morrow *et al.* 1971). It has also been detected in urine (Tripatziz and Horst, 1971). In Europe and America, however, there is no doubt that contamination of the skin by blood, blood products or parenteral inoculation are the commonest routes of transmission.

Congenital transmission has been considered (Turner *et al.* 1971). It is of interest, however, that an appreciable number of babies born in Papua, New Guinea, have detectable levels of Australia antibody in cord serum.

The antigen, however, was not detected in any sample (Woodfield, 1972). Tattooing, circumcision, and the possibility of intestinal parasites penetrating the skin and carrying the antigen from polluted soil has been favoured and rejected by different authors. The effect of possible transmission by circumcision of the first few weeks of life is of epidemiological interest in view of the possible high frequency of antibody in cord blood in tropical areas.

HAA has been detected in fibrinogen, thrombin and anti-haemophilic globulin (Zuckerman *et al.* 1971). The use of radio-iodinated fibrinogen in the diagnosis of deep-vein thrombosis may carry the danger of serum hepatitis.

Increased transmission is most likely to be the major factor in the high frequencies of Australia antigen found in the tropics, but on the other hand it has long been known that infective hepatitis was more common and severe in pregnancy—especially in the tropics (Edington and Gilles, 1969). An altered immunological reaction of the host which occurs in many tropical peoples subjected to multiple infections and infestations might well be an additional factor in the high frequencies of the infection recorded.

Detection of the Australia antigen and antibody*

Counter-immunoelectrophoresis is thought to be more sensitive than the immunodiffusion technique. It is of the same order of sensitivity as complement fixation but is less complicated (White *et al.* 1971). A radio-immuno-precipitation technique is, however, by far the most sensitive laboratory method (MacSween *et al.* 1973) but is complex, expensive and time-consuming. Counter-immunoelectrophoresis is the most widely used

---

* The following system of nomenclature of antigens associated with Viral Hepatitis Type B has been suggested (Morbidity and Mortality, 1974).

HB_sAg The hepatitis B antigen found on the surface of the Dane particle and on the unattached 20-nm particles.

HB_cAg The hepatitis B antigen found within the core of the Dane particle.

Dane particle   A current term for the 42-nm particle containing HB_cAg in its core and HB_sAg on its surface.

HBV   Reserved for hepatitis B virus. The Dane particle may turn out to be HBV.

HB_sAg/adr   Hepatitis B surface antigen manifesting the group-specific determinant, a, and subtype-specific determinants, d and r. All recognized subtypes are to be indicated to the right of the slash.

anti-HB_s Antibody to hepatitis B surface antigen. If the subtypic reactivity is known, the appropriate antigenic determinants are to be indicated to the right of a slash.

anti-HB_c Antibody to hepatitis B core antigen. If more than one core antigen is discovered, the corresponding antigens can be indicated.

The present use of HB Ab in designating the antibody to hepatitis B antigen should be abandoned.

technique as it is simple, sensitive and gives rapid results.
The two types of hepatitis are compared in Table 11.5.

TABLE 11.5. *Comparison of viral hepatitis type A and B*

	Viral hepatitis A	Viral hepatitis B
Contagious	Yes	? oro-faecal (Africa)
Route of infection	Oral and parenteral	Parenteral, ? oral, ? insect vector
Cause	? Virus A	Hepatitis-associated antigen (HBAg)
Age	Children and young adults	All ages
Incubation period	15–40 days	50–160 days
Onset	May be sudden	Insidious
Site of virus	Blood, faeces	Blood, faeces
Mode of infection	Water, faeces, shellfish	Transfusion, injections, faeces, ? insects
Smooth muscle antibody	Usually present	Usually present
Blood groups	?	? Excess Group O
Congenital transmission	Yes	?
Sequelae	Post-hepatitis syndrome	Post-hepatitis syndrome
	? Chronic persistent hepatitis	Chronic persistent hepatitis
	? Active chronic hepatitis	Active chronic hepatitis
	? Cryptogenic cirrhosis	Cryptogenic cirrhosis ? Hepatocellular carcinoma
Mortality	Low	May be high

Pathology of viral hepatitis types A and B

The discovery of the Australia (HAA) antigen has allowed the clinical differentiation of these two conditions but in the present state of knowledge the pathology will be considered similar and is discussed as one condition, although Iwarson *et al.* (1972) consider that patients with HBAg have more prominent hepatic parenchymal cell damage and Kupffer cell reaction with less cholestasis than is found in patients suffering from type A hepatitis.

Clinically, viral hepatitis may present in the following forms (Sherlock, 1963). (1) Acute icteric, (2) acute non-icteric, (3) relapsing hepatitis, (4) subacute hepatitis, (5) prolonged cholestatic type, and (6) fulminant. This last type is described on p. 585 when acute massive necrosis of the liver is discussed.

Infectious hepatitis may present acutely or insidiously with fever, anorexia, nausea, jaundice, tenderness over the liver, and biluria. The jaundice is hepatocellular in type and this is indicated by liver-function tests (see Table 11.6.)

TABLE 11.6. *Liver-function tests in jaundice*

	Haemolytic	Obstructive	Hepatocellular
Plasma or serum:			
Bilirubin	Increased	Increased	Increased
Diazo conjugated	Not increased	Increased	Increased ±
Unconjugated	Increased	Not increased	Increased ±
Albumin*	Normal	Normal	Low
Globulin (total)	Normal	Normal high	Increased
Globulin (fractions)	Normal	$\alpha_2\beta$ high	γ high
Flocculation tests	Negative	Negative	Positive
Alkaline phosphatase	Normal	> 30 K.A. units	< 30 K.A. units
Bromsulphthalein retention	Invalidated	Invalidated	Increased
Prothrombin time	Normal	Increased	Increased
Response to vitamin K	—	Yes	No
Aminotransferases:			
Alanine	Normal	Sometimes raised	Often raised
Aspartate	Normal	< 200 units	> 200 units
Ammonia	Normal	Normal	High
Cholesterol	Normal	Raised	Low

*The interpretation of serum proteins in some tropical communities is difficult because of the 'normal' high globulin and γ-globulin levels found.

The pathological changes in the liver are best seen in biopsy material as autolysis at post mortem markedly alters the histological findings, necrosis being much more widespread and the zonal distribution more marked. The liver cells vary in size, ballooning and feathery degeneration usually occurring throughout the lobule. Binucleated and multinucleated cells, mitotic figures, and enlarged nucleoli in the nuclei of the liver cells, are evidence of regenerative activity. Eosinophilic necrosis of individual cells with nuclear degenerative changes (pyknosis and karyolysis) occur throughout the lobule but are more marked in the central zone. Acidophilic structures representing remnants of liver cells may be seen in the Kupffer cells, whose cytoplasm may undergo a similar change. Rounded homogeneously eosinophilic structures with or without pyknotic nuclear material may also be seen lying free in the sinusoids. There is an associated intralobular focal infiltration of histiocytes, lymphocytes, and plasma cells with occasionally eosinophils and neutrophils present. There is a similar, sometimes intense, infiltrate in the portal tracts. Loss of liver cells may occur and is shown by collapse and condensation of the reticulin in central and periportal areas. Fatty change is rarely or never seen. Bile stasis may be prominent in the parenchymal cells, canaliculi, and Kupffer cells. Lipofuscin may be seen in the Kupffer cells and is thought to be related to the duration and severity of the process and to indicate liver-cell necrosis. It is a golden pigment on routine staining, argyrophilic, non-refractile, PAS-positive and gives a negative reaction to Perl's method for iron. Haemosiderin is inconstantly present. Gupta and Smetana (1957) described two forms of hepatitis in the Delhi outbreak of 1955–56. The 'standard' type showed the changes already described. The 'cholestatic' type showed feathery degeneration of the liver cells with no evidence of eosinophilic degeneration. Bile pigment was constantly present in the canaliculi and liver cells. An interesting feature was the gland-like arrangement of the hepatocytes around the bile thrombi in the canaliculi. This arrangement, even in the absence of bile thrombi, is common in our experience in West Africa and has also been noted by Edgcomb and Morrow (1963) in Ghana who also associated the cholestatic type with deficiency of the enzyme glucose-6-phosphate dehydrogenase in the erythrocytes. Morrow et al. (1968) have also reported an increased frequency of G6PD deficiency in patients suffering from hepatitis and noted that the condition tended to be more severe in these patients. Anti-smooth muscle and anti-mitochondrial antibodies have been reported in a high proportion of patients with acute viral hepatitis and have also been noted in yellow fever and primary liver cell carcinoma (Smith et al. 1972). An excess of blood group O has been described in acute viral hepatitis B and it was thought that the condition was more severe in these patients.

In rapidly fatal cases the appearances in the liver are those of massive liver-cell necrosis. Infectious hepatitis occurring in late pregnancy may result in miscarriage, premature delivery or stillbirth. In addition to the changes in the liver a rise in total serum globulin and in the immunoglobulin fraction accompanies both acute type A and type B hepatitis. A rise in IgM levels has been reported in acute hepatitis A but not B. A prodromal form of serum sickness with polyarteritis may occur in acute hepatitis B, and glomerulo-nephritis following infection has been described. In acute viral hepatitis changes in the mucosa of the small gut and kidney have been described. A haemolytic anaemia may occur in a small proportion of patients (Conrad, 1969). Depression of bone marrow function with leuco-penia thrombocytopenia and anaemia has also been reported.

The commonest sequel to acute viral hepatitis is the 'post-hepatitis syndrome' epitomized by malaise, fatigue, fat intolerance and right upper quadrant abdominal discomfort. Other sequelae are chronic persistent hepatitis, active chronic hepatitis and in some patients, cryptogenic cirrhosis and perhaps primary liver cell carcinoma. It would appear that the Australia antigen is associated more frequently with the latter four conditions and apart from chronic persistent hepatitis they are discussed separately below.

de Groote et al. (1962) have classified chronic hepatitis into chronic persistent and chronic aggressive. Chronic persistent hepatitis shows portal chronic inflammatory cell infiltration with preserved lobular archi-tecture and little or no fibrosis. Piecemeal necrosis is absent or slight. Features of acute hepatitis may be superimposed. Chronic aggressive hepatitis shows chronic inflammation in the portal tracts extending into the parenchyma with piecemeal necrosis and formation of intralobular septa. The lobular architecture is disturbed but there is no nodular regeneration. Features of acute hepatitis may be superimposed. Chronic aggressive hepatitis may simulate active chronic hepatitis—which condition the authors advise should be restricted to the clinical syndrome described below.

(II) ACTIVE CHRONIC HEPATITIS

Synonyms. Chronic active (lupoid) hepatitis; chronic liver disease in young women; plasma-cell hepatitis; active chronic viral hepatitis; lupoid hepatitis; active juvenile cirrhosis.

This is a condition in which signs of chronic hepatitis are associated with fever, arthralgia, splenomegaly, and hyperglobulinaemia, pericarditis, pleurisy, myocarditis, glomerulonephritis, thrombocytopenic purpura, endocrine changes and skin rashes.

Aetiology

Adolescents and young adults are mainly affected and the great majority are females. In about 25 per cent of patients the presenting feature is an attack of acute viral hepatitis. It may commence in pregnancy and it has been associated with ulcerative colitis, rheumatic fever and rheumatoid arthritis, spondylitis and Hashimoto's disease. In certain cases, it responds to corti-sone. L.E. cells are present in about 10 per cent of patients and an antinuclear factor has been detected in a high proportion of patients by an indirect immunofluorescence technique (Maclachan et al. 1965). Circulating anti-bodies to liver cells have also been demonstrated but are not specific. The evidence in favour of an auto-immune process in the aetiology is therefore considerable. On the other hand, chronic liver disease is not usual in the so-called collagen diseases including disseminated lupus erythematosus.

Pathology

The clinicopathological findings are those of parenchymal liver disease with the possible additional findings of L.E. cells and antinuclear factors enumerated above.

The parenchymal cells show ballooning, variation in size (even giant forms), and nuclear abnormalities in a focal fashion and mainly in the perilobular region. Individual cells may exhibit eosinophilic necrosis resembling the Councilman lesion (p. 222), but alcoholic hyaline and fatty change are not usually seen. In some lobules parts of the parenchyma are represented by condensed stroma. Kupffer cell proliferation is usual and bile stasis may occur. The portal tracts are infiltrated with lymphocytes, plasma cells, eosinophils, and occasional polymorphonuclear leucocytes. Bile ductular and pseudoductular proliferation may occasionally be seen. Intralobular and portal fibrous tissue proliferation with collapse eventually produce the histopathological picture of postnecrotic cirrhosis. There are changes in the liver function tests none of which are specific. The prothrombin time is seldom severely affected and jaundice is usually mild. There may be leucopenia and thrombocytopenia. The presence of antinuclear factor and serum antibodies to various tissue components has been mentioned above. The deposition of IgG in the liver has been described by Dawkins and Joske (1973). An abnormal cell mediated response to liver antigens has been reported. A definitive diagnosis cannot be made without a liver biopsy being performed to distinguish between acute viral hepatitis, persistent hepatitis, primary biliary cirrhosis, cholestatic hepatitis and pericholangitis.

(III) MASSIVE LIVER-CELL NECROSIS

Synonyms. Acute yellow atrophy; fulminant infectious hepatitis; massive cytolytic necrosis.

Massive liver-cell necrosis is an acute illness characterized by necrosis of all or nearly all the parenchymal cells in large areas of liver tissue, often more severe in the left lobe. Death may result rapidly from acute liver failure or, if sufficient parenchyma survives, scarring and hyperplasia may result in cirrhosis of the postnecrotic type.

Aetiology

In a number of instances the disease may occur in the absence of obvious aetiological factors. It occurs especially commonly in pregnancy and the puerperium in the tropics, and possible factors in these patients may be viral infections or the ingestion of herbal remedies containing hepatotoxic agents. The liver of the fetus, if stillborn, should always be examined for pathological changes. Chemical analysis of the liver in a few pregnant females dying of acute massive necrosis proved unfruitful in Ghana, and every effort should be made to investigate such cases thoroughly, as we are ignorant of their aetiology. Possible hepatotoxic agents are discussed on p. 557.

The condition may also be associated with surgical procedures, alcohol, drugs and infectious and homologous serum hepatitis (Rodgers *et al.* 1964). The sera of all cases should be screened for the presence of the Australia antigen (HAA).

It has been shown in experimental animals that dietary deficiencies, especially the sulphur-containing amino acids, cysteine and methionine, and vitamin E, may predispose to massive necrosis (Himsworth, 1950). In our experience massive necrosis appears to be more common in the tropics than in temperate climates but we have not been impressed by any greater incidence in malnourished subjects.

The fact that it occurs more frequently in pregnancy could be related to dietary, hormonal, or immunological factors. There is some evidence to suggest an altered immunological status in pregnancy, as malaria, pneumococcal meningitis, and possibly amoebic dysentery appear to be more frequent and severe in pregnancy than in non-pregnant adult females. Although it is possible that dietary deficiencies may predispose to massive necrosis, proof in man is still lacking.

Pathology

Clinically, patients may die within 2 or 3 days as a result of acute liver-cell failure. The progress may be so rapid that jaundice may be slight. On the other hand, there may be a more insidious course indistinguishable from severe infectious hepatitis and progressing gradually to signs and symptoms of cirrhosis. The liver-function tests exhibit changes similar to those of severe infectious hepatitis. Severe necrosis of liver cells causes disseminated intravascular coagulation with a severe haemorrhagic diathesis accentuated by the impaired synthesis of coagulation factors by the liver.

At autopsy, if death has occurred in a few days, the liver is uniformly yellow, is reduced in size and has a soft consistency. Histologically, all the parenchymal cells are affected, being swollen and granular and many of them are devoid of nuclei. The intralobular capillary walls are also affected. A rim of surviving liver cells may occasionally surround the portal tracts.

If death has occurred less rapidly the liver is small and soft and its capsule is wrinkled. On section, scattered throughout its substance, there are patchy areas of red, yellow, and brownish-green tissue, representing respectively congested areas of collapse of stroma where the liver cells have disappeared, areas of liver-cell necrosis, and areas of surviving liver tissue. Cellular infiltration in both instances is minimal. The left lobe is usually more severely affected.

If the patient survives, areas of collapse disappear with approximation of portal tracts and proliferation of bile duct and fibrous tissue. Eventually, greyish-white scars result. Hyperplasia of surviving liver cells leads to the formation of nodules. As the lesion was originally patchy in distribution the lobular pattern may be maintained in some areas. The scarring leads to interference with the blood supply and liver-function tests rarely return to normal. The eventual picture is described as postnecrotic cirrhosis (p. 547).

Associated changes in other organs

At autopsy the kidneys are bile stained and the cells of the proximal convoluted tubules show degenerative changes or even actual necrosis. Bile casts may be present. Whether these changes are due to toxic factors or hypotension is debatable. The urine is diminished in amount and contains bile, albumin, casts and excess amino acids. Crystals of leucine and tyrosine may be present. The ganglion cells in the brain may show acute non-specific degenerative changes. An associated pancreatitis and myocarditis has been described.

(IV) THE ACUTE FATTY LIVER OF PREGNANCY

This is a rare condition occurring in the last few weeks of pregnancy. Clinically, the patient presents with epigastric pain, vomiting, jaundice, and headache. Haematemesis may occur. The disease usually terminates in hepatic coma and death following premature labour with the delivery of a stillborn fetus. The fetal pathology has not been described.

The aetiology is unknown but a recent increase in incidence has been associated with tetracycline therapy (Duma *et al.* 1965).

The pathological changes in the liver are interesting and unusual. The liver cells, excluding these around the portal tracts, contain fine lipoid droplets. The nuclear changes are insignificant and there is no evidence of necrosis or a marked inflammatory reaction (Sheehan, 1940). There may be fatty change in the proximal convoluted tubules of the kidney and an acute haemorrhagic pancreatitis has been described in one case (Editorial, 1956).

Flocculation tests are normal. Serum bilirubin is raised and there is azotaemia and hypoprothrombinaemia. The alkaline phosphatase is high and the transaminases moderately increased.

(V) CONGENITAL DILATATION OF THE INTRAHEPATIC BILE
DUCTS

This is a developmental abnormality which may present at any age and
can cause multiple communicating cystic spaces in the hepatic parenchyma.
Cholangiocellular carcinoma may be a complication (Gallagher *et al.* 1972).

IX. TUMOURS OF THE LIVER

Simple tumours of the liver are rare. Adenomata and cavernous haemangiomas are the most frequently seen and do not differ from the well-described
features in standard textbooks. A giant haemangioma of the liver associated
with a micro-angiopathic haemolytic anaemia has been reported from Sri
Lanka (Prematilleke, 1972). Cysts may also occur in the liver and are usually
associated with congenital lesions in other viscera. Hamartomas are occasionally seen.

The malignant tumours of the liver can be classified as follows (Higginson
and Steiner, 1961).

A. *Epithelial tumours*
    1. Primary liver-cell carcinoma (synonyms: hepatocellular carcinoma,
       malignant hepatoma)
    2. Cholangiocellular carcinoma (synonyms: bile-duct carcinoma,
       malignant cholangioma)
    3. Hepatobiliary and mixed carcinomas
    4. Cholangiolocellular carcinoma
B. *Mesenchymal tumours* (sarcomas, angio-endotheliomas, etc.)
C. *Miscellaneous groups* including mixed epithelial and mesenchymal
   tumours
D. *Secondary tumours*

The classification of childhood hepatic tumours has recently been reviewed by Ishak and Glunz (1967) and Ito and Johnson (1969). The tumours
may be a hepatocellular carcinoma or a hepatoblastoma of epithelial or
mixed epithelial and mesenchymal type. Ultrastructurally the epithelial
cells are immature undifferentiated cells with scanty cytoplasm and poorly
developed organelles in contrast to the more differentiated cell seen in hepatocellular carcinoma. Foci of extra-medullary erythropoiesis may be present.
The liver cells are small, the cords are compact and resemble immature
or embryonal liver tissue.

A. PATHOLOGY OF EPITHELIAL TUMOURS OF THE LIVER

The classification of liver tumours is based essentially on histopathological
features. It is not usually difficult to distinguish liver-cell carcinoma from

cholangiocellular carcinoma. Occasionally, however, the former may exhibit an adenoid pattern and we have seen experienced pathologists misdiagnose this type as cholangiocellular. The presence of bile may be a helpful diagnostic feature and signifies that the tumour is of the liver-cell type. It is important to differentiate these two types as they most probably have different aetiological backgrounds. The common tumour in most areas of high liver cancer incidence is of liver-cell origin, whereas in areas in which clonorchiasis or opisthorciasis are endemic the more usual type is cholangiocellular. The pathology of the various types is described below.

(1) Primary liver-cell carcinoma

Macroscopically, the liver is always enlarged and the tumour may be nodular or massive (Berman, 1951). In the nodular type the liver is hard, scarred, and deformed, and studded with whitish-greyish or dark-green irregular nodular masses varying in size from a few millimetres to several centimetres. In the massive type there is a large tumour mass usually in the right lobe but multiple smaller growths may also be present in the left. Evidence of fatty change, haemorrhage and necrosis may be present in both types. Whether the tumour is unicentric or multicentric in origin is debatable. The intervening liver tissue will show evidence of cirrhosis, usually postnecrotic in type, in about 70–80 per cent of cases in the tropics. If siderosis is present the liver tissue is reddish-brown in colour (Fig. 11.7).

Histologically, various subgroups have been described, but variegated and mixed patterns are seen and the essential feature is the resemblance of the tumour cells to the parenchymal cells of the liver. The subgroups have been designated as (a) adenoid, (b) giant cell, (c) anaplastic, (d) pseudo-endothelial, and (e) miscellaneous.

The tumour cells are usually arranged in nodules of varying size with the cells in balls, cords, or trabeculae, which vary in thickness. They are surrounded by sinusoidal spaces containing blood and lined by endothelial-like cells often associated with reticulin septa. The nature of these cells is uncertain but true Kupffer cells and macrophages are not seen. Areas of necrosis are usual. The cells are usually large and polyhedral, and contain vesicular nuclei with a well-marked nucleolus, but occasionally they are small and have dense nuclei. The cytoplasm is eosinophilic but in liver biopsy material the cells may show ballooning and feathery degeneration. Bizarre mitotic figures and giant cells may be present. Bile canaliculi containing thrombi and bile pigment in the tumour cells may occur. The tumour cells may also contain glycogen. Alcoholic hyaline and fatty change, either as small droplets or large vacuoles, may occur in a focal fashion. It is said that haemosiderin deposition may also occur in tumour cells in siderotic livers but this has not been our experience, the non-pigmented malignant

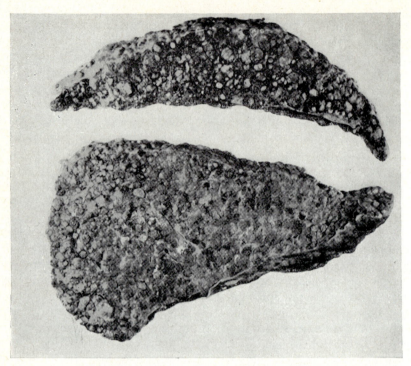

FIG. 11.7. Primary carcinoma of the liver. South African Zulu male aged 34 years. Liver shows coarse nodular cirrhosis many of the nodules are undergoing malignant change. (*From* Trowell, *Non-Infective Disease in Africa*, 1960. *Edward Arnold.*)

foci usually being in sharp contrast to the heavily pigmented 'normal' liver cells. Mucin secretion may occur in liver-cell carcinoma but is rare. The adenoid change which may occur has already been mentioned. A false ductular appearance may be formed by enlargement of a canaliculus in a trabeculum, by central degeneration in a group of cells, or by liver carcinoma cells lining a preformed space. Anaplastic forms occur and may present difficulties in diagnosis. We have never seen the pseudo-endothelial form but it is said to consist of numerous spindle cells with oval nuclei resembling fibroblasts. In liver-cell carcinoma the intervening liver tissue may show evidence of portal or postnecrotic cirrhosis, the latter being much more common. In the absence of cirrhosis the liver tissue is compressed and a fibrous reaction may be initiated at the periphery of the tumour. Signs of regenerative activity in the liver cells are usually marked and focal bile retention may be noted.

In liver-cell carcinoma there is clinically asthenia, jaundice, hepato-megaly, splenomegaly, ascites, and peripheral oedema. It is of interest that numerous asexual and sexual *P. falciparum* parasites have been reported in erythrocytes in ascitic fluid of a Gambian farmer suffering from primary liver cell carcinoma illustrating loss of immunity in this condition (Logie and Swanson Beck, 1970). A soft systolic murmur can sometimes be heard over the tumour nodules. Hypoglycaemic attacks and polycythaemia have been described by MacFadzean and Yeung (1969) in Hong Kong. The course in the tropics is rapid, with death occurring within a few months from hepatic coma, intercurrent infection, haemorrhage from ruptured oesophageal varices, or intraperitoneal haemorrhage from the tumour in the liver itself. The associated conditions described when the post-mortem findings in cirrhosis of the liver were being considered may be present.

Tumour thrombi may be seen in the portal or hepatic veins and may extend into the inferior vena cava and right side of the heart. Portal thrombosis sometimes occurs. Metastases are most frequently seen in the lungs and upper abdominal lymphatic glands, but tend to occur late. The hilar glands, diaphragm, ribs, gall bladder, mesentery, peritoneum, heart, skull, sternum, brain, and even the long bones, may also be affected by secondary deposits which in some instances may produce bile pigment. Cutaneous porphyria may be a rare complication (Thompson *et al.* 1970).

Diagnosis of liver-cell carcinoma

Diagnosis is usually made clinically supplemented by liver biopsy or cytological examination of ascitic fluid. The interpretation of the last technique is, however, not always easy as atypical cells may be found in the fluid in cirrhosis and other malignancies. Liver-function tests show abnorm-alities but are not specific. An anomalous serum protein has been reported in liver-cell carcinoma and hepatic metastases (Lippi *et al.* 1971). Its significance is not yet understood.

The serum IgA and IgM levels may be increased. The discovery of alpha-fetoprotein (discussed below) has produced a serological test which may detect the presence of liver-cell cancer in up to 80 per cent of patients in certain parts of Africa. Assay of serum proline hydroxylase may also prove to be a diagnostic aid of value and levels in the serum fall dramatically in patients responding to chemotherapy (Keiser *et al.* 1972). Abnormalities in the circulating fibrinogen have also been described (Felton *et al.* 1969) which may explain the prolonged thrombin times which are not always satisfactorily explained by the presence of circulating anticoagulants, in-creased fibrin degradation products or by fibrinogenopenia (Vogel and Linsell, 1972).

Alpha-fetoprotein (AFP)

Abelev in 1963 demonstrated a specific alpha-globulin of embryonic serum which was synthesized by mouse and rat hepatomas and secreted in the blood. This was also shown to occur in primary liver cell carcinoma in man by Tatarinov (1964). This work has been confirmed by workers in the U.S.S.R. and France (Abelev *et al.* 1967; Uriel *et al.* 1967). Antiserum to the alpha-fetoprotein was prepared and has been shown by numerous workers to detect the presence of AFP in the serum of 30–87 per cent of patients with hepatocellular carcinoma. It was also found in the serum of some patients with embryonal cell carcinoma of the testis and may occur in infants with severe hepatitis.

AFP is usually detected by double well diffusion in agar using specifically prepared anti-AFP antiserum.

All the above remarks, however, will require rethinking as a more sensitive technique (radioimmunoassay) has shown that AFP occurs in normal human serum and in all patients with primary liver cell carcinoma (Ruoslahti *et al.* 1972)—although in a number of these patients the values may be 'normal'. The highest frequency of elevated AFP in hepatomas is found in the tropical areas where its incidence is high and lower frequencies are found in Europe and the United States. AFP is normally synthesized by the fetal liver and yolk sac. In the fetus the highest serum concentration occurs during the 12–14th gestational week and begins to decrease around the 32nd week. High values are found until about 5 weeks post partum (Gitlin and Boesman, 1967). AFP can be detected in maternal serum by radioimmunoassay and increases during gestation. The highest levels are found during the mid-third trimester. Its estimation has been considered a method of predicting the outcome of threatened abortion, high levels being associated with intra-uterine fetal death (Seppala and Ruoslahti, 1972). By the indirect immunofluorescence technique it has been shown that in the neonate AFP is present predominantly in the periportal parenchymal cells of the liver and present in a focal fashion in the cytoplasm of malignant liver cells of patients whose sera contained high levels of AFP (Smith *et al.* 1971). AFP has also been detected in ascitic fluid, cerebrospinal fluid and bile from patients with AFP seropositive hepatocellular carcinoma (Smith *et al.* 1971a). Smith (1972) has also shown that AFP may be a factor necessary for the normal development of the embryo as anti-AFP antibodies injected into pregnant laboratory animals produced congenital abnormalities.

There is no doubt that the detection of AFP by the agar double diffusion method or counter-electrophoresis in serum are reliable tests for the presence of hepatocellular carcinoma in man. Patients under 25 years of age are almost universally positive in Africa. Patients over 60 years of age are rarely positive (Vogel and Linsell, 1972). A negative test does not, therefore, rule out the possibility of a hepatocellular carcinoma being present. It is of interest that the Australia antigen is found in greater frequency in patients with high levels of AFP in the serum when compared with controls (Prince et al. 1970; Vogel et al. 1972).

Quantitative AFP testing might serve as a marker of disease activity in treated patients. False-positive tests are very rare but in addition to embryonal cell carcinoma and infantile hepatitis mentioned above they have been reported in a few patients with gastric cancer and hepatic secondaries. Lastly the findings of Foy et al. (1970) should be mentioned.

AFP was detected in the sera of five out of ten baboons on a pyridoxine-free diet. The definitive pathology of the liver in these animals has still to be described. As the content of pyridoxine is marginal in the diet of most Africans this may be a factor which has to be considered seriously in the aetiology of hepatocellular carcinoma. It is of interest that the level of Vitamin B_{12} rose eight-fold in the pyridoxine-deprived animals.

Aetiology of liver-cell carcinoma in the tropics

Several factors have to be considered in the aetiology of liver-cell carcinoma in the tropics.

(a) Geographical distribution

The highest incidence rates of liver-cell carcinoma have been reported from Lourenço Marques (Prates and Torres, 1965) where the incidence in the 25- to 36-year-old age group is approximately 500 times that in North America. High incidence rates have also been reported in the South African Bantu (Higginson and Oettle, 1960), the Yoruba in Western Nigeria (Edington and Maclean, 1965), Uganda (Davies et al. 1965), and the Chinese living in Singapore (Muir and Shanmugaratnam, 1966). Post-mortem studies or relative ratio frequencies (i.e. the percentage of total malignancies) suggest that it is also very common in Senegal (Camain, 1954), Ghana (Edington, 1956), the Congo (Thijs, 1957), China (Tuan-Fu, 1959), Japan (Nori, 1966), and Papua-New Guinea (McGovern, 1966), Ethiopia (Pavlica and Samuel, 1970). In Ethiopia primary liver cell cancer was associated with cirrhosis in 94·7 per cent of patients studied (Pavlica and Samuel, 1970). Mycotoxins and herbal medicines (taenicides) were considered important aetiological agents. Shanmugaratnam and Tye (1970) have shown that immigrant Chinese in Singapore are more prone to develop liver cancer than Chinese born in Singapore.

The incidence is low in Egypt (Hashem, 1961), U.S. non-whites and whites (Dorn and Cutler, 1958), Brazil (Montenegro et al. 1958; de Carvalho, 1966), India (Paymaster, 1964), Japanese immigrants in Hawaii, Mexicans (Lopez-Corrella et al. 1968) (despite a high incidence of cirrhosis), Colombia

(Correa and Llanos, 1966), and in Jamaica (Bras *et al.* 1961). It is low in Indians or Malays in Malaya, although high in Chinese there (Marsden, 1958). The incidence in Thailand is probably intermediate between the areas of high and low incidence and, as in Hong Kong, liver flukes producing a cholangiocellular carcinoma complicate the picture.

From a study of the geographical distribution of liver-cell cancer it will be noted that there appears to be no consistent pattern in relation to the occurrence of malnutrition, schistosomiasis, or malaria and we would exclude them as agents directly responsible for a high liver-cell cancer incidence. Genetic and racial factors also do not appear to be important.

Cirrhosis and liver-cell carcinoma. In racial groups showing a high incidence of liver-cell cancer the incidence of cirrhosis may not be greatly increased but the striking feature is the number of cirrhotic livers which become malignant. This is a constant feature in all tropical areas from which figures are available. Fifty to eighty per cent of cirrhotic livers may become malignant, whereas in temperate climates and in Europeans living in South Africa (Becker and Chatgidikas, 1961) the figure varies from 2·5 to 15 per cent (Thomson, 1961). In Mexico a figure as low as 0·26 per cent has been quoted and the usual type of cirrhosis is micronodular. Carcinomatous change occurred in livers which were the seat of postnecrotic cirrhosis (Lopez-Corella *et al.* 1968). Similar findings have been reported from Chile (Velasco *et al.* 1971). There would appear therefore to be a relationship between liver-cell cancer and cirrhosis in certain areas of the tropics though cancer can occur in the absence of cirrhosis.

The type of cirrhosis is usually postnecrotic. Malignant change is not common in portal cirrhosis even with the presence of siderosis in South Africa. The association with postnecrotic cirrhosis suggests that liver-cell injury followed by regenerative hyperplasia is an aetiological factor. Anthony *et al.* (1973) have noted that liver-cell dysplasia (our regenerative activity, p. 548), defined as cellular enlargement, nuclear pleomorphism and multinucleation of liver cells, was not uncommon in postnecrotic and mixed forms of cirrhosis and very common in patients with cirrhosis and primary liver-cell carcinoma. There was a strong relationship between dysplasia and the presence of Australia antigen in the serum which suggested a possible carcinogenic mechanism for the serum hepatitis virus in some patients with liver-cell carcinoma. It was thought that liver-cell dysplasia identified a group of patients with a high risk of liver-cell carcinoma and that follow up by serial alphafetoprotein estimations would be of value. With this we would agree. It should also be noted that in these areas, with a high incidence of liver-cell cancer, cholangiocellular carcinoma and carcinoma of the gall bladder are no more common than they are in Europe, suggesting that the carcinogenic agent affects the liver cells themselves rather than the bile passages. It might perhaps be postulated that the cancer and the cirrhosis are two independent results of a single agent, rather than that the cirrhosis gives rise to the cancer. The evidence is equivocal. In laboratory animals cancer or cirrhosis may be initiated by the same agent depending upon dosage and method of administration. In man, therefore, it is possible that cirrhosis and cancer may be caused by the same agent or agents depending perhaps upon the strength of, and the time interval between, the stimuli to which the liver has been exposed.

(b) Sex

Males are affected four to five times as frequently as females, though the differential tends to narrow over the age of 55. The reason for this difference is obscure. Males may be more susceptible or undergo greater exposure to the environmental carcinogenic factor or factors. In laboratory animals challenged with various carcinogenic agents males are also usually more prone to develop malignant tumours and gonadectomy reduces the incidence in males and enhances the incidence in females. Hormonal factors may therefore be important in the differing sex ratio of liver-cell carcinoma in man although caution should be exercised in applying data obtained in laboratory animals to man. However, the sudden rise in incidence seen in menopausal women in Ibadan would suggest that sex hormones may play a part in the aetiology of the condition. Hyperoestrogenization has been described in males in Kampala, an area of high liver cancer (Davies, 1952), and feminization in West Africa (Dawson, 1966), and is discussed below. If this is a factor in the increased incidence of liver-cell carcinoma the lower rate in females is somewhat difficult to explain.

Enlargement of the male breast or *gynaecomastia* is common in many areas of the tropics. Incidence of 5 and 6 per cent have been given in parts of East and West Africa (Dawson, 1966). The high incidence has been associated with the 'oestrogenization' which is said to occur commonly in males, and an increased urinary excretion of oestrogen metabolites with a low androgen excretion has been shown in a number of peoples (Clifford and Bulbrook, 1966). Gynaecomastia is also very common in boys at the age of puberty in Britain but is not associated with increased urinary excretion of oestrogens. A raised excretion of oestrogens is not found frequently in adult patients with gynaecomastia in Britain (Jull *et al.* 1964). Controlled studies of this subject have not been done in the tropics so whether the relationship between oestrogenization and gynaecomastia is directly causal or not must remain conjectural. The cause of the oestrogenization itself is obscure. It seems unlikely that liver damage is so widespread that circulating oestrogens are not catabolized in large population groups. Gynaecomastia also occurs in many disease states (Editorial, 1964), the most common in the tropics being hepatic cirrhosis, leprosy, and malnutritional states. Drugs may also induce the condition.

The pathological findings are hyperplasia of the ducts and their lining epithelium, with a surrounding zone of oedematous fibrillary connective tissue. Lobules comparable with those of the female breast are not seen in the tropics but have been described in gynaecomastia associated with chromatin-positive Klinefelter's syndrome.

(c) Age

In areas of high incidence liver tumours are occasionally seen in children but the condition usually appears first in the 20-to 30-year-old age group. Its incidence rises steadily with age, but there may be some flattening of the incidence curve in the older age groups. It has been stated that in the elderly the proportion of cirrhotic livers which become malignant is low. This is explained as more probably due to a reduced intensity of exposure rather than to an occurrence in old people of many other forms of cirrhosis which may have lowered risks of malignant change (Oettle, 1965).

The average incidence of all types of cancer seen in this age group falls with increasing ages in a number of tropical areas (Edington and Maclean, 1965), but this does not occur with liver cancer. The age incidence curves differ remarkably from those seen in temperate climates, where liver-cell cancer is uncommon before the age of 50 years, and then rise steadily with age. The differing age structure would suggest that man in the tropics is exposed to a hepatic carcinogen at an earlier age and that possibly different aetiological agents are involved.

(d) Social class

In Nigeria, at present, social class would not appear a factor of importance but in other geographic areas the lower socio-economic groups are more frequently affected.

(e) Toxic and other factors

The geographical distribution of the high incidence of liver-cell carcinoma appears to exclude malnutrition in childhood, racial and genetic factors and parasite infestation as aetiological agents. Alcohol also can be dismissed as the carcinoma occurs in relatively young age groups, the type of cirrhosis is postnecrotic, and Moslems are affected. It has been suggested, however, that malnutrition may be a predisposing factor which, in the presence of an initiating factor (carcinogenic) and other promoting factors (co-carcinogenic), might lead to malignant change in the liver. This hypothesis is difficult to refute but, if correct, there must be carcinogenic factors and co-factors present in areas of Africa and China which are absent in India, North Africa, and South America, where protein-calorie deficiency diseases are common.

The effect of plant alkaloids on the liver has been discussed on p. 558. They are recognized as a cause of cirrhosis of the liver in the West Indies, but that is an area where the incidence of liver-cell carcinoma is not high.

The mycotoxins have also been discussed on p. 559. It is of interest that aflatoxin usually produces alpha-fetoprotein negative tumours in laboratory animals although AFP-positive tumours have been found in the rat. It is disappointing that the geographical distribution of liver-cell carcinoma has not shown a pattern conforming to low living standards, to humidity and temperature levels at which fungal contamination of staples is likely to occur. It is difficult to accept the possibility of mycotoxins being responsible for the occurrence of post necrotic cirrhosis and liver cancer when the incidence of both conditions is low in Brazil—the country from which the original ground-nut meal causing liver disease in turkeys emanated. However, as pointed out by Oettlé (1965), in humid areas where food is not stored long enough for mouldiness to develop, low rates of liver cancer may be found. Rate-incidence studies alone are therefore tenuous facts from which to draw conclusions. Sociological (including dietary) studies are required in areas where the incidence of liver cancer in high and in areas where it is low, but where the humidity and temperature levels are similar. Such studies might substantiate the attractive theory that mycotoxins are the aetiological agents responsible for the high incidence of carcinoma of the liver in many tropical areas. It is of interest, however, that Alpert *et al.* (1971) have found high levels of aflatoxin in foodstuff in Uganda, especially in provinces with a high hepatoma incidence.

(f) Viral hepatitis

Recent studies in Chile, Ghana, Greece, Kenya, Senegal, Uganda, U.K. and U.S.A. have shown a high prevalence (40 per cent) of Australia (HA) antigen (p. 578) in the serum of patients with hepatocellular carcinoma when compared with controls (Vogel and Linsell, 1972). Conflicting reports have, however, been received from Nigeria and Singapore. The HAA may be present in the serum of patients with hepatocellular carcinoma in the absence of cirrhosis. If, however, cirrhosis were present both in Uganda and Chile it was of macronodular type. In Uganda the HAA was not detected in patients with micronodular cirrhosis. No viral particles have, however, been noted in malignant liver cells studied ultrastructurally (O'Conor *et al.* 1972). The HAA has also been noted to be more prevalent in those patients with alpha-fetoprotein present in their serum when compared with AFP-negative hepatocellular cancer patients. In addition, when it is remembered that it has been reported that the antigen is associated with post-necrotic cirrhosis and with marked liver cell dysplasia, there is some reason for concluding that viral hepatitis B may be a factor in the development of post-necrotic cirrhosis and primary liver cell cancer in some patients. On the other hand the Australia antigen is detected frequently in patients with immunological deficiencies—leukaemia, leprosy, Hodgkins disease and Down's syndrome—so it is possible that patients with hepatocellular carcinoma may have an altered immunological status, thus rendering them more prone to infection by the antigen. Primack *et al.* (1973) investigated this problem and concluded that, with the tests employed, it appeared unlikely that generalized defects in host immune responses could account for the high incidence of persistent hepatitis B virus infection found in Ugandan patients with hepato-cellular carcinoma. We are not convinced that this is the true picture of host immune responses in cirrhosis as a heavy infection of *P. falciparum* malaria has been noted in the Gambia and pneumococcal peritonitis is a complication of the condition.

To sum up: viral hepatitis B may be an associated factor in the aetiology of some patients suffering from post-necrotic cirrhosis and hepatocellular carcinoma but this is, as yet, by no means proven. Much further work remains to be done on the problem and investigations on host immune deficiencies, mycotoxins, possible inheritable factors, dietary deficiencies and possible chemical carcinogens should not be neglected.

(2) Cholangiocellular carcinoma

This tumour varies in incidence, being much less frequent comparatively in areas where there is a high incidence of liver-cell cancer and common in certain areas where liver flukes are found. Macroscopically it cannot be differentiated with certainty from liver-cell carcinoma. It tends to be white in colour, may be single in the liver and there is no marked association with cirrhosis. Associated signs of parasitic infection and cholangitis may be present. The tumour arises from the intrahepatic bile ducts and the pathology has been described on p. 185, when its relationship with *clonorchiasis* was considered.

(3) Hepatobiliary and mixed carcinomas

In this tumour both liver-cell and cholangiocellular elements may be present. Care has to be taken to differentiate the cholangiocellular tissue from a pseudo-cholangiomatous arrangement due to adenoid change in a liver-cell carcinoma.

(4) Cholangiolocellular carcinoma

Histologically the cells lie in small simple cords, often containing a small canaliculus and separated by dense connective tissue. The cells are small and cubical with eosinophilic cytoplasm and dense hyperchromatic nuclei. They resemble the cells of the cholangioles (canals of Hering) from which the tumour is presumed to have arisen. Areas of liver-cell carcinoma or cholangiocellular carcinoma may be present.

B. MESENCHYMAL TUMOURS

These rarely occur in the liver but we have seen two well-differentiated fibrosarcomas, one with a similar tumour in the spleen, in young adults in Nigeria. Two extensive infantile haemangio-endotheliomas of the liver with associated lesions in skin and other viscera have also presented in infants in the last 2 years. Further information is required on the incidence of mesenchymal tumours of the liver in tropical areas.

C. MISCELLANEOUS

In the original classification (Higginson and Steiner, 1961), hepato-blastomas were included in this group. A rare tumour occurs in which there are malignant epithelial and mesenchymal elements.

D. SECONDARY TUMOURS OF THE LIVER

These are common and include metastases from carcinoma of the stomach, malignant melanoma, malignant disease of the trophoblast, and tumours of the reticulo-endothelial system including the Burkitt tumour.

X. DISEASES OF THE GALL BLADDER AND BILE DUCTS

In spite of the number of parasites and bacteria, including enteric organisms, which could affect the gall bladder cholecystitis is rare in many areas of the tropics. Serpeau *et al.* (1971) have demonstrated the presence of Australia antigen in gall-bladder bile. Caroli's disease is focal congenital dilatation of the intrahepatic bile ducts; the extrahepatic bile ducts are relatively normal thus differing from the dilatation of the ducts described in Asian countries. A cholangiocellular carcinoma has been reported in association with the condition (Jones and Shreeve, 1970). Chronic diseases affecting the intrahepatic bile radicles have been reviewed by Sherlock (1968).

An exception to this statement occurs in areas where the liver flukes are endemic. Cholangiohepatitis is one of the commonest surgical emergencies seen in Hong Kong. The patients present with acute abdominal pain, pyrexia and jaundice. Exacerbations and remissions are usual. Perforation of the gall bladder may occur. Strictures may form within the intrahepatic bile ducts with the formation of abscesses and the development of a cholangiocellular carcinoma may be a further complication. In Japan, pigmented calcium stores of parasitic origin are frequently found in the bile ducts and gall bladder and are considered to be due to the ova of *Ascaris lumbricoides*. The female preponderance noted in Western countries is lacking (Maki, 1961).

King (1971) has reported that biliary-tract disease requiring operation is common in Malaya and appears to be more common in Indians and Malays than in the Chinese. Two distinct patterns are encountered. The most common disease is similar to the Western type of cholelithiasis. The second which was termed 'Oriental cholangitis' was of a distinctly different pattern and was similar to the type seen in Hong Kong, Singapore, Korea, China and Japan and has been referred to as recurrent pyogenic cholangitis, cholangiohepatitis, Chinese biliary obstruction syndrome, and Japanese cholelithiasis (as described above). The sex incidence is equal or males may predominate. The condition occurred in Chinese, Indians and Malays in Malaya. Soft pigment stones and mud are found in the dilated intra- and extrahepatic bile ducts. Jaundice, fever and infected bile are usual. Enlargement of the gall bladder is common. Death may occur from renal failure or septicaemia. The aetiology is obscure. *Clonorchis sinensis* was detected in only one of the forty-four patients. Gastro-enteritis and intestinal parasites are possible factors. Young adults may be affected but the condition is usual in middle age.

The factors concerned in gall-stone formation are stasis, the composition of bile, and bacterial infection. Stones are formed of cholesterol, bile pigments, and lime salts. The mixed cholesterol and bile-pigment stone is the most common in temperate climates; the rare stones seen in tropical Africa are usually pigmentary and the pale-yellow cholesterol stone is never seen. Pigmentary stones are rarely seen in sickle-cell disease, although quite commonly reported in North America. A close association between opium addiction and cholelithiasis has been noted in the adult male Chinese in Singapore.

Carcinoma of the gall bladder

As gall stones are considered an important factor in the causation of this tumour it is not surprising that in tropical Africa especially it is not found in high incidence. The usual type of tumour is an adenocarcinoma.

12

The Nervous System

In few centres in the tropics has the study of neurology been pursued intensively: knowledge of diseases affecting the nervous system is therefore somewhat fragmentary. The effect of the various tropical diseases upon the nervous system is discussed when the individual conditions are considered in their appropriate text. A brief review of these conditions therefore is given in this chapter since the subject has been extensively reviewed in *Tropical Neurology* (Spillane, 1973). In certain areas of the tropics, however, recognized neurological conditions occur in high incidence, amyotrophic lateral sclerosis being an example and, in others, undescribed conditions in temperate climates, such as kuru (p. 262), have been noted. These two conditions and the neuropathic syndrome of unknown origin are therefore described in somewhat more detail.

Convulsions in children are common and the causes are multiple. Febrile convulsions are very common and may be complicated by traditional therapy—herbal remedies and the burning of feet and buttocks (Familusi and Sinnette, 1971). Cerebral malaria, gastro-enteritis, otitis media, hypoglycaemia—perhaps due to herbal remedies—and electrolyte imbalance are other causes. Meningitis and encephalitis should be excluded by examining the cerebrospinal fluid. The main problem in tropical neurology at the present moment is the control of such diseases as leprosy, beri-beri, parasitic infections and probably protein–calorie malnutrition.

CONGENITAL MALFORMATIONS

Anencephaly would appear to be rare in most parts of the tropics but encephalocoele, meningocoele, and meningomyelocoele are not uncommon (Odeku, 1967; Odeku *et al.* 1967). Hydrocephalus is seen but the relative importance of congenital and infective causes is not known. *Cysticercus cellulosae* and *Coenurus cerebralis* have been described as causal factors (Kuper *et al.* 1958). Dermoid cysts simulating a meningocele over the region of the anterior fontanelle are not uncommon in the neonate (Odeku, 1965).

Cerebral palsy, due to birth injury, and neonatal jaundice (often infective) are common. Anterior encephalocele is not uncommon in Bangkok and is more common than spina bifida aperta in contrast to the Western world (Spillane, 1972) and possibly in parts of Africa.

Congenital atlantoaxial dislocation is common in India (Wadia, 1967) and is epitomized by cervical pain and stiffness and transitory attacks of paralysis of short duration which may become progressively more severe. Young males are more frequently affected.

Frederick (1970) has shown that the incidence of anencephaly is negatively correlated with the total hardness, calcium content, pH, and to a certain extent the sodium content of the water supply in the United Kingdom. In the U.S.A. the death rate from spina bifida (a congenital abnormality generally considered to be aetiologically similar to anencephaly) was significantly lower in states with harder water when compared to those with soft water.

In Europe there are marked national variations in incidence in Northern Ireland, Wales, Scotland, England and France. Environmental influences are probably important.

The incidence among American negroes is one-third that of U.S. whites (Milic, 1969) and it was suggested that earlier uterine death and abortion particularly of the more vulnerable male fetus might account for the lower recorded incidence and for the preponderance of female anencephalic fetuses. Naggan (1971), has elaborated on the environmental hypothesis in Israel.

A low incidence of calcified pineal shadows has been reported in Fijians and Indians (McKay *et al.* 1973).

Mongolism and mental deficiency occur.

Mental deficiency is not uncommon in the tropics. There is little information on the rarer lipidoses, metabolic or endocrine disorders. These include amaurotic familial idiocy, Niemann–Pick's and Gaucher's diseases—although we have seen the last two in Nigeria and diseases due to the impaired metabolism of the mucopolysaccharides—Hurler's, Hunter's and Morquio's diseases. Galactosaemia, glycogenosis and the aminoacidurias are other metabolic causes. Histidinaemia has been described in a Negro child (Kappelman *et al.* 1971).

Chromasomal abnormalities and mongolism occur. Indeed the 'normal' chromasomal pattern has still to be assessed in children in areas of stable malaria. Pellagra and porphyria may cause mental upset. The heavy metals —copper in Wilson's disease and chronic manganese poisoning in Chilean miners (Mena, 1967)—may also injure the brain. Toxoplasmosis and syphilis are common in various regions. Probably the most common cause of mental deficiency is infection in the newborn causing kernicterus. The part that parasitic infection (including malaria) and malnutrition play in impaired intelligence in children in the tropics is uncertain and discussed when these subjects are considered.

BACTERIAL INFECTION

Cerebral abscesses due to trauma, extension of infection from the middle ear, or of haematogenous origin, are common.

Pyogenic meningitis (Lontie *et al.* 1973), especially pneumococcal and meningococcal, are problems of magnitude in the tropics. The latter two differ markedly in their incidence from that described in temperate climates and are dealt with below.

Tuberculous meningitis is extremely common in many areas of the tropics and tuberculomas may present as a space-occupying lesion (p. 396). Cerebrospinal fluid (C.S.F.) immunoglobulins vary in different types of meningitis—thus IgM values are raised in purulent meningitis and significantly lower in viral meningitis, while IgA and IgG levels are increased in the C.S.F. in all forms of acute meningitis (Smith *et al.* 1973).

Tetanus is a common cause of death. Cerebral symptoms may occur in typhoid fever, bartonellosis, plague, and melioidosis, and neurological complications may occur in bacillary dysentery.

Leprosy is peculiar in that it affects primarily the peripheral nerves, and the central nervous system is not involved. As there are probably 15 million lepers in the world (Editorial, 1965) it must be considered the most important single condition in tropical neurology.

Neurosyphilis is common in many areas, excluding those in which yaws is, or was until recently, endemic. The meningovascular and paretic are the most common forms. Tabes and Argyll–Robertson pupil are exceedingly rare in Africa (Hutton, 1956; Masawe and German, 1972). In Indonesia tabes dorsalis is a common cause of optic atrophy but the Argyll–Robertson pupil and lightening pains are unusual (Palthe, 1950). Purely spinal forms of neurosyphilis are not seen in Trinidad (Habib, 1962) but are common in Hyderabad (Rao, 1954).

PNEUMOCOCCAL MENINGITIS

Pneumococcal meningitis is a disease of world-wide distribution affecting both sexes and all age groups. Various workers have suggested that the African is peculiarly susceptible to pneumococcal infections. The pathology differs only in that primary pneumococcal meningitis occurs much more commonly than in temperate climates. The condition rarely occurs as secondary to middle-ear disease (Heffron, 1939; Hutton, 1956). Lucas (1964) showed that pregnant and puerperal women in Nigeria were more liable to pneumococcal meningitis than non-pregnant women. The cerebrospinal fluid is under pressure and presents varying degrees of turbidity. On microscopic examination numerous polymorphonuclear leucocytes are seen and smears may reveal the causative organism, *Str. pneumoniae*, as Gram-positive lanceolate, capsulated, and mostly extracellular diplococci.

In some cases culture may be necessary to recover the organism. The protein content of the fluid is raised and the sugar reduced or absent.

CEREBROSPINAL MENINGITIS

Cerebrospinal meningitis occurs in Africa in cycles of violent epidemics every 15–20 years. The cycles have always started in the Republic of the Sudan and spread westwards. The disease manifests itself in epidemic form during the dry season and is confined to the arid regions of tropical Africa (Waddy, 1957; WHO, 1973). Absolute humidity, the degree and duration of crowding, as well as inadequacy of ventilation are important epidemiological factors (Waddy, 1952). The meningococcus—the causative organism—most frequently inhabits the nasopharynx and is transmitted from person to person by droplet spread. The carrier rate increases prior to the onset of epidemics (Leading Article, 1974).

It should be remembered, however, that C.S.M. can very occasionally present as an acute septicaemia with shock and a generalized purpuric rash without evidence of meningitis. Adrenal haemorrhage may be found (the Waterhouse–Friderichsen syndrome). Subarachnoid haemorrhage has also been noted as a rare complication (Huskisson and Hart, 1969). The shock has been considered in some patients to be due to the adrenal haemorrhage, in others to disseminated intravascular coagulation demonstrated by fibrin thrombi at necropsy and by thrombocytopenia and diminished levels of fibrinogen and factors V and VIII in patients. If this is caused by a generalized Schwartzman reaction heparin would be useful in therapy.

If, on the other hand, the thrombosis is caused by direct involvement of the meningococci on the vessel wall as postulated by Hill and Kinney (1947) heparin might be harmful. Conflicting reports have been given on the use of steroids.

It is of interest that recently Whittle et al. (1973) have discussed the complications of arthritis, cutaneous vasculitis and episcleritis which occur in a small proportion of patients suffering from C.S.M. Histological and bacteriological study of the lesions of the arthritis and vasculitis suggested that they were not due to the infection itself but were probably due to an immune complex disease. Greenwood et al. (1973) demonstrated circulating meningococcal antigen at the time of presentation in four patients with these conditions. Circulating antibody was detected in three and a marked fall in the serum C_3 level occurred in two. Deposits of antigen, immunoglobulin, and C_3 were detected in synovial fluid, white cells and in one of three skin biopsies examined which was considered further evidence in favour of the lesion in the joints and skin having an immunological basis. Whittle et al. (1974) have devised a latex agglutination test for the rapid diagnosis of pyogenic meningitis.

The findings at necropsy are those described in standard textbooks. The diagnosis should always be confirmed by examination of the cerebrospinal fluid as isolated cases of pneumococcal meningitis can occur in cerebrospinal meningitis epidemics. The cerebrospinal fluid is under pressure, turbid, and frankly purulent. The cells and protein content are raised while the sugar is absent or greatly reduced. The causative organism—*Neisseria meningitides* —is seen on smears as a Gram-negative, oval, mostly intracellular diplococcus, or can be cultured.

VIRAL AND RICKETTSIAL DISEASES

Viral meningo-encephalitis is ubiquitous, poliomyelitis, dengue, and rabies being particularly widespread and common.

In the rickettsial diseases, vertigo, photophobia, meningism, and bulbar labiopharyngeal paralyses occur.

Post-measles encephalitis is an entity.

FUNGAL DISEASES

As yet, the systemic mycoses would not appear to be a common cause of disease of the nervous system in the tropics, although occasional cases have been described especially from Cuba (Hernandez *et al.* 1972). The possibility of a cryptococcal infection should be remembered in meningitis and occasional cases of cerebral mucormycosis have been reported.

THE PARASITIC DISEASES

It has been suggested that heavy parasitic infections may impair the mental capacity of children in the tropics, but further studies are required on this problem.

Cerebral malaria is still a problem in parts of the tropics. Whether residual brain damage occurs with any frequency is debatable. The presence of numerous other infections capable of affecting the brain in areas where malaria is prevalent renders diagnosis difficult.

Trypanosomiasis is still widespread in many parts of Africa and *Angiostrongylus cantonensis* has recently been shown to be an important cause of eosinophilic meningitis in the Far East. Hydatid disease and cysticercosis have a limited geographical distribution. Schistosomiasis can affect the brain or cord and *Toxocara canis* and toxoplasmosis produce cerebral symptoms. Primary amoebic meningo encephalitis has been described (p. 77; van den Driesche, 1973).

In the stage of migration many of the parasites of man may produce transitory acute cerebral symptoms. The possibility of a parasitic infection must always be considered as a possible cause of a neurological disorder in the tropics. Symptomatic epilepsy may be a complication of a number of parasitic diseases, e.g. cysticercosis (Powell *et al.* 1966). Idiopathic epilepsy is, however, common and accounts for the majority of cases (Levy *et al.* 1964; Dada and Odeku, 1966; Billingshurst *et al.* 1973). In Africa it occurs in children and adults usually below the age of 30 years, with males perhaps more frequently affected than females. The sociological aspects of the disorder are discussed by the above-mentioned authors. It should be noted that the epileptic is particularly prone to the complications of 'traditional' therapy. Epilepsy in Africa has been reviewed by Osuntokun and Odeku (1970). Before a diagnosis of idiopathic epilepsy is made infection, primary metabolic disorders, and intracranial lesions must be excluded.

VASCULAR DISEASE

The most common cause of cerebral vascular accidents is hypertension—either essential or secondary. Cerebral atherosclerosis is seen, but in its greatest severity is associated with hypertension, with the coronary arteries and aorta very much less affected. Cerebral thrombosis and haemorrhage associated with atheroma in the absence of hypertension is, in general, much less common. Senile dementia due to atherosclerosis is also not common. Cerebral vascular lesions, however, especially thrombosis, are common in West Central India and are found in the lower socio-economic groups (Dalal *et al.* 1968) and non-embolic ischaemic cerebrovascular disease is common in Nigeria (Osuntokun *et al.* 1969).

In the Indian sub-continent and parts of Africa arteriovenous malformations are a common cause of subarachnoid haemorrhage than aneurysms in contrast to the Western world. The aneurysms are not uncommon however in parts of West Africa (Collomb *et al.* 1966).

Cerebral venous and dural sinus thrombosis may occur secondarily to middle-ear or nasal sinus infection or primarily in malnourished children or adults. It is not recorded as a common complication in kwashiorkor. Cerebral thrombophlebitis in puerperal women has been described in West Africa (Payet and Armengaud, 1957).

Arteritis of obscure aetiology may cause cerebral and ocular symptoms or hypertensive encephalopathy.

Cerebral complications may also occur in sickle-cell disease, thrombocytopenic purpura, and other blood disorders.

TRAUMA

Traumatic lesions of the head and spinal cord are common in most areas of the tropics. Spinal injuries are particularly common in palm-wine tappers in West Africa. Cervical spondylosis is not as common in Bombay and Ibadan as it is in the Western World (Spillane, 1969).

DEGENERATIVE DISEASES

We have no information on the relative incidence of congenital spastic diplegia and birth palsy in the tropics. Spastic conditions do certainly occur in young children. Sydenham's chorea is not common. Tuberous sclerosis (Cosnett and Gibb, 1969; Olurin et al. 1971), progressive muscular atrophy, and amyotrophic lateral sclerosis have been recorded. The high incidence of the last condition in Guam is discussed below. Motor neurone disease is a disease of late middle life in the Western world but progressive muscular atrophy, amyotrophic lateral sclerosis and chronic bulbar palsy are seen in young adults in Southern India (Jaggannathan, 1972)—*juvenile motor neurone disease*. We have no information on the incidence of syringomyelia, Friedreich's ataxia or Alzheimer's disease. Parkinson's disease occurs and a parkinsonism–dementia complex, associated with the high incidence of amyotrophic lateral sclerosis, has been noted in Guam.

ENCEPHALOPATHY AND FATTY DEGENERATION OF THE VISCERA

This was first described by Brain et al. (1929). However, Reye et al. (1963) described the syndrome in twenty-three children in Australia aged 5 months to $8\frac{1}{2}$ years old. Fourteen were aged 2 years or less. Clinically there were profoundly disturbed consciousness, fever, convulsions, vomiting, disturbed respiratory rhythm, altered muscle tone, and altered reflexes. Hypoglycaemia was common, and the serum transaminases were raised. Ketones might be found in the urine and a neutrophil leucocytosis was usual. The blood urea may be raised. The pathological changes at post mortem were cerebral swelling, a slightly enlarged, firm and uniformly bright yellow liver and pallor and slight widening of the renal cortex. Histologically there was swelling of the cortical neurones. Others might be shrunken and deeply staining. The astrocytes and oligoglia were also swollen. In the liver all hepatocytes showed fatty degeneration, being packed with fatty droplets differing from the picture seen in kwashiorkor where a large fat globule fills the cell. There was no necrosis or other cellular changes excluding the occasional case in which a narrow zone of necrosis was seen about the portal tracts. In the kidney fatty degeneration occurred in the proximal tubules and loops of Henle. The glomeruli, vessels and interstitial tissue were normal. Fatty change also occurred in the myocardium and pancreas. No pathological changes were noted in the remaining organs. Reactive changes in lymphoid tissues have also now been noted. Sociological and toxicological studies revealed no evidence of any likely poisonous material. It differs from the vomiting sickness of Jamaica in that there is no necrosis of liver, kidney and pancreatic cells. Becroft (1966) reported the condition in nine children in New Zealand and noted that cases had been reported from Europe and South Africa.

The mortality would appear to be very high. Blood sugar levels and liver biopsy would appear to be most helpful in diagnosis. Olsen *et al.* (1970) have reported the condition endemic in North Eastern Thailand, an area in which rice is the staple, and cases of protein–calorie malnutrition, beri-beri, iron deficiency anaemia, Vitamin B_{12} deficiency and bladder stone are not uncommon.

Death frequently occurs within 48 hours of the onset. Survivors may show evidence of residual neurological defects. It has been suggested that aflatoxin may be concerned in the aetiology (Bourgeois *et al.* 1971; Becroft and Webster, 1972). If this is so the condition should occur in tropical Africa and India.

INFANTILE TREMOR SYNDROME

This has been described from various parts of India. The infants between the ages of 6 and 24 months show developmental retardation, apathy, hypokinesis and the sudden onset of tremors (Pownowalla *et al.* 1960; Sachdeva *et al.* 1965; Baipa *et al.* 1965). It differs from the tremors occasionally seen in children recovering from kwashiorkor. There are no particular reflex changes and it is usually self-limiting, but subsequent mental retardation is common. Anaemia is present. The C.S.F. is normal. The cause is unknown (Tandon and Bajpai, 1973).

AMYOTROPHIC LATERAL SCLEROSIS AND PARKINSONISM–DEMENTIA COMPLEX

The above two conditions have not been reported as common in any areas of the tropics, except in Guam and other Mariana Islands, in which a high incidence has been noted for decades. There are two other foci of high incidence of amyotrophic lateral sclerosis in the Pacific, in the Kii peninsula of Japan and in south-west New Guinea (Editorial, 1965). Other diseases such as gout, diaphyseal aclasis, diabetes, cirrhosis, and cancer of the liver are also found in high incidence in Guam.

The seeds of *Cycas circinalis* L. are ingested in this island as a source of carbohydrate, especially in times of famine. Neurological disorders have been produced in rhesus monkeys by feeding meal or leaves from *C. circinalis* and the water-soluble toxin, cycasin, produces a haemorrhagic centrilobular necrosis of the liver in laboratory animals. The part that the cycads play in the aetiology of any of these conditions in man is, as yet, unproven (Proceedings, 1964). Genetic transmission is thought unlikely as amyotrophic lateral sclerosis has been seen within the immigrant Carolinian community and both conditions have been noted in a few Filipinos and whites (Mathai, 1970). It was considered that the exogenous factor might be a virus. On the other hand an irregular autosomal dominant mode of inheritance has been suggested in the aetiology of A.L.S. in the mountainous Kii peninsula of Japan (Yase, 1970).

Pathology

Amyotrophic lateral sclerosis causes 10 per cent of adult deaths in Guam and the incidence is one hundred times that reported in any other population. It affects primarily the anterior horn cells in the cord and the pyramidal tracts, causing weakness, wasting, and fibrillary tremors in muscles. Wasting in the small muscles of the hand or spasticity of the lower limbs may be the presenting symptom. Bulbar palsy occurs terminally.

In the parkinsonism–dementia complex the involvement of the central nervous system manifests itself in the fifth and sixth decades. Motor neurone involvement is marked. Death occurs 3–5 years after onset. In the brain, cortical atrophy occurs and there is widespread ganglion-cell degenertion throughout the grey matter and basal nuclei of the cerebral hemispheres and brain stem.

DEMYELINATING DISORDERS

Post infectious encephalomyelitis is common but multiple sclerosis is rare in the tropics. The prevalence of multiple sclerosis in general increases with increasing distance from the equator. The relationship between diet and the geographical distribution of multiple sclerosis has been discussed by Agranoff and Goldberg (1974). It is uncommon in China, Japan, India, and Korea (Barlow, 1967). It is also rare in Israel, Mexico, and Africa, but increasing in South African whites (Bird and Kerrich, 1969). Three proven cases have been reported from Senegal (Collomb et al. 1970) and in 17 years two cases have been seen in Kenya (Foster and Harries, 1970). The clinical and diagnostic aspects of the disease have been reviewed by McAlpine (1973). Immigrants from a high-risk area to a low-risk area retain the prevalence rate of their source of origin and we have seen the condition first manifest itself in Europeans in West Africa who, however, annually visited Britain. It is somewhat less common in the American Negro than the white. Differences in the clinical expression have been noted in Northern- and Southern-born U.S. Negroes (Alter, 1962). It would appear that environmental rather than racial factors are important in the aetiology of the disease and Dean (1967) has suggested an infection in infancy may be responsible. Many virus antigens have been studied but significant prevalence of raised antibody titres has only been found to the measles virus. This is difficult to explain as in Africa measles is a common and severe infection whereas multiple sclerosis is rare. It may be, however, that the altered immunological status of the host in Africa, due to multiple infections and infestations, may prevent the formation of sufficient antibody to allow of antigen–antibody complexes to form—this must be regarded as purely speculative.

There is a condition which is known as demyelinating neuropathy (Trowell, 1960) which is relatively common in most tropical areas. Its relationship with a spastic type of neuropathy described in the West Indies (Montgomery *et al.* 1964) is obscure and both are described below. It should, however, be noted that demyelinating neuropathy may, in the future, have to be classified as a toxic neuropathy as there is evidence which suggests that dietary cyanide intoxication is an important factor in its causation (Monekosso and Wilson, 1966; Oshuntokun, 1968; *Lancet*, 1973).

Subacute myelo-optico neuropathy is a new neurological disorder described in Japan. It is mainly a disease of adults. Prodromal symptoms with pain and diarrhoea are usual. Sensory changes then occur with numbness and paraesthesia with a degree of ataxia. Paraplegia may occur. The optic nerve is involved in about 25 per cent of patients with complaints of loss of vision and optic atrophy in about 5 per cent. Mortality is about 4 per cent with blindness occurring in about 2 per cent of patients. Recovery is slow. There is segmental demyelinization of nerves in the posterior columns of the spinal cord, the pyramidal tracts and in the optic nerves and chiasma (Shiraki, 1971). A greenish fur on the tongue and greenish urine were noted in some patients. This was found to be due to the presence of the drug clioquinol. This drug is widely used throughout the world for various forms of diarrhoea. It belongs to the group of halogenated oxyquinolines. Due to the work of Tsubaki *et al.* (1971) the drug was banned in Japan and it would appear that the prevalence of the disease is diminishing. A few cases have also been noted in Australia. Clioquinol is widely used throughout the world in various forms of diarrhoea and it would appear that the disease is rare outside Japan. There is therefore possibly a further factor involved and this may be viral or genetic.

NEUROPATHIC SYNDROME OF UNCERTAIN ORIGIN

Synonyms. Tropical ataxic neuropathy; central neuritis; tropical nutritional ambylopia and retrobulbar neuritis; nutritional neuropathy of warm climates; demyelinating and spastic neuropathies.

A number of unusual degenerative neuropathies occur in the tropics. Sensory ataxia, optic atrophy, and nerve deafness are features of these syndromes, accompanied with or without mucocutaneous lesions suggesting vitamin B deficiencies (Money, 1959; Haddock *et al.* 1962). Cruickshank (1956) has described similar cases from the West Indies, but many of his patients showed evidence of an upper motor neurone lesion. In Nigeria, as in the West Indies, 'tropical amblyopia' is also common (Degazon, 1956;

Monekosso and Ashby, 1963). Reports indicate that the clinical picture may differ in the same place at different times (Rowland, 1963).

Spillane (1969) has reviewed the Jamaican, Nigerian and Senegalese neuropathies. Pyramidal signs are much more common in the Jamaican form. Few changes have been reported in the C.S.F. in this condition until recently when positive colloidal gold tests (paretic) have been noted in a third of patients. The part that treponemal infection plays in this neuropathy is controversial but the majority of workers on the evidence available consider it an unlikely aetiological agent.

Nerve deafness and retrobulbar neuropathy are more common in the Nigerian form and pyramidal signs much less common. There may be evidence of ariboflavinosis. There is no evidence of a syphilitic aetiology, a finding also present in the Senegalese form (Collomb et al. 1967).

The sex incidence is equal, and the age group 20–39 years in the poorer classes is most frequently affected. A familial incidence has occasionally been noted. Numerous factors—nutritional deficiencies, treponemal, or other infections, and neurotoxic substances—have been considered in the aetiology (Montgomery, 1965). Moore (1934) and Clark (1936) first suggested that cassava was related to the retrobulbar neuropathy seen in Nigeria and the latter author suggested that the toxic factor was cyanide. The aetiology of the Jamaican type of neuropathy is obscure but in Nigeria there is considerable evidence that chronic cyanide intoxication of dietary origin is the most important factor in its aetiology (Osuntokun and Aladetoyinbo, 1970; Monekosso and Wilson, 1966). Serum transferrin has been shown to be normal in these patients whereas serum caeruloplasmin is lower compared with normal controls (Osuntokun and Williams, 1970). In India, vitamin B_{12} has been considered an important aetiological agent (Jeejebhoy et al. 1967).

Pathology

The condition is rarely fatal and ataxia, paraesthesiae, weakness, clumsy hands, worsening vision, tinnitus, and deafness are slowly progressive. Deep reflexes are absent and associated signs of ariboflavinosis and malnutrition are common. Paraesthesiae include numbness and a burning sensation in the feet and lower legs.

Demyelinization of the optic, auditory, posterior column, and spinal nerves of the lower limbs are the main pathological findings. In the Nigerian neuropathy light and electron microscopy studies of peripheral nerves revealed a non-specific demyelinization as seen in other segmental demyelinative neuropathies. Similar changes were noted in the sciatic nerve of rats after injection of a single dose of potassium cyanide which was considered further evidence that cyanides may play a significant role in the pathogenesis of ataxic neuropathy in Nigerians (Williams and Osuntokun, 1969). The cerebrospinal fluid is usually normal, as are liver-function tests. Anaemia is not a marked feature and there is no evidence of vitamin-B_{12} deficiency in Africa or the West Indies.

In the West Indies and other areas of the tropics a spastic type of tropical neuropathy is common, with the associated syndrome, in many patients, of a demyelinating neuropathy (Montgomery *et al.* 1964). An older age group is usually affected and cerebrospinal fluid changes occur in about 40 per cent of patients and evidence of a treponemal infection is found in approximately 60 per cent. The pathological changes are those of a chronic inflammatory condition affecting the cord and to a lesser extent the brain. Patchy meningeal thickening, especially basal, may be noted. There is no endarteritis or thrombosis and the cellular exudate is predominantly lymphocytic with a few monocytes and plasma cells. There is a loss of myelin in the lateral pyramidal tracts and posterior columns of Gall. The spinothalamic and cerebellar tracts are occasionally affected. It is undecided whether these two conditions are separate entities or are manifestations of a similar disease process.

TOXIC, NUTRITIONAL, AND METABOLIC DISORDERS

The only important condition which occurs in the tropics and has not been dealt with elsewhere is lathyrism, and this is discussed in this section.

Alcoholic drinks, methyl alcohol, Indian hemp, lead, arsenic, carbon-monoxide poisoning, and the venom of certain snakes may affect the central nervous system. Ackee and other toxic substances, as well as hyper-insulinism, may cause hypoglycaemia with resulting cerebral anoxia. The effect of heatstroke and hyperpyrexia are dealt with on p. 735.

Pellagra, beri-beri, and Wernicke's encephalopathy are common in certain areas of the tropics. Subacute combined degeneration of the cord is generally considered to be rare. Hepatic coma, due to a high level of ammonia in the blood, occurs in diseases of the liver, especially cirrhosis. Severe protein deficiency causes pathological changes in the central nervous system but little is known of the long-term effects of these lesions in man.

Tay Sach's and Wilson's diseases are very rare, but porphyria and phenylketonuria occur. A case of Wilson's disease has been described in Senegal (Dumas *et al.* 1970).

Lathyrism

Human lathyrism occurs at times in India and occasional cases have been reported from Africa. It is caused by the ingestion of peas of the genus *Lathyrus*. Domestic animals may also be affected (Weaver and Spittell,

1964). The species which cause disease in man (*L. sativus*, *L. cicera*, and *L. clymenum*) are not toxic to rats. β amino proprionitrile isolated from other species of *Lathyrus*, however, causes lesions of elastic tissue with defective fibrogenesis in rats, mice, and chicks. In man there is an acute onset of weakness in the lower limbs at times preceded by pain and paraesthesia. A spastic paraplegia results. Spondylosis and other skeletal lesions follow from the resulting increased stress. The mechanism of the causation is unknown. Lathyrism usually occurs in times of famine and the possibility of its being a demyelinating (nutritional) neuropathy should be borne in mind (Trowell, 1960), but the former is usually a purely pyramidal tract disorder without the ocular and aural complications frequently seen in the latter.

DISORDERS OF THE CRANIAL AND PERIPHERAL NERVES

Retrobulbar neuritis is a relatively common condition. It is rare in childhood and the sexes are equally affected in adult life. It may progress to optic atrophy. A sudden or gradual onset of dimness of vision is the usual presenting complaint.

The aetiology is frequently obscure. Multiple sclerosis and syphilis should, of course, be excluded. It is a common finding in the demyelinating neuropathy of the tropics, and pellagra and beri-beri may be associated conditions. Toxic substances and drug therapy (tryparsamide, quinine, arsenic, and mepacrine) must always be considered. The condition does, however, occur in the professional classes in the tropics with no obvious background of infectious, toxic, or dietary factors. Steroid therapy in these circumstances has been helpful.

Colour blindness in many tropical peoples is surprisingly common.

Bell's palsy occurs but trigeminal neuralgia is thought to be rare.

Peripheral nervous disorders due to cervical spondylosis or vertebral disc lesions are uncommon and the carpal tunnel syndrome has not, to our knowledge, been described in the tropics.

Excluding leprosy, which has previously been mentioned, polyneuritis is still common. Standard textbooks of medicine and neurology enumerate almost a hundred possible causes but in spite of this in more than 50 per cent of clinical cases the aetiological factor or factors cannot be detected (Miller, 1966).

Toxic agents and diseases previously mentioned, vitamin deficiencies, tuberculosis, diabetes, and diphtheria, must be considered. In this connection it should be remembered that diphtheritic ulcers of the extremities may be responsible for localized nervous lesions.

It is strange that no mention of polyneuritis associated with malignant disease has yet appeared in tropical areas.

TUMOURS OF THE CENTRAL NERVOUS SYSTEM

Tumours of the central nervous system in the tropics would appear to be less common than in temperate zones. A report on their incidence in five continents (Doll *et al.* 1966) shows the incidence to be low in Uganda, Japan, Nigeria, Chile, the Chinese in Singapore, the Bantu in Johannesburg, and in the West Indies. In our experience caution should at present be exercised in completely accepting these findings, at least from Nigeria (where our own figures are low). The number of cerebral tumours detected is dependent upon the presence of adequate neurosurgical facilities and a recent report from Nigeria where these facilities have recently been instituted suggests that cerebral tumours are not uncommon (Odeku, 1965; Odeku and Janota, 1967). In this report gliomas were more frequent than meningiomas. This has also been shown in Uganda by a sudden rise in the diagnosis of intracranial tumours in the last few years (Bailly, 1973).

Tumours of the reticulo-endothelial system (including the Burkitt) frequently invade the meninges and cerebral cranial nerve and spinal cord tissue. Secondary deposits of chorion cancer are common in the brain and are not infrequently the presenting symptom. Metastases from the breast and lung are less commonly seen. Other space-occupying lesions such as the tuberculoma, gumma, and parasitic diseases are discussed in their appropriate context.

Simple tumours of the nerve roots and peripheral nerves are not uncommon in the tropics and include the schwannoma (neurilemmoma) and both solitary and generalized (von Recklinghausen's disease) neurofibromatous tumours.

Chordomas and teratomas occur and the retinoblastoma is common. A pinealoma is occasionally seen and it is of interest that pineal gland calcification which is common in adults in Western countries (50–70 per cent) has been found to be much less frequent in Fijians and Indians in Fiji (McKay, 1973).

Retinoblastoma

The tumour arises from the nuclear layers of the retina and is usually multifocal in origin. It may be inherited as an autosomal dominant characteristic with irregular penetrance or arise as a spontaneous mutation. It is bilateral in 20–39 per cent of patients. The incidence is considered to be in the region of 1 in 25,000 births. It would appear to be common in parts of Africa (Kodilinye, 1967) where the tumour is usually undifferentiated and frequently presents a diagnostic problem, as in small biopsies the resemblance to the Burkitt tumour and neuroblastoma may be close. Malignant cells have been seen in the cerebrospinal fluid. On phase contrast the cells are twice the size of lymphocytes, have pale nuclei with distinct nucleoli, and scanty cytoplasm containing fine granules and pseudopodia may be seen. In culture there is cohesion of cells in aggregates or in long, branching chains (Ifekwunigwe *et al.* 1966).

MENTAL ILLNESS

Although there is a shortage of trained psychiatrists in most areas of the tropics knowledge of psychiatric syndromes is gradually emerging—and transcultural psychiatry is fashionable. Its aim is to improve psychiatry in countries and cultures other than those in which the speciality originated. Existing assumptions are tested in a different environment and new theories necessarily developed (Murphy, 1973). It would appear that the well-known psychiatric syndromes occur in all areas. Depressive states and schizophrenia are common. The frequency of hysterical syndromes varies in different geographical areas—being uncommon in West Africa in contrast to parts of the Indian continent. Suicide is common in certain regions but said to be low in Mohammedan communities. Opium addiction occurs, and the taking of Indian hemp and amphetamines is causing concern, at least in West Africa. Traditional healers are frequently consulted but their success in therapy is unknown as only the disastrous effects or failures present themselves to the modern, trained psychiatrist. In any patient suffering from mental illness a complete investigation is indicated as we have seen inmates of asylums who have proved to be suffering from trypanosomiasis—to say nothing of a syphilitic infection.

13

The Urinary and Reproductive Systems

THE KIDNEY

There is little information available on normal kidney function in the tropics. In Nigerians in Lagos the blood urea levels are lower than comparable values in Europeans; this is not a genetic factor as urea levels were found to be at normal European levels in Nigerians in London (Kenney, 1953). Urea clearance and concentration tests have been shown to give low values and the specific gravity of the urine also tends to be low. Urinary pH values have been found to be higher in African women when compared with the values in Europeans and Asians in East Africa (Wing *et al.* 1971). An increased sensitivity of extracellular fluid volume which may be due to environmental temperature has been noted in Nigerians (Elebute, 1971). Hyposthenuria occurs in heterozygous and homozygous carriers of the sickle-cell gene (p. 430).

Congenital anomalies do not appear to differ in their incidence and types in tropical and temperate zones. The incidence of essential hypertension has already been discussed (p. 376) and the hypertensive kidney, either benign or malignant, is common in our experience. The senile arteriosclerotic kidney is not so common and reflects the age grouping of the population in the tropics and the relative mildness of atherosclerosis.

A. DISEASES OF THE GLOMERULI (GLOMERULONEPHRITIS)

The introduction of renal biopsy techniques has radically altered older concepts of glomerulonephritis. Clinical management in many patients depends upon renal histology.* A satisfactory classification of the pathology of glomerular lesions is therefore essential. Brewer (1964) has divided classifiers into those who recognize only a few divisions, 'the lumpers', and those who propose many, 'the splitters'. In temperate climates it is frequently impossible to specify the aetiological agent responsible for glomerular lesions—focal glomerulonephritis being a case in point. This problem is even more difficult in the tropics when the multiple infections and

*Studies on immunofluorescent techniques, levels of serum complement and renal clearance of plasma proteins are being pursued but none to date has proved more effective than biopsy.

616

infestations to which the population are exposed are remembered. It may well be, therefore, that in the tropics it will be found worthwhile for the pathologist to be a 'splitter' and to describe the pathology in detail, in the earnest hope that the clinician will undertake every possible laboratory test available to discover the underlying aetiology in individual patients.

Some definition of the terminology employed in glomerular lesions is necessary as there is considerable confusion in the literature (Mostofi, 1966). We have adopted the descriptive terms most frequently used in recent publications which alters the terminology we ourselves have used in the past. The term 'general' implies that the majority or all of the glomeruli are affected, and 'focal' that only some of the glomeruli are damaged and that others are normal. 'Diffuse' implies that the whole of the glomerular tuft and 'segmental' that only a part is involved.

Ellis type I and II nephritis are descriptive clinically but the expansion in knowledge of the pathological lesions seen in glomerulonephritis since they were first described renders them obsolete. A patient with the clinical type II presentation of Ellis may show the classical type I (proliferative) glomerular changes. In addition the 'minimal change' kidney with no lesions observable on light microscopy was not included in the Ellis classification. The term 'subacute nephritis' is not used here, as it is ambiguous and may convey different meanings to the clinician and the pathologist.

Glomerulonephritis is therefore not a single disease but a group of diseases and as the glomeruli receive a very high proportion of the cardiac output they are particularly susceptible to circulating pathogens. Some forms of glomerular damage are associated with systemic disease but in the great majority of cases the glomeruli are primarily involved. It is the latter group to which the term glomerulonephritis should be applied at least by the pathologist describing the histological appearances. Clinically the term 'nephritis' both acute and chronic may be preferable. Although an association between infection and immunity and glomerulonephritis has been postulated since the beginning of the century it is only within the last decade that rapid advances have been made in our knowledge as new immunological and bioassay techniques have been developed (Peters, 1974).

In man we have two forms of chronic nephritis in whom it has been established beyond reasonable doubt that chronic soluble complex deposition plays a major part in pathogenesis. These are the nephritis of systemic lupus erythematosis and the nephropathy associated with quartan malaria. The antigens (DNA and *P. malariae* respectively) have been detected in immune deposits within the glomeruli and specific antibody can be eluted from the renal tissue (Cameron, 1972). Antigens are being sought in other forms of glomerulonephritis associated with tumours (rare) and a number of infections including viral. It should not be forgotten that nephritis may be associated with mumps, measles, infectious hepatitis, E.C.H.O. and adenovirus infections and chickenpox. Australian antigen has also been implicated. An anti-kidney antibody has been detected in Goodpasture's syndrome and is probably an anti-glomerular-basement-membrane antibody. The glomeruli react in a number of ways to immunological insults, depending upon a number of factors, including host response and the antigen involved. It is thought that the deposition of antigen–antibody complexes in the kidney activate complement.

The activation of complement (which consists of nine main proteins and a number of associated ions and cofactors) produces a most involved chain reaction including the attraction of leucocytes, the release of vasoactive peptides and increased vascular permeability and the activation of the 'cascade' of coagulation with platelet aggregation and fibrin deposition that can lead to secondary fibrosis and scarring and possibly to the activation of specifically cytotoxic antibody (Cochrane and Dixon, 1968). The activation of complement may depress the C3 component (which is an excellent screening test for total complement) in the blood, measured as beta 1C globulin. These facts are leading to new thoughts in therapy which have been epitomized by Cameron (1972) in Table 13.1.

TABLE 13.1. *Possible levels of treatment for glomerulonephritis* (after Cameron, 1972)

	Mode of therapy	Application
Therapy directed at antigen	(1) Avoidance of antigen	*P. malariae*
	(2) Removal of antigen	Chemotherapy of infection. Removal of tumour
	(3) Induction of tolerance to antigen	? Cyclophosphamide
Therapy directed at antibody	(4) Suppression of antibody formation	Cytotoxic agents, corticosteroids
	(5) Inhibition of complement activity	Heparin
	(6) Inhibition of fibrin formation	Heparin, warfarin
Therapy directed at mediators of injury	(7) Inhibition of platelet aggregation	Corticosteroids, indomethacin, dypyridamole, heparin, aspirin
	(8) Inhibition and stabilization of leucocytes	Corticosteroids, indomethacin, aspirin
	(9) Inhibition of kinins, histamine, SRA ? A release	Cromoglycate, diethylcarbamazine

With this brief description of the immunological aspects of renal glomerular disease we proceed to the classification which is given below.

Classification of glomerulonephritis (Heptinstall, 1966)

1. Generalized acute diffuse glomerulonephritis.
2. Rapidly progressive glomerulonephritis.
3. Chronic glomerulonephritis including chronic lobular and chronic membranous forms.
4. Focal glomerulonephritis.
5. Forms of glomerulonephritis associated with the nephrotic syndrome. (These are described when conditions giving rise to the nephrotic syndrome are discussed.)

1. Acute diffuse proliferative glomerulonephritis

Acute diffuse proliferative glomerulonephritis and its sequelae occur in the tropics and its aetiology is related to streptococcal infection both tonsillar but most commonly probably cutaneous (Gallacher and Miller, 1967; Whittle *et al.* 1973). The latter authors noted an association with scabies and pyoderma with a seasonal incidence. Upper respiratory infections may also be followed by nephritis. In contrast to the continued prevalence of streptococcal M type 12 in many tonsillar and respiratory infections seven different M type strains have been associated at different times in Trinidad with acute glomerulonephritis associated with skin lesions (Potter *et al.* 1971). Whittle *et al.* (1973) noted a similar phenomenon in Nigeria. The latent period is usually 10 days following a throat infection but may be 3 weeks or longer with skin infections. It is of interest that the dermal nephritogenic streptococci are associated with little or no rheumatic fever (Bisno *et al.* 1970). This may be of epidemiological interest, as although rheumatic heart disease is common in many tropical areas as previously stated (p. 371), chorea and severe acute rheumatic fever are rarely diagnosed. It is possible that streptococcal skin lesions may be associated with a milder form of the condition affecting chronically the myocardium. Clinically the patient, usually a child aged 3 to 15 years, present classically with haematuria, malaise and periorbital oedema. In the tropics ascites and dependent oedema, simulating the nephrotic syndrome clinically, may be present, probably due to the anaemia and hypoalbuminaemia which is so common in children in many tropical areas. Hypertension and pulmonary congestion are usual with erythrocytes, leucocytes, casts and protein in a lowered, concentrated urinary output as additional findings. On the other hand it may present simply as haematuria with no other symptoms. The condition is usually benign, but heart failure, uraemia, and hypertensive encephalopathy can occur. No direct relationship with malaria or other tropical infection has been demonstrated in tropical populations but Berger *et al.* (1967) have reported occurrence of acute glomerulonephritis and the nephrotic syndrome in a small percentage of adult non-immunes suffering from *P. falciparum* malaria in Vietnam. Albuminuria and haematuria were not uncommon in these patients. The prognosis, however, was good.

Most attempts to demonstrate streptococcal antigens in renal lesions in post-streptococcal nephritis have been negative even although the lesions in the glomeruli on electron microscopy appear to be of the soluble complex type with 'lumpy deposits' seen on the epithelial surface of the glomerular capillary basement membrane as seen in the experimental type of soluble complex nephritis in laboratory animals. These 'humps' show the presence of Ig and complement by fluorescent antibody techniques and the pattern is granular, in contrast to the smooth linear pattern seen in Goodpasture's syndrome due to anti-kidney antibodies. The serum immunoglobulin is raised and the complement level is low as measured by BiC globulin during the first few weeks of the disease. If the complement level in the serum fails to rise after eight weeks following an attack of acute diffuse glomerulone-phritis a chronic renal disease should be suspected—probably membrano-proliferative glomerulonephritis.

Most patients recover completely but a proportion may develop the nephrotic syndrome and/or progress to chronic glomerulonephritis. The pathology of the kidney in the nephrotic syndrome is described on p. 625 as proliferative glomerulonephritis.

The pathology of the acute stage is as follows. All glomeruli show active endothelial and mesangeal cells proliferation within the tuft. The glomeruli are swollen and avascular. Fibrin thrombi may be seen in the capillaries and may be of prognostic value. In this connection Clarkson *et al.* (1971) have recently studied the serum and urine concentration of fibrin/fibrinogen degradation products (F.D.P.) in patients with glomerulonephritis by an immunoassay technique. It was considered that the urinary concentration provided a reliable and sensitive index of activity, progression and natural history in proliferative glomerulonephritis. The urinary F.D.P. content was thought to indicate lysis of intraglomerular fibrin deposits. Abnormal concentrations were present but much lower in patients with the minimal change kidney and membranous glomerulonephritis. Daily measurements of urinary F.D.P. concentration were thought to be of potential value in the differential diagnosis of patients with glomerulonephritis.

Erythrocytes may be present in Bowman's space and in the tubules. In a few patients an exudative lesion with necrosis and polymorphonuclear leucocytosis in the tuft may be seen. Fibrinoid necrosis and thrombosis of the afferent arteriole or glomerular capillaries can occur. On electron microscopy the capillary basement membrane shows electron dense deposits and the characteristic 'humps' are seen on the epithelial surface with focal fusion of the foot processes of the epithelial cells. Electron dense deposits are also seen in the mesangium. A case of glomerulonephritis associated with acute toxoplasmosis has been described (Ginsburg *et al.* 1974).

2. Rapidly progressive glomerulonephritis

Synonyms. Rapidly progressive type I of Ellis; subacute glomerulonephritis; active epithelial proliferative glomerulonephritis.

This has been well described by Heptinstall (1966). There may or may not be a history of streptococcal infection. An attack of acute nephritis is followed by increasing nitrogen retention and an increase in blood pressure. Hypoalbuminaemia may occur in some patients, resulting in a form of nephrotic syndrome. Red blood cells, granular, and white blood cell casts are present in the urine. Usually there is progressive deterioration in renal function, with death in renal failure some months after onset. Most patients are young adults.

It is considered that the condition may be due to the production of an anti-glomerular basement membrane antibody which cross-reacts with other basement membranes. In the kidney, IgG has been shown by fluorescent antibody techniques to be present in a smooth linear pattern along the glomerular basement membrane, and the antibody may be responsible for the associated pulmonary haemorrhages seen in Goodpasture's syndrome which is associated with this condition. This is a rare syndrome and has to be differentiated from other conditions in which pulmonary haemorrhage may be associated with glomerulonephritis. These include idiopathic pulmonary haemosiderosis, uraemic pneumonitis, acute glomerulonephritis with congestive cardiac failure, pneumonia complicated by nephritis, polyarteritis nodosa and Wegener's granulomatosis (Proskey *et al.* 1970).

Pathology

The kidneys are usually enlarged and pale and petechial haemorrhages may be present. The glomeruli stand out as grey, translucent dots.

The histopathological findings are those of a generalized diffuse exudative glomerulonephritis, with proliferation of the epithelial cells lining Bowman's capsule. The severity of the lesions in individual glomeruli varies. The 'crescents' may be cellular or collagenous. Lobulation and endothelial-cell proliferation may be marked in the tuft and hyalinization may have occurred in others. The tubules contain casts and red blood cells. Areas of interstitial fibrosis representing loss of tubules may be noted.

The vascular changes are variable and muscular hypertrophy of the arterioles with a variable degree of intimal proliferation and elastosis may be present. The interstitial tissue is oedematous with an infiltrate of lymphocytes and plasma cells present.

3. Chronic glomerulonephritis

Synonyms. The end-stage kidney.

Chronic nephritis is the end result of several different forms of glomerulonephritis. Some patients give a history of acute poststreptococcal glomerulonephritis, whereas in others the condition develops insidiously with no previous history of renal disease. A history of the nephrotic syndrome may be given in others and this is usual in chronic lobular and chronic idiopathic membranous glomerulonephritis, the pathology of which is described later.

The pathology of chronic glomerulonephritis is complicated by the vascular changes induced by the secondary hypertension which is a complication of the disease. It does not differ in temperate and tropical climates and is briefly described below. The kidneys are reduced in size. The capsules strip with difficulty and the subcapsular surface is granular. The cortex is narrowed and grey in colour with red mottling present. Yellowish streaking is inconstant and is more common in the other forms of chronic nephritis. The renal papillae are not blunted, and the pelves and calyces are normal. The arterial walls are thickened and the extra pelvic fat increased. Histologically, the majority of the glomeruli are abnormal and hyalinization of the tufts, either complete or with pseudotubule formation, is common. Other glomeruli may show segmental cellular proliferation, axial stalk thickening, adhesions, and segmental basement membrane thickening. Occasional cellular or fibroid epithelial crescents may be detected. Necrotizing lesions may be present if malignant hypertension has supervened. There is tubular loss and atrophy. Hyaline droplet degeneration and casts may be present. There is a fine fibrosis of the interstitial tissue infiltrated with lymphocytes and sometimes plasma cells. The arteries show intimal proliferation and fibroelastosis and fibrinoid necrosis may be present if malignant hypertension has occurred. At post-mortem, in addition to the renal pathology and hypertensive changes, other consequences of chronic renal failure may be present. There may be evidence of uraemia with haemorrhages, enteritis, pericarditis, and pulmonary changes. Renal osteodystrophy, metastic calcification, and even dwarfism may be noted. It is important to differentiate chronic glomerulonephritis from chronic pyelonephritis at necropsy, and the distinguishing features are emphasized below.

In chronic pyelonephritis there is usually a greater reduction in size in one kidney and deformity of the calyces is marked. Depressed areas are present on the granular cortex. Histologically, focal areas of scarring with many chronic inflammatory cells present, pericapsular fibrosis of some and destruction of other glomeruli with intervening areas of relatively normal renal tissue between may be seen. Dilated atrophic tubules containing colloid casts (thyroid areas) are present. Vascular changes of hypertension may occur, and complicate the pathology. In the severely affected kidney deformity of the calyces is probably the most reliable diagnostic sign (Rosenheim, 1967). Granular contracted kidneys may also result from essential hypertension in relatively young adults and are not uncommon in our material.

4. Focal glomerulonephritis

In focal glomerulonephritis only a proportion of the glomeruli are affected and the lesions in the glomeruli are focal or segmental. Focal lesions in subacute bacterial endocarditis, polyarteritis nodosa, systemic lupus erythematosis and those seen in Henoch–Schoenlein purpura should be excluded by appropriate clinical and laboratory procedures. In our experience only subacute bacterial endocarditis presents a differential diagnostic problem in the tropics. In most patients there is no evidence of any cause or history of streptococcal infection but an association with an upper respiratory tract infection has been noted in some patients and an allergic cause has been postulated.

The clinical presentation is variable. Haematuria and skin rashes are frequently present. Haemoptysis, joint symptoms, and hypertension may be associated conditions. Proteinuria may vary from a trace to gross, and in a proportion of patients the nephrotic syndrome may develop (Nagi *et al.* 1971). Complete recovery is said to occur in about one-third of patients.

Pathology

In the glomeruli focal segmental proliferative, necrotizing or hyalinized lesions are present. The hyalinized lesions are thought to be the result of the proliferative or necrotizing processes.

5. Pathological conditions giving rise to the nephrotic syndrome

The nephrotic syndrome can be defined as a condition in which there is massive proteinuria, hypoproteinaemia, generalized oedema, and hyperlipaemia, as shown by elevated levels of total lipids and cholesterol in the serum. In some patients haematuria, azotaemia, and/or hypertension may also be present. In parts of the tropics the levels of total lipids and cholesterol may not appear high if compared with the usual normal values in temperate climates, but it must be emphasized that the local 'normal' values may be low.

The condition is a symptom complex and is *not a specific disease* and several pathological conditions may give rise to the syndrome. Some of the more important are outlined below.

(a) Minimal change kidney (lipoid nephrosis).
(b) Proliferative glomerulonephritis (subsiding acute diffuse glomerulo-nephritis).
(c) Membrano-proliferative glomerulonephritis (lobular).
(d) Chronic glomerulonephritis.
(e) Membranous glomerulonephritis.
(f) Focal glomerulonephritis.
(g) Quartan malarial nephrosis.
(h) Other conditions—e.g. amyloidosis.

(a) Minimal change kidney (lipoid nephrosis)

In the 'minimal-change kidney', lesions in the glomeruli may not be observed by light microscopy. On electron microscopy, however, there is loss of the foot processes (podocytes) of the epithelial cells lying on the outer surface of the basement membrane of the glomerular capillaries. Thickening of the basement membrane and proliferation of endothelial cells may occur later. Hyaline-droplet degeneration is prominent in the proximal tubules. The proteinuria is usually highly selective, i.e. it consists mainly of low molecular weight proteins, notably albumin. It accounts for 18–30 per cent of adult cases of the nephrotic syndrome in temperate climates. The condition usually responds to steroids or cyclophosphamide if steroids fail. It may follow a respiratory viral illness or be found in patients with well developed specific allergies. It is of interest that Barr et al. (1972) have associated the use of mercury-containing skin-lightening creams with the minimal change nephrotic syndrome in females in East Africa. The prognosis is good.

Whereas, no 'abnormality' in the glomeruli on light microscopy is a common finding in children suffering from the nephrotic syndrome in temperate climates it has been rare in our renal biopsy material in Ibadan (Edington and Mainwaring, 1966) and has also been uncommon in Kampala, Uganda (Kibukamusoke and Hutt, 1967).

The low incidence of 'minimal change' in renal biopsies in children with the nephrotic syndrome in West Africa is borne out by the poor response to treatment and the progressive renal impairment seen on follow-up studies (Gilles, 1968). Generalized basement membrane thickening (membranous nephritis) is not thought to be a sequel, but the 'minimal change' appears to progress in some patients to sclerosis of the glomeruli. In some patients endothelial-cell proliferation (proliferative) may be associated with basement membrane thickening. It has been suggested that this type of lesion (in which haematuria, hypertension, or azotaemia may occur) is a disease entity unrelated to a streptococcal aetiology.

Only limited information is as yet available regarding the importance of 'minimal change kidney' in adults as a cause of the nephrotic syndrome in the tropics. IgE has been noted in the glomeruli but not IgG, IgM, IgA, or complement. The interpretation of this finding is at present obscure (Gerber and Paronetto, 1971), but may have an allergic aetiology. Intraglomerular fibrin and platelet aggregations may also be noted. The condition may progress to a chronic sclerosing glomerulonephritis in a few patients.

(b) Proliferative glomerulonephritis (subsiding acute diffuse proliferative glomerulonephritis)

In this condition there is a generalized diffuse glomerulonephritis. The severity of involvement may vary, however, in individual glomeruli. There is an increase of fibrillary PAS-positive material and of endothelial cells in the centre of the lobules (axial stalk lesions). A degree of lobulation may be present and segmental hyaline lesions may be seen. Adhesion of the tuft to Bowman's capsule is common, and gives rise to pseudotubule formation. An occasional epithelial crescent is not unusual. Hyaline droplet degeneration of the proximal tubules is prominent and an increase of interstitial fibrous tissue with tubular atrophy and chronic inflammatory cells present is usual. In a very few patients the histopathological findings described in the rapidly progressive type of glomerulonephritis may be seen.

A previous streptococcal infection is considered important in the aetiology of proliferative glomerulonephritis in temperate climates; it also occurs commonly in the tropics where the aetiology of proliferative glomerulonephritis is undecided.

(c) Membrano-proliferative glomerulonephritis (lobular)

This condition affects young adults and usually presents clinically as the nephrotic syndrome. Microscopic haematuria, azotaemia, and/or hypertension are common. There may, however, be only proteinuria and microscopic haematuria. In children, however, it usually presents as acute glomerulonephritis. On electron microscopy there are both subepithelial and subendothelial dense deposits as well as deposits in the basement membrane which may be diffusely affected. Immunofluorescence studies have revealed that the presence of immunoglobulin and complement do not always correlate with these electron dense alterations. The condition is chronic and progressive. There is reduced plasma levels of the C3 component of complement (hypocomplementaemia). Microscopically, the individual lobules of the glomerular tuft stand out prominently, like an outstretched hand, with endothelial-cell proliferation a marked feature. Segmental basement membrane thickening may be noted. Hyalinization of the lobules occurs centrally with eventually hyalinization of the tuft. Lobulation can, however, usually be distinguished. The condition is generalized and diffuse. Depending upon the stage of the process the kidneys may be enlarged, normal, or reduced in size. The subcapsular surface is smooth or finely granular. The cortex may be normal in thickness or reduced, and yellow flecking is common. Chronic inflammatory cells may be found in the interstitium and vascular changes of hypertension may be present. In some patients a previous history of acute diffuse glomerulonephritis associated with a streptococcal infection is obtained. Lobular glomerulitis occurs in the tropics but is not common either in Ibadan or Kampala.

(d) Chronic glomerulonephritis

In many children with the nephrotic syndrome in West Africa examination of renal biopsy specimens reveals the presence of chronic glomerulonephritis. A number of the tufts are hyalinized and shrunken. Bowman's space is prominent and epithelial cells surrounding the tuft and in the capsular membrane are prominent. Adhesions give marked pseudotubule formation, but capsular epithelial-cell proliferation is rare. The impression is given of a slowly progressive hyalinizing glomerular lesion. Hyaline droplet degeneration in the proximal tubules is common and the convoluted tubules show dilatation, atrophy and colloid casts. Loss of tubules is marked, with accompanying interstitial fibrosis and infiltration of chronic inflammatory cells. Vascular changes of hypertension are also a marked feature.

(e) Membranous glomerulonephritis

This condition usually presents insidiously as the nephrotic syndrome in young adults. No relationship with a streptococcal infection has been noted. There is uniform thickening of the basement membrane of the capillaries of the tuft in a generalized and diffuse fashion. It is not common in renal biopsies in West or East Africa, but is seen rather often in Chinese children in Hong Kong (Chan and Tsao, 1966). It occurs in systemic lupus erythematosus and diabetes mellitus. Lipoid-containing foam cells may be present in the interstitium. The prognosis is poor and the condition invariably progresses to the chronic form of membranous glomerulonephritis. At this stage the kidneys are normal or reduced in size and the surface is finely granular. Yellow flecking may be prominent in the cortex. The glomeruli are hyalinized, and basement membrane thickening can be noted in a few unsclerosed glomeruli. There are no normal or hypertrophied glomeruli. Tubules show degenerative changes and casts. Fibrosis and inflammatory changes are present in the interstitial tissue, and 'foamy macrophages' often occur there. Hypertensive vascular changes are common.

Electron microscopy in the early stages shows irregular dense deposits in the basement membrane. Later they form an almost continuous band.

There is also loss of epithelial cell foot processes. Silver staining reveals typical striations of bristle-like or club-like projections from the outer surface of the basement membrane, which contain gamma globulin and complement. Renal vein thrombosis may be an associated condition and it is responsible for about 20 per cent of primary adult nephrotic syndromes in temperate climates. A membranous nephropathy due to skin-lightening creams has been described by Kibukamusoke *et al.* (1974).

(*f*) *Focal glomerulonephritis*

The pathology of this condition has already been discussed (p. 623).

(*g*) *Quartan malarial nephrosis*

The relationship between the nephrotic syndrome and *P. malariae* has aroused interest for many years and reports of an association between the two conditions have been recorded from countries as wide apart as New Guinea in the east and Guyana in the west (Fig. 13.1). In endemic areas of malaria, *P. malariae* may be found in peripheral blood smears in about 30 per cent of children examined. It cannot therefore be accepted that every

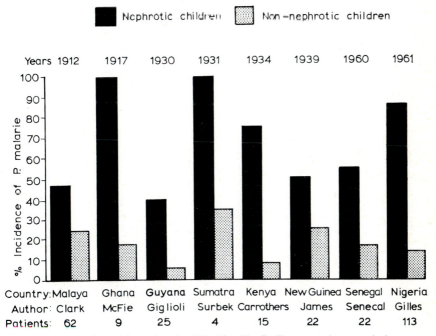

FIG. 13.1. Malarial nephrosis. World-wide findings on the association between *P. malariae* and the nephrotic syndrome.

child with the nephrotic syndrome and in whom parasites of *P. malariae* have been found is necessarily suffering from 'malarial nephrosis'. Unfortunately there is at present no certain way of differentiating a child suffering from 'malarial nephrosis' from one that has the nephrotic syndrome and an incidental *P. malariae* infection. Nevertheless, the relationship between the childhood nephrotic syndrome and *P. malariae* is so striking that it seems reasonable to conclude that 'malarial nephrosis' is a specific entity (Gilles, 1975). The relevant epidemiological features in favour of this concept are as follows: (1) the prevalence of *P. malariae* is significantly higher in children with the nephrotic syndrome than in sick or 'healthy' controls (Fig. 13.2), (2) there is a high incidence of cases in areas where *P. malariae* occurs (Kibuka-

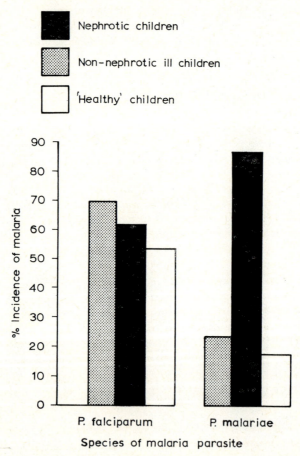

Fig. 13.2. Incidence of malaria in nephrotic and non-nephrotic Nigerian children (aged 2–10 years). (*By courtesy of the East African Medical Journal.*)

musoke, 1966), (3) the age at onset of childhood nephrosis is different from that encountered in Europe and America—i.e. the main peak of age-specific prevalence is at 5 years instead of 6 months to 2 years (Fig. 13.3), (4) the prognosis is poor in the tropics in contrast to the relatively favourable prognosis of childhood nephrosis in Europe and America, (5) most children with malarial nephrosis seem to have a poorly selective proteinuria and to be steroid-resistant (Soothill and Hendrickse, 1967), unlike their counterparts in Europe and America who respond well to steroid therapy, and (6) renal biopsies may reveal characteristic lesions.

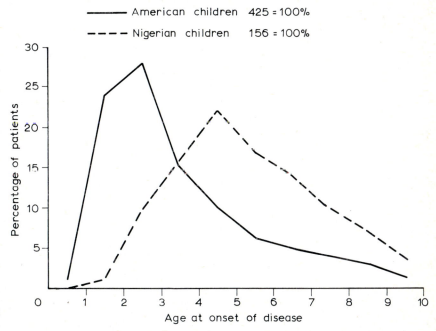

FIG. 13.3. Age at onset of the nephrotic syndrome in Nigerian and American children. (*By courtesy of the East African Medical Journal.*)

It has been suggested that repeated untreated attacks of *P. malariae* may provoke an abnormal immunological response in which the glomerular basement membrane is damaged by an antigen-antibody complex to which it has become sensitized (Hendrickse and Gilles, 1963). Fluorescent antibody studies have revealed heavy deposits of host gamma and β_{1C} globulins, suggesting an accumulation of immunological complexes at this site (Dixon, 1966). Granular, diffuse and mixed patterns of immunofluorescence occur. IgG is invariably present and IgM frequently. IgA has not been detected.

C3 is also frequently present and *P. malariae* antigen has been identified in the glomeruli of about 30 per cent of patients examined. *P. falciparum* antigen and streptolysin have not been detected. The proteinurea is usually poorly selective. The detection of well-defined immunofluorescence in children with minimal change differs from that found in temperate climates where immunoglobulin deposition is not usually described. It may be that the minimal change lesion with immunoglobulin deposition is the early stage of quartan malarial nephrosis—although the absence of quartan malarial antigen in the kidney noted in these patients is difficult to explain. It is not known, however, whether children with other types of malaria but without nephrosis also have such complexes in the kidneys.

We are doubtful if malarial nephrosis occurs in adults in West Africa because we have not been able to find any correlation with the presence of *P. malariae* in peripheral blood films. In addition the lesions seen in renal biopsies follow a somewhat different pattern, the most common condition being a generalized diffuse proliferative nephritis (Mainwaring, 1967, personal communication). However, we have seen a few biopsies from young adults which on light microscopy resembled the quartan malarial nephropathy which is described below. On the other hand, it is accepted in Uganda that the nephrotic syndrome in adults is associated with *P. malariae* infection (Kibukamusoke *et al.* 1967) but no evidence was found to support this in Nairobi (Rees *et al.* 1972).

Pathology

We have shown that acute diffuse glomerulonephritis is not rare in Ibadan and that the pathological lesions seen in proliferative glomerulo-nephritis are not uncommon in children with the nephrotic syndrome (Edington and Mainwaring, 1966), although a history suggestive of acute nephritis is unusual. In Jamaica where acute nephritis is common and *P. malariae* does not occur, the nephrotic syndrome is rarely a sequel of the acute attack. In some biopsies we have noted focal, segmental axial stalk lesions, focal endothelial-cell glomerulitis, focal increase of intracapillary PAS-positive material, lobular glomeritis, and capsular adhesions. These we would classify as proliferative glomerulonephritis. In the previous edition we described the majority of lesions seen in children in Ibadan with the nephrotic syndrome as focal segmental, proliferative and membranous glomerulonephritis with many of the glomeruli normal both on light and electron microscopy. It was a progressive lesion leading inexorably to chronic glomerulonephritis with hypertension and renal failure terminally. This lesion was thought to differ from the well-described lesions seen in Western countries but it was stated that final assessment should await further extended studies. These studies have now been undertaken by

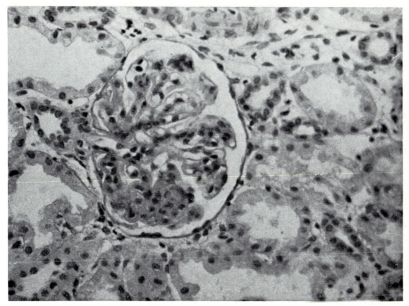

FIG. 13.4. Quartan malarial nephrosis. Glomerulus showing segmental endothelial cell proliferation and obliteration of capillary loops by PAS-positive material. Segmental basement membrane thickening is also present (PAS × 320).

workers in Ibadan and Birmingham (Hendrickse *et al.* 1972) and it has become apparent that the biopsy sections could not be assigned to any of the usual categories included in the classification for nephrotic children in temperate climates and the changes seen on renal biopsy were designated quartan malarial nephropathy. In the earliest lesions the capillary loops are dilated by the increase of PAS-positive material causes a 'haziness' or 'blurring' of the finer details in some of the glomeruli. There is thickening of the glomerular capillary wall which occurs in a focal and segmental fashion. The thickening affects the subendothelial aspect of the basement membrane, giving rise to a plexiform arrangement of PAS-positive, argyrophilic fibrils. With increasing severity more capillary loops and glomeruli are affected, and narrowing and obliteration of capillary loops occur. The sclerosing process also affects the mesangium and with increasing severity leads to total glomerular sclerosis. Mesangial cellular proliferation is not a marked feature in these biopsies but does occur. Fibro-epithelial crescents and glomerular adhesions are uncommon but also do occur.

Hyaline droplets in the proximal tubular epithelium are commonly seen. Tubular atrophy and interstitial changes are proportional to the glomerular

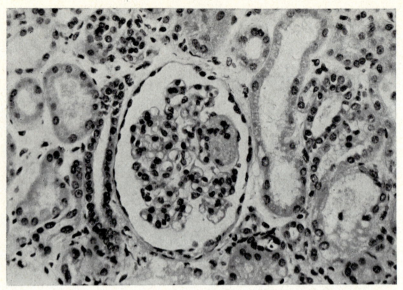

FIG. 13.5. Quartan malarial nephrosis. Glomerulus showing a segmental
hyalinized lesion (PAS × 320).

damage. For historical purposes it should be recorded that the first electron-
micrographic observations were reported on a single case by Herdson (1966)
who reported that some of the glomeruli look virtually normal whilst others
show distinct changes in some lobules. In the abnormal glomeruli epithelial
foot processes are fixed in some areas but not in others and in some regions
there is a zone of increased electron density within the epithelial cytoplasm
immediately adjacent to the basement membrane. The basement membrane
contains irregular deposits and there is quite an amount of basement
membrane-like material lying between the increased numbers of intracapillary cells. Many of these intracapillary cells show unusually prominent
rough endoplasmic reticulum.

In a larger series of cases ultramicroscopic findings show that the essential
abnormality is thickening of the capillary basement membrane in the subendothelial zone. Occasionally electron-dense material is seen within the
basement membrane itself. A constant feature is the presence of small
lacunae scattered throughout the basement membrane and was thought
to be a definitive criterion of diagnosis. Subepithelial 'humps' were not
seen although seen in other children with proliferative glomerulonephritis
in Ibadan (Hendrickse *et al.* 1972).

The appearances are not those usually described in a post-streptococcal
type of nephritis. They perhaps resemble more those described in the

advanced lesions of 'minimal-change kidney'. The lesions also differ from the membranoproliferative glomerulonephritis described in the nephrotic syndrome by McGovern (1964) in which the glomeruli are generally and not focally affected. The condition would appear to be a slowly progressive focal and hyalinizing lesion of the tuft (Fig. 13.6) which leads inexorably to chronic glomerulonephritis with hypertension and renal failure terminally. The changes of chronic glomerulonephritis are also seen in biopsy material from nephrotic children and in our post-mortem material.

Chronic glomerulonephritis is common in children in the tropics, and 30 per cent of deaths due to this cause occur under the age of 15 years in our

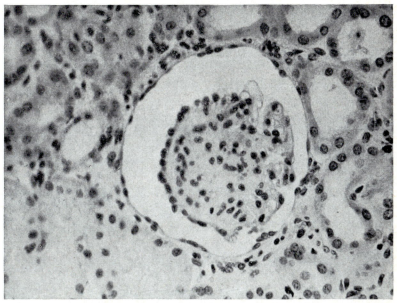

FIG. 13.6. Quartan malarial nephrosis. Partial hyalinization of the tuft with prominent glomerular epithelium and patent capsular space (H and E × 320).

post-mortem material. Thrombosis of the pulmonary arteries has been noted as a complication of the nephrotic syndrome in children treated with steroids (Levin et al. 1967) and changes in blood coagulation and fibrinolysis have been described (Thomson et al. 1974).

(h) Other conditions

With regard to other conditions giving rise to the nephrotic syndrome there is no evidence that their pathology differs markedly from that seen in temperate climates. In toxaemia of pregnancy the capillary endothelial cells are affected and cause narrowing of the capillary lumina. The changes are reversible following delivery. The condition does occur in the tropics but is probably less common than in temperate climates. In our experience lesions of the kidney tend to be less severe in diabetes mellitus in Africa, although they may be severe in Indians in India and Africa (Campbell, 1964). Disseminated lupus erythematosus and renal vein thrombosis are occasionally seen. Amyloidosis is discussed on p. 723 and the occasional complication of renal-vein thrombosis in this condition should be remembered. The nephrotic syndrome has also been described in sickle cell disease and the deposition of iron protein complexes in the kidney were thought to be concerned in the aetiology (McCoy, 1969).

B. DISEASES OF THE TUBULES

Acute renal failure is not uncommon in the tropics. Necrosis of proximal convoluted tubules may be caused by: (a) the direct toxic action of substances such as mercury or carbon tetrachloride on the tubular epithelium (some native medicines may act in this way), (b) renal ischaemia such as is seen in shock—(both traumatic and bacterial) and obstetric complications, especially accidental haemorrhage and abortion (Sheehan and Moore, 1952).

Lesions of distal convoluted tubules ('lower nephron nephrosis') may be caused by a combination of ischaemic and excretory factors, and blockage of the distal and collecting tubules by pigment or crystals may play a part. Examples of such conditions are blackwater fever, incompatible blood transfusion, myoglobinuria in crush injuries, haemolytic anaemias, and sulphonamides. The pathology was discussed when blackwater fever was considered, p. 463. We sometimes see sulphonamide crystals macroscopically in kidneys at post mortem.

Although low values of plasma and potassium are seen in kwashiorkor, the vacuolization of the proximal tubular epithelium described in hypokalaemia is rare in our experience. It has also been suggested that magnesium deficiency may be responsible for this type of lesion but once again we have not seen these lesions in kwashiorkor—a condition in which magnesium deficiency is thought to occur.

Tubular damage is common in many types of hepatic disease (the hepato-renal syndrome) and this is common in our experience. The kidneys are enlarged and usually jaundiced. Granular or amorphous deposits of green bile are found in the epithelium of the proximal and collecting tubules, the latter usually containing pigment casts. In the more severe cases there may be signs of tubular necrosis.

Uric-acid precipitates occur in the kidney in the neonate.

Bilateral renal cortical necrosis

Bilateral renal cortical necrosis occurs most frequently in the last trimester of pregnancy, particularly in association with accidental haemorrhage. It may, however, follow extensive burns associated with shock and bacterial toxaemia of staphylococcal origin. It is the most severe manifestation of the renal cortical ischaemia which in its milder forms causes tubular necrosis. It is invariably bilateral and may affect the entire renal cortex of both kidneys, which appear yellow and necrotic or it may be focal in distribution. The intralobular arteries show thrombosis and afferent glomerular arterioles may be necrotic. Microscopically the cortex appears to be infarcted, although some glomeruli may escape and show proliferative changes. We have seen reparative fibrosis of the cortex occur in these cases with the juxta-medullary glomeruli apparently intact. It is a rare condition in our experience.

C. INFECTIONS AND THE KIDNEY

Pyelonephritis is common in the tropics but in post-mortem material at Ibadan it is a less common cause of death than glomerulonephritis, in spite of the fact that urethral stricture, urinary schistosomiasis, and vesico-vaginal fistulae are common. Similar findings have been recorded in East Africa. The incidence of pyelonephritis as an incidental finding in post-mortem material has not been accurately assessed. The part that schistosomiasis plays in the aetiology of pyelonephritis and secondary hypertension is discussed on p. 160. The pathology of pyelonephritis would not appear to differ in tropical and temperate climates and has been briefly described. The back-pressure kidney with consequent hydro-and pyonephrosis is probably more common. In sickle-cell diseases the greater liability of the kidney to infection, necrosis of renal papillae, and haemorrhage is discussed on p. 441. Renal papillary necrosis may also be induced by the ingestion of drugs such as phenacetin and salicylates.

It should be remembered that urinary infection in young infants may be associated with jaundice, and blood culture should always be undertaken in young infants with unexplained jaundice. Intravenous pyelograms may be normal. Haemolysis may play a part in the aetiology and the presence of glucose-6-phosphate dehydrogenase in the red cells should be determined.

Pyaemic abscesses of the kidney are common findings in septicaemic conditions, including postabortive and puerperal sepsis.

Although pulmonary and abdominal tuberculosis is common in our material and miliary renal tuberculosis is seen, caseating renal tuberculosis is a rare finding in our experience, although not uncommon in India and China.

D. UROLITHIASIS

There is great variation in the incidence of stones in the urinary tract in the tropics. They are rare in West Africa, Rhodesia, and in the Bantu in Southern Africa, although not uncommon in the Indian population in the latter and in the Congo (Fain and Falaise, 1957). The incidence is, however, high in the Middle East, areas of India, North Thailand, and South China (Gershoff *et al.* 1963). Vesical calculi in temperate climates occur almost exclusively in elderly males, whereas in many areas of the tropics they are common in children, boys being more frequently affected than girls. This is explained by the short straight female urethra which permits the passage of crystalline aggregates which are retained in the male bladder and form centres for stone development. In the adult type, or urinary calculi common in Western countries, the stones are usually oxalate or phosphate and may be formed in the renal pelvis or bladder. Urinary obstruction and infection are common aetiological agents and occasionally a parathyroid tumour may be present. Hypercalcaemia with nephrocalcinosis (a deposition of calcium and phosphorous in the renal tubules or interstitial tissue) are also predisposing causes and in our material mild nephrocalcinosis in adults is not uncommon, although urinary calculi are rare. In adults in the tropics inadequate fluid consumption in hot dry climates may be a major aetiological factor.

It is of interest that the incidence of stone in men following different occupations varies greatly. The incidence is high in Czechoslovakian railway workers, officers in the U.S. army compared with other ranks and, in doctors in Scotland, surgeons and anaesthetists compared with general practitioners. Recurrence of the calculi is usual (Editorial, 1971). It has been said that in Fiji where the population is approximately half Indian and half Fijian that renal stones are very common in the Indian population but scarcely ever occur in Fijians. Spices in the diet of the Indians were thought in some way to be responsible (Holmes, 1971).

Calculi have been described in relation to haematobium infection in the urethra, bladder, ureter, and kidney and are found in up to 25 per cent of infected persons in Egypt, although rare in most other parts of Africa. The centre of these calculi consist of oxalate with an outer uric-acid layer frequently incorporating schistosome ova. Where the primary causative environmental factors for stone formation exist, *S. haematobium* infection and urinary stasis are most probably potent contributory factors. Vesical calculi are a not uncommon complication of vesicovaginal fistula.

Bladder stone disease in children

This used to be common in Europe but has disappeared with improved standards of living. In addition to the geographical areas outlined above the condition is common in parts of Iran (Sadre *et al.* 1973) and Israel. Children under 10 years of age are usually affected, the peak frequency being in the 2–5 year old age group although the condition has been reported in a child aged $4\frac{1}{2}$ months. Clinically dysuria and lower abdominal pain are usually the presenting symptoms. With regard to aetiology this probably varies in different regions, as in New Delhi there is no hypercalciuria whereas this has been reported from Northern Thailand in addition to oxaluria. In Northern Thailand the condition is associated with the practice of partly replacing breast feeds with premasticated glutinous rice from the early neonatal period. This increases the infant's intake of L-hydroxyproline which is a metabolic precursor of glyoxalate and hence of oxalate. The enzyme lactate dehydrogenase is concerned in this reaction. The intake of breast milk and thus of total fluids is reduced. There are increased oxalates, L-hydroxyproline and aggregated calcium oxalate crystals in the urine. The urinary excretion of phosphate is low and oral orthophosphate reduces the clumping of calcium oxalate crystals and the urine calcium concentration. (Dhanamitta and Valyasevi, 1972). There is no doubt that alterations in oxalate metabolism can cause renal calculi. Primary hyperoxaluria is a rare autosomal recessively inherited disorder in which the patients usually present during the first decade with recurrent urinary calculi and a sustained increase in urinary oxalate excretion. At post mortem deposits of calcium oxalate are found in the kidneys, myocardium, media of arteries and the rete testis (Watts, 1973), as well as signs of uraemia. Hyperoxaluria may also occur with extensive disease of the small intestine. Pyridoxine deficiency also increases oxalate excretion in laboratory animals and large doses may decrease the urinary oxalate excretion in man. Glycine is an important metabolic precursor of oxalate and dietary protein restriction has been used in the treatment of oxalosis which is strange when it is considered that protein deficiency has been considered an aetiological agent in bladder stone disease in childhood and in which growth failure is a feature clinically. Magnesium oxide and sodium orthophosphate inhibit oxalate crystallization clinically and magnesium deficiency has been mentioned as a possible aetiological agent in bladder stone disease in children.

In contrast to the oxaluria reported in Thailand in other regions ammonium acid urate stones may be more common.

In Thailand it is predominantly children in rural areas that are affected (Van Reen *et al.* 1970) whereas in Israel and New Delhi the condition occurs in both rural and urban areas in the lower socio-economic families (Stark, 1970; Aurora *et al.* 1970).

Vitamin A deficiency is frequently mentioned as a possible aetiological agent as it causes calculi in laboratory animals following keratinizing metaplasia of the transitional epithelium of the bladder. This change has not been reported in childhood calculi and the geographical distribution of the condition does not correspond with areas where Vitamin A deficiency is known to occur. With regard to infection, urine culture is sterile in the majority of the patients and infection probably follows ulceration caused by the trauma of the stone itself.

Further cultural studies, especially dietary, are indicated in other areas of the tropics where the frequency is high. It should be noted that recurrence following removal of the stone is rare and suggests that the aetiological factors, as in Thailand, are present in the early years of life.

Pathology

Bladder stones in children are commonly considered to be primary in contrast to adults in whom there is usually an underlying obstructive lesion in the lower urinary tract. In a study from New Delhi, however, in which voiding cystourethography, pyelography and endoscopy were employed Taneja et al. (1970) found evidence of ureteral reflux in 21 of 52 children and obstructive lesions such as valves, diverticulum or bladder neck contracture in $38 \cdot 5$ per cent.

The calculi may reach a size of 5 cm or more in diameter and are often irregular. Oedema, cystitis and ulceration of the bladder mucosa may occur with hydroureter, hydronephrosis and distortion of calyces and renal outline as further complications.

In India raised serum mucopolysaccharide levels have been reported with dark granular cells rich in PAS-positive material in the epithelium in bladder biopsies. The significance of these findings are as yet undecided (Aurora et al. 1970).

E. TUMOURS OF THE KIDNEY

Benign tumours are not, in our experience, common, excluding adenomas and angiomyolipomas. Renal-cell carcinoma (Grawitz tumour, hypernephroma) and Wilms' tumour are not uncommon.

URETER

The changes which occur in schistosomiasis have already been described. Dilatation of the ureters is common in gonococcal urethral stricture in males, and vesicovaginal fistula in females. Prostatic hypertrophy occurs and is discussed below. Inflammation and tuberculosis are not common lesions, nor are tumours, either benign or malignant. Ureteric calculi are common in Egypt, usually associated with schistosomiasis. 'Megaureter', a name given to a chronically dilated ureter in which no organic obstruction is evident, has been reported in a few children in India (Chatterjee, 1964).

BLADDER

Acute and chronic cystitis are common conditions. The immunological aspects of bladder cancer have recently been reviewed (Editorial, 1972). Rarely an interstitial cystitis, 'Hunner's ulcer', with diffuse fibrosis in the bladder wall may be a manifestation of an autoimmune disease. The trigone is not affected (Editorial, 1972). Malakoplakia is rare. This consists of soft yellowish to brown plaques measuring from 1 to 5 cm and histologically consisting of large eosinophilic cells with finely granular cytoplasm. They may contain intracytoplasmic inclusions. Tuberculosis of the bladder has not been common in our experience. The lesions which occur in schistosomiasis are described in that chapter, as are also tumours of the bladder. Tumours of the bladder are discussed on p. 166. Vesicovaginal fistulae are common and are most frequently the sequelae of obstetrical complications— and lymphogranuloma venereum.

URETHRA

By far the most common condition affecting the urethra is gonorrhoea due to *Neisseria gonorrhoea*. Its pathology in the tropics is similar to that seen in temperate climates but owing to lack of medical facilities it tends to be a much more serious and chronic condition. Urethral stricture in males is common in many parts of the tropics and special clinics may still be necessary for regular urethral dilatation. It is a common cause of hydroureter, hydronephrosis, and pyelonephritis. Cystitis is a common complication. Post-gonococcal strictures are situated in the penile and bulbar parts of the urethra since the basic pathology is in the corpus spongiosum in which fibrosis occurs following thrombophlebitis caused by extravasation of infected urine. Narrowing of the prostatic urethra may result from a gonococcal prostatitis. The prostate, seminal vesicles, epididymides and accessory urethral glands in the male, and Bartholin's and Skene's glands, cervix, and fallopian tubes in the female, are frequently infected. Pelvic inflammatory disease is a potent cause of sterility in the female. It should be noted that urethral and endocervical smears should be examined in the female. Fistulae are common and the watering-can scrotum due to multiple urethral strictures is not infrequently seen. Suppurative arthritis, bacterial endocarditis, and even meningitis are complications (Ikejiani, 1958). Skin lesions may be associated with pyrexia and joint lesions and the condition has been called benign gonococcaemia. Papules and pustules on the limbs occur in crops. The urethra is rarely involved in Schistosomiasis but stricture and periurethral abscesses can occur. Strictures due to trauma also occur.

Non-gonococcal urethritis due to viral, trichomonad, or amoebic infections occur and are described in their appropriate sections. Reiter's syndrome—urethritis, conjunctivitis, polyarthritis with cutaneous and visceral lesions—occurs, but there is little information on its frequency or geographical distribution. It has been reported from Papua (Editorial, 1971).

Tumours of the urethra are not common.

PENIS

Inflammation of the penis almost invariably involves the glans and prepuce and is common in areas where circumcision is not practised. The primary hard chancre of syphilis usually occurs on the glans or coronal sulcus. Chancroid, donovanosis (granuloma inguinale), and lymphogranuloma venerum are common in many areas of the tropics and are discussed in their appropriate text. Tuberculous ulceration can also occur but is rare (Walker and Jordan, 1968).

Cancer of the penis is usually of the squamous-cell type and affects the preputial sac. It is common in many Asian countries (Muir, 1962), parts of India (Mulay, 1963), South America (Riveros and Lebron, 1963), and Africa. The incidence is directly related to the circumcisional habits of the people. It is virtually absent in the Yorubas in Southern Nigeria where circumcision is practised in the first 2 weeks of life but is common in uncircumcised tribes in East Africa, (Dodge, 1965). Among Muslims in whom circumcision is performed at puberty the condition occurs but with less frequency than in the uncircumcised. Personal hygiene is an associated factor, frequent and thorough washing reducing the susceptibility in uncircumcised peoples. Metastases usually occur as a late manifestation of the disease, the inguinal glands, prostate gland, bladder, rectum, kidney, and testes being affected.

There is a condition called koro which is not uncommon amongst the Chinese and may also occur in Celebes and West Borneo (Mun, 1968). A case has been reported in Britain. There is a sudden feeling of retraction of the penis into the abdomen and if help is not available it is thought that the penis will disappear into the abdomen with a fatal outcome. It may occasionally assume epidemic proportions. It occurs in children and adolescents. Reassurance and mild sedation are effective in therapy.

THE PROSTATE GLAND

There are few anatomical studies of the gland in the tropics. Our own studies, however, and those of J. N. P. Davies in East Africa would suggest that in tropical Africa the weight of the gland is much less than that recorded in temperate climates.

Acute prostatitis certainly occurs in the tropics but its incidence is unknown. From a pathological point of view we have been impressed by the rarity of acute and chronic inflammatory lesions of the prostate seen in surgical biopsy specimens. Caution, however, is required in interpreting these results and until adequate surveys are undertaken to define the pathological conditions affecting the prostate gland in various areas of the tropics an open mind should be kept. It has frequently been stated that benign prostatic hyperplasia is uncommon in tropical areas but this is not so in our experience, a finding that would agree with the conclusions of Ahluwalia and Tandom (1965) in Northern India who also quote confirmatory findings from Indonesia. It is rare in our experience to diagnose schistosomiasis or other parasitic infections in surgical specimens, nor is it common to see tuberculous lesions. The absence of the latter condition may, however, be due to the more fulminating course of tuberculosis seen in tropical populations, the infection in the prostate and seminal vesicles being ignored or missed.

Although the highest incidence of cancer of the prostate is found in the American Negro the incidence is low in Nigeria as Fig. 13.7 shows. Similar findings to these have been recorded from Uganda and in the Johannesburg Bantu. The incidence is extremely low in the Japanese and higher in Japanese residents in the U.S.A. (Wynder *et al.* 1971). It would appear, therefore, that environmental factors are more important than racial in the aetiology.

Prostatic cancers are divided into clinical, latent and occult. Clinical prostatic cancer implies that the disease is producing symptoms and is diagnosed histologically. Latent cancers are those foci morphologically resembling prostatic cancer which do not produce symptoms and are found incidentally at prostatectomy or necropsy without dissemination having occurred. Occult cancers are those which produce metastases while the primary remains insignificant in size or hidden (Editorial, 1973). It is of interest that latent cancer in the Bantu in South Africa has been found in higher incidence than in the white although the incidence of cancer is very much less (Barnitson, 1954). Latent cancer has also been found in relatively high incidence in the Japanese who have a low incidence of clinical prostatic carcinoma. With regards to the aetiology it is our impression that benign prostatic hyperplasia is common in our material but that carcinoma of the prostate is found in low incidence and that this probably depends on hormonal factors—namely the oestrogen–androgen ratio. Oestrogenization has been reported in African males by a number of workers, and as oestrogen is utilized to suppress androgen stimulation in prostatic cancer it is reason-

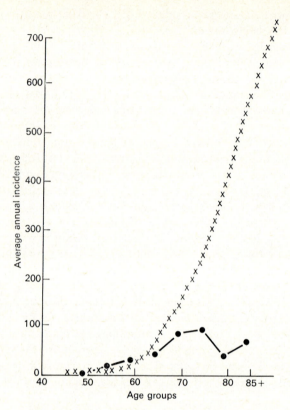

FIG. 13.7. Carcinoma of the prostate. Average annual age incidence.
●—● Ibadan. × × × × × New York State.

able to conclude that hormonal influences conditioned by environmental factors are the most likely aetiological agents in prostatic cancer.

THE TESTES

Scrotal swellings are common in the tropics, hydrocele, varicocele, and inguinal herniae being the usual causative factors. Tuberculosis of the epididymis occurs. Granulomatous fibrosing lesions of the peritesticular tissues are common and the aetiology is often obscure. We have seen one case of granulomatous orchitis, and torsion of the testis is not uncommon in adolescents (Nkposong, 1972). The latter condition has to be differentiated from torsion of a testicular appendage, acute mumps orchitis, epididymo-orchitis, idiopathic scrotal oedema of children, traumatic interstitial haematoma of the testis and traumatic hydrocele. Testicular calcification occurs (Priebe and Garbet, 1970). Lymphoedema due to parasitic or other infections must be considered and it should be remembered that bancroftian filariasis may present clinically as funiculitis. The effect of leprosy and cirrhosis on the testes and its association with gynaecomastia is discussed on p. 311. Testicular atrophy and fibrosis are common in male New Guineans (Kasiks and McGovern, 1971).

In children in the United States embryonal carcinoma is the most common tumour seen but the frequency is low in the Negro. In general, testicular tumours are uncommon in the tropics, especially in the African. Templeton (1972) analysed twenty-nine cases in Uganda and considered that there was a deficiency of seminomas and teratomas in the East African, orchioblastoma and interstitial cell tumours probably occurring in a similar frequency to that recorded in Caucasians. In an eleven-year period in Ibadan 40 tumours of the testes were recorded. The incidence was low as only 8 occurred in the Ibadan population, the remaining 32 coming from out-station hospitals. Seminomas and teratomas were the most frequent (20 and 10, respectively). There were 2 orchioblastomas, and lymphosarcoma and the Burkitt tumour were also seen. Connective tissue tumours may also occur. Mortality from malignant tumours of the testes has two age peaks—one in young adults and one in the elderly in Western countries and the incidence would appear to be rising, especially in adolescence in Denmark (Clemmeson, 1968).

GANGRENE OF THE SCROTUM

Fournier's idiopathic gangrene of the scrotum occurs in tropical areas, more often in patients who show no evidence of malnutrition, and the aetiology is unknown (Thomas, 1953). A filarial infection has been noted in some patients. It occurs between the ages of 20 and 40 years and an associated streptococcal infection or thrombosis of the scrotal arteries have also been noted. The lower two-thirds of the scrotal skin sloughs, leaving the testicles exposed. Healing by granulation occurs naturally. It has also been reported following vasectomy in the United Kingdom (Pryor et al. 1971).

THE OVARY

Acute and chronic oophoritis are common and are associated with infection in the Fallopian tubes and pelvic inflammatory disease. Ovarian cysts (follicular, dermoid, serous, and mucin-secreting) are common. There is a high incidence of the hormone-secreting granulosa and theca-cell tumours which cause dysfunctional bleeding. Malignant disease of the ovary in Africa occurs in a similar incidence to that seen in the Western world until the age of 60 years but is very rare over the age of 65.

The most common secondary tumours are malignant lymphomas (especially the Burkitt tumour in endemic areas) and Krukenberg tumours.

THE FALLOPIAN TUBES

Gonococcal and tuberculous salpingitis and pyo- and hydrosalpinx are common conditions. Schistosomal infection occurs, *S. mansoni* being more common than *haematobium*. Both the submucosa and muscularis may be involved with marked thickening and tortuosity of the tubes. The lumina usually remain patent although lower abdominal pain, menorrhagia and sterility have rarely been described. Ruptured ectopic pregnancies are common and in many instances there is no evidence of previous inflammatory disease.

THE UTERUS

Acute infections are common following abortions and childbirth, as are chronic infections with uterine displacement. Gonococcal and tuberculous infections are also common and prolapse is not uncommon in the older age groups. Metropathia haemorrhagica is in our experience uncommon, as is endometriosis. The incidence of endometriosis in the U.S. non-white is related to social status, being low in the lower socio-economic groups (Lloyd, 1964). The reason for the low incidence is obscure but may be related to early marriage, frequent pregnancies, and a high incidence of pelvic inflammatory disease. In the tropics there may be a lowered level of hormonal activity as indicated by a later age at menarche and a lowered frequency of post-menopausal oestrus. All the evidence would tend to show that increased standards of living lower the age at menarche.

Rupture of the uterus is a common complication of childbirth and is related to pelvic contractions and lack of adequate antenatal care (Cox, 1963).

Fibroids are extremely common in many areas of the tropics and sarcomatous change occurs in a small proportion. Although leiomyosarcoma of the uterus is said to be more common in the American Negro vis-a-vis the Caucasian it would not appear to be a commonly diagnosed tumour in the tropics. Mitotic counts accurately separate leiomyosarcoma from cellular leiomyoma, and Christopherson *et al.* (1972) found that no patient with fewer than 5 mitoses per 10 high-power fields died of the disease. Bizarre leiomyomas may have alarming histological and cytological features with a good prognosis. Adenocarcinoma would appear to be rare. Carcinoma of the uterus is considered on p. 646.

VAGINA

In the testicular feminizing syndrome congenital anomalies, especially atresia occur. Gynatresia is common in many parts of the tropics and may be congenital or acquired. The types of congenital malformations seen are similar to those described in standard text-books and have been discussed by Kanagasumtheram and Dassanayake (1958) in Sri Lanka. Acquired gynatresia may be due to ritual circumcision or to the use of caustic pessaries (Obasi, 1964). The pessaries may be used following labour, to procure criminal abortion, to cure infertility, to induce menses in menopausal women, or to prevent a threatened abortion. Trichomonal and monilial infections are common as are vesicovaginal and rectovaginal fistulae.

Anaerobic cocci have been found in high incidence in an area where the incidence of infertility was high and pelvic inflammatory disease common (Hare and Polunin, 1960). Other infections are discussed in their appropriate context.

Gonorrhoeal vulvovaginitis is not uncommon in children. In some areas of the tropics it is or was believed that gonorrhoea in the male could be cured by sexual contact with a virgin female child—with resulting vulvovaginitis.

Papillomas and benign connective tissue tumours occur. Primary epithelial tumours occur and adenocarcinoma in adolescent girls whose mothers were treated with stilboestral has been reported (Editorial, 1971). Mesodermal mixed tumours (sarcoma botryoides) also are seen. Deposits of chorion cancer are not unusual in surgical biopsy material.

VULVA

The usual conditions which are seen in temperate climates are present in the tropics. Gonorrhoea, syphilis, chancroid, lymphogranuloma venereum, amoebiasis, schistosomiasis, fungal infections, and elephantiasis have been discussed elsewhere. Kraurosis vulvae is relatively rare because of the age distribution in the tropics.

Female circumcisional mutilating operations or other tribal customs may cause stricture of the urethra and vagina, urinary retention, and gross deformities.

The circumcisional operations are of two types, (1) excision, and (2) infibulation (Hathout, 1963; Laycock, 1950). Excision or clitoridectomy is removal of part at least of the clitoris and adjacent tissue. Infibulation implies reducing the size of the orifice of the vulva by sutures. The operational procedures are usually undertaken between the ages of 1 and 14 years by native practitioners. Excision is practised in Africa, the East Indies, and South America, whereas infibulation is seen in East and Central Africa.

In other parts of the tropics substances (native medicines, cow dung, etc.) are introduced into the vagina following delivery, rock salt for instance being a common medicament in Arabia (Underhill, 1964). Tetanus, septicaemia, and gynatresia are common complications. The purpose of these customs is unclear and they appear to be practised as an immemorial custom.

Bartholin's cysts, papillomas, and condyloma acumination are common. Hydradenoma occurs, but by far the most common tumour is the squamous-cell carcinoma.

CARCINOMA OF THE CERVIX AND UTERUS

The various infections which affect the cervix, trichomonas, schistosomiasis, donovanosis, etc., have already been dealt with. Tuberculous cervicitis may mimic carcinoma and an associated inguinal adenitis is not uncommon. Elephantiasis of the labia and vulva may result. Chronic cervicitis with or without an erosion being present is common.

There is no doubt that squamous-cell carcinoma of the cervix is one of the most common tumours seen in many tropical areas. Females before the menopause are frequently affected and rarely the condition is seen in teenagers. Most of the data concerning incidence in the tropics are concerned with ratio frequencies and these are indeed high in most areas. Age specific rates in Africa compared with New York are shown in Fig. 16.3 on p. 693. The tumour is rare in virgins and the incidence is low in Jewish females and has been related to the habit of circumcision in their male partners. It is of interest, however, that somewhat similar incidences of cervical cancer occur in Ugandan and Yoruba women in Nigeria. In Uganda, male circumcision is not universally practised and penile cancer is common, whereas circumcision in the first two weeks of life is universal in the Yoruba and cancer of the penis is rare (Edington, 1970). Circumcision would not, therefore, appear to play a major aetiological role in cervical cancer in Africa. A high incidence is related to early marriage and repeated acts of sexual intercourse. Carcinoma of the cervix occurs in high incidence in prostitutes in temperate climates. It is also more common in divorced women. Poverty and poor personal hygiene have also been incriminated as possible aetiological agents. Recently it has been suggested that infection with *Herpevirus hominus* type 2 (HSV-2) may be associated with the condition (Editorial, 1972). This hypothesis arose from epidemiological studies, but serum antibody studies in patients and matched controls have as yet given conflicting results. It has been suggested that the virus may change the heredity of the cell by adding and incorporating virus genetic material (DNA) into that of the normal cell, thus initiating malignant change. In the tropics, the incidence of this tumour is likely to vary with the age of marriage, polygamy, and the sociological customs affecting pregnancy and intercourse and variations may be found to occur within relatively narrow geographical limits. The pathology is that of a squamous-cell carcinoma of varying degree of differentiation, and in our experience the majority of the tumours are of a high grade of malignancy. It is of interest that in Egypt schistosomiasis has been associated with the presence of a well-differentiated squamous cell carcinoma (Youseff *et al.* 1970) but no controlled studies have been undertaken. Epidermoid carcinoma, adenocarcinoma, undifferentiated carcinoma, and carcinosarcoma also occur probably in that order of frequency. Cervical smears in the tropics have also shown a much higher positivity rate than would be expected in Western communities and trichomonas and monilia infections are common (Trussel *et al.* 1968; Vaillant *et al.* 1968).

Carcinoma of the body of the uterus has been reported to be rare in all areas of the tropics in which figures are available, with the possible exception of the Sudan (Lynch *et al.* 1963). In temperate climates the ratio of carcinoma of the cervix to the corpus is about 2 to 1 (Editorial, 1966) whereas in most tropical areas it is 25 to 1. In contrast, chorioncarcinoma is extremely common in the tropics.

HYDATIDIFORM MOLE, CHORIONADENOMA DESTRUENS, AND CHORIONCARCINOMA

The modern tendency is to consider these three conditions under the title of malignant trophoblastic disease (M.T.D.). The following remarks apply to chorioncarcinoma. Hydatidiform mole and chorioadenoma destruens are described when the pathology is considered. Chorioncarcinoma is a malignant neoplasm of the embryonic chorion, both layers of the trophoblastic epithelium being involved. In some standard textbooks of pathology it is said to be a rarity, occurring once in approximately 160,000 pregnancies in Britain. This is certainly not true in the tropics; the incidence, for instance, in the Chinese in Hong Kong has been calculated as 1 in 1331 deliveries (Chan, 1967). The condition is common in West and East Africa, Madagascar (Dodin *et al.* 1962), southern India (Pai, 1967), Iraq, Indonesia, Philippines, Taiwan, Korea, and Java (Poen and Djojopranato, 1965). The age specific incidence of chorion cancer in Ibadan is shown in Fig. 16.4 on p. 694.

It is more common in multiparous and older patients in the tropics, in contrast to the oligoparity and youth in the Western world.

Lowered economic standards, undernourishment, and consanguinity have been suggested factors in the aetiology.

The trophoblastic elements are unique in that they are derived from the tissues of the patient and the husband. More and more attention is being paid to immunological factors in the genesis of the disease. Leucocyte antigens of husband and wife have been shown to be compatible and the patient has been shown to tolerate a skin graft from the husband to a greater extent than normal. The wife would appear to have developed immune tolerance against some of the husband's antigens (Robinson *et al.* 1963; Mathé *et al.* 1964). The absence of a mononuclear and lymphocytic response to the trophoblast, in contrast to syncytial endometritis, may indicate again immune tolerance in the host (Iliya *et al.* 1967). It has been suggested that the pregnant female fails to reject trophoblast as an allograft because there is a peritrophoblastic coat of sialomucin which has an electronegative surface charge and repels negatively-charged lymphocytes. Tumour antigens may escape recognition in a similar fashion (Currie and Bagshawe, 1967). An antiserum against the consort's seminal fluid prepared in rabbits has given encouraging results in therapy (Rider and Cinader, 1966). It is known that in pregnancy the effects of malaria in stable areas, infectious hepatitis, amoebic dysentery, and pneumococcal meningitis (Lucas, 1964) are much more severe when compared with non-pregnant females. This may be due to a generalized hormonal disturbance altering the immunological status of the host. It is, therefore, tempting to speculate that the relatively high incidence of chorioncancer in the areas described may be due to multiple infections and infestations altering the immunological status of the female and thus interfering with the normal 'reject mechanism' to a foreign antigen—namely trophobast (Edington, 1970).

Clinically, chorioncarcinoma presents as uterine haemorrhage following hydatidiform mole, abortion, or a normal pregnancy. Occasionally, pulmonary or vaginal deposits may be present with no demonstrable lesion in the uterus and we have seen the condition present as an intracranial space occupying lesion.

Pathology

There is confusion in the classification of hydatidiform mole, chorioadenoma destruens and chorioncarcinoma. A classification has been proposed by the International Union against Cancer as follows (Park, 1967).

A. Hydatidiform mole (*a*) non-invasive, (*b*) invasive.

B. Chorioncarcinoma.

C. Morphological diagnosis uncertain.

In hydatidiform mole the uterus is filled with white, grape-like structures representing degenerate chorionic villi. Microscopically the villi are large and consist of oedematous myxomatous stroma lacking the normal chorionic vessels. The surrounding trophoblastic epithelium may retain the two normal layers, the cells of Langhans and the syncytial cells, and is then regarded as a benign or non-invasive mole. The trophoblastic epithelium may, however, show proliferative activity. It may be several cells in thickness and the cells may show the atypia of malignancy and even invasive properties. This is the invasive mole, or chorioadenoma destruens. In choriocarcinoma no villi are detectable. Both cytotrophoblastic and syncytiotrophoblastic proliferation occur. Bizarre giant cells and mitotic figures may be numerous. Invasion is a marked feature and lakes of blood surround foci of malignant tissue and account for the haemorrhagic character of the tumours. Blood-vessel invasion occurs early and metastases are found in the lungs, brain, vagina, spleen, and other organs. Numerous tumour microemboli may be found in the pulmonary arterial system and may cause pulmonary hypertension with right-sided cardiac enlargement. Emphasis has been laid on the presence or absence of villi as a prognostic sign in the behaviour of the tumour, the presence of villi indicating a relatively good prognosis. We are not sure that we can fully agree with this as we have certainly seen the invasive mole metastasize to the lungs and brain. Lutein cysts may be an associated finding in the ovary. Thyrotoxicosis has been reported as a complication of hydatidiform mole and chorio-carcinoma and a thyroid-stimulating substance has been detected in these tumours just as it has also been described in the normal placenta and be responsible for the mild thyrotoxicosis which may occur in pregnancy (Editorial, 1971; Robson, 1971). Malignant trophoblastic disease is, therefore, another condition which may influence endocrine function in addition to tumours of the bronchus, sclerosing haemangiomas, testicular tumours, renal cysts and certain sarcomas.

It should be emphasized that trophoblast is a naturally invasive tissue and normally cells may be found in the deeper layers of the decidua, endometrium and myometrium. These large 'wandering cells' may cause the changes of syncytial endometritis. Endometrial blood vessels are also invaded to form lacunae—the forerunners of the intervillous spaces. It will be realized therefore that the histopathological diagnosis of M.T.D. may on occasions be extremely difficult. Some authorities consider the differentiation between invasive mole and chorioncarcinoma to be impracticable.

Recent advances in therapy and refined diagnostic techniques have rendered the histopathological diagnosis of M.T.D. of very much less importance than formerly.

Malignant trophoblastic disease can be diagnosed by percutaneous pelvic angiography and urinary gonadotrophin estimations in the absence of histopathological examination (Wide et al. 1961; Hendrickse et al. 1967). When it is remembered that curettage to obtain material for histopathological examination may cause dissemination of chorioncarcinoma and haemorrhage and sepsis are hazards and that the histopathological findings themselves may at times be equivocal, it can be understood why, in our experience, less and less material is being submitted for examination.

Pelvic angiography may show abnormalities with normal curettings. The contrast medium is seen to enter the defined irregular vascular spaces in the myometrium. Pregnancy, hydatidiform mole and other malignant lesions can be differentiated. In missed abortion, angiographic studies may be positive but the urinary gonadotrophin levels are normal. Extra-pelvic metastases may occur without evidence of a uterine primary source and in these patients the diagnosis rests on the urinary gonadotrophin levels. In all patients angiography should always be combined with gonadotrophin assays.

In pregnancy human chorionic gonadotrophin increases to a maximum between the fiftieth and seventieth days. It falls to normal (200 I.U. per litre of urine) 10–14 days after parturition. In M.T.D. the gonadotrophin levels can rise to 1,000,000 units per litre. Radio-immunochemical assays can detect as little as 0·001 I.U. per millilitre of urine and is more sensitive than the bioassay method.

Both these tests are complicated and are unlikely to be available in most areas of the tropics. The various tests in pregnancy have recently been reviewed (Editorial, 1967). In the absence of facilities the male toad pregnancy test can easily be performed by untrained personnel (Hughes, 1949). By the use of serial dilutions of urine high levels of gonadotrophin can be detected. Recently evolved, simple, commercially-available tests may be of value (Bosnes and Marney, 1967). A lymphopenia is usual and it has been suggested that the absolute lymphocyte count might be useful in assessing therapy—an increase denoting a favourable response.

BREAST

Inflammatory lesions of the breast occur—breast abscess, tuberculosis and, rarely, the primary chancre of syphilis. Fat necrosis is not uncommon. Gnathostomiasis and dracontiasis may simulate an inflammatory condition and elephantiasis may be a complication of filariasis. Spreading gangrene of the skin is a rare condition of unknown aetiology. The incidence of benign mammary dysplasia is not known in the tropics but it is not uncommon in our experience. Plasma cell mastitis occasionally occurs and supermammary breasts have been seen. Adenomas and fibroadenomas, sometimes of large size, are common simple tumours.

GYNAECOMASTIA

Gynaecomastia is common in 'healthy' African men but its aetiology remains uncertain (p. 595). It also occurs in association with testicular atrophy, hepatic disease, chronic renal failure, hormonal disturbances, leprosy, and nutritional deficiencies.

CARCINOMA OF THE BREAST

In many Western textbooks it is said that cancer of the breast is the commonest form of cancer in women (Lowe, 1974). This is not true in areas of the tropics where it may take second, third or even fourth place to cervix, skin and lymphoreticular tumours. The incidence is low in Nigeria, East Africa, the South African Bantu, the Singapore Chinese and in Asia (Segi, 1955).

In India the relative frequency of breast cancer varies in different ethnic groups, being more frequent than cervical cancer in Parsee women but much less frequent in the Hindu (Paymaster and Gangadbaran, 1972).

Breast cancer is the major cause of death from cancer in American women but the incidence in Negro women is 60 per cent less than that recorded in the white population (Wynder et al. 1960). These findings would support the view that early marriage, frequent pregnancies and prolonged lactation are factors which reduce the incidence of breast cancer. The earlier the menarche and the later the natural menopause, the greater the risk. The condition is said to be more common in the higher educational and socio-economic groups but this is probably related to the factors mentioned above. A familial factor has been considered. Single and infertile women are considered to be more liable to breast cancer as the oestrogen cycle of menstruation is not interrupted and a positive correlation between breast cancer and endometrial cancer has been postulated, in both of which oestrogen imbalance has been implicated. It is of interest that the frequency and incidence of endometrial cancer is extremely low in many parts of the tropics, thus supporting this hypothesis.

There is no evidence that carcinoma of the male breast is more common in the tropics apart from a report from Egypt in which hyperoestrogenism caused by hepatic damage due to bilharziasis was considered a possible aetiological agent (El-Gazayerli and Abdel-Aziz, 1963).

Pathology

Carcinoma of the breast is usually classified under five types, viz. scirrhous, medullary, adenocarcinoma, intraduct carcinoma, and Paget's disease. A more detailed classification has recently been evolved by Scarff and Torloni (1968). To all intents and purposes, however, cancer of the breast is an adenocarcinoma, which varies from the anaplastic to the well-differentiated with a varying fibrous tissue response. The intraduct carcinoma has the best prognosis. The methods of histological grading of primary tumours have recently been reviewed by Champion and Wallace (1971) and sinus histiocytosis in lymph nodes is thought to indicate a better prognosis (Black et al. 1953).

From the clinical point of view patients present in the late stages of the disease and the histopathological grading shows a poor prognosis in about 80 per cent of the patients (Pearson, 1963) in Nigeria. It is of interest that the undifferentiated carcinoma is the most common type seen in the American Negro (Leffall *et al.* 1963). Unfortunately, most patients in the tropics present with advanced disease and little can be done. The recently described method of Sonneland (1972), who reported the destruction of a fungating carcinoma of the breast by means of zinc chloride paste fixative, is perhaps worthy of further study in areas where radiotherapy is not available. Various types of sarcomas occur including sarcomatous change in the giant fibroadenoma (sarcoma phyllodes).

Massive infiltration of the breast by the Burkitt tumour can occur in pregnancy and other malignant lymphomas are occasionally seen.

BENIGN MAMMARY DYSPLASIA

Little information is available on the frequency of benign mammary dysplasia (B.M.D.) in the tropics, but Ellis (1937) considered the frequency in Nigeria to be greater than that recorded in Western communities although it is now known that carcinoma of the breast has a much lower incidence. B.M.D. has also been noted to be more common in Israeli-born and Orientals than in those of Western origin in Israel.

Benign mammary dysplasia, benign tumours, and carcinoma of the breast have recently been defined by Scarff and Torloni (1968). In benign mammary dysplasia there may be cysts, adenosis, epithelial proliferation in ducts or lobules, duct ectasia and/or fibrosclerosis. Malignant change may occur but probably infrequently.

14
The Endocrine Glands

It has been suggested that the endocrine pattern in some tropical populations—especially African—differs from that seen in Europe and America, but as yet there are few studies to confirm or refute this statement. Hyperoestrogenization in males would appear to be an entity in certain populations but whether this is due to genetic or pathological processes is uncertain, the latter being the most likely in our opinion. The endocrine patterns in the African have been reviewed by Adadevoh (1970) and in African children by Adadevoh *et al.* (1972).

THE PARATHYROID GLAND

Few studies have been made on the parathyroid gland in the tropics but disease of the gland would appear to be rare. Occasionally hyperparathyroidism due to an adenoma of the gland may be seen. Idiopathic hypoparathyroidism may rarely occur and tetany following thyroidectomy is an entity. Malabsorption and chronic renal disease may cause secondary or tertiary hyperparathyroidism (Editorial, 1968).

THE THYMUS GLAND

Although the thymus plays an essential role in the development of cellular immunity (delayed hypersensitivity) little information is available on the gland in the tropics.

Osunkoya (1967) has noted secondary thymic dysplasia characterized by gross atrophy, complete involution of the cortex, depletion of lymphocytes, and an abundance of spindle epithelial cells in the medulla at necropsy in children dying of Burkitt's lymphoma. Hassall's corpuscles showed wide variation in numbers and size from case to case and might be absent. These findings support the clinical observation that loss of cell-mediated immunity to autologous tumour antigens is a poor prognostic sign in Burkitt lymphoma patients. Whether the dysplasia precedes or is secondary to the development of the tumour is not known. Dysplastic changes in the thymus have also been noted in children dying of measles and kwashiorkor. Reports from temperate climates indicate that abnormalities occur in the autoimmune diseases and in certain forms of malignancy.

THE THYROID GLAND

In temperate climates the thyroid gland weighs between 20–30 g. In Iceland, East Africa, and Ibadan, Nigeria, the weight is very much less. In Ibadan, lymphocytic infiltration is a rare finding in all age groups (Taylor, 1968).

Excluding the presence of cretinism in areas of endemic goitre there is little information available on the congenital anomalies which may occur in the tropics. The relationship between deaf mutism, feeble mindedness, and endemic goitre is debatable (Scrimshaw, 1964).

Acute suppurative thyroiditis is not common but does occur (Adesola, 1962), usually in women with a pre-existing goitre, and there may be a greater susceptibility to the condition in pregnancy and the puerperium. The pneumococcus was the infecting organism in two of the three patients described by Adesola. De Quervains acute non-supperative thyroiditis has been described (Ekpechi, 1973). Chronic thyroiditis, including Hashimoto's disease, is rare in our experience. Hashimoto's disease is also less common in the American Negro than in the white and this has been considered evidence against an autoimmune aetiology in this condition, as disseminated lupus erythematosus is more frequent in the Negro (Editorial, 1965). We have little information on the incidence of autoimmune disease in the tropics. The rarity of pernicious anaemia and idiopathic Addison's disease in Africa would perhaps suggest that the incidence is low in Africa. Thyrotoxicosis is said to be more frequent in areas of endemic goitre but it is not common in West Africa and in most areas of the tropics. McGill (1971) has suggested that the low incidence of thyrotoxicosis in the African is related to an inability to form thyroid autoantibodies. The frequency in Africa has been reviewed by Lowenthal (1971). It has, however, been reported as common in the Congo (De Smet, 1954) and is known to be common in Chinese and Japanese. In the latter two races, and in Thais (Vejjajiva, 1972), the unusual complication of periodic paralysis has been reported (McFadzean and Yeung, 1967). Familial periodic paralysis, however, appears to be less common in these races than it is in the Western World. In thyrotoxicosis the occurrence of the paralysis is not related to the duration or severity of the disease. Hypokalaemia and retention of salt and water occur with an acute myopathy. On biopsy the muscle shows vacuolization. It should be noted that endemic goitre is rare in Japan and that thyrotoxicosis is also common in Iceland, where endemic goitre does not occur (Sigurjonsson, 1940). An association between the two conditions cannot, therefore, be accepted at present. It will, however, be interesting to note if thyrotoxicosis increases in West Africa if iodization of salt is introduced. Riedel's disease we have never seen.

The conditions affecting the thyroid gland in the tropics which appear worthy of further discussion are endemic goitre and carcinoma of the thyroid. Prior to discussing these a classification of thyroid disease is shown in Table 14.1.

ENDEMIC GOITRE

Endemic goitre is common in many areas of the tropics, including Africa, South America, India, Thailand and Indonesia (Miyasaki *et al.* 1967). The geographical distribution has been described by Kelly and Snedden (1960) and Scrimshaw (1964). New foci are, however, being reported (Nwokolo *et al.* 1966; Khodorovski, 1972; Stanbury, 1974) and, although the condition is recognized as one of the most widespread nutritional deficiency diseases in the world, the true extent of the problem in the tropics has not yet been sufficiently realized. In developing countries where the villagers tend to remain static and communications poor, many undiscovered endemic areas must still exist. The incidence of goitre varies in different districts and has been reported as high as 95 per cent in a village in Thailand (Fraser, 1964). In areas of low incidence females are affected more frequently than males, but in areas of high incidence males and females are affected equally. The stress of the menses, pregnancy, lactation and the menopause are considered to cause additional demands upon the thyroid and precipitate thyroxine lack.

The cause of endemic goitre is generally considered to be iodine deficiency in soil, food and water. Under the influence of the thyrotrophic hormone (TSH) of the anterior pituitary, the thyroid gland mobilizes iodine from the blood by means of an iodinase enzyme which can be blocked by thiocyanate. A peroxidase enzyme liberates the iodine and allows its linkage with tyrosine to form di-iodotyrosine. This step can be inhibited by certain organic sulphur compounds, such as thiouracil. Two molecules of di-iodotyrosine form tetraiodothyronine, known as thyroxine. Thyroxine is linked to thyroglobulin and stored as iodothyroglobulin (colloid) in the thyroid acini. Following release the colloid is converted by the liver and kidney to 3,5,3-iodothyronine. This substance, together with thyroxine, is found in the blood in loose combination with plasma proteins as the protein-bound iodine (PBI).

Although the cause of endemic goitre is generally considered to be dietary iodine lack, iodine supplementation of the diet in affected peoples does not always completely eliminate the condition, so other factors must be involved in a proportion of patients.

TABLE 14.1. *Classification of thyroid disease*

Condition	Cause
A. Conditions associated with hypothyroidism	
(a) Sporadic cretinism	Congenital hypoplasia of the thyroid
(b) Endemic cretinism	Lack of iodine in maternal diet or goitrogenic diet
(c) Primary myxoedema	Fibroid atrophy of the thyroid
(d) Secondary myxoedema	Following (i) Graves' disease, (ii) nodular goitre (iii) destruction of the pituitary (Simmonds'), (iv) operation, (v) drug intoxication, (vi) tumour
(e) Hashimoto's disease (struma lymphomatosa)	Lymphoid hyperplasia ? antigen–antibody reaction. Cause unknown
B. Usually normal thyroid function	
(a) Endemic goitre	Lack of iodine or goitrogenic diet
(b) Sporadic goitre	Hereditary (?), goitrogenic diet (?)
(c) Riedel's disease (invasive fibrous thyroiditis)	Cause unknown
C. Conditions associated with hyperthroidism	
(a) Exophthalmic goitre (Graves' disease)	Overactivity of thyrotrophic hormone and anterior pituitary
(b) Hyperthyroidism without exophthalmos	Nodular goitre—intermittent iodine lack
(c) Adenomata (see below)	
D. Inflammatory conditions of the thyroid gland	
(a) Acute thyroiditis and pyaemia	
(b) Tuberculosis and syphilis (rare)	
(c) Granulomatous thyroiditis (viral). Cause unknown	
E. Degenerative changes	
(a) Amyloid	
(b) Calcification	
F. Tumours of the thyroid gland	
(a) Simple: fibroma, osteochondroma, adenoma Adenomata: (i) fetal, (ii) colloid, (iii) papilliform, (iv) cystic	
(b) Malignant—carcinoma most common	
Other conditions	
Aberrant thyroid tissue	
Thyroglossal cysts	

Sporadic goitre occurs in low incidence throughout the world in the presence of an adequate intake of iodine and the iodine uptake of the gland has been shown to differ from that of endemic goitre (Fraser, 1964). The cause of the condition has been considered to be either an inherited enzyme defect or the long-term ingestion of weak antithyroid substances. In favour of a hereditary factor is the fact that there is a high incidence of individuals who cannot taste phenylthiocarbamide (PTC) in patients with nodular goitre in the United States. The ability to taste is inherited as a Mendelian dominant characteristic, whereas lack of ability to taste is a Mendelian recessive. It may be that in areas of endemic goitre a certain number of individuals have an inherited enzyme deficiency which is responsible for the lack of synthesis of thyroxine.

Other substances have been shown to be involved in the production of goitre. Radioactivity of the soil, bacterial infections, an increase of minerals in the diet, especially calcium and fluoride, and goitrogenic substances in the diet have been considered factors by various investigators. Steyn (1964) reviewed the subject and described a focus of goitre in South Africa which was considered to be due to a high fluoride content in the drinking water. There was no deficiency of iodine in the soil, plants, or water. A goitrogen has been detected in cow's milk which prevented a satisfactory response to iodine prophylaxis in children in goitrous areas (Clements and Wishart, 1956). The cattle had been feeding on kale, which contains a goitrogen. Clements (1960) classified food substances containing goitrogens into two groups:

(i) Those which prevent the uptake of iodine by the thyroid gland, e.g. thiocyanates present in certain foods.

(ii) Antithyroid compounds which block the organic binding of iodine, e.g. thio-oxazolidine (present in cabbages, cauliflower, brussels sprouts, etc.)

In Nigeria, where there are many foci of endemic goitre, environmental iodine deficiency has been considered the most important factor. Ekpechi (1964), however, has shown that cassava (manihot), which is widely consumed, has a mildly goitrogenic effect on rats. It is, therefore, possible in areas where the environmental iodine supply is marginal that the added presence of goitrogens in the diet may precipitate goitre. Amyloid change may rarely be noted.

Pathology

The low level of thyroxine in the blood in patients in endemic goitrous areas, whatever the cause, stimulates the anterior pituitary to liberate more TSH, which in turn produces thyroid hyperplasia with swelling of the gland. This is essentially a protective action and minimizes or prevents the development of hypothyroidism. Goitre is usually described as *colloid* when there is a marked increase in colloid in the acini or as *parenchymatous* when there is increased formation of acini with little colloid formation. Either may affect the gland in a diffuse or nodular fashion. It is doubtful, however, if this distinction is valid from an aetiological point of view.

The initial change in the thyroid is that of hyperplasia. The pure parenchymatous type of goitre is rarely seen but foci of hyperplasia alternating with atrophic and colloid areas are common. When iodine becomes available, colloid is formed and leads to enlargement. The gland is firm and has a translucent brownish appearance. The acini are distended with colloid and the epithelium is cubical. With excessive iodine intake signs of hyperthyroidism may occur, but this is rare in our experience. A varying intake of iodine leads to alternative episodes of hyperplasia and inactivity. Hyperplasia may be localized or generalized, and microfollicles or macrofollicles with unfolding walls lined by columnar or cubical epithelium are formed. The nuclei are regular in shape and size and mitotic figures are not seen. Scalloping of the colloid may be prominent. Nodule formation, difficult to distinguish from the adenoma, may also be prominent. In other areas the changes typical of the resting phase or phase of involution may be seen. These are acini with flattened epithelium distended by colloid which cannot be metabolized. The stroma is loose and fibrous or hyalinized. Vascular changes, hyperaemia, oedema and intra parenchymatous haemorrhage are marked. Siderophages and plasma cells may be prominent and siderofibrotic nodules may be formed. In our experience, lymphocytic infiltration with germinal centres is very rare. Areas of fibrosis and calcification are common. The overall picture is that of hyperplasia and involution with haemorrhage and repair the natural sequelae.

TUMOURS OF THE THYROID

Simple adenomas occur in the tropics and their pathology does not differ from that seen in temperate zones. It is frequently difficult to differentiate between an adenoma and a hyperplastic nodule in a goitre.

Malignant tumours

Carcinoma is by far the most common tumour seen. Adenomas, radiological examination of the neck region, and endemic goitre are considered important in its aetiology. Endemic goitre occurs in a district about 40 miles from Ibadan and goitre is a common condition in our surgical biopsy material. Carcinoma of the thyroid is also not uncommon, but, unfortunately, our incidence studies have been concerned with the defined Ibadan population in which goitre is not endemic. In a 3-year study

(Edington and Maclean, 1965) carcinoma of the thyroid was diagnosed in sixteen patients residing in Ibadan and in twenty-one from other areas. Only the former were included in the final rate incidences calculated. Our figures, therefore, cannot be taken as representative of an endemic goitrous area and this exemplifies the need for caution in interpreting rate-incidence studies in individual cancers. Excluding Cali, Colombia, Iceland, and Hawaii a low incidence of carcinoma of the thyroid has been recorded in five continents, females being more commonly affected than males (Doll *et al.* 1966). Endemic goitre is rare in Iceland. The incidence of carcinoma is low in Finland, where foci of endemic goitre exist. The relationship between endemic goitre and carcinoma of the thyroid is therefore uncertain and accurate surveys in endemic areas arc required to resolve this problem.

It has been suggested that papillary carcinoma of the thyroid is not related to endemic goitre whereas the follicular and anaplastic types may be. Uehlinger (1958) has stated that a haemangio-endothelioma of the thyroid is common in goitrous regions but this is a rare tumour in our experience.

The pathology of carcinoma of the thyroid with the relatively few examples we have examined would appear to conform to the usual types described in temperate climates. The follicular type of carcinoma is more common than the mixed, papillary, or undifferentiated types. Malignant change can occur in a nodular goitre and may present one of the most difficult diagnoses confronting a pathologist. Medullary carcinoma which arises from parafollicular or C cells, consists of sheets of polyhedral cells separated by fibrous strands containing amyloid. This tumour is often associated with phaeochromocytoma, parathyroid adenoma, and multiple mucosal neuromata. Severe diarrhoea may be a symptom. The tumour may rarely be familial. The cells secrete a serum calcium lowering hormone—calcitonin—and may also secrete 5-hydroxy-tryptamine, corticotrophin and prostaglandins.

Spindle-cell sarcomas and malignant haemangio-endotheliomas occasionally are seen and tumours of the lymphoreticular tissues (including the Burkitt tumour) are found not uncommonly in the thyroid gland at autopsy. Metastases from cancer of the lung, breast, kidney, and malignant melanoma occur.

THE PITUITARY AND HYPOTHALAMUS

Little information is available on the normal structure and function of the pituitary gland in the tropics. The part that the gland plays in malnutritional syndromes is unclear. Atrophy, colloid cysts, and vacuolation of the basophilic cells have been described in adult pellagrins (Gillman, 1942).

The dwarfism which has been reported in areas of endemic onchocerciasis (Raper and Ladkin, 1950) is probably due to some disturbance of the hypothalamus, but pathological details are lacking. Involvement of the pituitary in trypanosomiasis most probably explains the panhypopituitarism which may be seen terminally (Gallais and Badier, 1952). Partial degrees of hypopituitarism are probably much more common than realized as, in addition to typanosomiasis and tumours, granulomas, trauma, and meningitis may be aetiological agents. Cases of acromegaly and gigantism occur (Sankale *et al.* 1958).

In spite of the frequency of severe post-partum haemorrhage and of seeing post-partum necrosis of the anterior pituitary at post mortem, Simmonds' disease or Sheehan's syndrome would appear to be rare in our experience. Sheehan has suggested that the apathy which these patients exhibit may prevent their attendance at clinics and hospitals and cases may well be being missed. A number of cases have indeed been recently reported —one being a complication of haemoglobin SC disease (Adadevoh, 1970). Amenorrhoea with prolonged lactation following childbirth (Chiari-Frommel syndrome) which may respond to gonadotrophin has also been reported. Diabetes insipidus is rarely diagnosed.

TUMOURS OF THE PITUITARY GLAND

In our experience chromaphobe adenomas are not rare and eosinophil adenomas and acromegaly occur. We have also seen a number of craniopharyngiomas occasionally associated with dwarfism. Rarely a pinealoma may be seen. Further information on the types of pituitary tumours seen in Africa is to be found in the *African Journal of Medical Science* (1973).

THE ADRENAL GLAND

There is some evidence that the adrenal cortex may be smaller in East African and West Indian males than in North American males (Trowell, 1960). The output of 17-ketosteroids and 17-ketogenic steroids has been shown to be low in Bantu males (Trowell, 1960), French West Africans (Monnet *et al.* 1952), West Africans both in Nigeria and London (Barnicott and Wolffson, 1952; Edozien, 1960), Malayans (Lugg and Bowness, 1954), Egyptians (Awad, 1958), and Indians (Friedmann, 1954). The response to ACTH was less than expected in Nigeria. It is possible that there are minor degrees of cortical hypoactivity in areas of the tropics. It is also known that Africans over the age of 30 years may excrete higher amounts of oestrogen in the urine than is recorded in temperate climates, the oestrogen-androgen ratio being high, which would suggest that there is either overproduction by the testis, inefficient degradation by the liver, or perhaps a diminished amount of binding protein in the sera. The exact significance of these findings is not fully understood and the possible effects of 'oestro-genization' in African males are discussed on p. 595. Associated abnormalities of salt and water metabolism, renal function, carbohydrate and protein metabolism, and response to 'stress' have not, however, been noted in association with the lowered urinary steroid output.

Acute adrenal insufficiency occurs most commonly in children, following haemorrhage into the gland. It occurs most frequently in meningococcal infections but can occur in other severe infections and follow abdominal injury. It is characterized by profound shock, with oliguria and anuria ensuing. Cortisol is essential in therapy. It is also a common finding in necropsies on stillbirths and babies who die soon after birth but generally produces little or no metabolic upset in the infant as the adrenal is in a state of acute involution, secondly the functions of the adrenal medulla are largely performed outside the adrenal at this age, and lastly the active subcapsular cells that are going to form the definitive cortex can be largely vascularized through the capsule. The finding of calcified foci in the adrenals of older children would suggest that perinatal haemorrhages are common and usually symptomless. Thrombosis of the renal vein, the inferior vena cava or mesenteric veins may, however, be serious complications (Editorial, 1973).

Addison's disease due to 'idiopathic' atrophy of the adrenal cortex would appear to be rare in the tropics. Addison's disease due to tuberculosis occurs, and is perhaps not as uncommon as some writers have postulated (Bagshawe and Forrester, 1966). It would not appear to be common in West Africa and occurs more frequently in amyloidosis complicating tuberculosis (Brew, 1962). Pigmentation is said to be more obvious on the palms of the hands than in the buccal mucosa in Africans (Bagshawe and Forrester, 1966).

Occasional cases of Cushing's syndrome have been reported and pseudo-hermaphoditism occurs. Primary aldosteronism has rarely been reported. The changes in the gland in malnutrition are discussed on p. 679.

TUMOURS OF THE ADRENAL GLAND

Neuroblastoma would appear to be not uncommon. The tumour consists of small round or oval cells with little protoplasm round the nucleus and may show differentiation into rings or rosettes, the centre of the ring being occupied by a large number of fine fibrils. The cells are radially arranged and the fibrils emanate from them. In the absence of rosettes a biopsy may be difficult to distinguish from the Burkitt tumour, and this is discussed on p. 509.

Phaeochromocytoma and medulloblastomas are not common tumours but do occur.

Secondary growths occur and the Burkitt tumour is the most frequent in our experience.

DIABETES MELLITUS

Diabetes mellitus associated with calcification of the pancreas and African siderosis are dealt with on pp. 665 and 571. There is much evidence to suggest that with advancing 'civilization' and the increased consumption of refined sugar products the incidence of diabetes mellitus increases.

A WHO Expert Committee (1965) recommended that diabetes should be classified as follows:

(1) Infantile or childhood diabetes between 0 and 14 years. The initial symptoms are usually severe and the patients rapidly become insulin-dependent. It is a rare condition in the tropics.

(2) Young diabetics between 15 and 24 years. The onset is usually acute and most patients become insulin-dependent. In the tropics, however, diabetics in this age group may resemble the adult type.

(3) Adult diabetics between 25 and 64 years. In this group the patients are much less insulin-dependent.

(4) Elderly diabetics over the age of 65 years. These patients can often be controlled without insulin.

Other types of diabetes are recognized. The juvenile type are diabetics of any age group who require insulin and are prone to attacks of ketosis. Brittle diabetics are juvenile types who are difficult to stabilize alternating between hyperglycaemia and ketosis on the one hand and hypoglycaemia on the other. Insulin-resistant diabetic patients are those who require more than 200 units of insulin daily. Pancreatic diabetics are those in whom the disordered carbohydrate tolerance can be attributed directly to destruction of the gland by surgery, calcification, or other means. Endocrine diabetics are those in whom the disease is attributable to endocrinological disease such as acromegaly. Finally, iatrogenic diabetes mellitus is recognized.

The incidence of diabetes in the tropics is generally considered to be low and it is rare in children in the first decade (Tulloch, 1962; Dodu, 1967; King et al. 1968; Steel and Hugola, 1974). It has been reported to be rare in New Guinea but a high prevalence has been reported in Indians in Natal, being at least ten times the incidence found in Indians in India (Campbell, 1964). Pancreatic calcification is rare in this area. Insulinopenia has been reported in the general African population in Salisbury and was considered to be due to the high proportion of unrefined carbohydrates (maize meal), in the diet (Wicks and Jones, 1973). It was also thought to explain the comparative rarity of typical non-insulin dependent diabetes mellitus. On the other hand the fasting blood sugar is low in many areas of the tropics.

Changes in growth hormone secretion and in serum lipids were similar to those found in Europeans.

The condition occurs most frequently between 15 and 64 years. Elderly diabetics are not commonly seen and this reflects the age structure of the population at risk. Excluding areas in which African siderosis occurs, females are more frequently affected than males. It has been said that the lower social classes are more frequently affected. It is difficult to assess the part that heredity plays as family histories are difficult to obtain. No association with the ABO blood groups or with deficiency of the enzyme glucose-6-phosphate dehydrogenase has been noted in South Africa (Seftel *et al.* 1963). Husband and wife diabetic pairs occur. The incidence is higher in urban than in rural areas and this has been related to a greater food intake, obesity, and sedentary habits. With increasing urbanization and the greater ingestion of refined sugar products it has been suggested that the incidence of diabetes should increase. Adi (1974) reported nine cases of diabetes mellitus associated with an epidemic of infectious hepatitis. He suggested that the virus may have damaged pancreatic islet cells to cause an acute remittant form of diabetes mellitus.

Ketosis and infection are the main causes of death. Tuberculosis and pyogenic infections (expecially of the urinary tract) are common complications. Mucormycosis may occasionally occur.

Pathology

There is evidence that the pathology differs in tropical and temperate climates, mainly in the lowered incidence of vascular lesions.

In a study of 240 diabetics in Nigeria, Greenwood and Taylor (1968) noted the following: retinopathy 3·3 per cent; ischaemic heart disease 0·4 per cent; cataracts 12·5 per cent; hypertension 12·5 per cent; peripheral vascular disease 1·7 per cent. Pancreatic carcinoma occurred in three of these patients, one with associated calcification. An examination of the dermal capillaries showed some thickening of the basement membrane but it was never severe and there was little endothelial proliferation in the capillaries or arterioles. Nodular glomerulosclerosis was not common. The low morbidity noted was considered to be due to the mildness of the vascular changes, most probably due to a low intake of animal fats. The cholesterol values were low. However, the difficulty of ensuring adequate therapy in the tropics in semi-literate peoples must be borne in mind and early death from the disease or from infective or other causes may be a factor in limiting the severity of the vascular lesions. It is of interest that injection abscesses are not common in patients undergoing therapy in Ibadan.

In contrast to these findings peripheral neuropathy was found in 58·3 per cent of patients and in 15 per cent of a control group. It was rarely severe and it was considered that, in diabetes, metabolic factors were more important in the aetiology of this condition in Ibadan than disease of the vasa vasorum.

The low incidence of myocardial infarction, retinopathy, peripheral vascular disease, and gangrene accords with findings elsewhere in the tropics, excluding the Indian population in Natal. Gupta (1964) has recorded renal changes in a high proportion of diabetics in India, whereas the incidence is low in most parts of Africa. There is some evidence that the incidence of these conditions is increasing in the Bantu in South Africa. A relationship between diabetes and carcinoma of the body of the uterus has been suggested but has not been evident as yet in our material in Ibadan.

Excluding the differences in the complications and the occurrence of calcification and siderosis of the pancreas the pathology of diabetes is similar to that recorded in temperate climates. In the pancreas no one lesion is characteristic of the disease. It may be reduced in size with a diminished number of islets. In a few cases a chronic interstitial pancreatitis may be present. The islets may be replaced by hyaline refractile material. In the juvenile type there may be glycogenic vacuolation of the islets. The diagnosis at post mortem is difficult in the absence of ante-mortem biochemical findings. Samples of urine and cerebrospinal fluid should be tested for the presence of sugar and ketone bodies. Glycogenic vacuolation of the islets and nuclei of the liver are helpful if present. Glycogenic and fatty vacuolation of the renal tubules are more reliable indicators. The typical nephropathy may be present.

THE PANCREAS

Most of the conditions which affect the pancreas in temperate zones are seen in the tropics but their frequency varies. Cystic fibrosis (mucoviscidosis) is rare in Negroes, Indians, Asians and Australian aborigines. This may be factual or due to early death in hot climates due to electrolyte imbalance. The condition occurs in about 1 in 2500 births in Britain. Only one case has been reported from the Orient (Wang et al. 1968), a few from Africa (Levin et al. 1967) and India (Reddy et al. 1970). Clinically, in the early stages the condition may be suspected if the submaxillary salivary glands are enlarged, the abdomen distended and the liver easily palpable. Signs of respiratory involvement may be present and nasal polyps are present in about 10 per cent of children. Meconium ileus may be present at birth. A rapid screening test of neonates has been evolved (Deall, 1971) and it application in tropical areas should confirm or otherwise the rarity of the condition. Acute haemorrhagic or suppurative pancreatitis and chronic relapsing pancreatitis are uncommon in our experience. Chronic pancreatic disease presenting with the malabsorption syndrome, diabetes mellitus and abdominal pain is, however, not uncommon in Uganda (Owor, 1972) and alcohol is an aetiological agent in the chronic pancreatitis seen in Cape Town (Jackson *et al.* 1968). Calcification occurs late in the latter area. Diabetes is common in India (Patel and Talwalkar, 1968) and Geevargese and Pitchumoni (1968) described pancreatic diabetes in 325 patients in Kerala. All the patients had calculi which were thought to be the sequelae of chronic pancreatitis and occurred in young patients. This is discussed when calcification of the pancreas is considered. Deposits of iron pigment may be seen in African siderosis or in haemochromatosis.

Atrophy of the pancreas may be the most marked finding in protein calorie deficiency diseases. Ascites due to pancreatitis or pseudocysts due to injury has been reported (Gunstone *et al.* 1971).

CALCIFICATION OF THE PANCREAS

Fibrosis and calcification of the pancreas has been described not infrequently in Indonesia, West and East Africa, the Congo Republic, Malaya, Jamaica, and southern India.

Concomitant fibrosis and calcification of the pancreas has been described as a common cause of diabetes mellitus in patients under the age of 30 years in many areas of the tropics. It may also present clinically in young children as a malabsorption syndrome with steatorrhoea (Zuidema, 1959; Shaper, 1960; Bourgoignie *et al.* 1962; Kinnear, 1963; Stein *et al.* 1965; Sonnet *et al.* 1966; Varhese, 1966).

The aetiology in temperate climates where the condition is uncommon may be associated with long-standing hyperparathyroidism or secondary to a duct obstructing carcinoma or to chronic pancreatitis associated with alcoholism. A familial form has been described which is rare. In the tropics the aetiology is obscure, and has generally been ascribed to protein malnutrition in childhood in which marked atrophy of the pancreas occurs. We have seen severe fibrosis and calcification of the pancreas in a child aged 4 years in whom the clinical diagnosis during life had been kwashiorkor. In many areas in which protein malnutrition in childhood is common, however, calcification of the pancreas would appear to be rare; thus it has not been reported as common in South Africa or Brazil. In the tropics ascaris infection has been implicated as a cause of pancreatitis, but we consider this an unlikely cause, at least in West Africa. We have no evidence that it is a hereditary form of pancreatitis. The possibility of viral diseases which affect the pancreas (cytomegalic inclusion disease, mumps, etc.) acting on a background of enzyme depletion should also be considered in the aetiology. There is no doubt that mumps can cause pancreatitis in children (Messaritakis *et al.* 1971) and virus-induced diabetes has been reported in cattle and laboratory animals. It should be noted that neither the function of the parathyroid glands nor the osseous changes described in chronic pancreatitis in temperate zones (Serle *et al*. 1965) have been adequately investigated in calcification of the pancreas in the tropics.

There is no evidence that in the tropics the incidence of pancreatic calcification increases with age; and whatever the aetiology of the condition it is clear that neither alcoholic pancreatitis nor protein calorie malnutrition adequately explains the recorded incidence of pancreatic calcification in some tropical countries (Shaper, 1964).

Pathology

The condition may be diagnosed fortuitously on radiological examination of the abdomen for other suspected conditions or the patient may present with diabetes mellitus or, less commonly, with steatorrhoea.

Males are more frequently affected than females. There is no evidence of a hereditary disposition. Radiologically there may be a fine disseminated calcification in the body or tail of the pancreas or large discrete calculi may be seen (Fig. 14.1).

There is intralobular, perilobular, and perivascular fibrosis with disappearance of the islets of Langherhans. Calcification is said first to appear in the ducts and ductules. Eventually the pancreas is represented by a fibrous cord encrusted with calcium salts (Fig. 14.1). Cirrhosis of the liver is not a usual complication although hepatic fibrosis has been described (Stin *et al*. 1965). Theoretically, siderosis should be a complication but has not as yet been considered a problem in the condition.

All diabetics or patients with steatorrhoea in the tropics should have a

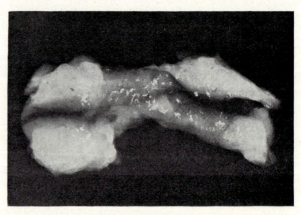

FIG. 14.1. Calcification of the pancreas. Bissected pancreas removed at post mortem, showing diffuse calcification (child of 4 years).

straight X-ray of the abdomen to exclude the possibility of pancreatic calcification. The intestinal enzymatic activity of the pancreas is said to disappear late in the disease and is therefore not of much help in diagnosis.

TUMOURS OF THE PANCREAS

The Zollinger–Ellison syndrome in which there is a non-β-islet cell tumour associated with intractable peptic ulceration has been seen in West Africa and in the Bantu (Banks and Marks, 1965). Cancer of the pancreas is not found in high incidence in the tropics although diabetics have a significantly increased risk of death from this tumour. The ratio frequency in our material was 1 per cent with a sex ratio of males:females of 1·4:1. The crude annual rate incidences in males and females were 0·7 and 0·4 per 100,000, respectively, which are similar to the figures recorded in East and South Africa and are much lower than those recorded in New York and England and Wales. Pancreatic atrophy in kwashiorkor, calcification of the pancreas in younger age groups and schistosomiasis would not, therefore, appear to be important agents in the aetiology of pancreatic carcinoma. In men in the U.S.A. there is a significant association with cigarette smoking and a suggested association with cigar smoking. In females there is a significant relationship to early-onset diabetes and a suggestive association with a history of cholecystectomy (Wynder et al. 1973).

15
Disorders of Nutrition

In large areas of the tropics, malnutrition, especially that affecting young children, is one of the principal causes of morbidity and mortality. In 1966, of the estimated 667 million children in the developing countries about 270 million suffered from protein-calorie malnutrition (PCM) and, if present conditions persist, about 330 million of the 815 million children in these countries by 1975 will not have enough to eat (WHO, 1968). Much research is being undertaken on this problem, and populations are being studied. The biochemical parameters which are considered best to assess the adequacy of protein-calorie intake are the plasma amino acid ratio (non-essential to essential), the urea nitrogen:creatinine ratio and the inorganic sulphate sulphur:creatinine ratio (Simmons and Bohdal, 1970). Five forms of malnutrition are distinguished (Jelliffe, 1973):

(i) Imbalance, of which the most common form is a deficiency of dietary protein in the presence of a normal or excessive intake of carbohydrate and is exemplified clinically by the condition known as kwashiorkor.

(ii) Undernutrition, which implies a deficiency of total calories on a balanced diet and clinically is exemplified most frequently by marasmus in the infant.

(iii) Specific deficiency, which includes the various vitamin deficiencies.

(iv) Overnutrition.

(v) Toxic factors.

For obvious reasons we shall only concern ourselves in this section with the first three forms. Human malnutrition is an ecological problem and the following intimately related factors may be involved in its pathogenesis, (i) bacterial, viral, and parasitic infections, (ii) food consumption, (iii) cultural influences, (iv) socio-economic factors (Ransome-Kuti, 1972), (v) food production, (vi) psychological trauma, (vii) medical and education services (Bengoa, 1940 and 1974; Scrimshaw, 1964; Gopalan, 1967; WHO, 1972a, b). In a recent provocative and stimulating article McLaren (1974a) has attempted to debunk the 'protein gap'. This has led to a constructive exposition view which has emphasized the complex pathogenesis of nutritional disorders (McLaren, 1974b; Brock and Henson, 1974; Rivers *et al.* 1974; Stewart, 1974). Rao (1974) has recently reviewed the problem of malnutrition in the Eastern Mediterranean Region. It has been suggested that the difference between kwashiorkor and marasmus results not from a difference in the diet but in the capacity of the child to adapt (Gopalan, 1968). Waterlow (1974a, b), however, has adduced evidence in support of the classical theory (see below); and has reviewed the subject of childhood malnutrition as a public health problem.

PROTEIN-CALORIE MALNUTRITION OF EARLY CHILDHOOD

Synonyms. Protein-calorie deficiency disease (Waterlow, 1973).

Protein-calorie malnutrition of early childhood (PCM) is a generic term which is exemplified at one end of the spectrum in its more severe form as marasmus, which implies a deficiency of total calories on a balanced diet, and at the other by kwashiorkor, which implies a deficiency of dietary protein in the presence of a normal or high carbohydrate intake. One form may merge imperceptibly into the other, and the term marasmic kwashiorkor has been used. It must be emphasized that the most common form of protein-calorie deficiency disease in the tropics is retarded growth in the 6 months to 5-year-old age group. These children are living on a protein borderline deficiency and any reduction of dietary protein or the stress of an infection, the most common being gastro-enteritis, malaria, measles, and tuberculosis, may precipitate frank signs of disease (Vahlquist, 1973). Thus, PCM is a metabolic breakdown in the young child occurring at a time when his nutritional needs are high and his vulnerability to infections and parasites is great. Shakir (1973) has pointed out that the Quack stick assessment of protein-calorie malnutrition—arm circumference for height—is as satisfactory as that of weight for age. It has many practical advantages, especially under field conditions.

I. KWASHIORKOR

Synonyms. Enfants rouges; culebrilla; boufissure d'Annam; syndrome pigmentation oedeme; fatty-liver disease; dystrofia pluricarencial; nutritional oedema syndrome; malignant malnutrition.

The word 'kwashiorkor' was used by the Ga tribe of Accra (Ghana) and the first clinical description of the condition was given by Cicely Williams in 1933. It is an extreme form of PCM with a peak incidence in early childhood (1–4 years) although it can occur in infancy and rarely in adult life. The aetiology is multifactorial although the principal cause is nutritional imbalance with a diet low in protein and containing a normal or high proportion of carbohydrate especially during the weaning period. It is found all over the tropical belt amongst under privileged sections of the community, particularly those who subsist mainly on cereal staples such as maize, rice, yams, cassava, and plantain, and amongst whom the consumption of protein foods is very low.

The clinical picture is variable but certain constant features are found. These are: oedema, growth retardation, muscle wasting with retention of some subcutaneous fat and psychomotor changes. Certain other features are usually but not invariably present either singly or in combination, e.g. diarrhoea, hair changes (Bradfield and Jelliffe, 1974), diffuse depigmentation of the skin, moon-face, and anaemia. Occasional signs are: flaky-paint rash, hepatomegaly, indolent sores, fissures, and a 'moist' groin rash (Trowell *et al.* 1954). It has been claimed that in Peruvian and West Indian children of African extraction atrophy of the hair root bulb is one of the first signs of protein deficiency (Bradfield *et al.* 1969; Bradfield and Jelliffe, 1970). Associated vitamin deficiencies vary from area to area. Thus riboflavin and folic acid are frequently deficient in many parts of Africa while vitamin A is deficient in India and Indonesia and vitamin D in Ethiopia. Xerophthalmia complicating PCM with vitamin A deficiency is a frequent cause of blindness.

Concomitant acute infections, e.g. tuberculosis, measles, salmonellosis, and urinary infection, are not uncommon (Phillips and Wharton, 1968). Boys and girls are equally affected.

It has been shown that protein-deficient children have a marked impairment in antibody production to yellow-fever vaccine (Brown and Katz, 1966) while they seem to respond normally to vaccinia virus challenge (Brown and Katz, 1966). Mathews *et al.* (1972) have shown that in New Guinean school children protein supplementation of the diet produced an augmented antibody response and more rapid growth over an 8-month period when compared with controls. The implications of this to developing nations are obvious.

Induction of delayed hypersensitivity to dinitrofluorobenzene (DNFB) is impaired in children with PCM (Edelman *et al.* 1973); while similar children do not develop a proper tuberculin response after BCG vaccination (Katz and Brown, 1973).

They also show a high frequency of delayed cell-mediated immunity and a low lymphocyte transformation after phytohaemagglutinin stimulation which correlates with the severity of the disease and improves on therapy (Geefhuysen *et al.* 1971). This may contribute to the high frequency and severity of infection in these children. Chandia (1974) has shown that the frequency of rosette-forming thymus-dependent lymphocytes was reduced in the peripheral blood of malnourished infants and children. Shousha and Kamel (1972) have shown by the nitro-blue tetrazolium test that neutrophils in children with kwashiorkor may have a decreased bactericidal activity.

Metabolic changes

Metabolic changes are pronounced in kwashiorkor since the severe deficiency of amino acids that occurs (see later) has a marked effect on the composite enzymes systems of the individual. Smith (1966) utilizing titriated thymidine to evaluate nucleic-acid synthesis in short-term tissue-marrow cultures in groups of children with severe PCM demonstrated the inhibiting effect on the mitotic index of severe nutritional deficiency. There is thus interference with the metabolism of protein, fat, and carbohydrate and a marked fall in serum proteins. Hypothermia may occur in mal-nourished children even in tropical climates and may be an adaption to conserve calories. A high-calorie diet rapidly restores the temperature to normal (Brooke, 1972). Hypothermia itself may cause oedema and paralytic ileus and inhalation of the subsequent vomitus may cause intrapulmonary haemorrhage. Fat necrosis along the pancreas which is often found in adult cases is slight or absent.

a. Protein

Total plasma proteins and plasma-albumin concentrations are low in kwashiorkor and have for many years been used for the evaluation of the status of protein nutrition in a community (Whitehead et al. 1973). They are not of much value, however, for detecting mild to moderate cases and their interpretation in many tropical populations possessing high γ-globulin levels requires careful reappraisal. Alpha globulin and β globulin are also reduced in kwashiorkor but γ-globulin synthesis in children with compli-cating infections has been reported raised to three times normal value and it has been suggested that the cells which synthesize γ-globulin may prefer-entially utilize available amino acids, thus precipitating the clinical syndrome of kwashiorkor in children on a marginal protein diet (Cohen and Hansen, 1962). Amino-acid metabolism is altered in kwashiorkor and the levels of essential amino acids in the blood (leucine, isoleucine, valine, methionine, lysine, etc.) are reduced, while relatively normal or even elevated levels are found for the non-essential amino acids (glycine, serine, glutamine, taurine, etc.). The ratio of dispensable to indispensable amino acids has been used as a diagnostic test for subclinical kwashiorkor (Whitehead, 1964). It is high (5–10) in kwashiorkor and low (< 2) in healthy children. A ratio above 3 is considered abnormal. This subject has been reviewed by Simmons (1970). The plasma amino acid ratios are of no value for the assessment of marasmus. The pattern of free amino acids in the plasma of kwashiorkor patients is a uniform one, regardless of the diet of the country of origin (Holt *et al.* 1963) and the metabolism of several of the individual amino acids has been studied. The biochemical changes in the skin have been investigated by Vasantha *et al.* (1970). Total nitrogen was low and there was a significant reduction in the hydroxyproline content of the dermis with a rise in the arginine and ammonia content. A reduction in the amino acid content of the dermis was thought to account for the skin lesions. Histidine is broken down by the action of histidase to urocanic acid, which is in turn acted upon by urocanase to eventually form FIGLU, which is found in the urine of folic-acid-deficient individuals and is a glutamate precursor. FIGLU excretion is used normally as an index of folate deficiency. In severe kwashiorkor, however, urocanic acid may be found in the urine which is an intermediary in the breakdown of histidine to FIGLU and is probably due to the absence of urocanase. The FIGLU excretion test is not therefore an accurate method of assessing folic-acid deficiency in protein-deficiency states—or indeed in liver disease. Patel and Bunger (1973) have used a radioimmunoassay technique for estimating circulating T_3 in plasma of children with kwashiorkor, but this method has been recently criticized by Westhuyzen (1973). Disturbances in phenylalanine and tyrosine have also been described with the excretion of abnormal nitrogenous substances in the urine. The hydroxylation of phenylalanine is interfered with and phenylalanine and tyrosine are excreted in excess in the urine. Tyrosine is concerned in the synthesis of melanin, noradrenaline, the catecholamines and thyroid hormones and its deficiency is probably responsible for the dyspigmentation of the hair which is such a striking feature of so many kwashiorkor patients.

In addition to the serum proteins and amino acids being reduced in the serum, the level of most enzymes is also low; thus alkaline phosphatase, pseudocholinesterase, and serum amylase are all depressed. Abnormalities in protein metabolism are further evidenced by low urea and cholesterol values with a high ratio of free to esterified fatty acids. The basal metabolic rate is low. Whitehead (1965) has introduced a test for marginal PCM based on the urinary excretion of hydroxyproline. In Malaysia the 'hydroxyproline index' was generally lower in hospitalized than in normal children (Chandrasekharan and Candlish, 1973).

b. Carbohydrate

The fasting blood sugar and fasting plasma insulin are low. There is diminished glucose tolerance, due to insulin hypersensitivity, and poor pancreatic response to intravenous glucose (Baig and Edozien, 1965). Severe hypoglycaemia may occur. The exact biochemical mechanisms are not clear. There are usually adequate amounts of glycogen in the liver, blood insulin levels are rarely high and contains raised levels of growth hormone and cortisol, all of which would favour maintenance of the blood glucose level. Lactase deficiency is discussed on p. 533.

c. Fat

There is diminished activity of lipase, amylase, and trypsin in the duodenal and pancreatic secretions and gut. One of the features of kwashiorkor is the marked fatty change which occurs in the liver. The presence of this excessive fat in the liver has been attributed to a number of factors. It has been suggested that it arises from adipose tissue and is transferred as free fatty acids to the liver which is unable to dispose of this excessive input in the absence of lipotropic factors (Lewis et al. 1964). Others have suggested that the fat arises in the liver from synthesis of dietary glucose (Macdonald et al. 1963). In the liver, glucose-6-phosphatase is reduced and glycogen is increased, suggesting that the liver is unable to secrete glucose. Dietary carbohydrate is continuously being transported to the liver where some is stored as glycogen and the remainder is converted to fat (Fletcher, 1966). This latter hypothesis is borne out by the low blood glucose and perhaps by the considerable amount of depot fat seen at post mortem. It could be argued, however, that lipogenesis is occurring in the depots as well as in the liver and that a dual process is probably going on. Another explanation is that excessive fat synthesized from dietary carbohydrate is being stored in the liver, where, because of a deficiency of the lipotropic factors methionine and choline, the fat cannot be oxidized or incorporated with the plasma lipoproteins. Truswell and Hansen (1969) considered that reduced hepatic synthesis of the protein moiety of β-lipo protein was the major factor in causing the fatty liver of kwashiorkor. Serum triglyceride and β-lipoprotein cholesterol were lowest in children with the most severe fatty livers. They also found that the serum phosphatidyl choline (lecithin) was not reduced more than other lipid classes as would be expected if the lipotropic factors methionine and choline were deficient. This was considered evidence against lipotropic factor deficiency. Low serum cholesterol and low albumin are the standard tests which suggest a fatty liver. The estimation of serum β-lipoprotein and triglyceride should increase diagnostic accuracy.

Although extreme fatty infiltration of the liver is a constant necropsy finding, considerable clinical enlargement of this organ only occurs in certain parts of the world, e.g. in the West Indies and Indonesia (Waterlow, 1948; Oomen, 1957). Although in general the levels of enzymes are low this statement may not hold for those enzymes which leak into the serum with cell damage. For instance alanine amino transferase (AIAT) may be raised in the serum and in patients with high values the prognosis is poor (McLean, 1966). Isocitrate dehydrogenase and lactate dehydrogenase may also be increased.

In India raised serum levels and increased urinary excretion of the lysosomal enzyme arylsulphatase were noted by Ittyerah *et al.* (1967). Infection, however, also causes raised values.

Serum cholinesterase, a protein derived from the liver, and creatine kinase are reduced, the latter being thought to reflect the reduction in muscle mass. Hypothermia is common in kwashiorkor and marasmus.

d. Electrolytes

After potassium, magnesium is the most abundant cation in the cells of the body, and is deficient in severe kwashiorkor (Hassanein *et al.* 1972). It has been claimed that magnesium is essential in the therapy of severe PCM and improves the electrocardiographic changes and significantly reduces the mortality (Caddell, 1967). In South Africa, however, magnesium was not found helpful in the therapy of kwashiorkor (Rosen, 1971). Measurement of magnesium is best carried out by atomic absorption spectrophotometry which gives very accurate results which are necessary as the plasma levels are normally low. The existence of subacute or chronic magnesium deficiency is difficult to diagnose. The hypomagnesia seen in both adults and children with cirrhosis is most likely related to secondary hyperaldosteronism and the deficiency can be corrected by an aldosterone antagonist (spironolactone). Changes may occur in the cardiovascular, renal, and neuromuscular systems.

There may be marked *potassium* depletion and values as low as 1 mEq/litre have been recorded. *Sodium* and *chloride* are retained with increase in total body water; serum *calcium* is low (Smith and Waterlow, 1960).

e. Anaemia

Protein is required for the synthesis of haemoglobin and a mild anaemia is usual in kwashiorkor.

It is normocytic, hypo-, or normochromic, and the red cell precursors are normoblastic. It should be noted, that the presence of anaemia may be masked by the haemoconcentration which has occurred in the presence of severe oedema, and significant degrees of anaemia may occur when treatment is instituted. The reticulocyte and platelet counts may be reduced. It is generally considered that the anaemia is mainly due to the lowered dietary-protein intake limiting erythroid activity (Ghitis *et al.* 1963; Allen and Dean, 1965; Adams *et al.* 1967). If the degree of anaemia is severe, contributing factors such as malaria or hookworm infection should be suspected. The life of the red blood cell itself is also shortened and returns to normal with treatment. In many areas of the tropics the danger of folic-acid deficiency is real and in some series megaloblastic change has been noted in up to 17 per cent of patients. Iron deficiency may be present and in these instances the iron-binding capacity of the serum is low. The MCHC is also low and there is an absence of stainable iron in the bone marrow, in which malarial pigment will usually be noted in areas of stable malaria. In the later stages of the disease, copper, manganese, cobalt, pyridoxine, or enzymatic deficiencies may play a part. Siderophilin levels are depressed and the iron-binding capacity is also lowered. Serum transferrin values have been reported to be low and are thought to provide an accurate index of the severity, prognosis and response to treatment. A consistent haematological response to treatment with vitamin E has been reported (Marvin and Audu, 1964; Whitaker *et al.* 1967). The levels of copper, zinc and magnesium in tissues including the heart and liver have been shown by atomic absorption spectrophotometry to be significantly lower than in controls (Lehmann *et al.* 1971). The levels in brain tissue were normal as were the levels in marasmic children. Vacuolization of early erythroblasts in the marrow has been described but it is doubtful if this is a specific finding. Infection may play a role in the pathogenesis of the anaemia and it should be noted that the white cell count may be low, thus showing a slight response to the infection.

There is little information available on the factors concerned with coagulation in kwashiorkor. Thrombotic phenomena do occur although their incidence is probably not as high as would be expected in the malnourished European child.

Necropsy changes

As would be expected, at post mortem the most marked changes are seen in the enzyme-secreting organs, but every tissue in the body is affected and the protoplasm of most cells is reduced. The striking features at necropsy are the relatively normal quantities of depot fat and the markedly fatty liver. In contrast the muscles are pale, greyish-red and show marked loss of substance. This persistence of fat in the depots may mask, in life, the muscular wasting which has occurred and is one of the features which distinguishes kwashiorkor from marasmus. J. N. P. Davies, who was one of the first writers to describe the pathology of kwashiorkor in detail, emphasized the importance of pancreatic atrophy as one of the first demonstrable pathological changes.

The pancreas

Profound hypoglycaemia may occur with fatal results and is usually associated with hypothermia, coma and severe infections (Wharton, 1970). Moderate hypoglycaemia (a blood glucose level above 20 mg per 100 ml) is common and not of great clinical significance. Chromium deficiency may also influence glucose utilization in both marasmus and kwashiorkor (Gurson and Saner, 1971).

The pancreas is pale and markedly atrophic. Histologically there is atrophy and vacuolization of the acinar cells with reduction of the zymogen granules. Much of the cytoplasm may be lost and the structure may be difficult to detect. French writers have described the appearance as 'sarcomatous' (Fig. 15.1). Pancreatic fibrosis and calcification have also been attributed to kwashiorkor and this has been discussed on p. 665. The levels of serum amylase and lipase are reduced and accompanied by a reduced output of pancreatic enzymes into the gut. Children may present with the

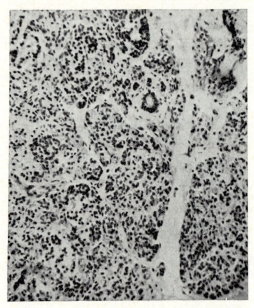

FIG. 15.1. Kwashiorkor. Pancreas, showing marked atrophy of the acinar cells (H and E × 120).

paradoxical condition of hypoglycaemia with reduced glucose tolerance (Waterlow, 1971).

The peripheral utilization of glucose and insulin secretion have been noted to be low in both malnourished and recovered children suggesting, perhaps, that malnutrition may cause long-lasting metabolic changes.

The liver

The liver is yellow in colour, firm in consistency and greasy on section. Massive fatty change in the parenchymal cells which commences in the periportal regions is seen. The liver cell consists of a fat globule with the nucleus flattened against the cell membrane on one side. Every cell in the lobule may be so affected. The cell membrane may be somewhat thickened on electron microscopy. The mitochondria are swollen and there is a decrease in endoplasmic reticulum (Camain *et al.* 1959; Chaudhuri *et al.* 1972). Focal areas of necrosis may occur but are rare in our experience and are a complication of an associated infection. Alcoholic hyaline is never seen.

The portal tracts are somewhat thickened and strands of reticulin may radiate into the lobule itself and along the perilobular areas, giving the

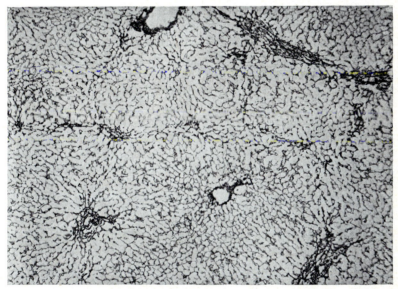

FIG. 15.2. Kwashiorkor. Reticulin stain of the liver, illustrating 'stellate fibrosis' (Reticulin × 80).

picture of stellate fibrosis (Fig. 15.2). A cellular infiltrate (lymphocytes and monocytes) is usual and malarial pigment lying free or in histiocytes in the portal tracts with lesser amounts in the Kupffer cells is a constant finding in areas of stable malaria. Retention of bile pigment in any appreciable quantity does not occur. In spite of the intense fatty change, liver-function tests in kwashiorkor are usually normal, although in a small proportion of children changes suggestive of liver-cell necrosis may be found. At one time it was considered that this intense fatty change and stellate fibrosis was the precursor of the cirrhosis which is so commonly found in many areas of the tropics but this is not now considered to be so and is discussed more fully when the aetiology of cirrhosis is considered (p. 553). The possibility that prolonged untreated kwashiorkor may proceed to cirrhosis cannot, however, be ruled out (Ramalingaswami, 1964). Moreover, there is evidence that liver pathology may vary in different areas. Thus in New Guinea, atrophy and vacuolization of parenchymal cells are more obvious than the fatty infiltration which is so consistently found in Africa (Bailey, 1966).

The heart

The heart is undoubtedly affected in kwashiorkor. Clinically the electrocardiogram shows a low amplitude of all deflections and there are alterations in the ST segment and T and V waves. A number of factors are concerned in the pathology of the heart, the most important being the effect of protein deficiency on the myofibrils themselves, hypoproteinaemia, electrolyte imbalance (especially potassium and magnesium deficiency), and the presence of anaemia. Raised levels of the first band of the lactate dehydrogenase isoenzymes may be noted in some children and it is considered evidence of heart damage (Wharton *et al.* 1969). In addition a systemic infection may be present. Sudden death may occur in the process of recovery and may be due to haemodynamic factors associated with an expanding plasma volume.

The examination of the heart may be unrewarding with the techniques at present employed. It is usually reduced in size but whether this is due solely to atrophy of the myofibrils or to a reduction in their number is undecided. On the other hand, oedema may mask the reduction in muscle mass (Swanepoel *et al.* 1964). Changes reminiscent of the adult type of idiopathic cardiomegaly have been described, namely: venous congestion, interstitial oedema, interstitial collections of lymphocytes and macrophages, and vacuolization and variation in size of the myofibrils with nuclear aberrations. Apical mural thrombi are, however, never seen and endocardial changes are unusual. It is tempting to speculate on the probable association of these changes with certain forms of heart disease seen in tropical areas but, at present, there is no evidence to suggest that permanent damage to the heart follows, or is associated with, protein-calorie deficiency in childhood.

The alimentary system

Diarrhoea is a common problem and in a few children may be due to enteric infection. Sugar intolerance may be a factor mainly due to lactose but others may be involved. If reducing substances are found in the stool of a child on a milk diet a diet based on sucrose should be substituted and if intolerance persists a fructose diet should be given (Wharton *et al.* 1968). In India, in 100 malnourished infants, intolerance to lactose, sucrose, and maltose was noted (Chandra *et al.* 1968). In the colon there is surface epithelial atrophy, an infiltration of plasma cells and a disorganized vascular pattern, all of which improve on therapy (Redmond *et al.* 1971).

There is atrophy of the salivary glands and the enzyme-secreting glands of the gastro-intestinal tract. Parotid-gland enlargement is discussed on p. 516. The intestine at necropsy is paper-thin and white. Mild congestion of the Peyer's patches is usual and the mesenteric glands are usually slightly enlarged and hyperaemic. Stanfield and his colleagues (1965) have described changes in the mucosa of the jejunum on biopsy. The changes are non-specific and resemble those described in malabsorption states. Broadening and atrophy of the villi with fusion were noted in association with an increase of inflammatory cells in the lamina propria and a decrease in the height of the epithelial cells. Disaccharidase was also found to be deficient in the affected intestine and was considered a possible factor in the aetiology of the diarrhoea seen in these patients. Similar changes in the jejunal mucosa have been described in coeliac disease, hookworm anaemia, strongyloidiasis, giardiasis, and sprue, and also in normal adult Ugandans and South Indians.

These changes in the jejunum did not return to normal within 1 year of a favourable clinical response to treatment, but others have reported a return to relative normality with longer follow-up (Cook and Lee, 1966), although the lactase levels remained low. Apart from secondary deficiency of the disaccharidases, lactase deficiency may be hereditary and also rarely sucrase and isomaltase. In sugar intolerance the pH of the stool is low (below 6) and a reducing substance can be demonstrated with a Clinitest tablet.

Kumar *et al.* (1971) have noted values of the intestinal dipeptide hydrolase enzymes which cleave dipeptides into amino acids in undernourished children with diarrhoea. It was suggested therefore that hydrolysed proteins or simple amino acid mixtures should be utilized in the treatment of such children.

However, Prinsloo *et al.* (1971) in Bantu children noted that glucose tolerance tests and serum insulin levels returned to normal with recovery. In view of this, and in view of the low incidence of diabetes mellitus recorded in the Bantu, the authors were doubtful that permanent impairment of pancreatic endocrine function resulted from protein–calorie malnutrition. We would agree with this view but it should be remembered that the question of the aetiology of calcification of the pancreas and its relationship with PCM has finally to be assessed.

The endocrine glands

Atrophy of the endocrine glands has been reported but accurate descriptions of most are lacking. Attention has mostly been focused on the adrenal, and adrenocortical insufficiency has been reported in malnutrition.

Necrosis, haemorrhage, small infarctions, and incomplete involution of the foetal cortex have been noted (Chatterjee and Sen Gupta, 1960) and there is cortical atrophy with absence of lipid. Plasma growth hormone levels are high in kwashiorkor whereas they are low in marasmus and respond poorly to arginine stimulation (Beas *et al.* 1971). Information regarding the thyroid gland is conflicting. A defective ^{131}I uptake has been reported from Egypt whereas normal activity was found in Jamaica.

The lungs

The findings in the lungs are non-specific and bronchopneumonia is a usual complication.

The kidneys

Pyelonephritis may be present. Mild albuminuria occurs in about 18 per cent of children with kwashiorkor but usually disappears rapidly on treatment. Fairly severe histopathological changes have been described by various authors but this has not been our experience and it is considered that a positive correlation between malnutrition and renal lesions has still to be proven. Low potassium values are usual but tubular vacuolization is rarely seen. On the other hand, glomerular filtration rate and renal plasma flow are often reduced and tubular function is diminished. The causes of this impaired renal function have not been well defined but they may be related to potassium and magnesium deficiencies (Alleyne, 1967).

The central nervous system

Mental changes are among the most constant of all findings in kwashiorkor, and abnormalities in the electroencephalogram have been noted (Cravioto, 1966). Atrophic degeneration, chromatolysis, cytoplasmic vacuolation, and disorganization of the neurofibrils in the motor cells of the spinal cord have been produced in experimental protein-calorie deficiency in animals (Platt *et al.* 1964). In spite of the widely held view that malnutrition in early life jeopardizes mental development, the evidence to support this opinion—especially that from studies in man—is scanty (WHO, 1974; Valman, 1974; Waterlow, 1973; Osuntokun, 1972*a* and *b*; Fisher *et al.* 1972; Birck *et al.* 1971; Cravioto and Delicardie, 1970). The relationship of protein–calorie malnutrition to intellectual performance in childhood has been reviewed by Osuntokun (1973). Drowsiness and stupor might be hepatic in origin but this was thought unlikely in Uganda and cerebral oedema due to electrolyte imbalance was thought a more likely cause. Garrow (1967) has shown a low concentration of potassium in the brain at post mortem. Motor nerve conduction velocity has been shown to have low values in kwashiorkor and to return to normal with treatment. In fatal cases very low values were recorded. Histopathological examination of the peripheral nerves revealed no evidence of demyelinization (Osuntokun, 1971).

The reticulo-endothelial system

The changes in the bone marrow and the presence of malarial pigment in the reticulo-endothelial system in areas of stable malaria have already been remarked upon. Severe atrophy of the thymus and lymphocyte depletion of the paracortical areas of lymph nodes in addition to atrophy of the lymphoid follicles of the spleen and appendix have been reported. It was considered that these findings indicated an immunological deficiency which might account for the increased susceptibility of children suffering from kwashiorkor to secondary infection (Mugerwa, 1971).

II. NUTRITIONAL MARASMUS

Nutritional marasmus is due to severe undernutrition from a continued restriction of both calories and proteins as well as of all other nutrients. In contrast to kwashiorkor it chiefly affects infants (first year of life) and in many parts of the world, e.g. most of the Near and Far East, in North Africa, and much of Latin America, it dominates the picture of PCM (Mönckeberg, 1966). Marasmus has a complex aetiology (McLaren and Read, 1972) and the following factors play a major role in the epidemiology of the disease: (1) urbanizing influences, (2) rapid succession of pregnancies, (3) early abrupt weaning, (4) dirty and nutritionally unsound artificial feeding, e.g. very dilute milk, (5) repeated infections, especially gastro-enteritis and tuberculosis, and (6) starvation therapy for these infections (McLaren, 1966a).

The two constant features of nutritional marasmus are growth retardation and wasting of muscle and of subcutaneous fat. More occasional signs are hair changes and associated vitamin deficiencies, especially angular stomatitis and keratomalacia. Oedema is absent and psychomotor changes are uncommon. Disturbances in metabolism have been reported; thus the albumin half-life was found to be significantly longer in marasmic infants than in normal ones, implying a decrease in the catabolism of albumin in the infant with severe marasmus (Donoso et al. 1965). In general serum enzymes may be normal or reduced but not to the low levels found in kwashiorkor. The activity of enzymes in serum is the resultant of two opposing factors, viz: protein deficiency tending to lower the levels and calorie deficiency tending to increase them (Waterlow, 1971). The immediate survival of the child with marasmus is linked primarily to the success of rehydration and restoration of the electrolyte balance consequent on his gastro-enteritis.

In marasmic children who have been successfully treated there is no gross evidence of retarded development, mental or physical, beyond failure to catch up completely in height and weight. The mortality from marasmus is very variable; in South Africa it was about three times as high as for kwashiorkor in the same hospital, while in Jamaica no significant difference was found (Pretorius and Novis, 1965; Garrow, 1966).

Necropsy changes

The body is that of an emaciated infant. The liver shows only slight or no fatty changes, in marked contrast to the findings in kwashiorkor. Slight atrophy of the pancreatic acinar cells may be found, and there may be slight atrophy of the myocardial fibres. Evidence of bronchopneumonia is often present in the lungs (Pretorius and Novis, 1965).

Undernutrition in adults

Adults are the least vulnerable segments of the population and only uncommonly—famines, concentration camps, etc.—exhibit signs of under-nutrition. In our experience most cases of PCM in adults have had some serious underlying disease such as tuberculosis, and we would like to stress that the presence of other disease processes should be excluded before a diagnosis of 'adult kwashiorkor' is ever made.

VITAMIN DEFICIENCIES

Nutritional disorders attributable to deficiencies of vitamin A, vitamin D, thiamine, riboflavine, and niacin occur widely in many tropical countries. Their incidence and degree of severity vary from place to place but they occur predominantly among population groups of low socio-economic status living on defective diets in poor sanitary environments (WHO, 1967). The clinical and pathological features of the vitamin deficiencies are thoroughly covered in general textbooks of pathology and nutrition (Davidson and Passmore, 1966). In this section we shall merely attempt to indicate the magnitude of the problem in the tropics and to define some of the most striking manifestations of the various conditions encountered. It must be stressed from the outset that vitamin deficiencies are usually multiple and those which predominate determine the character of the salient clinical manifestations. Folic acid and vitamin B_{12} deficiencies have been discussed on p. 408.

VITAMIN A

The mammalian form of this fat-soluble vitamin is known as vitamin A, or retinol. Its provitamins are a group of carotene and carotenoid pigments occurring as yellow and orange pigments in fruit, green leafy vegetables, and red palm oil. Thus carrots, mangoes, and papayas, which are common foods in many tropical areas, are good sources of the vitamin, as is red palm oil, which is responsible for the peculiar orange-yellow tint of West African sera and fat. Vitamin A is stored in the liver and a direct assessment of body reserves can be made on liver biopsy material. Serum vitamin A levels can be estimated biochemically and are more commonly used, since low levels reflect not only inadequate recent intake but depletion of liver reserves. The infant derives its supply from milk hence the mother will require a supplement during lactation.

Vitamin A is transported in the form of lipoprotein. Thus in PCM the blood level will fall, and rise when protein is increased provided stores are available in the liver.

The earliest manifestation of deficiency is a defect in dark adaption leading to light blindness. Epithelial surfaces are affected with conversion of mucous surfaces to stratified squamous epithelium thus being more liable to infection. Urinary calculus formation is a complication. Hypervitaminosis A is a danger in some developed countries. It has teratogenic effects. Papilloedema and optic atrophy can occur in adults.

Vitamin A deficiency is particularly common in South and East Asia (Sinha and Bang, 1973), but the condition is also prevalent in Latin America, the Near East, North Africa, and Africa south of the Sahara (Oomen et al. 1964; Korte and Wiersinga, 1972). It is hardly ever found by itself; thus low levels of serum vitamin A are found in acute infections (McLaren et al. 1966) and in kwashiorkor; they are probably due to liver dysfunction and impaired blood transport (Arroyave et al. 1965). Keratomalacia—the most dangerous manifestation of vitamin A deficiency—principally affects the pre-school child and infections (shigellosis, measles, tuberculosis, etc.) are precipitating factors. Another invariable accompaniment of the more severe ocular manifestations of hypovitaminosis A is some degree of PCM.

The signs of vitamin A deficiency vary with age and are (i) Bitot's spots, (ii) conjunctival xerosis—both these signs are commonly seen in school children, (iii) corneal xerosis, (iv) keratomalacia—usually seen in infants and pre-school children, and (v) xerosis of the skin and follicular hyperkeratosis (McLaren, 1963).

A mortality of nearly 30 per cent has been reported in young children suffering from keratomalacia, due to intercurrent infections and possibly adrenal cortical failure; of those who survive it is estimated that 25 per cent become totally blind and vision is reduced in one or both eyes in about 60 per cent. After PCM vitamin A deficiency is probably the most important world problem in nutrition (WHO, 1965).

THE B GROUP VITAMINS

This is a complex group of vitamins derived from yeast, liver, green vegetables, wheat germ, and rice polishings. They can be divided into two large groups—those concerned with the intracellular metabolism of carbohydrates, fats and proteins, and those concerned with haemopoiesis. The latter include Vitamin B_{12} (cyanocobalamin) and folic acid, and have already been discussed.

Thiamine deficiency

The importance of this vitamin to the nervous and cardiovascular system is well known and considerable information is available concerning the role of thiamine in intermediary metabolism. The intake of this vitamin, as with niacin and riboflavine, is related to energy metabolism and hence their needs are expressed in terms of 1000 calories consumed. Thiamine is synthesized to form a coenzyme for carboxylase which is concerned with pyruvic acid metabolism and helps the synthesis of fat from carbohydrate. With deficiency, pyruvate accumulates and carbohydrate metabolism is interfered with.

Thiamine deficiency occurs essentially in countries in which rice is the main staple and hence beriberi occurs most frequently in south-east Asia. Two forms of beriberi are described, infantile beriberi and adult beriberi. Possibly the best test for assessing thiamine deficiency is the thiamin pyrophosphate stimulatory effect on the activity of erythrocyte transketolase which is low in thiamin deficiency. Urinary thiamin can also be estimated and the clinical response to specific therapy in florid cases is diagnostic (Tanphaichitr et al. 1970; Dewhurst and Morgan, 1970).

Infantile beriberi

This condition develops suddenly and unexpectedly and can kill an infant in 24–48 hours. It occurs as a result of thiamine deficiency in the mother, reflected in a low thiamine level in her milk (Simpson and Chow, 1956). The clinical picture is one of convulsions and acute heart failure in the early months of life. It has been shown that infantile beriberi is an important cause of death between 2 and 5 months of age in some parts of south-east Asia (Aykroyd and Krishnan, 1941).

Adult beriberi

This condition is not uncommonly found in the Philippines, Vietnam, Thailand, and Burma, as well as in other countries of south-east Asia. Suggestive signs are referable to cardiovascular function and the central nervous system. There may thus be oedema, cardiac enlargement, tachycardia, loss of ankle and knee jerks, motor weakness, calf-muscles tenderness, and sensory loss (Smith and Woodruff, 1951). Cerebral beriberi (Wernicke's encephalopathy occurs).

Beriberi can occur with alcoholism and as a complication of pregnancy. Urinary excretion of thiamine reflects the intake of this nutrient. A review of the Japanese literature on beriberi and thiamine over the past 20 years has recently been produced (Shimazono and Katsura, 1965) and should be consulted by interested readers.

Pathology

The changes in the heart are not specific for beriberi (Rowlands and Vilter, 1960) and have been described on p. 380. The brain is oedematous and there is engorgement of the meningeal vessels. There may be degeneration in the column of Goll in the spinal cord. Haemorrhagic lesions in the paraventricular grey matter, in the mamillary bodies, in the corpora quadrigemina, and in the ependymal lining of the fourth ventricle may occur. Microscopically, there may be ring haemorrhages in the part of the brain affected. In the spinal cord, there is demyelination of the posterior columns of Goll and also at times of the lateral and anterior pyramidal tracts. The ganglia of the anterior horn show degenerative changes. The peripheral nerves show demyelination, as evidenced by the appearance of fat within the medullated fibres, followed by disruption of the Schwannian membrane. The interstitial connective tissue of the nerve is oedematous and is infiltrated by mononuclear phagocytes. Later, complete destruction of axis cylinders occurs. An inflammatory cellular infiltrate is absent.

Riboflavine deficiency

Riboflavine is widely distributed in plant and animal foods, e.g. milk, eggs, fish, and growing leafy vegetables. Cereals and legumes provide much of the riboflavine of human diets in the tropics due to the large quantities that are consumed of these substances. Milling of grains—a common practice in the tropics—deprives the flour of much of the vitamin, because most of the riboflavine is in the germ and bran.

Manifestations of riboflavine deficiency are more widespread though less serious than those of thiamine deficiency. They have been reported from south-east Asia, Africa, and Latin America. Suggestive signs are: angular stomatitis, cheilosis, magenta tongue, atrophic lingual papillae, dyssebacea, scrotal dermatosis, and corneal vascularization. Some of these manifestations are not specific for hyporiboflavinosis. A case of the burning feet syndrome associated with malabsorption responded to riboflavine (Lai and Ransome, 1970). Riboflavine levels may be determined in a single random urine specimen (Morell and Slater, 1946).

Niacin deficiency

The amino acid tryptophan serves as a precursor of niacin in man and any consideration of niacin metabolism must include this potential source of niacin. Thus, milk and eggs provide little niacin but are not pellagragenic because of their high tryptophan content (60 mg tryptophan = 1 mg niacin). Moreover, niacin can exist in certain cereals in the bound form 'niacytin' (Kodicek, 1962). Niacin deficiency results in pellagra which is still endemic in the Near East, Africa and south-east Europe. It also occurs in non-maize-eating countries such as India, Cuba, and Brazil. It is interesting that in Central America, where maize is one of the staples, pellagra is rare. This has been attributed to lime treatment of maize in Central America and in the other areas to the consumption of other sources of niacin such as beans, coffee, and local beverages—pulque and kaffir beer. The main manifestations of pellagra are dermatoses in the exposed parts of the body, scarlet and raw tongue, atrophic lingual papillae, tongue fissuring, and malar and supra-orbital pigmentation (Pene and Sankale, 1960). In pellagrinous children a greater degree of impairment of lactose absorption and intestinal lactase levels were seen than in kwashiorkor (Prinsoloo et al. 1971). Psychiatric symptoms may be noted and defective intestinal absorption may occur Mehtra et al. 1972).

Vitamin D deficiency

Vitamin D nutrition is related to intake as well as exposure of the skin to sunlight, since body synthesis of the vitamin can occur in this way (Kodicek, 1974; Brit. med. J. 1973). Deficiency of vitamin D results in rickets in young children and osteomalacia in adult women. Rickets is common in both tropical and subtropical countries but its distribution is very patchy. It occurs in Singapore (Williams, 1946), Johannesburg (Feldman, 1950), Manila (Stransky and Ocampo, 1958), and is very common in Ethiopia (Mannheimer, 1966). It also occurs in West and Central Africa but seems uncommon in Uganda. In Calcutta it was found among the children of wealthy Gujarati merchants but not among Bengali children who are put out in the sun, their skin being protected by oil (WHO, 1966). The highest prevalence of rickets is in the group 0–1 year. Cultural reasons, e.g. keeping the skin fair or avoiding the 'evil eye', play an important part in the epidemiology of rickets in some parts of the tropics (Cook et al. 1974). Vitamin D deficiency has been reported among Asian immigrants to Britain (Preece et al. 1973). Rickets and osteomalacia are not uncommon in the Pakistani and Indian communities in the United Kingdom and neonatal rickets has been described (Ford et al. 1973).

Active rickets in young children is manifested by a combination of any of the following signs: painless epiphyseal enlargement, bending of ribs, persistently open anterior fontanelle, craniotabes, and muscular hypotonia. None are specific and direct assessment of rickets is based on the presence of at least three of the above signs supported by a high serum-alkaline-phosphatase level and by radiological examination of the wrists (Winter, 1954). In active rickets the normally smooth and slightly convex lower borders of the radius and ulna become frayed, broadened, and concave (cupping). The distance between the diaphysis and the metacarpal bones is increased because the metaphysis consists largely of non-radio-opaque uncalcified osteoid tissue. The shafts of the long bones in all but the mildest cases show rarefaction and increased trabeculation from decalcification.

Osteomalacia

Softening of bone is an acquired systemic disorder of bone in which there is a decrease or absence of mineralization of bone matrix.

It is the adult form of rickets and may be caused by a number of factors.

1. *Dietary deficiency of vitamin D.*

This occurs in India and parts of Asia, and has been noted in immigrants in Britain (Kendall, 1966). It is most commonly detected in Hindu and Chinese women in pregnancy and deficiency of calcium is an additional factor.

2. *Decreased absorption of calcium or vitamin D* (e.g. malabsorption syndromes, see p. 526.

3. *Renal tubular acidosis.*

There is a group of renal lesions that affect the urinary excretion of calcium and cause demineralization of bone (renal rickets).

This condition is occasionally seen in chronic glomerulonephritis, chronic pyelonephritis, and polycystic kidneys. We have seen this condition in children in West Africa. There is a second group of conditions in which there are tubular defects which cause an increased loss of calcium. Renal rickets due to tubular defects would appear to be rare in the tropics.

Hereditary disorders

These include familial vitamin-D-resistant rickets and the Fanconi syndrome. Hypophosphatasia is said to be an extremely rare disorder in which the activity of alkaline phosphatase is depressed in the serum and tissues. Bone formation is grossly affected and the radiological findings are characteristic. We have seen this condition twice in stillborn children in West Africa. There are probably between 100 and 1000 of these diseases which are rare—alkaptonuria, galactosaemia and phenylketonuria being the best known. The problem of these diseases has been reviewed by Raine (1972).

The pathology of these conditions is dealt with in the standard textbooks and is not considered further.

Other vitamin deficiencies

Pyridoxine deficiency has been described in association with isoniazid treatment of tuberculosis and has resulted in myelopathy (Money, 1959). It has also been associated with a rare form of hypochromic anaemia in which iron stores are plentiful. The part that it may play in primary liver cell carcinoma has been mentioned on p. 593. *Vitamin-E* deficiency has been suggested as a possible aetiological factor in the anaemia of kwashiorkor (Marvin and Audu, 1964; *Lancet*, 1974). The complaint of burning pain in the feet has been reviewed in an Editorial (1972) and may occur in many conditions—acute polyneuritis, diabetes, subacute combined degeneration of the cord, and ergotism. *Pantothenic acid* may be involved in the pathogenesis of the 'burning feet' syndrome, and a case of this syndrome has been described from Ghana in association with optic neuropathy (Dodu and Pobee, 1962). Finally a 'tarsal tunnel syndrome' may be responsible.

Vitamin-C deficiency is relatively uncommon in the tropics; when it occurs it presents with the well-known classical features of lassitude, anaemia, haematoma formation, painful epiphyseal enlargement, petechiae, spongy bleeding gums. The predominant manifestations will vary according to the age of the patient. It is of interest that a deficiency of ascorbic acid has been thought to be a contributory factor in the development of myocardial, aortic and cerebral atherosclerosis (Shaffer, 1970). Scurvy has very occasionally been reported in children in Africa, India and Malaysia (Maclean and Kamath, 1970).

Vitamin K. This vitamin is fat soluble and necessary for the production of prothrombin and normal blood clotting. With deficiency hypoprothrombinaemia results. Vitamin K deficiency may occur in any condition in which fat absorption is interfered with especially in obstructive jaundice. Prothrombin is formed in the liver, so with severe liver damage, hypoprothrombinaemia may be found which is not corrected by Vitamin K administration. It may also occur in the neonate due to (1) the maternal stores being low, (2) malabsorption due to inadequate bile formation by the neonatal liver, (3) inadequate formation of prothrombin by a premature liver, and (4) inadequate production of Vitamin K by the small number of intestinal bacteria present.

UNCOMMON DISORDERS OF NUTRITION

Alkaptonuria is a rare hereditary inborn error of metabolism usually associated with ochronosis or deposition of pigment in cartilage. It is due to a defect in the metabolism of phenylalanine and tyrosine resulting in the excretion of homogentisic acid in the urine. It has been reported in the American Negro and in the Bantu (Baldachin and Rothman, 1959).

Zinc deficiency

Nutritional deficiency of *zinc* in the Middle East has been thought to produce severe growth retardation, hypogonadism, roughened skin, general lethargy and an oral glucose tolerance test suggestive of delayed absorption. In patients with repeated infections, cirrhosis of the liver and malabsorption poor wound healing may be the primary feature (Prasad and Oberleas, 1970). These conclusions were based on the facts that zinc concentrations in plasma, red cells and hair were decreased and that radioactive zinc-65 studies showed that the plasma-zinc turnover rate was greater in these patients.

16

Miscellaneous Disorders

In this section the following conditions are described: (1) malignant disease in the tropics; (2) malignant diseases in children in the tropics; (3) diseases of immune origin; (4) diseases of bone; (5) diseases of joints; (6) diseases of muscle; (7) disorders of calcium metabolism with particular reference to tumoral calcinosis; (8) fluorosis; (9) amyloidosis; (10) venomous bites and stings; (11) tropical ulcers; (12) keloid; (13) rhinoscleroma; (14) heat disorders; (15) pregnancy in the tropics as well as a few interesting conditions which were found difficult to classify such as ainhum, porocephalosis, familial Mediterranean fever, myasis, tunga penetrans, and poisoning. Finally, we include two small sections on the rather specialized but important subjects of eye diseases and skin disease in the tropics.

MALIGNANT DISEASE IN THE TROPICS

The public health importance of cancer in a community can be measured by ratio frequencies and/or age specific and crude incidence rates. Prior to 1960 our knowledge of cancer in the tropics was limited to ratio frequency studies, i.e. the percentage of a tumour type related to the total number of tumours diagnosed. These findings were usually compiled from biopsy material received in a central laboratory or from hospital statistics. Although the fallacies of ratio frequencies are well known they have proved surprisingly accurate in defining the cancer patterns in Africa (Edington, 1955) and indeed throughout the tropics (Dunham and Bailar, 1968) when supporting incidence studies have become available. Age specific and crude incidence rates of cancer, the former being the frequency with which a particular type of cancer occurs in each age group in a given population in a specified period of time and usually expressed in terms of 100,000 of the population per year, are, however, by far the most accurate methods of comparing cancer data throughout the world.

Not long ago it was thought that malignant disease was rare in the tropics. Recent rate-incidence studies have shown this to be untrue (South Africa,

Higginson and Oettle, 1960; Jamaica, Bras and Watler, 1965; Uganda, Davies *et al.* 1965; Nigeria, Edington and Maclean, 1965; Portuguese East Africa, Prates and Torres, 1965; Colombia, Correa and Llanos, 1966; Singapore Chinese, Muir and Shanmugaratnam, 1966; Chile, Doll *et al.* 1966; Hawaii, Batten, 1966; Bombay, Jusawalla, 1966). Doll *et al.* (1966) in their survey of cancer incidence in five continents have made available the findings of most of these surveys in tropical areas and comparable findings from temperate climates are included. In most areas of the tropics the incidence of cancer is less than half that recorded in temperate zones and the cancer pattern differs markedly not only between tropical and temperate zones but within areas of the tropics. Marked variations in the pattern may be seen in territories only a few hundred miles apart and, indeed, are also seen in different races with different sociological customs living in the same territory. Cancer of the penis may be common in a tribe and rare in a neighbouring one, depending upon circumcisional custom, and cancer of the oesophagus has a focal distribution in Central, East and South Africa. The cancer pattern differs in Caucasians and Hawaiians in Hawaii; and in the Bantu, Coloured, Indian and white populations of South Africa. This does not imply that cancer patterns are racial, indeed the reverse is true, and the different patterns in these groups are due to sociological or reactional differences to environment. The low incidence of primary liver-cell cancer in the South African white in contrast to the Bantu is a case in point. The pattern and incidence of cancer in the American Negro is much closer to the U.S. white population than to West African populations. There are differences in the pattern of cancer in the Japanese population and their descendants in Hawaii. There is therefore little evidence to incriminate race as an aetiological agent in cancer, excluding, of course, the greater liability to skin cancer of non-pigmented peoples exposed to the ultraviolet light of the sun's rays, mentioned above, and perhaps also a greater liability of the Chinese to suffer from nasopharyngeal cancer. The evidence for the latter, however, is tenuous. Most cancers are probably associated with environmental factors: cancer of the lung and cigarette smoking, melanoma of the sole of the foot and trauma in some instances, clonorchiasis and carcinoma of the bile ducts, etc. Intensive studies on possible environmental factors in almost all types of cancer are being undertaken throughout the world, including the tropics. The factors possibly concerned are discussed when the various tumours are considered in their appropriate sections of the text. Although in the tropics attention is usually directed to tumours found in high incidence, attention should also be paid to those that are rare or absent although not uncommon in temperate zones, as this implies that they are probably preventable if the correct factors could be identified, carcinoma of the lung being by far the best example.

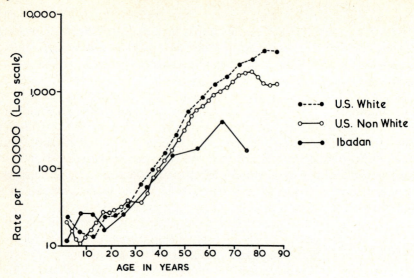

FIG. 16.1. Cancer incidence (all sites) by age groups in Ibadan. U.S. white and non-white males. (*By courtesy of British Journal of Cancer.*)

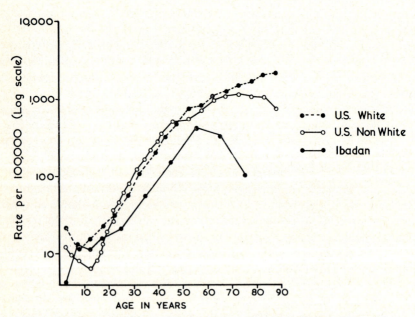

FIG. 16.2. Cancer incidence (all sites) by age groups in Ibadan. U.S. white and non-white females. (*By courtesy of British Journal of Cancer.*)

Age and cancer in the tropics

One of the striking features of cancer incidence-rate surveys in the tropics is the rarity of malignant disease in the older age groups, and this is illustrated in Fig. 16.1 and 16.2. It should be noted that the rate-incidence in this chart is plotted on a logarithmic scale and the differences between the U.S.A. and Ibadan figures may be more than tenfold in the older age groups. Professor J. N. P. Davies first noted this discrepancy in East Africa and suggested that, from the evidence in Africa, there need not necessarily be an association between cancer and the biological effect of ageing. In the tropics there is a tremendous mortality in childhood and few live to more than 55 years. Population 'pyramids' differ markedly in the tropics from those seen in temperate climates (Colbourne *et. al.* 1950). Crude rate-incidence of cancer or mortality figures cannot therefore be used to compare the incidences of cancer in tropical and temperate zones (Figs. 16.3–16.5). The tremendous

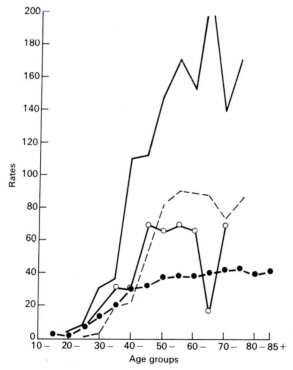

FIG. 16.3. Age specific rates of cancer of the cervix in the South African Bantu (Higginson and Oettlé, 1966), Ibadan (Edington and Hendrickse, 1966), Kyando, Uganda (Davies and Knowelden, 1966), and New York (Handy and Burnett, 1966). – – – Ibadan. ●——● New York. ○ – – – ○ Uganda. —— Bantu.

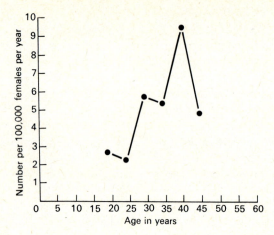

FIG. 16.4. Age specific rate incidence of chorion cancer per 100,000 of the female population per year in Ibadan.

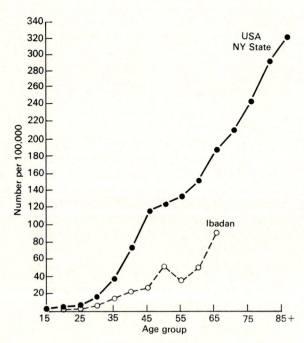

FIG. 16.5. Carcinoma of the breast. Age specific rate/100,000 of the female populations in U.S.A. and Ibadan.

loss of life in childhood and the paucity of elderly people in the tropics makes these figures meaningless. Cancer incidence in the tropics can be compared with that pertaining in temperate zones in a number of ways. The actual number of cancers seen in a defined population can be expressed as the number seen per 100,000 of the population in specific age groups; this is illustrated in Fig. 16.6 for cancer of the stomach. Alternatively the method of indirect standardization may be applied. In this latter method reliable age-specific rates from temperate areas are applied to a known tropical population. The number of cancers expected in each age group can be calculated and compared with the actual numbers seen (Fig. 16.7).

All the available data would suggest that in tropical areas the incidence of

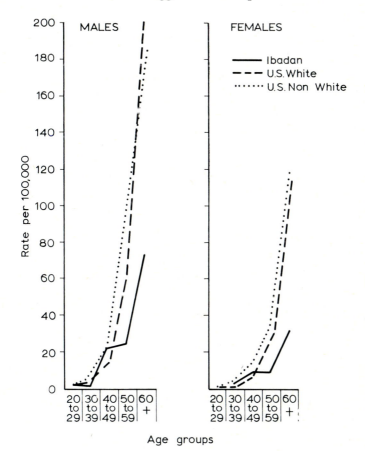

FIG. 16.6. Carcinoma of the stomach. Age-specific rates in the Ibadan population (Nigeria) U.S. whites and non-whites. (*By courtesy of British Journal of Cancer.*)

cancer in the elderly is indeed low. The reason for this is obscure and the following hypotheses have been postulated (Figs. 16.6 and 16.7).

(1) There is an absence in the tropics of the common tumours affecting the elderly, namely: lung, large bowel, and probably prostate. This to a certain extent is true, but liver cancer shows an increasing incidence with age.

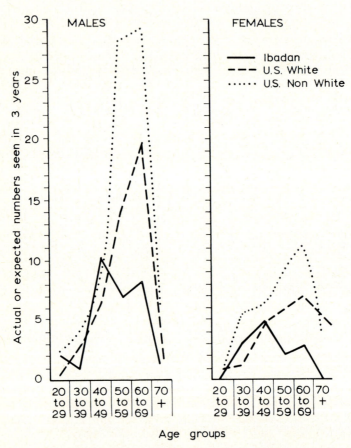

FIG. 16.7. Carcinoma of the stomach. Method of indirect standardization.
(*By courtesy of British Journal of Cancer*.)

(2*a*) The early exposure to carcinogens (e.g. the Burkitt tumour and liver cancer in young adults) may eliminate the 'cancer-prone' members of the community.

(2*b*) A 'precancerous state' may predispose to death in the presence of multiple infections and infestations in childhood. Those that survive may have a natural immunological resistance to many diseases including cancer. There is no evidence in favour of this theory as the changing status of infectious diseases has not been shown to influence the incidence of malignant disease in temperate climates. It is, however, interesting that the incidence of lung cancer would appear to vary inversely with the decreasing incidence of pulmonary tuberculosis in many areas of the world.

(3) Genetic differences may be responsible. There is no evidence to substantiate this. The pattern of cancer in developing countries of differing genetic composition tends to be similar. The pattern of cancer in the U.S. non-white closely approaches that of the U.S. white population.

(4) Lastly, and most important, it has been suggested that sociological factors may be involved. Do the elderly in developing countries accept modern medicine and attend hospital when sick? Little work has been done on this problem. In a general survey it was found in Ibadan that the majority of the population would eventually attend hospital if chronically sick (Edington and Maclean, 1965) but the attitude of the family with special regard to its aged members was not specifically investigated. In our experience, having seen elderly patients brought many hundreds of miles for 'terminal' therapy, we would conclude that this 'falling off' in the incidence of malignant disease in the elderly in tropical countries probably reflects a low incidence of malignant disease in this age group, but we would emphasize that sociological investigations into this problem are required.

Immunological aspects of cancer

It is now generally recognized that most, and perhaps all, neoplasms are antigenic in relation to the host in which they originate. It is therefore virtually certain that immunity plays some role in carcinogenesis and that certain forms of cancer may result from a breakdown of the body's immunologic surveillance (Prehn, 1972). The possible role of immunology in some tumours is shown by:

(1) Spontaneous regression,
(2) Failure of circulating cancer cells to form new growths,
(3) Regression of metastases after removal of the primary growth,
(4) Regression of the tumour with minimal chemotherapy,
(5) Increased tumour incidence after immunosuppressive therapy, and
(6) Patients with congenital immunologic deficiencies are at a sharply increased risk of developing cancer.

Both cellular and humoral immunity play important roles in the immune response to tumours. The cellular immune response (via lymphocytes) is perhaps of greatest importance in killing tumour cells.

Lymphoid infiltrates in the primary tumour and sinus histiocytosis of the regional lymph nodes have been said to prognosticate prolonged survivals without regard to the differentiation of the primary tumour (Black, 1965).

The possible breakdown of immunological surveillance due to multiple infections and infestations and the part that it may play in the occurrence of lymphoreticular tumours and malignant trophoblastic disease have already been discussed.

Immune surveillance is, however, probably only one of a number of defence mechanisms against neoplasia and may vary from individual to individual and probably also with regard to different types of neoplastic cells (Weiss, 1973).

Alterations to cell-mediated immunity have been noted in patients with a number of tumours.

The Mantoux response has been reported as depressed in patients with primary carcinoma of the gastro-intestinal tract, breast and prostrate prior to resection but not in bronchial carcinoma. The response returned to normal following resection (Steward, 1973). Similar findings have been reported in some lymphoreticular tumours. Lymphocytes from tumour-bearing donors are often cytotoxic *in vitro* against cultured tumour cells from the same individual. If, however, the tumour cells are exposed to the serum of homologous tumour-bearing hosts the cytotoxic effects of the lymphocytes are lost. The serum of the tumour-bearing host would appear to contain factors which interfere with cell-mediated immunity. The mechanism of the blocking of lymphocyte-mediated cytotoxicity is unknown. The serum-blocking activity is rapidly lost following removal or regression of the tumours (Baldwin *et al.* 1973).

Immune responses by the host against tumour-associated antigens have been shown by various methods particularly in Burkitt's lymphoma, nasopharyngeal carcinoma, osteogenic sarcoma, malignant melanoma, neuroblastoma and carcinoma of the colon and bladder (Klein, 1970).

Certain fetal antigens may be found to be increased in malignant tumours and may be detected in the serum and other body fluids by a variety of techniques utilizing specifically prepared antisera. Alphafetoprotein has already been discussed and the subject has been reviewed by Alexander (1972). Carcino-embryonic antigen (CEA) should however be mentioned. The term CEA was used by Gold and Freedman in 1965 to describe a substance detected by the use of heterologous antiserum in all adenocarcinomas of the human digestive tract but in no benign tumours. CEA was also detected in the digestive organs of human fetuses. It has also been found to be raised in other malignant tumours outside the gastro-intestinal tract, including neuroblastoma, breast and bronchus. Raised values may also be found in inflammatory conditions or with regeneration. The finding of raised plasma levels, therefore, lacks specificity. Effective surgical therapy, however, restores high CEA levels to normal and the test may be useful in prognosis or in detecting a recurrence of the malignancy. Its presence in the urine is of value in the detection and follow-up of tumours of the urinary system. It may be found in raised amounts in the faeces in colonic cancer. Its level in various disease states has been described by Khoo and Mackay (1973).

It is of interest that Makari (1955) was able to detect the presence of circulating carcinoma-specific antigens in the serum of patients with carcinoma. Later the polysaccharide nature of the antigens was discovered and a skin test was developed based on the immediate type of cutaneous autohypersensitivity in subjects with early cancer (Makari, 1960). The autohypersensitivity is directed against antigen–antibody complexes formed by tumour polysaccharide substance (TPS) and serum antibodies from the subject being tested. The incidence of positive tests decreases with the advancing stage of the carcinoma and a negative test may have prognostic significance in proven cancer. The Makari tumour skin test has been evaluated by Tee (1973), Honda et al. (1973) and Boisivon (1973). The test was positive in 100 per cent of patients with early cancer. False positive results may be got in patients with inflammatory conditions of the digestive system or with benign tumours. It is considered that the test will be useful in detecting early cancer.

Caspary and Field (1971) have described the cytopherometric method of assessing lymphocytic sensitization. Sensitized lymphocytes react with a specific antigen to liberate a substance which has the property of slowing the electrophoretic migration of normal macrophages. It is claimed that lymphocytes from patients with malignant neoplasia generally produce a 15–20 per cent macrophage speed reduction with an extraction of brain tissue used as the antigen (encephalitogenic factor) as compared with less than 5 per cent in normal subjects. Comparable reduction occurs when tumour basic protein is substituted for the brain extract. It is suggested that a common antigen is present in human malignant growths manifesting itself by specific lymphocyte sensitization. This may prove a useful screening test for cancer if this hypothesis is proven.

Endocrine and metabolic manifestations of cancer

This subject has been reviewed by Ross (1972) and many cancers cause endocrine and metabolic disturbances in the host and these are illustrated in Table 16.1.

Neurological complications of cancer are common and are shown in Table 16.2.

TABLE 16.1. *Hormones secreted by malignant cells, their principal sites of origin, and the chief metabolic abnormality of diagnostic significance* (from Ross 1972, *Brit Med. J.*, 1, 735)

Hormone	Principal cancers concerned	Principal metabolic (or clinical) abnormality
Corticotrophin	Bronchus (oat-cell) Pancreas (islet-cell) Thymoma Thyroid (papillary and medullary) Stomach Pancreas Ovary	Hypokalaemic alkalosis (weakness, thirst, polyuria)
α- and β-melanocyte stimulating hormone	Bronchus (oat-cell)	(Pigmentation)
Vasopressin	Bronchus (oat-cell) Duodenum Cerebellar haemangioblastoma Lymphoma, Hodgkin's disease	Dilutional hyponatraemia (drowsiness)
Parathormone	Bronchus (squamous cell) Bladder Uterus Vulva	Hypercalcaemia (vomiting, constipation, psychosis)
Thyroid-stimulating hormone	Choriocarcinoma Hydatidiform mole Embryoma of testis Bronchus	Hypermetabolism (tachycardia)
Gonadotrophin	Hepatoma Bronchus	Increased androgen production (precocious puberty)
Luteinizing hormone	Trophoblast tumour in women Teratocarcinoma Bronchus	Increased oestrogen production (gynaecomastia)
Gastrin	Pancreas (α-cell)	High gastric acidity (peptic ulceration)
5-hydroxytryptamine (serotonin)	Carcinoid of Small intestine Caecum Appendix	(Diarrhoea, abdominal cramps, cyanotic flushes)
5-hydroxytryptophan histamine	Carcinoid of bronchus	(Tachycardia, flushing, hypotension)

TABLE 16.2. *Other manifestations of cancer* (from Ross, 1972, *Brit. Med. J.*, **1**, 735)

Complications	Neoplasms commonly concerned
Neurological	Bronchus
Myopathy	Breast
Polymyositis	Cervic
Myasthenia	Ovary
Dermatomyositis	Colon
Neuropathy	
Sensory	
Mixed sensori-motor	
Encephalopathy	
Myelopathy	
Dermatological	Lymphomas
Acanthosis nigricans	Breast
Ichthyosis	Stomach
Hypertrichoris	Uterus
Dermatitis herpetiformis	Ovary
Herpes zoster (dermatomyositis)	
Vascular	Pancreas
Thrombophlebitis	Ovary
Arterial thrombosis	Cervix
	Breast
	Hypernephroma
Haematological	Breast
Leukoerythroblastic and leukaemoid reactions	Prostate
Eosinophilia	Thymus
Red cell aplasia	Hypernephroma
Erythrocytosis	
Intravascular coagulopathy	
Proteinopathies	Most cancers
Hypoalbuminaemia	
Hyper γ_2 globulinaemia	
Amyloidosis	
Cryofibrinogenaemia	
Skeletal	Bronchus
Clubbing	
Hypertrophic osteoarthropathy	
Renal	
Nephrotic syndrome (membranous glomerulonephritis)	

Histology of cancer in the tropics

In general, the histology of the various types of tumours seen in the tropics resemble those described in standard textbooks of pathology.

Differences when they exist are mentioned, the frequency of squamous-cell carcinoma of the bladder associated with *S. haematobium* infection being an example. It is felt by some that the incidence of anaplastic malignant tumours *vis-à-vis* the well-differentiated is greater in tropical areas and this is our impression in breast and large bowel cancers. Whether the fact that patients in the tropics usually present at a late stage of the disease plays a part in this observation is debatable. It is more likely that the relatively younger age of the patient presenting with cancer in the tropics and the paucity of cancer in the older age groups, which also tends to be less florid, are responsible for this finding.

Common tumours seen in the tropics

The majority of these have already been discussed in some detail (the Burkitt tumour, liver-cell carcinoma, carcinoma of the bile ducts, oral, nasopharyngeal and oesophageal carcinoma, carcinoma of the penis, and chorioncarcinoma). The occurrence of malignant change in tropical ulcers was only briefly mentioned, as it is a squamous-cell carcinoma with no remarkable features. The differing pattern of cancer in childhood in Africa has been remarked upon, the high incidence of the Burkitt tumour being in contrast to the low incidence of acute leukaemia. Wilms' tumour and the retinoblastoma are also not uncommon tumours in childhood. Cancers of the nervous system are also seen (Collomb *et al.* 1971).

There are a number of common tumours which have not yet been dealt with (a number of types of skin malignancy and Kaposi's sarcoma) and these are discussed on the following pages.

CANCER OF THE SKIN

Rates of skin cancer are high in non-pigmented peoples in Australia, New Zealand, and South Africa. Camain *et al.* (1972) have compared the pattern of skin cancer in Africa, Asia and Europe. Squamous-cell carcinoma is the most frequent type in Asia and Africa and relatively much less prevalent among the Caucasians of the United States and Australia. Basal-cell carcinoma prevails in white populations. It occurs less often in Asians and is rare in Africans.

The rarity of basal-cell carcinoma in the African has been considered to be due to two factors. Basal-cell carcinomas may arise from the pilary and sebaceous apparatus under some stimulation, probably ultraviolet light. The density of the pilary system is less in Africans and hair growth is slow; melanin prevents sunburn and cancer formation by absorbing ultraviolet radiation. In addition to basal cell carcinoma keratoacanthoma is also seldom seen. In our practice in West Africa if basal carcinoma is diagnosed the patient is expected to be a Caucasian or an albino. Albinism is inherited as an auto-somal recessive metabolic defect. The estimated gene frequency is 0·033 in the Bantu, which is much higher than the incidence recorded in Caucasians or in the Japanese (Oettle, 1962). The reason for this high frequency is unknown. It may be due to a higher mutation rate or it may be that the heterozygotes enjoy a selective advantage. In the albino, melanocytes are present in normal numbers and premelanosomes and melanosome struc-tures can be seen by electron microscopy. There is, however, defective synthesis of tyrosinase which catalyses the hydroxylation of the melanin precursor tyrosine to dioxyphenylalanine (DOPA). A primary dysfunction of platelet adenosine diphosphate release with a hereditary mild bleeding disorder has been described in a few patients. The bleeding time is prolonged (Logan *et al.* 1971). Squamous- and basal-cell carcinomas are common in albinos and melanomas, and sweat-gland carcinoma can occur (Kennedy and Zelickson, 1963). In India basal cell carcinoma is common and forms 30·3 per cent of skin tumours (Paymaster *et al.* 1971). Apart from the peculiar forms of squamous cell carcinoma described below it is an ex-tremely common tumour in many parts of the tropics as about 9 per cent of tropical ulcers are considered to exhibit malignant change. It is of interest that an enhanced frequency of squamous-cell carcinoma of the skin has been noted in patients on immunosuppressive therapy (Walder *et al.* 1971), perhaps suggesting that immunological surveillance may be important in its aetiology. Malignant melanoma is considered separately on p. 707.

The role of arsenic in Taiwan and the environmental factors concerned in Kangri and Dhoti cancer are discussed below. No obvious racial differ-ences have been noted in adnexal tumours of the skin.

It should be noted that mortality rates cannot be utilized in comparing the incidence of skin cancers in tropical and temperate zones, as the result of therapy readily available in the latter is likely to markedly influence mortality. Morbidity studies are the only valid criteria of comparison.

Kangri cancer

Kangri cancer is a squamous-cell carcinoma which occurs usually on the abdomen and thighs and is seen in Kashmir. It is associated with the habit of carrying an earthenware pot covered with wicker-work and containing burning charcoal to protect the individual from the cold. The pot is carried against the abdomen when walking or between the thighs when squatting. Chronic dermatitis, burns, and scars eventually lead to cancer, more commonly in males, in the sixth decade. The combustion products of live coal and the dried leaves of the Chinas tree used to keep the coal alive are probably carcinogenic (Gothoskar and Ranadive, 1966).

Dhoti cancer

This occurs in Bombay, India, and is due to the pressure and irritation of the loin cloth on the loins, right groin, inner surface of the right buttock and posteriorly along the midline behind the sacrum. Associated factors are dust, sweat, and poor hygiene. A squamous-cell carcinoma may develop in any of the sites quoted above.

Cancer associated with arsenical dermatitis

Epidermoid or basal-cell carcinomas have been shown to occur in high incidence in areas of Taiwan where there is a high content of arsenic in water and chronic arsenical intoxication occurs.

KAPOSI'S SARCOMA

Synonym. Idiopathic multiple haemorrhagic sarcoma.

Kaposi's sarcoma usually presents as nodules in the subcutaneous tissue of the lower limb, frequently symmetrical, and associated with lymphoedema. The lesions, however, may be widespread and mucous membranes or

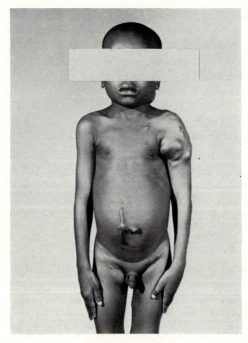

FIG. 16.8. Kaposi's sarcoma in a child, 9 years old, showing gross lymphadenopathy.

viscera may be primarily affected—including the cervical lymph nodes in children. Regression of subcutaneous lesions with the spontaneous occurrence of fresh lesions are features of the disease.

Epidemiology

The condition is common in Jews living in Eastern Europe and in the African in South, East, Central and parts of West Africa. It is not common in the American Negro, in the West Indian, or in the Indians, Coloureds, or whites in South Africa.

Although Maclean (1963) noted no variation in frequency in differing areas of Nigeria, Oluwasanmi and Osunkoya (1969) noted a high frequency in the Mid-Western State of Nigeria and all 29 cases were males. The usual male:female sex ratio is 12:1 (Slavin *et al.* 1969; Baddeley, 1974).

The lesions were mainly on the limbs and occupation exposure was considered a possible explanation. All age groups are affected but lymph gland involvement is usual in children, usually with a rapidly fatal course. It has been seen in association with lymphoreticular tumours and has occurred in association with immunosuppressive therapy (Haim *et al.* 1972). Herpes-type viruses have been observed in cultures from the tumour from different geographical regions (Giraldo *et al.* 1972). The condition is rare in the American Negro. These observations would suggest environmental factors are important in the aetiology of Kaposi's sarcoma and that perhaps an alteration of the immunological surveillance of the host is important. However, the relatively high incidence of the condition in the Johannesburg Bantu contrasts with the low incidence of the Burkitt and other lymphoreticular tumours in that population poses an interesting epidemiological problem which has still to be solved.

No variation in incidence has been noted in Nigeria in differing areas with marked climatic variations in temperature and humidity (Maclean, 1963). Genetic factors would appear to be eliminated and occupation, diet, social, and infective factors require further investigation. All age groups are affected and males are more frequently affected than females. The incidence rises steadily with age. In the Caucasian an association with tumours of lymphoreticular tissue has been noted.

Pathology

Kaposi's sarcoma presents first as macular then as nodular circumscribed ulcerating skin lesions affecting the limbs, trunk, head, and neck or scrotum. The intestine, bones, or lymph nodes may be primarily involved. The course may be rapid with widespread metastases in the internal organs or relatively benign, the patient surviving many years with little disability.

The histological features vary considerably even in different lesions in the same patient, as involution may occur spontaneously in individual lesions with the formation of dense collagenous tissue. The striking feature is proliferating spindle cells with numerous spaces present containing red blood cells, and the resemblance to a haemangiomatous tumour may be marked (Fig. 16.9). The spindle cells may be narrow and filiform, with dense hyperchromatic nuclei and few or no mitoses, or large plump cells, with active mitoses present (Murray and Lothe, 1962). In some cases globules

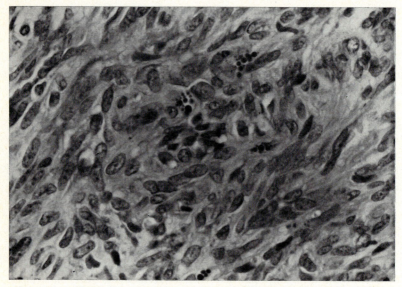

Fig. 16.9. Kaposi's sarcoma showing proliferating spindle cells and globules of cosmophilic material (Phloxine tartrazine × 800).

of eosinophilic material (well shown by the phloxine tartrazine stain) have been observed both intra- and extra-cellularly. Large, well-formed vessels may be present in the tumour and thrombosis of blood vessels and vasculitis are occasionally seen. Foci of necrosis are also occasionally present. Haemorrhages may occur and lead to siderotic pigmentation. The neoplastic nodules are well defined and may have a pseudocapsule or infiltrate the surrounding connective tissue, which is, as are the trabeculae traversing the tumour, infiltrated by lymphocytes, histocytes, and plasma cells. Dilatation of lymphatics may be marked.

The origin of the spindle cells is debatable and they have variously been considered fibroblasts, smooth-muscle cells, and endothelial cells. Electron microscopy studies have shown that the vascular spaces have no endothelial lining and that the spindle cells are most probably derived from Schwann cells (Pepler and Theron, 1962). The literature has recently been reviewed by Reynolds *et al.* (1965).

Lesions have been described in lymph glands, tongue, oesophagus, gastro-intestinal tract, pancreas, suprarenal glands, thyroid, heart, lungs, bone, liver, voluntary and smooth muscle. Very occasionally, lesions may be found in the central nervous system.

Radiological examination may reveal (*a*) cortical erosion of bone due to soft tissue tumour pressure, (*b*) cysts arising centrally in the marrow cavity, or (*c*) areas of rarefaction (Palmer, 1962). Tumours may be outlined in soft tissues with scattered calcification present.

Peripheral arteriography shows the blood supply of the tumour and can demonstrate previously unsuspected lesions.

MALIGNANT MELANOMA

The incidence of malignant melanoma is lowest in the pigmented races and appears to occur most frequently where the pigment is least, the sole of the foot being the most common site in Africa. Other areas which may be affected are the nail matrix, conjunctiva, and the nasal and oral cavities. Occasionally the anorectal region is affected and rarely in Africa an intra-ocular melanoma may be seen, in contrast to some European countries in which this site is frequently affected. Rarely, the central nervous system may be primarily involved (Odeku and Janota, 1965). In Caucasians the head and neck are most frequently affected, although it has been shown in England and Wales that the incidence of malignant melanoma of the lower limb in females is high and that they have high death rates compared to other sites and to the rates for the lower limb in males. The excess mortality is at a maximum at ages 40–44. This has been associated with exposure resulting from modern dress. The most common form of malignant melanoma of the lower limb in females is the superficial spreading (Lee, 1970). (See below)

In Caucasians it is not uncommon for the tumour to arise in junctional naevi. Naevi are common and it has been estimated that there are about 10–30 per person whereas in the American Negro the figure is two. There was an average figure of 11 naevi present on adult Ugandans—the figure being higher in females. They were more common on the lower extremity than on the head and neck, in contrast to the findings in the U.S.A. (Lewis and Johnson, 1968).

Trauma has long been considered an aetiological agent in the frequency with which the sole of the foot is affected in Africa but this site is also commonly affected in the Bantu in the urbanized townships of South Africa, and in the American Negro.

An association between malignant melanoma and exposure to sunlight has also long been suspected in Caucasians, especially in people whose tanning response is poor. The incidence varies with latitude, mortality in Caucasians increasing as the equator is approached. This is, however, not entirely a direct effect of sunlight since all areas of the body are affected, not just the exposed areas. It has been suggested that lentigo, malignant melanoma and superficial spreading melanoma (see below) on exposed sites are likely to be a direct result of sunlight trauma whereas nodular melanoma of non-exposed sites is more likely to be due to the effect of materials released by sunlight-influenced skin causing malignant change in melanocytes remote from the damaged area. A viral aetiology has also been postulated and the rarity of the tumour before puberty suggests hormonal influences may also be factors. It is of interest that the tumour behaves 'normally' in pregnant women. In the non-pigmented conjunctiva all racial groups should be equally at risk to the carcinogenic effects of solar rays but intraocular melanomas, possibly the result of indirect solar exposure, should be rare in the melanin-shielded Negro—as indeed is the case. Spontaneous regression occasionally occurs and immunological factors have been considered in the behaviour of the tumour. Two types of antibodies have been reported in sera of patients with malignant melanoma—one directed against the cytoplasmic contents and the other against the surface membrane of melanoma cells (Lewis and Phillips, 1972).

Bluming et al. (1972) have described cutaneous reactivity to extracts of autologous melanoma cells but no correlation with prognosis, such as has been described in the Burkitt tumour, was noted.

It is of interest to note that there is said to be no significant difference in the number of melanocytes (the cell from which the tumour arises) in whites, Negroes, and albinos, and a malignant melanoma can arise in an albino (Kennedy and Zelickson, 1963). The physiology of melanin production has been reviewed by Wasserman (1965). The tumour occurs in adults of any age but is rare in childhood. In Uganda three clinical types of malignant melanoma have been delineated (Lewis and Kiryabwire, 1968) in 200 patients. Group 1 (40 per cent) consisted of patients with a relatively long history of a localized tumour, usually on the sole of the foot, with no metastases. Group 2 (48 per cent) included patients with a primary lesion with regional or distant metastases and a short clinical history. Group 3 (12 per cent) consisted of patients presenting with metastatic melanoma in whom no primary lesion could be found. There were no distinguishing histological features among the three groups, and the authors suggested that a difference might exist in the host response to this tumour. Lewis (1967) also demonstrated an *in vitro* cytotoxic effect of autologous serum against melanoma cells of Group 1 but not Group 2 patients, suggesting possible immunological differences.

Three basic types of melanoma have been described by Clark *et al.* (1969) as: *the lentigo*, a flat, pigmented patch occurring on the face of elderly people which slowly advances to tumour formation; *the superficial spreading type*, normally slowly growing and metastasizing somewhat late; and the more actively growing *nodular type* of tumour, which carries a greater risk of spread. These are sub-divided into five categories according to depth of dermal invasion.

The usual type in our experience in Africa is an ulcerated nodular type. The cells in the tumour vary from round to spindle-shaped forms. There may be a diverse nuclear pattern with frequent mitoses. Multinucleated giant cells may be present. Pigment is usually increased and is liberated and taken up by phagocytes. Rarely in our experience the pigment may be difficult to detect (amelanotic melanoma). The pigment gives a negative Prussian-blue reaction, reduces silver salts (Fontana's stain) and can be bleached by hydrogen peroxide and potassium permanganate.

Spread of the tumour is usually first by the lymphatics, but latterly widespread haematogenous dissemination occurs.

MALIGNANT DISEASE IN CHILDREN IN THE TROPICS

In Ibadan 582 tumours were recorded in children under the age of 15 years in a total of 4514 malignant tumours seen in the years 1960–66. The most common tumours are shown in Table 16.3.

TABLE 16.3

Type of tumour	Number	R.R.F.
Burkitt tumour	321	55·2
Tumours of connective tissue	37	6·4
Wilm's tumour	33	5·7
Leukaemia	31	5·3
Retinoblastoma	25	4·3
Hodgkin's disease	19	3·3
Tumours of bone	16	2·7
Neuroblastoma	14	2·4
Cerebral tumours	14	2·4
Liver cancer	8	1·4
Ameloblastoma	6	1·0
Reticulum cell sarcoma	6	1·0

The average annual incidences of the Burkitt tumour, leukaemia and Wilm's tumour were 8·5, 1·7 and 1·1 per 100,000 children respectively. Wilms tumour would appear to be more common and leukaemia less common in Nigeria than in temperate climates. Hodgkin's disease and retinoblastoma would also appear to be slightly increased in the Ibadan population.

In Jamaica, childhood malignancy accounted for 2·9 per cent of all malignancies in contrast to the 12·9 per cent in Ibadan. This is almost entirely due to the almost total absence of the Burkitt tumour (Bras *et al.* 1969). The tumour pattern in Jamaica largely resembled that in the United States and Western Europe and contrasted significantly with tropical Africa, although over 90 per cent of the Jamaican population is either pure Negro or of predominantly Negro descent.

In Brazil there would appear to be higher frequencies of adrenal cortical tumours and renal carcinomas in addition to Hodgkin's disease which has already been discussed (p. 498) (Marigo *et al.* 1969). In Central India a high frequency of Hodgkin's disease, chronic leukaemia, retinoblastoma and oropharyngeal carcinoma have been noted (Grover and Hardas, 1972). It would thus appear that environmental factors are important in a number of childhood malignancies. Although not shown in Table 16.3 sacrococcygeal teratoma are common in Ibadan and a number may show malignant tendencies (Williams *et al.* 1970). A papillary carcinomatous pattern is not unusual.

DISEASES OF IMMUNE ORIGIN

There are five main classes of immunoglobulins IgG, IgA, IgM, IgD and IgE, which migrate on serum electrophoresis mostly as gammaglobulins. The structure of the antibody molecule consists of two pairs of polypeptide chains linked by disulphide bonds. One pair are called light chains and two types, K and λ, can be distinguished with specific antisera. The other pair of chains are twice as large (heavy chains). Five main immunological classes, each with certain specific properties corresponding with the five main immunoglobulins have been identified. Cellular factors however are possibly of more fundamental importance than antibodies in protecting the individual from infections. The cells concerned are the thymus-dependent T lymphocytes and the 'bursa equivalent' or B lymphocytes which turn into plasma cells and make antibodies. The T cells can be non-specifically stimulated in culture by mitogens such as phytohaemagglutinin and also by contact with a specific antigen in a previously sensitized individual. They have a long life span and are probably cytotoxic for target cells. They also release a number of soluble factors which are chemotactic for mononuclear cells and increase vascular permeability, and are thus important in cell-mediated immunity which can be assessed by (a) the delayed-type skin reactions, (b) *in vitro* stimulation of lymphocytes to divide and form blast cells, and (c) the release from lymphocytes of the macrophage migration inhibition factor. Defects in these two systems can occur and cause the 'combined immune deficiency syndrome', or cellular immunity and antibody synthesis can be affected separately. The frequency of these syndromes is not high and are likely to be rapidly fatal in the tropical environment. Neonates are liable to develop generalized vaccinia if inoculated soon after birth so theoretically immuno-globulins should be estimated at three months of age before embarking on immunization programmes—a procedure unlikely to be practical in the tropics. Primary immunodeficiencies have been reviewed by WHO (1971). In the light of our present knowledge the classification of diseases of immune origin is difficult and is attempted below:

(a) Primary or acquired immuno-deficiencies (hypogammaglobulinaemia or a reduction in cell-mediated immunity as seen in many conditions).

(b) Neoplasia or overactivity:
Myeloma (Light chain disease),
Waldenstrom's macroglobulinaemia,
Heavy chain disease (Editorial, 1968).

(c) Hypersensitivity reactions (Type I).
IgE, the reagenic antibody, becomes attached to cells and reacts with circulating antigen with the release of vasodilator substances, histamine, serotonin, and bradykinin. Complement is not fixed and the reaction occurs rapidly. Drugs and chemicals may act as haptens.
Anaphylaxis (systemic or localized),
Hay fever and asthma,
Some forms of allergic dermatitis.

(d) Cytotoxic antibody reactions (Type II).
The antigen present on the surface of cells combines with circulating antibody (usually IgG or IgM) and fixes complement which can cause lysis of cells or increased phagocytosis.
Autoimmune haemolytic anaemia,
Transfusion reactions,
Idiopathic thrombocytopenic purpura (in some instances),
Certain types of nephritis in which anti-basement membrane antibody is present.

(e) Immune complex reactions (Type III).

> Antigen and antibody are free in the circulation and complexes are formed with the fixation of complement—usually with antigen excess. The deposition of these complexes and the activation of complement can cause lesions in various organs.
>
> Serum sickness,
> Arthus type of reaction,
> Quartan malarial nephrosis and other types of nephritis,
> Henoch–Schonlein purpura,
> Reactional states in leprosy.

(f) Cell-mediated immune reactions (Type IV):

> Specifically sensitized lymphocytes react to an introduced foreign antigen,
> Delayed hypersensitivity skin reactions,
> Rejection of homografts,
> Contact dermatitis,
> Reactions in certain infections such as tuberculosis.

(g) Diseases with complex immune responses:

> Systemic autoimmune diseases,
> Systemic lupus erythematosis,
> Rheumatoid arthritis,
> Polyarteritis nodosa,
> Polymyositis,
> Scleroderma and dermatositis,
> Sjorgen's syndrome,
> Goodpasture's syndrome.

ORGAN SPECIFIC IMMUNO-DEFICIENCIES

Organ	Disease
Central nervous system	Encephalitis, demyelinating diseases
Endocrine	Addison's disease, hypoparathyroidism, thyroiditis
Gastro-intestinal	Pernicious anaemia, regional ileitis, ulcerative colitis.
Liver	Chronic active hepatitis, biliary cirrhosis, cryptogenic cirrhosis (in some cases)
Muscle	Myasthenia gravis
Heart	Rheumatic fever
Eye	Uveitis, ? unilateral ophthalmoplegia
Skin	Pemphigus
Fibrous tissue	? Retroperitoneal fibrosis

A few of these conditions have already been discussed—namely quartan malarial nephrosis, rheumatic fever, and forms of anaemia. The part that the possible altered immunological status of the host due to multiple infections and infestations may play in the disease pattern and the possible altered immunological surveillance in malignancy has also been mentioned (pp. 498 and 499). As diseases in which autoimmune processes are thought to be involved are uncommon in parts of the tropics (Greenwood, 1968) the reader is advised to consult standard text books on the other conditions. There is no doubt that Hashimoto's thyroiditis, thyrotoxicosis, myxoedema, and pernicious anaemia are uncommon in parts of tropical Africa. On the other hand asthma is common. Rheumatoid arthritis is less common and would appear to run a milder course although rheumatoid factor in sera shows a higher prevalence than that found in the United Kingdom—as also pertains in the rural populations of Southern Nigeria as a whole—possibly due to the presence of stable malaria (Muller *et al.* 1972; Greenwood *et al.* 1971).

In spite of the different patterns of rheumatoid arthritis in adults, Still's disease in children with a similar pattern to that seen in the United Kingdom is not uncommon. A form of acute tropical arthritis has been described which would appear to differ from the usual forms described in temperate climates. It has been shown that malaria infection can suppress autoimmune disease in mice (Greenwood *et al.* 1970) and as autoimmune disease is seen frequently in the American Negro it would appear that environmental factors are important in the prevalence and pattern of certain of these diseases.

Tropical populations characteristically have elevated serum gamma globulin concentrations and this may affect IgG, IgM, IgD or IgE. There seems little doubt that multiple parasitic infestations provide the major stimulus to increased immunological production. High IgM concentrations have been observed in individual cases of a number of tropical diseases including trypanosomiasis, leishmaniasis, leprosy, hepatic cirrhosis, and splenomegaly of obscure cause but are regularly only associated with trypanosomiasis and the tropical splenomegaly syndrome (Crane *et al.* 1971). In Nigeria, however, a heterophile agglutinin (an IgM macroglobulin) is also commonly found in sera unassociated with trypanosomiasis (Adeniyi-Jones, 1967). In areas of stable malaria higher IgM values are found in adults than in children and are higher in females. In areas of unstable malaria children have higher values than in areas of stable and the mean adult level is twice that found in stable areas. In African populations autoantibodies to heart, stomach and thyroid have also been noted to be raised (Shaper *et al.* 1968).

In India significantly lower serum albumin and higher gamma- and beta-globulin values were obtained than in Europeans and was thought to be due mainly to environmental factors (Saha and Banerjee, 1970). All these findings would tend to prove that the immunological status of the host is altered in the tropics but the degree will vary in different geographical regions according to environmental and genetic factors.

DISORDERS OF BONE

Achrondroplasia, spina bifida, talipes equinovarous, and polydactyly are common in our experience. A high incidence of carpal fusion has been recorded in Africa (Cockshott, 1963). Congenital dislocation of the hip and marble-bone disease are rare. The reason for the rarity of congenital dislocation of the hip may be genetic as it is especially common in certain racial groups (Richards, 1971). Dislocations of the hip occurring in association with other congenital defects such as arthrogryposis multiplex are, however, seen and also following septic arthritis in young children. Congenital dislocation of the knee is occasionally seen. Madelung's deformity (a disorder of the development of the radius) is not uncommon in Africans and usually presents in adolescence. Osteogenesis imperfecta and diaphyseal aclasia also occasionally are diagnosed. Genu valgum and varum are common.

With regard to diseases of bone, only disorders of calcium metabolism, tumoral calcinosis, osteoporosis and osteomalacia (p. 718) are discussed in any detail. Those associated with specific disorders (tuberculosis, smallpox, typhoid, etc.) are mentioned in their appropriate context. Acute and chronic osteomyelitis are common and excluding the salmonellae associated with sickle-cell disease the usual organism is the *Staphylococcus pyogenes*. In non-sickle-cell disease the metaphysis is the usual primary site with secondary involvement of the epiphysis of the lower and upper ends of the femur common in small children. The diaphysis is usually involved in sickle-cell disease. Large sequestrae are not the rarities they now are in temperate zones. Gout may be missed if its possible occurrence is not kept in mind, since there are marked racial differences in its prevalence. Blood uric-acid levels are highest in certain Pacific races and lowest in Caucasians, with Negroes having intermediate levels. Paget's disease is not common but does occur in Africa (Bohrer, 1970) although rare in Asian countries.

Fractures of bone are extremely common and many hospitals in the tropics are finding it increasingly difficult to cope with the rising incidence of road accidents. Fracture of the spine is a hazard of palm wine tappers and fracture of the upper cervical spine may occur in the 'porter's neck' syndrome which occurs in labourers carrying heavy head loads (Levy, 1968). Benign tumours of bone are common. Ameloblastoma has already been discussed (p. 535). Fibrous dysplasia has been discussed by Odeku *et al.* (1969). It may affect one (monostotic) or several (polyostotic) bones. In its severe form the triad of Albright is seen with associated cutaneous pigmentation and endocrine disorders. The last is rare in our experience. The bones of the face and skull are most frequently affected in Nigeria with the maxilla predominating. The condition occurs in Negroes in North America, in Indians and in Sudanese and Egyptians. Race would not appear to be a factor nor does it bear any relationship to keloid formation. The patients are usually young adults. Giant cell tumours are also common and have an equal sex incidence in the age group 17–45 years. A considerable proportion may exhibit histological features of malignancy. The upper end of the tibia and the lower ends of the femur and radius are the usual sites. Osteochondromas are also fairly common but chondromas and osteoid osteomas are not. Aneurysmal bone cysts occur. We have little information on epiphyseal chondroblastoma or chondromyxoid fibroma.

With regard to malignant tumours of bone their incidence would not appear to vary greatly throughout the world but the striking feature in Africans, in Jamaicans and the U.S. Negro is their absence in the older age, groups in contrast to the findings in South African whites, in Cali, Colombia, in temperate climates and in Indians in Bombay. In Ibadan 63 per cent of the tumours occurred under the age of 30 years. It is of interest that evidence is now accumulating which suggests that osteosarcoma should be included among the growing list of neoplasms such as melanoma, neuroblastoma and Burkitt's tumour that possess specific tumour-associated antigens. An antibody has been found in the serum directed against sarcoma-specific antigens and a viral aetiology has been postulated (Editorial, 1973). If this is so, a detailed study of the incidence of osteosarcoma in different geographic areas should help to confirm or refute this theory. Primary reticulum-cell sarcoma has been described from India (Potdar, 1970) as being more frequently seen in adult males and most commonly in the femur.

Ewing's sarcoma has been reported to be rare in the U.S. Negro (Fraumeni and Glass, 1970; Jensen and Drake, 1970). It is also rare in Nigeria (Edington et al. 1970) and probably in other parts of tropical Africa. On the other hand it is common in Bombay Indians. It would thus appear that Negroes are genetically resistant to Ewing's sarcoma.

Malignant lymphomas, including the Burkitt tumour, are common primary or secondary tumours of bone in many parts of the tropics. Epithelial secondary tumours are not as common as they would be in temperate climates because of the differing cancer patterns.

DISEASES OF JOINTS

Arthropathies are common and the causes are multifactorial. The classification has been reviewed by Hart (1971). Rheumatoid arthritis and Still's disease have already been mentioned. Acute arthritis secondary to other infections, especially gonococcal, is common and chronic arthritis also occurs especially tuberculous. Viral diseases including rubella, Chikungunya and O'nyong-Nyong fevers are other common causes in certain areas. Guineaworm arthritis especially of the knee joint is an entity. Osteo-arthritis would not appear to be common but may reflect the differing age structure in the tropics. Charcot's joints are still seen and marked destruction of the distal joints of the limbs may occur in leprosy. Marked changes in the joints may occur in sickle-cell disease and haemophilia should not be forgotten. Reiter's disease may follow dysentery, gonorrhoea or non-specific urethritis and presents as a rash, urethral discharge and arthritis. Marfan's syndrome has occasionally been mentioned in the differential diagnosis of cardiac and aortic disease in the tropics. It is a disorder of connective tissue inherited as an autosomal dominant. It affects the media of large arteries, the chordal tendineae, mitral and aortic valves, the suspensory ligament of the lens of the eye and joint capsules and tendons. There is increased excretion of hydroxyproline in the urine. Malignant involvement of joints occasionally occurs. Tenosynovitis, bursitis and ganglia are common as are giant cell tumours of tendon sheaths. The malignant synovomia is occasionally seen. Acute tropical arthritis is described below.

ACUTE TROPICAL ARTHRITIS

An unusual form of acute polyarthritis has been described in tropical Africa (Greenwood, 1969) and New Guinea (Jeremy, 1969) and has been called 'acute non-specific arthritis in the African' or acute tropical arthritis. The patients are febrile and one or more of the larger joints usually the knee, ankle or wrist are affected. Both sexes are affected in the age group 20 to 62 years. Pain and swelling are complained of and the ESR is raised. Antistreptolysin titres are not raised nor do the patients develop a chronic condition. Rheumatoid or antinuclear factors are not found. The radiological findings are normal. The synovial fluid may contain polymorphonuclear leucocytes and lymphocytes but no crystals and bacteriological examination is negative. There is a mild lymphocytic and plasma cell infiltration in the synovium with polymorphonuclear leucocytes occasionally present. The aetiology is unknown.

DISEASES OF MUSCLE

In Africa, at least, tropical pyomyositis is much the most common primary disease of muscle and is described separately below. Specific conditions such as trichinosis, Bornholm disease caused by viruses of the Coxsackie group, leprosy, etc., are discussed in their appropriate context. Familial periodic paralysis has been mentioned in connection with thyrotoxicosis on p. 654. Alcohol and chloroquine may cause a myopathy. Muscular dystrophies occur and the clinical presentations are in no way different from those described for Caucasian patients but parents in the tropics may fail to recognize the symptoms and often attribute the weakness of the patient to laziness (Osuntokun, 1971).

McArdle's disease in which the patients experience painful cramps on exercise due to the hereditary absence of myophosphorylase is rarely seen. Polymyositis and myasthenia gravis occur (Greenwood and Francis, 1967; Harries, 1969).

Myasthenia gravis is now considered to be an autoimmune disorder. Antibodies to muscle have been detected in the serum and antigenic cross-reaction has been noted between them and myoid cells in the thymus. Thymectomy is beneficial. Thymic extracts injected into animals produce a myasthemia gravis like disease. It is thought that following antibody stimulation the thymus produces excessive amounts of 'thymin' which reduces the amount of acetylcholine in the end-plate potentials. Histologically secondary degenerative changes in voluntary muscle and collections of lymphocytes (lymphorrhages) are seen. Neoplastic change or lymphoid germinal centres in the medulla are changes which occur in the thymus. Giant cell myocarditis may be a rare complication and an association with other autoimmune manifestations has been noted.

Crush injuries are common but we have no information on the frequency of myoglobinaemia or myoglobinuria in the tropics. It should certainly be looked for in tetanus. Immunofluorescent techniques are available (Kagen, 1970). In the diagnosis of primary muscle disease from those conditions secondary to denervation electromyography, serum enzyme estimations and muscle biopsy are most helpful. The serum creatine kinase level is the most sensitive indicator of primary muscle disease.

The most suitable muscles for biopsy are the quadriceps and the deltoid or biceps in the upper limb. The biopsy should be taken in the long axis of the muscle. The local anaesthetic should surround the biopsy area to avoid artefact. Trauma to the biopsy should also be avoided. The best fixative is Heidenhain's Susa fluid.

Benign and malignant tumours of muscle are relatively common the rhabdomyosarcoma being especially so in our experience. They have been described in the upper respiratory tract (Williams et al. 1968) and orbital region (Olurin, 1969) in Ibadan. It is interesting that the two orbital rhabdomyosarcomas were in pregnant women and the tumours grew rapidly.

TROPICAL PYOMYOSITIS

Tropical pyomyositis has been reported from widely scattered parts of the tropics, including various parts of West Africa, East Africa, Malaya, Dutch East Indies, Pacific islands, Brazil, and the West Indies (Traquair, 1947). It consists essentially of deep-seated large abscesses, single or multiple, in voluntary muscles, any of which may be affected. Various organisms have been isolated from the pus but by far the most frequently reported has been *Staphylococcus aureus*, and in Uganda, phage-typing showed that 60 per cent of the pyomyositis strains belonged to phage Group II. Subsequent contractures are very rare.

The source of the infecting staphylococcus is not known.*

Histologically there are areas of focal muscle necrosis with mononuclear cell infiltration; the regional lymph glands are rarely affected (Leedham-Green and Evans, 1943). Subcutaneous abscesses in man in Trinidad and Dutch Guiana have been attributed to *Lagochilascaris minor*.

DISORDERS OF CALCIUM METABOLISM

Disorders of calcium metabolism would not, in general, in the tropics appear to differ greatly from the descriptions given in standard textbooks but their differing incidence in geographical areas is marked. There is, however, a condition, known as tumoral calcinosis, which appears to be not uncommon in our experience in West Africa and is also present in East and South Africa (Palmer, 1966) which is not usually mentioned when these conditions are described. A classification of disorders of calcium metabolism (modified after Robbins, 1962) is given in Table 16.4.

TABLE 16.4. *Disorders of calcium metabolism*

(i) *Derangements due to calcium imbalance*	(ii) *Hypocalcaemia*
Metastatic calcification	Hypoparathyroidism
Dystrophic calcification	Vitamin-D deficiency
Calcinosis:	Chronic renal disease
(i) universalis	Decreased absorption of calcium
(ii) circumscripta	Osteoporosis
(iii) localisata	
(iv) tumoral	
Arterial calcification	
Heterotopic bone formation	
Lithiasis	

*An association with filarial infection has been suggested.

Metastatic calcification is associated with hypercalcaemia which may be caused by hyperparathyroidism, neoplasms involving bone, hypervitaminosis D, chronic nephritis, bone atrophy, or an excessive intake of milk and antacids. Calcification occurs in areas of local alkalinity, namely: the gastric mucosa, kidney, and lung.

In dystrophic calcification, calcium is deposited in injured, degenerative or dead tissues. The serum calcium is not affected and local anoxia and alkalinitiy are important factors. Calcification is frequently seen in degenerate tissue in benign and malignant tumours, in abscesses, fetal tissues, parasites, tuberculous foci, areas of fat necrosis and following pericarditis, valvulitis, and, possibly, pancreatitis.

In calcinosis universalis there are small, hard, calcified nodules and plaques in the skin, subcutaneous tissues, and superficial muscle layers. Children are most frequently affected and muscle atrophy, contractures, and ankylosis of joints are usual. Scleroderma is frequently an associated condition and the prognosis is poor.

Calcinosis circumscripta affects an older age group. Small nodules and streaks of calcium are located about flexor tendon sheaths in the hands, wrists, elbows, or knees. It is associated with Raynaud's disease or a collagen disease in about 40 per cent of patients, and has been described in the scrotum in onchocerciases.

Calcinosis localisata occurs in areas of trauma, the tendon insertion of the supraspinatous muscle being frequently affected.

Tumoral calcinosis is thought to be a separate entity and is described below.

Arterial calcification requires no comment and heterotopic bone formation may occur in any tissue, including the heart. Myositis ossificans is a separate entity.

Stones in the urinary tract, salivary ducts, and gall bladder are discussed elsewhere. It is of interest to note that tumoral calcinosis occurs in areas where gall stones, salivary and urinary calculi are considered rare, although pancreatic calcification is relatively common (p. 665).

Conditions causing hypocalcaemia are discussed when vitamin-D deficiency and steatorrhoea are considered.

TUMORAL CALCINOSIS

Synonyms. Lipocalcinogranulomatosis; calcifying collagenolysis.

Tumoral calcinosis is a condition in which, in otherwise apparently healthy patients, radio-opaque tumours are noted, most usually in the vicinity of the hip or elbow joints. The tumours are composed mainly of calcium phosphate and have a characteristic histopathology. It has also been reported in immigrants to the U.K. and in three indigenes—two of whom, however, were in chronic renal failure—and the condition has been reported in Papua–New Guinea (Cooke, 1969) and Zaire (Jacquerye *et al.* 1974).

Epidemiology

The condition was first described at the end of the nineteenth century in France and called tumoral calcinosis. Lafferty *et al.* (1965) reviewed the findings in the eighteen patients reported in the literature up until 1965, and Palmer (1966) reported a further fifty cases from Africa. It occurs in Caucasians but is more common in the Negro race and in the age group 6–25 years, although it does occur in the elderly. Males are more frequently affected than females and a familial incidence has been noted in a few cases. There is some evidence to suggest that there may be a disturbance of phosphorus metabolism (Lafferty *et al.*, 1965). Others have suggested fat necrosis as the underlying lesion and Thomson (1966), from purely histological studies, considered the basic lesion was digestion of collagen with subsequent calcification. There is no evidence to suggest that an increased intake of vitamins, milk, or antacids is an important aetiological agent nor have trauma or the collagen diseases been associated factors. The condition occurs in Africa in areas where urinary calculi and gall stones are rare.

Pathology

The tumours may be single or bilateral and multiple and are most frequently noted in the hip or elbow region but have been reported in the lateral and superior aspect of the shoulder, buttocks, in the scapular region, where they may be retroscapular, in the acromioclavicular, sacral and ischial regions or lateral aspects of the feet. They are slow growing and may attain a size of 20 cm in diameter. Disability is minimal in the early stages. Pain is experienced if pressure is exerted on nerves. The swelling is rubbery in consistency, lobulated, and mobile. Later it becomes fixed to skin, fascia, muscle, or tendon and may ulcerate, with the formation of sinuses discharging a chalky fluid.

The excised tumour consists of fibrous septa separating clumps of calcium or cystic spaces containing milky or pasty white fluid which is alkaline and consists almost entirely of tribasic calcium phosphate (Fig. 16.10). The cystic spaces are lined by mononuclear cells and multinucleated giant cells. Calcium phosphate is formed in the mitochondria of the mononuclear cells, which are rich in alkaline phosphatase. Cartilage and enchondral bone have very rarely been noted. There are no constant biochemical changes in the blood but exhaustive investigations in only one patient were suggestive of deranged calcium and phosphorus metabolism (Lafferty *et al.* 1965).

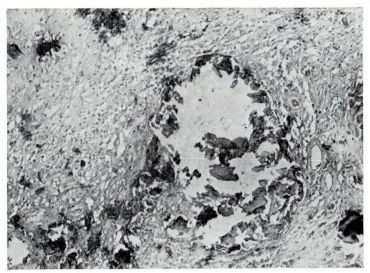

FIG. 16.10. Tumoral calcinosis. Section shows deposits of calcium in collagenous tissue and a cystic space containing flakes of calcium (H and E × 100).

The serum phosphorus has been noted to be sightly raised in a number of patients.

No association with other conditions has been noted apart from the fortuitous presence of amyloidosis in one patient.

OSTEOPOROSIS

The condition has been defined as a disorder in which there is too little bone of normal composition, and has recently been reviewed by Dent and Watson (1966). It is common in old age but bone steadily loses density from the age of 20 onwards, both in the Negro and white races (Trotter *et al.* 1960). Apart from idiopathic osteoporosis, which includes senile, post-menopausal, adult idiopathic and juvenile idiopathic, osteoporosis occurs as a complication of at least twenty other conditions, hormonal, nutritional, and disuse being the most common. It is a common complication in patients with rheumatoid arthritis receiving corticosteroid therapy.

Severe spinal osteoporosis has been described as common in middle-aged Bantu males, many of whom exhibited the features of classical acute scurvy, and severe siderosis was also almost invariably present. Alcoholism was an associated condition (Seftel *et al.* 1966). The condition is disabling and vertebral collapse occurs. One similar case has been reported from Zambia (Lowenthal *et al.* 1967).

Pathology

The bony trabeculae are decreased in number and markedly attenuated, with the marrow spaces enlarged. Fibrous replacement is unusual. Osteoclastic and osteoblastic activity is decreased. Deposits of haemosiderin in the marrow are present in the Bantu patients, with the associated signs of scurvy and siderosis. The only biochemical abnormality in a proportion of these patients was a low urinary excretion of calcium.

FLUOROSIS

Chronic toxic effects of fluoride on the skeletal system have been reported from India, Sri Lanka (Senewiratne *et al.* 1974), Japan, South Africa, North Africa, Argentina, the Middle East, the United States, Canada and Europe. In this condition the teeth are first affected by white opacities and very faint yellow lines across the enamel. Later a distinct brown stain appears with lastly considerable pitting all over the enamel. The incidence in the Punjab in children was $22 \cdot 6$ per cent. Clinically young adults are usually affected and the complaints are vague pains in the small joints of the hands and feet, the knee joints, lower limbs and spine. Later stiffness of the spine and kyphosis develop. Neurological complications develop at a late stage. Secondary hyperparathyroidism has also been described (Teotia and Teotia, 1973).

Pathology

The bones are irregular. There are multiple exostoses at the site of muscle and tendon inertions. Irregular deposits of bone are found in joint capsules and interosseous membranes. Calcification of the spinal ligaments and enlarged vertebral bodies with marked lipping occur. The vertebrae may also be fused in many places. The margins of the foramen magnum are irregular and narrow. On X-ray the spinal column and pelvis show roughening and blurring of the trabeculae. Later the trabeculae merge and the bone has a diffuse structureless appearance. Latterly the bones appear marble white with irregular periosteal thickening and the changes outlined above.

On histological examination the compact bone shows disordered lamellar orientation and an enlarged poorly formed Haversian system. Irregular deposits of osteoid tissue extend into attached muscle. Fluorosis would appear to stimulate osteoblastic activity with resulting exostosis and extensive production of new bone. In the late stages crippling deformities occur such as kyphosis and flexion deformities of the limbs with quadriplegia and other neurological manifestations. Diagnosis is made by clinical and radiological examination. The urinary excretion of fluoride may be increased (normal $< 0 \cdot 185$ mg per cent).

AMYLOIDOSIS

Primary amyloidosis is said to be a rare disease (Editorial, 1966) and secondary amyloidosis is a disappearing disease in Western countries (Patrassi, 1965; Kennedy *et al.* 1974). In the tropics primary amyloidosis is not uncommon and secondary amyloidosis in association with tuberculosis is a problem of some magnitude (Edington and Mainwaring, 1964). Its relative rarity in leprosy is discussed on p. 312. Various writers have classified amyloidosis on organ distribution and staining reactions into primary, secondary (including amyloidosis associated with multiple myeloma), localized, and familial. We have no experience of localized amyloidosis which affects the larynx, lung, or bladder, nor has, to our knowledge, the familial type (Gafni and Sohar, 1960) been described in the tropics, except in Israel. However, if an unexplained lower limb neuropathy occurs sural nerve biopsies should be examined for the presence of amyloid (Thomas, 1973). Amyloidosis, frequently with a concomitant giant-cell reaction, is not uncommon in multiple myelomatosis in West Africa. We have been unable to differentiate primary amyloidosis, which occurs in relatively young age groups in the tropics, from secondary amyloidosis associated with tuberculosis, by organ distribution or staining reactions. Primary amyloidosis, therefore, does not differ greatly from secondary, the differentiating feature being the absence of an obvious chronic disease process which should always be carefully searched for as there is some evidence that amyloid may occasionally regress if the chronic infective process is successfully treated. In the tropics the tongue, heart, muscles, and joints are rarely severely involved and the kidney, adrenals, and spleen are the site of the heaviest deposits, renal-vein thrombosis being a not uncommon complication. We have seen one adult female with a cardiomyopathy due to amyloidosis. The liver tends to be minimally affected. Amyloidosis most frequently presents clinically as the nephrotic syndrome.

The aetiology of the condition is obscure. Amyloid is a glycoprotein-sulphated nucopolysaccharide complex. There are thought to be three types: type A proteins found with perireticulin distribution secondary to chronic sepsis or some inborn error of the lymphoreticular system; type B proteins mainly found with pericollagen distribution secondary to myelomatosis and other paraprotein disorders or some inborn error; Type C proteins which are formed locally with certain tumours, e.g. bladder, kidney, and thyroid (Hobbs, 1973).

The view is steadily gaining ground that amyloid arises from the immunoglobulins—in myelomatosis as a result of plasma cell dyscrasia, in primary amyloidosis from some lesser form of reticulo-endothelial abnormality and in secondary amyloid as a result of chronic antigenic stimulation by the inflammatory process. Paraproteins should always be looked for in the plasma and urine of patients with primary amyloidiosis. Changes in the plasma proteins are usual and alphaglobulin is constantly raised, beta occasionally raised and gamma usually lowered.

In the tropics it affects most frequently the capillary basement membrane of the glomeruli of the kidney and renal tubules and the walls of blood vessels and reticulin framework of the adrenal and other organs. The malphighian corpuscles of the spleen (sago spleen) are not usually involved and only the vascular tissue in the liver and heart are usually affected.

Amyloidosis is considered to be the result of a profound disturbance of protein metabolism and perhaps a manifestation of an immunological reaction.

Amyloid on routine H and E stains is a homogeneous, translucent, acidophilic material resembling hyaline but gives a khaki colour with van Gieson. Methyl violet stains amyloid tissue red, Congo red stains it pink and gives an apple green birefringence under polarized light while thioflavine T produces fluorescence when viewed by ultra-violet microscopy. The most specific histological method, however, is electron microscopy in which its fibrillary structure is characteristic. Fluorescence microscopy using thioflavine T provides an even more sensitive method. It stains a mahogany-brown colour in post-mortem specimens treated with an aqueous solution of iodine. Hepatic, renal, and gingival biopsy have been used in diagnosis and rectal biopsy has been advised as the method of choice in temperate climates; its comparative value in the tropics however has yet to be evaluated. The Congo red test is a useful diagnostic method for amyloid disease. In a normal individual, 10–30 per cent of intravenously injected Congo red (15 ml of a 0·75 per cent solution) disappears within an hour, but in the presence of amyloid 40–60 per cent of the dye may disappear. Anaphylactic reactions to the drug may occur.

VENOMOUS BITES AND STINGS

Venomous bites and stings occur throughout the world but are more common in the tropics. Poisoning can occur either through the bite or stings of a variety of animals, e.g. venomous fish, bees, and wasps; scorpions and spiders; and certain species of centipedes. The properties of cantharadin and its occurrence in 'Spanish flies' and widely-distributed genera of 'blister beetles' (*Mylabris, Epicauta, Cyanolytia,* and *Cercoctis*) are recognized by orthodox toxicologists, and by witch-doctors in some African countries (Gelfand, 1948), and accidental poisoning by percutaneous absorption of this substance has been described (Browne, 1960). An epidemic of vesicular dermatitis due to *Paederus* beetles has been described in Okinawa. The lesions may be mistaken for herpes zoster and are caused by the toxic substance named pedarin (Armstrong and Winfield, 1969). Beetle dermatitis is common in Java, tropical Africa, India, and South America; various moths may cause irritating lesions either by powder from the dorsal surfaces of the wings or by the detachment of hairs with hooklets which become embedded in the skin. Keegan (1969; Reid, 1975) has reviewed in some detail the lesion caused by insects and venomous arachnids. Scorpion stings are not uncommon and are painful but do not usually cause severe symptoms. Deaths, however, due to myocarditis, neurotoxicity and acute pancreatitis have been described (Poon-King, 1963).

Snake-bite is the most important in this group and will be described in a little more detail; it is an occupational hazard for farmers, fishermen, etc. (Reid *et al.* 1963a). The front-fanged poisonous snakes can be detected as follows:

1. Viperidae—found in the Old World.
2. Crotalidae (pit vipers)—found in the New World and Asia.
3. Elapidae—found in all tropical countries.
4. Hydrophidae (sea snakes)—found in the Indian and Pacific Ocean.

Pathology of land-snake poisoning

The classical studies of Reid and his colleagues (1963b, c) on patients bitten by the Malayan pit viper, *Ancistrodon rhodostoma*, are detailed and comprehensive and should be read in the original by those interested in the subject of snake poisoning. The laboratory and necropsy findings have recently been extensively reviewed by Reid (1968 and 1972) and are summarized below.

Local tissue necrosis may be extensive in bites by certain vipers and cobras. In cobra bites with severe poisoning, there is an initial leucocytosis and a moderate haemolytic anaemia, while in systemic viperine poisoning the paramount laboratory findings are due to haemorrhage and a prolonged coagulation defect resulting from defibrination (Reid, 1967). It is important to distinguish between disseminated intravascular coagulation and primary fibrinolysis. They can be distinguished by performing a platelet count, the serial thrombin time, the euglobulin lysis time and estimating the plasma fibrinogen levels. In the defibrination syndrome thrombocytopenia, hypofibrinogenaemia and a prolonged serial thrombin time occur. Weiss *et al.* (1969), however, noted afibrinogenaemia following a rattlesnake bite with a normal platelet count. The venom converted fibrinogen to fibrin directly. Proteinuria is common in both cobra and viperine poisoning and renal failure may occur. At necropsy there are no changes characteristic of elapid poisoning. In viperine poisoning, haematomata and abrasions may be seen over the scalp, the bitten limb is swollen, and the subcutaneous tissues packed with blood. Severe necrosis of muscle (rhabdomyolysis) may occur and has also been described following hornet stings (Shilkin *et al.* 1972). Haemorrhages may occur in the dura, subarachnoid space, brain, and other organs. Histological examination may reveal centrilobular degeneration and necrosis in the liver. Using an immunodiffusion technique Greenwood *et al.* (1974) made a positive species diagnosis of snake bite in 40 out of 101 patients.

Pathology of sea-snake poisoning

The main pathological lesions are to be found in the skeletal muscles, kidney, and liver (Marsden and Reid, 1961). Macroscopically the liver may be pale and brown, and black urine is found in the bladder, since myoglobinuria is a prominent feature of sea-snake bite. Histologically, there are widespread hyaline necroses in skeletal muscles; the whole kidney is engorged but the boundary zone is intensely congested and stands out prominantly. There are a few granular myoglobin casts in the tubules and distal tubular necrosis is commonly found. Acute renal failure is not infrequently the cause of death.

Centrilobular degeneration of the liver with a round-or mixed-cell infiltration of the portal areas is seen and the serum transaminases are often raised.

TROPICAL ULCERS

The high incidence of tropical ulcers in the tropics and subtropics is due to a combination of factors such as poor environmental hygiene, paucity of medical facilities, frequency of and neglect of minor trauma. The ulcers may reach enormous size, thus causing considerable morbidity from immobility, and loss of earnings. Complications such as tetanus, gas gangrene, and malignant transformation may occur (Ngu, 1967).

I. TROPICAL PHAGEDENIC ULCER

The tropical phagedenic ulcer must be distinguished from ulcers due to pyogenic infection and specific tropical conditions. The Veld sore is also a separate entity.

The ulcer occurs in the lower limbs, most frequently in hot damp climates. The exact cause of the lesion is not known but it is associated with the presence of the organisms *Fusiformis fusiformis* and *Borrelia vincenti* (see p. 516). These organisms are found as commensals in the mouth and were present in the mouth in 32 per cent of ulcer patients (Ngu,

1960). It is possible that the organisms are introduced into minor injuries by the application of saliva. This, however, does not explain the predilection of the lesion for the lower leg, as saliva is applied indiscriminately to lesions in any part of the body. It is not transmissible and it is generally considered that predisposing factors are necessary. It can occur in almost epidemic proportion in labour forces and in troops subjected to arduous campaigns in the tropics. Low standards of hygiene, multiple infections, and dietary deficiencies contribute to the high incidence in tropical areas. The condition has, however, been seen in healthy European males. Minor trauma and its neglect are probably the most important precipitating factors.

Pathology

The lesion commences as a bleb which ruptures with the formation of a rapidly-spreading ulcer covered by an ash grey, foul-smelling, moist slough. The ulcerative process may extend rapidly laterally and in depth to involve skin, subcutaneous tissue, muscle, tendon, nerves, and even bone. The slough separates, leaving an ulcer with a raised, frequently depigmented, firm edge. With healing, papery-thin, white, fibrous scars eventuate and if the lesion has been extensive deformities may be great.

The histology is that of any chronic infection, showing a coagulation necrosis on the surface with meshed fibrin enclosing large numbers of necrotic polymorphs and Vincent's organisms. The epithelium is acanthotic at the periphery of the lesion and the corium is infiltrated with lymphocytes and plasma cells. Dense fibrosis surrounds the lesion. In long-standing ulcers pseudo-epitheliomatous hyperplasia may simulate epidermoid carcinoma. Squamous-cell carinoma may occur in 9 per cent of chronic tropical ulcers and tetanus and gas gangrene are complications. Malignant transformation is rare before the age of 20 and may develop in as short a time as 3 months or as long as 50 years (Camain *et al.* 1972).

Diagnostic pathology

The organisms can be seen on dark-ground examination or on staining scrapings from the ulcer base by Gram's method. The spirochaete measures 5–10 μm and has a wavy spiral appearance. *F. fusiformis* is cigar-shaped, 5–12 μm in length, and has a banded appearance.

Secondary infection is usually present and bacteriological investigations and antibiotic sensitivity tests should be undertaken where facilities exist. Radiological examination may reveal an underlying periosteal reaction with new bone formation. Deformity and bowing of the lower leg may occur (Kolawole and Bohrer, 1970).

If malignant change has occurred the edge of the ulcer becomes hard, rolled, and everted, and surgical biopsy is necessary to arrive at a diagnosis.

2. VELD SORE

Synonym. Desert sore.

Ulceration of the skin associated with the presence of *Corynebacterium diphtheriae* occurs in North India, Assam, Chittagong, the Pacific area, the Middle East, North Africa, North Australia, and probably widely in Africa.

The ulcers may be single or multiple and are shallow, punched-out, and circular. The margins are thickened, indurated, and occasionally undermined. The base is grey or grey-green with an adherent membrane. They rarely exceed 5 cm in diameter. The exposed parts are affected, the hands, forearms, elbow, or knee joint being the most common sites. The diphtheria bacillus can be isolated in the acute stage but may not be detected in the chronic when secondary infection has occurred. The histopathology is non-specific but Gram-positive bacilli may be seen in appropriately stained sections.

Diphtheritic pareses may occur in up to 25 per cent of patients, usually commencing in anatomical relationship with the ulcer. General pareses and polyneuritis are seen. Blurring of vision, tingling, and numbness of the extremities may be complained of. The gait may be ataxic.

The cranial nerves are not commonly affected but palatal paralysis and changes in the cerebrospinal fluid have been described. Myocarditis is a rare complication. Auto-infection of the nasopharynx can occur.

The ulcers are much more commonly recorded in immigrants than in the indigenous populations. Large numbers of troops in the Middle East and Pacific, for instance, were affected. The incidence is out of all proportion to the incidence of faucial diphtheria. There must be a reservoir of cutaneous diphtheria in natives in areas of the tropics and its presence probably accounts for the gradual immunization of the population in early life (Liebow *et al.* 1946). This statement is probably true in West Africa where diphtheria was considered to be rare until recently and where immunity was shown to be high by Schick testing (Cauchi and Smith, 1964). It is interesting to note in this respect that Senecal *et al.* (1962) have remarked that in Senegal diphtheria is more and more frequently being diagnosed in children aged 1–4 years. Deaths from faucial diphtheria (about two or three per year) have also occurred in Ibadan. The number of cases seen at post mortem is not as high as might be expected in a population which is not actively immunized.

3. MYCOBACTERIAL SKIN ULCERS DUE TO MYCOBACTERIUM
ULCERANS (**Synonym.** Buruli ulcer)

Mycobacterioses are slender rods occurring mostly in pairs or small clumps. Once stained they resist decolorization with acid (acid-fast). They are non-motile, non-capsulated and non-sporing. Their growth is usually slow and aerobic. All forms of animal life may be affected by various species of these bacteria. The most important are *Mycobacterium tuberculosis* and *Mycobacterium leprae*. The former is discussed in the chapter on the respiratory system (Chapter 9) and the latter on p. 297. Mycobacteria, however, also cause ulcerative skin lesions. *Mycobacterium ulcerans* was reported from Australia in 1948 (McCallum *et al.* 1948) and *Mycobacterium balnei* from Sweden (Linell and Norden, 1954). Various other species may cause ulcers and all biopsies or smears from non-specific ulcers in the tropics should always be routinely stained by Ziehl–Neelsen. These, however, may be negative if due to *Mycobacterium balnei* and culture on Lowenstein–Jensen's medium at 31 °C is necessary for diagnosis.

Skin ulcers caused by acid-fast bacilli have been reviewed by Janssens (1972) and described separately as the Bairnsdale, Kakerifu, Kasongo, and the Buruli and Orebro ulcers.

Necrotizing skin ulcers with a characteristic histopathology in which numerous acid-fast bacilli are present have been reported from Australia (MacCallum *et al.* 1948), Zaire (van Oye and Ballion, 1950; Meyers *et al.* (1974); Mexico (Aguilar *et al.* 1953), Uganda (Clancey *et al.* 1961), Gabon (Woringer *et al.* 1961), and Nigeria (Gray *et al.* 1967).

We have seen a number of biopsies from patients with this condition from the River States in Eastern Nigeria and in Ibadan where infection was considered to arise from a fish pond. The disease was first recognized in Australia by MacCallum *et al.* (1948). The acid-fast bacilli were cultured and produced ulcers in rats, and the organism was named *Mycobacterium ulcerans*.

Janssens *et al.* (1959) reviewed 170 cases from the Kakerifu and Kasongo areas of the Congo. There appeared to be differences in the strains of the acid-fast bacilli recovered from the lesions in the two areas. Clancey (1964) described the bacteriological characteristics of the Uganda strain. In the most recent survey from Uganda (Connor and Lunn, 1966) where the literature is reviewed the similarity of the organism and ulcers found in Uganda to those found in Australia and the Congo is stressed.

The term Buruli was first used in 1961 by Clancey and his colleagues pending a more detailed bacteriological investigation. If the causative organism is now thought to be *Myco. ulcerans* the eponym Buruli is really no longer valid.

In the Congo, Uganda, and Eastern Nigeria the infection would appear to occur in individuals living in riverine areas. There is no evidence of contagion nor have insect vectors been incriminated. A history of trauma is not usual. The possibility of infection from water has been discussed by Connor and Lunn (1966) and the occurrence of a somewhat similar mycobacterial disease in fish described by Parisot and Wood (1960) mentioned.

The lesions bear a slight resemblance to 'swimmers' granuloma' due to *Myco. balnei* described in Sweden by Linell and Norden (1954). It is interesting that this infection occurs in water, the bacterium being found in swimming-pool sediment. Extensive necrosis is, however, not seen in this condition. Infection has also been acquired from aquaria and following a dolphin bite (Mansson, 1970; Flowers, 1970).

Mycobacterium ulcerans

The acid-fast bacilli are rod-shaped, straight or slightly curved organisms measuring 1–4 μm in length and 0·3–0·6 μm in breadth. They occur in oval or rounded masses in the necrotic tissue in the ulcer. They can be grown on Lowenstein–Jensen's glycerine agar or Petragnani's medium incubated at 30–33 °C. Growth above or below this temperature range is poor or absent. Primary culture takes 6–8 weeks. The organisms are sensitive to streptomycin *in vitro* but resistant to isoniazid. The rat is a susceptible laboratory animal. Intravenous inoculation leads after some weeks to lesions of the tail, followed later by swelling and ulceration of the scrotum and lesions on the peripheral hairless parts of the body (Fenner, 1956).

Pathology

The ages of the patients range from 18 months to middle age, with the majority in the 5- to 15-year-old age group. The lesion commences as an indurated nodule which in some weeks breaks down and ulcerates. The ulcer is usually single and the most common sites are the lower limbs and arms. The margin of the ulcer is undermined and the surface consists of a yellowish necrotic slough. The original lesion is in the subcutaneous fat but muscle and bone may occasionally be affected (Janssens *et al.* 1959). The surrounding skin is hyperpigmented. The ulcers are chronic and indolent and tend to heal naturally over a period of years. They spread distally down the limb, healing tending to occur proximally. There is no general reaction, the patients usually being otherwise well. Tenderness is absent unless secondary infection occurs and lymph gland involvement is unusual.

In the small, non-ulcerated lesion the main feature is an extensive necrosis of the lower dermis and subcutaneous fat (Dodge and Kirk, 1962). The necrotic area is almost acellular and consists of fibrillary eosinophilic debris. In caseous-like material are large numbers of extracellular acid-fast bacilli and basophilic deposits of calcium salts. The absence of an inflammatory infiltrate is remarkable. The restriction of the lesion to the subcutaneous fat has been tentatively explained by the temperature limits of the optimal growth of the bacillus. It is unable to multiply at 37 °C but may be able to cause pathological lesions in tissues at lower temperatures which are poor conductors of heat. There is no satisfactory explanation which accounts for the presence of the bacilli in the tissues. It is not known whether they multiply in viable tissue or antecedent necrosis is necessary for infection to be established.

As the lesion enlarges an inflammatory reaction occurs and a few giant cells appear. Vesiculation of the epidermis with rupture occurs and an ulcer is formed. Necrosis extends in the dermis and subcutaneous fat and the edges are undermined With possibly increasing immunity, lymphocytes, plasma cells, and macrophages become prominent at the periphery of the lesion. Superficially, there may be secondary infection with fibrin deposition and leucocytic infiltration. Granulation tissue showing repair may be seen at the periphery of the ulcer and giant-cell systems due to fat necrosis, a reaction to keratin or medicaments or tuberculous-like follicles may occur. The underlying muscles may show necrosis or degenerative changes and bacilli may be present in areas of bone necrosis.

Diagnostic Pathology

In our limited experience, the histopathological picture of acellular necrosis of the subcutaneous tissues reminiscent of an infarct has always suggested the diagnosis which has been confirmed by the finding of numerous acid-fast bacilli by the Ziehl–Neelsen stain. In a few instances, however, other workers have reported that mycobacteria may not be seen in biopsy specimens. In these patients direct smears from the lesion or culture on Lowenstein–Jensen's medium at 31 °C have shown the presence of acid-fast bacilli.

Radiological examination may show the presence of fine calcium deposits in the subcutaneous tissue. Reactive periosteal lesions may also be seen in a small proportion of patients. The Mantaux test may be negative and BCG vaccination may be protective. The Mantaux test in *Myco. balnei* infections is positive.

KELOID

A keloid is an overgrowth of fibrous tissue, occurring usually in response to injury, and tends to recur when removed surgically. There may be a familial or racial susceptibility and the condition is more common in women.

Negroes and pigmented races are especially prone. Keloids are seen in tribal markings, pierced ears, in healed ulcers, and surgical scars.

They represent an 'overhealing' phenomenon with an over-production of fibrous tissue. It has been suggested that the skin of the Negro and Polynesian may have a 'fibroblastic diathesis'. The skin of the majority of Africans, however, reacts normally to trauma—but there is no doubt that, in a percentage, keloid formation, even with minor trauma, occurs. Whether this is a familial or individual susceptibility is unknown. Genetic factors have not been studied. The action of steroids in treatment or prevention following surgical procedures has not been found to be satisfactory in West Africa.

It is interesting to note that Caucasians who reside for long periods in tropical areas are thought to be more liable to the condition than those residing in temperate climates. The keloid itself consists of dense collagenous tissue arising in the dermis and subcutaneous tissues underlying an atrophic epidermis with loss of rete pegs. The growth is slow. Sarcomatous change has rarely been described. Further investigations on the serum protein, genetic, and immunological aspects of the condition are indicated.

RHINOSCLEROMA

Synonym. Scleroma.

Rhinoscleroma, as the name implies (rhin : nose; sclera : hard), is a condition in which there are hard plaques in the nasal mucosa. The disease may spread to the pharynx, larynx, and trachea. The condition has been reviewed by Hoffmann (1967). The disease rarely may originate in the larynx. It may spread from the nasal cavity to the lips, palate, pharynx, larynx and trachea, Clinically it usually presents as rhinitis leading to granulomatous infiltration and finally scarring.

Epidemiology

The distribution is world-wide but the greatest incidence is found in Eastern Europe, North Africa, Indonesia, and Central and South America (Kerdel-Vegas *et al.* 1963; Fisher and Dimling, 1964). Both sexes and all age groups are affected, with the greatest incidence in the 16- to 35-year-olds. The disease is associated with poverty.

A Gram-negative diplobacillus, *Klebsiella rhinoscleromatosis* (the von Frisch bacillus), is always present in the lesions, but the disease has never been produced experimentally and the organism may be found in normal nasal mucosa.

Pathology

The diagnosis is made on biopsy material. There is a profusion of plasma cells, Russell bodies, and the characteristic foamy cells of Mikulicz, with occasional lymphocytes and eosinophils (Figs. 16.11 and 16.12).

The Russell body is a circular degenerate plasma cell measuring 20–40 μm in diameter. The cytoplasm is homogeneous, brilliantly eosinophilic and light refractile. There is usually no nucleus. The Mikulicz's cell is a large, round, histiocyte measuring up to 100 μm or more. The cytoplasm is foamy or reticulated and the nucleus is displaced to one side. Fat is absent. Short, Gram-negative rods can be demonstrated in the cytoplasm by Gram's method. Giemsa's stain and silver impregnation methods are valuable

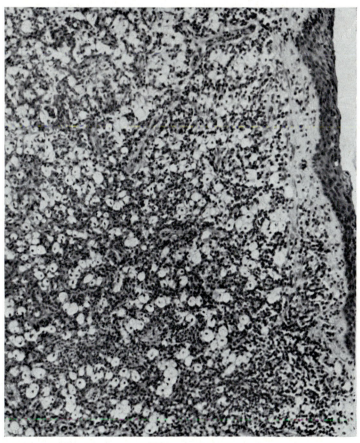

FIG. 16.11. Rhinoscleroma. Numerous plasma cells and large, pale Mikulicz cells are demonstrated. The epithelium covering the nodule is rarely ulcerated (H and E × 250). (*By courtesy of Professor M. S. R. Hutt.*)

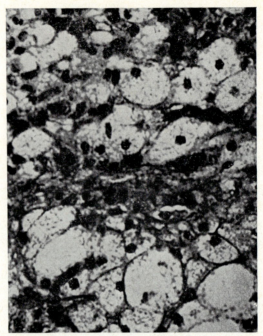

FIG. 16.12. Rhinoscleroma. Mikulicz cells are demonstrated; note the small nucleus and foamy cytoplasm. The von Frisch bacilli can be seen faintly in the haematoxylin and eosin section (H and E × 250). (*By courtesy of Professor M. S. R. Hutt.*)

diagnostic aids. The bacilli can also be identified on smears or they can be cultured. There is an absence of obliterative vascular lesions, and muscle, cartilage, and bone are not usually involved in the inflammatory process. Fibrosis is marked in the later stages of the disease.

HEAT DISORDERS

Heat illness results from both disordered function and failure of thermo-regulation. Existing classifications are unsatisfactory and the important heat disorders can conveniently be listed as follows (Leithead, 1964):

1. Heat stroke and heat hyperpyrexia.
2. Heat syncope (heat collapse, exercise-induced heat exhaustion).
3. Heat oedema.
4. Water-depletion heat exhaustion.
5. Salt-depletion heat exhaustion (heat exhaustion type I).

6. Heat cramps (mill cramps; miners', stokers', cane-cutters' or firemen's cramps).

7. Prickly heat (miliaria rubra; lichen tropicus; heat rash).

8. Anhydrotic heat exhaustion (thermogenic anhydrosis; tropical anhidrotic asthenia; heat exhaustion type II).

With the exception of heat stroke, most of the above conditions are only rarely fatal, and when death does occur the changes are few and non-specific. The pathogenesis of the various disorders has been fully dealt with by Leithead and Lind (1964).

Heat disorders have a world-wide distribution. They are more frequent in regions which are consistently hot and dry (Friend, 1932) and are an important cause of morbidity in the annual pilgrimages to Mecca (Halawani, 1964). Heavy industry and certain occupations, e.g. crews of ships sailing in the Persian Gulf, are frequently associated with heat illness (Caplan, 1944; Wyndham, 1961; Leithead et al. 1958). An irregular prolonged fever due to inadequate water intake occurs in infants and has been described from Kuwait (Shaker, 1966), while some of the problems of fluid and electrolyte requirements of patients convalescing from surgery in hot and humid atmospheres have been investigated by Tinckler (1966). In this section we shall only describe in some detail heat stroke and heat hyper-pyrexia.

HEAT STROKE AND HEAT HYPERPYREXIA

Heat stroke is the term usually used for patients presenting with convulsions or coma, generalized anhydrosis, and hyperpyrexia (rectal temperature above 40·6 °C, 105 °F); while in heat hyperpyrexia (rectal temperature above 40·6 °C) the patient is conscious and sweating may be present. Among the many factors of aetiological significance the following are particularly relevant: (1) environmental temperatures, (2) occupation, (3) inadequate acclimatization, (4) intercurrent febrile illnesses, e.g. tetanus, meningitis, malaria, etc., (5) clothing, (6) administration of drugs which inhibit sweating, (7) age (infants and the elderly being more susceptible), (8) build, (9) alcohol, (10) miscellaneous factors, e.g. history of previous heat disorder, congenital ectodermal dysplasia, ignorance of the dangers of heat stress, etc., (11) strenuous physical activity.

It has recently been pointed out that patients with heat stroke may sweat freely and that the arbitrary temperature reading of 40·6°C is not invariably applicable (Shibolet et al. 1967).

Pathology

The pathological changes have been described by Malamud et al. (1946), and are considered to be due to shock and some impairment of the coagulability of the blood. Degenerative changes in the megakaryocytes have been reported.

The most striking changes are in the central nervous system. The meninges are congested and confluent or petechial haemorrhages may be present. Neuronal degeneration is marked in the cerebellum, cerebral cortex, and basal ganglia, and petechial haemorrhages occur in the region of the third ventricle, aqueduct, and fourth ventricle. Although dysfunction of the hypothalamic centre has been suggested as a cause of the cessation of sweating which often occurs, no characteristic histopathological changes have been described. Residual neuropsychiatric complications, cerebellar ataxia, right-sided hemiparesis, and mental deterioration have been described by Salem (1966).

Haemorrhages may occur in any of the other organs, including the skin, lungs, subendocardium, and subepicardium. Blood-stained effusions are usual in the serous cavities. Areas of necrosis may be found in the adrenal cortex, centrilobular regions of the liver, and myocardium. Myocardial damage has been noted in the few young adults in whom electrocardiograms have been performed. Hepatocellular damage as shown by alteration of liver function tests is constant but only severe in a small proportion of patients, congestion and centrilobular necrosis with cholestasis occurring. Haemo-concentration is usual in the early stages and raised values of serum lactic dehydrogenase isoenzyme patterns have been noted. Hypokalaemia may be an additional complication.

The changes in renal function and structure were described by Kew *et al.* (1967) in twenty Bantu gold miners. Variable renal damage was present in all the patients. Some had mild functional disturbances with normal histology or rapidly reversible tubular degeneration, others had moderate impairment of renal function associated with mild degenerative changes in the tubules, glomerular basement membrane thickening, and slight interstitial fibrosis. Seven patients developed acute renal failure which was characterized pathologically by acute tubular necrosis and slight glomerular basement membrane thickening. A few patients may develop chronic interstitial nephritis. Gram-negative sepsis and endotoxic shock may be a complication (Graber *et al.* 1971).

In addition to the changes induced by heat stroke, precipitating factors such as degenerative cardiovascular disease or obesity may be present.

Diagnostic pathology

The laboratory findings in heat stroke and heat hyperpyrexia depend upon the degree and duration of the changes in the various organs. Leucocytosis and thrombocytopenia are common and the latter partly accounts for the bleeding tendency often observed in patients with heat stroke. In addition, prolonged bleeding and clotting times and afribrinogenaemia have also been reported (Shibolet *et al.* 1962). The haemoglobin red-cell count and packed cell volume are variable (Ferguson and O'Brien, 1960). Red-cell survival is decreased in the majority of patients, implying a haemolytic anaemia which becomes manifest in the week following successful treatment (Halden *et al.* 1955). There are no consistent changes in the concentration of potassium, sodium, and chloride in the plasma. The blood urea nitrogen is often elevated while proteinuria, granular and cellular casts, and increased urinary excretion of erythrocytes and leucocytes are common. There is a marked rise in the serum transaminases and lactic dehydrogenase (Kew *et al.* 1967). In the cerebrospinal fluid there may be a rise in pressure and in protein concentration (Austin and Berry, 1956).

PREGNANCY IN THE TROPICS

The relationships of various conditions to pregnancy have been discussed in their appropriate context. A number of diseases would appear to be more severe in pregnancy including malaria, pneumococcal meningitis, infectious hepatitis, amoebiasis and smallpox. In addition chest diseases are common, especially lobar and bronchopneumonia. A fulminating form of the Burkitt tumour has been described. In this connection it is interesting that cellular immunity as measured by the phytohaemagglutin induced lymphocyte transformation rate and the tuberculin reaction have been noted to be reduced in pregnancy (Finn *et al.* 1972). It was considered that a reduction in T-cell activity during pregnancy might help to protect the fetus from rejection by the mother's immunological mechanisms. The reduction in cellular immune activity may be due to an inhibitory serum factor (St. Hill *et al.* 1973).

Pregnancy is hazardous in many parts of the tropics as conception usually occurs at an early age, multiple infections and infestations are common, strenuous physical work has to be undertaken, iron deficiency and megaloblastic anaemias are common, there may be a high incidence of the abnormal haemoglobin diseases and lastly medical care with adequate antenatal supervision is lacking.

Rupture of the uterus as has been previously mentioned is a common complication in Africa, India and Asia and usually occurs in the third or fourth pregnancy. Fibrous scarring of the cervix due to trauma in previous pregnancies may be an important aetiological agent. Cephalo–pelvic disproportion, traumatic rupture due to obstetrical procedures and rupture of a scar due to a previous caesarean section are the usual predisposing factors. The associated perinatal mortality is exceedingly high.

The frequency of toxaemia of pregnancy is generally low in the tropics but convulsions occur at a relatively low blood pressure level. It is most common in primigravida and especially so in the first 24 hours of the puerperium. Hyperpyrexia is a particular hazard. Maternal and fetal case mortality is relatively low in West Africa (Lawson, 1961) but high in Hong Kong. It is of interest that the frequency of fetal abnormalities, including anencephaly, has been noted to be high in the latter area. Cardiomyopathies are also common especially in the puerperium. Gas gangrene has been reported in intra-uterine and extra-uterine pregnancies (Kolawole and Akande, 1971). Septicaemia may lead to circulatory failure and death. Other complications are peritonitis, emphysematous vaginitis, thrombophlebitis, lymphangitis and renal failure.

There is a high frequency of twinning in parts of the tropics and this is due to the increase in the dizygotic twinning rate, the monozygotic rate being similar to that recorded in temperate climates (Nylander, 1969). The greater the parity the greater is the likelihood of a multiple pregnancy.

Abortion (both natural and criminal) is common in the tropics. The part that malaria may play has already been discussed. Ectopic pregnancies are also common. Culdocentesis (needle aspiration of the Pouch of Douglas) performed as a side-room procedure can be helpful in diagnosis (Editorial, 1970), and autotransfusion is useful in therapy. The Arias-Stella phenomenon in uterine curettings has also been found to be of value in the diagnosis of ectopic pregnancy. In this condition there is focal enlargement of glandular epithelial cells with hypertrophic, hyperchromatic nuclei and proliferation of atypical masses of epithelial cells. A striking feature is the presence of glands lined by very tall epithelium with strikingly clear foamy cytoplasm and large irregular nuclei.

Lithpedions occur in about 2 per cent of extra-uterine pregnancies and may be classified as follows (Onifade et al. 1970):

1. Lithokelyphos in which the membranes alone are calcified.
2. True lithopedion where only the fetus is calcified.
3. Lithokelyphopedion where both the fetus and the membranes are calcified.

Infection of the calcified mass may occur and the patient may present many years following the calcification of the dead fetus with septicaemic symptoms.

AINHUM

Ainhum is a slowly progressive fibrous constriction involving usually the digito-plantar fold of the fifth toe.

The condition is found in its highest incidence in Africa but also occurs in those of Negro descent in South and Central America and in the West Indies. A few cases have been reported in India (Aggarwal and Singh, 1963). It is an acquired disease (in contrast to congenital annular constriction of the digits) and the over-production of fibrous tissue in response to repeated infection or injury is considered important in its aetiology (Browne, 1965). The fibroblastic diathesis thought to be common in the African and discussed when keloids are considered (p. 732) may be an associated factor. The fifth toe is usually affected but the fourth and third can also be involved. The condition is frequently bilateral. Plantar keratosis is usual and yaws may be a complicating condition in some patients. Over the age of 6 years all age groups are affected, with males predominating.

The fibrous constriction causes rarefaction and absorption of the phalanges. The toe may become a mass of fibro fatty tissue covered by a fibrotic dermis and hyperkeratotic epidermis. Spontaneous separation may occur. Occasionally, ainhum of the finger also occurs (Browne and McLoughlin, 1962).

POROCEPHALOSIS (PENTASTOMIASIS)

The adults of the species of the genus *Porocephalus* (class—pentastomida) are parasitic in the lungs of large snakes, crocodiles, and other carnivora. The larvae and nymphs of *P. armillatus* may be found in the liver, intestinal mucosa, lung, and peritoneal cavity of man in Africa and the Middle East. In Asia the larvae and nymphs of *P. moniliformis* occasionally occur in man, while *Linguatula serrata* has been reported as being found with relative frequency (4 per cent) in human necropsies in Chile. Prathap *et al.* (1969) have described the presence of the nymph in 45·4 per cent of 30 consecutive autopsies performed on Malaysian Aborigines. The liver and lungs were the viscera most frequently infected and three types of lesions were seen, viz.: the encysted nymph, the necrotic granuloma, and the 'cuticle' granuloma. Infection was thought to be caused by either drinking water contaminated with the secretions of infected snakes or eating partially cooked snake meat. Gill *et al.* (1968) have noted the occurrence of *Linguatula* infection in sheep, goats, buffaloes and the rabbit in India.

The eggs containing a developed larva are passed with the bronchial secretions of the snakes and are ingested with contaminated leaves, food or water, by monkeys and occasionally by man, especially in areas where snake meat is consumed as a source of food. The larvae penetrate the liver or other organs, undergo a protracted period of development (about 2 years) and finally encyst (nymph). The calcified nymphs have been observed repeatedly in X-ray films of man in Africa. Loehleim (1912) reported infestation rates of about 8 per cent in a study of post-mortem material in the Cameroons, while Van Wymeersch (1954) in the Congo found three infected patients among 70,000 patients examined by X-ray, Lindner (1965) showed that in 1000 randomly-selected abdominal X-ray films taken in Ibadan 1·4 per cent showed calcified nymphs of *Porocephalus*. The most common localization was the right upper quadrant of the abdomen. The literature on these little-known parasites was fully reviewed in 1942 by Cannon and by Self *et al.* (1972).

Pathology

The encysted nymphs are not infrequently found incidentally at necropsy. They are about 8–10mm in diameter, the wall is transparent, and white, coiled-up bodies about 5mm in diameter can be seen within. Others may be firm, white and structureless, due to fibrosis and partial or complete calcification. They are usually few in number and are most commonly found in the peritoneal surface of the abdominal organs, especially the intestine and liver, and are well demarcated and raised from the surface. They have been described in the pleura and parenchyma of the lung,

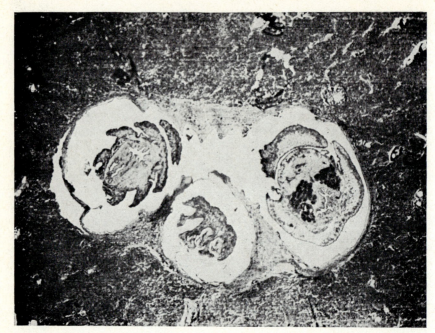

FIG. 16.13. Porocephalosis. Section of porocephalus nymph in liver
(H and E × 10).

the meninges, the parenchyma of the liver, the bile ducts, and hepatic vein, the mesenteric glands and in the mucosa of the intestinal wall (Fig. 16.13).

No information is available regarding the pathology of the migratory stage in man, and histologically when encysted they appear to excite no tissue reaction apart from surrounding fibrosis.

They are usually considered to be harmless but have been thought to cause meningitis (Fornara, 1924), intestinal obstruction (Cannon, 1942), acute abdominal symptoms (Manuwa, 1935, 1947), other surgical complications (Buchanan, 1967), and pulmonary collapse (Stock, 1946) in individual patients.

FAMILIAL MEDITERRANEAN FEVER

This is a genetic disorder with complete autosomal recessive inheritance. It affects mainly two ethnic groups, the Sephardic Jews and Armenians. Most cases have been reported from Israel but it occurs rarely and sporadically in families in Europe, the Mediterranean littoral, the U.S.A. and Canada (Brickman and Feldman, 1969).

It is due to an inborn error of metabolism. A low-fat diet may help in treatment. It is characterized by short, sharp attacks of serositis with fever, abdominal, joint and chest pains. Pericarditis is uncommon. Amyloidosis is a complication in about 30 per cent of patients and may be the presenting symptom. It commences in infancy and continues throughout life. Eclampsia and amyloidosis have been reported in association with FMF in pregnancy. Diagnosis is usually made on family and clinical histories, ethnic background and exclusion of other conditions.

MYIASIS

Myiasis is the invasion of living tissue by the larvae of certain species of flies. Two main forms are recognized, (*a*) external, and (*b*) internal. Children are particularly affected. It is occasionally seen in Britain as an imported disease (*B.M.J.* 1972).

External or dermal myiasis in man usually results from invasion of the skin, mucous membrane, or conjunctiva by larvae of the following species of flies: *Calliphora*, *Chrysomyia*, *Cordylobia*, *Dermatobia*, and *Wohlfahrtia*. Internal myiasis may be of intestinal or genito-urinary origin and may be caused by many different species of the larvae, including those responsible for external myiasis.

In genito-urinary myiasis, the larvae enter a genital or urinary orifice and ascend the genital or urinary tract, while intestinal myiasis is usually caused by the ingestion of eggs or larvae of food-frequenting flies. Larvae may be found at post mortem and may be difficult to identify. They should be reared to adult stage by transferring to decaying meat in a gauze-covered jar with a sanded bottom. The hatched flies should be killed with ether or chloroform and correct identification can then be undertaken (Chinery and Christian, 1972). Tumbu fly dermal myiasis is common in Africa (Gunther, 1967).

TUNGA PENETRANS (JIGGER FLEA)

Tunga penetrans is a flea, the pregnant female of which invades the feet, thighs, perineum, or external genitalia of man, causing itching, inflammation, swelling, and later ulceration and secondary sepsis of the affected parts. The risk of tetanus following invasion by the jigger flea must be borne in mind. It occurs in South America, tropical Africa, and in many other parts of the tropics.

POISONING

Accidental poisoning is common in the tropics in our experience—mainly in children, although lead poisoning has been reported in Gurkha soldiers due to the contamination of chilli powder with lead chromate (Power *et al.* 1969). Therapeutic overdose in children with many drugs occurs due either to inexperienced or careless dispensers or to the over-enthusiastic attitude of the mothers to the medicines prescribed. All children's prescriptions in the tropics should be most carefully considered to ensure that no accidents can occur. Kerosine poisoning is common (Baldachin and Melmed, 1964) and aspiration causes severe pulmonary symptoms. Gastric lavage is not advised as it will be associated with some aspiration of kerosine into the lungs. Olive oil should be administered orally. In different areas of the tropics native medicines of varying types may also be implicated, for example 'cows' urine' in West Africa and 'waragi' (a local alcoholic drink) in East Africa (Bwibo, 1969). An outbreak of poisoning caused by bread in which the flour used had been contaminated by an insecticide (*Endrin*) occurred in Arabia. The symptoms were abdominal pain, vomiting, mental confusion and convulsions. Over 800 patients were affected with 29 deaths (WHO, 1968). Similar incidents have occurred with parathion in Singapore and Mexico.

Lead poisoning

In developed countries **lead poisoning** is now an uncommon condition, although it can still arise as an industrial hazard. In tropical areas it may be more common in some areas than is at present suspected. In addition to the usual causes (paint, lead water pipes, etc.) in India it may be caused by a mascara-like substance applied to the eyelids containing a high content of lead sulphide (Warley *et al*. 1968). Clinically the major lesions are found in the haemopoietic, gastro-intestinal and nervous systems. Stippling of the red cells, the lead line in the mouth and increased radiographic density of the epiphyseal ends of the bones in children establish a diagnosis which can be confirmed by estimating the lead content in the blood and urine.

THE EYE IN THE TROPICS

This subject is briefly discussed—not because it is thought to be un-important—indeed we believe it is of major importance—but because it is largely a specialized field. This is also unfortunate, as in many areas of the tropics some knowledge of ophthalmic surgery is essential if the health of the population is to be efficiently maintained. Ventigataswamy (1972) has for instance estimated that there are 10 million Indians in that country suffering from cataract and that blindness shortly leads to death. Wilson (1972) stated that there were millions of blind in the developing countries whose sight even now could be restored by surgery.

Blindness rates are in general around or below 200 per 100,000 population in America and Europe, but in Africa and Asia the rates are much higher and reach values above 1000 (WHO, 1973). The principal causes listed are the infectious diseases (gonorrhoea, smallpox, syphilis, trachoma and onchocerciasis) which of course will vary in different geographic regions. For instance, in some villages of Upper Volta and Ghana where oncho-cerciasis is endemic the prevalence of blindness in adult males may reach 30–40 per cent. Xerophthalmia is a common cause of blindness in children in the Far East and is closely related to infectious disease in childhood, especially measles and diarrhoea.

Some causes of eye diseases in the tropics are listed in Table 16.5. It should, however, be emphasized that in addition to diseases exclusive to the tropics most of the conditions seen in temperate climates also occur in an identical fashion. Diseases of the eye are therefore a problem of magnitude. Many of the diseases listed in Table 16.5 have been dealt with previously and will not be considered further.

TABLE 16.5. *Some diseases of the eye in the tropics*

Cause	Disease
Hereditary	Dahlak blindness, Pingelap blindness, sickle-cell disease, albinism, colour blindness, retinitis pigmentosa
Viral	Measles, haemorrhagic dengue, smallpox, trachoma, inclusion conjunctivitis, kerato-conjunctivitis, cytomegaloverus infection, ? epidemic conjunctivitis
Bacterial	Gonorrhoea, staphylococcal conjunctivitis in the newborn, brucellosis, treponehatoses, post-meningitis, leprosy
Protozoal	Malaria and fevers (cortical blindness), toxoplasmosis, South American trypanosomiasis
Helminthic	Toxocariasis, trichinellosis, loiasis, onchocerciasis, cysticercosis, hydatid disease, coenuris cerebralis, sparganosis
Nutritional	Xerophthalmia, retrobulbar neuritis, keratomalacia
Climatic	Solar retinopathy, melanoma, pterygium
Autoimmune	? Ophthalmoplegia, sympathetic ophthalmia
Others	Blister beetle, myiasis, cobra venom, mites

Hereditary conditions

A high incidence of hereditary blindness (4–10 per cent) occurs in the Pingelap people of the Eastern Caroline Islands. It is inherited as an autosomal recessive and manifests itself in the first two months of life (Brody *et al.* 1970). Bilateral cystic corneal degeneration is of unknown aetiology.

It occurs in the population of the Dahlak Islands in the Red Sea and accounts for 52 per cent of the blindness prevalence rate of 4000 per 100,000 population. Dahlak blindness affects in some degree or another 50 per cent of the men and women living on the islands. Cataract is also common (Rodger, 1971). It has also been noted in the Nama people of South West Africa (Freedman, 1972). Amblyopia, which is defined as reduced visual acuity in an eye without ophthalmoscopically detectable anomalies of the fundus in patients with or without strabismus, is common in children in many parts of the tropics. In Egypt the visual acuity and field of vision of urban and rural Egyptians decreases markedly at about 45 years of age. The loss of visual acuity is more marked in rural areas and in females when compared to males (Said *et al.* 1969). The causes are probably environmental.

In albinism there is deficiency of pigment in the uveal tract which causes severe photophobia and, if the retina is affected, causes defective vision. Nystagmus is very common. The iris is pink in colour in complete albinism or pale blue if partial. Retinitis pigmentosa occurs and colour blindness may be common.

DISEASES OF THE EYELIDS

The usual infective diseases are seen usually with more severe manifestations owing to the late presentation of the patient and the climatic factors of dust and heat. The toxin of the blister beetle can cause lesions of the eyelid and conjunctivitis and mites can cause a blepharitis (English, 1969). Entropion (a rolling in of the eyelid margin) is a problem of magnitude in some areas of the tropics especially in dry hot dusty climates—usually initiated by trachoma. Corneal injury with ulceration and permanent opacities or worse ensues. Ectropion (eversion of the eyelid) also occurs with resulting ocular inflammation. The chalazion is a tough elastic nodule which develops in the eyelid and is a tuberculoid non-caseating granuloma. The tumours most frequently seen are haemangioma, papilloma, dermoid cyst, pleomorphic adenoma and squamous cell carcinoma. Basal cell carcinoma, so common in temperate climates, is rare in the heavily pigmented peoples.

LACRIMAL GLAND

The condition we have most frequently seen affecting the lacrimal gland is the pleomorphic adenoma. Adenoid cystic carcinoma and adenocarcinomas also occur.

DISEASE OF THE CONJUNCTIVA

Neonatal conjunctivitis is common. The infecting organisms are usually staphylococci or gonococci. Inclusion conjunctivitis also occurs. Trachoma has already been discussed (p. 242). Epidemic kerato-conjunctivitis due to a viral infection occurs in humid parts of the tropics.

An epidemic of acute conjunctivitis was reported in Ghana in June 1969 and spread rapidly throughout the country within a month. In September it spread to Lagos, Nigeria. The lay public named it 'Apollo 11 disease'. There is an acute conjunctivitis with haemorrhage and secondary infection may occur. The prognosis is good. A viral aetiology (adenovirus) is suspected (Chatterjee *et al.* 1970). Steroids are contraindicated in therapy. Phlyctenular kerato-conjunctivitis occurs

Conjunctivitis may also be caused by the instillation of native medicine in the eye. The larvae of certain flies may develop in the conjunctival sac (Myiasis) and cause conjunctivitis. The larvae may burrow through the conjunctiva and even through the sclera as an intraoccular parasite leading to destruction of the eye (Somerset, 1968).

Pterygium is common in parts of the tropics especially in areas with hot dry climates. Its highest prevalence is found close to the equator. Sunlight irritation and perhaps a hereditary factor are thought to be aetiological agents. There is collagenous thickening extending from usually the nasal or much less commonly the temporal bulbar conjunctiva onto the cornea in a pyramidal fashion with the apex towards the cornea. It invades the cornea deep to the epithelium and destroys Bowman's membrane. Pseudo-elastic tissue may be present (Ansari *et al.* 1970).

Benign tumours are not uncommon. We have seen Bowen's disease (intraepithelial carcinoma) but the most common malignant tumour is the squamous cell carcinoma, especially in hot dusty dry climates. A melanoma occasionally and lymphocytic tumours rarely occur. Kaposi's disease has also been described in children (Seavin *et al.* 1970).

DISEASES OF THE CORNEA

Xerophthalmia is common in areas where Vitamin A deficiency occurs. The basic pathology is atrophy of columnar epithelium with a substitution of stratified keratinizing epithelium, which occurs in the conjunctiva and lacrimal glands. The eye is dry. The cornea becomes ulcerated and infected. It may become softened and perforate which is known as keratomalacia and has already been mentioned (p. 683).

Keratitis and iritis are complications of many of the tropical diseases listed in Table 16.5. Leprosy and onchocerciasis are probably of major importance. Corneal opacities are frequently seen and there is a widespread need for keratoplasty. Corneal ulceration is common and staphyloma with protrusion of cornea, iris and inflammatory tissue occurs as does pan-ophthalmitis. Trauma is also a potent cause of panophthalmitis and enuclea-tion.

It is of interest that arcus senilis is common in certain racial groups in the tropics and is not related to atherosclerosis, coronary artery disease, or raised serum cholesterol (Bersohn *et al.* 1969; Hearn, 1970).

Benign tumours, squamous cell carcinoma and melanoma are reported but spread from the conjunctiva is usual.

There are many causes of inflammation of the uveal tract including autoimmune disease, bacterial disease, viruses and many tropical conditions. The precise cause in many cases is uncertain as organisms are not usually present. A sensitivity reaction is postulated. Sympathetic ophthalmitis is the inflammation of the uveal tract of the contralateral eye following similar inflammation in the other as a result of a penetrating injury. The inflammation is granulomatous with eosinophils prominent. A malignant melanoma may arise from the uveal tract. The choroid is the commonest site of melanoma in the Western world but it is rare in the African.

Cataract

Cataract is a common cause of blindness in parts of India and Kenya but would appear to be much less so in Japan and Ghana. Prevalence studies in the Punjab have confirmed the high figures. Sunlight has been implicated as a contributory cause in cataract in some parts of the world and it is of interest that no difference in prevalence has been noted by some investigators in diabetics and non-diabetics—though it is known to develop rapidly in some young diabetics.

Glaucoma

Primary claucoma excluding congenital glaucoma is the second commonest cause of blindness in eye-clinic patients in Ibadan. Many of the patients are below 21 years of age. The patients suffer severe loss of vision as they present late as the gradual loss of vision and field is not sufficiently severe to bring them to hospital at an early stage. Primary acute congestive glaucoma which causes pain and so brings patients for early treatment in other countries is seldom encountered in Nigerians (Olurin, 1972).

Epidemic dropsy glaucoma

The disease is seen in India, Fiji and Mauritius and is due to the adulteration of mustard oil with oil from the seeds of the *Argemone mexicana* plant. Poisoning produces peripheral oedema with intestinal disturbance, fever and perhaps evidence of a myocarditis. A small proportion of cases are complicated by glaucoma (Somerset, 1968).

THE RETINA

There is absence of pigment in albinism. Retrolental fibroplasia was a major cause of blindness in children in developed countries. The administration of oxygen to the premature neonate was considered causal and restriction of oxygen therapy dramatically decreased the incidence. This, however, has led to a marked increase in the respiratory distress syndrome which is of course common in developing countries. With increasing wealth and medical facilities oxygen is now becoming available in certain centres in the tropics and no doubt will be administered to premature babies and neonates with the syndrome. The possible occurrence of retrolental fibro-plasia, which is at present rare, may thus occur in certain regions. The retino-pathies associated with vascular and renal disease and diabetes mellitus have already been discussed. The retinoblastoma is a common tumour of childhood. There is a hereditary factor in some patients. The differential diagnosis from the Burkitt tumour is discussed on p. 510. Tuberous sclerosis and neurofibromatosis may occasionally involve the retina.

Solar retinopathy

Short exposure of the retina to the sun may result in serious damage such as severe macular burns (Ridgway, 1967). Solar retinopathy has been reported among Punjabis who look at the sun for religious reasons and in temperate climates following the observation of the eclipse of the sun or rarely following sunbathing (Ridgway, 1967). The only safe way of observing the sun is to project the sun's image on to a screen.

THE OPTIC NERVE

Optic atrophy is associated with many diseases. In many cases of primary optic atrophy, however, the cause is not immediately apparent. In Nigeria, excluding tropical ataxic neuropathy, the commonest causes of bilateral primary optic atrophy were acute bilateral retrobulbar neuritis retinitis pigmentosa, onchocercal infection, idiopathic choroidoretinal degeneration, trauma, unidentified toxins, post-meningitic, pituitary tumours and maturity onset diabetes in that order of importance (Osuntokun et al. 1972). The patients with preceding bilateral retrobulbar neuritis probably had a form of neuromyolitis optica, which is not uncommon in Nigerians. Multiple sclerosis the most probable cause in temperate zones is rarely if ever seen in Nigeria. Toxoplasmosis was not diagnosed as a cause of chor-oidoretinal degeneration in the series listed above. In a previous investigation the Sabin–Feldman dye test for toxoplasmosis was found to be as frequently positive in normal adult Nigerians as in those with choroidoretinitis (Osuntokun et al. 1972). Tumours of the optic nerve are not common but fibroma and glioma are described.

CORTICAL BLINDNESS

Cortical blindness due to a defective blood supply to the occipital cortex may occur in children following convulsions and fever. The prognosis is usually good and full vision is restored. Causes of cortical blindness are birth trauma, meningitis, trauma, encephalitis, cardiac arrest, malaria and other pyrexias of unknown origin (Olurin, 1970).

PROPTOSIS

Retrobulbar haemorrhage may cause proptosis in the neonate (Quar-coopome, 1970). A unilateral painful ophthalmoplegia occurs in Southern India and as isolated cases in other parts of the world, with diplopia and ptosis as the symptoms. The third, fourth and sixth cranial nerves may be involved. Males are more commonly affected than females, and young adults and the middle-aged are the age groups involved. It may be due to a periarteritic carotid lesion due possibly to an immunoallergic disturbance. It responds dramatically to steroids but may recur (Mathew and Chandy, 1970). In the Western world the usual cause is an intracranial aneurysm. Inflammation of neighbouring sinuses or invasion of the orbit by parasites or fungi are other causes. Pseudotumour of the orbit is not uncommon and the clinical findings are similar to an orbital tumour. It is probably secondary to an orbital infection. Necrosis of orbital fat with inflammation and fibrosis occur. The condition responds to steroids and antibiotics. Orbital haemangioma occurs.

The tumours usually causing proptosis are fibrous dysplasia of the neighbouring bones, Burkitt's lymphoma, retinoblastoma, chloroma and the pleomorphic adenoma (Templeton, 1971; Olurin and Williams, 1972). In the United States rhabdomyosarcoma has been stated to be the most common primary malignant orbital tumour of childhood (Porterfield and Zimmerman, 1962), whereas in Nigeria Burkitt's lymphoma is much the commonest and rhabdomyosarcoma of the orbit in children would appear to be less common. The tumour types seen will, therefore, depend upon the specific geographical area being considered.

SKIN DISEASE IN THE TROPICS

Dermatology in the tropics does not basically differ from that seen in temperate climates but the frequency of the dermatoses differ in different geographical areas and are influenced by sociological and environmental factors, race, age, and climate. Findlay and Park (1969), for instance, have drawn up frequency charts by race and age for the common skin diseases seen in the Transvaal. In children in the Bantu patients scabies, impetigo, papular urticaria (including insect bites) tinea capitis, ecthyma and seborrhoeic eczema were the most common diseases. In Indian children impetigo, constitutional eczema, eczema and pityriasis alba, took pride of place whereas in white children constitutional eczema, eczematides and pityriasis alba, and fourthly impetigo were most common. In adolescents in all races acne was common, although said to be uncommon in the African. It is also uncommon in the Japanese. This illustrates the differing disease pattern that may be seen in different races living in the same geographic area. The skin diseases seen in the tropics have been described by Marshall (1964) in Africa and in essays on tropical dermatology by Simons and Marshall (1969) and Marshall (1972).

The pathology of the dermatological changes seen in most tropical diseases have already been described in their appropriate context and the list is long, viz.: leishmaniasis, leprosy, creeping eruption, amoebiasis, the treponematoses, onchocerciasis, the mycoses, protein calorie malnutrition, cancrum oris, filariasis, myiasis, dracontiasis, vitamin deficiencies and granuloma multiforme, to name but a few.

Many authors have written on the geographical frequency of skin diseases in the tropics but it must be emphasized that this will vary even within a few hundred miles depending upon the presence of such conditions as onchocerciasis and leishmaniasis as examples. It has been said, however, that in the tropics, the common skin diseases are the mycoses, pyodermas, parasitoses, the treponematoses and leprosy. We still believe that no dogmatic statements can be made. In our experience in Zaria (Nigeria), tropical phagedenic ulcer is by far the most frequent skin condition received in the Department of Pathology—frequently with malignant change—in contrast to the situation in Ibadan. It is realized, of course, that such conditions as scabies and pyoderma which are common in Zaria will not be biopsied for diagnosis, and thus will not be considered in our studies.

Xeroderma pigmentosum is common in North Africa but rare in the African although it has been described. Hyperpigmentation and atrophy of the skin with telangiectases, warty and finally malignant growths occur. It commences in early childhood. Photophobia with keratitis and corneal opacities occur (Harris and Keet, 1960).

There is no doubt, however, that pigmentation confers a high degree of protection against light-induced degenerative changes. Excluding chronic discoid lupus erythematosis, pellagra and some drug eruptions, diseases due to photosensitivity are uncommon in pigmented peoples. Solar dermatoses are rare and this was discussed when cancer of the skin was considered.

Pigmented peoples would appear to be less liable to eczema, seborrhoeic dermatitis, prickly heat, familial baldness, naevi, alopecia areata, rosacea and varicose ulcer. Psoriasis, also thought to be rare, has, however, been reported as common in Kenya and of higher prevalence in Africans than in Caucasians (Verhagen and Koten, 1967) whereas it is uncommon in Nigeria and in the American Negro. Although chronic actinic damage hardly occurs in Africans (keratosis senilis and basal-cell carcinoma) sun-influenced diseases such as chronic actinic cheilitis, chronic lupus erythematosis, and chronic polymorphic light eruption are common in Africans living in the Highlands of Kenya. Eczema and psoriasis are said to be increasing in frequency in urbanized Africans.

It is obviously impossible in a text such as this to describe the pathology of all skin diseases which are adequately described in textbooks so we limit ourselves below to a few conditions which are relevant to the tropics.

DRUGS

Fixed eruptions especially due to phenolphthalein and dapsone treatment in leprosy are common (Browne, 1964).

IMMUNOLOGICAL DISORDERS OF THE SKIN

The part that multiple infections and infestations play in the pattern of skin disease in the tropics, if any, has still to be elucidated. Cell mediated immunity is known to be important in leprosy, leishmaniasis and certain fungal diseases.

OCCUPATIONAL DERMATOSES

These are said to be uncommon but this probably represents a lack of medical investigation into the problems. We have seen severe superficial fungal infections in washermen. Pineapple dermatosis has been described in workers in pineapple factories who cut the raw fruit. Superficial raw areas occur on the fingertips and are thought to be due to contact with a proteolytic enzyme, bromelin, in the pineapple (Polunin, 1951).

Sabra dermatitis is an acute papulopustular itching dermatitis which affects workers handling the prickly pear—a cactus named *Opuntia ficus indica*—which grows in Mexico, Morocco, Tunisia and Italy.

TUBERCULOSIS

In our experience the tuberculous chancre is rare, although not uncommon in Asia. Scrofuloderma would appear to be uncommon in West Africa although common in some other areas of the tropics. An indolent warty lesion (prosector's wart) may affect the buttocks and legs by squatting on infected material in India and the Far East. The epidermis shows pseudo-epitheliomatous hyperplasia. There is a dermal infiltrate of neutrophils and lymphocytes. Giant cells are frequently seen but typical tubercles are uncommon. Bacilli are scanty. Lupus vulgaris is not uncommon and histologically may be confused with sarcoid. It can be differentiated from tuberculoid leprosy by lack of nervous involvement. Tuberculides are not common in our experience although, as the histopathology may be non-specific, some cases may well be being missed. Localized subcutaneous tuberculous abscesses with the absence of pain, tenderness and signs of inflammation can occur. They do not appear to have any deep connections nor serious significance. They may occur on the trunk or limbs. An active pulmonary lesion may or may not be present. The diagnosis is confirmed by aspiration but frequently in our experience surgical biopsy or excision is performed. Indeed excision and primary suture is a recognized form of treatment (Editorial, 1971).

LEPROSY

In the differential diagnosis of leprosy, fungal infections especially pityriasis versicolor and tinea marginatum, fixed drug eruptions (Browne (1964), macular hypochromia of unknown aetiology, vitiligo and ichthyosis have to be considered. Granuloma multiforme has already been discussed (p. 313). Systemic sclerosis which produces hypopigmentation and some clawing of the fingers has also been mistaken for leprosy (Addy, 1971).

CLIMATIC DISORDERS

These seldom affect pigmented peoples. Tropical anhidrotic asthenia is caused by excessive sweating followed by loss of sweating over the body. There may be continued abundant perspiration from the face and neck. Due to fluid and electrolyte imbalance weakness, vertigo, headache, exhaustion, and palpitation occur. The skin of the body becomes dry and warm with fine scaling and a heat rash occurring.

Prickly heat (*Milaria Rubra*) is the effect of hyperhidrosis and blocking of the sweat ducts by plugs of keratin. There is periductal acute inflammation and oedema which is probably the primary cause induced by friction or solar damage.

OTHER CONDITIONS

Lichen planus is common and the histopathology is similar to that seen in the Western world. Eczema occurs and the causes are multifactorial. Close cooperation between the dermatologist and pathologist are necessary to elucidate the aetiology. In any non-specific dermatitis in the tropics it is essential that special stains be employed in biopsy material. The most useful in our experience are the Ziehl–Neelson, Giemsa and methenamine silver stains combined with a periodic acid Schiff technique. The tendency of pigmented peoples to form keloids has already been mentioned. Phrynoderma is a particular type of follicular hyperkeratosis seen in tropical countries. The elbows, thighs and buttocks are characteristically affected. The follicles contain large keratin plugs and the adjacent skin is usually darker than normal. Deficiency of the B group of vitamins has been suggested (Shrank, 1966). Toxic epidermal necrolysis was first described by Lyell (1956) and has been reviewed in an Editorial (1971) as the scalded skin syndrome. It was reported in Africa by Browne and Ridge (1961). We have seen one or two cases and it can be puzzling if not known to the physician. The aetiology may be unknown (idiopathic) but staphylococci, drugs and other factors have been incriminated. The patients present with erythema, flaccid bullae, or desquamation of the skin in sheets and the differential diagnosis will include bullous erythema multiforme or pemphigus. Histologically there is complete necrosis of the epidermis with very little abnormality of the underlying dermis.

The 'Velvet Leg' syndrome has been described by Clarke (1952) in West Africa and consists of hyperpigmented widespread diffuse areas of hyperkeratosis on the legs, usually on the shins. The surface is thick, tough, deep black in colour and of rough consistency. The lesions are dry and there is never ulceration. There may be pruritus. An eosinophilia is usual.

Histologically there is marked keratosis with plugging of follicles, acanthosis and papilliferous proliferation of the epidermis. The upper dermis and papillae are collagenous with atrophy of the adnexal structures which may be surrounded by a minimal plasma cell and lymphocytic infiltrate. Brazilan foliaceous pemphigus is endemic in certain areas of Brazil. Fever and crusted bullae are usual involving the whole body but not the mucous membranes. The endocrine glands may be affected. Acantholysis is a constant diagnostic feature. It resembles closely dermatitis herpetiformis (Azulay, 1969).

We have occasionally seen dwarfism associated with skin lesions of undetermined aetiology. Adamson (1973) has described icthyosis linearis circumflexa in association with idiopathic dwarfism.

Dermatitis papulosa nigra appears to occur only in Negroes.

Dermatitis cruris pustulosa et atrophicans, an infective dermatitis of the skin, is common in tropical Africa (Clarke, 1952) and is resistant to treatment.

Some Laboratory Diagnostic Methods

with the assistance of

J. E. FRIEND, A.I.S.T.

Senior Demonstrator and Tutor, Liverpool School of Tropical Medicine

CONTENTS

A. Parasitological techniques:
    (1) Faeces
    (2) Blood
B. Laboratory detection of abnormal haemoglobins
C. Blood transfusion methods
D. Histological methods
E. Miscellaneous

A. PARASITOLOGICAL TECHNIQUES

I. EXAMINATION OF FAECES FOR PROTOZOA AND HELMINTHS

No technique is claimed to be 100 per cent successful for the detection of parasites by a single stool examination. Cysts tend to be excreted in 'showers' and it is generally accepted that five of more serial stools must be examined before an individual is considered free from an intestinal protozoal infection. It is obviously of assistance to know what one is expecting to find, but often parasites unsuspected from the clinical history are found in routine examination.

Naked-eye appearances

(a) *Blood and mucus present:* examine microscopically for trophozoites of amoebae (or rarely *Balantidium*) not for cystic forms. Ova of *S. mansoni* or *S. japonicum* may be found.

(b) *Loose stools without blood or mucus:* examine microscopically for trophozoites of amoebae, flagellates, and their cysts.

(c) *Formed stools:* examine microscopically for cysts. If present, *Taenia* segments and *Enterobius* can be seen with the unaided eye.

1. Direct examination in saline

This is the only method except culture for detection of motile amoebae or flagellates. Protozoa and helminth ova if present in moderate numbers will be detected but if scanty concentration methods will be required.

Method. A small amount of faeces is emulsified in a drop of physiological saline on a slide and a cover glass is then applied to the smear. Examine immediately and also note the type of exudate.

It must be noted that *Taenia* ova are found in only about 20 per cent of patients passing segments.

2. Direct examination in iodine

Used only after cysts have been found in saline or by concentration.

(a) *Lugol's iodine*, 1 per cent (this is the formula given in British textbooks and differs from that used in MIF stain, see below):

Iodine	1 g
Potassium iodide	2 g
Distilled water	100 ml

Dissolve the salt in 10 ml of distilled water, then add iodine crystals. Shake until iodine dissolved, then add remainder of water.

For staining amoebic cysts a small amount of faeces is emulsified in a drop of this iodine and examined immediately.

(b) *Merthiolate-Iodine-Formalin* (MIF), Sapero and Lawless (1953).

Mix 1 drop of Lugol's iodine less than 3 weeks old;
   1 drop of Formalin (40 per cent Formaldehyde);
   8 drops of Merthiolate tincture, in tube.

To use, place a drop of distilled water on a slide and add an equal volume of MIF. Emulsify faeces in this mixture.

Staining occurs in two stages: (1) initial iodine stage in which cysts and trophozoites stain a yellowish-green to a yellowish-brown; (2) subsequent eosin stage gradually replaces iodine and is permanent. Nuclear elements of human intestinal protozoa, except *Dientamoeba*, are well-defined.

3. Concentration

The aim is to separate protozoan cysts and helminth ova from faecal material through differences in specific gravity. Methods fall into two types, sedimentation and flotation. With sedimentation, cysts (and ova) which are denser than the suspending fluid are concentrated in the bottom of the tube. With flotation the use of denser liquids is involved, the parasites less dense than the liquid rising to the surface. The methods mentioned below are used in many medical laboratories.

(a) *Zinc sulphate flotation* (Faust, 1939), for cysts, and ova exclusive of trematode.

(1) Emulsify about 1 g of faeces in water; strain into 17 × 111 mm tube through a wire or nylon sieve having 40 meshes to the linear inch. A tea strainer is a good substitute, most having 30 meshes to the linear inch.

(2) Centrifuge, decant supernatant, add fresh water, shake; centrifuge until supernatant clear (centrifuge for 2 min at 1200–1800 rpm 2 or 3 times).

(3) Decant supernatant, half fill tube with 1·180 sp.gr. zinc sulphate solution, shake, fill tube to 5 mm of brim with zinc sulphate and spin at 2500 rpm for 1 min ($ZnSO_4$ 331 g in 1 l H_2O; test with hydrometer).

(4) Transfer surface scum by loop to slide and examine, add iodine if necessary. Or, with the addition of a further step, pipette 3 ml of supernatant into a clean centrifuge tube, fill with water, shake, centrifuge, and examine deposit.

(*b*) *Flotation in brine* (method for qualitative examination of stools for light infestations of *Ascaris* and hookworm ova).

(1) Emulsify 1–2 g of faeces through fine sieve with saturated salt solution, sp.gr. 1·200.

(2) Pour suspension into straight-walled tube about 25 mm high until meniscus forms at brim; apply coverslip.

(3) Leave 10–20 min, remove coverslip vertically and quickly, place on slide and examine.

(*c*) *Formol-ether*, after Ridley and Hawgood (1956), for cysts and ova including trematodes.

(1) Emulsify 1–2 g of faeces in 7–10 ml of 10 per cent formol-saline, strain through wire gauze (40 mesh) into a centrifuge tube.

(2) Add 3 ml ether and shake vigorously for 1 min.

(3) Centrifuge, set regulator at 2000 rpm. Switch off after one and a half minutes, and allow tube to come to rest.

(4) Loosen debris on the surface and at the interface between the two liquids with a swab stick. Pour away the supernatent together with the debris. Wipe the upper inside part of the tube clean.

(5) Shake up the small deposit and examine. Concentration of cysts and ova should be 20–30 times.

(*d*) *Saline or glycerol sedimentation, for S. mansoni and S. japonicum.*

Emulsify 1–2 g of faeces in 100 ml of either 0·9 per cent saline or 0·5 per cent glycerol; strain through a 40 mesh sieve into conical urine glass.

Leave in subdued light for about 20 min., when ova will have settled. Examine deposit.

Filtration-ninhydrin (Bell, 1963). This technique was first used by Bell as an accurate and sensitive method for counting schistosome eggs in faeces. It is undoubtedly the most sensitive method available when used in conjunction with the saline or glycerol sedimentation method but has the disadvantage of being time-consuming. The method is, however, readily adapted for use with urine and it is this method that is described and recommended.

Method for use with urine (*S. haematobium*). For maximum diagnostic efficiency a 24-hr specimen should be used. If random samples are used, those collected around the middle of the day (10 a.m.–2 p.m.) are most likely to contain the most eggs.

To prevent hatching, the specimen should be kept in a refrigerator (hatching in urine is very unusual unless water is added or the specimen is very dilute). A preservative, iodine, may be used which kills the eggs and so prevents hatching and also has the advantage of acting as a mordant to the ninhydrin reaction.

A saturated solution of iodine in potassium iodide is added at the rate of 4 ml/l of urine (gross excess of iodine has no adverse effect to the reaction).

Filter the urine through a filter paper (Whatman 541 is best) in a suitable device to prevent the escape of eggs round the sides of the paper. The stainless steel Buchner funnel (Gallenkamp FD 704) which takes a 6·5 cm filter paper is suitable for large specimens and the millipore funnel (Millipore (U.K.) Ltd.) which takes a filter paper about 4·7 cm is suitable for specimens of under 1 litre.

Filtration is achieved by vacuum, and the funnel top well washed to carry all the eggs on to the paper. If the paper becomes blocked by either phosphates or urates wash the paper through with hot water and dilute acetic acid.

After the paper has been rinsed with water it is removed from the filter support and placed in a small amount of saturated aqueous ninhydrin so that the solution soaks into the paper. The colour is then developed by incubating the paper at 37 °C for 2 hr or 60 °C for 1 hr or at any convenient temperature between these limits. The colour will only develop when the paper is dry, the miracidium inside the egg will stain a deep purple, the egg shell will be seen as a refractile halo.

The papers are examined wet after mounting in a few drops of water. It is more convenient to bisect the paper for examination and mount on a 75×50 mm slide. The papers are relatively opaque, so a fairly intense light-source is necessary. A suitable magnification is about 30 overall, as the use of higher magnifications makes scanning unreasonably slow. It is the fact that the eggs stand out as brilliantly purple objects against a predominantly brown faecal background that makes the scrutiny at low magnification possible.

If iodine has been used the colour will persist even after repeated moistening of the filter paper.

4. Permanent staining

(a) *Heidenhain's*, by short or long procedure, is the classical method.

Iron-haematoxylin stain (Heidenhain, 1892) staining of faecal smears. The following solutions are required:

(1) Schaudinn's fluid:

Acetic acid glacial	1 ml
Ethyl alcohol absolute	33 ml
Mercuric chloride saturated aqueous solution	66 ml

(2) Ferric ammonium sulphate (iron alum)   4 g
Distilled water   100 ml

(3) Haematoxylin   1 g
Ethyl alcohol 95 per cent   10 ml
Distilled water   100 ml

Dissolve the haematoxylin in the alcohol with gentle heat and then add 90 ml of the distilled water. Store in well-stoppered bottle for 1 week to ripen, then add 100 ml distilled water, mix well, filter. The ripe brown-coloured solution is now ready for use.

(4) Ferric ammonium sulphate   2 g
Distilled water   100 ml

Method. Prepare several thin, wet, faecal smears in coverslips and place while still wet into solution (1) to fix for 15 min. Transfer to 70 per cent alcohol (in which the specimens will keep indefinitely).

Transfer to 70 per cent alcohol to which Lugol's iodine has been added to make the solution a light brown colour. Leave for 10 min to remove the mercuric chloride from the smear. Transfer to clean 70 per cent alcohol for 10 min and then to distilled water for 10 min.

Place smear in solution (2) and leave 6–24 hr. Note time in this mordant. Wash smear in distilled water for 30 sec and place into solution (3) to stain. Leave in stain for the same time as the smear was in solution (2). Remove the smears from the stain and place in water. Decolorize the smears one at a time by placing them in solution (4). Remove the smear after 30 sec, wash in water and examine under a microscope to check differentiation. Continue this process until the nuclear structure is clearly visible; it may be necessary to replace the smear in solution (4) several times. The time for this step varies with each smear. When differentiation is complete wash the smear for 20 min in gently running water. Dehydrate in ascending grades of alcohol, clear in xylol and mount on a slide using a suitable neutral mounting media.

Result—nuclei: blue-black; cytoplasm and debris: grey or bluish-grey.

The time taken by the standard method may be reduced if the temperature of solutions (2) and (3) is raised to 50 °C and the time reduced to 10 min in each solution.

Note. The smear must not be permitted to dry at any stage.

(b) *MIF for preservation of specimens*

(1) Stock 'MF' solution (stable):

Distilled water	50 ml
Formaldehyde 40 per cent	5 ml
Tincture of Merthiolate★ (1 : 1000)	40 ml
Glycerine	1 ml

Store in brown bottle.

(2) Add 2·35 ml 'MF' stock to 0·15 ml Lugol's iodine (less than 3 weeks old) *immediately before use*, as prior addition of the iodine causes a dense precipitate to be formed and the iodine fails to act satisfactorily on the protozoa.

(3) Thoroughly mix a portion of the faeces about the size of a pea in the MIF solution. It is important not to use too much faeces. For larger samples, use increased amounts of MIF.

(4) To examine, take a drop of fluid from the top of the sedimented faeces and place on a slide, giving a preparation roughly comparable in density to a direct smear. Cysts, trophozoites and ova tend to collect in the upper layers.

(5) This preserved specimen can be used for concentration by the formol-ether technique.

Lugol's iodine 5 per cent B.P. for MIF

Iodine	5 g
Potassium iodide	10 g
Distilled water	100 ml

Tincture of Merthiolate No. 99 1 : 1000 Lilly is a trade preparation for skin asepsis; it is coloured with eosin.

5. Quantitative egg-count techniques

Three methods are commonly used for the quantitative assessment of helminth ova.

(a) *Stoll's method* (Stoll and Hausheer, 1926).

(1) Weigh out 3 g of faeces.

(2) Fill a stoppered bottle with 42 ml of water (N/10 NaOH is better than water and must be used if faeces hard, allow to soften for several hours).

(3) Add faeces and some glass beads and shake until faeces thoroughly comminuted.

(4) Pipette 0·15 ml on to a glass slide and cover with a coverslip. Count total number of eggs in sample including any in fluid exuded from sides of coverslip.

Eggs counted were present in $\dfrac{3 \times 0\cdot 15}{45}$ g of faeces or 0·01 g.

Eggs counted × 100 gives numbers per gram.

Note. Counts of most types of ova can be made by this method.

★(Thiomersal) International Non-property Name.

(b) *McMaster's method* (Gordon and Whitlock, 1949)

(1) Mix 2 g of faeces in 28 ml of saturated salt solution.
(2) Pass the mixture through a sieve, and wash the retained debris with a further 30 ml of saturated salt solution.
(3) Thoroughly mix the suspension and fill both chambers of a McMaster slide by means of a pipette.
(4) Count the total number of eggs in both chambers.

Each chamber has an area of 1 cm² and a depth of 1·55 mm. The volume in each chamber is therefore 0·15 ml, 60 ml of the original suspension contained 2 g of faeces, and so 0·3 ml of the suspension (the contents of the two chambers) contains 0·01 g of faeces. Hence the total number of eggs counted in both chambers × 100 equals the number of eggs per gram of faeces.

The morphological appearances of some of the more common helminth ova are shown in Fig. A2.

(c) *Kato's method (1954). Modified by Martin and Beaver (1968).*

Materials required
  Glass microscope slides.
  Cellophane 'coverslips' (22 mm × 30 mm strips of wettable cellophane of medium chickness).
  Glycerin–malachite green solution (100 ml pure Glycerin 100 ml water and 1 ml 3 per cent aqueous malachite green).

Method. Place 50–60 mg of faeces on a clean glass slide, cover with strip of cellophane (previously soaked in the glycerin–malachite green solution for at least 24 hr).

Invert the preparation and press it against a flat absorbent surface (filter paper on bench) until the faecal mass almost covers the area of the cellophane.

Allow the smear to stand for about 1 hr at room temperature or for 20 min at 34–40 °C. This clears the faeces but leaves helminth eggs uncleared.

Examine the smear immediately it clears as overclearing will cause hookworm eggs to disappear and sometimes causes schistosome eggs to become indistinct. Examine the entire film under low power magnification (×60) using higher magnification to confirm identification.

Specimens of faeces that contain an excessive amount of fibrous material may be passed through a wire sieve before placing on slide.

II. EXAMINATION OF BLOOD FOR PARASITES

The following procedures are employed in the various conditions listed below.

(a) *Malaria*

Thin- and thick-blood film stained by a Romanowsky stain.

(b) *Trypanosomiasis*

(1) Fresh blood preparation examined for motile trypanosomes.
(2) Thin- and thick-blood film stained by a Romanowsky stain.
(3) Triple centrifugation of citrated or heparinized blood.
(4) Fresh preparation of gland aspirate examined for motile trypanosomes.
(5) Centrifuged deposit of cerebral spinal fluid examined for motile trypanosomes.
(6) Inoculation of laboratory animals.
(7) Xenodiagnosis (*T. cruzi*).
(8) Culture. Not generally accepted as a means of diagnosis, except in *T. cruzi*.

(c) *Leishmaniasis*
  (1) Serological tests.
  (2) Film obtained from marrow, spleen puncture or ulcer stained by a Romanow-sky stain.
  (3) Culture on blood agar media (NNN) at room temperature or 25 °C.

(d) *Toxoplasmosis*
  (1) Serological tests. Sabin-Feldman dye test and CFT.
  (2) Centrifuged deposit of cerebrospinal fluid stained by a Romanowsky stain.
  (3) Inoculation of laboratory animals.

(e) *Spirochaetes*
  (1) Fresh blood preparation examined will show disturbance of red cells; organisms are very difficult to detect.
  (2) Fresh blood preparation examined by dark ground, organism visible.
  (3) Thin- and thick-blood film stained by a Romanowsky stain will show some species.
  (4) Thin film stained by negative staining (film made from a mixture of blood and Indian ink).

(f) *Microfilariae*
  (1) Fresh blood preparation examined for motile microfilariae.
  (2) Thick-blood film stained by haemalum or Giemsa.
  (3) Blood laked with formalin and centrifuged deposit examined.
    W. bancrofti and *B. malayi*, nocturnal:
      Blood collected preferably between 10 p.m. and 2 a.m.
    L. loa, diurnal:
      Blood collected preferably between 10 a.m. and 2 p.m.
    A. perstans and *M. ozzardi*:
      Non-periodic.

(g) *Examination of skin for microfilariae*
  The technique for the performing a skin snip is shown in Fig. A1.
  (1) Skin snip teased in saline and examined.
  (2) Drop of serum added to teased skin, allowed to dry, fixed and stained with haemalum (p. 620).

III. PREPARATION AND STAINING OF THIN AND THICK BLOOD FILMS

(a) *Thin blood films*

In an adequately-prepared film, cells should be discretely separated and not distorted.

Method. Clean puncture site (either finger, lobe of ear or, in the case of small children, the heel) with 70 per cent alcohol, wipe dry. Prick the skin, using a sterile needle with a cutting edge. Gently squeeze until a globule of blood exudes. By touching with the end of a glass slide, transfer to the slide a small drop of blood. Using another glass slide as a spreader place the edge in contact with the blood slide at an angle of about 30°, and move it back into the drop of blood. The blood will run along the back edge of the spreader. When it has run about two-thirds of the slide width, push the spreader forwards, taking the trailing blood with it along the slide. Dry the film quickly by waving in the air. Protect the film from flies and air-borne contamination.

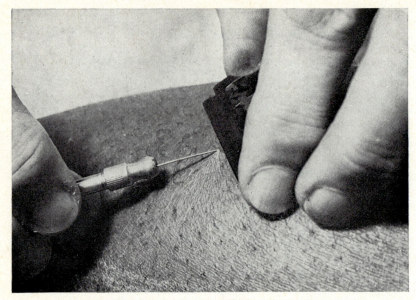

FIG. A1. Technique of skin snip for onchocerciasis.

Delay the spreading of very anaemic blood for a few moments to obtain a satisfactory film.

The ideal thin film should cover less than the full width and about two-thirds
of the length of the slide.

In humid atmospheres dry the slide thoroughly by any convenient means before
taking blood otherwise lysis may occur. Parasitized red cells tend to roll to the edge
and to be carried to the tail of the blood film, so examine these areas for malarial
parasites. Haemoglobin is retained during staining, so parasites appear framed in
red blood cells.

(b) Thick blood film

Method. Transfer blood to glass slide as for thin film but using 2 to 3 drops.
Spread rapidly and evenly with a needle or the corner of another slide into an area
about 2 cm in diameter, or into a rectangle 1·5 cm × 0·75 cm in the centre of the
slide. The film should not be so thick that the hands of a watch cannot be seen
distinctly through it. Dry as rapidly as possible, preferably at 37 °C, keeping the film
horizontal. Make the film quickly and do not stir, undue delay may lead to fibrin
formation and promote auto-agglutination of red cells in anaemic cases.

The thick film, being opaque to transmitted light, is made transparent by removal
of haemoglobin, hence is not fixed in alcohol. Lysis and staining are simultaneous in
water stains. The outline of red blood cells is usually not apparent.

(c) Labelling

Thin films. When dry, write name and date with graphite pencil or needle on the
spread blood.

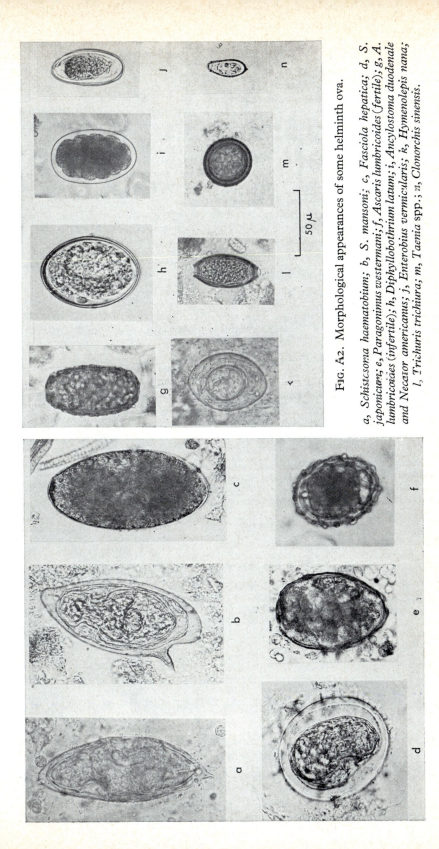

Fig. A2. Morphological appearances of some helminth ova.

a, Schistosoma haematobium; b, S. mansoni; c, Fasciola hepatica; d, S. japonicum; e, Paragonimus westermani; f, Ascaris lumbricoides (fertile); g, A. lumbricoides (infertile); h, Diphyllobothrium latum; i, Ancylostoma duodenale and Necator americanus; j, Enterobius vermicularis; k, Hymenolepis nana; l, Trichuris trichiura; m, Taenia spp.; n, Clonorchis sinensis.

Thick film. The same method can be used but is likely to give difficulties with artefacts during examination. Two thick films can be made on the same slide and one labelled in pencil, or use a grease pencil or writing diamond on the slide itself.

(d) Method of storing films

Thin or thick films made for diagnostic purposes are stained the same day.

Batches of unstained films can be kept for teaching purposes for up to 6 months by packing them together immediately after the films are dry, and wrapping them tightly in several thicknesses of polythene secured with elastic bands. Store at 4 °C until required. After removal from refrigerator allow packet to reach room temperature (half an hour). Haemolysis of thin films due to condensation will occur if slides are unwrapped and exposed immediately to room temperature. Alternatively, thin films can be fixed in methyl alcohol and preserved at room temperature.

(e) Stains for blood protozoa

Several combinations of original polychromed methylene blue and eosin (Romanowsky stain) may be used, e.g. Leishman, Giemsa, Field, Wright, and JSB. The basic methylene blue and oxidized azures combine with the acid eosin in water solution and stain chromatin reddish-purple and cytoplasm of the parasite grey-blue.

The various methods of preparing Romanowsky stains are legion. The method first described is both time-saving and efficient, and is recommended.

Method (Walker). The measured quantity of dry dye is added directly to a hard glass ('Pyrex') bottle containing alcohol or alcohol-glycerol mixture and at least 50 clean glass beads of about 5 mm in diameter. The bottle is tightly stoppered immediately to keep out any moisture. Allow a few minutes for the dye to sink, then shake the bottle thoroughly for a few minutes and leave on the laboratory bench. Repeat the shaking process 6–10 times at half-hourly intervals.

Stains prepared in this way will be found ready for use within 24 hr,[*] although Walker recommends shaking 6–10 times a day for a minimum of 3 days.

Keep stock solution in well-stoppered glass bottle in subdued light or stain rapidly deteriorates. In the tropics, keep in a refrigerator if one is available.

(i) **Leishman's stain.** Thin films only

    Leishman powder   0·15 g
    Methyl alcohol   100 ml

Prepare by Walker's method.

It should be noted that the stain contains alcohol and that prior fixing of the smear is unnecessary. The stain is also, therefore, unsuitable for use with thick films.

Two pipettes are required, one graduated to deliver 0·5 ml and one to deliver 1·5 ml.

(1) Pipette 0·5 ml stain on to a horizontal slide, film upwards. This fixes the film in 30 sec.
(2) Add 1·5 ml buffered water pH 7·0–7·2. Mix and leave staining, 10 min for malarial parasites, spirochaetes or trypanosomes, 15–20 min for L-D bodies and tissue smears.
(3) Flood the staining mixture off with running water for a few seconds. Avoid prolonged washing.
(4) Place slide at an angle to dry. Do not blot.

[*]*Laboratory Technique for the Study of Malaria,* 2nd Ed. 1966. Shute-Maryon.

(ii) Giemsa stain. Thin and thick films

Giemsa powder	3·8g
Glycerol, pure	250ml
Methyl alcohol (Analar)	250ml

Prepare by Walker's method.

Thin film

(1) Fix film in methyl alcohol 30 sec.
(2) Dilute stain 1:10 with buffered water pH 7·0–7·2.
(3) Run stain under slide placed film downwards on curved staining plate or, for large numbers of slides, use a staining trough. Stain for 20–30min, wash away stain rapidly. Place slide at an angle to dry. Do not blot.

Thick film

(1) Dilute stain 1:30 with buffered water pH 7·0–7·2.
(2) Stain as in thin film but for 1 hr.
(3) Wash away stain rapidly and gently. Place at an angle to dry. Do not blot.

Thick films must not be fixed, lysis of red cells and staining of the parasites occur simultaneously.

(iii) Field's stain

Suitable only for thick films. This is the most rapid method for clinical use. Two solutions A and B:

Stain A

Methylene blue (medicinal)	0·8g
Azure 1	0·5g
Disodium hydrogen phosphate (anhydrous)	5·0g
Potassium dihydrogen phosphate	6·25g
Distilled water	500ml

Field A. If bacteria become troublesome discard and make up fresh stain. An oxidation scum will appear if the stain in the jar is used infrequently and should be removed by drawing filter paper across the surface.

Stain B

Eosin, water soluble	1·0g
Na_2HPO_4	5·0g
KH_2PO_4	6·25g
Distilled water	500ml

Field B. Change when it becomes a greenish colour.

If heat is used to dissolve the phosphate salts the solution should be cool before adding the dyes, which may be in some of the buffered water. The stain is now left for 24hr, then filtered before use. Lysis and staining occur simultaneously.

Method. (1) Dip film into Stain A for 5 sec. Avoid agitation of stain since bacteria which may grow in the solution and collect at the bottom will be dispersed and adhere to the wet film.

(2) Wash in jar of clean tap water for 5 sec or until haemoglobin starts to run.
(3) Dip film into Stain B for 3 sec.
(4) Wash in jar of tap water for 5 sec.

Place at an angle to dry. Do not blot.

Times given are approximate, varying with batches of stain and thickness of film. The film is usually of varying thicknesses which take up the stain at different rates, the acid dyes not penetrating into the thicker parts of the film. The optimum staining of parasites, usually near edges of film, occurs when nuclei of leucocytes are stained a rich purple colour.

When staining large numbers of slides, more uniform results are obtained by staining a number of films individually in Stain A, washing and allowing them to drain, thus giving a longer period for lysis, before putting them successively through Stain B. The time in Stain B should be reduced.

Phosphate buffered water. With Giemsa and Leishman's stains phosphate buffered water pH 7·0–7·2 should be used.

Stock solutions

M/15 NA$_2$HPO$_4$ (disodium hydrogen phosphate): 9·5 g/l.
M/15KH$_2$PO$_4$ (potassium dihydrogen phosphate): 9·07 g/l.

	M/15 NA$_2$HPO$_4$	M/15 KH$_2$PO$_4$	Distilled water
pH 7·0	61·1 ml	38·9 ml	900 ml
pH 7·2	72·0 ml	28·0 ml	900 ml

The solutions should be stored in hard glass ('Pyrex') stoppered bottles. The pH should be tested with a comparator and adjusted if necessary.

(f) Preservation of Romanowsky-stained films

Immersion oil is removed carefully with xylol. When dry apply a drop of neutral mounting media and cover with a No. 1 coverslip. This will preserve the film from dust and scratching.

Deterioration may occur quickly in the tropics. Films should not be left exposed to sunlight.

(g) Preparation of film and staining of microfilariae

(i) Mayer's acid haemalum

Haematoxylin	2 g
Aluminium potassium sulphate	50 g
Sodium iodate	0·2 g
Distilled water	1000 ml
Thymol: a crystal	

Dissolve the haematoxylin crystals in 10 ml absolute alcohol. Dissolve the aluminium potassium sulphate in water by warming, add haematoxylin and sodium iodate.

When cool add 20 ml glacial acetic acid.

Method. Dehaemoglobinize a thick blood film in water. Allow to dry and fix in methyl alcohol for 1 min. Flood the slide with stain and heat until steam rises. Keep the stain hot for 3–10 min (do not allow the stain to boil or to dry on the slide). Wash stain off by plunging slide into water. Prolong the washing to blue the nuclei.

(ii) Giemsa

Dilute stain 1:50 with buffered water pH 7·0–7·2. Stain for 1 hr as previously described under Giemsa thick film. This method is useful where a single species (*bancrofti*) or *bancrofti* and *malayi* are endemic. Differential staining of these species occurs (see p. 123).

IV. CONCENTRATION OF TRYPANOSOMES (TRIPLE CENTRIFUGATION)

(1) Centrifuge 5–10 ml of citrated blood at 2000 rpm to pack the red cells.
(2) Transfer the plasma and white cell layer with a pasteur pipette to a clean tube.
(3) Centrifuge for a short period to deposit any red cells carried over.
(4) Transfer supernatant with a pasteur pipette to a clean tube.
(5) Centrifuge for 10 min at 5000 rpm. Remove supernatant and examine deposit.

V. CONCENTRATION OF MICROFILARIAE (KNOTT'S METHOD)

Centrifuge 1 ml blood laked in 9 ml 1 per cent formalin and examine deposit. Addition of a drop of 1 per cent methylene blue will render microfilariae more obvious.

VI. COUNTING METHODS

(a) Malarial parasite counts

Several methods are available for assessing the density of malaria parasites. A useful and practical method is to count the number of parasites per 100 fields using a 2 mm oil immersion lens. By dividing by 100 the number of parasites per oil immersion field is obtained. The following is a useful guide in assessing the severity of an infection in a thick blood film:—

(i) less than 10 parasites per oil immersion field—mild infection;
(ii) 10–50 parasites per oil immersion field—moderate infection;
(iii) over 50 parasites per oil immersion field—severe infection.

For more accurate assessment the number of parasites can be counted against 400 WBC, a white blood cell count having been done. The result is expressed as number of parasites per cubic millimetre.

VII. INDIRECT FLUORESCENT TECHNIQUE FOR MALARIA ANTIBODY

The principles of this technique are as follows:
Patient's serum is pipetted on to a dehaemoglobinized thin blood film containing malaria parasites, allowed to react, washed in saline, and fluorescent-labelled anti-human globulin is then applied. Examination by fluorescence microscopy reveals specifically stained parasites. By testing individual serum dilutions on separate slides, the antibody titre can be determined (Voller, 1964).

VIII. CULTURE MEDIA FOR LEISHMANIA

Novy, MacNeal and Nicolle (NNN)
Agar, shredded   14 g (or powdered agar 8 g)
Sodium chloride   6 g
Distilled water   900 ml
Sterile, fresh, or defibrinated rabbit blood

Dissolve the agar and salt in the water by heating, distribute 5 ml amounts into 25 ml screw-capped bottles. Autoclave at 15 lb (121 °C) for 20 min. Cool to 48 °C and add aseptically 15 drops of rabbit blood. Rotate the bottles between the hands to mix, avoiding frothing the blood. Allow the media to solidify in a slightly sloped position. When solid, place the bottles in an incubator at 37 °C for 24 hr to sweat and produce water of condensation, an abundance of which is essential (if water of condensation is scanty add a few drops of sterile distilled water and allow 24 hr for it to become isotonic). Discard any bottles showing contamination. Store at 4 °C (will keep for up to 6 months). Immediately before use add penicillin and streptomycin (100 units/ml of each) and inoculate into water of condensation. Incubate at 15–25 °C.

IX. METHOD OF COUNTING SCHISTOSOME OVA IN TISSUE

The following method has been described by I. O. Nwabuebo.

A known weight of tissue (about 20 g) is well minced, and about 5 ml of 6 per cent KOH is added for each gram.

The minced preparation is digested at 60 °C for 10-12 hr and allowed to cool. The digest is transferred to a 1-l graduated container. Tap water is added gradually with thorough mixing until the volume reaches 10 ml/g of tissue. 10 ml of the digest mixture is taken into each of three graduated centrifuge tubes. The tubes are centrifuged at 1500 rpm for 3 min. The supernatant is drawn off with a pipette, leaving 0·2 ml in each tube*. Deposit is mixed thoroughly. From each of the three tubes 0·05 ml (50 mm³) is pipetted on to a separate slide and covered with a 22 mm × 26 mm coverslip. The number of ova under each coverslip is counted using the strip-count method. The average of the three counts is taken. The number obtained is multiplied by 4 to give the number of ova per gram of tissue.

B. LABORATORY DETECTION OF ABNORMAL HAEMOGLOBINS

A manual on techniques for studying abnormal haemoglobins has been prepared by Jonxis and Huisman (1958) and by Lehmann and Ager (1960); some of the methods are briefly described below.

1. The Sickling test

One drop of blood is mixed on a slide with 3 drops of freshly prepared 2 per cent sodium metabisulphite ($Na_2S_2O_5$) and the preparation is covered with a coverslip. Sickle cells, if present, will be seen after 15 min.

2. Preparation of oxyhaemoglobin solution

Wash the red cells obtained from unclotted blood at least twice in 0·9 per cent NaCl solution by centrifuging, and on the final occasion with 1·25 per cent saline. To the packed cells add one volume of distilled water and half a volume of carbon tetrachloride, toluene, or chloroform. Shake the tube manually, then centrifuge it at 3000 rpm for 15–20 min. Separate the clear haemoglobin solution and filter it through two layers of No. 1 Whatman filter paper, lightly moistened with distilled water beforehand. The filtrate is virtually pure haemoglobin solution.

3. Estimation of foetal haemoglobin (alkali-resistant haemoglobin)

The most convenient method of estimation is that of Singer *et al.* (1951) and referred to as the 'One Minute Alkali Denaturation Test'. Adult haemoglobin is denatured by alkali but haemoglobin F is unaffected. The denatured haemoglobin is removed by precipitation with ammonium sulphate and the remaining haemo-globin is measured photometriallly.

Reagents. N/12 NaOH or KOH. Ammonium sulphate solution: 76g dissolved in distilled water to give a final volume of 200ml with 0·5ml 10 N HCl added.

*If the deposit is greater than 0·2ml, 0·5ml should be left and the average of the three counts multiplied by 10.

Test. The reagents should be kept at 20 °C and the test should be performed at a temperature between 18° and 25 °C. 0·2 ml oxyhaemoglobin solution (10 g/100 ml prepared as described above) is added to 3·2 ml N/12 alkali. It is thoroughly mixed and left for 1 min precisely (use a stop watch). 6·8 ml ammonium sulphate reagent are then added. It is inverted several times and after waiting about 1 min the mixture is filtered through a No. 42 Whatman filter paper. If the filtrate is colourless, it signifies that no measurable amount of haemoglobin F is present; otherwise 0·1 ml of the original haemoglobin solution should be added to 5 ml ammoniated water and the filtrate should be compared with this solution of untreated haemoglobin photometrically. Use a spectrophotometer with a narrow wavelength band at 540 nm., e.g. Unicam S.P. 600. Results below 1·7 per cent 'alkali-resistant haemoglobin' are of no diagnostic significance.

4. Paper electrophoresis

Paper electrophoresis by the vertical (hanging strip) method is the most satisfactory for routine use (Lehmann and Smith, 1954).

Buffers:

1. Standard barbiturate. pH 8·6; ionic strength 0·05. This is made up as follows:

Sodium diethylbarbiturate	10·3g
Diethylbarbituric acid . , ...	1·84g
Distilled water to	1 litre

2. Tris. pH 8·9. This is used for the demonstration of haemoglobin A_2.

Tris-(hydroxy-methyl)-amino-methane	50·4g
Ethylene-diamine-tetra-acetic acid	5·0g
Boric acid	3·8g
Distilled water to	1 litre

3. *Phosphate.* pH 6·5; ionic strength 0·1. This enables the differentiation of haemoglobin C from haemoglobin E. It is also useful for distinguishing other fast-moving haemoglobins from each other.

KH_2PO_4	3·11g
$NA_2HPO_4–2H_2O$	1·87g
Distilled water to	1 litre

Method. Cut out Whatman No. 3MM filter paper into sheets 18 cm. × 38 cm. and fold gently at the midline. Mark the position of the haemoglobin solution and its identification mark with pencil. Soak the paper in diluted buffer. Streak with a fine Pasteur pipette, oxyhaemoglobin solution along the marked line. Place the filter paper in position, the ends dipping into the barbiturate buffer present in the electrode compartments. At about 200 volts, electrophoresis should be carried out over 12–18 hr. The haemoglobin S band is identified, if present, by comparison against an oxyhaemoglobin solution from a known sickler and electrophoresed simultaneously on the same sheet of paper. Blot the paper, after the current is switched off, and dry it in an oven in front of a fan. Unless a room temperature of about 20 °C is available all through the electrophoretic run, it is advisable to carry out the run in a refrigerator at about 5 °C to avoid artefacts from heat denaturation of the oxyhaemoglobin (Vella, 1963).

5. Solubility test

The relative degree of solubility of haemoglobins is a further method used for differentiating various forms of sickle-cell disease (Itano, 1953).

Reagents. 2·4M phosphate buffer pH 6·8. Sodium dithionite ($Na_2S_2O_4$) 100 mg (also called sodium hydrosulphite).

The blood specimen is prepared as for haemoglobin electrophoresis above.

Method. Weigh 100 mg of sodium dithionite carefully into a 100 ml volumetric flask.

Add 8·0 ml of 2·4M phosphate buffer.

Layer on 0·5 ml distilled water and carefully add exactly 50 mg of haemoglobin without shaking (if the oxyhaemoglobin solution contains 10g/100ml, this amount of haemoglobin will be contained in 0·5 ml).

Make to volume with distilled water and incubate flask for 15 min in a 25 °C water bath.

Mix, carefully, by inversion. Compare against standards of *AA, AS, AC,* and *SS*.

Result

(1) Haemoglobin SS is completely insoluble and therefore opaque.

(2) Haemoglobins SC and AS are partially soluble and therefore translucent.

(3) Haemoglobins AA, AC, and CC are totally soluble and therefore transparent.

6. Test for inclusion bodies: haemoglobin H

Vital staining reveals inclusion bodies in haemoglobin H disease (Gouttas *et al.* 1955).

Drops of blood are mixed in a small tube containing 0·5 ml 1 per cent cresyl blue in citrate saline. The blood is allowed to stand for a few hours at room temperature. Blood films are then made and examined for inclusion bodies in the red cells.

7. Sending of haemoglobin and blood samples

If local facilities for investigation of the abnormal haemoglobins are not available samples can be prepared in a variety of ways and shipped to other investigators, e.g. M.R.C. Haemoglobin Reference Laboratory, Cambridge.

(1) Solutions of oxyhaemoglobin kept cold in a thermos flask (0–4 °C) can be sent by airmail.

(2) Washed red cells in a frozen state can be similarly despatched or washed red cells suspended in ACD solution (acid citrate dextrose).

(3) Uncoagulated red blood cells (unwashed) can also be sent in a thermos flask kept at (0–4 °C.)

8. Screening procedures for G-6-PD

The three most commonly used methods for screening populations are (1) the brilliant cresyl blue dye test (Motulsky and Campbell-Kraut, 1961), (2) the methaemoglobin reduction test (Brewer *et al.* 1962), and (3) the MTT-linked spot test (Faubanks and Beutler, 1962). These and other more sophisticated tests have been recently described in detail (WHO, 1967).

Brilliant cresyl blue dye test

Method. Add 0·02 ml whole blood to 1·9 ml distilled H_2O in a test tube. Then mix with:

0·1 ml sodium G-6-P (825 mg/100 ml)

0·1 ml NADP (50 mg/100 ml) [Nicotinamide-adenine-dinucleotide-phosphate]

0·18 ml BCB (32 mg/100 ml)

0·2 ml tris buffer (pH 8·5): 8·96 g/97 ml + 3 ml concentrated HCl.

Top the tube with liquid paraffin or oil and incubate at 37 °C preferably in a water bath. Observe the disappearance of the blue colour. Normal specimens will usually decolorize by 65 min. The blood of enzyme-deficient subjects will decolorize between 100–180 min or more.

C. BLOOD TRANSFUSION METHODS

1. Preparation of solutions and blood bottles

A. Normal saline

Dissolve 9·0 g of sodium chloride in distilled water and make up to 1 litre.

B. Acid citrate dextrose (ACD)

	For 120 ml	For 1000 ml
Disodium hydrogen citrate	2 g	16·6 g
Dextrose (glucose)	3 g	25 g
Pyrogen-free distilled water to	120 ml	to 1000 ml

C. Preparation of components for blood collection

(1) Single-holed metal caps and rubber liners to fit MRC bottles, metal rings, pilot bottles. Metal caps and rubber liners to fit pilot bottles are soaked and boiled in soapy water.

(2) Wash scrupulously with wire or hand brush and transfer to a solution of Pyroneg (or other suitable detergent) overnight.

(3) Wash in tap water and rinse 2 or 3 times in pyrogen-free distilled water.

(4) Dry all materials except rubber liners in hot air oven. Rubber liners are dried at 60–70 °C.

(5) Dispense 1 ml ACD into each pilot bottle and replace rings, caps and liners.

D. Bottles for blood collection

(1) Blood bottles (MRC bottles) are similarly treated with Pyroneg solution, water and pyrogen-free distilled water.

(2) Invert bottles in wire-cages to drain and dry in oven.

(3) Into each MRC bottle dispense 120 ml. ACD solution.

(4) Replace caps and liners.

(5) Sterilize at 126 °C for 45 min at 15 lb pressure *or* 10 lb for 1 hr.

E. Precautions

(1) Pyrogen-free distilled water must be used.

(2) After sterilization, culture to check sterility.

2. Emergency ABO and Rhesus grouping

A. Emergency ABO grouping

(1) Mark out a grouping tile as shown below in the diagram.

	A cells 1 drop	B cells 1 drop	O cells 1 drop	Patient's cells 1 drop
1 drop Anti-A				
1 drop Anti-B				
1 drop Anti-A+B				
1 drop patient's serum				

(2) Centrifuge the clotted specimen from the patient. *Collect patient's serum* into a separate tube. Obtain *patient's cells* by gently releasing some cells from the clot, and re-suspending them in saline (0·90 g NaCl per cent) so as to obtain a cell suspension of approximately 25 per cent.

(3) Add 1 drop of serum and 1 drop of cell suspension to each square as indicated.

(4) Mix the contents of each square using separate corners of a microscope slide for each.

(5) Compare the patient's cell and serum grouping with the controls after 5–10 min.

		A cells	B cells	O cells	Pt. cells	
Example:	Anti-A	+	−	−	−	
	Anti-B	−	+	−	+	
	Anti-(A+B)	+	+	−	+	
	Patient's Serum	+	−	−	−	Patient's group is B

Notes. (1) It is always advisable to perform both cell and serum grouping, as indicated here. The known A, B, and O cells can usually be obtained from members of staff who belong to these groups, and are best washed once with normal saline and then made up to a 25 per cent suspension.

(2) The rate of error, if this test is performed by an experienced worker, is less than 1 per cent.

(b) Emergency rhesus grouping

(1) Lay out a heavy glass slide (which has been warmed in an incubator at 37 °C) in the manner described in the diagram.

Anti-D 1 drop	Anti-D 1 drop	Anti-D 1 drop	Patient's Serum 1 drop
O+ cells 1 drop	AB− cells 1 drop	Patient's cells 1 drop	Patient's cells 1 drop
Positive control	Negative control	Test	'Auto' control

(2) Add 1 drop of serum and 1 drop of packed cells as indicated.

(3) Mix each square with a separate corner of a microscope slide.

(4) Leave in the incubator (in a covered box) at 37 °C for 5 min and compare test with controls.

Notes. (1) *False positives* may occur if temperature is below 37 °C.

(2) *False negatives* may occur if dilute cells are used instead of packed cells.

(3) The rate of error in experienced hands is less than 5 per cent, provided a potent complete anti-D is used. Most Rh sera come with specific instructions as to their use. These instructions should be followed exactly. The method above is only for use with the dried 'saline' or complete Rh-grouping sera obtainable from the Lister Institute, London.

3. Cross-matching

Four tests are always set up;

(1) Saline tube test at room temperature.

(2) Saline tube test at 37 °C.

(3) Albumin tube test at 37 °C.

(4) Indirect Coombs test at 37 °C.

Method:

The cross-matching of three donors A, B, and C against the serum of one patient is described below.

(1) Arrange the tubes in a rack or wooden block as shown below with patient's serum added as indicated.

(2) Row 1: Washed donor's red cells are prepared by removing a small amount of blood from the appropriate pilot bottle by a sterile needle and syringe and adding 4 drops to a Kahn tube full of normal saline appropriately labelled. Invert twice to mix. Centrifuge and discard the supernatant. Refill tube with saline and repeat the procedure. Washed donor's packed cells are now available.

(3) Row 2: Add 1 drop of washed packed cells to 5 drops of the patient's serum. Incubate at 37 °C. for ½ to 2 hr. Following this procedure an indirect Coombs' test is performed as outlined below.

	A	B	C	
Washed donor's red cells	◯	◯	◯	1 (Kahn tube)
Patient's serum 5 drops	◯	◯	◯	2 For indirect Coombs' test (Kahn tube)
Patient's serum 1 drop	○	○	○	3 For 'albumin' test at 37 °C (precipitin tube)
Patient's serum 1 drop	○	○	○	4 For 'saline' test at 37 °C (precipitin tube)
Patient's serum 1 drop	○	○	○	5 For 'saline' test at room temp. (precipitin tube)

(4) The remainder of the washed packed cells in tubes in Row 1 are now diluted with normal saline to give an approximate red cell suspension of 2–4 per cent. One drop of this suspension is pipetted into the appropriate tubes in Rows 3–5 containing 1 drop of the patient's serum.

(5) The tubes in Row 3 are incubated at 37 °C for $1\frac{1}{2}$ hr. One drop of 30 per cent bovine albumin is then added and incubation continued for a further $\frac{1}{2}$ hr. The bovine albumin should be allowed to run gently down the inside of the tube forming a layer over the red cells. DO NOT MIX. The sediment should be examined for agglutination after 2 hr but in an emergency the first incubation period can be reduced to 15 min, when, following centrifugation, the albumin can be added and left for 10 min before reading. With this emergency method the blood is utilized on the doctor's own responsibility.

(6) The tubes in Row 4 are incubated at 37 °C for 2 hr. In cases of emergency the incubation period can be shortened to 5–15 min and the mixture centrifuged at 1000 rpm for 1 min before examination. The blood must then be taken on the doctor's own responsibility.

(7) The tubes in Row 5 are left at room temperature for 2 hr.

(8) At the end of 2 hr remove sample gently with a Pasteur pipette from the tubes in Rows 3, 4, and 5 on to glass slides and examine for agglutination macroscopically and microscopically.

Interpretation

Agglutination in any of the tubes usually means that the blood is not compatible, and therefore cannot be transfused.

No agglutination in any tube means the blood is compatible in 99 per cent of the cases.

If the patient has received previous transfusions, or has obstetrical history suggestive of immunization, it is strongly indicated to perform in addition the indirect Coombs' Test, as follows:

(a) Following incubation, fill tube in Row 2 with saline and resuspended cells. Centrifuge and remove supernanant.

(*b*) This washing procedure is repeated 3 more times. Remove last supernatant and add to cells 1 drop of saline. This should yield a cell suspension about 40 per cent.

(*c*) On a glass tile (washed with soap and brush and wiped with clean towel) lay out the protocol as shown.

	Test cells	Positive control cells	Negative control cells
Anti-human globulin			
Saline			

(*d*) Add cells, anti-human globulin (Coombs' serum) and saline as indicated and mix well using corner of microscope slides.

(*e*) After 7 min read the test comparing with both positive and negative controls.

Notes.

(1) If Coombs' test is positive, blood is not compatible.

(2) The Coombs' test, in its DIRECT form, is very useful in the diagnosis of haemolytic disease of newborn due to blood group incompatibility (except in the ABO system). The DIRECT Coombs' test is performed by washing 4 times the patient's cells as described and then adding the anti-human globulin as described.

(3) The controls are essential for getting reliable results in the Coombs' test. A positive control can be obtained by incubating known Rh-positive cells with an incomplete anti-D and a negative control by incubating Rh-negative cells with an incomplete anti-D. The cells are then washed and processed like the test cells.

4. Investigation of group O donors

Whenever possible, blood of the same ABO and Rhesus group should be selected. When one is forced to administer O blood to a recipient of another group, it is important to rule out the presence of a strong haemolytic anti-A and/or anti-B in the donor's serum. It should be noted that the incidence of these haemolytic antibodies is very high (at least 56 per cent) in Nigeria. This can be done as follows:

(1) To each of two precipitin tubes (7 mm × 50 mm) add 1 drop of donor's **fresh** serum. **Fresh** = not more than 12 hr old and kept throughout at 4 °C.

(2) To the first tube add 1 drop of a 4 per cent suspension of A cells in saline.

(3) To the second tube add 1 drop of a 4 per cent suspension of B cells in saline.

(4) Incubate for 2 hr at 37 °C.

(5) Read for haemolysis. If there is no haemolysis all red cells will be clumped at the bottom of the tube and the supernatant fluid will be clear. If there is haemolysis all the fluid will be pink-red and there will be few or no cells at the bottom.

5. Choice of blood for cross-matching for babies under 6 months

(1) Group both mother and child as in method (2).

(2) Cross-match bottle which is **compatible both with mother and child using mother's serum.**

EXAMPLE: (a) Mother: A, Rhesus positive.
    Child: B, Rhesus positive.
    Compatible blood is O, Rh positive, without haemolysins.
(b) Mother: A, Rhesus negative.
    Child: B, Rhesus positive.
    Compatible blood is O, Rh negative, without haemolysins.
(c) Mother: AB, Rhesus positive.
    Child: B, Rhesus positive.
    Compatible blood is B, Rh positive.

D. HISTOLOGICAL METHODS

(a) Fixation, preservation and storage of tissue

10 per cent neutral-buffered formalin:

Sodium dihydrogen phosphate (anhydrous)	3·5 g
Disodium hydrogen phosphate (anhydrous)	6·5 g
Concentrated formaldehyde solution (40 per cent)	100 ml
Distilled water	900 ml

Method. Combine the formaldehyde solution with the water and add the two salts, making sure that the first salt has dissolved before adding the second.

Small blocks of tissue about 0·5 cm. in thickness should be placed in 25 times their volume of the buffered formalin solution as soon as possible. The nature of the specimen and the type of preservative used should be written in pencil on paper and placed inside the bottle with the specimen, which should then be dispatched to the laboratory.

(b) Sellers' technique in rabies

Sellers' technique has proved accurate, quick, and economical in the laboratory diagnosis of rabies.

Stock solution

(1) Methylene blue	10 g
Methanol (absolute acetone-free) up to	1000 ml
(2) Basic fuchsin	5 g
Methanol (absolute acetone-free) up to	500 ml

Staining solution

Methylene blue (stock solution No. 1)	2 parts	
Basic fuchsin (stock solution No. 2)	1 part	

After preparing smears or impressions of the brain, the slides *while still moist*, are immersed in the staining solution for 1–5 sec. They are then rinsed quickly in running water, and air dried without blotting. The negri bodies stain deep magenta red against the blue violet of the neurones.

E. MISCELLANEOUS

(a) Diagnosis of pinworm/threadworm/enterobius vermicularis

The adult females are sometimes seen in the faeces or on the perinaeum but the most satisfactory method of diagnosis is the recovery of the eggs. The eggs are rarely found in faeces but may be recovered from the perinaeum by the use of the 'Scotch tape' method (Graham). A piece of Scotch tape is placed sticky side down on to a microscope slide. The tape should overlap the slide by half an inch at each end. At one end the tape is wrapped round the end of, and on to the reverse (under) side of the slide. The overlap at the other end is turned back on to itself to form a nonsticky tab.

Method. Pull the Scotch tape from the slide using the tab, leaving the tape on the underside of the slide still attached, the weight of the slide still attached will stop the tape from curling up. Place the finger on the non-sticky side of the tape and press the sticky side on to the skin in several areas of the perianal region. Replace the tape on to the slide as before so as it forms its own coverslip. Examine the slide for the characteristic eggs.

The specimen should be collected first thing in the morning.

(b) Examination of sputum for parasites

Thoroughly mix the whole specimen with an equal volume of 3 per cent sodium hydroxide solution and centrifuge at 3000 rpm for 30 min. Decant the supernatant, and examine the deposit.

Should the sputum contain pus from a suspected amoebic source examine a direct preparation of the sputum keeping it warm (37 °C) and search for active trophozoites of *E. histolytica*.

(c) Examination for superficial fungi

Scrape skin at spreading edge of skin lesion. Place scraping on a glass slide in a drop of 10 per cent NaOH or KOH. Heat gently over a low flame. Apply coverslip and examine under low-power objective. The fungal mycelia and spores are easily seen.

(d) Eosinophils

It is useful to obtain a thin blood smear stained by one of the Romanowsky methods, p. 762, to detect a possible increase in eosinophils.

(e) Protection of optical instruments in tropical climates

Two adaptations of established methods of protecting optical instruments in tropical climates have recently been devised by Payne (1966) and are summarized below.

Heat cabinets

The heat cabinet is simplified into a metal hood which can be placed over the microscope in its normal position on the laboratory bench. The heat required for the hood can be supplied from the microscope illuminator lamp, or more economically from an ordinary 10- or 15-watt bulb built into the metal hood. No additional electric source is required as the normal a.c. socket provided for the microscope illuminator may be used. The hood can be readily fabricated at a nominal cost by any village tinsmith from old kerosene cans. The size of the hood is dictated by the dimensions of the microscopes to be protected.

The principle of the heat hood is the same as that of the heat cabinet, i.e. of lowering the relative humidity by raising the temperature with an internal heat source. By maintaining this elevated temperature, and largely preventing air entry, condensation is prevented and thus corrosion and fungus propagation inhibited. As a broad generalization it may be expected that the heat hood with a 15-watt bulb will cause rise of about 10 °C over an ambient temperature of 32 °C, and the effect on the relative humidity will be to reduce it by 15–30 per cent; the greatest reduction occurring at the higher end of the relative humidity range. The heat hood cannot be recommended for instruments with Canada balsam-mounted lenses when the ambient temperature is consistently considerably higher than 30 °C. It is particularly useful in laboratories when instruments are constantly in use—itself a protective measure.

Desiccators

The principle employed in the standard glass, plastic, or metal desiccator is different from that of the heat cabinet in that the drying of the air is brought about by the physical or chemical removal of the water from the air by drying agents; there is no rise in temperature. In this way condensation is prevented and thus corrosion and propagation of fungus inhibited.

A recent development of this principle is a refrigerated coil which is used to cool the air drawn over it by a fan. On cooling, the air gives up its moisture and this is collected in a container for disposal. With a machine designed for this purpose (*called a dehumidifier*) an entire room can be used as a dry storage room, enabling several hundred instruments to be stored in a relatively small space under closely controlled conditions of relative humidity. Hawker (1950) has shown experimentally that the principal lens-affecting fungi—*Aspergillus* and *Pencillium*—have optimum propagation and growth in the temperature range 18–35 °C and relative humidity 81 per cent. On the basis of these criteria a desiccation system using the dehumidifier becomes feasible providing that the volume of the dehumidified room is equal to, or less than, the rating of the machine as given by the manufacturer; the windows and any ventilation openings are sealed, and any doors fitted with draught excluders. The interior of the room is fitted with open racks or shelves of wire mesh to keep equipment off the floor and away from the walls so that efficient circulation of the air is ensured. Under these conditions the dehumidifier should maintain the relative humidity of the room at a mean of 50 per cent or below throughout the year.

(f) Preparation of specimens for transmission to laboratories

General

Send specimens by hand without delay (if possible), labelled clearly with the patient's name, type of specimen, time collected, preservatives used, if any, type of examination required. Include short clinical and geographical history.

Should it be necessary to send specimen through the post, the postal regulations of the country concerned should be consulted. They are usually identical to the regulations in the U.K. Specimens must be sent by the quickest service, i.e. letter post, **not** by parcel post, packed in a watertight container with sufficient absorbent material to soak up any leakage. Package labelled **Pathological specimen with care.**

Faeces

For microscopic examination send roughly a tablespoonful including portions showing blood and mucus. Collect in clean screw-capped container. Never fill the container or use corked tubes.

For bacterial examination collect as above in sterile container if possible. Add to specimens likely to be delayed, 2 volumes of 30 per cent neutral glycerol in 0.6 per cent saline. In cases of suspected cholera use alkaline peptone water.

Rectal swabs must reach laboratory within 6 hr. In possibility of delay emulsify in nutrient broth or a transport medium.

Blood

For blood culture collect 10 ml venous blood and add aseptically to special blood culture bottle. If blood culture bottles are not available, send clotted blood in sterile tube, but if sending through the post, the blood should be allowed to clot and the serum separated off into another sterile tube before posting.

Most biochemical tests can be performed on serum collected as above.

Specimens for blood alcohol and alkali reserve, fill the tube to the stopper with blood or serum. Tests for glucose require special tubes. Test for methaemalbumin and fibrinogen collected in oxalated blood.

Haematology specimens should be collected ETDA (Sequestrine) bottles. For abnormal haemoglobins and red cell fragility collect in heparinized tube. Bloods for prothrombin collected in special tubes. Blood films should be packed so that they do not touch each other and wrapped in a plastic bag.

Urine

For routine examination collect early morning specimen. If urinary schisto-somiasis is suspected collect specimen between 10.00 hours and 14.00 hours. If this is not possible, a random specimen should be sent. (**Note:** Exercise does **not** increase egg yield.)

For bacteriological examination collect urine (mid-stream) into sterile screw-capped bottle.

(g) Notes on laboratory procedures

It is not proposed to deal extensively with this subject as all necessary procedures are adequately dealt with in standard text books.*

A. Sampling of bone marrow

Bone marrow puncture is performed with the aid of trocars which vary from country to country, the most usual being the Mallarme, Salah and Klima. The cannula possesses a horizontal guard forming a rest for the operator's index and middle finger and is fitted with a bevelled stilette. The size of the trocars vary depending upon the bones to be punctured and the age of the patient. Powerful aspiration syringes, clean microscopic slides, and watch glasses should be available. The latter is used to allow the residue of the marrow to clot for fixation in formol saline or other fixative if paraffin sections are required. The sternum, iliac crest and tibia are the most usual sites of puncture.

*The most useful in our experience is *Practical Haematology* by J. V. Dacie and S. M. Lewis, Churchill, London (1968), which is available in an English Language Book Society edition.

Sternal puncture

The patient lies on his back with the head resting flat. The skin over the first segment of the body of the sternum is disinfected with alcohol. The trocar should be inserted into the right- or left-half segment between the margin and the median line.

If a local anaesthetic (1 per cent novocaine) is used the periosteum should be infiltrated. Pierce the skin and approach the periosteum at right angles. Thrust the trocar into the bone. Once the resistance of the bone has been overcome, the cannula will remain fixed at right angles to the chest wall. Withdraw the stilette. Mount the syringe and apply strong suction. The patient will experience some pain. A mixture of blood and marrow will be drawn into the syringe and should be transferred to slides and smears made. As much blood as possible should be drawn into the syringe to ensure a maximum concentration of bone marrow cells. Complications are unusual but prosternal or retrosternal haematomas may occur.

Iliac puncture

The trocars should be strong, long and of large calibre. The iliac bone can be punctured at several sites. A good site is the iliac crest about 5 cm posterior to the anterior superior iliac spine. Here the bone can be 'held' between thumb and index finger of the left hand and then entered by applying the trocar (with the right hand) exactly between the two fingers perpendicular to the skin and into the thickness of the crest.

Tibial puncture

This is performed only in young infants and in the newborn.

Puncture biopsy

This is usually performed when marrow puncture has been unsatisfactory. A satisfactory technique has been described by Dacie and Lewis (1968).

Haemophilia, major defibrination syndromes, thrombocytopenia and other thrombopathies are contra indications. As it is likely that this procedure will only be undertaken at the larger centres it is not further discussed.

Samples of lymph node tissue

Lymph node puncture

Powerful aspiration syringes and needles 35–40 mm in length with a small internal diameter (0·6–0·8 mm) should be used. If there is polyadenopathy a 'medium' sized node most characteristic of the suspected disease should be chosen. The skin should be sterilized. Immobilize the lymph node between two fingers and pierce the skin and capsule. Strong suction is necessary. The tissue usually remains within the needle. Withdraw the needle and syringe and detach the latter. Fill with air and eject the fragment on to a clean glass slide. Prepare smears in the usual way. Complications are rare but mild syncope may follow puncture of a jugular lymph node in the area of the carotid sinus.

Lymph node biopsy

A suitable lymph node should be chosen and the inguinal and axillary sites avoided if possible as due to repeated minor infections reactive hyperplasia and fibrosis are most usual in these areas and may obscure the diagnosis. The disposal of the lymph node depends upon the facilities available. Where facilities are limited it is useful to make an 'imprint' or 'touch' preparation. The node should be bisected and one half immediately placed in fixative, the other being utilized for imprints prior to fixation. In layer centres portions may be sent for additional bacteriological and/or phase contrast examination, tissue culture, electron microscopy studies, etc.

(h) A simplified technique for electron microscopy in a routine laboratory by J. Oguigo

It is proposed to give a simple technique which a busy pathology department can carry out along with routine surgical histology and post-morten materials. This technique is also intended for the final embedding of specimens in Araldite in pathology departments which have no electron microscopy available for their own micrographs or even an ultramicrotome to cut their own sections. Such embedded blocks could be forwarded to larger units having these facilities.

As the success of good slides for light microscopy depends on good processing of the tissues, so also in electron microscopy good micrographs are the result of good enbedding techniques.

Essential requirements

(a) Glutaraldehyde.
(b) Osmic acid.
(c) Casting resin mixture (Araldite, DDSA, DMP).
(d) Embedding oven set at 60 °C.
(e) pH meter.

Other requirements include reagents and apparatus one would normally expect to have in a routine histology laboratory, e.g. refrigerator, chemicals and other facilities.

Fixation, unlike fixation for light microscopy where a few minutes between removal from the host body and placing in fixative may not cause significant cellular changes, fixation for electron micrographs **must** be effected within seconds. This is also because the tissue is usually very small, e.g. liver or renal biopsy and autolysis will be rapid and more pronounced.

The specimen must not be allowed to be dry at any stage. Fixation to final dehydration is best done under cold conditions preferably on ice blocks in a beaker.

The most widely used fixative is 1 per cent osmic acid at pH 7·4.

Osmic acid (osmium tetroxide) is sold in ampoules of 0·5 or 1·0 g. It is a very toxic chemical and must not be allowed to touch the skin. Its vapour causes sinusitis and conjunctivitis. The working solution is given separately below.

Stock solution of osmic acid 2 per cent

The procedure for making the solution is as follows: Wash off the labels and other wrappings using distilled water. Rinse again with distilled water and dry. In order to minimize reduction of osmic acid to osmium dioxide, the solution is stored in a brown bottle in a refrigerator.

There are two methods which may be used in preparing the fluid:

(a) One method is to place the 1·0 g ampoule of osmic acid in a thick-walled brown reagent bottle. Add about 25 ml distilled water, stopper and shake vigorously to break the ampoule thus releasing the osmic acid crystals. The broken pieces are left in the bottle. Make up to the required concentration by adding the remaining 25 ml distilled water.

(b) The other method is to slightly file a 1 g ampoule with a glass file after washing off the labels with distilled water and drying the ampoule with a clean tissue paper. Hold the ampoule between the thumbs and forefingers, carefully break as when breaking glass tubing, using a pad of clean linen or lint to prevent accident. Both halves of the ampoule with the contents are carefully dropped into 50 ml distilled water in the brown reagent bottle. This latter method, though workable in expert hands, is not recommended for beginners.

Phosphate buffer

This is made in distilled water from these two stock solutions:

（1）2·2 per cent $Na_2PO_4.H_2O$
（2）2·52 per cent NaOH.

Mix 83 ml solution (1) with 17 ml solution (2). The pH should work out to be about 7·4. If not, add either solution (1) or (2) to adjust to this pH. Store in the refrigerator.

The third stock solution is a 10 per cent sucrose in distilled water. Store also in the refrigerator.

The complete working fixative

To 10 ml of the 2 per cent osmic acid, add in the following order: 9 ml of the phosphate buffer; 1 ml of 10 per cent sucrose.

Any left over from the above could be stored for use for up to 3 months. It should be stored in brown bottle also in the refrigerator and discard when there is decoloration.

The above fixative has its bases on 'Millonig's Fixative'.

When this fixative is used, it is advisable that the whole processing should be completed the same day.

Three per cent glutaraldehyde in phosphate buffer pH 7·4

Glutaraldehyde is obtained commercially as a 25 per cent concentration. A 3 per cent concentration in phosphate buffer pH 7·4 is used in fixing materials for electron microscopy. Tissues can be left in glutaraldehyde for a much longer time, up to 4 weeks, without much harm. It can be used alone or, as in most cases, used as a primary fixative followed by secondary fixation in osmic acid. Its disadvantage compared with osmic acid is that while the latter gives a good contrast in micrograph, the sections from the former are usually stained with other metals to effect this contrast.

Procedure

Requirements

Clean double-edge blade free from packing grease.
Dental-wax slab.
Tooth-picks.
Beaker with ice blocks.
Pasteur pipette of fairly wide bore.
Bijou bottle with about 5 ml of the fixative.

Introduce the specimen, i.e. liver or renal biopsy, on to the clean dental wax slab. Using the Pasteur pipette, cover up the specimen immediately with drops of the fixative. Break the double-edge blade into two and using one half, cut the specimens into cubes about 1 mm or less.

The 'cutting up' should be a direct vertical movement of both hands. The pieces so cut **must** be covered by the fluid fixative and **not** allowed to be dried up.

Transfer the small pieces of specimen into the specimen bijou bottle using the wide-bore pipette or a tooth-pick and leave in the fixative for the appropriate time on ice blocks.

If osmic acid is used, fix for a maximum of $1\frac{1}{2}$ hr, but if it is glutaraldehyde, the pieces could be left in it much longer, up to four weeks.

Dehydration clearing and impregnation and embedding

Fixation in osmic acid 1 per cent	1 hour at 0 °C
50 per cent ethyl alcohol	15 min
70 per cent ethyl alcohol	15 min (could be stored in the refrigerator for a longer time—1 week)
95 per cent ethyl alcohol	15 min
Absolute ethyl alcohol (1)	20 min
Absolute ethyl alcohol (2)	20 min
Absolute ethyl alcohol (3)	20 min
Toluene (1)	30 min
Toluene (2)	30 min
Toluene/Araldite 50/50	30 min
Araldite (1)	60 min at 60 °C
Araldite (2)	60 min at 60 °C
Araldite (3)	60 min at 60 °C

Embed in Araldite, and polymerize at 60 °C for 11 hr.

Important notes

Tissues fixed in glutaraldehyde can be osmium fixed and the steps followed will thereafter be as when initially fixed in osmic acid.

It is necessary to start dehydration in low ethyl-alcohol concentration (50 per cent ethyl alcohol in some cases), otherwise 70 per cent ethyl alcohol is used. Tissues can be stored in 70 per cent ethyl alcohol in the fridge. The absolute ethyl alcohol **must** be absolute. Open a fresh bottle for the purpose of the three changes in absolute ethyl alcohol and make sure the bottle is tightly stoppered after use in order to maintain some degree of purity.

During processing occasional shaking of the specimen is necessary to enhance the infiltration of the solution into the tissue.

Polymerization for exactly 11 hr produces good blocks especially with the brand of Araldite mixture we are using in this Department (Araldite 6005, DDSA and DMP30).

From the table below the correct quantity of Araldite mixture is given in order to avoid wastage.

In compiling the table below, a rough estimate of about 4 ml of mixture per tissue vial of an average of about 10 pieces of tissue, using 1 ml for embedding in the beem capsule is used. For loss in drainage an additional 8 ml is added. The correct volume required is calculated from this. The total quantity of Araldite mixture could be worked out from the table below. The constituents of the Araldite mixture are very viscoid and care and patience must be exercised to make sure of complete drainage into the mixing vessel. Small beakers can be used, but where a large quantity is required, measuring cylinders are better. The mixture should be homogeneous and

Araldite mixtures for various volumes rounded up to one decimal place

Total vol.	Casting resin (Araldite 6005)	DDSA (dodecyryl sucrinic anhydridge)	DMP 30 (catalyst)
17·2	10·0	7·0	0·24
25·9	15·0	10·5	0·36
34·5	20·0	14·0	0·48
43·1	25·0	17·5	0·60
51·7	30·0	21·0	0·72
60·3	35·0	24·5	0·84
69·0	40·0	28·0	0·96
77·6	45·0	31·5	1·08
86·2	50·0	35·0	1·20
94·8	55·0	38·5	1·32
103·4	60·0	42·0	1·44

for this purpose a stout glass rod with one flattened end is a useful instrument for stirring continuously for ten minutes. After stirring, allow the mixture to drain off the rod completely. If not used immediately the mixture can be properly covered and stored in the refrigerator.

Caution: Araldite has been known to cause dermatitis and so contact with the skin should be avoided. Wash very well after use.

Infiltration of the specimens with Araldite mixture is usually carried out in polyethylene cups for the purpose of easy cleaning. Approximately 1 ml of the mixture per one tissue vial is used. During changing, the tissue is rolled over fluffless blotting paper using tooth-picks to get rid of excess of Araldite mixture before the next stage.

'Beem' capsules are used for the final embedding, although gelatin capsules can also be used. Where these facilities are not available, aluminium foil boats can be made and the tissues embedded flat in about 3 mm of Araldite. The tissues are spaced out in such a way that each can be subsequently 'sawed' out and fastened to wooden pegs by means of sealing wax. These pegs fit into the microtone chuck holder.

The Beem/gelatin capsules are arranged vertically in rolls using a paper rack device made from microscope slide-paper boxes. Fill up with the Araldite mixture and with a tooth-pick, introduce the tissue, to be embedded at the bottom of the capsule. Place in the oven at 60 °C and examine after about 30 min to ensure the correct positioning of the tissue. Finally leave in the oven for the full period for polymerization.

Using the Araldite mixture given here polymerization is complete after 11 hr in the oven at 60 °C. It should be noted that the smallest variations in the ratio of the reagents, the curing time or the oven temperature will produce unsatisfactory plastic blocks, and microtomy will be difficult.

References

ABDALLA, A., et al. (1963). *J. Egypt med. Ass.* **46**, 544.

ABDALLA, R. E. (1974). Filariasis in the Sudan. *Trans. roy. Soc. trop. Med. Hyg.*, **68**, 53.

ABDEL-HAKIM, M. (1965). Parasite lung disease. *Dis. Chest*, **48**, 580–583.

ABDEL-HAKIM, M. and ELWI, A. M. (1963). Bronchopulmonary schistosomiasis: report of a case. *Dis. Chest*, **43**, 317.

ABDEL-MONEIM, R. I. (1972). Rupture of the spleen in rural parts of Egypt. *Amer. J. Surg.*, **123**, 674.

ABELEV, G. (1963). Study on the antigenic structure of tumours. *Acta Un. Int. Cancr.*, **19**, 80.

ABELEV, G., et al. (1967). Embryonal serum alpha-globulin in cancer patients— diagnostic value. *Int. J. Cancer*, **2**, 551.

ABIOYE, A. A. (1967). Interstitial plasma cell pneumonia (*Pneumocystis carinii*) in Ibadan: report of a case. *W. Afr. med. J.*, **16**, 130.

ABIOYE, A. A. and EDINGTON, G. M. (1972). Prevalence of amoebiasis at autopsy in Ibadan. *Trans. roy. Soc. trop. Med. Hyg.*, **66**, 754.

ABRAHAMS, D. G. (1959). An unusual form of heart-disease in West Africa. Its relation to endomyocardial fibrosis. *Lancet*, **2**, 111.

ABRAHAMS, D. G., ALELE, C. A. and BARNARD, B. G. (1960). The systemic blood pressure in a rural West African community. *W. Afr. med. J.*, **9**, 45.

ABRAHAMS, D. G. and COCKSHOTT, W. P. (1962). Multiple non-leutic aneurysms in young Nigerians. *Brit. Heart J.*, **24**, 83.

ABRAHAMS, D. G., et al. (1962). Annular subvalvular left ventricular aneurysms. *Quart. J. Med.* (n.s.), **31**, 345.

ABRAHAMS, D. G. and PARRY, E. H. O. (1963). The mechanism of arterial oxygen desaturation in right ventricular endomyocardial fibrosis. Evidence in favour of the existence of an azygos/pulmonary venous shunt. *Clin. Sci.*, **24**, 69.

ABRAMSON, R. K., RUCKNAGEL, D. L. and SHREFFLER, D. C. (1970). Homozygous Hb J Tongariki. *Science*, **169**, 194.

ACHAR, S. T., RAJU, V. B. and SRIRAMACHARI, S. (1960). Indian childhood cirrhosis. *J. Pediat.*, **57**, 744.

ACHESON, E. D. and TRUELOVE, S. C. (1961). Early weaning in the aetiology of ulcerative colitis: a study of feeding in infancy in cases and controls. *Brit. med. J.*, **2**, 929.

ACKERMAN, L. V. and MURRAY, J. F., eds. (1963). Symposium on Kaposi's sarcoma. Karger, Basel, New York. (Reprinted from *Acta Un. int. Cancr.*, 1962, **18**.)

ADADEVOH, B. K. (1970). Endocrine patterns in the African. *Trop. geogr. Med.*, **22**, 125.

ADADEVOH, B. K., FRANCIS, T. I. and AJAYI, O. O. A. (1972). Endocrine disorders in African children. *Nig. med. J.*, **2**, 2.

ADAM, M., et al. (1973). Hyperinfection syndrome with *Strongyloides stercoralis* in malignant lymphoma. *Brit. med. J.*, **1**, 264.

ADAMS, E. B., WRIGHT, R., BERMAN, E. and LAURENCE, D. R. (1959). Treatment of tetanus with chlorpromazine and barbiturates. *Lancet*, **1**, 755.

ADAMS, E. R., *et al.* (1967). Observations on the aetiology and treatment of anaemia in kwashiorkor. *Brit. med. J.*, **3**, 451.

ADAMSON, J. E. B. (1973). Icthycosis linearis circumflexa and Netherton's Syndrome with idiopathic dwarfism. *Proc. roy. Soc. Med.*, **66**, 624.

ADDAE, S. and KONOTEY-AHULU, F. I. D. (1971). Lack of diurnal variations in sodium potassium and osmolal excretion in the sickle-cell patient. *Afr. J. med. Sci.*, **2**, 349.

ADDY, J. (1971). Systemic sclerosis masquerading as leprosy in Ghana. *Ghana med. J.*, **10**, 218.

ADELOYE, A., LUZZATTO, L. and EDINGTON, G. M. (1971). Severe malarial infection in a patient with sickle-cell anaemia. *Brit. med. J.*, **2**, 445.

ADELOYE, A. and ODEKU, E. L. (1970). The nervous system in sickle-cell disease. *Afr. J. med. Sci.*, **1**, 33.

ADENIYI-JONES, C. (1967). Agglutination of tanned sheep erythrocytes by serum from Nigerian adults and children. *Lancet*, i, 188.

ADESOLA, A. O. (1962). Acute suppurative thyroiditis. *W. Afr. med. J.*, **11**, 248.

ADI, F. C. (1963). Endomyocardial fibrosis in two brothers. *Brit. Heart J.*, **25**, 684.

ADLER, S. (1964). *Leishmania. Advances in Parasitology*, **2**, 35. Academic Press, New York and London.

ADNER, M. M., ALSTATT, L. B. and CONRAD, M. E. (1968). Coombs' positive haemolytic disease in malaria. *Ann. intern. Med.*, **68**, 33.

ADOLPH, P. E., KAGAN, I. G. and MCQUAY, R. M. (1962). Diagnosis and treatment of *Acanthocheilonema perstans* filariasis. *Amer. J. trop. Med. Hyg.*, **11**, 76.

AFRICA, C. H., DE LEON, W. and GARCIA, E. Y. (1936). Heterophyidiasis: 111. Ova associated with a fatal haemorrhage in the right basal ganglia of the brain. *J. Philipp. med. Ass.*, **16**, No. 1, 22.

— (1937). Heterophyidiasis: VI. Two more cases of heart failure associated with the presence of eggs in sclerosed valves. *J. Philipp. med. Ass.*, **17**, No. 10, 605.

— (1937). Heterophyidiasis: V. Ova in the spinal cord in man. *Philipp. J. Sci.*, **62**, No. 3, 393.

AGER, J. A. M. and LEHMANN, H. (1957). Haemoglobin L: a new haemoglobin found in a Punjabi Hindu. *Brit. med. J.*, **2**, 142.

— (1958). Observations on some 'fast' haemoglobins: K, J, N, and 'Bart's.' *Brit. med. J.*, **1**, 929.

AGER, J. A. M., LEHMANN, H. and VELLA, F. (1958). Haemoglobin 'Norfolk': a new haemoglobin found in an English family, with observations on the naming of new haemoglobin variants. *Brit. med. J.*, **2**, 539.

AGGARWAL, N. D. and SINGH, H. (1963). Ainhum. *J. Bone Jt Surg.*, **45**, 376.

AGRANOFF, B. W. and GOLDBERG, D. (1974). Diet and the geographical distribution of multiple sclerosis. *Lancet*, **2**, 1061.

AGUILAR, P. L., ITURRIBARRIA, F. M. and MIDDLEBROOK, G. (1953). Un caso de infeccion hummana por mycobacterium ulcerans en et hemisferio occidental nota previa. *Int. J. Leprosy*, **21**, 469.

AHLUWALIA, M. S. and TANDON, H. D. (1965). Nodular hyperplasia of the prostate in N. India. *J. Urol.*, **93**, 94.

AHSAN, I. and RAHMAN, H. (1967). Volvulus of the sigmoid colon among Pathans. *Brit. med. J.*, **1**, 29.

AIDAROS, S. M. and SOLIMAN, L. A. M. (1961). Portal vascular changes in human bilharzial cirrhosis. *J. Path. Bact.*, **82**, 19.

AJAYI, O. O. A., *et al.* (1969). Hirschprung's disease in the monate presenting as caecal perforation. *Pediatrics*, **43**, 102.

AKBARIAN, M., YANKOPOULOS, N. A. and ABELMANN, W. H. (1966). Hemodynamic studies in beriberi heart disease. *Amer. J. Med.*, **41**, 197.

AKINKUGBE, O. O. (1967). Renal papillary necrosis in sickle-cell haemoglobinopathy. *Brit. med. J.*, **3**, 283.

AKINLADE, N. O. (1967). A case of Sasswood poisoning. *W. Afr. med. J.* (n.s.), **16**, 63.

AKINOSI, J. O. and WILLIAMS, A. O. (1969). Ameloblastoma in Ibadan, Nigeria. *Oral. Surg.*, **27**, 257.

AKISADA, M. and TANI, S. (1970). Lymphangioadenopathy of filariasis. *Trans. roy. Soc. trop. Med. Hyg.*, **64**, 885.

AKSOY, M. (1959). Abnormal haemoglobins in Turkey. In *Abnormal Haemoblogins—A Symposium*, p. 216. Blackwell Scientific Publications, Oxford.

ALBERT, J. P., *et al.* (1972). Contribution à l'étude de l'épidemiologie de la tuberculose humaine en Afrique occidentale. *Ann. Soc. belge Méd. trop.*, **52**, 75.

ALCORN, M. O., JR., and KOTCHER, E. (1961). Secondary malabsorption syndrome produced by chronic strongyloidiasis. *Sth. Med. J.*, **54**, 193.

ALEXANDER, P. (1972). Foetal 'antigens' in cancer. *Nature*, **235**, 137.

ALEXOPOULOS, C. J. (1962). *Introductory Mycology*. John Wiley, New York and London.

AL-HASANY, M. and MOHAMED, A. S. (1970). Veno-occlusive disease of the liver in Iraq. *Arch. Dis. Childh.*, **45**, 722.

ALICATA, J. E. (1953). Human fascioliasis in the Hawaiian Islands. *Hawaii med. J.*, **12**, 196.

— (1962). *Angiostrongylus cantonensis* (Nematoda: Metastrongylidae) as a causative agent of eosinophilic meningoencephalitis of man in Hawaii and Tahiti. *Canadian J. Zool.*, **40**, 5.

ALICATA, J. E. and BROWN, R. W. (1962) Observations on the method of human infection with *Angiostrongylus cantonensis* in Tahiti. *Canadian J. Zool.*, **40**, 755.

ALJEBOORI, T. I. and IVEY, M. H. (1970). An improved haemagglutination technique for detecting antibody against *Toxocara canis*. *Amer. J. trop. Med. Hyg.*, **19**, 244.

ALLAN, N., BEALE, D., IRVINE, D. and LEHMANN, H. (1965). Three haemoglobins K: Woolwich, and abnormal, Cameroon and Ibadan, two unusual variants of human haemoglobin A. *Nature (Lond.)*, **208**, 658.

ALLEN, D. M. and DEAN, R. F. A. (1965). The anaemia of kwashiorkor in Uganda. *Trans. roy. Soc. trop. Med. Hyg.*, **59**, 326.

ALLEN, D., *et al.* (1960). Iron in experimental malaria: relation to the histological technique. *Ann. trop. Med. Parasit.*, **54**, 272.

ALLEN, D., EDINGTON, G. M. and SCHNIEDEN, H. (1960). Iron in experimental malaria. Relation to the histological picture. *Ann. trop. Med. Parasit.*, **54**, 272.

ALLEN, J. R., CARSTENS, L. A., and KATAGIRI, G. J. (1969). Hepatic veins of monkeys with veno-occlusive disease. *Arch. Path.*, **87**, 279.

ALLEYNE, G. A. O. (1967). The effect of severe protein calorie malnutrition on the renal function of Jamaican children. *Pediatrics*, **39**, 400.

ALLISON, A. C. (1954). Protection afforded by sickle-cell trait against subtertian malarial infection. *Brit. med. J.*, **1**, 290.

ALLISON, A. C., BLUMBERG, B. S. and REES, W. (1958). Haptoglobin types in British, Spanish Basque and Nigerian African populations. *Nature (Lond.)*, **181**, 824.

ALMEIDA, J. D. (1971). Electron microscopic observations and speculations on Australia antigen. *Postgrad. med. J.*, **47**, 484.

ALP, M. H. and HISLOP, I. G. (1969). The effect of *Giardia lamblia* infestation on the gastro-intestinal tract. *Aust. Ann. Med.*, **18**, 232.

ALPERS, M. P. (1967). *Symposium on geographical pathology*. International Academy of Pathology, Washington.

ALPERS, M. P. (1970). Kuru in New Guinea. *Amer. J. trop. Med. Hyg.*, **19**, 133.

ALPERT, M. E., *et al.* (1971). Association between aflatoxin content of food and hepatoma frequency in Uganda. *Cancer (Philad.)*, **28**, 253.

ALTER, M. (1962). Multiple sclerosis in the Negro. *Arch. Neurol.*, **7**, 83.

ALTMAN, H. and STEIN, H. (1956). Idiopathic hypertrophy of the heart in African children: a report of four cases. *Brit. med. J.*, **1**, 1207.

ALTMANN, G. and BUBIS, J. J. (1959). A case of multiple infection with *Taenia saginata*. *Israel med. J.*, **18**, 35.

ALTON, G. G. and JONES, L. M. (1967). Laboratory techniques in brucellosis. *W.H.O.*, *Monogr. Ser.* No. 55.

AMENT, M. E. and RUBIN, C. E. (1972). Relation of giardiasis to abnormal intestinal structure and function in gastrointestinal immunodeficiency syndromes. *Gastroenterology*, **62**, 216.

AMLA, I., *et al.* (1971). Cirrhosis in children from peanut meal contaminated by aflatoxin. *Amer. J. clin. Nutr.*, **24**, 609.

ANAND, S. S. (1956). 50 cases of hypertrophic ileocaecal tuberculosis. *Ann. roy. Coll. Surg. Engl.*, **19**, 205.

ANAND, S. S. and PATHAK, K. (1961). Surgical treatment of abdominal tuberculosis with special reference to ileocaecal tuberculosis. *J. Ind. med. Ass.*, **37**, 423.

ANAND, S. U. and DAVEY, W. W. (1965). Surgery of the spleen in Nigeria. *Brit. J. Surg.*, **52**, 335.

ANDERSON, C. R. (1963). Recent advances in arthropod-borne virus research in India. *Bull. Nat. Inst. Sci. India*, No. 24, 205.

ANDERSON, C. R. and WATTLEY, G. H. (1955). The isolation of yellow fever virus from human liver obtained at autopsy. *Trans. roy. Soc. trop. Med. Hyg.*, **49**, 580.

ANDERSON, C. R., *et al.* (1957). The isolation of St. Louis virus from Trinidad mosquitoes. *Amer. J. trop. Med. Hyg.*, **6**, 688.

— (1957). Mayaro Virus: A new human disease agent. II. Isolation from blood of patients in Trinidad, B.W.I. *Amer. J. trop. Med. Hyg.*, **6**, 1012.

ANDERSON, I. F. (1965). Takayasu's arteritis. *S. Afr. med. J.*, **39**, 374.

ANDERSON, J. and FUGLSANG, H. (1973). Variation in numbers of microfilariae of *Onchocerca volvulus* in the anterior chamber of the human eye. *Trans. roy. Soc. trop. Med. Hyg.*, **67**, 544.

ANDERSON, J., *et al.* (1974). Studies on onchocerciasis in the United Cameroon Republic. *Trans. roy. Soc. trop. Med. Hyg.*, **68**, 190.

ANDERSON, M., *et al.* (1959). Chemical and pathological studies on aortic atherosclerosis. *Arch. Path.*, **68**, 380.

ANDERSON, R. E., *et al.* (1970). Geographic aspects of malignant lymphoma and multiple myeloma. *Amer. J. Path.*, **61**, 85.

ANDERSON, R. I. (1960). Serologic diagnosis of *Schistosoma mansoni*. Infections. 1. Development of a cercarial antigen slide flocculation test. *Amer. J. trop. Med. Hyg.*, **9**, No. 3, 299.

ANDRADE, S. G. and ANDRADE, Z. A. (1966). Chagas's disease and neuronal changes in the Auerbach Plexus (experimental study in mice). *Rev. Inst. Med. trop. S. Paulo*, **8**, 219.

ANDRADE, Z. A. (1965). Hepatic schistosomiasis. *Progr. Liver Dis.*, **2**, 228.

ANDRADE, Z. A. and ABREU, W. N. (1971). Follicular lymphoma of the spleen in patients with hepatosplenic *schistosomiasis mansoni*. *Amer. J. trop. Med. Hyg.*, **20**, 237.

ANDRADE, Z. A. and ANDRADE, S. G. (1966). New aspects of the pathology of kala azar (Morphological study of 13 cases at necropsy). *Rev. Inst. Med. trop. S. Paulo*, **8**, 259.

— (1967). The heart in the 'megas' of the digestive tract. *Hospital (Rio de J.)*, **71**, 719.

ANDRADE, Z. A., ANDRADE, S. G. and SADIGURSKY, M. (1971). Renal changes in patients with hepatosplenic schistosomiasis. *Amer. J. trop. Med. Hyg.*, **20**, 77.

ANDRADE, Z. A. and CHEEVER, A. W. (1971). Alterations to intrahepatic vasculature in hepatosplenic schistosomiasis mansoni. *Amer. J. trop. Med. Hyg.*, **20**, 425.

ANDRE, R., *et al.* (1957). Cutaneous leishmaniasis, cutaneous-glandular leishmaniasis and transfusional kala azar. *Bull. Mém. Soc. méd. Hôp. Paris*, Nos. 25/26, 854.

ANDREWS, P. S. and MARMION, B. P. (1959). Chronic Q fever. 2. Morbid anatomical and bacteriological findings in a patient with endocarditis. *Brit. med. J.*, **2**, 983.

ANG, P. L., TAY, J. S. H. and LOH, T. F. (1974). Hospital mortality in a Singapore Paediatric Unit—a 10-year review. *J. Singapore paediat. Soc.*, **16**, 9.

ANGEL, C. R., GUERRA, R., MARTINEZ, J. and PLOUGH, I. C. (1963). Malabsorption of xylose in Puerto Rico. *Fed. Proc.*, **22**, 550.

ANNAMUNTHODO, H. (1962). Rectal lymphogranuloma venereum in Jamaica. *W. Indian med. J.*, **11**, 73.

ANSARI, M. W., RAHI, A. H. S. and SHUKLA, B. R. (1970). Pseudoclastic nature of ptery-gium. *Brit. J. Ophthal.*, **54**, 473.

ANSELMI, A. and MONEIRO, F. (1974). *Pathogenetic Mechanisms in Chagas' Cardio-myopathy. Trypanosomiasis and Leishmaniasis*. Ciba Foundation Symposium 20 (new series). Associated Scientific Publishers, Amsterdam.

ANTHONY, P. P. and DRURY, R. A. B. (1970). Elastic vascular sclerosis of mesenteric blood vessels in argentaffin carcinoma. *J. clin. Path.*, **23**, 110.

ANTHONY, P. P., VOGEL, C. L. and BARKER, L. F. (1973). Liver cell dysplasia; a pre-malignant condition. *J. clin. Path.*, **26**, 217.

ANTHONY, P. P., *et al.* (1973). Hepatitis—Associated antigen and antibody in Uganda. *Brit. med. J.*, **1**, 403.

ANTIA, A. V., COCKSHOTT, W. P. and THORPE, G. J. (1969). Idiopathic cardiomegaly in Nigerian children. *Brit. Heart J.*, **31**, 178.

ANTIA, F. P., *et al.* (1966). Giardiasis in adults. Incidence, symptomatology and absorption studies. *Indian J. med. Sci.*, **20**, 471.

ARABATZIS, G. and PAPAPANAGIOTOU, J. (1963). Laboratory tests in hydatid disease: a comparison of the indirect haemagglutination, complement-flxation and intra-dermal tests. *Bull. Wld Hlth Org.*, **28**, 266.

ARCHAMPONG, E. Q. (1969). Operative treatment of typhoid perforation of the bowel. *Brit. med. J.*, **3**, 273.

ARCHIBALD, H. M. (1956). The influence of malarial infection of the placenta on the incidence of prematurity. *Bull. Wld Hlth Org.*, **15**, 842.

AREÁN, V. M. (1956). Manson's schistosomiasis of the female genital tract. *Amer. J. Obstet. Gynec.*, **72**, 1038.

— (1956). Lesions caused by *Schistosoma mansoni* in the genitourinary tract of men. *Amer. J. clin. Path.*, **26**, 1010.

— (1958). Ascaridic granuloma: an experimental study. *A.M.A. Arch. Path.*, **66**, 427.

— (1966). Schistosomiasis: a clinicopathologic evaluation. *Path. A.*, **1**, 68.

AREÁN, V. M. and KOPPISCH, E. (1956). Balantidiasis: a review and report of cases. *Amer. J. Path.*, **32,** 1089.

ARENDS, T. (1967). High concentration of haemoglobin A_2 in malaria patients. *Nature (Lond.)*, **215,** 1517.

ARENDS, T. and GALLANGO, M. L. (1962). Frecuencia de Haptoglobinas en varias poblaciones Suramericanas. *Acta cient. venez.* **13,** 116.

ARIZTIA, A., *et al.* (1957). Interstitial plasma cell pneumonia and pneumocystis carinii. *J. Pediat.*, **51,** 634.

ARMSTRONG, R. K. and WINFIELD, J. L. (1969). *Paederus fuscipes* dermatitis. *Amer. J. trop. Med. Hyg.*, **18,** 147.

ARNIM, K. (1966). Histopathological aspects and frequency of lesions of lymphoid tissue in Iranians. *Proc. Int. Acad. Path. Kyoto, Japan,* 176.

ARRIBADA, A. and ESCOBAR, E. (1968). Cardiomyopathies produced by *Toxoplasma gondii. Amer. Heart J.* **76,** 329.

ARRIBALZAGA, R. A. (1955). Una neuva enfermedad epidémica a germen desconocido: Hipertermia nefrotóxica, leucopénica y enantemática. *Día méd.*, **27,** 1204.

ARROYAVE, G., WILSON, D., CONTRERAS, C. and BÉHAR, M. (1963). Alterations in serum concentration of vitamin A associated with the hypoproteinemia of severe protein mulnutrition. *J. Pediat.*, **62,** 920.

ARTIGAS, J. and BEAVER, P. C. (1961). Salmon diet in relation to amebic colitis in the dog. *Amer. J. trop. Med. Hyg.*, **10,** 812.

ASBELL, M. B. (1964). Orthodontic aspects of Cooley's Anaemia. *Ann. N.Y. Acad. Sci.*, **119,** 694.

ASH, J. E. and SPITZ, S. (1945). *Pathology of Tropical Diseases: An Atlas.* Saunders, Philadelphia and London.

ASHBY, B. S., APPLETON, P. J. and DAWSON, I. (1964). Eosinophilic granuloma of gastro-intestinal tract caused by herring parasite eustoma rotundatum. *Brit. med. J.*, **1,** 1141.

ASHCROFT, M. T., MILNER, P. F. and WOOD, C. W. (1969). Haemoglobin concentration, eosinophilia and intestinal helminths in children in rural Jamaica. *Trans. roy. Soc. trop. Med. Hyg.*, **63,** 811.

ASHCROFT, M. T. (1972). Cardiac enlargement in Jamaicans. *Bull. med. J.* **2,** 655.

ASHLEY, D. J. B. (1965). Two cases of clostridial hepatitis. *J. clin. Path.*, **18,** 170.

ASHTON, N. (1960). Larval granulomatosis of the retina due to *Toxocara. Brit. J. Ophthal.*, **44,** 129.

ASSAAD, F. and COCKBURN, W. C. (1972). Four-year study of WHO virus reports on enteroviruses other than poliovirus. *Bull. Wld Hlth Org.*, **46,** 329.

ASSOKU, R. K. G. (1972). Evidence for the immunological basis of anaemia of acute gram-negative bacterial infection. *Ghana med. J.*, **11,** 101.

ASTALDI, G., MEARDI, G. and LISINO, T. (1966). The iron content of jejunal mucosa obtained by Crosby's biopsy in hemachromatosis and hemosiderosis. *Blood*, **28,** 70.

ATALA, A. and ZAHER, M. F. (1969). Bilharzial calcification of renal capsule. *J. Urol.*, **101,** 125.

ATALA, A., ZAHER, M. F. and RAGU, I. (1969). Bilharzial bladder outlet obstruction. *J. Urol.*, **101,** 183.

ATKINSON, L., CHESTER, I. C., SMYTH, F. G. and TEN SELDAM, R. E. S. (1964). Oral cancer in New Guinea: a study in demography and etiology. *Cancer, N.Y.*, **17,** 1289.

ATWATER, J., SCHWARTZ, I. R. and TOCANTINS, L. M. (1960). A variety of human hemoglobin with 4 distinct electrophoretic components. *Blood*, **15,** 901.

AURORA, A. L., TANEJA, O. P. and GUPTA, D. N. (1970). Bladder stone disease of childhood. *Acta paediat. scand.*, **59**, 385.

AUDY, J. R. and HARRISON, J. L. (1951). A review of investigations on mite typhus in Burma and Malaya, 1945–1950, *Trans. roy. Soc. trop. Med. Hyg.*, **44**, 371.

AUSTIN, M. G. and BERRY, J. W. (1956). Observations on 100 cases of heatstroke. *J. Amer. med. Ass.*, **161**, 1525.

AUSTEN, W. G. and BLENNERHASSETT, J. B. (1965). Giant-cell aortitis causing an aneurysm of the ascending aorta and aortic regurgitation. *New Engl. J. Med.*, **272**, 80.

AWAD, N. A. (1958). Urinary 17-ketosteroid excretion, blood eosinophil level and adrenocortical function in adult male Egyptians. *J. trop. Med. Hyg.*, **61**, 204.

AYKROYD, W. R. and KRISHNAN, B. G. (1941). Infantile mortality in the beriberi area of the Madras Presidency. *Indian J. med. Res.*, **29**, 703.

AYREY, F. (1948). Outbreaks of sprue during the Burma campaign. *Trans. roy. Soc. trop. Med. Hyg.*, **41**, 377.

AZIMI, P. H., CRAMBLETT, H. G. and HAYNES, R. E. (1969). Mumps meningoencephalitis in children. *J. Amer. med. Ass.*, **207**, 509.

AZULAY, R. D. (1969). Brazilian foliaceous pemphigus. In: *Essays on Tropical Dermatology*, ed. R. D. G. Ph. Simons and J. Marshall, p. 49. Excerpta Medica Foundation, Amsterdam.

BAAR, H. S. and GALINDO. J. (1965). Ossifying pulmonary granulomatosis due to larvae of *Ascaris. J. clin. Path.*, **18**, 737.

BABB, R. R., *et al.* (1971). Giardiasis: a cause of traveler's diarrhoea. *J. Amer. med. Ass.*, **217**, 1359.

BABERO, B. B., AL-DABAGH, M. A., AL-SAFFAR, A.S. and ALI, F. M. (1963). The zoonosis of animal parasites in Iraq. VIII: Hydatid disease. *Ann. trop. Med. Parasit.*, **57**, 499.

BABUDIERI, B. (1953). Epidemiology, diagnosis and prophylaxis of Q fever. In Advances in the Control of Zoonoses. *Monogr. Ser.* No. 19, p. 157. Geneva, *W.H.O.*

BACHMANN, F. and MARTI, H. R. (1962). Hemoglobin Zürich. II: Physicochemical properties of the abnormal hemoglobin. *Blood*, **20**, 272.

BACK, E. H. and DEPASS, E. E. (1957). Acute rheumatic fever in Jamaican children. *W. Indian med. J.*, **6**, 98.

BADDELEY, H. (1974). Kaposi's sarcoma. *Proc. roy. Soc. Med.*, **67**, 866.

BADOE, E. A. (1965). Acute intestinal obstruction in Accra, Ghana (a review of 628 cases). *Ghana med. J.*, **4**, 128.

— (1967). Acute appendicitis in Accra. *Ghana Med. J.*, **6**, 69.

BAGLIONI, C. (1963). Correlations between genetics and chemistry of human hemoglobins. In *Molecular Genetics*, ed. J. H. Taylor, **1**, 405. Academic Press, New York and London.

— (1963). A child homozygous for persistence of foetal haemoglobin. *Nature (Lond.)*, **198**, 1177.

BAGSHAWE, A. F. and FORRESTER, A. T. T. (1966). Addison's disease in Kenya. *E. Afr. med. J.*, **43**, 21.

BAGSHAWE, A. and NGANDA, T. N. (1973). Hepatitis B antigen in a rural community in Kenya. *Trans. roy. Soc. trop. Med. Hyg.*, **67**, 663.

BAHARY, C. M., OVADIA, Y. and NERI, A. (1967). Schistosoma mansoni of the ovary. *Amer. J. Obstet. Gynec.*, **98**, 290.

BAIG, H. A. and EDOZIEN, J. C. (1965). Carbohydrate metabolism in kwashiorkor. *Lancet*, **2**, 662.

BAILENGER, J., CAILLAU, M. and PAUTRIZEL, R. (1960). La distomatose. I: Etat actual de son épidémiologie dans le sud-ouest de la France. *Rev. Hyg. Méd. soc.*, **8**, 603.

BAILEY, K. V. (1966). Liver pathology in malnourished New Guineans. *Med. J. Aust.*, **1**, 572.

BAILEY, N. M., *et al.* (1967). The indirect fluorescent antibody technique applied to dried blood, for use as a screening test in the diagnosis of human trypanosomiasis in Africa. *Trans. roy. Soc. trop. Med. Hyg.*, **61**, 696.

BAILLY, I. C. (1973). Pituitary tumours in Kampala, Uganda. *Afr. J. med. Sci.*, **4**, 171.

BAJPAI, P. C., *et al.* (1965). Infantile Tremor Syndrome. *Acta neurol. scand.*, **41**, 473.

BAKER, D. H. (1964). Roentgen manifestations of Cooley's anaemia. *Ann. N. Y. Acad. Sci.*, **119**, 641.

BAKER, J. R. (1974). *Epidemiology of African Sleeping Sickness. Trypanosomiasis and Leishmaniasis.* Ciba Foundation Symposium 20 (new series). Associated Scientific Publishers, Amsterdam.

BAKER, R. D., Editor (1971). *Human Infection with Fungi, Actinomycetes and Algae.* Springer Verlag, New York.

BAKER, S. J. (1957). Idiopathic tropical steatorrhea: a report of sixty cases. *Indian J. med. Sci.*, **11**, 687.

BAKER, S. J., IGNATIUS, M., MATHAN, V. I., VAISH, S. K. and CHACKO, C. C. (1962). Intestinal biopsy in tropical sprue. In *Intestinal Biopsy, Ciba Foundation Study Group Report* No. 14: ed. G. E. W. Wolstenholme and M. P. Cameron, p. 84. Churchill, London.

BAKINOSI, J. O. and WILLIAMS, A. O. (1968). Adamantinoma in Ibadan, Nigeria. *W. Afr. Med. J.*, **17**, 45.

BAKKER, A. W., BLIEK, A. and LUYKEN, R. (1957). The serum proteins of malaria-free inhabitants of Central Netherlands, New-Guinea. *Docum. Med. geogr. trop.* (Amst.), **9**, 1.

BALDACHIN, B. J. and ROTHMAN, W. T. (1969). Alkaptonuric arthritis. *Cent. Afr. J. Med.*, **5**, 287.

BALDACHIN, B. J. and MELMED, R. N. (1964). Clinical and therapeutic aspects of kerosine poisoning. *Brit. med. J.*, **2**, 28.

BALDWIN, R. W., EMBLETON, M. J. and ROBINS, R. A. (1973). Humoral factors influencing cell-mediated immune responses to tumour-associated antigens. *Proc. roy. Soc. Med.*, **66**, 466.

BALL, J. D. and TREU, R. (1950). Tropical pulmonary eosinophilia. *Trans. roy. Soc. trop. Med. Hyg.*, **44**, 237.

BALL, P. A. J. (1966). The relationship of host to parasite in human hookworm infection. *The Pathology of Parasitic Diseases.* Fourth Symposium of the British Society for Parasitology. Blackwell Scientific Publications, Oxford.

BALL, P. A. J., VOLLER, A., TAFFS, L. F. (1971). Hypersensitivity to some nematode antigens. *Brit. med. J.*, **1**, 210.

BANDEIRA, V. and CARVALHO, A. (1958). Adult *Schistosoma mansoni* worms in veins of the oesophageal plexus. *An. Fac. Med. Recife*, **18**, 17.

BANKS, S., *et al.* (1965). Malignant Zollinger–Ellison syndrome in a Bantu woman with a prolonged remission after gastric radiotherapy. *Gut*, **6**, 279.

BANTI, G. (1894). Splenomegaly with cirrhosis of the liver. *Med. Week, Paris*, **2,** 364. (Reprinted in *Med. Classics*, (1937) **1,** 907.)

— (1937). Splenomegaly with cirrhosis of the liver. *Med. Classics*, **1,** 899.

BANWELL, J. G. (1962). Report from meeting of Association of Physicians of East Africa. *E. Afr. med. J.*, **39,** 506.

BANWELL, J. G., HUTT, M. S. R. and TUNNICLIFFE, R. (1964). Observations on jejunal biopsy in Ugandan Africans. *E. Afr. med. J.*, **41,** 46.

BANWELL, J. G., *et al.* (1967). Hookworm infection and intestinal absorption amongst Africans in Uganda. *Amer. J. trop. Med. Hyg.*, **16,** 309.

BARKHAN, P., STEVENSON, M. E., PINKER, G., DANCE, N. and SHOOTER, E. M. (1964). Haemoglobin Lepore trait: an analysis of the abnormal haemoglobin. *Brit. J. Haemat.*, **10,** 437.

BARLOW, J. S. (1967). Multiple sclerosis in North Korea and China. *Neurology*, **17,** 802.

BARNES, D. E., ADKINS, B. L. and SCHAMSCHULA, R. G. (1970). Etiology of caries in Papua New Guinea. *Bull. Wld Hlth Ord.*, **43,** 769.

BARNES, R. and MCKAY, J. (1962). Report of a case of a flagellate causing a urinary infection. *Med. J. Aust.*, **2,** 913.

BARNETT, R. N., *et al.* (1969). Pneumocystis carinii in lymph nodes and spleen. *Arch. Path.*, **88,** 175.

BARNICOT, N. A. and KARIKS, J. (1960). Haptoglobin and transferrin variants in peoples of New Guinea Highlands. *Med. J. Aust.*, **11,** 359.

BARNICOT, N. A. and WOLFFSON, D. (1952). Daily urinary 17-ketosteroid output in African Negroes. *Lancet*, **1,** 893.

BARNITSON, J. (1954). L'epithelioma latent de la prostate. *Arch. Anat. path.*, **30,** 129.

BARR, R. (1966). Human trichinosis: report of four cases, with emphasis on central nervous system involvement, and a survey of 500 consecutive autopsies at the Ottawa Civic Hospital. *Canadian med. Ass. J.*, **95,** 912.

BARR, R. D., *et al.* (1972). Nephrotic syndrome in Adult Africans in Nairobi. *Brit. med. J.*, **2,** 131.

BARR, R. D., ROY, A. D. and MILLER, J. R. M. (1972). Idiopathic gangrene in African adults. *Brit. med. J.*, **4,** 273.

BARRETT-CONNOR, E. and CONNOR, J. D. (1970). Extraintestinal manifestations of Shigellosis. *Amer. J. Gastroent.*, **53,** 234.

BARRETT, G. S. and MACDERMOTT, J. (1972). Breast abscess—a rare presentation of typhoid. *Brit. med. J.*, **2,** 628.

BARTELLONI, P. J. (1967). Combined therapy for chloroquine-resistant *Plasmodium falciparum* infection. *J. Amer. med. Ass.*, **199,** 173.

BARTEN, J. (1973). Neonatal tetanus in Indonesia. *Trop. Doc.*, **3,** 3, 107.

BARTLETT, A. and BALL, P. A. J. (1972). *Nematospiroides dubius* in the mouse as a possible model of endemic human hookworm infection. *Ann. trop. Med. Parasit.*, **66,** 129.

BARTON, E. G. and CAMPBELL, W. G. (1967). Further observations on the ultrastructure of Pneumocystis. *Arch. Path.*, **83,** 527.

BARTON, J. C. (1961). Tuberculosis of the vault of the skull. *Brit. J. Radiol.*, **34,** 286.

BASU, A. K. (1965). Tropical surgery. In *Clinical Surgery*. Butterworths, London.

BASU, A. K. and AIKAT, B. K. (1963). *Tropical Splenomegaly*. Butterworths, London.

BATES, L. E., THØGER BUSK and PALMER, C. E. (1951). Tuberculin sensitivity at different altitudes of residence. *Publ. Hlth. Rep. (Wash.)*, **66,** 1427.

BATTEN, G. H. (1966). Incidence of cancer in U.S.A., Hawaii. In *Cancer Incidence in Five Continents*, ed. R. Doll, P. Payne and J. Waterhouse, chapter IV, p. 204.

BAYLISS, T. M. and ROSENSWEIG, N. S. (1966). A racial difference in incidence of lactase deficiency: a survey of milk intolerance and lactase deficiency in healthy adult males. *J. Amer. med. Ass.*, **197**, 968.

BEAER, P. C., FALLON, M. and SMITH, G. N. (1971). Pulmonary nodule caused by a living Brugia Malayi-like filaria in an artery. *Amer. J. trop. Med. Hyg.*, **20**, 661.

BEAL, C. B., *et al.* (1970). A new technique for sampling duodenal contents. *Amer. J. trop. Med. Hyg.*, **19**, 349.

BEALE, P. J., CORMACK, J. D. and OLDREY, T. B. N. (1972). Thrombocytopenia in malaria with immunoglobulin (IgM) changes. *Brit. med. J.*, **1**, 345.

BEARCROFT, W. G. C., PORTERFIELD, J. S. and SUTTON, R. N. P. (1963). The isolation and identification of Ukauwa, a Bunyamwera group virus, from Nigeria. *Trans. roy. Soc. trop. Med. Hyg.*, **57**, 308.

BEAS, F., *et al.* (1971). Growth hormone in infant malnutrition. *Brit. J. Nutr.*, **26**, 169.

BEATTIE, C. P. (1963). Immunity to *Toxoplasma*. In *Immunity to Protozoa*, ed. P. C. C. Garnham, A. E. Pierce and I. Roitt, p. 253. Blackwell, Oxford.

BEAVER, P. C. (1956). Larva migrans. A review. *Exp. Parasit.*, **5**, 587.

BEAVER, P. C. (1959). Visceral and cutaneous larva migrans. *Publ. Health Rep.* (*Wash.*), **74**, 328.

— (1964). Cutaneous larva migrans. *Industr. Med. Surg.*, **33**, 319.

BEAVER, P. C. and DANARAJ, T. J. (1958). Pulmonary ascariasis resembling eosinophilic lung. Autopsy report with description of larvae in the bronchioles. *Amer. J. trop. Med. Hyg.*, **7**, 100.

BEAVER, P. C., YASHIDA, Y. and ASH, L. R. (1964). Mating of *Ancylostoma caninum* in relation to blood loss in the host. *J. Parasit.*, **50**, 286.

BEAVER, P. C., *et al.* (1952). Chronic eosinophilia due to visceral larva migrans. *Pediatrics*, **9**, 7.

BECHELLI, L. M., *et al.* (1973). Some epidemiological data on leprosy collected in a mass survey in Burma. *Bull. Wld Hlth Org.*, **48**, 3, Article 3014.

BECK, E., *et al.* (1966). Experimental 'kuru' in chimpanzees. A pathological report. *Lancet*, **2**, 1056.

BECKER, B. J. P. (1963). Idiopathic mural endocardial disease in South Africa. *Med. Proc.*, **9**, 147.

BECKER, B. J. P. and CHATGIDAKIS, C. B. (1961). Primary carcinoma of the liver in Johannesburg. *Acta Un. int. Cancr.*, **17**, 650.

— (1961). Cirrhosis of the liver in Johannesburg. *Acta Un. int. Cancr.*, **17**, 639.

BECKER, B. J. P., CHATGIDAKIS, C. B. and VAN LINGEN, B. (1953). Cardiovascular collagenosis with parietal endocardial thrombosis: a clinicopathologic study of forty cases. *Circulation*, **7**, 345.

BECKER, W. (1966). Herpes virus infection in three racial communities in Cape Town. *S. Afr. J. Lab. clin. Med.*, **12**, 109.

BECROFT, D. M. O. and WEBSTER, D. R. (1972). Aflatoxins and Reye's Disease. *Brit. med. J.*, **4**, 117.

BECROFT, D. M. O. (1966). Syndrome of encephalopathy and fatty degeneration of viscera in New Zealand children. *Brit. med. J.*, **2**, 135.

BEDDOE, H. L. (1956). Peritoneal granuloma due to *Enterobius vermicularis*. *A.M.A. J. Dis. Child.*, **91**, 577.

BEESON, P. B. (1941). Factors influencing the prevalence of trichinosis in man. *Proc. roy. Soc. Med.*, **34**, 585.

BEET, E. A. (1946). Sickle cell disease in the Balovale district of Northern Rhodesia. *E. Afr. med. J.*, **23**, 75.

— (1948). Pigmentation of the tongue in African children. *E. Afr. med. J.*, **25**, 433.

— (1956). Rheumatic heart disease in Northern Nigeria. *Trans. roy. Soc. trop. Med. Hyg.* **50**, 587.

BEGGS, W. A. and FISCHMAN, A. (1970). A preserved antigen for the hydatid fluorescent antibody and other tests utilizing scolices. *Bull. Wld Hlth Org.*, **42**, 331.

BEGHIN, I. D. (1973). Central American Symposium on measles and its vaccination. *Ann. Soc. belge Méd. trop.*, **53**, 57.

BEHAR, M., ASCOLI, W. and SCRIMSHAW, N. S. (1958). An investigation into the causes of death in children in four rural communities in Guatemala. *Bull. Wld Hlth Org.*, **19**, 1093.

BEHEYT, P. and VANDEPITTE, M. (1958). Heart aneurysms. *Acta Cardiol. (Brux.)*, **13**, 419.

BEHL, P. N. (1962). *Practice of dermatology*. Allied Pacific Private Ltd, Bombay.

BEKER, G. S., *et al.* (1963), Strongyloidiasis in Venezuela. *G.E.N. (Caracas)*, **17**, 285.

BEKER, S., RIVAS GÓMEZ, A., VALENCIA-PARPARCÉN, J. and MONCADA, P. R. (1963). Strongiloidiasis intestinal en Venezuela. *G.E.N. (Caracas)*, **17**, 285.

BELDING, D. L. (1965). *Textbook of Clinical Parasitology*. Third edition. Appleton-Century-Crofts, New York.

BELL, D. R. (1964). Diet and therapy in bilharzia. *Lancet*, **1**, 643.

— (1967). Membrane filters and microfilariae: a new diagnostic technique. *Ann. trop. Med. Parasit.*, **61**, 220.

BELL, S. (1953). Predisposing factors in tick-borne relapsing fever in Meur district. Kenya. *Trans. roy. Soc. trop. Med. Hyg.*, **4**, 309.

— (1956). The Meru people of Kenya. Part VII. Relapsing fever. *J. trop. Med. Hyg.*, **59**, 82.

BELL, T. M., MASSIE, A., ROSS, M. G. R. and WILLIAMS, M. C. (1964). Isolation of a reovirus from a case of Burkitt's lymphoma. *Brit. med. J.*, **1**, 1212.

BELTRAN, G., BAEZ, A. and CORREA, P. (1966). Burkitt's lymphoma in Colombia. *Amer. J. Med.*, **40**, 211.

DI BELLO, R. (1955). Diagnosis and clinical patterns of cardiac echinococcosis. *An. Fac. Med. Montevideo*, **40**, 93.

BELZER, M., *et al.* (1965). Salmonella infections of the kidney. *J. Urol.*, **94**, 23.

BENDALL, R. (1966). Osteomalacia in Asian immigrants. (Correspondence.) *Brit. med J.*, **2**, 300.

BENGOA, J. M. (1940). *Medicina social en el medio rural Venezolano*. Litografia del Comercio, Caracas.

— (1974). The problems of malnutrition. *WHO Chron.*, **28**, 3.

BENNETT, J. H. (1961). Haptoglobin types in natives from the kuru region and other parts of Melanesia. *Brit. med. J.*, **2**, 428.

BENNETT, M. A., HESLOP, R. W. and MEYNELL, M. J. (1967). Massive haematuria association with sickle-cell trait. *Brit. med. J.*, **1**, 677.

BENSTER, B. and CAUCHI, M. N. (1972). Haemoglobin A_2 level in pregnancy. *J. clin. Path.*, **23**, 538.

BENYAJATI, C. (1966). Experimental cholera in humans. *Brit. med. J.*, **i**, 140.

BENZER, S., INGRAM, V. M. and LEHMANN, H. (1958). Three varieties of human haemoglobin D. *Nature (Lond.)*, **182**, 852.

BERGER, M., BIRD, L. M. and CONTE, N. F. (1967). The nephrotic syndrome secondary to acute glomerulonephritis during falciparum malaria. *Ann. intern. Med.*, **67**, 1163.

BERGHOUT, E. (1973). Onchocerciasis and glaucoma in the forest area of Ghana. *Trop. geogr. Med.*, **25**, 233.

BERGMAN, F. and VAN DER LINDEN, W. (1965). The association of peptic ulcer with cirrhosis of the liver: an analysis of an autopsy series. *Acta path. microbiol. scand.*, **65**, 161.

BERGNER, J. F., NEAVE, C. and TANTALO, H. F. (1964). A parasitologic-epidemiologic study in Hapung aborigine village, Taiwan. *Chin. med. J.*, Republic of China, **11**, 177.

BERMAN, C. (1951). *Primary Carcinoma of the Liver.* H. K. Lewis, London.

BERRY, A. (1966). A cytopathological and histopathological study of bilharziasis of the female genital tract. *J. Path. Bact.*, **91**, 325.

BERSOHN, I., POLITZER, W. M. and BLUMSOHN, D. (1969). Arcus senilis cornear. *S. Afr. med. J.*, **43**, 1025.

BERTHELOT, P., WALKER, J. G., SHERLOCK, S. and REID, L. (1966). Arterial changes in the lungs in cirrhosis of the liver—lung spider nevi. *New Engl. J. Med.*, **274**, 291.

BESKIN, C. A., COLVIN, S. H. JR. and BEAVER, P. C. (1966). Pulmonary dirofilariasis cause of a pulmonary nodular disease. *J. Amer. med. Ass.*, **198**, No. 7, 665.

BEUTLER, E. (1960). Drug-induced hemolytic anemia (primaquine sensitivity). In *The Metabolic Basis of Inherited Disease.* Eds. J. B. Stanbury, J. B. Wyngaarden, and D. S. Fredrickson, p. 1031. McGraw-Hill, New York.

— (1970). Annotation: glucose-6-phosphate dehydrogenase deficiency. *Brit. J. Haemat.*, **18**, 117.

BHAMARAPRAVATI, N. and NIMSOMBURANS, P. (1963). Geographic pathology of cirrhosis and carcinoma of the liver in Thailand. *Proc. 16th Ass. Japan Med. Congress*, **3**, 376.

BHAMARAPRAVATI, N. and VIRRANUVATTI, V. (1966). Liver diseases in Thailand. An analysis of liver biopsies. *Amer. J. Gastroent.*, **45**, 267.

BHAMARAPRAVATI, N., et al. (1967). Pathology of Thailand haemorrhagic fever: a study of 100 autopsy cases. *Ann. trop. Med. Parasit.*, **61**, 500.

BHAMARAPRAVATI, N., et al. (1967). Pathology of abnormal hemoglobin diseases seen in Thailand. I. Pathology of β-thalassemia hemoglobin E disease. *Amer. J. clin. Path*, **47**, 745.

BHATNAGAR, B. N. S., DUBE, B. and SHUKLA, A. P. (1970). Testicular histology in tropical vaginal hydrocele. *Int. Surg.*, **53**, 167.

BHUYAN, U. U., et al. (1965) Effect of dietary protein on carbon tetrachloride induced hepatic fibrogenesis in albino rats. *Lab. Invest.*, **14**, 184.

BIAGI, F. F. and BELTRAN, F. (1969). The challenge of amoebiasis: understanding pathogenic mechanisms. *Int. Rev. trop. Med.*, **3**, 219.

BIAGI, F. F. and TAY, J. (1958). A precipitation reaction for the diagnosis of cysticercosis. *Amer. J. trop. Med. Hyg.*, **7**, No. 1, 63.

BIAGI, F. F., TAY, J. and MARTINEZ MURRAY, R. (1964). The immunofluorescence test in the diagnosis of Chagas's disease. *Bol. Ofic. sanit. panamer.*, **57**, 237.

BIANCO, I., MODIANO, G., BOTTINI, E. and LUCCI, R. (1963). Alteration in the α-chain of haemoglobin L$_{Ferrara}$. *Nature (Lond.)*, **198**, 395.

BICKERS, W. M. (1970). Hydatid disease of the female pelvis. *Amer. J. Obstet. Gynec.*, **107**, 477.

BIENZLE, U., et al. (1972). Glucose-6-phosphate dehydrogenase and malaria. *Lancet*, **1**, 107.

BIGGART, J. H. (1937). Human infestation with *Fasciola hepatica*. *J. Path. Bact.*, **44,** 488.

BIGUET, J., *et al.* (1964). A study of precipitating antibody in persons suffering from onchocerciasis. *Bull. Soc. Path. exot.*, **57,** 1098.

BILLINGHURST, J. R. and WELCHMAN, J. M. (1966). Idiopathic ulcerative colitis in the African: a report of four cases. *Brit. med. J.*, **1,** 211.

BILLINGS, F. T., WINKENWERDER, W. L. and HUNNINEN, A. V. (1946). Studies on acute schistosomiasis japonica in the Philippine Islands. I: A clinical study of 337 cases with a preliminary report on the results of treatment with fuadin in 110 cases. *Bull. Johns Hopk. Hosp.*, **78,** 21.

BILLINGHURST, J. R., GERMAN, G. A. and ORLEY, J. H. (1973). The pattern of epilepsy in Uganda. *Trop. geogr. Med.*, **25,** 226.

BINZ, G. and WATSON, H. J. C. (1973). Observations on the patterns of blood IgM levels in the populations of endemic and nonendemic sleeping sickness areas in Kenya. *Bull. Wld Hlth Org.*, **47,** 6, Article 2961.

BIRCH, H. G., *et al.* (1971). Relation of kwashiorkor in early childhood and intelligence at school age. *Pediat. Res.*, **5,** 579.

BIRD, A. C., *et al.* (1970). Nematode optic neuritis. *Amer. J. Ophthal.*, **69,** 72.

BIRD, A. V. (1965). Spinal cord complications of bilharziasis. *S. Afr. med. J.*, **39,** 158.

BIRD, A. V. and KERRICH, J. E. (1969). Multiple sclerosis in South Africa. *S. Afr. med. J.* **43,** 1031.

BIRD, G. W. G. and MENON, K. K. (1961). Survival of *Microfilaria bancrofti* in stored blood. *Lancet*, **2,** 721.

BIRD, T., ENNIS, J. E., WORT, A. J. and GARDNER, P. S. (1963). Disseminated herpes simplex in newborn infants. *J. clin. Path.*, **16,** 423.

BISNO, A. L., *et al.* (1970). Contrasting epidemiology of acute rheumatic fever and acute glomerulonephritis. *New Engl. J. Med.*, **283,** 561.

BLACK, M. M. (1965). Reactivity of the lymphoreticuloendothelial system in human cancer. *Prog. clin. Cancer*, Grune & Stratton, New York, 26.

BLACK, M. M., KERPE, S. and SPEER, F. D. (1953). Lymphnode structure in patients with cancer of the breast. *Amer. J. Path.*, **29,** 505.

BLACK, W. C. and HAFFNER, H. F. (1968). Diffuse hyperplasia of gastric argyrophil cells and multiple carcinoid tumours. *Cancer*, **21,** 1080.

BLACKLOCK, D. B. and GORDON, R. M. (1925). Malaria infection as it occurs in late pregnancy; its relationship to labour and early infancy. *Ann. trop. Med. Parasit.*, **19,** 327.

BLACKMAN, V. (1962). Target cells in East African anaemias. *E. Afr. Med. J.*, **39,** 565.

BLACKWELL, R. Q., HUANG, J. T. H. and CHIEN, L. C. (1965). Haemoglobin E in Vietnamese. *Nature (Lond.)*, **207,** 768.

BLAND, K. G. and GELFAND, M. (1970). The influence of urinary bilharziasis on vesicovaginal fistula in relation to causation and healing. *Trans. roy. Soc. trop. Med. Hyg.*, **64,** 588.

BLASTOMYCOSIS. (1964). *Amer. Rev. resp., Dis.*, **89,** 659.

BLISS, B. P., RHODES, J. and RAINS, A. J. H. (1963). Cystic myxomatous degeneration of popliteal artery. *Brit. med. J.*, **2,** 847.

BLOOMFIELD, D. K. and LIEBMAN, J. (1963). Idiopathic cardiomyopathy in children. *Circulation*, **27,** 1071.

BLUMBERG, B. S., ALTER, H. J. and VISNICH, S. (1965). A 'new' antigen in leukaemia sera. *J. Amer. med. ass.*, **191,** 541.

BLUMBERG, B. S., DRAY, S. and ROBINSON, J. C. (1962). Antigen polymorphism of a low density beta-lipoprotein. *Nature*, **194**, 656.

BLUMBERG, B. S., SUTNICK, A. I. and LONDON, W. T. (1970). Australia antigen as a hepatitis virus. *Amer. J. Med.*, **48**, 1.

BLUMING, A. Z., et al. (1972). Delayed cutaneous sensitivity reactions to extracts of autologous malignant melanoma. *J. nat. Cancer Inst.*, **48**, 17.

BOBOWSKI, S. J. and REED, W. G. (1958). Toxoplasmosis in an adult, presenting as a space-occupying cerebral lesion. *A.M.A. Arch. Path.*, **65**, 460.

BOERMA, F. W. and HUISMAN, T. H. J. (1964). Serologic investigations of human hemoglobins. II: Antibodies produced by isolated human hemoglobin types with known structural differences. *J. Lab. clin. Med.*, **63**, 264.

BOHM, G. M. (1968). Quantative study of the intrinsic inervation of the heart in endomyocardial fibrosis and the African idiopathic cardiopathies. *Rev. Inst. Med. trop. S. Paulo*, **10**, 84.

BÖHM, G. M., and SMITH, B. (1966). Pathology of an East African megacolon. *Gut*, **7**, 662.

BOHRER, S. P. (1966). Typhoid perforation of the ileum. *Brit. J. Radiol.*, **39**, 37.

— (1970). Osteitis deformans in Nigerians. *Afr. J. med. Sci.*, **1**, 109.

— (1970). Acute long bone diaphyseal infarcts in sickle cell disease. *Brit. J. Radiol.*, **43**, 685.

BOISIVON, A. (1973). Clinical investigations with the Makari tumour skin test in France. *Trans. N.Y. Acad. Sci.*, **35**, 380.

BOISSON, C., et al. (1965). Electron microscopic study of the flagellum of *Trypanosoma gambiense*. *C. R. Soc. Biol. (Paris)*, **159**, 228.

BOLIO-CICERO, A., AGUIRRE, J. and PEREZ-TAMAYO, R. (1961). Malignant peritoneal mesothelioma. *Amer. J. clin. Path.*, **36**, 417.

BONOMO, L., TURSI, A., TRIMIGLIOZZI, G. and DAMMACCO, F. (1965). L. E. cells and antinuclear factors in leprosy. *Brit. med. J.*, **2**, 689.

BONSNES, R. W. and MARNEY, A. F. (1967). Accuracy of passive hemagglutination inhibition method for the determination of chorionic gonadotropin in the urine. *Amer. J. Obstet. Gynec.*, **98**, 208.

BOON, W. H. (1973). Mild Beta-thalassaemia major in Singapore. *J. Singapore paediat. Soc.*, **15**, 18.

BOOTH, C. C. (1965). Nutritional problems associated with small intestinal disease. In *Symposium on Advanced Medicine, London*, 1964, ed. N. Compston, p. 184. Pitman Medical, London.

BOOTH, C. C. and MOLLIN, D. L. (1964). Chronic tropical sprue in London. *Amer. J. dig. Dis.*, **9**, 770.

BORELL, U., FERNSTRÖM, I., LINDBLOM, K. and WESTMAN, A. (1952). The diagnostic value of arteriography of the iliac artery in gynaecology and obstetrics. *Acta radiol. (Stockh.)*, **38**, 247.

BORRERO, J. et al. (1961). Clinical and laboratory studies on hookworm disease in Colombia. *Amer. J. trop. Med. Hyg.*, **10**, 735.

BOSHELL, J. (1969). Kyasanur forest disease. *Amer. J. trop. Med. Hyg.*, **18**, 67.

BOTHA, D. J. (1963). Bilharzial cholecystitis with calculus. *Brit. J. Surg.*, **50**, 543.

BOTHWELL, T. H. and BRADLOW, B. A. (1960). Siderosis in the Bantu. *A.M.A. Arch. Path.*, **70**, 279.

BOURGEOIS, C. H., et al. (1971). Acute aflatoxin B_1 toxicity in the Macaque and its similarities to Reye's syndrome. *Lab. Invest.*, **24**, 206.

BOURGOIGNIE, J., SONNET, J. and DECHEF, G. (1962). Etude clinique du diabète sucré du Bantou de la région de Léopoldville. *Ann. Soc. belge. Méd.. trop.*, **42**, 261.

BOYD, J. F. and NEDELKOSKA, N. (1964). Inclusion-bearing cells in urinary sediment in infectious diseases. *J. Path. Bact.*, **88**, 115.

BOYD, W. C. (1958). *Genetics and the Races of Man*, Boston University Press.

BOYER, J. L., *et al.* (1967). Idiopathic portal hypertension. *Amer. J. Int. Med.*, **66**, 41.

BOYLAND, E., ROE, F. J. C., GORROD, J. W. and MITCHLEY, B. C. V. (1964). The carcinogenicity of nitrosoanabasine, a possible constituent of tobacco smoke. *Brit. J. Cancer*, **18**, 265.

BOYLES, P. W. and CURRIE, J. (1958). Classic haemophilia in a Negro infant. *Amer. J. med. Sci.*, **235**, 452.

BRADFIELD, R. B., CORDANO, A. and GRAHAM, G. G. (1969). Hair root adaption to marasmus in Andean Indian children. *Lancet*, **2**, 1169.

BRADFIELD, R. B. and JELLIFFE, E. F. P. (1970). Early assessment of malnutrition. *Nature*, **225**, 283.

— (1974). Hair-colour changes in Kwashiorkor. *Lancet*, **1**, 461.

BRADLEY, D. J. (1965). The measurement of bilharziasis. Prevalence and schistosomal egg output. Aims and techniques, with an account of a field method. *Bull. Wld Hlth Org.*, Geneva, **33**, No. 4, 503.

BRADLEY, D. J. and MCCULLOUGH, F. S. (1973). Egg output stability and the epidemiology of *Schistosoma haematobium*. II. An analysis of the epidemiology of endemic *S. haematobium*. *Trans. roy. Soc. trop. Med. Hyg.*, **67**, 4, 491.

BRAIMBRIDGE, M. W., *et al.* (1967). Possibility of a new infective aetiological agent in congestive cardiomyopathy. *Lancet*, **1**, 171.

BRAIN, M. C. and VELLA, F. (1958). Haemoglobin H trait in a Nepalese-Gurkha woman. *Lancet*, **1**, 192.

BRAIN, W. R., HUNTER, D. and TURNBULL, H. M. (1929). Acute meningo-encephalo-myelitis of childhood. *Lancet*, **1**, 221.

BRANDBORG, L. L., *et al.* (1970). Human coccidiosis—a possible cause of malabsorption: the life cycle in small bowel mucosal biopsies as a diagnostic feature. *New Engl. J. Med.*, **283**, 1306.

BRANDBORG, L. L., *et al.* (1967). Histological demonstration of mucosal invasion by *Giardia lamblia* in man. *Gastroenterology*, **52**, 143.

BRAS, G. (1952). The morbid anatomy of smallpox. *Docum. Med. georg. trop.*, **4**, 303.

— (1952). Observations on formation of smallpox scars. *Arch. Path.*, **54**, 149.

BRAS, G., BROOKS, S. E. H. and WATLER, D. C. (1961). Cirrhosis of the liver in Jamaica. *J. Path. Bact.*, **82**, 503.

BRAS, G., IRVINE, R. A., RICHARDS, R. C., MILNER, P. F. A. and RAGBEER, M. M. S. (1964). Infection with *Strongyloides stercoralis* in Jamaica. *Lancet*, **2**, 1257.

BRAS, G., WATLER, D. C. and ASHMEADE-DYER, A. (1965). The incidence of malignant neoplasms in Jamaica. *Brit. J. Cancer*, **19**, 681.

BRAS, G., *et al.* (1969). Report on 141 childhood malignancies observed in Jamaica. *J. nat. Cancer Inst.*, **43**, 417.

BRASS, K. (1955). Statistische Untersuchungen über die idiopathische Myokarditis im Raum Valencia (Venezuela). *Frankfurt Z. Path.*, **66**, 77.

BRAY, R. S. (1974). *Epidemiology of Leishmaniasis: Some Reflections on Causation. Trypanosomiasis and Leishmaniasis.* Ciba Foundation Symposium 20 (new series). Associated Scientific Publishers, Amsterdam.

BRAY, R. S. and LAINSON, R. (1965). The immunology and serology of leishmaniasis. I. The fluorescent antibody staining technique. *Trans. roy. Soc. trop. Med. Hyg.*, **59**, 535.

BRAY, R. S., ASHFORD, R. W. and BRAY, M. A. (1973). The parasite causing cutaneous Leishmaniasis in Ethiopia. *Trans. roy. Soc. trop. Med. Hyg.*, **67**, 345.

BRAY, R. S., RAHIM, G. A. F. and TAJELDIN, S. (1967). The present state of Leishmaniasis in Iraq. *Protozoology*, **2**, 171.

BRAY, R. S., *et al.* (1973). Studies on the immunology and serology of leishmaniasis. IX. Serological investigation of the parasite of Indian kala-azar and Indian post-kala-azar dermal leishmaniasis. *Trans. roy. Soc. trop. Med. Hyg.* **67**, 1, 125.

BREM, T. H. and KONWALER, B. E. (1955). Fatal myocarditis due to emetine hydrochloride. *Amer. Heart J.*, **50**, 476.

BRETLAND, P. M. (1962). *Armillifer armillatus* infestation: radiological diagnosis in two Ghanaian soldiers. *Brit. J. Radiol.*, **35**, 603.

BREW, D. ST. J. (1962). *A review of 183 autopsies of patients with tuberculosis.* Health and Tuberculosis Conference. Chest and Heart Association, London. 165.

BREW, D. ST. J. and EDINGTON, G. M. (1965). Haemoglobins S and C in post mortem material in Ibadan, Nigeria. In *Abnormal haemoglobins in Africa*, ed. J. H. P. Jonxis, p. 213. Blackwell, Oxford.

BREWER, D. B. (1964). *Renal Biopsy.* Edward Arnold, London.

BRICKMAN, H. F. and FELDMAN, W. (1969). Familial Mediterranean fever in Canada. *Canad. med. Ass. J.*, **100**, 938.

BRIERS, P. J. (1974). Schistosomiasis with particular reference to pulmonary and abdominal lesions (Abridged). *Proc. roy. Soc. Med.*, **67**, 861.

BRIGDEN, W. and ROBINSON, J. (1964). Alcoholic heart disease. *Brit. med. J.*, **2**, 1283.

BRINK, A. J., LEWIS, C. M. and WEBER, H. W. (1965). Myocardiopathy in *Argemone mexicana* poisoning. *S. Afr. med. J.*, **39**, 108.

BRINK, A. J. and WEBER, H. W. (1963). Fibroplastic parietal endocarditis with eosinophilia: Löffler's endocarditis. *Amer. J. Med.*, **34**, 52.

BRITISH MEDICAL BULLETIN (1967). Intestinal absorption, **23**, No. 3.

BRITISH MEDICAL JOURNAL (1954). Trichinosis (Leading article) **1**, 1025.

— (1962). Geographical distribution of ulcerative colitis. (Leading article) **2**, 36.

— (1964). Carcinogen in groundnuts. (Leading article) **2**, 204.

— (1964). Onchocerciasis in Britain. (Leading article) **1**, 1133.

— (1966). Recent research on Burkitt's tumour: conference at Kampala, Uganda. **1**, 1043

— (1967). Tropical splenomegaly syndrome. **4**, 614.

BRITISH MEDICAL ASSOCIATION (1973). Broadsheet No. 77. *Assoc. clin. Path.* (Published by BMA).

DE BRITO, T., *et al.* (1965). Electron microscopy of the biopsied kidney in human leptospirosis. *Amer. J. trop. Med. Hyg.*, **14**, 397.

BROADSHEET (1973). No. 77 Ass. clin. Path. B.M.A. House, Tavistock Sq., London.

BROCK, J. F. and HANSEN, J. D. L. (1974). Protein requirement. *Lancet*, **2**, 712.

BROCKINGTON, I. F. and EDINGTON, G. M. (1972). Adult heart disease in W. Nigeria. *Amer. Heart J.*, **83**, 27.

BROCKINGTON, I. F., LUZZATTO, L. and OSUNKOYA, B. O. (1970). The heart in eosinophilic leukaemia. *Afr. J. med. Sci.*, **1**, 343.

BROCKINGTON, I. F., OLSEN, E. G. J. and GOODWIN, J. F. (1967). Endomyocardial fibrosis in Europeans resident in tropical Africa. *Lancet*, **1**, 583.

BRODY, J. A., YASE, Y., CHEMIER, G. and PHILIPPE, Y. (1969). Hyperreflexia and spastic paralysis among New Caledonian leprosy patients. *Amer. J. trop. Med. Hyg.*, **18**, 132.

BRODY, J. A., *et al.* (1970). Hereditary blindness among Pingelapese people of Eastern Caroline Islands. *Lancet*, **1**, 1253.

BRONTE-STEWART, R. (1965). Epidemiology and dietary factors in occlusive vascular disease. *Ann. roy. Surg. Eng.*, **36**, 206.

BROOKE, O. G. (1972). Influence of malnutrition on the body temperature of children. *Brit. med. J.*, **1**, 331.

BROOKS, S. E. N., *et al.* (1970). Acute veno-occlusive disease of the liver. *Arch. Path.*, **89**, 507.

BROWN, A., MOHAMED, S. D., MONTGOMERY, R. D., ARMITAGE, P. and LAURENCE, D. R. (1960). Value of a large dose of antitoxin in clinical tetanus. *Lancet*, **2**, 227.

BROWN, G. W. (1974). *Schistosoma mansoni* infection with portal hypertension (Symmers' fibrosis). *Proc. roy. Soc. Med.*, **67**, 1027.

BROWN, H. W. and PERNA, V. P. (1958). An overwhelming *Strongyloides* infection. *J. Amer. med. Ass.*, **168**, 1648.

BROWN, J. and JACOBS, L. (1956). Adult toxoplasmosis: report of a case due to laboratory infection. *Ann. intern. Med.*, **44**, 565.

BROWN, J. A. K., STONE, M. M. and SUTHERLAND, I. (1966). B.C.G. vaccination of children against leprosy: first results of a trial in Uganda. *Brit. med. J.*, **1**, 7.

BROWN, J. B., CREAN, G. P. and GINSBURG, J. (1964). Oestrogen metabolism and excretion in liver disease. *Gut*, **5**, 56.

BROWN, J. E. (1943). Pelvic phleboliths. *E. Afr. med. J.*, **20**, 122.

BROWN, K. N., *et al.* (1967). Heterophile antibody in trypanosomiasis. *Trans. roy. Soc. trop. Med. Hyg.*, **61**, 147.

BROWN, R. E. and KATZ, M. (1966). Failure of antibody production to yellow fever in children with kwashiorkor. *Trop. geogr. Med.*, **18**, 125.

— (1966). Smallpox vaccination in malnourished children. *Trop. geogr. Med.*, **18**, 129.

BROWN, W. R., *et al.* (1972). Clinical, microbiological and immunological studies in patients with immunoglobin deficiencies and gastrointestinal disorders. *Gut*, **13**, 441.

BROWNE, S. (1973). The epidemiology of leprosy. *Z. Tropenmed. Parasit.* **24**, Suppl. 1, 1.

BROWNE, S. G. (1960). Cantharidin poisoning due to a 'Blister Beetle'. *Brit. med. J.*, **2**, 1290.

— (1960). Onchocercal depigmentation. *Trans. roy. Soc. trop. Med. Hyg.*, **54**, 325.

— (1960). Some clinical features of Bancroftian filariasis among adult males in an unreported focus in the Belgian Congo. *Cent. Afr. J. Med.*, **6**, 513.

— (1962). Calcinosis circumscripta of the scrotal wall: the etiological role of *Onchocerca volvulus*. *Brit. J. Derm.*, **74**, 136.

— (1962). *Leprosy: lecture notes for medical students and practitioners*. Dept. of Medicine, University College, Ibadan, Nigeria.

— (1962). Present perspectives in leprosy. *Scot. med. J.*, **7**, 446.

— (1964). The liver in leprosy: a review. *W. Afr. med. J.* (n.s.), **13**, 35.

— (1964). Fixed eruption in deeply pigmented subjects. *Brit. med. J.*, **2**, 1041.

— (1965). True ainhum: its distinctive features. *J. Bone Jt Surg.*, **47**, 52.

— (1966). Localized bacilliferous skin lesions appearing in patients with quiescent lepromatous leprosy. *Int. J. Leprosy*, **34**, 289.

BROWNE, S. G. and MCLOUGHLIN, D. (1962). A case of ainhum of the finger. *W. Afr. med. J.*, **11**, 168.

BROWNE, S. G. and RIDGE, E. (1961). Toxic epidermal necrolysis. *Brit. med. J.*, **1**, 550.

BROWNING, D. and GROSS, S. (1968). Epidemiological studies of acute childhood leukaemia. *Amer. J. Dis. Child.*, **116**, 576.

BRUCE-CHWATT, L. J. (1952). Malaria in African infants and children in Southern Nigeria. *Ann. trop. Med. Parasit.*, **46**, 173.

— (1956). Biometric study of spleen- and liver-weights in Africans and Europeans, with special reference to endemic malaria. *Bull. Wld Hlth Org.*, **15**, 513.

— (1959). Birth weight and prematurity, Tanganyika. *Trans. roy. Soc. trop. Med. Hyg.*, **53**, 363.

— (1967). Malaria in Africa. *Brit. med. J.*, **2**, 311.

BRUMPT, L. C. and BRUMPT, V. (1958). Resistance against malaria and the abnormal haemoglobins (especially haemoglobin E). *Bull. Soc. Path. Exot.*, **51**, 217.

BRUMPT, L. C. and HO THI SANG (1955). *Bull. Soc. Path. exot.*, **48**, 46.

BRYCESON, A. and LEITHEAD, C. S. (1966). Diffuse cutaneous leishmaniasis in Ethiopia. *Ethiopian Med. J.*, **5**, 31.

BRYCESON, A. et al. (1970). Louse-borne relapsing fever. *Quart. J. med.*, **39**, 129.

BRYCESON, A. and PFALTZGRAFF, R. E. (1973). *Leprosy for Students of Medicine*. Churchill-Livingstone, Edinburgh.

BRYCESON, A. D. M. (1974). Immune response to parasitic infection. *Tropical Doctor*, **4**, 99.

BUCHANAN, G. (1967). Surgical aspects of porocephalosis. (Correspondence.) *Trans. roy. Soc. trop. Med. Hyg.*, **61**, 746.

BUCHANAN, W. N. (1970). Peritonitis and Bantu siderosis. *S. Afr. med. J.*, **44**, 43.

BUCHNER, A. and SREEBNY, L. M. (1970). Effect of prolonged food reduction on the rat parotid gland and exocrine pancreas. *J. Nutr.*, **100**, 655.

BUCK, A. A., et al. (1972). Microfilaruria in onchocerciasis: a clinical and epidemiological follow-up study in the Republic of Chad. *Bull. Wld Hlth Org.*, **45**, 353.

BUCK, A. A. (1974). Onchocerciasis. Symptomatology, pathology, diagnosis. World Health Organisation, Geneva.

BUCKLEY, J. J. C. (1958). Occult filarial infections of animal origin as cause of tropical pulmonary eosinophilia. *E. Afr. m. J.*, **35**, 492.

BUCKLEY, S. M. and CASALS, J. (1970). Lassa fever, a new virus disease of man from West Africa. *Amer. J. trop. Med. Hyg.*, **19**, 680.

BUCKLEY, S. M., CASALS, J. and DOWNS, W. G. (1970). Isolation and antigenic characteristics of Lassa virus. *Nature*, **227**, 174.

BUDDEN, F. H. (1958). The aetiology of the ocular lesions associated with onchocerciasis. *Trans. roy. Soc. trop. Med. Hyg.*, **52**, 500.

— (1963). Comparative study of ocular onchocerciasis in savannah and rain forest. *Trans. roy. Soc. trop. Med. Hyg.*, **57**, 64.

BUGHER, J. C. (1951). The pathology of yellow fever. In *Yellow Fever*, ed. Strode, G. K., p. 137. McGraw-Hill, New York and Maidenhead.

BUNNAG, T., COMER, D. S. and PUNYAGUPTA, S. (1970). Eosinophilic Myeloencephalitis caused by *Gnathostoma spinigerum*. *J. neurol. Sci.*, **10**, 419.

BUNNAG, T., PUNYAGUPTA and JUTTIJUDATA, P. (1967). *Clinical manifestations and pathological findings in eosinophilic meningoencephalitis due to Gnathostoma spinigerum*. SEAMES, Third Conference on Parasitic Diseases. Abstracts of Papers, p. 115.

BURCH, G. E. and GILES, T. D. (1972). The role of viruses in the production of heart disease. *Amer. J. Cardiol.*, **96**, 231.

BURGANINON, G. C. (1937). Fatal case of hepatitis with massive localisation of microfilariae in liver. *Ann. belges Méd. trop.*, **17**, 1.

BURKE, J. (1973). About congenital African trypanosomiasis. *Ann. Soc. belge Méd. trop.*, **53/1**, 63.

BURKITT, D. (1958). A sarcoma involving the jaws in African children. *Brit. J. Surg.*, **46**, 218.

— (1962). Determining the climatic limitations of a children's cancer common in Africa. *Brit. med. J.*, **2**, 1019.

BURKITT, D. and WRIGHT, D. (1966). Geographical and tribal distribution of the African lymphoma in Uganda. *Brit. med. J.*, **1**, 569.

BURKITT, D. P. (1952). Acute abdomens—British and Baganda compared. *E. Afr. med. J.*, **29**, 189.

— (1964). *Symposium on Lymphoreticular Tumours in Africa. Paris 1963.* p. 119. S. Karger, Basel.

— (1972). Varicose veins, deep vein thrombosis and haemorrhoids: epidemiology and suggested aetiology. *Brit. med. J.*, **2**, 556.

BURKITT, D. P., WILSON, A. M. M. and JELLIFFE, D. B. (1964). Subcutaneous phycomycosis. *Brit. med. J.*, **1**, 1669.

BURLINGAME, P. L. and CHANDLER, A. C. (1941). Host-parasite relations of *Moniliformis dubius* (Acanthocephala) in albino rats, and the environmental nature of resistance to single and superimposed infections with this parasite. *Amer. J. Hyg.*, **33**, D, 1.

BURRELL, R. J. W. (1962). Esophageal cancer among Bantu in the Transkei. *J. nat. Cancer Inst.*, **28**, 495.

BURRELL, R. J. W., ROACH, W. A. and SHADWELL, A. (1966). Esophageal cancer in the Bantu of the Transkei associated with mineral deficiency in garden plants. *J. nat. Cancer Inst.*, **36**, 201.

BUSUTTIL, A. (1974). Kala-azar in the Maltese Islands. *Trans. roy. Soc. trop. Med. Hyg.*, **68**, 236.

BUTCHER, G. A. and COHEN, S. (1972). Antigenic variation and protective immunity in *Plasmodium knowlesi* malaria. *Immunology*, **23**, 4, 503.

BUTLER, T., *et al.* (1973). Chloramphenicol-resistant typhoid fever in Vietnam associated with R factor. *Lancet*, **2**, 983.

— (1973). Chronic splenomegaly in Vietnam. *Amer. J. trop. Med. Hyg.*, **22**, 1.

BUTT, E. M. and HIGGINSON, J. (1957). Trace element pattern in liver disease and liver carcinoma. *Acta Un. int. Cancr.*, **13**, 599.

BWIBO, N. O. (1969). Accidental poisoning in children in Uganda. *Brit. med. J.*, **4**, 601.

CABANNES, R. and BUHR, L. (1955). Une nouvelle fraction hémoglobinique humaine à migration électrophorétique plus rapide que l'hémoglobine A et moins rapide que l'hémoglobine H: note préliminaire. *Pédiatrie*, **10**, 888.

CADDELL, J. L. (1965). Magnesium in the therapy of protein-calorie malnutrition of childhood. *J. Pediat.*, **66**, 392.

CAHILL, K. M. (1965). Filarial chyluria: a biochemical and radiological study of five patients. *J. trop. Med. Hyg.*, **68**, 27.

CAMAIN, R. (1954). Aperçus sur le cancer en A.O.F. *Bull. Soc. Path. exot.*, **47**, 614.

— (1954). Apercus sur le cancer on A.O.F. *Bull. méd. Afrique*, **ii**, 203.

— (1957). Symposium of primary cancer of the liver in Africa: report. *Acta Un. int. Cancr*, **13**, 617.

CAMAIN, R., ROUILLER, C. and DUPIN, H. (1959). Évolution de la stéatose hépatique dans le kwashiorkor sous l'influence du régime hyperprotidique: étude en microscopie normale et électronique. *Ann. Anat. path.*, **4**, 220.

CAMAIN R., *et al.* (1964). Les hemato-sarcomes de la face chez l'enfant en Afrique Occidentale et Centrale francophone—Histopathologie, tentatives de culture et autres examens biologiques. *Symposium on Lymphorecticular Tumors in Africa.* p. 256. S. Karger, Basel, New York.

CAMAIN, R., *et al.* (1972). Cutaneous cancer in Dakar. *J. Nat. Cancer Inst.*, **48**, 33.

CAMERON, G. L. and STAVELY, J. M. (1957). Blood group P substance in hydatid cyst fluids. *Nature (Lond.)*, **179**, 147.

CAMERON, J. L., MADDREY, W. C. and ZUIDEMA, G. D. (1971). Biliary tract disease in sickle cell anaemia. *Ann. Surgery*, **174**, 702.

CAMERON, J. S. (1970). Glomerulonephritis. *Brit. med. J.*, **4**, 285.

— (1972). Bright's disease today. *Brit. med. J.*, **4**, 217.

CAMPBELL, A. M. G. (1969). Herpes encephalitis. *Postgrad. med. J.*, **45**, 382.

CAMPBELL, G. D. (1964). Some thoughts on the syndrome of diabetes in Indian people in Natal. *Leech (Johannesburg)*, **34**, 125.

CAMPBELL, G. D. and WEBB, W. R. (1964). Eosinophilic pleural effusion. *Amer. Rev. resp. Dis.*, **90**, 194.

CAMPBELL, J. H. and CUMMINS, S. D. (1951). Priapism in sickle cell anaemia. *J. Urol.*, **66**, 697.

CAMPBELL, T. C., CAEDO, J. P., BULATAO-JAYME, J., SALAMAT, L. and ENGEL, R. W. (1970). Aflatoxin M_1 in human urine. *Nature*, **227**, 403.

CANFIELD, C. J. (1969). Renal and haematologic complications of acute falciparum malaria in Vietnam. *Bull. N.Y. Acad. Med.*, **45**, 1043.

CANNON, D. A. (1942). Linguatulid infestation of man. *Ann. trop. Med. Parasit.*, **36**, 160.

CANNON, D. S. H. (1958). Malaria and prematurity in the Western Region of Nigeria. *Brit. med. J.*, **2**, 877.

CAPLAN, A. (1944). A critical analysis of collapse in underground workers on the Kolar gold field. *Trans. Instn Min. Metall. (Lond.)*, **53**, 95.

CARDIGAN, F. C., *et al.* (1972). The effect of habitat on the prevalence of human scrub typhus in Malaysia. *Trans. roy. Soc. trop. Med. Hyg.*, **66**, 582.

CAREY, D. E., *et al.* (1972). Lassa fever. Epidemiological aspects of the 1970 epidemic. Jos, Nigeria. *Trans. roy. Soc. trop. Med. Hyg.*, **66**, 402.

CARPENTER, C. C. J., *et al.* (1965). Clinical evaluation of fluid requirements in Asiatic cholera. *Lancet*, **1**, 726.

CARPENTER, C. M., MILLER, J. N. and BOEK, R. A. (1960). A 'triple-test plan' for the serological diagnosis of syphilis. *New Engl. J. Med.*, **263**, 1016.

CARROLL, D. G. (1946). Cerebral involvement in schistosomiasis japonica. *Bull. Johns Hopk. Hosp.*, **78**, 219.

CARSTENS, P. H. B. (1969). Pulmonary bone marrow embolism following external cardiac massage. *Acta path. microbiol. scand.*, **76**, 510.

CARTER, P. K., SCHOEN, I. and MUJAHIRA, T. (1970). Quantitation of a slide test (Mono-test) for infectious mononucleosis. *J. clin. Path.*, **23**, 700.

CARTER, R. and MCGREGOR, I. A. (1973). A. Enzyme variation in *Plasmodium falciparum* in the Gambia. *Trans. roy. Soc. trop. Med. Hyg.*, **67**, 6, 830.

CARTER, R. and VOLLER, A. (1973). Enzyme typing of malaria parasites. *Brit. med. J.*, **1**, 149.

CARTER, R. C. (1972). Primary amoebic meningo-encephalitis. An appraisal of present knowledge. *Trans. roy. Soc. trop. Med. Hyg.*, **66**, 193.

CARTER, R. F. (1972). Primary amoebic meningo-encephalitis. *Trans. roy. Soc. trop. Med. Hyg.*, **66**, 193.

DE CARVALHO, A. R. L. (1966). Cancer distribution in the tropical area of N.E. Brazil. *Int. Canc. Congress, Tokyo*, 736.

CASALS, J. and WHITMAN, L. (1961). Group C, a new serological group of hitherto undescribed arthropod-borne viruses. Immunological studies. *Amer. J. trop. Med. Hyg.*, **10**, 250.

CASPARY, E. A. and FIELD, E. J. (1971). Specific lymphocyte sensitisation in cancer. *Brit. med. J.*, **2**, 613.

CATHIE, I. A. B. (1954). *Toxoplasma* adenopathy in a child with isolation of the parasite. *Lancet*, **2**, 115.

CATTOIR, E. and MARILL, F. G. (1950). Vue d'ensemble sur les splénomégalies chroniques dites 'algériennes'. *Cah. méd. Un. fr.*, **5**, 585.

CAUSEY, O. R. (1966). Arbovirus Research Project, University of Ibadan. Annual Report.

CAUSEY, O. R., *et al.* (1961). The isolation of arthropod-borne viruses, including members of two hitherto undescribed serological groups, in the Amazon region of Brazil. *Amer. J. trop. Med. Hyg.*, **10**, 227.

CAVE, L., *et al.* (1963). Radiological and pathogenetic studies on arterial lesions in leprosy. *Bull. Soc. med. Afr. noire Langue franç.*, Dakar, **8**, 67.

CELLE, P. L. L. and WEED, R. I. (1971). *The Contribution of Normal and Pathologic Erythrocytes to Blood Rheology in Progress in Haematology*, p. 1. Heinemann, London.

CEPPELLINI, R. (1959). L'emoglobina normale lente A_2. Symposium Geneticae Haematologicae. *Acta Genet. Med. (Roma)*, Suppl. **2**, 47.

CHAFFEE, E. F., BAUMAN, P. M. and SHAPILO, J. J. (1954). Diagnosis of schistosomiasis by complement-fixation. *Amer. J. trop. Med. Hyg.*, **3**, No. 5, 905.

CHAI and CH'EN WANG SHAN-CHI (1957). Acute colonic obstruction in schistosomiasis japonica. *Chin. med. J.*, **75**, 517.

CHAIT, A. and GANNON, W. E. (1969). Schistosomiasis of the spinal cord. *Amer. J. Roentgenol.*, **105**, 400.

CHALFIN, D. and HOLT, P. R. (1967). Lactase deficiency in ulcerative colitis, regional enteritis, and viral hepatitis. *Amer. J. dig. Dis.*, **12**, 81.

CHAMBON, L., *et al.* (1967). Une épidémie de fièvre jaune en Sénégal en 1965. L'épidémie humaine. *Bull. Wld Hlth Org.*, **36**, 113.

CHAMPION, H. R. and WALLACE, I. W. J. (1971). Breast cancer grading. *Brit. J. Cancer*, **25**, 441.

CHAN, D. P. (1967). *Choriocarcinoma*, p. 37. Springer-Verlag, Berlin and New York.

CHAN, T. K. (1972). G-6-PD Deficiency, typhoid and co-trimoxazole. *Lancet*, **2**, 1258.

CHAN, T. K., TODD, D. and LAI, M. C. S. (1972). Glucose-6-phosphate dehydrogenase: Identity of erythrocyte and leukocyte enzyme with report of a new variant in Chinese. *Biochem. Genet.*, **6**, 119.

CHAN, T. K., TODD, D. and WONG, C. C. (1964). Erythrocyte glucose-6-phosphate dehydrogenase deficiency in Chinese. *Brit. med. J.*, **2**, 102.

CHAN, T. K., *et al.* (1971). The survival of glucose-6-phosphate dehydrogenase-deficient erythrocytes in patients with typhoid fever on chloramphenicol therapy. *J. Lab. clin. Med.*, **77**, 177.

CHAN, T. K. and MACFADZEAN, A. J. S. (1974). Haemolytic effect of trimethoprim-sulphamethoxazole in G-6-PD deficiency. *Trans. roy. Soc. trop. Med. Hyg.*, **68**, 61.

CHAN, W. C. and TSAO, Y. C. (1966). Diffuse membranous glomerulonephritis in children. *J. clin. Path.*, **19**, 464.

CHANCE, M. L., *et al.* (1973). A comparative study of DNA in the genus *Leishmania*. *Trans. roy. Soc. trop. Med. Hyg.*, **67**, 24.

CHANDER, K., MAIR, H. J. and MAIR, N. S. (1968). Case of toxoplasma polymyositis. *Brit. med. J.*, **1**, 158.

CHANDLER, A. C. (1943). Studies on the nutrition of tapeworms. *Amer. J. Hyg.*, **37**, 121.

CHANDLER, R. L. (1958). Studies on the tolerance of N'Dama cattle to trypano-somiasis. Reprinted from *J. comp. Path.*, **68**, 253.

CHANDRA, R. K. (1970). Immunological picture in Indian childhood cirrhosis. *Lancet*, **1**, 537.

— (1974). Rosette-forming T lymphocytes and cell-mediated immunity in malnutrition. *Brit. med. J.*, **3**, 608.

CHANDRA, R. K., PAWA, R. R. and GHAI, O. P. (1968). Sugar intolerance in malnourished infants and children. *Brit. med. J.*, **4**, 611.

CHANDRASEKHARAN, N. and CANDLISH, J. K. (1973). The urinary 'hydroxyproline index' in hospitalized and normal Malaysian children. *Trop. geogr. Med.*, **1**, 71.

CHANG, H. T., WANG, C. W., YÜ, C. F., HSÜ, C. F. and FANG, J. C. (1958). Paragonimiasis: a clinical study of 200 adult cases. *Chin. med. J.*, **77**, 3.

CHANG, Y. C., CHU, C. C. and FAN, W. K. (1957). Cerebral schistosomiasis: an observation of forty-five cases. *Chin. med. J.*, **75**, 892.

CHANMUGAM, D. and WANIGANETTI, A. (1969). Guillain-Barré syndrome associated with typhoid fever. *Brit. med. J.*, **1**, 95.

CHAPADEIRO, E., LOPES, E. R. and MESQUITA, P. M. (1965). Primary hydatid cysts of the heart. *J. trop. Med. Hyg.*, **68**, 9.

CHAPUIS, Y. (1973). Acute Chagas' disease in children in Cochabamba (Bolivia). *Ann. Soc. belge Méd. Trop.*, **53**, 6, 581.

CHARACHE, S. and CONLEY, C. L. (1964). Rate of sickling of red cells during deoxygenation of blood from persons with various sickling disorders. *Blood*, **24**, 25.

CHARACHE, S. and RICHARDSON, S. N. (1964). Prolonged survival of a patient with sickle cell anemia. *Arch. intern. Med.*, **113**, 844.

CHARLES, E. D. B. and GRANT, L. S. (1962). Poliomyelitis in Jamaica, W.I. *W. Indian med. J.*, **11**, 203.

CHARLES, L. J. and SMITHERS, B. T. (1959). Hereditary elliptocytosis in two Nigerian families. *W. Afr. med. J.* (N.S.), **8**, 102.

CHARMOT, G. and VARGUES, R. (1963). Les macroglobulinemies en Afrique. *Ann. Soc. belg., Méd. trop.*, **43**, 487.

CHARMOT, G., *et al.* (1966). A report on 50 cases of glucose-6-phosphate dehydrogenase deficiency observed in hospital in Tananarive, Madagascar. *Bull. Soc. Path. exot.*, **59**, 400.

CHARTERS, A. D. and MANSON-BAHR, P. E. C. (1946). Epidemic thrombophlebitis in the East Africa Command. *Lancet*, **2**, 333.

CHARTRES, J. C. and COCKSHOTT, P. (1961). Radiological aspects of some parasitic diseases: porocephalosis. In *Tropical radiology*, ed. H. Middlemiss, p. 119. Heinemann, London.

CHATTERJEA, J. B. (1959). Haemoglobinopathy in India. In *Abnormal Haemoglobins: Symposium*, p. 322. Blackwell Scientific Publications, Oxford.

— (1964). Some aspects of iron-deficiency anaemia in India. *Iron Metabolism—An International Symposium*, p. 219. Springer-Verlag, Berlin and New York.

— (1967). Nutritional megaloblastic anaemia in tropical zones. *J. Indian med. Ass.*, **48**, 51.

CHATTERJEA, J. B., *et al.* (1963). Haematological and biochemical studies in Kyasanur Forest disease. *Indian J. med. Res.*, **51**, 419.

CHATTERJEE, A. and CHOWDHURY, A. B. (1964). Sex dependence of microfilaraemia in infection with *Wuchereria bancrofti*. *Bull. Calcutta Sch. trop. Med.*, **12**, 3.

CHATTERJEE, S. K. (1964). Giant megaureter. *Brit. J. Urol.*, **36**, 406.

CHATTERJEE, S., QUARCOOPOME, C. O. and APENTENG, A. (1970). An epidemic of acute conjunctivitis in Ghana. *Ghana med. J.*, **9**, 9.

CHATTERJI, A. and SEN GUPTA, P. C. (1960). Adrenals in malnourished and under-nourished infants. *Indian J. Pediat.*, **27**, 353.

CHAUDHURI, A., *et al.* (1972). The liver in pre-kwashiorkor and kwashiorkor-marasmus syndromes. *Trans. roy. Soc. trop. Med. Hyg.*, **66**, 258.

CHAUDHURI, A. K. R. and MCKENZIE, P. (1970). Peripheral gangrene after measles. *Brit. med. J.*, **4**, 679.

CHAUDHURI, R. N. (1956). Tropical eosinophilia. *J. Indian med. Ass.*, **27**, 195.

CHAUDHURI, R. N., *et al.* (1956). Chronic splenomegaly. *Indian J. med. Res.*, **44**, 305.

— (1964). Calcutta hemorrhagic fever. *Bull. Calcutta Sch. trop. Med.*, **12**, 1.

CHAVES, E. (1966). Necrotizing and healing pulmonary arteritis in schistosomal cor pulmonale: a retrospective study of ten cases. *Amer. J. trop. Med. Hyg.*, **15**, 162.

CHAVES, E. and PALITOT, P. (1964). Schistosomiasis. *Amer. J. Obstet. Gynec.*, **89**, 1000.

CHEETHAM, H. D., HART, J., COGHILL, N. F. and FOX, B. (1970). Rabies with myocarditis. *Lancet*, **1**, 921.

CHEEVER, A. W. and ANDRADE, Z. A. (1967). Pathological lesions associated with *Schistosoma mansoni* infection in man. *Trans. roy. Soc. trop. Med. Hyg.*, **61**, 626.

CHEEVER, A. W. and WELLER, T. H. (1958). Observations on the growth and nutritional requirements of *Schistosoma mansoni in vitro*. *Amer. J. Hyg.*, **68**, No. 3, 322.

CH'EN, M. C., HU, J. C., CHIANG, P. Y., CHUANG, C. Y., TS'AU, P. F., CHANG, S. H., WANG, F. P., CH'EN, T. L. and CHOU, S. C. (1965). Pathogenesis of carcinoma of the colon and rectum in schistosomiasis japonica: a study of 90 cases. *Chin. med. J.*, **84**, 513.

CH'EN, M. D. and CH'EN, W. S. C. (1957). Acute colonic obstruction in *schistosomiasis japonicum*. *Chin. med. J.*, **75**, 517.

CHEN, T. H. and MEYER, K. F. (1966). An evaluation of *Pasteurella pestis* fraction-1-specific antibody for the confirmation of plague infections. *Bull. Wld Hlth Org.*, **34**, 911.

CHEN, T. H. (1971). Schistosomiasis in mainland China. *Amer. J. trop. Med. Hyg.*, **20**, 26.

CHERRY, J. K. T. (1959). Adenolymphocoele and elephantiasis in onchocerciasis. *E. Afr. med. J.*, **36**, 224.

CHHETRI, M. K., *et al.* (1970). Endocardial lesions in a case of takayasu's arteriopathy. *Brit. Heart J.*, **32**, 859.

CHIEN TEH and LIU YU-K'UN (1957). Clinical analysis of one hundred and seventy fatal cases observed during antimony treatment. *Chinese J. Int. Med.*, **5**, 524.

CHING-FAN, C. (1957). *Schistosoma japonicum* of the colon associated with carcinoma. *Chin. Med. J.*, **75**, 500.

CHILD, L. P., MACKENZIE, R. B., VALVERDE, L. R. and JOHNSON, K. M. (1967). Bolivian haemorrhagic fever. *Arch. Path.*, **83**, 434.

CHILDS, B. and ZINKHAM, W. H. (1959). The genetics of primaquine sensitivity of the erythrocytes. In: *Biochemistry of Human Genetics*, p. 76. Eds: Wolstenholme, G. E. W. and O'Connor, C. M., Little, Brown & Company, Boston.

CHINERY, W. A. and CHRISTIAN, E. C. (1972). Myiasis fly larvae in the 'liver' of adult Ghanaian. *Ghana med. J.*, **11**, 186.

CHISLER, E., *et al.* (1965). Annular subvalvular left ventricular aneurysms in the South African Bantu. *Circulation*, **32**, 43.

CHITWOOD, M. B., *et al.* (1968). Capillaria Philippinensis Sp. N (Nematoda: Trichinellida) from the intestine of man in the Philippines. *J. Parasit.*, **54**, 368.

CHOREMIS, C., *et al.* (1966). Viral hepatitis in G-6-Pd deficiency. *Lancet*, **1**, 269.

CHOWDHURY, A. B. and SCHAD, G. A. (1972). *Ancylostoma ceylanicum:* A parasite of man in Calcutta and environs. *Amer. J. trop. Med. Hyg.*, **21**, 3, 300.

CHOYCE, D. P. (1964). Ocular onchocerciasis in Central America, Africa and British Isles (with a note on equine periodic ophthalmia). *Trans. roy. Soc. trop. Med. Hyg.*, **58**, 11.

— (1964). The eyes in leprosy. In *Leprosy in Theory and Practice*, ed. R. G. Cochrane and T. F. Davey, 2nd ed., p. 310.

— (1972). Kerato-uveal changes in leprosy and onchocerciasis: a question of immunity. *Proc. roy. Soc. Med.*, **65**, 955.

CHRISTOPHERSON, W. M., WILLIAMSON, E. O. and GRAY, L. A. (1972). Leiomyosarcoma of the uterus. *Cancer*, **29**, 1512.

CHUNG, H. L. and CH'EN, H. C. (1957). Primary carcinoma of liver : a clinical analysis of 107 cases. *Chin. med. J.*, **75**, 295.

CHUTTANI, H. K., *et al.* (1967). Hookworm disease and duodenal ulceration. *Gut*, **8**, 69.

— (1967). Ulcerative colitis in the tropics. *Brit. med. J.*, **4**, 204.

CIFERRI, F., *et al.* (1965). Immunologic studies in onchocerciasis and bancroftian filariasis. I. Intracutaneous tests with antigens extracted from *Onchocerca* and *Dirofilaria*. *Amer. J. trop. Med. Hyg.*, **14**, 263.

CIFUENTES, E., CALDERON, E. and BIJLENGA, G. (1971). Rabies in a child diagnosed by a new intra-vitam method. The cornea test. *J. trop. Med. Hyg.*, **74**, 23.

CLANCEY, J. K. (1964). Mycobacterial skin ulcers in Uganda: description of a new *Mycobacterium (Mycobacterium buruli) J. Path. Bact.* **88**, 175.

CLANCEY, J. K., *et al.* (1961). Mycobacterial skin ulcers in Uganda. *Lancet*, **2**, 951.

CLARK, A. W., LLOYD-MOSTYN, R. H. and SADLER, M. R. DE C. (1972). 'Ischaemic' colitis in young adults. *Brit. med. J.*, **4**, 70.

CLARK, B. M. and EDINGTON, G. M. (1971). In *Human Infection with Fungi, Actinomycetes and Algae*, p. 684. Springer Verlag, New York.

CLARK, B. M. and GREENWOOD, B. M. (1968). Pulmonary lesions in African histoplasmosis. *J. trop. Med. Hyg.*, **71**, 4.

CLARK, W. H., *et al.* (1969). The histogenesis and biologic behaviour of primary human malignant melanomas of the skin. *Cancer Res.*, **29**, 705.

CLARKE, A. (1936). Report on the effects of certain poisons contained in food-plants of West Africa upon the health of the native races. *J. trop. Med. Hyg.*, **39**, 269.

CLARKE, G. H. (1959). *Skin Diseases in the African*. H. K. Lewis, London.

CLARKE, G. H. V. (1952). A note on dermatitis cruris pustulosa et atrophicans. *Trans. roy. Soc. trop. Med. Hyg.*, **46**, 558.

— (1952). The velvet leg syndrome. *W. Afr. med. J.* (N.S.), **1**, 134.

CLARKE, V. de V. (1966). Evidence of the development in man of acquired resistance to infection of *Schistosoma* spp. *Cent. Afr. J. Med.*, **12**, No. 1, 1.

CLARKE, V. de V., WARBURTON, B. and BLAIR, D. M. (1970). The Katayama syndrome: report on an outbreak in Rhodesia. *Cent. Afr. J. Med.*, **16**, 123.

CLARKSON, A. R., *et al.* (1971). Serum and urinary fibrin/fibrinogen degradation products in glomerulonephritis. *Brit. med. J.*, **3**, 447.

CLEAVE, T. L., CARPBELL, G. D. and PAINTER, N. S. (1967). *Diabetes, coronary thrombosis and the Saccharine Disease*. John Wright, Bristol.

CLEGG, J. A., SMITHERS, S. R. and TERRY, R. J. (1970). Host antigens associated with schistosomes: observations on their attachment and their nature. *Parasitology*, **61**, 87.

— (1971*a*). Concomitant immunity and host antigens associated with schistosomiasis. *Int. J. Parasit.*, **1**, 43.

— (1971*b*). Acquisition of human antigens by *Schistosomiasis mansoni* during cultivation *in vitro*. *Nature (Lond.)*, **232**, 653.

CLEMENTS, F. W. (1960). Naturally occurring goitrogens. *Brit. med. Bull.*, **16**, 133.

CLEMENTS, F. W. and WISHART, J. W. (1956). A thyroid-blocking agent in the etiology of endemic goiter. *Metabolism*, **5**, 623.

CLEMMESEN, J. (1968). A doubling of morbidity from testis carcinoma in Copenhagen. *Acta path. microbiol. scand.*, **72**, 348.

CLIFFORD, P. (1965). Carcinoma of the nasopharynx in Kenya. *E. Afr. med. J.*, **42**, 373.

CLIFFORD, P. and BULBROOK, R. D. (1966). Endocrine studies in African males with nasopharyngeal cancer. *Lancet*, **1**, 1228.

COADY, A. (1964). Aflatoxin. (Correspondence.) *Brit. med. J.*, **1**, 1510.

COATNEY, G. R. (1968). Simian malarias in man. *Amer. J. trop. Med. Hyg.* **17**, 147.

COCHRAN, R. T. (1963). Hyposthenuria in sickle cell states. *Arch. intern. Med.*, **112**, 222.

COCHRANE, C. G. and DIXON, F. J. (1968). *Textbook of Immunology*, eds. P. A. Miescher and H. J. Muller-Eberhard, p. 94. Grune and Stratton, New York.

COCHRANE, R. G. and DAVEY, T. F., eds. (1964). *Leprosy in Theory and Practice*. 2nd ed. Wright, Bristol.

COCKSHOTT, P. (1961). Splenic abscesses. In *Tropical Radiology*. Ed. by H. Middlemiss, p. 205. Heinemann, London.

COCKSHOTT, W. P. (1963). Carpal fusions. *Amer. J. Roent. genol.*, **89**, 1260.

— (1965). Some radiological aspects of the S haemoglobinopathies as seen in Ibadan. In *Abnormal Haemoglobins in Africa*, ed. J. H. P. Jonxis, p. 131. Blackwell, Oxford.

— (1965). Radiological aspects of Burkitt's tumour. *Brit. J. Radiol.*, **38**, 172.

— (1965). Angiocardiography of endomyocardial fibrosis. *Brit. J. Radiol.*, **38**, 192.

COCKSHOTT, W. P. and LUCAS, A. O. (1964). Histoplasmosis duboisii. *Quart. J. Med.*, **33**, 223.

COCKSHOTT, P. and MCGREGOR, M. (1958). Osteitis variolosa. *Quart. J. Med.*, **27**, 639.

COCKSHOTT, W. P. and WEAVER, E. J. M. (1962). Primary tropical splenic abscess: a misnomer. *Brit. J. Surg.*, **49**, 665.

COGHLAN, J. D. and WEIR, D. M. (1967). Antibodies in human brucellosis. *Brit. med. J.*, **2**, 269.

COHEN, M. H., *et al.* (1970). Infectious mononucleosis followed by Burkitt's Tumour. *Ann. intern. Med.*, **73**, 591.

COHEN, S. and HANSEN, J. D. L. (1962). Metabolism of albumin and gamma globulin in kwashiorkor. *Clin. Sci.*, **23**, 351.

COHEN, S., MCGREGOR, I. A. and CARRINGTON, S. (1961). Gamma-globulin and acquired immunity to human malaria. *Nature (Lond.)*, **192**, 733.

COHEN, N. A. (1963). Myocarditis in prodromal measles. *Amer. J. clin. Path.*, **40**, 50.

COLBOURNE, M. J., EDINGTON, G. M. and HUGHES, M. H. (1950). A medical survey in a Gold Coast village. *Trans. roy. Soc. trop. Med. Hyg.*, **44**, 271.

COLE, A. C. F., RIDLE, D. S. and WOLFE, H. R. I. (1965). Bowel infection with *Histoplasma duboisii*. *J. trop. Med. Hyg.*, **68**, 92.

COLE, G. J. (1965). A review of 436 cases of intestinal obstruction in Ibadan. *Gut*, **6**, 151.

COLES, R. M. and DAVIES, J. N. P. (1959). The normal heart weight of Uganda Africans: Mulago Hospital post-mortem studies, no. XII. *E. Afr. med. J.*, **36**, 76.

COLLARD, P. (1962). Antibodies against brucellae in the sera of healthy persons in various parts of Nigeria. *W. Afr. med. J.* (n.s.), **11**, 172.

COLLARD, P. and UDEOZO, I. O. K. (1959). Serological evidence of the existence of Q-Fever in Ibadan. *W. Afr. Med. J.* **8**, 137.

COLLIER, L. H., DUKE-ELDER, S. and JONES, B. R. (1958). Experimental trachoma produced by cultured virus. *Brit. J. Ophthal.*, **42**, 705.

COLLIER, L. H. and SOWA, J. (1958). Isolation of trachoma virus in embryonate eggs. *Lancet*, **1**, 993.

COLLINS, W. E., et al. (1966). Fluorescent antibody studies in human malaria. IV. Cross-reactions between human and simian malaria. *Amer. J. trop. Med. Hyg.*, **15**, 11.

COLLINS, J. R. (1965). Small intestinal mucosal damage with villous atrophy. *Amer. J. clin. Path.*, **44**, 36.

COLLOMB, H., DUMAS, M., LEMERCIER, G. and GIRARD, P. L. (1970). Sclérose en Plaqeus Au Sénégal. *Afri. J. med. Sci.*, **1**, 257.

COLLOMB, H., GIRARD, P.-L., DUMAS, M. and COURSON, B. (1971). Cancers en neurologie. *Méd. Afr. noire*, **18**, 539.

COLLOMB, H., et al. (1966). La part des malformations vasulaires dans les accidents hémorragiques cérébraux. *Bull. Soc. méd. Afr. noire Langue franç.* **11**, 243.

COLLOMB, H., et al. (1967). Les neuropathies dites nutritionnelles au Sénégal. *J. neurol. Sci.*, **5**, 159.

COMMUNICABLE DISEASE CENTER (ATLANTA) (1966). *Leptospiral Serotype Distribution Lists according to Host and Geographic Area*. U.S. Department of Health, Education, Welfare, Public Health Service.

COMTE, H., MARTIN, L. A. and OURADOU, J. (1960). A propos de 42 cas d'artérite dite juvénile. *Arch. Inst. Pasteur Maroc*, **6**, 85.

CONLEY, C. L. (1964). Pathophysiological effects of some abnormal hemoglobins. *Medicine (Baltimore)*, **43**, 785.

CONNOR, D. H. and LUNN, H. F. (1966). Buruli ulceration. *Arch. Path.*, **81**, 183.

CONRAD, M. E. (1969). Persistent haemolysis after infectious hepatitis. *Gut*, **10**, 516.

CONSTANTOPOULOS, A., et al. (1973). Fulminant diarrhoea and acute haemolysis due to G-6-PD. Deficiency in salmonellosis. *Lancet*, **1**, 1522.

CONTACOS, P. G. and COLLINS, W. E. (1973). Malaria relapse mechanism. *Trans. roy. Soc. trop. Med. Hyg.*, **67**, 4, 617.

CONVIT, J., ARVELO, J. J. and MENDOZA, S. (1960). Lepromatous myositis. *Int. J. Leprosy*, **28**, 417.

CONVIT, J. and KERDEL-VEGAS, F. (1965). Disseminated cutaneous leishmaniasis: innoculation [*sic*] to laboratory animals, electron microscopy and fluorescent antibodies studies. *Arch. Derm.*, **91**, 439.

CONVIT, J., REYES, O. and KERDEL, F. (1957). Disseminated anergic American leishmaniasis: report of three cases of a type clinically resembling lepromatous leprosy. *A.M.A. Arch. Derm.*, **76**, 213.

CONVIT, J. E. and PINARDI, M. E. (1974). *Cutaneous Leishmaniasis: the Clinical and Immunopathological Spectrum in South America. Trypanosomiasis and Leishmaniasis*. Ciba Foundation Symposium 20 (new series). Associated Scientific Publishers, Amsterdam.

COOK, G. C. (1967). Lactase activity in newborn and infant Baganda. *Brit. med. J.*, **1**, 527.

COOK, G. C. and HUTT, M. S. R. (1967). The liver after kwashiorkor. *Brit. med. J.*, **3**, 454.

COOK, G. C. and KAJABI, S. K. (1966). Tribal incidence of lactase deficiency in Uganda. *Lancet*, **1**, 725.

COOK, G. C. and LEE, F. D. (1966). The jejunum after kwashiorkor. *Lancet*, **2**, 1263.

COOK, J. (1963). Pyomyositis. *E. Afr. med. J.*, **40**, 574.

COOK, J., MCFADZEAN, A. J. S. and TODD, D. (1963). Splenectomy in cryptogenetic splenomegaly. *Brti. med. J.*, **2**, 337.

COOK, P. (1971). Cancer of the oesophagus in Africa. *Brit. J. Cancer*, **25**, 853.

COOKE, R. A. (1969). Tumoral calcinosis. *Brit. med. J.*, **4**, 174.

COOKE, W. T., *et al.* (1974). Rickets, growth and alkaline phosphatase in urban adolescents. *Brit. med. J.*, **2**, 293.

COOPER, L. Z., *et al.* (1969). Rubella: clinical manifestations and management. *Amer. J. Dis. Child.*, **118**, 18.

COORAY, G. H. (1960). Some observations on filarial infection in Ceylon with special reference to its histopathology. *Indian J. Malar.*, **14**, 617.

CORNBLATH, M., ROSENTHAL, I. M. and REISNER, S. H. (1963). Hereditary fructose intolerance. *New Eng. J. Med.*, **269**, 1271.

CORNIOU, B., *et al.* (1972). First isolation of a South American strain of Eastern Equine virus from a case of encephalitis in Trinidad. *Trop. geogr. Med.*, **24**, 162.

CORREA, P. and LLANOS, G. (1966). Morbidity and mortality from cancer in Cali, Colombia. *J. nat. Cancer Inst.*, **36**, 717.

CORREA, P., RESTREPO, C., GARCIA, C. and QUIROZ, A. C. (1963). Pathology of heart diseases of undetermined etiology which occur in Cali, Colombia. *Amer. Heart J.*, **66**, 584.

CORTNER, J. A. (1959). Giardiasis, a cause of celiac syndrome. *A.M.A. J. Dis. Child.*, **98**, 311.

COSNETT, J. E. and GIBB, B. H. (1969). Tuberous sclerosis and cardiac arrhythmia in three Zulu patients. *Brit. med. J.*, **2**, 672.

COTTENOT, F. (1964). Quantitative appreciation of serum antibodies in human leprosy, with the use of Murine leprosy bacillus. *C. R. Soc. Biol. (Paris)*, **158**, 1004.

COURDURIER, J. and BRYGOO, E. (1947). The blood sedimentation rate in Africans. *Med. trop., Marseilles.* **7**, 254.

COURT BROWN, W. M. and DOLL, R. (1961). Leukaemia in childhood and young adult life. Trends in mortality in relation to aetiology. *Brit. med. J.*, **1**, 981.

COWPER, S. G. and JACKSON, H. (1964). Onchocercal hydrocoele without cutaneous manifestations. *J. trop. Med. Hyg.*, **67**, 69.

COX, M. L. (1963). Contracted pelvis in Nigeria. *J. Obstet. Gynaec. Brit. Cwlth.*, **70**, 487.

COX, P. S. V. (1965). Six cases of sparganosis from South Karamoja. (Correspondence). *E. Afr. med. J.*, **42**, 319.

— (1966). Brucellosis: a survey in south Karamoja. *E. Afr. med. J.*, **43**, 43.

CRAIL, N. W., ALT, H. I. and NADLER, W. H. (1948). Myelofibrosis associated with tuberculosis. *Blood*, **3**, 1426.

CRANE, G. G. (1972). The tropical splenomegaly syndrome in New Guinea—a review. *Papua N. Guinea med. J.*, **15**, 3.

CRANE, G. G., HUDSON, P. and HUDSON, B. E. T. (1973). The effect of suppressive antimalarial therapy in tropical splenomegaly syndrome in New Guineans. *Papua N. Guinea med. J.*, **16**, 46.

CRANE, G. G., WELLS, J. V. and JONES, P. (1974). The role of plasma proteins in chronic expansion of plasma volume in tropical splenomegaly syndrome. I. Metabolism of ^{131}I-labelled albumin. *Trans. roy. Soc. trop. Med. Hyg.*, **68**, 246.

CRANE, G. G., *et al.* (1971). Immunoglobulin levels in the Kaiapit and Upper Watut areas of New Guinea. *Trans. roy. Soc. trop. Med. Hyg.*, **65**, 795.

— (1972). Humoral immune responses in the tropical splenomegaly syndrome in New Guinea. *Clin. Sci.*, **43**, 869.

— (1972). Tropical splenomegaly syndrome in New Guinea. I. Natural history. *Trans. roy. Soc. trop. Med. Hyg.*, **66**, 724.

— (1972). Tropical splenomegaly syndrome in New Guinea. II. Long term results of splenectomy. *Trans. roy. Soc. trop. Med. Hyg.*, **66**, 733.

CRANE, P. S., PAK, Y. H. and LEE, H. K. (1965). Surgical complications of massive infestations with *Ascaris lumbricoides*. *Ann. Surg.*, **162**, 34.

CRAVIOTO, J. (1966). Malnutrition and behavioural development in the pre-school child. In *Pre-school child malnutrition: ... an international conference on prevention of malnutrition in the pre-school child, Washington, D.C., December 7–11, 1964,* p. 74. Nat. Acad. Sci.—Nat. Res. Coun., Washington.

CRAVIOTO, J. and DELICARDIE, E. R. (1970). Mental performance in school age children. *Amer. J. Dis. Child.*, **120**, 404.

CRAWFORD, M. A. (1963). Endomyocardial fibrosis and carcinoidosis: a common denominator? *Amer. Heart J.*, **66**, 273.

CROCE, E. J., MacGILLIVRAY, W. F. and MURPHY, C. J. Salpingitis due to *Enterobius vermicularis*. Report of a case. *New Engl. J. Med.*, **254**, 67.

CROFTON, J. W., *et al.* (1952). Pulmonary eosinophilia. *Thorax*, **7**, 1.

CROSBY, W. H. (1969). Haemochromatosis and venesection. *Brit. med. J.*, **4**, 109.

CROSS, J. H. (1969). Fasciolopsiasis in S.E. Asia and the Far East: A review. In *Proceedings of the 4th S.E. Asian Seminar on Parasitology and Tropical Medicine, Schistosomiasis and other snail-transmitted helminthiasis*, p. 177. Manila.

CROSS, J. H., *et al.* (1972). Studies on the experimental transmission of *Capillaria philippinensis* in monkeys. *Trans. roy. Soc. trop. Med. Hyg.*, **66**, 819.

CRUICKSHANK, E. K. (1956). A neuropathic syndrome of uncertain origin. *W. Indian med. J.*, **5**, 147.

CRUICKSHANK, J. G., BEDSON, H. S. and WATSON, D. H. (1966). Electron microscopy in the rapid diagnosis of smallpox. *Lancet*, **2**, 527.

CUADRA, C. M. (1956). Salmonellosis complication in human bartonellosis. *Texas Rep. Biol. Med.*, **14**, 97.

CUATRECASAS, P., LOCKWOOD, D. H. and CALDWELL, J. R. (1965). Lactase deficiency in the adult. *Lancet*, **1**, 14.

CUNNINGHAM, M. P., *et al.* (1967). The estimation of IgM immunoglobulin in dried blood, for use as a screening test in the diagnosis of human trypanosomiasis in Africa. *Trans. roy. Soc. trop. Med. Hyg.*, **61**, 688.

CURRIE, G. A. and BAGSHAWE, K. D. (1967). The masking of antigens on trophoblast and cancer cells. *Lancet*, **1**, 708.

CURZEN, P. (1964). Sickle cell disease with 'leather pouch' uterus. *Brit. med. J.*, **1**, 1360.

CVJETANOVIC, B., *et al.* (1972). Epidemiological model of tetanus and its use in the planning of immunization programmes. *Int. J. Epidem.*, **1**, 2, 125.

— (1972). Epidemiological model of typhoid fever and its use in the planning and evaluation of antityphoid immunization and sanitation programmes. *WHO Bull.*, **45**, 1.

DACIE, J. V. (1970). Auto immune haemolytic anaemia. *Brit. med. J.*, **2**, 381.

— (1974). The hereditary haemolytic anaemia: The Croonian Lecture 1973. *J. roy. Coll. Phycns Lond.*, **8**, 206.

DACIE, J. V., et al. (1969). Non-tropical idiopathic splenomegaly. *Brit. J. Haemat.*, **17**, 317.

DA COSTA, L. R. (1971). Small intestinal cell turnover in patients with parasitic infections. *Brit. med. J.*, **3**, 281.

DADA, T. O. and ODEKU, E. L. (1966). Epilepsy in the Nigerian patient: a review of 234 cases. *W. Afr. med. J.*, **15**, 153.

DAENGSVANG, S., et al. (1964). Epidemiological observations on *Gnathostoma spinigerum* in Thailand. *J. trop. Med. Hyg.*, **67**, 144.

DAFTARY, V. G. and BHENDE, Y. M. (1956). *Postgrad. med. J.*, **2**, 44.

DAGUET, G. L. and LANGUILLON, J. (1961). Serological tests in 150 cases of leprosy. *Brit. J. vener. Dis.*, **37**, 282.

DALAL, P. M., SHAH, P. M., AIYAR, R. R. and KIKANI, B. J. (1968). Cerebrovascular diseases in West Central India. *Brit. med. J.*, **3**, 769.

DALGAARD, O. Z. (1957). Bilateral polycystic disease of the kidneys: a follow-up of two hundred and eighty-four patients and their families. *Acta med. scand.*, **158**, suppl. 328.

DALGLEISH, P. G. and ANSELL, B. M. (1950). Anaphylactoid purpura in pulmonary tuberculosis. *Brit. med. J.*, **1**, 225.

DALLDORF, G. (1951). The sparing effect of coxsackie virus infection on experimental poliomyelitis. *J. exp. Med.*, **94**, 65.

DAMLUJI, S. F., AL-KHOURY, M. and JOHNSTONE, R. M. (1964). Cor pulmonale due to chronic infestation with *Schistosoma haematobium*. *J. trop. Med. Hyg.*, **67**, 220.

DANARAJ, T. J. (1958). Treatment of eosinophilic lung (tropical eosinophilia) with diethylcarbamazine. *Quart. J. Med.*, **27**, 243.

DANARAJ, T. J., de SILVA, L. S. and SCHACHER, J. F. (1959). Serological diagnosis of eosinophilic lung (tropical eosinophilia) and its etiological implications. *Amer. J. trop. Med.*, **8**, 151.

DANARAJ, T. J. and ONG, W. H. (1959). Primary arteritis of abdominal aorta in children causing bilateral stenosis of renal arteries and hypertension. *Circulation*, **20**, 856.

DANARAJ, T. J., WONG, H. O. and THOMAS, M. A. (1963). Primary arteritis of aorta causing renel artery stenosis and hypertension. *Brit. Heart J.*, **25**, 153.

DANARAJ, T. J., et al. (1966). The etiology and pathology of eosinophilic lung (tropical eosinophila). *Amer. J. trop. Med. Hyg.*, **15**, 183.

DANCE, N. and HUEHNS, E. R. (1962). A haemoglobin containing only δ-chains. *Biochem. biophys. Res. Commun.*, **7**, 444.

DANE, D. S., CAMERON, C. H. and BRIGGS, M. (1970). Virus-like particles in serum of patients with Australia-antigen associated hepatitis. *Lancet*, **1**, 695.

DANIEL, P. M. (1971). Transmissible degenerative diseases of the nervous system. *Proc. roy. Soc. Med.*, **64**, 787.

DAO, C., FU, F. Y. and CH'I, W. L. (1956). Pulmonary manifestations in schistosomiasis following tartar emetic therapy. *Chin. med. J.*, **74**, 268.

DAS, G. C. and SEN, S. B. (1968). Chylous arthritis. *Brit. med. J.*, **2**, 27.

DAS, R. K. and SEIDELIN, R. (1972). Blood dyscrasias and myocarditis in infectious mononucleosis. *Brit. med. J.*, **1**, 289.

DA SILVA, L., et al. (1970). Kidney biopsy in the hepatosplenic form of infection with *Schistosoma mansoni* in man. *Bull. Wld Hlth Org.* **42**, 907.

DA SILVA, L. C., DE BRITO, T., CAMARGO, M. E., DEBONI, D. R., LOPES, J. D. and GUNJI, J. (1970). Kidney biopsy in the hepatosplenic form of infection with *Schistosoma mansoni* in man. *Bull. Wld Hlth Org.*, **42**, 907.

DAVEY, T. F., DREWETT, S. E. and STONE, CYNTHIA. (1958). Tuberculin and lepromin sensitivity in E. Nigeria. *Leprosy Rev.* **29**, 81.

DAVEY, W. W. and DICKSON, J. A. S. (1964). Stomal ulcer in Nigeria. *J. roy. Coll. Surg. Edinb.*, **9**, 300.

DAVEY, W. W. and PEARSON, J. B. (1965). Obstruction of the third part of the duodenum. *Brit. J. Surg.*, **52**, 189.

DAVID, H. L. and EDESON, J. F. B. (1965). Filariasis in Portuguese Timor, with observations on a new microfilaria found in man. *Ann. trop. Med. Parasit.*, **59**, 193.

DAVIDSON, C. S. (1963). Fungal toxins in the etiology of human and animal diseases. *Med. Sci.*, **14**, 32.

DAVIDSON, SIR S. and PASSMORE, R. (1966). *Human Nutrition and Dietetics*. 3rd ed. Livingstone, London, Edinburgh.

DAVID-WEST, A. S. (1974). Relapses after withdrawal of Proguanil treatment in tropical splenomegaly syndrome. *Brit. med. J.*, **3**, 499.

DAVID-WEST, T. S. (1972). The use of mouse embryo cell cultures in primary isolation of Chikungunya virus. *Bull. Wld Hlth Org.*, **45**, 487.

DAVIES, J. N. P. (1948). Pathology of Central African natives. Causes of sudden death in Africans. *E. Afr. med. J.*, **25**, 322.

— (1948). Endocardial fibrosis in Africans. *E. Afr. med. J.*, **25**, 10.

— (1952). Primary carcinoma of the liver in Uganda Africans. *W. Afr. med. J.* (n.s.), **1**, 141.

— (1956). Endomyocardial fibrosis in Uganda. *Central Afr. J. med.*, **2**, 323.

— (1965). Leukaemia in children in tropical Africa. *Lancet*, **2**, 65.

DAVIES, J. N. P. with the assistance of COLES, R. M. (1960). Some considerations regarding obscure diseases affecting the mural endocardium. *Amer. Heart J.*, **59**, 600.

DAVIES, J. N. P., KNOWELDEN, J. and WILSON, B. A. (1965). Incidence rates of cancer in Kyadondo County, Uganda, 1954–1960. *J. nat. Cancer Inst.*, **35**, 789.

DAVIES, J. N. P. and OWOR, R. (1965). Chloromatous tumours in African children in Uganda. *Brit. med. J.*, **2**, 405.

DAVIES, J. N. P. *et al.* (1964). Cancer in an African community, 1897–1956: an analysis of the records or Mengo Hospital, Kampala, Uganda. Parts 1, 2. *Brit. med. J.*, **1**, 259, 336.

DAVIES, P. R. and ROWLAND, H. A. K. (1965). Vertebral fractures in West Africans suffering from tetanus: a clinical and osteological study. *J. Bone Jt Surg.*, Brit. ed., **47**, 61.

DAVIS, A. (1973). Drug treatment in intestinal helminthiases, WHO, Geneva.

DAVIS, C. M. (1970). Granuloma inguinale. *J. Amer. med. Ass.*, **211**, 632.

DAWKINS, R. L. and JOSKE, R. A. (1973). Immunoglobulin deposition in liver of patients with active chronic hepatitis and antibody against smooth muscle. *Brit. med. J.*, **2**, 643.

DAWSON, J. (1945). Cancrum oris. *Brit. dent. J.*, **79**, 151.

DAWSON, J. L. M. (1966). Kwashiorkor, gynaecomastia, and feminization processes. *J. trop. Med. Hyg.*, **68**, 175.

DEALL, A. M. (1971). Diagnosis of cystic fibrosis. *Brit. med. J.*, **3**, 639.

DEAN, G. (1967). Annual incidence, prevalence, and mortality of multiple sclerosis in white South-African-born and in white immigrants to South Africa. *Brit. med. J.*, **2**, 724.

DEANE, L. M. and DEANE, M. P. (1964). Visceral leishmaniasis in South and Central America. *Arq. Hig. Saúde Públ.*, **29,** 89.

DE CARNERI, I., *et al.* (1973). Subcutaneous dirofilariasis in man—not so rare. *Trans. roy. Soc. trop. Med. Hyg.*, **67,** 887.

DEEGAN, T., GILLES, H. M. and MCGREGOR, I. A. (1956). Observations on the erythrocyte sedimentation rates and blood protein patterns of Gambian Africans. *Ann. trop. Med. Parasit.*, **50,** 451.

DEEGAN, T. and MAEGRAITH, B. G. (1956). Studies on the nature of malarial pigment (Haemozoin). II : The pigment of the human species, *Plasmodium falciparum* and *Plasmodium malariae. Ann. trop. Med. Parasit.*, **50,** 212.

DEGAZON, D. W. (1956). Tropical amblyopia in Jamaica. *W. Indian med. J.*, **5,** 223.

DEGEN, J. A. (1937). Visceral pathology in measles. *Amer. J. med. Sci.*, **194,** 104.

DE GROOTE, J., *et al.* (1968). A classification of chronic hepatitis. *Lancet*, **2,** 626.

DEGROOTE, V. (1960). Note préliminaire sur les flèches empoisonnées et les poisons de flèches au Congo belge. *Ann. Soc. belge Méd. trop.*, **40,** 97.

DE GRUCHY, G. C. (1966). *Clinical Haematology in Medical Practice.* 2nd ed. Blackwell, Oxford.

DE GRUCHY, G. C. and GRIMES, A. J. (1968). Haemolytic anaemias associated with abnormalities of the Embdenmeyerhof pathway. Recent Advances in Clinical Pathology, p. 241. J. & A. Churchill, London.

DE LEON, E. P. and PARDO DE TAVERA, M. (1968). Pulmonary schistosomiasis in the Philippines. *Dis. Chest*, **63,** 154.

DE LEON, J. R. and DUKE, B. O. L. (1966). Experimental studies on the transmission of Guatemalan and West African strains of *Onchocerca volvulus* by *Simulium ochraceum*, *S. metallicum* and *S. callidum. Trans. roy. Soc. trop. Med. Hyg.*, **60,** 735.

DELLER, J. J. JR., *et al.* (1967). Malaria hepatitis. *Milit. Med.*, **132,** 614.

DEMISSIE, A. and SVEDMYR, A. (1968). Age Distribution to antibodies to Burkitt cells. *Acta. path. microbiol. Scand.*, **73,** 653.

DE MOOR, P. P. and STEFFENS, F. E. (1970). A computer-simulated model of an arthropod-borne virus transmission cycle, with special reference to Chikungunya virus. *Trans. roy Soc. trop. Med. Hyg.*, **64,** 927.

DENNIS, L. H., EICHELBERGER, I. W., INMAN, M. M. and CONRAD, M. E. (1967). Depletion of blood coagulation factors in drug resistant *P. falciparum* malaria. *Blood*, **29,** 713.

DENNIS, L. H., *et al.* (1966). A coagulation defect and its treatment with heparin in *Plasmodium knowlesi* malaria in rhesus monkeys. *Research in Malaria.* Suppl. *Milit. Med.*, **131,** 1107.

DENTON, J. G. (1970). Fatal pulmonary oedema as a complication of acute falciparum malaria. *Amer. J. trop. Med. Hyg.*, **19,** 196.

DE QUADROS, C. C. A., *et al.* (1972). Epidemiology of variola minor in Brazil based on a study of 33 outbreaks. *Bull. Wld Hlth Org.*, **46,** 165.

DE RAADT, P. (1974). *Immunity and Antigenic Variation: Clinical Observations Suggestive of Immune Phenomena in Trypanosomiasis.* Ciba Foundation Symposium 20 (new series). Associated Scientific Publishers, Amsterdam.

DERN, R. J., *et al.* (1954). The hemolytic effect of primaquine. I. The localization of the drug-induced hemolytic defect in primaquine-sensitive individuals. *J. Lab. clin. Med.*, **43,** 303.

DE ROEVER-BONNET, H. (1972). Toxoplasmosis in tropical Africa. *Trop. geogr. Med.*, **24,** 7.

DERRICK, E. H. (1948). A fatal case of generalized amoebiasis due to a protozoon closely resembling, if not identical with, *Iodamoeba butschlii*. *Trans. roy. Soc. trop. Med. Hyg.*, **42**, 191.

— (1964). *The Query Fever*. The Elkington Oration. Queensland Health. **1**, 1.

DESAI, H. G. and JEEJEEBHOY, K. N. (1967). Jejunal mucosa and absorption studies in tropical malabsorption syndrome. *Indian J. Path. Bact.*, **10**, 107.

DESAI, H. G., et al. (1967). Intestinal disaccharidasas in tropical sprue. *Gastroenterology*, **53**, 375.

DESAI, S. C. (1963). Mycotic infection as a world problem. *Proc. 12th Int. Cong. Dermat.* **2**, Excerpta Medica Foundation, Amsterdam.

DESCHIENS, R. and COURDURIER, J. (1966). Observations on eosinophilic meningitis caused by *Angiostronylus*. *Bull. Soc. Path. exot.*, **59**, 349.

DE SILVA, K. (1970). Intraperitoneal rupture of an amoebic liver abscess in a pregnant woman at term. *Ceylon med. J.*, **15**, 51.

DESMONTS, G., COUVREUR, J., ALISON, F., BAUDELOT, J., GERBEAUX, J. and LELONG, M. (1965). Étude épidémiologique sur la toxoplasmose: de l'influence de la cuisson des viandes de boucherie sur la fréquence de l'infection humaine. *Revue franç. Étude. clin. biol.*, **10**, 952.

DESOWITZ, R. S. (1959). Studies on immunity and host parasite relationships. I. The immunological response of resistant and susceptible breeds of cattle to trypanosome challenge. *Ann. trop. Med. Parasit.*, **53**, 293.

DESOWITZ, R. S. and SAAVE, J. J. (1965). The application of the haemagglutination test to a study of the immunity to malaria in protected and unprotected population groups of Australian New Guinea. *Bull. Wld Hlth Org.*, **32**, 149.

DE TAVERA, M. P. and DE LEON, E. P. (1967). Tuberculosis of the lymphatics in children, its relation to spinal tuberculosis. *Dis. Chest*, **52**, 469.

DETELS, R., et al. (1969). An epidemic of intestinal capillariasis in man. *Amer. J. trop. Med. Hyg.*, **18**, 676.

DEVAKUL, K., AREEKUL, S. and VIRAVAN, C. (1967). Vitamin B_{12} absorption test in amoebic liver abscess. *Ann. trop. Med. Parasit.*, **61**, 29.

DEVAKUL, K., GARBY, L. and HARINASUTA, T. (1966). Erythrocyte destruction in *Plasmodium falciparum* malaria: effects of erythrocyte glucose-6-phosphate dehydrogenase deficiency. *Ann. trop. Med. Parasit.*, **60**, 432.

DEVAKUL, K., et al. (1966). ^{125}I-Labelled fibrinogen in cerebral malaria. *Lancet*, **2**, 886.

DEVI, P. K. (1966). Observations on anaemia of pregnancy in India. *Israeli J. Med. Sci.*, **2**, 494.

DEWHURST, W. G. and MORGAN, H. G. (1970). Importance of urine volume in assessment of Thiamin deficiency. *Amer. J. clin. Nutr.*, **23**, 379.

DEWITT, W. B., OLIVER-GONZALEZ, J. and MEDINA, E. (1964). Effects of improving the nutrition of malnourished people infected with *Schistosoma mansoni*. *Amer. J. trop. Med. Hyg.*, **13**, No. 1, Pt. 1, 25.

DHANAMITTA, S. and VALYASEVI, A. (1972). WHO Symposium on vesical calculus. Bangkok, Thailand.

DHARMENDRA. (1966). Some recent trends in leprosy. *Leprosy in India.*, **38**, 159.

DHAYAGUDE, R. G. and AMIN, B. M. (1942). Microfilarial granulomata of the spleen. *Amer. J. Path.*, **18**, 351.

DI BELLO, R., ABO, J. C. and BORGES, U. L. (1970). Hydatid constrictive pericarditis. *J. thorac. cardiovasc. Surg.*, **59**, 530.

DIBLE, J. H. (1951). Degeneration, necrosis, and fibrosis in the liver. *Brit. med. J.*, **1**, 833.

DICK, G. W. A. (1947). Aortic size in East African natives. *Ann. trop. Med. Parasit.*, **41**, 52.

DICK, G. W. A. and HADDOW, A. J. (1952). Uganda S. virus. A hitherto unrecorded virus isolated from mosquitoes in Uganda. I. Isolation and pathogenicity. *Trans. roy. Soc. trop. Med. Hyg.*, **46**, 600.

DIEHL, V., *et al.* (1969). Infectious mononucleosis in E. Africa. *E. Afr. med. J.*, **46**, 410.

DIETRICK, R. B. and LEE, M. H. (1965). Intussusception: a different clinical entity in Korea. *Surgery*, **57**, 651.

DIGGS, L. W. (1965). Sickle cell crises. *Amer. J. clin. Path.* **44**, 1.

DIGGS, L. W., KRAUS, A. P., MORRISON, D. B. and RUDNICKI, R. P. T. (1954). Intraerythrocytic crystals in a white patient with hemoglobin C in the absence of other types of hemoglobin. *Blood*, **9**, 1172.

DIMMETTE, R. M., ELWI, A. M. and SPROAT, H. F. (1956). Relationship of schistosomiasis to polyposis and adenocarcinoma of large intestine. *Amer. J. clin. Path.*, **26**, 266.

DIXON, C. W. (1962). *Smallpox*. Churchill, London.

DIXON, F. J. (1966). Comments on immunopathology. *Research in Malaria*. Suppl. *Milit. Med.*, **131**, 1233.

DIXON, H. B. F. and HARGREAVES, W. H. (1944). Cysticercosis (*Taenia solium*). A further ten years' clinical study covering 284 cases. *Quart. J. Med.* (n.s.), **13**, No. 52, 107.

DIXON, H. B. F. and LIPSCOMB, F. M. (1961). Cysticercosis: an analysis and follow-up of 450 cases. *Spec. Rep. Ser. med. Res. Coun.* (*Lond.*), **299**, vi + 58.

DJABANOR, F. F. T. (1972). The sickling of erythrocytes. *Ghana med. J.*, March 29.

DOBSON, C. and WELCH, J. S. (1974). Dirofilariasis as a cause of eosinophilic meningitis in man diagnosed by immunofluorescence and Arthus hypersensitivity. *Trans. roy. Soc. trop. Med. Hyg.*, **68**, 223.

DOBY, J. M., DOBY-DUBOIS, M. and DEBLOCK, S. (1957). Incidence of taeniasis due to *Taenia saginata* in 3,000 children of the Yaounde region (Cameroons) detected by the Graham method. *Bull. Soc. Path. exot.*, **50**, 929.

DOCQUIER, J., DESTOMBES, P. and GIGASE, P. (1974). African histoplasmosis in the Republic of Niger. *Ann. Soc. belge Méd. trop.*, **54**, 61.

DODGE, O. G. (1965). Carcinoma of the penis in East Africans. *Brit. J. Urol.*, **37**, 223.

DODGE, O. G. and KIRK, R. (1962). Buruli ulcer: a mycobacterial skin ulcer in a Uganda child. *J. trop. Med. Hyg.*, **65**, 139.

DODIN, A., RANDRIANARIVO, P. and BRYGOO, E. R. (1963). Moles hydatidiformes et chorio-epitheliomes a Madagascar. *Arch. Inst. Pasteur Madagascar*, **32**, 67.

DODSWORTH, H. and BURNS, A. (1971). Disseminated intravascular coagulation complicating infectious mononucleosis. *Brit. med. J.*, **4**, 466.

DODU, S. R. A. (1958). Diabetes and haemosiderosis—haemochromatosis—in Ghana. *Trans. roy. Soc. trop. Med. Hyg.*, **52**, 425.

— (1967). Diabetes in the tropics. *Brit. med. J.*, **2**, 747.

DODU, S. R. A. and POBEE, J. O. M. (1962). A case of burning (or painful) feet syndrome—without obvious dietary deficiency. *Ghana med. J.*, **1**, 50.

DOEGE, T. C. and NORTHROP, R. L. (1974). Evidence for inapparent rabies infection. *Lancet*, **2**, 826.

DOGRA, J. R. (1940). Studies on peptic ulcer in South India. *Indian. J. med. Res.*, **28**, 481.

DOLL, R., PAYNE, P. and WATERHOUSE, J., eds. (1966). *Cancer Incidence in Five Continents: A Technical Report.* International Union Against Cancer. Springer Verlag, Berlin, Heidelberg, New York.

DE DOMINICIS, A., BALESTRIERI, A. and ASSUMMA, M. (1966). Tests with radioisotopes in the diagnosis of infective and parasitic diseases of the liver. *Arch. ital. Sci. med. trop.*, **47**, 215.

DONALDSON, G. W. K., *et al.* (1969). Coagulation factors in chronic liver disease. *J. clin. Path.*, **22**, 199.

DONALDSON, J. R. and ANGELO, T. A. (1961). Quadriplegia due to guinea worm abscess. *J. Bone J. Surg.*, **43-A**, 197.

DONIACH, D. (1970). The concept of an 'auto allergic' hepatitis. *Proc. roy. Soc. Med.*, **63**, 527.

DONOHUGH, D. L. (1963). Tropical eosinophilia. An etiologic inquiry. *New Engl. J. Med.*, **269**, 1357.

DONOSO, G., BRUNSER, O. and MÖNCKEBERG, F. (1965). Metabolism of serum albumin in marasmic infants. *J. Pediat.*, **67**, 306.

DORFMAN, R. F. (1965). Childhood lymphosarcoma in St. Louis, Missouri, clinically and histologically resembling Burkitt's tumor. *Cancer*, **18**, 418.

DORN, H. F. and CUTLER, S. J. (1958). Morbidity from cancer in the United States. *Publ. Hlth Monogr.*, No. 56.

DOULL, J. A. (1962). The epidemiology of leprosy. Present status and problems. *Int. J. Leprosy*, **30**, 48.

DOWNIE, A. W. (1971). Tanapox: a new disease caused by a pox virus. *Brit. med. J.*, **1**, 363.

DOWNIE, A. W. and MACCALLUM, F. O. (1967). *Virus and Rickettsial Diseases of Man*, p. 374. Arnold, London.

DOWNS, E. F. (1964). Nutritional dwarfing: a syndrome of early protein-calorie malnutrition. *Amer. J. clin. Nutr.*, **15**, 275.

DOXIADES, T., *et al.* (1961). Chronic diffuse non-suppurative amoebic hepatitis. *Brit. med. J.*, **1**, 460.

DOXIADIS, S. A., FESSAS, P. and VALAES, T. (1961). G-6-Pd deficiency. A new aetiological factor of severe neonatal jaundice. *Lancet*, **1**, 297.

DRONFIELD, M. W., FLETCHER, J. and LANGMAN, M. J. S. (1974). Coincident salmonella infections and ulcerative colitis: problems of recognition and management. *Brit. med. J.*, **1**, 99.

DUBIN, H. V., COURTER, M. H. and HARRELL, E. R. (1971). Toxoplasmosis. *Arch. Derm.*, **104**, 547.

DUBOIS, A., JANSSENS, P. G., BRUTSAERT, P. and VANBREUSEGHEN, P. (1952). Un cas d'histoplasmose africaine. *Ann. Soc. Belge Med. Trop.*, **32**, 569.

DUDGEON, J. A. (1968). Rubella. *Recent Advances in Clinical Pathology*, p. 59. J. A. Churchill, London.

— (1970). *Modern Trends in Medical Virology*, p. 78. Butterworth, London.

DUGDALE, A. E. and EDKINS, E. (1964). Unirary urea/creatinine ratio in healthy and malnourished children. *Lancet*, **1**, 1062.

DUGGAL, K., TANDON, H. D., KARMARKER, M. G. and RAMALINGASWAMI, V. (1966). Diffuse intimal thickening of the aorta in India and its relation to atherosclerosis. *J. Path. Bact.*, **92**, 49.

DUKE, B. O. L. (1957). A case of 'streptocerciasis' in a European. *Ann. trop. Med. Parasit.*, **51**, No. 4, 364.

— (1973). Studies on factors influencing the transmission of onchocerciasis. VIII. The escape of infective *Onchocerca volvulus* larvae from feeding 'forest' *Simulium damnosum. Ann. trop. Med. Parasit.*, **67**, 95.

DUKES, D. C., MACDOUGALL, B. R. D., ORNE-GLIEMANN, R. H. and DAVIDSON, L. (1967). Urinary leucocyte excretion in African subjects: its relation to bacteriuria and the passage of bilharzial ova in urine. *Brit. med. J.*, **4**, 537.

DUKES, D. C. *et al.* (1968). Cerebral filariasis due to *A. perstans. Cent. Afr. J. Med.* **14**, 21.

DUKES, H. M. and MYNORS, J. M. (1970). Obstructive renal failure in Bilharziasis. *Brit. J. Surg.*, **57**, 347.

DUMA, M., *et al.* (1965). Acute fatty liver of pregnancy. *Ann. intern. Med.*, **63**, 851.

DUMAS, M., GIRARD, P. L., JACQUIN-COTTON, L. and KONATE, S. (1970). Premier cas de maladie de Wilson au Sénégal. *Bull. Soc. méd. Afr. noire Langue franç*, **15**, 96.

DUNHAM, L. J. and BAILAR, K. C. (1968). World maps of cancer mortality rates and frequency ratios. *J. nat. Cancer Inst.*, **41**, 155.

DUNN, J. M. and HAYNES, R. L. (1967). Sickle cell thalassemia in pregnancy. *Amer. J. Obstet. Gynec.*, **97**, 574.

DUNN, M. I. (1969). Alterations of red blood cell sodium transport during malarial infection. *J. clin. Invest.*, **48**, 674.

DUONG-HONG-MO and TRAN-HIEP-CUONG. (1967). A typical case of melioidosis in South Vietnam. *Milit. Med.*, **132**, 98.

DU PLESSIS, L. S., NUNN, J. R. and ROACH, W. A. (1969). Cancer—carcinogen in a Bantu food additive. *Nature*, **222**, 1198.

DUTTA, N. K. and OZA, N. B. (1963). The effect of gastrointestinal enzymes on cholera toxin *Bull. Wld Hlth Org.*, **28**, 307.

DUTTA, N. K., PANSE, M. V. and KULKARNI, D. R. (1959). Role of cholera toxin in experimental cholera. *J. Bact.*, **78**, 594.

DUTZ, W., SAIDI, F. and KOHOUT, E. (1970). Gastric anthrax with massive ascites. *Gut*, **11**, 352.

DUXBURY, R. E. and SADUN, E. H. (1964). Fluorescent antibody test for the serodiagnosis of visceral leishmaniasis. *Amer. J. trop. Med. Hyg.*, **13**, 525.

DYSON, B. C. and DECKER, J. P. (1958). Endocardial fibroelastosis in the adult. *A.M.A. Arch. Path.*, **66**, 190.

DZBENSKI, T. H. (1966). Immuno-fluorescent studies on *Balantidium coli. Trans. roy. Soc. trop. Med. Hyg.*, **60**, 387.

EARLE, K. M. and DUPONT, J. R. (1966). Negri bodies in human rabies. *Tex. Rep. Biol. Med.*, **24**, 317.

EATON, J. W. and MUCHA, J. J. (1971). Increased fertility in males with the sickle cell trait. *Nature*, **231**, 456.

EDELMAN, R., *et al.* (1973). Mechanisms of defective delayed cutaneous hypersensitivity in children with protein–calorie malnutrition. *Lancet*, **1**, 506.

EDEN, M., *et al.* (1973). Feasibility of computer screening of blood films for the detection of malaria parasites. *Bull. Wld Hlth Org.* **48**, 2 (2998).

EDESON, J. F. B. and WILSON, T. (1964). The epidemology of filariasis due to *Wuchereria bancrofti* and *Brugia malayi. A. Rev. Ent.*, **9**, 245.

EDGCOMB, J. H. and JOHNSON, C. M. (1970). Natural infection of *Rattus rattus* by *Trypanosoma cruzi* in Panama. *Amer. J. trop. Med. Hyg.*, **19**, 767.

EDGCOMB, J. H. and MORROW, R. H. (1963). Histopathological characteristics of infectious hepatitis in Accra, 1962/63. *Ghana med. J.*, **2**, 111.

EDGE, J. R. (1946). Myocardial fibrosis following arsenical therapy: report of a case. *Lancet*, **2**, 675.

EDINGTON, G. M. (1953). Significance of the target cell (leptocyte) in peripheral blood smears of the Gold Coast African. *Trans. roy. Soc. trop. Med. Hyg.*, **47**, 401.

— (1954). Haemosiderosis and anaemia in the Gold Coast African. *W. Afr. med. J.* (n.s.), **3**, 66.

— (1954). Cerebral malaria in the Gold Coast African: four autopsy reports. *Ann. trop. Med. Parasit.*, **48**, 300.

— (1955). The Pathology of sickle cell disease in West Africa. *Trans. roy. Soc. trop. Med. Hyg.*, **49**, 253.

— (1956). Malignant disease in the Gold Coast. *Brit. J. Cancer*, **10**, 595.

— (1956). Some observations on blood transfusion in the Gold Coast. *W. Afr. med. J.* (n.s.), **5**, 71.

— (1957). Schistosomiasis in Ghana with special reference to its pathology. *W. Afr. med. J.* (n.s.), **6**, 45.

— (1959). Nutritional siderosis in Ghana. *Cent. Afr. J. Med.*, **5**, 186.

— (1963). The abnormal haemoglobins in West Africa. *Ghana med. J.*, **2**, 83.

— (1964). Phycomycosis in Ibadan, Western Nigeria. *Trans. roy. Soc. trop. Med. Hyg.*, **58**, 242.

— (1966). Tumours of the gastrointestinal tract in Africa. *Activ. Rep. Un. int. Cancr.*, 1962–66, 25.

— (1967). Pathology of malaria in West Africa. *Brit. med. J.*, **1**, 715.

— (1970). Cancer of the uterus in the Western State of Nigeria. *Afr. J. med. Sci.*, **1**, 67.

— (1971). African histoplasmosis (Part I). In *Human Infection with Fungi, Actinomycetes and Algae*, p. 139. Springer Verlag, New York.

EDINGTON, G. M., BOHRER, S. P. and MIDDLEMISS, J. H. (1970). Ewing's sarcoma in negroes. *Lancet*, **1**, 1171.

EDINGTON, G. M. and DODU, S. R. A. (1957). The diagnosis of haemosiderosis by sternal marrow puncture. *Trans roy. Soc. trop. Med. Hyg.*, **51**, 429.

EDINGTON, G. M. and EASMON, C. O. (1967). Incidence of cancer of the alimentary tract in Accra, Ghana, and Ibadan, Western Nigeria. *Nat. Cancer Inst. Monogr.*, No. 25, 17.

EDINGTON, G. M. and GILLES, H. M. (1969). *Pathology in the Tropics*. 1st Ed. Edward Arnold, London.

EDINGTON, G. M. and JACKSON, J. G. (1963). The pathology of heart muscle disease and endomyocardial fibrosis in Nigeria. *J. Path. Bact.*, **86**, 333.

EDINGTON, G. M. and LAING, W. N. (1957). Relationship between haemoglobins C and S and malaria in Ghana. *Brit. med. J.*, **2**, 143.

EDINGTON, G. M. and LEHMANN, H. (1954). Haemoglobin G, a new haemoglobin found in a West African. *Lancet*, **2**, 173.

EDINGTON, G. M. and LEHMANN, H. (1955). Expression of the sickle-cell gene in Africa. (Correspondence.) *Brit. med. J.*, **2**, 1328.

EDINGTON, G. M. and MACLEAN, C. M. U. (1964). Incidence of the Burkitt tumour in Ibadan, Western Nigeria. *Brit. med. J.*, **1**, 264.

— (1965). A cancer rate survey in Ibadan, Western Nigeria, 1960–63. *Brit. J. Cancer*, **19**, 471.

EDINGTON, G. M. and MAINWARING, A. R. (1964). Amyloidosis in Western Nigeria. *Path. Microbiol.*, **27**, 841.

— (1966). Nephropathies in West Africa. *The Kidney*. International Academy of Pathology Monograph, No. 6, 488.

EDINGTON, G. M., OSUNKOYA, B. O. and HENDRICKSE, M. (1973). Histologic classification of Hodgkins disease in the Western State of Nigeria. *J. nat. Cancer Inst.*, **50**, 1633.

EDINGTON, G. M. and SARKIES, J. W. R. (1952). Two cases of sickle-cell anaemia associated with retinal microaneurysms. *Trans. roy. Soc. trop. Med. Hyg.*, **46**, 59.

EDINGTON, G. M. and SHEIHAM, A. (1966). Salivary gland tumours and tumours of the oral cavity in Western Nigeria. *Brit. J. Cancer*, **20**, 425.

EDINGTON, G. M. and WHITE, H. A. (1972). The pathology of lassa fever. *Trans. roy. Soc. trop. Med. Hyg.*, **66**, 381.

EDINGTON, G. M., *et al.* (1970). Pathologic effects of schistosomiasis in Ibadan, Western State of Nigeria. *Amer. J. trop. Med. Hyg.*, **19**, 982.

EDINGTON, G. M., *et al.* (1970). Pathological effects of schistosomiasis in Ibadan, Western State of Nigeria. *Amer. J. trop. med. Hyg.*, **19**, 928.

EDITORIAL (1954). Trichinosis. *Brit. med. J.*, **1**, 1025.

— (1956). Acute yellow atrophy. *Lancet*, **1**, 847.

— (1956). Obstetric acute yellow atrophy. *Lancet*, **1**, 847.

— (1961). The Madras experiment. *Lancet*, **2**, 532.

— (1964). Infected ascitic fluid in cirrhosis. *Brit. med. J.*, **2**, 774.

— (1965). Blood tests for syphilis. *Brit. med. J.*, **1**, 76.

— (1965). Hashimoto's disease. *Brit. med. J.*, **2**, 380.

— (1965). Transfusion and severe anaemia. *Brit. med. J.*, **1**, 744.

— (1965). Tropical neurology. *Lancet*, **1**, 149.

— (1965). Mycoplasmas. *Brit. med. J.*, **2**, 1549.

— (1966). Aberdeen typhoid outbreak of 1964. *Brit. med. J.*, **2**, 601.

— (1966). Carcinoma of the uterus. *Brit. med. J.*, **1**, 247.

— (1966). Chromosomes and leukaemia. *Brit. med. J.*, **2**, 719.

— (1966). Diagnosis of amyloidosis. *Brit. med. J.*, **2**, 1090.

— (1966). Diagnosis of variola minor. *Brit. med. J.*, **2**, 255.

— (1966). Rubella virus in giant cell hepatitis. *Lancet*, **1**, 293.

— (1967). Paterson/Brown Kelly syndrome. *Brit. med. J.*, **1**, 258.

— (1968). Amoebiasis. *Lancet*, **1**, 77.

— (1968). Diseases caused by cytomegaloviruses. *Brit. med. J.*, **1**, 72.

— (1968). Infective hepatitis. *Lancet*, **1**, 79.

— (1968). Measles in Africa. *Lancet*, **1**, 239.

— (1968). Heavy chain disease. *Brit. med. J.*, **4**, 403.

— (1968). Leucocyte alkaline phosphatase and Hodgkin's Disease. *Brit. med. J.*, **3**, 390.

— (1968). Nasal cancer in wood workers. *Brit. med. J.*, **2**, 572.

— (1968). Pulmonary calcification after chickenpox. *Brit. med. J.*, **2**, 68.

— (1968). Renal damage in chicken pox. *Brit. med. J.*, **3**, 264.

— (1968). Varieties of hyperparathyroidism. *Brit. med. J.*, **2**, 389.

— (1969). Antiglobulin tests. *Brit. med. J.*, **1**, 593.

— (1969). Bone and joint changes in haemochromatosis. *Brit. med. J.*, **3**, 191.

— (1969). Chronic cyanide neurotoxicity. *Lancet*, **2**, 942.

— (1969). Diverticular disease of the colon. *Brit. med. J.*, **3**, 311.

— (1970). Amoebic meningitis. *Lancet*, **1**, 184.

— (1970). Burkitt's lymphoma and malaria. *Lancet*, **2**, 300.

— (1970). Crohn's disease and its consequences. *Brit. med. J.*, **2**, 65.

— (1970). Culdocentesis and ectopic pregnancy. *Brit. med. J.*, **1**, 187.

— (1970). Gastric ulcer and gastric cancer. *Brit. med. J.*, **2**, 250.

— (1970). Genital herpes and cervical cancer. *Brit. med. J.*, **4**, 256.

— (1970). Laboratory diagnosis of rubella. *Brit. med. J.*, **3**, 237.

— (1970). Melioidosis, *Lancet*, **1**, 761.

— (1970). Oxygen tension in the gut. *New Engl. J. Med.*, **282**, 1039.

— (1970). Septic shock. *Brit. med. J.*, **1**, 3.

— (1970). Glucose-6-phosphate dehydrogenase deficiency and age. *Lancet*, **1**, 1329.

— (1971). Cytomegalovirus infection. *Brit. med. J.*, **1**, 687.

— (1971). Genitourinary tuberculosis. *Brit. med. J.*, **2**, 183.

— (1971). Hepatic vein occlusion. *Brit. med. J.*, **3**, 550.

— (1971). Hydatidiform mole and hyperthyroidism. *Brit. med. J.*, **2**, 606.

— (1971). New-style cold abscesses. *Brit. med. J.*, **1**, 247.

— (1971). Pneumonia in atypical measles. *Brit. med. J.*, **2**, 235.

— (1971). Pulmonary aspergilloma. *Brit. med. J.*, **2**, 124.

— (1971). Rabies diagnosis. *Brit. med. J.*, **2**, 483.

— (1971). Reiter's disease. *Brit. med. J.*, **3**, 387.

— (1971). Renal stones in top people. *Brit. med. J.*, **2**, 668.

— (1971). Scalded skin syndrome. *Brit. med. J.*, **4**, 66.

— (1971). Stilboestrol and cancer. *Brit. med. J.*, **3**, 593.

— (1971). Tanapox. *Brit. med. J.*, **1**, 358.

— (1971). The kveim controversy. *Lancet*, **2**, 750.

— (1971). The Masai's cholesterol. *Brit. med. J.*, **3**, 262.

— (1971). Tuberculous meningitis in children. *Brit. med. J.*, **1**, 1.

— (1971). Tularaemia. *Brit. med. J.*, **4**, 4.

— (1971). EB virus, Burkitt lymphoma and nasopharyngeal carcinoma. *Lancet*, **i**, 218

— (1972). Blackfat tobacco smokers lung. *Brit. med. J.*, **1**, 393.

— (1972). Burning feet. *Brit. med. J.*, **3**, 193.

— (1972). Carcinoma of the cervix and herpesvirus. *Brit. med. J.*, **2**, 548.

— (1972). Cardiac biopsy. *Brit. med. J.*, **2**, 420.

— (1972). Immunological characteristics of bladder cancer. *Brit. med. J.*, **4**, 502.

— (1972). Influenza, pregnancy and leukaemia. *Brit. med. J.*, **2**, 477.

— (1972). Interstitial cystitis. *Brit. med. J.*, **1**, 644.

— (1972). Pulmonary veno-occlusive disease. *Brit. med. J.*, **3**, 369.

— (1972). Radical treatment of acute leukaemia in childhood. *Lancet*, **2**, 910.

— (1972). Sarcoid heart disease. *Brit. med. J.*, **4**, 627.

— (1972). Viral hepatitis. *Brit. med. J.*, **2**, 669.

— (1972). New light on cholera. *Lancet*, **ii**, 167.

— (1972). Lassa fever. *Brit. med. J.*, **4**, 253.

— (1972). Transmission of cholera. *Brit. med. J.*, **4**, 626.

— (1973). Adrenal haemorrhage in the new born. *Brit. med. J.*, **3**, 120.

— (1973). Carcinoma of the prostrate. *Brit. med. J.*, **2**, 566.

— (1973). Herpes hepatitis in adults. *Brit. med. J.*, **1**, 248.

— (1973). Immunological aspects of osteosarcoma. *Brit. med. J.*, **1**, 502.

— (1973). Liver injury by salicylates. *Brit. med. J.*, **2**, 732.

— (1973). Monkey pox. *Brit. med. J.*, **1**, 3.

— (1973). Subtypes of Australian antigen. *Brit. med. J.*, **1**, 127.

— (1973). Pathogenesis of measles. *Brit. med. J.*, **3**, 187.

— (1973). Venezuelan encephalitis. *Lancet*, **1**, 29.

— (1973). Snow (1849) on cholera (1973). *Lancet*, **2**, 601.
— (1973). The cardiomyopathies. *Brit. med. J.*, **2**, 434.
— (1973). Rabies. *Lancet*, **2**, 545.
— (1973). Animal reservoirs of rabies. *Lancet*, **1**, 89.
— (1973). Chloramphenicol resistance in typhoid. *Lancet*, **2**, 1008.
— (1973). New ideas on vitamin D. *Brit. med. J.*, **1**, 629.
— (1973). Chronic cassava toxicity. *Lancet*, **2**, 245.
— (1973). Blood-transfusion and tropical disease. *Lancet*, **1**, 32.
— (1974). Deep seated and systemic mycoses. *Brit. med. J.*, **1**, 252.
— (1974). Chronic brucellosis. *Brit. med. J.*, **1**, 299.
— (1974). Sleeping sickness. *Brit. med. J.*, **2**, 236.
— (1974). Vitamin E in clinical medicine. *Lancet*, **1**, 18.
— (1974). Smallpox target zero ? *Lancet*, **1**, 295.
— (1974). Kuru, Creutzfeldt-Jakob, and Scrapie. *Lancet*, **2**, 1551.
— (1974). Screening for sickle-cell disease. *Brit. med. J.*, **3**, 701.
— (1974). Meningococcal infections. *Brit. med. J.*, **3**, 295.
— (1974). Onchocerciasis—river blindness. *Brit. med. J.*, **2**, 401.
— (1974). Rodent control and lassa fever. *Lancet*, **2**, 632.
EDOZIEN, J. C. (1958). Chemical evaluation of hepatic function in Nigerians. *J. clin. Path.* **11**, 437.
— (1960). Biochemical normals in Nigerians. Urinary 17-oxosteroids and 17-oxogenic steroids. *Lancet*, **1**, 258.
EDOZIEN, J. C. (1965). Establishment of a biochemical norm for the evaluation of nutritional status in West Africa. *J. West Afr. sci. Ass.*, **10**, 3.
EDOZIEN, J. C., BOYO, A. E. and MORLEY, D. C. (1960). The relationship of serum gamma-globulin concentration to malaria and sickling. *J. clin. Path.*, **13**, 118.
EDOZIEN, J. C., GILLES, H. M. and UDEOZO, I. O. K. (1962). Adult and cord-blood gamma-globulin and immunity to malaria in Nigerians. *Lancet*, **2**, 951.
EDWARDS, L. B. and PALMER, C. E. (1953). Geographic variation in naturally acquired tuberculin sensitivity. *Lancet*, **1**, 53.
EHRENFORD, F. A. (1957). Canine ascariasis as a potential source of visceral larva migrans. *Amer. J. trop. Med. Hyg.*, **6**, 166.
EHRENKRANZ, N. J., *et al.* (1963). Arthropod-borne virus disease in Florida. Report of a 1958 outbreak in Miami and a serologic survey of Miami residents. *Amer. J. Med.*, **35**, 673.
EISERT, J., HANNIBAL, J. E., JR. and SANDERS, S. L. (1959). Fatal amebiasis complicating corticosteroid management of pemphigus vulgaris. *New Engl. J. Med.*, **261**, 843.
EKPECHI, O. L. (1973). De quervains acute non-suppurative thyroiditis in Nigeria. *Trop. geogr. Med.* **25**, 223.
EL BADAWI, A. A. (1960). Bilharzial polypi of the urinary bladder. *Brit. J. Urol.*, **38**, 24.
EL-BEDRI, L. (1958). Ectopic pregnancy caused by *Schistosoma haematobium* infection of the fallopian tube : a case report. *Amer. J. Obstet. Gynec.*, **76**, 515.
ELDER, G. H., GRAY, C. H. and NICHOLSON, D. C. (1972). The porphyrias. *J. clin. Path.*, **25**, 1013.
ELEBUTE, O. (1971). Renal response to salt load in nosmotensive and hypertensive Nigerian males. *Afr. J. med. Sci.*, **2**, 367.
EL-GAZAYERLI, M. M. and ABDEL-AZIZ, A. S. (1963). On bilharziasis and male breast cancer in Egypt. *Brit. J. Cancer*, **17**, 566.
EL HASHMI, W. (1971). Charcot leyden crystals. *Amer. J. Path.*, **65**, 311.

EL-HASSAN, A. M. and WASFI, A. (1972). Cardiovascular disease in Khartoum. *Trop. geogr. Med.*, **24**, 118.

ELISBERG, B. L. and BOZEMAN, F. L. (1966). Serological diagnosis of Rickettsial diseases by indirect immunofluorescence. *Arch. Inst. Pasteur Tunis*, **43**, 193.

ELKINGTON, S. G., MCBRIEN, D. J. and SPENCER, H. (1963). Hepatoma in cirrhosis. *Brit. med. J.*, **2**, 1501.

ELLIOTT, W. G. (1970). Placental toxoplasmosis. *Amer. J. clin. Path.*, **53**, 413.

ELLIS, M. (1937). Chronic mastitis in the African native. *Brit. J. Surg.*, **25**, 39.

ELLIS, M. (1937). A case of porocephalosis. *W. Afr. med. J.*, **9**, 41.

ELLMAN, B., MCLEOD, I. N. and POWELL, S. J. (1965). Diagnostic pneumoperitoneum in amoebic liver abscess. *Brit. med. J.*, **2**, 1406.

ELMES, B. G. T. (1958). Forensic medicine in Uganda. *E. Afr. med. J.*, **34**, 41.

ELTON, N. W., RONERO, A. and TREJOS, A. (1955). Clinical pathology of yellow fever. *Amer. J. clin. Path.*, **25**, 135.

EL-ZAWAHRY, M. (1965). Schistosomal granuloma of the skin. *Brit. J. Derm.*, **77**, 344.

EMMONS, C. W., BINFORD, C. H. and UTZ, J. P. (1963). *Medical Mycology*. Kimpton, London.

EMSLIE, H. D. (1963). Cancrum oris. *Dent. Practit. dent. Rec.*, **13**, 481.

ENDERS, J. F. (1962). Measles virus. Historical review, isolation, and behavior in various systems. *Am. J. Dis. Child.*, **103**, 282.

ENGLAND, J. M. and FRASER, P. M. (1973). Differentiation of iron deficiency from thalassaemia trait by routine blood-count. *Lancet*, **1**, 449.

ENGLE, M. A. (1964). Cardiac involvement in Cooley's anemia. Problems in Cooley's anemia. *Anns. N.Y. Acad. Sci.*, **119**, 694.

ENGLISH, J. M. (1970). Infectious mononucleosis followed by Hodgkin's disease. *Lancet*, **1**, 948.

ENTICKNAP, J. B. and SMITHER, W. J. (1964). Peritoneal tumours in asbestosis. *Brit. J. indust. Med.*, **21**, 20.

EPIDEMIOLOGY (1972). Tambu fly. *Brit. med. J.*, **2**, 58.

EPSTEIN, M. A., ACHONG, B. G. and BARR, Y. M. (1964). Virus particles in cultured lymphoblasts from Burkitt's lymphoma. *Lancet*, **1**, 702.

ERHARDT, A., GERMER, W. D. and HOINING, B. (1962). Opistorchiasis due to *Opistorchis felineus*. *Parasit. SchrReihe*, No. 15, 171.

ERLICK, D. and REITLER, R. (1960). Intrahepatic typhoid infection as cause of the carrier state. *Lancet*, **1**, 1216.

ESSENFELD, E. and FENNELL, R. H., JR. (1964). Immunofluorescent study of experimental *Trypanosoma cruzi* infection. *Proc. Soc. exp. Biol.*, **116**, 728.

ESSIEN, E. M. (1973). Leukaemia in Nigeria (in press).

ESSIEN, E. M. and ADELOYE, A. (1972). Intracranial haemorrhage in haemophilia in Nigerians. *Trans. roy. Soc. trop. Med. Hyg.*, **66**, 255.

ESSIEN, E. M., FOLAMI, A. O. and LUZZATTO, L. (1970). Haemophilia in Nigeria. *Trop. Geogr. Med.*, **22**, 403.

ESSIEN, E. M., *et al.* (1973). The normal platelet count and platelet factor 3 availability in some Nigerian population groups. *Scand. J. Haemat.*, **10**, 378.

EVANS-AMFON, E. (1963). Intestinal perforation. *Ghana Med. J.*, **2**, 99.

EVANS, K. T., COCKSHOTT, W. P. and HENDRICKSE, P. DE V. (1965). Pulmonary changes in malignant trophoblastic disease. *Brit. J. Radiol.* (n.s.), **38**, 161.

EVANS, T. S., DE LUCA, V. A. and WATERS, L. L. (1952). The association of miliary tuberculosis of the bone marrow and pancytopenia. *Ann. intern. Med.*, **37**, 1044.

EVELAND, W. C., OLIVER, W. J. and NEEL, J. V. (1971). Characteristics of *Escherichia coli* serotypes in the Yanomama, a primitive Indian tribe of S. America. *Infect. Immunity*, **4**, 753.

EZEILO, G. C. (1972). Non-genetic neutropenia in Africans. *Lancet*, **2**, 1003.

EZZAT, E., *et al*. (1974). The association between *Schistosoma haematobium* infection and heavy proteinuria. *Trans. roy. Soc. trop. Med. Hyg.*, **68**, 315.

FACEY, R. V. and MARSDEN, P. D. (1960). Fascioliasis in man: an outbreak in Hampshire. *Brit. med. J.*, **2**, 619.

FAIN, A. (1956). Cénurose chez l'homme et les animaux due à *Taenia brauni* Setti au Congo belge et au Ruanda-Urundi. I: La cénurose chez les animaux sauvages, avec existence de localisations cérébrales. *Ann. Soc. belge Méd. trop.*, **36**, 673.

FAIN, A. and FALAISE, A. (1957). Calculose vésicale et avitaminose A chez les enfants au Ruanda-Urundi. *Ann. Soc. belge. Méd. trop.*, **37**, 136.

FAIN, A., VANDEPITTE, J. and WERY, M. (1974). Microfilaraemia due to *Onchocerca volvulus*. *Ann. Soc. belge Méd. trop.*, **54**, 121.

FAIN, A., *et al*. (1974). The human filariases in the Mayumbe region and adjacent areas (Zaire Republic). Evaluation of the microfilarial density. *Ann. Soc. belge Méd. trop.*, **54**, 5.

FAMILUSI, J. B. and MOORE, D. L. (1972). Isolation of a rabies related virus from the cerebrospinal fluid of a child with aseptic meningitis. *Afr. J. med. Sci.*, **3**, 91.

FAMILUSI, J. B. and SINNETTE, C. N. (1971). Febrile convulsions in Ibadan childen. *Afr. J. med. Sci.*, **2**, 135.

FARAGO, C. (1964). Bilateral parotid gland enlargement in a tropical country, the territory of Papua and New Guinea. *Med. J. Aust.*, **2**, 218.

FARBER, S., *et al*. (1940). Encephalitis in infants and children caused by the virus of the eastern variety of equine encephalitis. *J. Amer. med. Ass.*, **114**, 1725.

FARIA, J. L. (1954). Pulmonary vascular changes in schistosomal cor pulmonale. *J. Path. Bact.*, **68**, 589.

FARIA, L., *et al*. (1959). Pulmonary schistosomatic arteriovenous fistulas producing a new cyanotic syndrome in Manson's schistosomiasis. *Amer. Heart J.*, **58**, 556.

FARID, Z., *et al*. (1972). Chronic salmonellosis, urinary schistosomiasis and massive proteinuria. *Amer. J. trop. Med. Hyg.*, **21**, 5, 578.

FARIS, A. A., GUTH, C., YOUMANS, R. A. and POSER, C. M. (1964). Internal carotid artery occlusion in children: diagnosis by arteriography. *Amer. J. Dis. Child.*, **107**, 188.

FARRER-BROWN, G. and TARBIT, M. H. (1972). What is the spectrum of endomyocardial fibrosis? *Trop. geogr. Med.*, **24**, 208.

FASS, L., HERBERMAN, R. B. and ZEIGLER, J. (1970). Delayed cutaneous hypersensitivity to Burkitt lymphoma cells. *New Engl. J. Med.*, **282**, 776.

FAUST, E. C. (1948). An inquiry into the ectopic lesions in schistosomiasis. *Amer. J. trop. Med.*, **28**, 175.

— (1929). What is *Sparganum mansoni*? *J. trop. Med. Hyg.*, **32**, 76.

— (1957). Human infection with species of *Dirofilaria*. *Z. Tropenmed. Parasit.*, **8**, Nos. 1/2, 59.

FAUST, E. C. and MELENEY, H. E. (1924). Studies on schistosomiasis japonica. VI: The pathological anatomy of the disease. *Monogr. Ser. Amer. J. Hyg.*, **3**, 174.

FAWDRY, A. L. (1955). Syndrome of splenomegaly, anaemia, and hepatomegaly often left-lobed, in south Arabia. *Trans. roy. Soc. trop. Med. Hyg.*, **49**, 387.

FEINSTONE, S. M., KAPIKIAN, A. Z. and PURCELL, R. H. (1973). Hepatitis. A: A detection by immune electron microscopy of a virus-like antigen associated with acute illness. *Science*, **182**, 1026.

FEJFAR, Z. (1968). Idiopathic Cardiomegaly. *Bull. Wld Hlth Org.*, **38**, 979.

FELDMAN, N. (1950). Infantile rickets: its occurrence in non-Europeans in Johannesburg. *S. Afr. med. J.*, **24**, 1053.

FELSENFELD, O., *et al.* (1966). Relationship of some vibrio antibodies in serum immune globulins in man and in *Cercopithecus aethiops. J. infect. Dis.*, **116**, 329.

FELTON, A., VON STRAUB, P. W. and FRICK, P. G. (1969). Dysfibrinogenemia in a patient with primary hepatoma. *New Engl. J. Med.*, **280**, 405.

FEMI-PEARSE, D. and OLOWU, A. O. (1971). Myositis ossificans—a complication of tetanus. *Clin. Radiol.*, **22**, 89.

FENDALL, N. R. E. and GROUNDS, J. G. (1965). The incidence and epidemiology of disease in Kenya. *J. trop. Med. Hyg.*, **68**, 77.

FENNELLY, J., FRANK, O., BAKER, H. and LEEVY, C. M. (1964). Peripheral neuropathy of the alcoholic. I: Aetiological role of aneurin and other B-complex vitamins. *Brit. med. J.*, **2**, 1290.

FENNER, F. (1956). The pathogenic behavior of *Mycobacterium ulcerans* and *Mycobacterium balnei* in the mouse and the developing chick embryo. *Amer. Rev. Tuberc.*, **73**, 650.

FERGUSON, J. C., MACKAY, N. and MCNICOL, G. P. (1970). Effect of feeding fat on fibrinolysis, Stypven time and platelet aggregation in Africans, Asians and Europeans. *J. clin. Path.*, **23**, 580.

FERGUSON, M. and O'BRIEN, M. M. (1960). Heat stroke in New York City. *N.Y. St. J. Med.*, **60**, 2531.

FERIA-VELASCO, A. and TREVINO, N. (1972). The ultrastructure of trophozoites of *Entamoeba histolytica* with particular reference to spherical arrangements of osmiophilic cylindrical bodies. *J. Protozool.*, **19**, 200.

FERNANDO, D. B. and THANABALASUNDERAM, R. S. (1951). Infective hepatitis and cirrhosis of the liver. *Quart. J. Med.* (n.s.), **20**, 403.

FERRANS, V. J., HIBBS, R. G., WEILBAECHER, D. G., BLACK, W. C., WALSH, J. J. and BURCH, G. E. (1965). Alcoholic cardiomyopathy: a histochemical study. *Amer. Heart J.*, **69**, 748.

FESSAS, P. (1959). Thalassaemia and alterations in the haemoglobin pattern. In *Abnormal Haemoglobins: Symposium*, p. 134. Blackwell Scientific Publications, Oxford.

— (1961). Haemoglobin H and Bart's. In *Haemoglobin Colloquium, Vienna,* ed. Lehmann H. and Betke K, p. 90. George Thieme Verlag, Stuttgart.

— (1963). Inclusions of hemoglobin in erythroblasts and erythrocytes of thalassemia. *Blood*, **21**, 21.

— (1967). Thalassaemia clinical and patho-physiological considerations. *Trans. roy. Soc. trop. Med. Hyg.*, **61**, 164.

FESSAS, P., DOXIADIS, S. A. and VALAES, T. (1962). Neonatal jaundice in glucose-6-phosphate-dehydrogenase deficient infants. *Brit. med. J.*, **2**, 1359.

FESSAS, P., KARAKLIS, A. and GNAFAKIS, N. (1961). A further abnormality of foetal haemoglobin. *Acta haemat.*, **25**, 62.

FESSAS, P., MASTROKALOS, N. and FOSTIROPOULOS, G. (1959). New variant of human foetal haemoglobin. *Nature (Lond.)*, **183**, 30.

FESSAS, P. and PAPASPYROU, A. (1957). New 'fast' hemoglobin associated with thalassemia. *Science, N.Y.*, **126**, 1119.

FIALKOW, P. J., KLEIN, G., GARTLER, S. M. and CLIFFORD, P. (1970). Clonal origin for individual Burkitt tumours. *Lancet*, **1**, 384.

FINCH, J. T. and PERUTZ, M. F. (1974). Structure of sickle-cell haemoglobin. *Trans. roy. Soc. trop. Med. Hyg.*, **68**, 79.

FINDLAY, G. H. and PARK, R. G. (1969). Common skin diseases in the Transvaal. *S. Afr. med. J.*, **43**, 590.

FINDLAY, G. M. (1948). Infective hepatitis in West Africa. *Mth. Bull. Minist. Hlth*, **7**, 2, 32.

FINKELSTEIN, R. A. and GOMEZ, C. Z. (1963). Comparison of methods for the rapid recognition of cholera vibrios. *Bull. Wld Hlth Org.*, **28**, 327.

FINKELSTINE, R. A., *et al.*, (1966). Pathogenesis of experimental cholera: biologic activities of purified prochloragen A. *J. Immunol.*, **96**, 440.

FINLAY-JONES, L. R. (1964). Fatal myocarditis after vaccination against smallpox: report of a case. *New Engl. J. Med.*, **270**, 41.

FINLEY, K. H., *et al.* (1955). Western equine and St. Louis encephalitis. Preliminary report of a clinical follow-up study in California. *Neurology*, **5**, 223.

FINN, R., *et al.* (1972). Immunological responses in pregnancy and survival of fetal homograft. *Brit. med. J.*, **3**, 150.

FISCHMAN, A. (1960). A rapid latex test for hydatid disease. *N.Z. med. J.*, **59**, 485.

FISCHMAN, A. and SKOREPOVA, G. (1973). Serology of yaws. *Trans. roy. Soc. trop. Med. Hyg.*, **67**, 3, 421.

FISHER, A. C. (1941). Acute thrombophlebitis of unknown origin. *S. Afr. med. J.*, **15**, 131.

FISHER, A. C., FISHER, M. M. and TENDREN, A. C. (1946). Tropical primary phlebitis. *J. Path. Bact.*, **59**, 405.

FISHER, E. R. and DIMLING, C. (1964). Rhinoscleroma. *Arch. Path.* **78**, 501.

FISHER, M. M., *et al.* (1971). Malnutrition and reasoning ability in Zambian school children. *Trans. roy. Soc. trop. Med. Hyg.*, **66**, 471.

FISTEIN, B. (1960). Toxic hypoglycaemia (Jamaican vomiting sickness): first case reported from the territory of Trinidad and Tobago. *W. Indian med. J.*, **9**, 62.

FLATZ, G., PIK, C. and SUNDHARAGIATI, B. (1964). Malaria and haemoglobin E in Thailand. *Lancet*, **2**, 385.

FLATZ, G. and SRINGAM, S. (1963). Malaria and glucose-6-phosphate dehydrogenase deficiency in Thailand. *Lancet*, **2**, 1248.

FLECK, D. (1972). The seroepidemiology of toxoplasma infection in man. *Proc. roy. Soc. Med.*, **65**, 1002.

FLECK, D. G. and LUDLAM, G. B. (1965). Indications for laboratory tests for toxoplasmosis. *Brit. med. J.*, **2**, 1239.

FLEMING, A. F. (1970). Seasonal incidence of anaemia in pregnancy in Ibadan. *Amer. J. clin. Nutr.*, **23**, 224.

— (1972). Urinary excretion of folate in pregnancy. *J. Obstet. Gynaec. Brit. Cwlth.*, **79**, 916.

FLEMING, A. F. and ALLAN, N. C. (1969). Severe haemolytic anaemia in pregnancy in Nigerians treated with prednisolone. *Brit. med. J.*, **4**, 461.

FLETCHER, A. and MAEGRAITH, B. G. (1972). The metabolism of the malaria parasite and its host. *Advanc. Parasit.*, **10**, 31.

FLETCHER, G. H. (1966). Sarcoidosis in miners in the Republic of Zambia. *Cent. Afr. J. Med.*, **12**, 29.

FLETCHER, K. (1966). Observations on the origin of liver fat in infantile malnutrition. *Amer. J. clin. Nutr.*, **19**, 170.

FLETCHER, S. (1965). Indirect fluorescent antibody technique in the serology of *Toxoplasma gondii. J. clin. Path.*, **18**, 193.

FLORENTIN, R. A., *et al.* (1963). Geographic pathology of arteriosclerosis: A study of the age of onset of significant coronary arteriosclerosis in adult Africans and New Yorkers. *Exp. molec. Path.*, **2**, 103.

FLOWERS, D. J. (1970). Human infection due to *Mycobacterium marinum* after a dolphin bite. *J. clin. Path.*, **23**, 475.

FLUCK, D. J., *et al.* (1973). Ultrastructure of the hepatic sinusoids in the tropical splenomegaly syndrome. *Trans. roy. Soc. trop. Med. Hyg.*, **67**, 638.

FODOR, J., MIALL, W. E., STANDARD, K. L., FEJFAR, Z. and STUART, K. L. (1964). Myocardial disease in a rural population in Jamaica. *Bull. Wld Hlth Org.*, **31**, 321.

FONG, Y. L., CADIGAN, F. C. and COATNEY, C. R. (1971). A presumptive case of naturally occurring *Plasmodium knowlesi* malaria in man in Malaysia. *Trans. roy. Soc. trop. Med. Hyg.*, **65**, 840.

FORBES, C. D., MACKAY, N. and KHAN, A. A. (1966). Christmas disease and haemophilia in Kenya. *Trans. roy. Soc. trop. Med. Hyg.*, **66**, 777.

FORD, J. A., *et al.* (1973). Neonatal rickets in Asian immigrant population. *Brit. med. J.*, **3**, 211.

FORFAR, J. O., MILLER, R. A., BAIN, A. D. and MACLEOD, W. (1964). Endocardial fibroelastosis. *Brit. med. J.*, **2**, 7.

FORNARA, L. (1924). Note sur un cas de localisation sous-arachnoïdienne d'une larve de porocéphale. *Ann. Soc. belge Méd. trop.*, **3**, 233.

FORREST, C. R., *et al.* (1967). Vi reaction in Hong Kong. *Brit. med. J.*, **2**, 472.

FORSYTH, D. M. and MACDONALD, G. (1965). Urological complications of endemic schistosomiasis in schoolchildren. Part 1. Usagara School. *Trans. roy. Soc. trop. Med. Hyg.*, **59**, No. 2, 171.

— (1966). Urological complications of endemic schistosomiasis in schoolchildren. Part 2. Donge School, Zanzibar. *Trans. roy. Soc. trop. Med. Hyg.*, **60**, No. 5, 568.

FOSSATI, C. J. (1970). Las parasitosis respiratorias halladas en pacientas arabolibicos de Cirenaica. (Libya), en los ultimos diez anos. II. Hidatidosis toracica. *Rev. ibér. Parasit.*, **30**, 587.

FOSTER, R., BIRCH, N. H. and URASA, J. (1965). A case of sparganosis from Tanzania (Tanganyika). *E. Afr. med. J.*, **42**, 74.

FOSTER, R. M. and HARRIES, J. R. (1970). Multiple sclerosis in the African. *Brit. med. J.*, **3**, 628.

FOSTER, S. O., *et al.* (1972). Human monkeypox. *Bull. Wld Hlth Org.*, **46**, 569.

FOULK, W. T., BUTT, H. R., OWEN, C. A., WHITCOMB, F. F. and MASON, H. L. (1959). Constitutional hepatic dysfunction (Gilbert's disease): its natural history and related syndromes. *Medicine (Baltimore)*, **38**, 25.

FOUNTAIN, J. R. (1954). Blood changes associated with disseminated tuberculosis. *Brit. med. J.*, **2**, 76.

FOUQUES, M., *et al.* (1972). Les lymphangiectasies de la filariose de Bancroft et leur traitement chirurgical. *Premières Journées Médicales de la Polynésie Française*, **2**, 83.

FOURNIER, J. (1965). Epidemiological and taxonomic discussion on melioidosis and Whitmore's bacillus. *Bull. Soc. Path. exot.*, **58**, 753.

FOWLER, M. (1947). A clinico-pathological study of two cases of idiopathic cardiac hypertrophy with congestive failure. *Med. J. Aust.*, **1**, 672.

FOWLER, M. and ROBERTSON, E. G. (1959). Observations on kuru. III. Pathological features in five cases. *Aust. Ann. Med.*, **8**, 16.

FOWLER, N. O. (1964). Classification and differential diagnosis of the myocardiopathies. *Progr. cardiovasc. Dis.*, **7**, 1.

FOX, W. (1962). The chemotherapy and epidemiology of tuberculosis. Some findings of general applicability from the tuberculosis chemotherapy centre, Madras. *Lancet*, **2**, 473.

— (1963). Ambulatory chemotherapy in a developing country: clinical and epidemiological studies. *Adv. Tuberc. Res.* **12**, 28.

FOY, H. and KONDI, A. (1956). Anaemias in Africans. *Cent. Afr. J. of Med.*, **2**, 254.

— (1956). Nutritional and intestinal factors and iron losses in the genesis of tropical anaemias. *Lancet*, **1**, 423.

FOY, H., *et al.* (1970). Positive alpha-fetoprotein tests in pyridoxine deprived baboons. *Nature*, **225**, 952.

FRAME, J. D., BALDWIN, J. M., GOCKE, D. J. and TROUP, J. M. (1970). Lassa fever, a new virus disease of man from West Africa. *Amer. J. trop. Med. Hyg.*, **19**, 670.

FRANCIS, T. I. (1972). Abdominal tuberculosis in Nigerians, a clinico-pathological study. *Trop. geogr. Med.*, **24**, 232.

FRANCIS, T. I., MOORE, D. L., EDINGTON, G. M. and SMITH, A. J. (1972). A clinico-pathological study of human yellow fever. *Bull. Wld Hlth Org.*, **46**, 659.

FRASER, P. M. and FRANKLIN, D. A. (1974). Mathematical models for the diagnosis of liver disease. *Quart. J. Med.*, **43**, 73.

FRASER, R. (1964). Endemic and non-endemic goitre. *The Leech*, **34**, 114.

FRAUMENI, J. F. and GLASS, A. G. (1970). Rarity of Ewings tumour in Negroes. *Lancet*, **1**, 777.

FRAUMENI, J. H. and MILLER, R. W. (1967). Epidemiology of human leukaemia: recent observations. *J. Nat. Cancer Inst.*, **38**, 593.

FREDRICK, J. (1970). Anencephalus and the local water supply. *Nature*, **227**, 176.

FREEDMAN, J. (1972). Dahlak blindness. *Brit. med. J.*, **1**, 379.

FREIMAN, I., SCHMAMAN, A., ZAMIT, R. and APPLEBERG, M. (1968). Veno-occlusive disease of the liver. *S. Afr. med. J.*, **42**, 126.

FRESH, J. W., VERSAGE, P. M. and REYES (1964). Intestinal morphology in human and experimental cholera. *Arch. Path.*, **77**, 529.

FRICK, P. G., HITZIG, W. H. and BETKE, K. (1962). Hemoglobin Zürich. I: A new hemoglobin anomaly associated with acute hemolytic episodes with inclusion bodies after sulfonamide therapy. *Blood*, **20**, 261.

FRIEDMANN, H. C. (1954). 17-Ketosteroid excretion in Indian males. *Lancet*, **2**, 262.

FRIEND, N. B. (1932). The geographical distribution and meteorological aspect of hyperpyrexial heatstroke. *Med. J. Aust.*, **1**, 233.

FRIPP, P. J. (1965). Bilharziasis and bladder cancer. *Brit. J. Cancer*, **19**, 292.

FUGLSANG, H. and ANDERSON, J. (1973). *Onchocerca volvulus* microfilariae in urine. *Lancet*, **2**, 321.

FULLERTON, W. T. and TURNER, A. G. (1962). Exchange transfusion in treatment of severe anaemia in pregnancy. *Lancet*, **1**, 75.

FULLERTON, W. T. and WATSON-WILLIAMS, E. J. (1962). Haemoglobin SC disease and megaloblastic anaemia of pregnancy. *J. Obstet. Gynaec. Brit. Cwlth.*, **69**, 729.

FULTON, J. D. (1963). Serological tests in toxoplasmosis. In *Immunity to protozoa*, ed. P. C. C. Garnham, A. E. Pierce and I. Roitt, p. 259. Blackwell, Oxford.

— (1965). Micro-agglutination test for *Toxoplasma* antibodies. *Immunology*, **9**, 491.

FULTON, J. D., JOYNER, L. P. and PRICE, I. N. O. (1951). Studies on protozoa. Part IV. A complement-fixation test for amoebiasis. *J. trop. Med. Hyg.*, **54**, 27.

GAFNI, J. and SOHAR, E. (1960). Rectal biopsy for the diagnosis of amyloidosis. *Amer. J. med. Sci.*, **240**, 332.

GAJDUSEK, D. C. (1963). Motor-neuron disease in natives of New Guinea. *New Engl. J. Med.*, **268**, 474.

GAJDUSEK, D. C., GIBBS, C. J., JR. and ALPERS, M. (1966). Experimental transmission of a kuru-like syndrome to chimpanzees. *Nature*, **209**, 794.

GAJDUSEK, D. C. and ZIGAS, V. (1957). Degenerative disease of the central nervous system in New Guinea. The endemic occurrence of 'Kuru' in the native population. *New Engl. J. Med.*, **257**, 974.

GAJDUSEK, D. C., *et al.* (1972). Persistence of viruses of Kuru and Creutzfeldt–Jakob disease in tissue cultures of brain cells. *Nature (Lond.)*, **235**, 104.

GALINDO, L., VON LICHTENBERG, F. and BALDIZÓN, C. (1962). Bancroftian filariasis in Puerto Rico: infection pattern and tissue lesions. *Amer. J. trop. Med. Hyg.*, **11**, 739.

GALINDO, P., DE RODANICHE, E. and JOHNSON, C. M. (1959). St. Louis encephalitis in Panama. I. Isolation of the virus from forest mosquitoes and human blood. *Amer. J. trop. Med. Hyg.*, **8**, 557.

GALL, E. A. (1960). Posthepatic, postnecrotic, and nutritional cirrhosis: a pathologic analysis. *Amer. J. Path.*, **36**, 241.

GALL, J. C., JR., BREWER, G. J. and DERN, R. J. (1965). Studies of glucose-6-phosphate dehydrogenase activity of individual erythrocytes: the methemoglobin-elution test for identification of females heterozygous for G6PD deficiency. *Amer. J. hum. Genet.*, **17**, 359.

GALLACHER, B. A. and MILLER, C. G. (1967). Acute glomerulonephritis in Jamaican children. *W. Indian med. J.*, **16**, 17.

GALLAGHER, P. J., MILLIS, R. R. and MITCHINSON, M. J. (1972). Congenital dilatation of the intrahepatic bile ducts with cholangiocarcinoma. *J. clin. Path.*, **25**, 804.

GALLAIS, P. and BADIER, M. (1952). Recherches sur l'encephalite de la trypanosomiase humain Africain. *Méd. trop.*, **12**, 633.

GAN, E., *et al.* (1972). Filter paper collection of blood for use in a screening and diagnostic test for scrub typhus using the IFAT. *Trans. roy. Soc. trop. Med. Hyg.*, **66**, 588.

GALTON, M. M., *et al.* (1962). *Leptospirosis: Epidemiology, Clinical Manifestations in Man and Animals, and Methods in Laboratory Diagnosis*. U.S.P.H.S. Publication No. 951. U.S. Government Printing Office, Washington D.C.

GANS, J. C. and KARBAAT, J. (1967). Histoplasmosis in Dutch servicemen returning from Surinam. *Trop. geogr. Med.*, **19**, 177.

GARA, A. C. and SUBRAMANIAN, R. (1964). Autopsy study of atherosclerosis at Madras, South India. *Circulation*, **29**, 546.

GARCIA LOPEZ, G., MILANES, F., SPIES, T. D., LOPEZ TOCA, R., ARAMBURU, T. and LOPEZ, H. (1949). The association of hypoproteinemia with severe tropical sprue. *Amer. J. med. Sci.*, **218**, 660.

GARCIA-PALMIERI, M. R. (1962). Rheumatic fever and rheumatic heart disease as seen in the tropics. *Amer. Heart J.*, **64**, 577.

GARDINER, M. R., ROYCE, R. and BOKOR, A. (1965). Studies on *Crotalaria crispata*, a newly recognised cause of Kimberley horse disease. *J. Path. Bact.*, **89**, 43.

GARDNER, F. H. (1958). Tropical sprue. *New Engl. J. Med.*, **258**, 791.

GARDNER, P. S., BLACK, M. M. and RICHARDSON, J. (1968). The rapid diagnosis of *Herpes virus hominus* infections. *Brit. med. J.*, **4**, 89.

GARNHAM, P. C. C. (1936). A case of congenital relapsing fever. *E. Afr. med. J.*, **13**, 50.

— (1949). Malarial immunity in Africans: effects in infancy and early childhood. *Ann. trop. Med. Parasit.*, **43**, 47.

GARNHAM, P. C. C., BAKER, J. R. and BIRD, R. G. (1962). Fine structure of cystic form of *Toxoplasma gondii. Brit. med. J.*, **1**, 83.

GARNHAM, P. C. C., *et al.* (1969). Human Babesiosis in Ireland: Further observations and the medical significance of this infection. *Brit. med. J.*, **4**, 768.

GARRATT, E. I. (1945). Clinical filariasis due to *Acanthocheilonema (Filaria) perstans. Trans. roy. Soc. trop. Med. Hyg.*, **38**, 287.

GARRET, G., HAY, W. J. and RICKARDS, A. G. (1959). Familial cardiomegaly. *J. clin. Path.*, **12**, 355.

GARRET, R. (1962). Chronic diffuse giant cell mesaortitis, with dissecting aneurysm and rupture. *Amer. J. clin. Path.*, **38**, 406.

GARROW, J. S. (1966). Protein-calorie malnutrition. (Correspondence.) *Lancet*, **2**, 592.

— (1967). Loss of brain potassium in kwashiorkor. *Lancet*, **2**, 643.

GAULT, E. W., JOB, C. K. and WEBB, J. K. G. (1960). Aetiology of tropical eosinophilia. *Indian J. Malar.*, **14**, 633.

GEAR, J. H. S., GORDON, F. B., JONES, B. R. and BELL, S. D., JR. (1963). Nomenclature of isolates of virus from trachoma and inclusion blennorrhea. *Nature, (Lond.)* **197**, 26.

GEBBIE, D. A. M., *et al.* (1964). Malarial antibodies in idiopathic splenomegaly in Uganda. *Lancet*, **2**, 392.

GEEFHUYSEN, J., *et al.* (1971). Impaired cellular immunity in kwashiorkor with improvement after therapy. *Brit. med. J.*, **4**, 527.

GEEVARGHESE, P. J. and PITCHUMONI, C. S. (1968). *Pancreatic Diabetes in Kerala.* Diabetic association of India, p. 223. Bombay.

GEIGY, R. and MOSSER, H. (1955). Studies on the epidemiology of African relapsing fever in Tanganyika. *J. trop. Med. Hyg.*, **58**, 199.

GEIGY, R., *et al.* (1972). Additional animal reservoirs of *T. rhodesiense* sleeping sickness. *Acta trop. Basel*, **29**, 199.

GELDERMAN, A. H., *et al.* (1971). A comparison of genome sizes and thermal-denaturation-derived base composition of DNAs from several members of *Entamoeba* (histolytica group). *J. Parasit.*, **57**, 912.

GELFAND, M. (1947). Symmetrical gangrene in the African. *Brit. med. J.*, **1**, 847.

— (1948). *The Sick African.* 2nd ed. Stewart Printing Co., Cape Town.

— (1949). Some peculiar cases of gangrene and their possible relationship to tropical phlebitis. *Trans. roy. Soc. trop. Med. Hyg.*, **43**, 75.

— (1950). *Schistosomiasis in South Central Africa: A Clinico-Pathological Study.* Post-Graduate Press, Cape Town and Johannesburg.

— (1952). Cardiac and vascular disorders in the African. *W. Afr. med. J.* (n.s.), **1**, 91.

— (1957). *The Sick African: A Clinical Study.* 3rd ed. Juta, Cape Town.

— (1961). The clinical aspects of cirrhosis and primary carcinoma of the liver in the African of the Central African Federation of Rhodesia and Nyasaland. *Acta Un. int. Cancr.*, **17**, 604.

— (1961). *Medicine in Tropical Africa.* Livingstone, London.

— (1972). Haemoglobinuria due to typhoid and paratyphoid fever. *Trop. geogr. Med.*, **24**, 18.

GELFAND, M. and BERNBERG, H. (1959). Tropical eosinophilic syndrome: a clinical description of the disorder as seen in S. Rhodesia. *Cent. Afr. J. Med.*, **5**, 405.

GELFAND, M. and HAMMAR, B. (1966). Acute intestinal obstruction from a granuloma due to *Schistosoma haematobium* in the large intestine. *Trans. roy. Soc. trop. Med. Hyg.*, **60**, 231.

GELFAND, M., WEINBERG, R. W. and CASTLE, W. (1967). Relation between carcinoma of the bladder and infestation with *Schistosoma haematobium*. *Lancet*, **1**, 1249.

GELFAND, M. and WESSELS, P. (1964). *Acanthocheilonema perstans* in a European female: a discussion of its possible pathogenicity and a suggested new syndrome. *Trans. roy. Soc. trop. Med. Hyg.*, **58**, 552.

GELFAND, M., *et al.* (1970). Schistosomiasis of the male pelvic organs. *Amer. J. trop. Med. Hyg.* **19**, 779.

GELPI, A. P. (1966). Q Fever in Saudi Arabia. *Amer. J. trop. Med. Hyg.*, **15**, 785.

GELPI, A. P. and MUSTAFA, A. (1968). Ascaris pneumonia. *Amer. J. Med.*, **44**, 377.

GERALD, P. S. and DIAMOND, L. K. (1958). A new hereditary hemoglobinopathy (the Lepore trait) and its interaction with thalassemia trait. *Blood*, **13**, 835.

GERBAUX, A., GARIN, J. P. and LENÈGRE, J. (1957). Cardiopathy and filariasis. *Bull. Soc. méd Hôp. Paris.*, nos. 25/26, 873.

GERBER, M. A. and PARONETTO, F. (1971). IgE in glomeruli of patients with nephrotic syndrome. *Lancet*, **1**, 1097.

GERBER, P., *et al.* (1968). Infectious mononucleosis: complement fixing antibodies to herpes like virus associated with Burkitt lymphoma. *Science (Washington)*, **161**, 173.

GERLE, P. D., WALKER, L. A., ACHORD, J. L. and WEENS, H. S. (1965). Osseous changes in chronic pancreatitis. *Radiology*, **85**, 330.

GERMAN, L. J., MCCRACKEN, A. W. and WILKIE, K. MCD. (1968). Outbreak of febrile illness associated with ECHO virus type 5 in a maternity unit in Singapore. *Brit. med. J.*, **1**, 742.

GERSHOFF, S. N., PRIEN, E. L. and CHANDRAPANOND, A. (1963). Urinary stones in Thailand. *J. Urol.*, **90**, 285.

GHITIS, J., *et al.* (1963). Cali–Harvard nutrition project. II. The erythroid atrophy of kwashiorkor and marasmus. *Amer. J. clin. Nutr.*, **12**, 445.

GHONEIM, M. A., ASHAMALLAH, A. and KHALIK, M. A. (1971). Bilharzial strictures of the ureter presenting with anuria. *Brit. J. Urol.*, **43**, 439.

GIBLETT, E. R. and CHASE, J. (1959). Js a 'new' red cell antigen found in Negroes, evidence for an eleventh blood group system. *Brit. J. Haemat.*, **5**, 319.

GIBSON, J. A. (1973). Granulomatous liver disease and portal hypertension. *Proc. roy. Soc. Med.*, **66**, 502.

GIBSON, J. B. (1960). Chiari's disease and the Budd-Chiari syndrome. *J. Path. Bact.*, **79**, 381.

GIBSON, J. B. and SUN, T. (1965). Chinese liver fluke—*Clonorchis sinensis*: its occurrence in Hong Kong. *Int. Path.*, **6**, 94.

GIDEL, R., LEFÈVRE, M. and ATHAWET, B. (1966). An enquiry by sampling on the epidemiology of rickettsial infections in rural districts of the Ivory Coast. *Méd. Trop.*, **26**, 649.

GILBERT, C. and GILLMAN, J. (1963). Yams and liver necrosis. *Nature (Lond.)*, **198**, 196.

GILBERTSON, A. A. (1965). Anaesthesia in West African patients with sickle-cell anaemia, haemoglobin SC disease, and sickle-cell trait. *Brit. J. Anaesth.*, **37**, 614.

GILL, H. S., RAO, B. V. and CHHABRA, R. C. (1968). A note on the occurrence of *Lingatula serrata* (Frohlich, 1789) in domesticated animals. *Trans. roy. Soc. trop. Med. Hyg.*, **62**, 506.

GILLANDERS, A. D. (1951). Nutritional heart disease. *Brit. Heart J.*, **13**, 177.

GILLES, H. M. (1957). The development of malarial infection in breast-fed Gambian infants. *Ann. trop. Med. Parasit.*, **51,** 58.

— (1961). The natural history of 'stable' falciparum malaria in the pre-school child. *W. Afr. med. J.*, **10,** 293.

— (1967). *Akufo. An Environmental Study of a Nigerian Village Community.* p. 80. University of Ibadan Press.

— (1967). Medical care in developing countries. A review and commentary. *Lancet*, **1,** 718.

— (1968). *Proceedings of a Tropical Medicine Conference held at the Royal College of Physicians of London,* 1967, p. 29. Pitman Medical, London.

— (1971). *Management and Treatment of Tropical Diseases,* eds. Maegraith and Gilles. Blackwell, Oxford.

— (1974). Aspects of Tropical Medicine: Malaria. *Medicine:* A monthly add-on series of practical general medicine, 1972–74. 1522. Published by Medical Education (International) Ltd., London.

— (1975). Ecology of disease in the tropics., *Ann. N.Y. Sci.*, (in press).

— (1975). *Quartan malaria and childhood nephrosis.* Medical Surveys and Clinical trial. 3rd Ed. Oxford University Press.

GILLES, H. M. and BALL, P. A. J. (1964). Guinea-worm infection and gastric function. *Ann. trop. Med. Parasit.*, **58,** No. 1. 78.

GILLES, H. M. and IKEME, A. C. (1960). Haemoglobinuria among adult Nigerians due to glucose-6-phosphate dehydrogenase deficiency with drug sensitivity. *Lancet*, **2,** 889.

GILLES, H. M. and MCGREGOR, I. A. (1959). Studies on the significance of high serum gamma-globulin concentrations in Gambian Africans. I. Gamma-globulin concentrations of Gambian children in the first two years of life. *Ann. trop. Med. Parasit.*, **53,** 492.

— (1961). Studies on the significance of high serum gamma-globulin concentrations in Gambian Africans. III. Gamma-globulin concentrations of Gambian women protected from malaria for two years. *Ann. trop. Med. Parasit.*, **55,** 463.

GILLES, H. M. and TAYLOR, B. G. (1961). The existence of the glucose-6-phosphate dehydrogenase deficiency trait in Nigeria and its clinical implications. *Ann. trop. Med. Parasit.*, **55,** 64.

GILLES, H. M., WATSON WILLIAMS, E. J. and BALL, P. A. J. (1964). Hookworm infection and anaemia. *Quart. J. Med.* (n.s.), **33,** 1.

GILLES, H. M., WATSON-WILLIAMS, J. and TAYLOR, B. G. (1960). Glucose-6-phosphate dehydrogenase deficiency trait in Nigeria. *Nature (Lond.)*, **185,** 257.

GILLES, H. M., WILLIAMS, E. J. W. and BALL, P. A. J. (1964). Hookworm infection and anaemia. *Quart. J. Med.*, **33,** 1.

GILLES, H. M., *et al.*, (1967). Glucose-6-phosphate dehydrogenase deficiency, sickling, and malaria in African children in South Western Nigeria. *Lancet*, **1,** 138.

— (1969). Malaria, anaemia and pregnancy. *Ann. trop. Med. Parasit.*, **63,** 2.

— (1973). Results of a 7-year snail control project on the endemicity of *Schistosoma haematobium* infection in Egypt. *Ann. trop. Med. Parasit.*, **67,** 1, 45.

GILLMAN, T. (1942). *The cytology of the anterior lobe of the human (Bantu) pituitary gland.* M.Sc. Thesis, Johannesburg.

GILLMAN, J. J. and GILLMAN, T. (1951). *Perspectives in Human Malnutrition.* Grune and Stratton, New York.

GILMAN, R. H. and PRATHNAP, K. (1971). Acute intestinal amoebiasis proctoscopic appearances with histopathological correlation. *Ann. trop. Med. Parasit.*, **65,** 359.

GILMORE, H. R., JR., KEAN, B. H. and POSEY, F. M., JR. (1942). A case of sarcosporidiosis with parasites found in Heart. *Amer. J. trop. Med.*, **22**, 121.

GINGER, C. D. and KATZ, F. E. (1970). Separation of relapsing fever spirochaetes from blood by DEAE cellulose anion exchanger. *Trans. roy. Soc. trop. Med. Hyg.*, **64**, 700.

GINSBURG, B. E., WASSERMAN, J. and HULDT, A. B. (1974). Case of glomerulonephritis associated with acute toxoplasmosis. *Brit. med. J.*, **3**, 664.

GIRALDO, G., et al. (1972). Kaposi's sarcoma. *J. nat. Cancer Inst.*, **49**, 1495.

GIRAUD, R. M. A. and LUKE, I. (1969). Crohn's disease in the Transvaal Bantu. *S. Afr. med. J.* **43**, 610.

GIRDWOOD, R. W. (1963). Deficiency of folic acid and vitamin B_{12} in man. *Ghana med. J.*, **2**, 93.

GIUSTRA, F. X. (1954). Final report on a case of myocarditis following measles. *Amer. J. Dis. Child.*, **87**, 615.

GLOVER, W. E. (1928). *Porocephalus armillatus.* (Correspondence.) *W. Afr. med. J.*, **2**, 107.

GODAL, T., et al. (1971). Characterization of the cellular immune defect in lepromatous leprosy: a specific lack of circulating *Mycobacterium leprae*—reactive lymphocytes. *Clin. Exp. Immunol.*, **9**, 821.

GODFREY, M. F. (1937). Hydatid disease: clinical, laboratory and roentgenographic observations. *Arch. intern. Med.*, **60**, 783.

GOLD, P. and FREEDMAN, S. O. (1965). Specific carcinoembryonic antigens of the human digestive system. *J. exp. Med.*, **122**, 467.

GOLDBERG, G. M. (1962). A study of malignant lymphomas and leukaemias. *Cancer*, **15**, 869, 882.

GOLDBERG, G. M. and SAPHIR, O. (1959). Follicular lipidosis of the spleen. *Amer. J. Path.*, **34**, 1123.

GOLDBERG, M. A. and SCHWARTZ, S. O. (1954). Mediterranean anemia in a Negro complicated by pernicious anemia of pregnancy. *Blood*, **9**, 648.

GOLDBERG, M. F. (1972). Retinal detachment associated with proliferative retinopathies. *Israel J. med. Sci.* **8**, 1447.

GOLDEN, H. D., et al. (1971). A filterable agent in throat washings of patients with infectious mononucleosis. *J. infect. Dis.*, **124**, 422.

GOLDSMITH, R. S., et al. (1965). Haemorrhagic fever in Singapore. A changing syndrome. *Lancet*, **1**, 333.

GOLDSTEIN, H. B., DALE, B. N. and FELSENFELD, O. (1966). A study of gamma globulins in cholera. *Proc. Soc. exp. Biol.*, **121**, 425.

GOLDWASSER, R. A. and KISSLING, R. E. (1958). Fluorescent antibody staining of street and fixed rabies virus antigens. *Proc. Soc. exp. Biol.*, **98**, 219.

GOMPERTS, E., et al. (1969). Von Willebrand's disease in the Bantu. *South Afr. med. J.*, **43**, 1107.

GONZALEZ-CORTES, A., et al. (1973). Water-borne transmission of chloramphenicol-resistant *salmonella typhi* in Mexico. *Lancet*, **2**, 605.

GOODALE, F., LEE, K. T., SCOTT, R. F., EDINGTON, G. M., SNELL, E. S. and DAVIES, J. N. P. (1964). Geographic pathology of arteriosclerosis: a study of disease patterns in autopsied individuals from Kampala, Uganda; Ibadan, Nigeria; and Albany, New York. *Exp. molec. Path.*, **3**, 148.

GOODALL, H. B. (1973). Giant nuclear masses in the lungs and blood in malignant malaria. *Lancet*, **2**, 1124.

GOODHEART, C. R. (1970). Herpes viruses and cancer. *J. Amer. med. Ass.* **211**, 91.

GOODMAN, G., VON SALLMANN, L., and HOLLAND, M. G. (1967). Ocular manifestations of sickle-cell disease. *A.M.A. Arch. Ophthal.*, **58**, 655.

GOODWIN, J. F. (1964). Cardiac function in primary myocardial disorders. *Brit. med. J.*, **1**, 1527, 1595.

GOODWIN, L. G. (1974). *The African Scene: Mechanism of Pathogenesis in Trypanosomiasis.* Ciba Foundation Symposium 20 (new series). Associated Scientific Publishers, Amsterdam.

GOONERATNE, B. W. M. (1966). Massive generalized alopecia after poisoning by *Gloriosa superba. Brit. med. J.*, **1**, 1023.

GOPALAN, C. (1967). Malnutrition in childhood in the tropics. *Brit. med. J.*, **4**, 603.

— (1968). *Calorie Deficiency and Protein Deficiency.* Ed. McCance and Widdowson. London, p. 49.

GORDON, J. E., BEHAR, M. and SCRIMSHAW, N. S. (1964). Acute diarrhoeal disease in less developed countries. *Bull. Wld Hlth Org.*, **31**, 1.

GORDON, R. M. and LAVOIPIERRE, M. M. J. (1962). *Entomology for Students of Medicine.* Blackwell Scientific Publications, Oxford.

GORE, I. and SAPHIR, O. (1947). Myocarditis: a classification of 1402 cases. *Amer. Heart J.*, **34**, 827.

GORE, R. W., SADUN, E. H. and HOFF, R. (1970). *Echinococcus granulosus* and *E. multilocularis:* soluble antigen fluorescent antibody test. *Exp. Parasit.*, **2**, 272.

GORMAN, J. G. (1964). Selection against the Rh-negative gene by Malaria. *Nature (Lond.),* **202**, 676.

GOTHOSKAR, S. V. and RANADIVE, K. J. (1966). Experimental studies on the aetiology of 'kangri cancer'. *Brit. J. Cancer*, **20**, 751.

GOUDIE, R. B., MACSWEEN, R. N. M. and GOLDBERG, D. M. (1966). Serological and histological diagnosis of primary biliary cirrhosis. *J. clin. Path.*, **19**, 527.

GOUTTAS, A., *et al.* (1955)..Description d'une nouvelle variété d'anémie hémolytique congénitale. (Étude hématologique, électrophorétique et génétique.) *Sang*, **26**, 911.

GOVAN, A. D. T. (1962). Tuberculous endometritis. *J. Path. Bact.*, **83**, 363.

GRABER, C. D., *et al.* (1971). Fatal heat stroke. *J. Amer. med. Ass.*, **216**, 1195.

GRACE, H. and WASSEF, S. A. (1969). Juxta-intestinal cystic schistosomal granuloma. *J. Path.*, **99**, 176.

GRAFF, G. and GRAFF, M. (1971). Famileal Mediterranean fever, amyloidosis and eclampsia. *J. Obstet. Gynaec. Brit. Cwlth.*, **78**, 284.

GRAHAM, G. G., CORDANO, A., BAERTL, J. M. and MORALES, E. (1966). Programs for combatting malnutrition in the pre-school child in Peru. In *Pre-school child malnutrition: . . . an international conference on prevention of malnutrition in the pre-school child*, Washington, D.C., 7th–11th December, 1964, 163. Nat. Acad. Sci.—Nat. Res. Counc. Washington.

GRANICK, S. (1964). A test for detection of porphyria-inducing drugs. (Correspondence.) *J. Amer. med. Ass.*, **190**, 475.

GRAY, H. H., KINGMA, S. and KOK, S. H. (1967). Mycobacterial skin ulcers in Nigeria. *Trans. roy. Soc. trop. Med. Hyg.*, **61**, 712.

GRAY, I. R. (1951). Endocardial fibrosis. *Brit. Heart J.*, **13**, 387.

GRAY, J. A. (1973). Mumps. *Brit. med. J.*, **1**, 338.

GREEN, R. L., HUNTSMAN, R. G. and SERJEANT, G. R. (1971). The sickle-cell and attitude. *Brit. med. J.*, **4**, 593.

GREENHOUGH, W. B. (1965). Pancreatic and hepatic hypersecretion in cholera. *Lancet*, **2**, 991.

GREENWOOD, B. M. (1967). Acute intermittent porphyria in Nigerians. *Trop. geogr. Med.*, **19**, 289.

— (1968). Autoimmune disease and parasitic infections in Nigerians. *Lancet*, **2**, 380.

— (1969). Acute tropical polyarthritis. *Quart. J. Med.*, **28**, 295.

— (1974). Possible role of a B-cell mitogen in hypergammaglobulinaemia in malaria and trypanosomiasis. *Lancet*, **1**, 435.

GREENWOOD, B. M., BRANDLEY-MOORE, A. M., PALIT, A. and BRYCESON, A. D. M. (1972). Immunosuppression in children with malaria. *Lancet*, **1**, 169.

GREENWOOD, B. M., HERRICK, E. M. and VOLLER, A. (1970). Suppression of auto-immune disease in NZB and (NZBX NZW)F, hybrid mice by infection with malaria. *Nature*, **226**, 266.

GREENWOOD, B. M., MULLER, A. S. and VALKENBURG, H. A. (1971). Rheumatoid factor in Nigerian sera. *Clin. exp. Immunol.*, **8**, 161.

GREENWOOD, B. M. and TAYLOR, J. R. (1968). The complications of diabetes in Nigerians. *Trop. geogr. Med.*, **20**, 15.

GREENWOOD, B. M. and WHITTLE, H. C. (1973). Cerebrospinal-fluid IgM in patients with sleeping sickness. *Lancet*, **1**, 525.

GREENWOOD, B. M., WHITTLE, H. C. and BRYCESON, A. D. M. (1973). Allergic complications of meningococcal disease. *Brit. med. J.*, **2**, 737.

GREENWOOD, B. M., *et al.* (1972). Immunosuppression in children with malaria. *Lancet*, **1**, 169.

— (1973). Immunosuppression in Gambian trypanosomiasis. *Trans. roy. Soc. trop. Med. Hyg.*, **67**, 6, 846.

— (1974). Immunodiagnosis of snake bite. *Brit. med. J.*, **4**, 743.

GRIFFITH, R. L. (1952). Condition of the heart following beriberi and malnutrition. *Arch. intern. Med.*, **89**, 743.

GRIMES, A. J. and MEISLER, A. (1962). Possible cause of Heinz bodies in congenital Heinz-body anaemia. *Nature (Lond.)*, **194**, 190.

GRITSAY, M. K. and YAKUBOV, T. G. (1970). On peculiarities of epidemiology and epizootiology of opisthorchiasis in the Ukraine (Russian). *Med. Parazit. (Mosk.)*, **39**, 534.

GROB, P. J. and JEMELKA, H. (1971). Faecal S.H. (Australia) antigen in acute hepatitis. *Lancet*, **1**, 206.

GRODE, H. E. and LASZLO, J. (1966). Sickle cell trait, refractory anemia, and nutritional anemia with variable expression of A and S hemoglobin. *Ann. intern. Med.*, **65**, 321.

GROLL, A. and SMITH, J. (1965). A case of disseminated typhoid osteitis. *S. Afr. med. J.*, **39**, 417.

GROSFELD, J. L., *et al.* (1970). Primary non-specific ileal ulcers in children. *Amer. J. Dis. Child.*, **120**, 447.

GROUD, P. (1951). Les Rickettsioses in Afrique equatoriale. *Bull. Wld Hlth Org.*, **4**, 535.

GROVER, S. and HARDAS, U. D. (1972). Childhood malignancies in central India. *J. nat. Cancer Inst.*, **49**, 953.

GUINTO, R. S., *et al.* (1954). The trend of leprosy in Cordova and Talisay, Cebu Province., Philippines. *Int. J. Leprosy*, **22**, 409.

GUIOT, G. (1964). An outbreak of Q fever in Tulear, Madagascar. *Méd. trop. Marseilles*, **24**, 66.

GUNSTONE, R. F., *et al.* (1971). Pancreatic ascites. *Brit. med. J.*, **1**, 536.

GUNTHER, S. (1967). Furuncular tumbu fly myiasis of man in Gabon. *J. trop. Med. Hyg.*, **70**, 169.

GUPTA, D. N. and SMETANA, H. F. (1957). The histopathology of viral hepatitis as seen in the Delhi epidemic (1955–56). *Indian J. med. Res.*, **45**, suppl., 101.

GUPTA, O. P. (1964). *Diabetic nephropathy. A clinical and histological study by renal biopsy*. Joint Ann. Conf. Ass. of Phys. of India, Patiala.

GUPTA, P. S., GUPTA, G. D. and SHARMA, M. L. (1963). Veno-occlusive disease of liver. *Brit. med. J.*, **1**, 1184.

GURSON, C. T. and SANER, G. (1971). Effect of chromium on glucose utilization in marasmic protein–calorie malnutrition. *Amer. J. clin. Nutr.*, **24**, 1313.

GUTMAN, A., *et al.* (1973). An outbreak of tick typhus in the coastal plain of Israel. 13 cases from the Sharon area. *Trans. roy. Soc. trop. Med. Hyg.*, **67**, 112.

HABIB, G. B. (1962). Neurosyphilis (clinical experience in the diagnosis and treatment). *W. Indian med. J.*, **11**, 100.

HACKETT, C. J. (1963). On the origin of the human treponematoses. *Bull. Wld Hlth Org.*, **29**, 7.

— (1967). Yaws eradication. *Trans. roy. Soc. trop. Med. Hyg.*, **61**, 148.

HACKETT, C. J. and LOEWENTHAL, L. J. A. (1960). *Differential Diagnosis of Yaws*. W.H.O., Geneva.

HADDOCK, D. R. W. (1967). The pattern of leukaemia in Accra, Ghana. *J. trop. Med. Hyg.*, **70**, 60.

HADDOCK, D. R. W., EBRAHIM, G. J. and KAPUR, B. B. (1962). Ataxic neurological syndrome found in Tanganyika. *Brit. med. J.*, **2**, 1442.

HADDOW, A. J. (1964). Age incidence in Burkitt's lymphoma syndrome. *E. Afr. med. J.*, **41**, 1.

HADDOW, A. J., DAVIES, C. W. and WALKER, A. J. (1960). O'nyong-nyong fever: an epidemic virus disease in East Africa. I. Introduction. *Trans. roy. Soc. trop. Med. Hyg.*, **54**, 517.

HADEN, R. F. and LANGSJOEN, P. H. (1961). Manifestations of myocardial involvement in acute reactions to penicillin. *Amer. J. Cardiol.*, **8**, 420.

HAENZEL, W. and KURIHARA, M. (1968). Studies of Japanese migrants. *J. nat. Cancer Inst.*, **40**, 43.

HAHN, R. G. and BUGHER, J. C. (1953). Observations during an outbreak of infectious hepatitis in British West Africa. *Trans. roy. Soc. trop. Med. Hyg.*, **47**, 77.

HAIM, S., *et al.* (1972). Kaposi's sarcoma in association with immunosuppressive therapy. *Israel J. med. Sci.*, **8**, 1993.

EL HALAWANI, A. W. (1964). Heat illness during the Mecca pilgrimage. *W.H.O. Chron.*, **18**, 283.

HALDEN, E. R., *et al.* (1955). Haematologic studies in heat stroke: the anaemia of heat stroke with emphasis on a haemolytic component. *Amer. J. Med.*, **19**, 141.

HALL, E. W. and PARRY, E. H. O. (1963). Lobar pneumonia with jaundice in adult Nigerians. *Trans. roy. Soc. trop. Med. Hyg.*, **57**, 206.

HALL-CRAGGS, M., MARSDEN, P. D., RAPER, A. B., LEHMANN, H. and BEALE, D. (1964). Homozygous sickle-cell anaemia arising from two different haemoglobins S: interaction of haemoglobins S and Stanleyville-II. *Brit. med. J.*, **2**, 87.

HALSTEAD, C. L. (1970). Oral manifestations of haemoglobinopathies. *Oral Surg.*, **30**, 615.

HALSTEAD, S. B., YAMARAT, C. and SCANION, J. E. (1963). The Thai hemmorhagic fever epidemic of 1962. *J. Med. Ass. Thailand*, **46**, 449.

HAMILTON, P. J. S., *et al.* (1967). Splenectomy in 'big spleen disease'. *Brit. med. J.*, **3**, 823.

HAMMON, W. MCD., RUDNICK, A. and SATHER, G. E. (1960). Viruses associated with epidemic hemorrhagic fevers of the Philippines and Thailand. *Science*, **131**, 1102.

— (1961). Identification and classification of the dengue group of viruses. In *Symposium on Haemorrhagic Fever*, SEATO Med. Res. Monograph No. 2, 30.

HAMMON, W. MCD., *et al.* (1941). Isolation of the viruses of western equine and St. Louis encephalitis from *Culex tarsalis* mosquitoes. *Science*, **94**, 328.

HAMMOND, J. A. (1974). Human infection with the liver fluke *Fasciola gigantica*. *Trans. roy. Soc. trop. Med. Hyg.*, **68**, 253.

HANADA, M. and RUCKNAGEL, D. L. (1964). The characterization of hemoglobin Shimonoseki. *Blood*, **24**, 624.

HANNE, O. H. (1964). Lung abscess due to *S. typhi*. *Amer. Rev. resp. Dis.*, **89**, 566.

HARADA, Y. and MORI, O. (1951). *Igaku to Seitbutsugaku*, **20**, 65 (in Japanese).

HARE, R. and POLUNIN, J. (1960). Anaerobic cocci in the vagina of native women in British North Borneo. *J. Obstet. Gynaec. Brit. Emp.*, **67**, 985.

HARINASUTA, C. (1969). Opisthorchiasis in Thailand: a review. In *Proceedings of the 4th S.E. Asian Seminar on Parasitology and Tropical Medicine*, Schistosomiasis and other snail-transmitted helminthiasis. Manila, 1969, p. 253.

HARINASUTA, C., JATSNASEN, S., IMPAND, P. and MAEGRAITH, B. G. (1967). *Investigation on the health problems in association with the construction of the dams in Northeast Thailand. A preliminary survey on the status of health in the population.* SEAMES. The First Southeast Asian Regional Seminar on Tropical Medicine. Abstracts of Papers, p. 157.

HARINASUTA, C. and VAJRASTHIRA, S. (1960). Opisthorchiasis in Thailand. *Ann. trop. Med. Parasit.*, **54**, 100.

HARLING, D. S. MARSDEN, P. D. and RIDLEY, D. S. (1965). Some observations on the pattern of heart disease in the Gambia. *Trans. roy. Soc. trop. Med. Hyg.*, **59**, 628.

HARRIES, J. R. (1964). Tropical sprue in the African. *E. Afr. med. J.*, **41**, 180.

HARRIES, J. R. (1969). Myasthenia gravis in Kenya. *Trans. roy. Soc. trop. Med. Hyg.*, **63**, 680.

HARRIS, L. C. and KEET, M. P. (1960). Xeroderma pigmentosum. *J. Pediat.*, **57**, 759.

HARRISON, C. V., ed. (1960). *Recent Advances in Pathology*. 7th ed. Churchill, London.

HARRISON, D. F. N. (1964). Snuff—its use and abuse. *Brit. med. J.*, **2**, 1649.

HARRISON, E. G., JR. and THOMPSON, J. H., JR. (1965). Dirofilariasis of human lung. *Amer. J. clin. Path.*, **43**, No. 3, 224.

HARRISON, K. A. (1967). Blood-volume changes in severe anaemia of pregnancy. *Lancet*, **1**, 20.

HARRISON, K. A. and LAWSON, J. B. (1966). Ethacrynic acid in blood transfusion. *Lancet*, **2**, 905.

HARROW, B. R., SLOANE, J. A. and LIEBMAN, N. C. (1963). Roentgenologic demonstration of renal papillary necrosis in sicke-cell trait. *New Engl. J. Med.*, **268**, 969.

HART, F. D. (1971). Classification of the arthropathies. *Brit. med. J.*, **2**, 210.

HARTLEY, W. J. (1966). A review of the epidemiology of toxoplasmosis. *Med. J. Aust.*, **1**, 232.

HARTZ, P. H. (1946). Human strongyloidiasis with internal autoinfection. *Arch. Path.*, **41**, 601.

— (1950). Filarial orchitis. *Docum. neerl. indones. Morb. trop.*, **2**, 170.

— (1958). The incidence of carcinoma of the oesophagus in the Caribbean region and in Venezuela, compared with that of gastric cancer. *Acta Un. int. Cancr.*, **14**, 548.

HARVEY, P. W. and KERSHAW, W. E. (1964). Low incidence of latent trichinosis near Blackpool compared with incidence elsewhere in England and Wales. *Brit. med. J.*, **2**, 1632.

HARVEY, W. P., SEGAL, J. P. and GUREL, T. (1964). The clinical spectrum of primary myocardial disease. *Progr. cardiovasc. Dis.*, **7**, 17.

HASHEM, M. (1947). The etiology and pathogenesis of the endemic form of spleno-megaly: Egyptian splenomegaly. *J. Egypt. med. Ass.*, **30**, 48.

HASHEM, M., ZAKI, S. A. and HUSSEIN, M. (1961). The bilharzial bladder cancer and its relation to schistosomiasis: a statistical study. *J. Egypt. med. Ass.*, **44**, 579.

HASSAN, M. A., RAHMAN, E. A. and RAHMAN, I. A. (1973). Postoperative deep vein thrombosis in Sudanese patients. *Brit. med. J.*, **1**, 515.

HASSAN, M. M. (1960). Kwashiorkor in Sudanese children (clinical notes). *J. trop. Pediat.*, **6**, 98.

HASSANEIN, E. A., *et al.* (1972). Serum ketone bodies, pyruvic acid, lactic acid and serum electrolytes in protein-calorie malnutrition. *Trop. geogr. Med.* **24**, 76.

HATHOUT, E. S., EL-GHAFFAR, A. Y. and AWYNY, A. Y. (1967). Salmonellosis complicat-ing schistosomiasis in Egypt. A new clinical appreciation. *Amer. J. trop. Med. Hyg.*, **16**, 462.

HATHOUT, S. E., *et al.* (1966). Relation between urinary schistosomiasis and chronic enteric urinary carrier state among Egyptians. *Amer. J. trop. Med. Hyg.*, **15**, 156.

HAWKING, F. (1940). Distribution of filariasis in Tanganyika Territory, East Africa. *Ann. trop. Med. Parasit.*, **34**, 107.

— (1952). A histological study of onchocerciasis treated with hetrazan. *Brit. med. J.*, **1**, 992.

— (1964). Recent work on *T. cruzi* in Brazil and Central America. *J. trop. Med. Hyg.*, **67**, 214.

— (1965). Advances in filariasis especially concerning periodicity of microfilariae. *Trans. roy. Soc. trop. Med. Hyg.*, **59**, 9.

HAWKING, F. and GREENFIELD, J. G. (1941). Two autopsies on *rhodesiense* sleeping sickness: visceral lesions and significance of changes in cerebrospinal fluid. *Trans. roy. Soc. trop. Med. Hyg.*, **35**, 155.

HAYASHI, A., SHIMIZU, A., YAMAMURA, Y. and WATARI, H. (1966). Hemoglobins M: identification of Iwate, Boston, and Saskatoon variants. *Science, N.Y.*, **152**, 207.

HAYES, J. A. and LOVELL, H. G. (1966). Heart weight of Jamaicans: autopsy study of normal cases and cases of hypertension and chronic lung disease. *Circulation*, **33**, 450.

HAYES, J. A. and RICHARDS, R. (1964). Cor pulmonale due to uncommon forms of lung fibrosis. *W. Indian med. J.*, **13**, 73.

HAYES, J. A. and SUMMERELL, J. (1963). Emphysema in Jamaica: a preliminary report. *W. Indian med. J.*, **12**, 34.

HAYNES, M. E., HAYNES, D. W. G. and WILLIAMS, R. (1972). Cytoplasmic particles in hepatocytes of patients with Australia antigen-positive liver disease. *J. Clin. Path.*, **25**, 403.

HEADINGTON, J. T., *et al.* (1967). Segmental infarcts of the small intestine and mesenteric adenitis in Thai children. *Lancet*, **1**, 802.

HEARN, C. E. D. (1970). Racial differences in the prevalence of corneal arcus. *Arch. environ. Hlth.*, **20**, 506.

HEATH, D. D. and SMYTH, J. D. (1970). *In vitro* cultivation of *Echinococcus granulosus*, *Taenia hydatigena*, *T. ovis*, *T. pisiformis* and *T. serialis* from oncosphere to cystic larva. *Parasitology*, **61**, 329.

HEATON, F. W., PYRAH, L. N., BERESFORD, C. C., BRYSON, R. W. and MARTIN, D. F. (1962). Hypomagnesaemia in chronic alcoholism. *Lancet*, **2**, 802.

HECHT, V. (1910). Die Riesenzellenpneumonie in Kindesalter. *Beitr. path. Anat.*, **48**, 263.

HEDENBURG, F., *et al.* (1958). Haemoglobin H and inclusion body anaemia in a Swedish family. *Acta Paediat. (Uppsala)*, **47**, 652.

HEFFRON, R. (1939). *Pneumonia*. Commonwealth Fund, London.

HEGGTVEIT, H. A. (1965). Alcohol and the heart. *Amer. Heart J.*, **69**, 422.

HEISCH, R. B. (1950). Studies in East African relapsing fever. *E. Afr. med. J.*, **17**, 1.

HEISCH, R. B., *et al.* (1958). The isolation of *Trypanosoma rhodesiense* from a bushbuck. *Brit. med. J.*, **2**, 1203.

HELIN, M., SAVOLA, J. and LAPINLEIMU, K. (1969). Cardiac manifestations during Coxsackie B5 epidemic. *Brit. med. J.*, **2**, 97.

HENDERSON, B. E., GARY, G. W., KISSLING, R. E., FRAME, J. D. and CAREY, D. E. (1972). Lassa fever. Virological and serological studies. *Trans. roy. Soc. trop. Med. Hyg.*, **66**, 409.

HENDERSON, R. J. and HILL, D. M. (1972). Subclinical Brucella infection in man. *Brit. med. J.*, **3**, 154.

HENDRICKSE, J. P. DE V. (1972). Pregnancy in abnormal haemoglobins CC S-thalassaemia, SF, CF, double heterozygotes. *J. Obstet. Gynaec. Brit. Cwlth*, **79**, 410.

HENDRICKSE, J. P. DE V., *et al.* (1972). Pregnancy in homozygous sickle-cell anaemia. *J. Obstet. Gynaec. Brit. Cwlth.*, **79**, 396.

HENDRICKSE, J. P. DE V., COCKSHOTT, W. P. and JAMES, D. M. (1967). *Choriocarcinoma*, p. 98. Springer-Verlag, New York.

HENDRICKSE, R. G. (1965). The effect of malaria chemoprophylaxis on spleen size in sickle-cell anaemia. In *Abnormal Haemoglobins in Africa*, ed. J. H. P. Jonxis, p. 445. Blackwell, Oxford.

— (1972). Quartan malarial nephrotic syndrome. *Lancet*, **1**, 1143.

HENDRICKSE, R. G. and GILLES, H. M. (1963). The nephrotic syndrome and other renal diseases in children in Western Nigeria. *E. Afr. med. J.*, **40**, 186.

HENDRICKSE, R. G. and SHERMAN, P. M. (1965). Morbidity and mortality from measles in childhood seen at U.C.H. Ibadan. *Arch. ges. Virusforsch.*, **16**, 27.

HENDRICKSE, R. G., *et al.* (1960). Studies on the haemoglobins of newborn Nigerians. *Brit. med. J.*, **1**, 611.

— (1964). Studies on measles vaccination in Nigerian children. *Brit. med. J.*, **2**, 470.

— (1971). Malaria in early childhood. An investigation of 500 seriously ill children in whom a 'clinical' diagnosis of malaria was made on admission to the Children's Emergency Room at University College Hospital, Ibadan. *Ann. trop. Med. Parasit.*, **65**, 1, 1.

— (1972). Quartan malarial nephrotic syndrome. *Lancet*, **1**, 1143.

HENLE, G. and HENLE, W. (1970). Observations on childhood infections with the Epstein–Barr virus *J. Infect. Diseases*, **121**, 303.

HENLE, G., HENLE, W. and DIEHL, W. (1968). Relation of Burkitt's tumour associated herpes-type virus to infectious mononucleosis. *Proc. nat. Acad. Sci. (Wash.)*, **59**, 94.

HENLE, W. and HENLE, G. (1969). The relation between the Epstein-Barr virus and infectious mononucleosis, Burkitt's lymphoma and cancer of the postnasal space. *E. Afr. med. J.* **46**, 402.

HENRY, J. D., *et al.* (1966). Echinococcal disease of the kidney. *J. Urol.*, **96**, 431.

HENRY, W. J. (1963). Multiple aneurysm formation in a young man: a case report. *Ann. Surg.*, **158**, 1043.

HENSHAW, J. E. (1959). Observations on the chronicity of pulmonary tuberculosis in Africans. *W. Afr. med. J.*, **8**, 229.

HEPTINSTALL, R. H. (1966). *Diseases of the Kidney*. Churchill, London.

HERNANDEZ, O., *et al.* (1972). Mycosis of the central nervous system. *Rev. cuba. Med. Trop.*, **24**, 5.

HERRICK, J. B. (1910). Peculiar elongated and sickle-shaped red blood corpuscles in a case of severe anaemia. *Arch. intern. Med.*, **6**, 517.

HERSKO, C. and VARDY, P. A. (1967). Haemolysis in typhoid fever in children with G-6-Pd deficiency. *Brit. med. J.*, **1**, 214.

HEWETSON, J. F., GOTHASKAR, B. and KLEIN, G. (1972). Radioiodine-labelled antibody test for the detection of membrane antigens associated with the Epstein–Barr virus. *J. nat. Cancer Inst.*, **48**, 87.

HIGGINSON, J. (1963). Geographical pathology of primary liver cancer. *Cancer Res.*, **23**, 1624.

HIGGINSON, J., GILLANDERS, A. D. and MURRAY, J. F. (1952). The heart in chronic malnutrition. *Brit. Heart J.*, **14**, 213.

HIGGINSON, J., ISAACSON, C. and SIMSON, I. (1960). The pathology of cryptogenic heart disease: a study of the pathological pattern in eighty cases of obscure heart failure in the South African Bantu negro. *Arch. Path.*, **70**, 497.

HIGGINSON, J. and OETTLÉ, A. G. (1960). Cancer incidence in the Bantu and 'Cape colored' races of South Africa: report of a cancer survey in the Transvaal (1953–55). *J. nat. Cancer Inst.*, **24**, 589.

HIGGINSON, J. and STEINER, P. E. (1961). Definition and classification of malignant epithelial neoplasms of the liver. *Acta. Un. int. Cancr.*, **17**, 593.

HILKOVITZ, G. and JACOBSON, A. (1961). Hepatic dysfunction and abnormalities of the serum proteins and serum enzymes in sickle-cell anemia. *J. Lab. clin. Med.*, **57**, 856.

HILL, K. R. (1960). Section of comparative medicine: Discussion on seneciosis in men and animals. *Proc. roy. Soc. Med.*, **53**, 281.

HILL, K. R. and BRAS, G. (1957). *Hepatitis Frontiers*, ed. F. W. Hartman, G. A. Logrippo, J. G. Mateer and J. Barron, p. 51. Churchill, London.

HILL, K. R., RHODES, K., STAFFORD, J. L. and AUB, R. (1953). Serous hepatosis: a pathogenesis of hepatic fibrosis in Jamaican children: preliminary report. *Brit. med. J.*, **1**, 117.

HILL, K. R., STEPHENSON, C. F. and FILSHIE, I. (1958). Hepatic veno-occlusive disease produced experimentally in rats by the injection of monocrotaline. *Lancet*, **1**, 623.

HILL, M. J., *et al.* (1971). Bacteria and aetiology of cancer of large bowel. *Lancet*, **1**, 95.

HILL, W. R. and KINNEY, T. D. (1947). The cutaneous lesions in acute meningo-coccemia. *J. Amer. med. Ass.*, **134**, 513.

HIMSWORTH, H. P. (1950). *The Liver and its Diseases*. 2nd ed. Blackwell Scientific Publications, Oxford.

HIRSH, J. and DOERY, J. C. G. (1971). Platelet function in health and disease. *Progress in Hematology*, I, p. 185. Heinemann, London.

HOARE, C. A. (1949). *Handbook of Medical Protozoology*. Baillière, Tindall and Cox, London.

HOBBS, J. R. (1973). An ABC of amyloid. *Proc. roy. Soc. Med.*, **66**, 705.

HOEPPLI, R. (1932). Histological observations in experimental schistosomiasis japonica. *Chin. med. J.*, **46**, 1179.

— (1933). Histological changes in the liver of sixty-six Chinese infected with *Clonorchis sinensis. Chin. Med. J.*, **47**, 1125.

HOFFMAN, E. O. (1967). The etiology of rhinoscleroma. *Internal Path.*, Oct., 74.

HOGARTH-SCOTT, R. S. (1966). Visceral larva migrans—An immunofluorescent examination of rabbit and human sera for antibodies to the ES antigens of the second stage larvae of *Toxocara canis, Toxocara cati* and *Toxascaris leonina* (Nematoda). *Immunology*, **10**, 217.

HOGARTH-SCOTT, R. S., *et al.* (1969). Antibodies to *Toxocara* in the sera of visceral larva migrans patients: the significance of raised levels of IgE. *Clin. exp. Immunol.*, **5**, 619.

HOLLAND, J. F. and HRESHCHYSHYN, M. M., eds. (1967). *Choriocarcinoma: Transactions of a Conference of the International Union against Cancer.* Springer, Berlin, Heidelberg, New York.

HOLMES, E. G., STAMIER, M. W. and THOMPSON, M. D. (1955). The serum protein pattern of Africans in Uganda: relation to diet and malaria. *Trans. roy. Soc. trop. Med. Hyg.*, **49**, 376.

HOLMES, G. (1971). Worcestershire sauces and the kidneys. *Brit. med. J.* **3**, 252.

HOLT, L. E. (1963). The plasma aminogram in kwashiorkor. *Lancet*, **2**, 1343.

HOMEWOOD, C. A. and JEWSBURY, J. M. (1971). Comparison of malarial and schistosomal pigment. *Trans. roy. Soc. trop. Med. Hyg.*, **65**, 1.

HOMEWOOD, C. A., *et al.* (1975). Purification and some properties of malarial pigment. *Ann. trop. Med. Parasit.*, **69**, (in press).

HONDA, K., *et al.* (1973). Studies with the makari tumour skin test in Japan. *Trans. N.Y. Acad. Sci.*, **35**, 368.

HO PING KONG, H. and ALLEYNE, G. A. O. (1969). Acid-base status of adults with sickle cell anaemia. *Brit. med. J.*, **3**, 271.

HÖRLEIN, H. and WEBER, G. (1948). Uber chronische familiäre Methämoglobinämie und eine neue Modifikation des Methämoglobins. *Dtsch. med. Wschr.*, **73**, 476.

HORSFALL, F. L. and TAMM, I. (1965). *Viral and Rickettsial Infections of Man.* 4th. ed. Pitman Medical, London.

HOTCHIN, J. (1971). *Persistent and Slow Virus Infections.* S. Karger, London.

HOU, P. C. (1955). The pathology of *Clonorchis sinensis* infestation of the liver. *J. Path. Bact.*, **70**, 53.

— (1956). The relationship between primary carcinoma of the liver and infestation with *Clonorchis sinensis. J. Path. Bact.*, **72**, 239.

HOU, P. C. and PANG, L. S. C. (1964). *Clonorchis sinensis* infestation in man in Hong Kong. *J. Path. Bact.*, **87**, 245.

HSU, F. H. (1962). Clinical observation on 110 cases of *Ascaris* invasion into the biliary tract. *Nagoya J. med. Sci.*, **24**, 215.

HSU, S. Y. LI, HSU, H. F., CHU, K. Y., TSAI, C. T. and EVELAND, L. K. (1966). Immunization against *Schistosoma haematobium* in Rhesus monkeys by administration of cercariae of *Schistosoma bovis. Z. Tropenmed. Parasit.*, **17**, No. 4, 407.

HSUECH, C. H. and WU, Y. H. (1963). Endocrine disturbances in late schistosomiasis: a clinical study of 17 cases. *Chin. med. J.* **82**, 519.

HSUEH-LI, C. and NAO-CHU, C. (1957). Primary carcinoma of the liver. *Chin. Med. J.* **75**, 295.

HUANG, C. T., *et al.* (1969). Post-mortem and laboratory examinations for human intestinal helminths in Hong Kong, *Trop. Med.*, **11**, 136.

HUCKSTEP, R. L. (1962). *Typhoid Fever*, p. 180. Livingstone, London.

HUDSON, E. H. (1965). Treponematosis in perspective. *Bull. Wld Hlth Org.*, **32**, 735.

HUDSON, R. E. B. (1965). *Cardiovascular Pathology*. 2 vol. Edward Arnold, London.

HUEHNS, E. R. (1965). Abnormal haemoglobins causing haemolytic anaemia. *Proc. roy. Soc. Med.*, **58**, 514.

HUEHNS, E. R. and SHOOTER, E. M. (1965). Human haemoglobins. *J. med. Genet.*, **2**, 48.

HUGHES, J. T., *et al.* (1959). Leukaemoid reaction in disseminated tuberculosis. *J. clin. Path.*, **12**, 307.

HUGHES, M. H. (1954). Some observations on the pathology of onchocerciasis. *W. Afr. med. J.*, **3** (n.s.), 157.

HUGHES, R. A. C., *et al.* (1970). A case of fatal peri-partum cardiomyopathy. *Brit. Heart J.*, **32**, 272.

HUISMAN, T. H. J. (1960). Genetic aspects of two different minor haemoglobin components found in cord blood samples of Negro babies. *Nature (Lond.)*, **188**, 589.

HUISMAN, T. H. J., DOZY, A. M., HORTON, B. E. and WILSON, J. B. (1965). A fetal hemoglobin with abnormal γ-polypeptide chains: hemaglobin Warren. *Blood*, **26**, 668.

HUISMAN, T. H. J., HORTON, B. and SEBENS, T. B. (1961). Identity of the α-chains of the minor human haemoglobin components A_2 and $A_{2'}$ with the α-chains of human haemoglobin A and F. *Nature (Lond.)*, **190**, 357.

HUISMAN, T. H. J. and LEE, R. C. (1965). Two δ-chain abnormal hemoglobins in one individual. *Blood*, **26**, 677.

HUNT, A. H., PARR, R. M., TAYLOR, D. M. and TROTT, N. G. (1963). Relation between cirrhosis and trace metal content of liver, with special reference to primary biliary cirrhosis and copper. *Brit. med. J.*, **2**, 1498.

HUNTLEY, C. C., COSTAS, M. C. and LYERLY, A. (1965). Visceral larva migrans syndrome: clinical characteristics and immunologic studies in 51 patients. *Pediatrics, Springfield*, **36**, 523.

DE HURTADO, I. and LAYRISSE, M. (1968). Epidemiologic role of skin hypersensitivity in hookworm disease. *Amer. J. trop. Med. Hyg.*, **17**, 72.

HUSKISSON, E. C. and HART, F. D. (1969). Fulminating meningococcal septicaemia presenting with subarachnoid haemorrhage. *Brit. med. J.*, **2**, 231.

HUTCHINSON, M. P. (1953). The epidemiology of human trypanosomiasis in British West Africa. I and II: The Gambia. *Ann. trop. Med. Parasit.*, **47**, 156.

HUTCHISON, R. M., MERRICK, L. V. and WHITE, J. M. (1973). Fat embolism in sickle cell disease. *J. clin. Path.*, **26**, 620.

HUTCHISON, W. M., *et al.* (1970). Coccidian-like nature of *Toxoplasma gondii*. *Brit. med. J.*, **1**, 142.

— (1970). Coccidian-like nature of *Toxoplasma gondii*. *Brit. med. J.*, **1**, 142.

— (1972). Cats as a source of toxoplasmosis. *Proc. roy. Soc. Med.*, **65**, 1001.

HUTT, M. S. R., FERNANDES, B. J. J. and TEMPLETON, A. C. (1971). Myospherulosis. *Trans. roy. Soc. trop. Med. Hyg.*, **65**, 182.

HUTT, M. S. R. and LOWENTHAL, N. M. (1974). Chronic splenomegaly in the tropics. *Tropical Doctor*, **4**, 51.

HUTTON, P. W. (1956). Neurological disease in Uganda. *E. Afr. med. J.*, **33**, 209.

HWANG, W. and LIV, L. S. (1962). Constrictive arteritis of the aorta and its main branches. *Clin. med. J.*, **81**, 526.

IBER, F. L. and MADDREY, W. C. (1965). Familial hepatic diseases with portal hypertension with or without cirrhosis. In *Progress in Liver Diseases*, ed. H. Popper and F. Schaffner, **2**, 290. Heinemann, London.

IDSOE, O., *et al.* (1973). Venereal disease and treponematoses—the epidemiological situation and WHO's control programme. *WHO Chronicle*, **27**, 10, 410.

IFEKWUNIGWE, A. B. and LUZZATTO, L. (1966). Kernicterus in G-6-Pd deficiency. *Lancet*, **1**, 667.

IFEKWUNIGWE, A. E., PULVERTAFT, R. J. and WILLIAMS, A. O. (1966). The cerebrospinal fluid in retinoblastoma. *Brit. J. Cancer*, **20**, 250.

IKEJIANI, O. (1958). Gonococcal meningitis: A review of literature and report of a case. *W. Afr. med. J.* (n.s.), **7**, 139.

ILIYA, F. A., WILLIAMSON, S. and AZAR, H. A. (1967). Choriocarcinoma in the Near East: consanguinity as a possible etiologic factor. *Cancer, N.Y.*, **20**, 144.

IMPERIAL, E. S. and FELARCA, A. (1963). Autopsy study of heart disease in the Phillipines General Hospital, Based on a review of 6,000 consecutive cases. *Amer. Heart J.*, **66**, 470.

INDIAN COUNCIL OF MEDICAL RESEARCH (1957). Infectious hepatitis in Delhi (1955–56). A crucial study. *Indian J. med. Res.*, Suppl., **45**.

INGRAM, V. G., *et al.* (1966). Diarrhea in children of West Pakistan: occurrence of bacterial and parasitic agents, *Amer. J. trop. Med. Hyg.*, **15**, 743.

INGRAM, V. M. (1956). A specific chemical difference between the globins of normal human and sickle-cell anaemia haemoglobin. *Nature (Lond.)*, **178**, 792.

— (1957). Gene mutations in human haemoglobin: the chemical difference between normal and sickle cell haemoglobin. *Nature (Lond.)*, **180**, 326.

— (1959). Constituents of human haemoglobin: separation of the peptide chains of human globin. *Nature (Lond.)*, **183**, 1795.

INTERNATIONAL COLLOQUIUM OF LEPTOSPIROSIS (1966a). *Ann. Soc. belg. Med. trop. Parasit.*, **1**, 9.

— (1966b). *Ann. Soc. belg. Méd. Trop. Parasit.*, **2**, 135.

IRVINE, R. A., GRANT, L. S. and BELLE, E. A. (1963). Acute viral encephalitis in Jamaica. *Amer. J. trop. Med. Hyg.*, **12**, 916.

ISAACSON, C. (1961). An idiopathic aortitis in young Africans, *J. Path. Bact.*, **81**, 69.

ISAACSON, C. and WAYBURNE, S. (1957). Malignant hypertension in a child due to unilateral kidney disease. *Arch. Dis. Childh.*, **32**, 106.

ISHAK, K. G. and GLUNZ, P. R. (1967). Hepatoblastoma and hepatocarcinoma in infancy and childhood. *Cancer*, **20**, 396.

ISLAM, N. (1967). Splenic abscess, *J. trop. Med. Hyg.*, **70**, 153.

ISRAEL, M. S. (1959). The nodule in onchocerciasis *Trans. roy. Soc. trop. Med. Hyg.*, **53**, 142.

ISRAELS, L. G., YAMAMOTO, T., SKANDERBEG, J. and ZIPURSKY, A. (1963). Shunt bilirubin: evidence for two components. *Science, N.Y.*, **139**, 1054.

ITANO, H. A. (1951). A third abnormal hemoglobin associated with hereditary hemolytic anemia. *Proc. nat. Acad. Sci. (Wash.)*, **37**, 775.

ITANO, H. A., BERGREN, W. R. and STURGEON, P. (1954). Identification of a fourth abnormal human hemoglobin. *J. Amer. chem. Soc.*, **76**, 2278.

ITANO, H. A. and NEEL, J. V. (1950). A new inherited abnormality of human hemoglobin. *Proc. nat. Acad. Sci. (Wash.)*, **36**, 613.

ITANO, H. A. and ROBINSON, E. (1959). Properties and inheritance of haemoglobin by asymmetric recombination. *Nature (Lond.)*, **184**, 1468.

ITANO, H. A. and SINGER, S. J. (1958). On dissociation and recombination of human adult hemoglobins A, S, and C. *Proc. nat. Acad. Sci. (Wash.)*, **44**, 522.

ITO, J. and JOHNSTON, W. W. (1969). Hepatoblastoma and hepatoma in infancy and childhood. *Arch. Path.*, **87**, 259.

ITTYERAH, T. R., DUMM, M. E. and BACHHAWAT, B. K. (1967). Urinary excretion of lysosomal arylsulfatases in kwashiorkor. *Clin. chim. Acta*, **17**, 405.

IVE, F. A., *et al.* (1967). Endomyocardial fibrosis and filariasis. *Quart. J. Med.*, **36**, 495.

IWARSON, S., LUNDIN, P. and HERMODSSON, S. (1972). Liver morphology in acute viral hepatitis related to the hepatitis B antigen. *J. Clin. Path.*, **25**, 850.

IYER, C. G. S., *et al.* (1959). Kyasanur Forest disease. VI. Pathological findings in three fatal human cases of Kyasanur Forest disease. *Indian J. med. Sci.*, **13**, 1011.

JACKSON, J. G. and BREW, D. ST. J. (1961). Aortic aneurysm: a report of two cases of unknown cause. *W. Afr. med. J.* (n.s.), **10**, 47.

JACKSON, R. C. and WOODRUFF, A. W. (1962). The artificial kidney in malaria and blackwater fever. *Brit. med. J.*, **2**, 1367.

JACKSON, W. P. U., MARKS, I. N. and BANKS, S. (1968). *Chronic Pancreatitis and Diabetes in the Cape of Goodhope*, p. 230. Diabetic Assoc. of India, Bombay.

JACOBS, A. (1963). Epithelial changes in anaemic East Africans. *Brit. med. J.*, **1**, 1711.

JACOBS, A., *et al.* (1972). Ferritin in the serum of normal subjects and patients with iron deficiency and iron overload. *Brit. med. J.*, **4**, 206.

JACOBS, L. (1963). Chronic toxoplasmosis: latency and activity relative to serological findings. *Proc. 7th int. Congr. trop. Med. Malar., Rio de Janeiro*, **2**, 335.

— (1963). Toxoplasma and toxoplasmosis. *Ann. Rev. Microbiol.*, **17**, 429.

JACOBS, L., FAIR, J. R. and BICKERTON, J. H. (1954). Adult ocular toxoplasmosis: report of a parasitologically proved case. *A.M.A. Arch. Ophthal.*, **52**, 63.

JACOBS, P. A., TOUGH, I. M. and WRIGHT, D. H. (1963). Cytogenetic studies in Burkitt's lymphoma. *Lancet*, **2**, 1144.

JACQUERYE, L., *et al.* (1974). Tumoral calcinosis. Two cases observed in Shaba, Zaire Republic. *Ann. Soc. belge Méd. trop.*, **54**, 209.

JADIN, J. M. and CREEMERS, J. (1966). The ultrastructure of rosette forms of *Leishmania tropica*. *Ann. Soc. belge Méd. trop.*, **46**, 349.

JAFFÉ, E. R. and HELLER, R. (1964). Methemoglobinemia in man. *Prog. Hemat.*, **4**, 48.

JAFFÉ, L. (1954). Nasal leishmaniasis americana in Panama. *Arch. Otolaryng.*, **60**, 601.

JAFFE, R., *et al.* (1961). Observations on the pathogenesis of Chagas's disease. *Z. Tropenmed. Parasit., Stuttgart*. **12**, 137.

JAGANNATHAN, K. (1973). Juvenile motor neurone disease. In *Tropical Neurology*. Ed. J. D. Spillane, p. 127. Oxford University Press, London.

JAIN, R. C. and GUPTA, O. P. (1966). Electrophoretic pattern of serum proteins in dracunculosis. *Indian J. Med. Sci.*, **20**, No. 10, 713.

JANIS, B., *et al.* (1971). A new method for detecting plasmodia. *Milit. Med.*, **136**, 1, 23.

JANOTA, I. (1966). Involvement of the nervous system in malignant lymphoma in Nigeria. *Brit. J. Cancer*, **20**, 47.

JANSSENS, P. G. (1965). Les symptômes de la strongyloïdose. *Ann. Soc. belge Méd. trop.*, **45**, 131.

— (1964). *Dipetalonema perstans* est-elle pathogene pour l'homme? (Is *perstans* pathogenic for man?) *Ann. Soc. belge Méd. Trop.*, **44**, No. 6, 989.

— (1972). Skin ulcers caused by acid-fast bacilli. In *Essays on Tropical Dermatology*, ed. R. D. G. Ph. Simons, and J. Marshall, p. 264. Excerpta Medica Foundation, Amsterdam.

JANSSENS, P. G. and MUYNCK, A. DE. (1966). Appendicular pathology in the African Negro. *Trop. geogr. Med.*, **18**, 81.

JANSSENS, P. G., VAN BOGAERT, L. and HAYMAKER, W. (1956). Pathology of the peripheral nervous system in African trypanosomiasis: a study of seven cases. *J. Neuropath. exp. Neurol.*, **15**, 269.

JANSSENS, P. G., *et al.* (1959). Necrotic tropical ulcers and mycobacterial causative agents. *Trop. geogr. Med.*, **2**, 293.

JARPA, G. A. (1966). Coccidiosis humana. *Biologica (Santiago)*, **39**, 3.

JARRETT, E. E. E. and URQUHART, G. M. (1971). *Int. Rev. trop. med.*, **4**, 53.

JARUMILINTA, R. and MAEGRAITH, B. G. (1961). The patterns of some proteolytic enzymes of *Entamoeba histolytica* and *Acanthamoeba* spp. II. The action of *E. histolytica* and *Acanthamoeba* spp. on various synthetic substrates. *Ann. trop. Med. Parasit.*, **55**, 518.

JASIM, K. A. and TAHA, I. (1971). Toxoplasmic lymphadenitis in Iraq. *Trans. roy. Soc. trop. Med. Hyg.*, **65**, 790.

JAVETT, S. N., *et al.* (1956). Myocarditis in the newborn infant. *J. Paediat.*, **48**, 1.

JAYARATNAM, F. J., *et al.* (1967). Pernicious anaemia among Asians in Singapore. *Brit. med. J.*, **3**, 18.

JEANES, A. L. (1966). Indirect fluorescent antibody test in diagnosis of hepatic amoebiasis. *Brit. med. J.*, **1**, 1464.

JEEJEEBHOY, K. N., DESAI, H. G. and VERGHSE, R. V. (1964). Milk intolerance in tropical malabsorption syndrome. Role of lactase malabsorption. *Lancet*, **2**, 666.

JEEJEEBHOY, K. N. WADIA, N. H. and DESAI, H. G. (1967). Role of Vitamin B_{12} deficiency in tropical 'nutritional' neuromyelopathy. *J. neurol. neurosurg. Psychiat.*, **30**, 7.

JELLIFFE, D. B. (1951). Blackwater fever in African children. *Brit. med. J.*, **1**, 1117.

— (1952). *Ascaris lumbricoides* presenting through the umbilicus. *W. Afr. med. J.*, **1**, 183.

— (1954). The racial incidence of umbilical hernia. *J. trop. Med. Hyg.*, **57**, 270.

— (1963). The incidence of protein-calorie malnutrition of early childhood. *Amer. J. publ. Hlth*, **53**, 905.

— (1966). The assessment of the nutritional status of the community (with special reference to field surveys in developing regions of the world). *W.H.O. Monogr. Ser.*, No. 53.

— (1967). The assessment of nutritional status: an author introduces his book. *W.H.O. Chron.*, **21**, 127.

— (1973). Classification of malnutrition. *Lancet*, **2**, 905.

JEREMY, R., *et al.* (1969). Clinical and laboratory studies of a distinctive type of arthritis observed in New Guinea. *Med. J. Aust.*, **1**, 1273.

JINDRÁK, K. and ALICATA, J. E. (1965). A case of parasitic meningo-encephalitis in Vietnam probably caused by *Angiostrongylus cantonensis*. *Ann. trop. Med. Parasit.*, **59**, 294.

JOB, C. K. (1961). Gynecomastia and leprous orchitis: a preliminary study. *Int. J. Leprosy*, **29**, 423.

— (1963). Pathology of leprous osteomyelitis. *Int. J. Leprosy*, **31**, 26.

— (1970). *Mycobacterium leprae*—nerve lesions in lepromatous leprosy. *Arch. Path.*, **89**, 195.

JOFFE, N. (1965). Aortitis of obscure origin in the African. *Clin. Radiol.*, **16**, 130.

JOHNSON, D. W. (1960). The Australian leptospiroses. *Med. J. Aust.*, **2**, 724.

JOHNSON, K. M., HALSTEAD, S. B. and COHEN, S. N. (1967). Haemorrhagic fevers of S.E. Asia and South America. *Progr. med. Virol.*, **9**, 105.

JOHNSON, K. M., *et al.* (1965). Virus isolations from human cases of haemorrhagic fever in Bolivia. *Proc. Soc. exp. Biol. (N.Y.)*, **118**, 113.

JOHNSON, P. N., FORREST-HAY, I. and GILES, C. (1969). Vitamin B_{12}, serum-folate and hypochronic anaemia. *Brit. med. J.*, **1**, 643.

JOLLY, S. S., *et al.* (1968). Epidemiological, clinical and biochemical study of endemic dental and skeletal fluorosis in Punjab. *Brit. med. J.*, **4**, 427.

JOLY, B. M. (1956). Peptic ulcer in W. Nigeria and Southern United States. *W. Afr. med. J.* (n.s.), **5**, 55.

JOLY, B. M. and THOMAS, H. O. (1954). Non-infantile idiopathic intussusception in Western Nigeria (with a report of 33 cases). *W. Afr. med. J.* (n.s.), **3**, 3.

JONES, A. W. and SHREEVE, D. R. (1970). Congenital dilatation of intrahepatic biliary ducts with cholangiocarcinoma. *Brit. med. J.*, **2**, 277.

JONES, C. A. (1950). Clinical studies in human strongyloidiasis. I: Semeiology. *Gastroenterology*, **16**, 743.

JONES, R. T., *et al.* (1959). Gross structure of hemoglobin H. *J. Amer. chem. Soc.*, **81**, 3161.

JONES, S. R., BINDER, R. A. and DONOWHO, E. M. (1970). Sudden death in sickle-cell trait. *New Engl. J. Med.*, **282**, 323.

JORDAN, P. (1960). Bancroftian filariasis in Tanganyika: observations on elephantiasis, microfilarial density, genital filariasis and microfilaraemia rates. *Ann. trop. Med. Parasit.*, **54**, 132.

— (1966). Recent advances in knowledge of schistosomiasis in East Africa, medical aspects. *Trans. roy. Soc. trop. Med. Hyg.*, **60**, 294.

JORDAN, P., COOK, J. A. and DAVIS, A. (1974). *Schistosoma haematobium* infection. Immunity or concomitant immunity? *Trans. roy. Soc. trop. Med. Hyg.*, **68**, 340.

JORDAN, P., TRANT, M. H. and LAURIE, W. (1956). Non-bancroftian elephantiasis in Tanganyika. *Brit. med. J.*, **1**, 209.

JOSHI, R. A. (1967). Total granulomatous infarction of testes due to *S. haematobium*. *J. clin. Path.*, **20**, 273.

JOSHI, S. G. (1953). Submucous fibrosis of the palate and pillars. *Indian J. Otolarying.*, **4** (3), 1.

JUEL-JENSEN, B. E. (1973). Herpes simplex and zoster. *Brit. med. J.*, **1**, 406.

JULL, J. W., BONSER, G. M. and DOSSETT, J. A. (1964). Hormone excretion studies of males with gynaecomastia, *Brit. med. J.*, **2**, 797.

JUMINER, B. (1960). Anti-rickettsial agglutinins in *Rattus norvegicus* in Tunis in June to August 1959. *Bull. Soc. Path. exot.*, **53**, 85.

JUNG, R. C. and JELLIFFE, D. B. (1952). The clinical picture and treatment of whipworm infection. *W. Afr. med. J.*, **1**, 11.

JUSWALLA, D. J. (1966). *Cancer in Greater Bombay, 1964*. Indian Cancer Society, Bombay.

KAGAN, I. G. (1960). Trichinosis: a review of biologic, serologic and immunologic aspects. *J. infect. Dis.*, **107**, 65.

— (1963). A review of immunologic methods for the diagnosis of filariasis. *J. Parasit.*, **49**, 773.

KAGAN, I. G. and NORMAN, L. (1963). The isolation and characterization of two host antigens in hydatid fluid of *Echinococcus granulosus*. *Amer. J. trop. Med. Hyg.*, **12**, 346.

KAGAN, I. G., OSIMANI, J. J., VARELA, J. C. and ALLAIN, D. S. (1966). Evaluation of intradermal and serologic tests for the diagnosis of hydatid disease. *Amer. J. trop. Med. Hyg.*, **15**, 172.

KAGAN, I. G. and PELLEGRINO, J. (1961). A critical review of immunological methods for the diagnosis of bilharziasis. *Bull. Wld Hlth Org.*, **25,** Nos. 4/5, 611.

KAGEN, L. J. (1970). Immunofluorescent demonstration of myoglobin in the kidney. *Amer. J. med.*, **48,** 649.

KALLICHURUM, S. (1969). Thrombo-embolic corpulmonale in the Bantu in Durban. *S. Afr. med. J.*, **43,** 291.

— (1969). Venous thromboembolisms in the Bantu. *S. Afr. med. J.*, **43,** 358.

— (1972). Major aetiological types of heart failure in the Bantu in Durban. *S. Afr. med. J.*, **43,** 250.

KALRO, R. H. and STEWART, J. S. (1974). Chronic tropical sprue and penicious anaemia in a young Indian man. *Proc. roy. Soc. Med.*, **67,** 1021.

KALTREIDER, H. B. and TALAL, N. (1969). Bilateral parotid gland enlargement and Hyperlipo proteinaemia. *J. Amer. med. Ass.* **210,** 2067.

KANAGASUNTHERAM, R. and DASSANAYAKE, A. G. S. (1958). Nature of the obstructing membrane in primary cryptomenorrhoea. *J. Obstet. Gynaec. Brit. Emp.*, **65,** 487.

KANANI, S. R. and KNIGHT, R. (1969). Relapsing amoebic colitis of 12 years standing exacerbated by corticosteroids. *Brit. med. J.*, **2,** 613.

KAPLAN, H. S. (1971). Role of immunologic disturbance in human ocogenesis. *Brit. J. Cancer*, **25,** 620.

KAPOOR, O. P., *et al.* (1972). Amoebic peritonitis; a study of 73 cases. *J. trop. Med. Hyg.*, **75,** 11.

KAPPELMAN, M., THOMAS, G. H. and HOWELL, R. R. (1971). Histidinemia in a Negro child. *Amer. J. Dis. Child.*, **122,** 212.

KARAKLIS, A. and FESSAS, P. (1963). The normal minor components of human foetal haemoglobin. *Acta haemat.*, **29,** 267.

KARAT, A. B. A., JOB, C. K. and RAO, P. S. S. (1971). Liver in leprosy. *Brit. med. J.*, **1,** 307.

KARIKS, J. and MCGOVERN, V. J. (1971). Impaired spermatogenesis and tubular fibrosis in testis of New Guineans. *Pathology*, **3,** 13.

KASS, E. H., ANDRUS, S. B., ADAMS, R. D., TURNER, F. C. and FELDMAN, H. A. (1952). Toxoplasmosis in the human adult. *A.M.A. Arch. intern. Med.*, **89,** 759.

KASS, L., *et al.* (1971). Blastoid transformations of lymphocytes in falciparum malaria. *Amer. J. trop. Med. Hyg.*, **20,** 195.

KATZ, M. and BROWN, R. E. (1973). Cutaneous hypersensitivity in protein–calorie malnutrition. *Lancet*, **1,** 779.

KAUR, B. and METSELAAR, D. (1967). Poliomyelitis in Kenya—the 1965–66 epidemic. *E. Afr. med. J.*, **44,** 74.

KEEGAN, H. L. (1969). Some medial problems from direct injury by arthropods. *Int. Path.*, **10,** 35.

KEEGAN, H. L., RADKE, M. G. and MURPHY, D. A. (1970). Nasal leech infestation in man. *Amer. J. trop. Med. Hyg.*, **19,** 1029.

KEISER, H. R., VOGEL, C. L. and SADIKALI, F. (1972). Protocollagen proline hydroxylase in sera in Ugandans with hepatocellular carcinoma. *J. nat. Cancer Inst.*, **49,** 1251.

KELLER, A. E., LEATHERS, W. S. and BISHOP, E. L. (1932). A state-wide study of the human intestinal helminths in Tennessee. *J. prev. Med.*, **6,** No. 3, 161.

KELLERMEYER, R. W. and GRAHAM, R. C. (1968). Kinins—possible physiologic and pathologic roles in man. *New Engl. J. Med.*, **279,** 754, 802 and 859.

KELLY, F. and SNEDDEN, W. W. (1960). Prevalence and distribution of endemic goitre. *W.H.O. Monogr. Ser.* No. 44, p. 27.

KENG, C. B. and KHOO, T. K. (1970). Liver in haemoglobin H disease. *Gut*, **11,** 423.

KENNEDY, A. C., BURTON, J. A. and ALLISON, M. E. M. (1974). Tuberculosis as a continuing cause of renal amyloidosis. *Brit. med. J.*, **3**, 795.

KENNEDY, B. J. and ZELICKSON, A. S. (1963). Melanoma in an albino. *J. Amer. med. Ass.*, **186**, 839.

KENNEY, R. A. (1957). Some observations on the renal function of the male. *W. Afr. J. trop. Med. Hyg.*, **60**, 79.

KERDEL-VEGAS, F., et al. (1963). *Rhinoscleroma*. C. C. Thomas, Springfield.

KERR, D. N. S., HARRISON, C. V., SHERLOCK, S. and WALKER, R. M. (1961). Congenital hepatic fibrosis. *Quart. J. Med.* (n.s.), **30**, 91.

KERR, W. R., et al. (1968). Techniques and interpretations in the serological diagnosis of Brucellosis in man. *J. med. Microbiol.*, **1**, 181.

KERSHAW, W. E., DUKE, B. O. L. and BUDDEN, F. H. (1954). The distribution of the microfilariae of *Acanthocheilonema streptocerca* in the skin of man. *Trans. roy. Soc. trop. Med. Hyg.*, **48**, 287.

KERSHAW, W. E., ST. HILL, C. A., SEMPLE, A. B. and DAVIES, J. B. M. (1956). The distribution of the larvae of *Trichinella spiralis* in the muscles, viscera and central nervous system in cases of trichinosis at Liverpool in 1953, and the relation of the severity of the illness to the intensity of infection. *Ann. trop. Med. Parasit.*, **50**, 355.

KESSEL, J. F., et al. (1965). Indirect hemaglutination and complement fixation tests in amebiasis. *Am. J. trop. Med. Hyg.*, **14**, 540.

KESSLER, R. E., AMADEO, J. H., TICE, D. A. and ZIMMON, D. S. (1970). Filtration of schistosomes in unanaethetized man. *J. Amer. med. Ass.*, **214**, 519.

KHAFAGY, H. and KHALIL, H. M. (1970). The schistosomal circumoval precipitin tests in cases of chronic prostatis. *Trans. roy. Soc. trop. Med. Hyg.*, **64**, 909.

KHALEQUE, K. A. and ALAM, K. S. (1963). Hepatic granuloma caused by *Ascaris* ova. *J. trop. Med. Hyg.*, **66**, 249.

KHANOLKAR, V. R. (1964). Pathology of leprosy. In *Leprosy in Theory and Practice*, ed. R. G. Cochrane and T. F. Davey, 2nd ed., p. 125. Wright, Bristol.

KHODOROVSKI, G. I. (1972). Goitre survey in Chief Mungule's area of Zambia. *Trop. geogr. Med.*, **24**, 86.

KHOO, S. K. and MACKAY, I. R. (1973). Carcinoembryonic antigen in serum in diseases of the liver and pancreas. *J. clin. Path.*, **26**, 470.

KIBUKAMUSOKE, J. W. (1966). The nephrotic syndrome in Lagos, Nigeria. *W. Afr. med. J.*, **15**, 213.

KIBUKAMUSOKE, J. W., DAVIES, D. R. and HUTT, M. R. S. (1974). Membranous nephropathy due to skin-lightening cream. *Brit. med. J.*, **2**, 646.

KIBUKAMUSOKE, J. W. and HUTT, M. S. R. (1967). Histological features of the nephrotic syndrome associated with quartan malaria. *J. clin. Path.*, **20**, 117.

KIBUKAMUSOKE, J. W., HUTT, M. S. R. and WILKS, N. E. (1967). The nephrotic syndrome in Uganda and its association with quartan malaria. *Quart. J. Med.* (n.s.), **36**, 393.

KIDSON, C. and GORMAN, J. G. (1962). A challenge to the concept of selection by malaria in glucose-6-phosphate dehydrogenase deficiency. *Nature (Lond.)*, **196**, 49.

KILGOUR, V. and GODFREY, D. G. (1973). *Nature New Biology*, **244**, 69.

KIM, E. H. and BAHK, Y. W. (1964). Intracranial calcifications in cerebral paragonimiasis. *Brit. J. Radiol.*, **37**, 670.

KIM, K. H., et al. (1972). Histologic types of gastric carcinoma among Koreans. *Cancer*, **29**, 1261.

KIM, S. K. and WALKER, A. E. (1961). Cerebral paragonimiasis. *Acta psychiat. scand.*, **36**, suppl. 153, 1.

848 REFERENCES

KINARE, S. G., PARULKAR, G. B. and SEN, P. K. (1962). Constrictive pericarditis resulting from dracunculosis. *Brit. med. J.*, **1**, 845.

KING, M. S. (1971). Biliary-tract disease in Malaya. *Brit. J. Surgery.* **58**, 829.

KINMONT, P. D. and MCCALLUM, D. I. (1965). The aetiology, pathology and course of giant-cell arteritis: the possible role of light sensitivity. *Brit. J. Derm.*, **77**, 193.

KINMONTH, J. B., TAYLOR, G. W., TRACY, G. D. and MARSH, J. D. (1957). Primary lympho-edema: clinical and lymphangiographic studies of a series of 107 patients in which the lower limbs were affected. *Brit. J. Surg.*, **45**, 1.

KINNEAR, T. W. G. (1963). The pattern of diabetes mellitus in a Nigerian teaching hospital. *E. Afr. med. J.*, **40**, 288.

KITIKOON, V., *et al.* (1973). Mekong schistosomiasis. *Southeast Asian J. trop. Med. Pub. Hlth.*, **4**, 350.

KITIKOON, V., SCHNEIDER, C. R. and SORNMANI, S. (1973). Mekong schistosomiasis. 2. Evidence of the natural transmission of *Schistosoma japonicum*, Mekong strain, at Khong Island, Laos. *S.E. Asian J. trop. Med. publ. Hlth.* **4**, 3, 350.

KLATZO, I., GAJDUSEK, D. C. and ZIGAS, V. (1959). Pathology of kuru. *Lab. Invest.* **8**, 799.

KLEIHAUER, E., BRAUN, H. and BETKE, K. (1957). Demonstration von fetalem Hämo-globin in den Erythrocyten eines Blutausstrichs. *Klin. Wschr.*, **35**, 637.

KLEIN, G. (1970). Immunological factors affecting tumour growth. *Brit. med. J.*, **4**, 418.

— (1971). Immunological studies on Burkitt's lymphoma. *Postgrad. med. J.* **47**, 141.

KLEMME, W. (1966). Cerebral paragonimiasis: a case report. *Arch. Neurol. (Chic.)*, **15**, 185.

KLINGBERG, M. A., JASINSKA-KLINGBERG, W. and GOLDBLUM, N. (1959). Certain aspects of the epidemiology and distribution of immunity of West Nile virus in Israel. *Proc. 6th Int. Congr. trop. Med. Malar.*, **5**, 132.

KLIPSTEIN, F. A., SAMLOFF, I. M. and SCHENK, E. A. (1966). Tropical sprue in Haiti. *Ann. intern. Med.*, **64**, 575.

KODILINYE, H. C. (1967). Retinoblastoma in Nigeria: problems of treatment. *Amer. J. Ophthal.*, **63**, 469.

KNOTT, J. (1939). A method for making microfilarial surveys on day blood. *Trans. roy. Soc. trop. Med. Hyg.*, **33**, 191.

KNOX-MACAULEY, H. H. M., *et al.* (1973). Thalassaemia in the British. *Brit. med. J.*, **3**, 150.

KOBAYASHI, S. (1929). *Sang*, **3**, 129.

KOBERLE, F. (1963). Enteromegaly and cardiomegaly in Chagas disease. *Gut*, **4**, 399.

— (1968). The pathology of American trypanosomiasis. *Advances in Parasitology* (6), p. 63. Academic Press, London.

KOBERNICK, S. D., MANDELL, G. H., ZIRKIN, R. M. and HASHIMOTO, Y. (1963). Succinic dehydrogenase deficiency in idiopathic cardiomegaly. *Amer. J. Path.*, **43**, 661.

KOCHAR, V. K., *et al.* (1974). *Medical Anthropology*, ed. Grollig and Hayley. Hague, Monton.

KODICEK, E. (1974). The story of vitamin D from vitamin to hormone, *Lancet*, **1**, 325.

KOEZE, T. H. and KLINSON, G. H. (1964). Acquired toxoplasmosis. *Arch. Neurol.*, **11**, 191.

KOFFLER, D. (1964). Giant cell pneumonia. *Arch. Path.*, **87**, 267.

KOJIMA, S., *et al.* (1972). Raised levels of serum IgE in human helminthiases. *Amer. J. trop. Med. Hyg.*, **21**, 6, 913.

KOKERNOT, R. H., *et al.* (1957). Studies on arthropodborne viruses of Tongaland. VIII. Spondweni virus, an agent previously unknown, isolated from *Taenior-hynchus (Mansonioides) uniformis* Theo. *S. Afr. J. med. Sci.*, **22**, 103.

— (1960). Further isolations of Wesselsbron virus from mosquitoes. *S. Afr. med. J.*, **34**, 871.

KOLAWOLE, M. T. and AKANDE, E. O. (1971). Pyogaseous infection in pregnancy. *Brit. med. J.*, **3**, 620.

KOLAWOLE, T. M. and BOHRER, G. P. (1970). Ulcer osteoma—bone response to tropical ulcer. *Amer. J. Roentgenol.*, **109**, 611.

KONOTEY-AHULU, F. I. D. (1971). Treatment and prevention of sickle cell crisis. *Lancet*, **2**, 1255.

KONSTAM, P. G. (1955). Gastric acidity in Nigerian peptic ulcer. *W. Afr. med. J.*, **4**, 203.

— (1963). Spinal tuberculosis in Nigeria. *Ann. roy. Coll. Surg. Engl.*, **32**, 3.

KORTE, R. and WIERSINGA, A. (1972). Deficiency in male prisoners reflecting border-line vitamin A intake in the population of Kenya. *Trop. geogr. Med.*, **24**, 339.

KORTMAN, H. F. C. M. (1972). Malaria and pregnancy (Thesis), 118 pp. Drukkerij Elinkwijk, Utrecht.

KOZHEVNIKOV, P. V. (1958). Classification of manifestations of cutaneous leishmania-sis (Borovsky's disease) based upon the state of reactivity of the patient's organism. *Med. Parazit. (Mosk.)*, **27**, 387.

KOZMA, C. (1962). Specific cardiac auto-antibodies in the myocarditis of Chagas's disease. *Z. Tropenmed. Parasit., Stuttgart*, **13**, 175.

KROHN, K., et al. (1970). Electron microscopical and immunological observations on the serum-hepatitis (SH) antigen in primary biliary cirrhosis. *Lancet*, **2**, 379.

KRUATRACHUE, M. and HARINASUTA, T. (1970). Erythrocyte morphology in black-water fever. *Amer. J. trop. Med. Parasit.*, **64**, 73.

KRUATRACHUE, M., KLONGKUMNUANHARA, K. and HARINASUTA, C. (1966). Infection-rates of malarial parasites in red blood-cells with normal and deficient glucose-6-phosphate dehydrogenase. *Lancet*, **1**, 404.

KRUATRACHUE, M., et al. (1961). Haemoglobin E and malaria in South-East Thailand. *Ann. trop. Med. Parasit.*, **55**, 468.

KRUPP, I. M. (1966). Immunoelectrophoretic analysis of several strains of *Entamoeba histolytica*. *Amer. J. trop. Med. Hyg.*, **15**, 849.

KUANG, WU. (1937). Deux nouvelles plantes pouvant transmettre le *Fasciolopsis buski*. Revue generale. (Two new plants on which infection with *F. buskii* may be transmitted.) *Ann. Parasit., Hum. Comp.* **15**, No. 5, 458.

KUIPERS, F. C. et al. (1960). Eosinophilic phlegmon of the alimentary canal caused by a worm. *Lancet*, **2**, 1171.

KULKA, F. and BARABAS, M. (1955). Clinical aspects of X-ray diagnosis of paragoni-miasis. *Acta med. Acad. Sci. hung.*, **7**, Nos. 3/4, 371.

KUMAR, V., GHAI, O. P. and CHASE, H. P. (1971). Intestinal dipeptide hydrolase activities in undernourished children. *Arch. Dis. Childh.* **46**, 801.

KUPER, S., MENDELOW, H. and PROCTOR, N. S. F. (1958). Internal hydrocephalis caused by parasitic cysts. *Brain.* **81**, 235.

KURBAN, A. K., MALAK, J. A., FARAH, F. S. and CHAGLASSIAN, H. T. (1966). Histopathology of cutaneous leishmaniasis. *Arch. Derm.*, **93**, 396.

LAFFERTY, F. W., REYNOLDS, E. S. and PEARSON, O. H. (1965). Tumoral calcinosis: a metabolic disease of obscure etiology. *Amer. J. Med.*, **38**, 105.

LAGRAULET, J., MONJUSIAU, A. and DURAND, B. (1964). A study of the location of nodules in onchocerciasis and their relationship to the sites of biting of *Simulium* flies. *Méd. trop., Marseilles*, **24**, 566.

LAGUNDOYE, S. B. (1970). Radiological features of sickle-cell anaemia and related haemoglobinopathies in Nigeria. *Afr. J. med. Sci.*, **1**, 315.

LAGUNDOYE, S. B., EDINGTON, G. M. and IBEACHUM, G. (1975). Post-mortem coronary arteriography in Nigerians. (in press)

LAI, C. S. and RANSOME, G. A. (1970). Burning-feet syndrome. *Brit. med. J.* **2**, 151.

LAINSON, R. and SHAW, J. J. (1972). Leishmaniasis in the New World: taxonomic problems. *Brit. med. Bull.*, **28**, 44.

LAINSON, R. and STRANGWAYS-DIXON, J. (1963). *Leishmania mexicana*: The epidemiology of dermal leishmaniasis in British Honduras. I. The human disease. *Trans. roy. Soc. trop. Med. Hyg.*, **57**, 242.

— (1964). The epidemiology of dermal leishmaniasis in British Honduras: Part II. Reservoir hosts of *Leishmania mexicana* among the forest rodents. *Trans. roy. Soc. trop. Med. Hyg.*, **58**, 136.

LAL, D. (1953). Diffuse oral submucous fibrosis. *J. All-India dent. Ass.*, **26**, 1.

LAMBOTTE, C. (1974). Sickle-cell anaemia and childhood in black Africa. *Ann. Soc. belge Méd. trop.*, **54**, 177.

LANCASTER, M. C., JENKINS, F. P. and PHILP, J.MCL. (1961). Toxicity associated with certain samples of groundnuts. *Nature (Lond.)*, **192**, 1095.

LANCET (1965). New light on Chagas' disease. (Leading article.) **1**, 1150.

— (1974). Epidemic Giardiasis. (Leading article) **2**, 1493.

LANDAU, J. W. and NEWCOMER, V. D. (1962). Acute cerebral phycomycosis (mucormycosis). *J. Pediat.*, **61**, 363.

LANGEN, C. D., DE (1928). Anguillosis en het ziektebeeld van de 'Idiopathische Hypereosinophilie'. *Geneesk. T. Ned.-Ind.*, **68**, 973.

LAQUEUR, G. L., MICKELSEN, O., WHITING, M. G. and KURLAND, L. T. (1963). Carcinogenic properties of nuts from *Cycas circinalis* L. indigenous to Guam. *J. nat. Cancer Inst.*, **31**, 919.

LARGE, S. E. (1964). Tuberculosis in the Gurkhas of Nepal. *Tuberculosis (Lond.)*, **45**, 321.

LARIZZA, P. (1961). Enzymopenic hemolytic anemias. *Folia haemat. Frankf.*, **6**, 19

LARRACILLA, A. J., *et al.* (1971). Amoebiasis intestinal en los tres primeros meses de la vida. *Salud. publ. Mex.*, **13**, 79.

LASSMAN, P. (1939). The blood sedimentation rate of the natives of the Congo. *Ann. Soc. belge Méd. trop.*, **19**, 557.

LATIF, B. M. A. and ADAM, K. M. G. (1973). *Bull. Wld Hlth Org.*, **48**, 401.

LAUCKNER, J. R. (1959). The treatment of tuberculosis in the tropics. *J. trop. Med. Hyg.*, **62**, 1.

LAVIER, G. and DESCHIENS, R. (1956). Les distomatoses hépatiques en France, leur traitement. *Bull. Soc. Path. exot.*, **49**, 541.

LAWSON, J. B. (1961). Pre-eclampsia and eclampsia in Nigeria. *Path. et Microbiol.* (Basel), **24**, 478.

— (1962). *Health and Tuberculosis Conference, Nigeria*, p. 197. Chest and Heart Association. London.

— (1963). Lymphopathia venereum in Nigerian women. *W. Afr. med. J.*, **12**, 89.

LAWSON, J. B. and STEWART, D. B. (1967). *Obstetrics and Gynaecology in the Tropics and Developing Countries.* Edward Arnold, London.

LAYCOCK, H. I. (1950). Surgical aspects of female circumcision in Somaliland. *E. Afr. med. J.*, **27**, 445.

LEATHER, H. M. (1961). Portal hypertension and gross splenomegaly in Uganda. *Brit. med. J.*, **1**, 15.

LEATHERWOOD, et al. (1965). Dental caries and dental fluoroses in Thailand. *Amer. J. publ. Hlth*, **55**, 1792.

LE BOUVIER, G. L. (1972). Subspecificities of the Australia antigen complex. *Amer. J. Dis. Child.*, **123**, 420.

LEDINGHAM, J. G. G. (1964). Ethacrynic acid parenterally in the treatment and prevention of pulmonary oedema. *Lancet*, **1**, 952.

LEE, J. A. H. (1970). Fatal melanoma of the lower limbs and other sites. *J. nat. Cancer Inst.*, **44**, 257.

LEE, K. T., et al. (1964). Geographic pathology of myocardial infarction. *Amer. J. Cardiol.*, **13**, 30.

LEE, V. H., et al. (1974). Arbovirus studies in Nupeko Forest, a possible natural focus of yellow fever virus in Nigeria. II. Entomological investigations and viruses isolated. *Trans. roy. Soc. trop. Med. Hyg.*, **68**, 39.

LEECH, R. B. and WRIGHT, F. J. (1944). Intussusception in typhoid fever. *E. Afr. med. J.*, **21**, 340.

LEEDHAM-GREEN, J. C. and EVANS, W. (1943). Myositis tropica. *Trans. roy. Soc. trop. Med. Hyg.*, **36**, 359.

LEFFALL, L. D., WHITE, J. R. and EWING, J. (1963). Cancer of the breast in Negroes. *Surg. Gynec. Obstet.*, **117**, 97.

LEHMAN, J. S., FARID, Z., BASSILY, S., HAXTON, J., WANAB, M. F. A. and KENT, D. C. (1970). Intestinal protein loss in schistosomal polyposis of the colon. *Gastroenterology*, **59**, 433.

LEHMANN, B. N., HANSEN, J. D. L. and WARREN, P. J. (1971). The distribution of copper, zinc and manganese in various regions of the brain and in other tissues of children with protein calorie malnutrition. *Brit. J. Nutr.*, **26**, 197.

LEHMANN, D. L. (1961). Attempts at the selective cultivation of *Trypanosoma rhodesiense*, *T. brucei* and *T. congolense*. *Ann. trop. Med. Parasit.*, **55**, 440.

LEHMANN, H. (1974). Some aspects of the haemoglobinopathies. *Trans. roy. Soc. trop. Med. Hyg.*, **68**, 92.

LEHMANN, H. and HUNTSMAN, R. G. (1966). *Man's Haemoglobins, including the Haemoglobinopathies and their Investigation*. North-Holland Publ. Co., Amsterdam.

LEIFER, E., GOCKE, D. J. and BOURNE, H. (1970). Lassa fever, a new virus disease of man from West Africa. *Amer. J. trop. Med. Hyg.*, **19**, 677.

LEIKER, D. L., KOK, S. H. and SPRAS, J. A. J. (1964). Granuloma multiforme a new skin disease resembling leprosy. *Int. J. Leprosy*, **32**, 368.

LEINBACH, G. E. and RUBIN, C. E. (1970). Eosinophilic gastroenteritis. *Gastroenterol.*, **59**, 874.

LEITHEAD, C. S. (1964). Heat illness and some related problems. *W.H.O. Chron.*, **18**, 288.

LEITHEAD, C. S. and LIND, A. R. (1964). *Heat Stress and Heat Disorders*. Cassell, London.

LEITHEAD, C. S., et al. (1958). Incidence, aetiology and prevention of heat illness on ships in the Persian Gulf. *Lancet*, **2**, 109.

LEJKINA, E. S. (1965). Research on ascariasis immunity and immunodiagnosis. *Bull. Wld Hlth Org.*, **32**, 699.

LENNOX, B. (1948). Acute parietal endocarditis in a case of status asthmaticus: a possible early stage of Löffler's endocarditis parietalis fibroplastica with eosinophilia. *J. Path. Bact.*, **60**, 621.

LEPTOSPIRAL SEROTYPE DISTRIBUTION TESTS (1966). U.S. Department of Health, Education, and Welfare, Public Health Service. National Communicable disease Centre, Atlanta, Georgia, pp. 1–125.

LETAC, R., MAWUPE VOVOR, V. and CABANNE, F. (1958). De la rareté de la pathologie veineuse des membres inférieurs en Afrique noire. *Schweiz. Z. allg. Path.*, **21**, 587.

LETAC, R., *et al.* (1953). Les thromboses cardiaques chirurgicales. *Bull. méd. A.O.F.*, **10**, 215.

LEVERE, R. D., LICHTMAN, H. C. and LEVINE, J. (1964). Effect of iron-deficiency anaemia on the metabolism of the heterogenic haemoglobins in sickle cell trait. *Nature (Lond.)*, **202**, 499.

LEVIN, R. L. and ARMSTRONG, D. E. (1970). Human infection with *Entamoeba polecki*. *Amer. J. clin. Path.*, **54**, 611.

LEVIN, S. E. (1967). Haemolysis in typhoid fever. *Brit. med. J.*, **2**, 175.

LEVIN, S. E., ZAMMIT, R. and SCHMAMAN, A. (1967). Thrombosis of the pulmonary arteries and the nephrotic syndrome. *Brit. med. J.*, **1**, 153.

LEVIN, S. E., *et al.*, (1967). Mucoviscidosis in Bantu twin neonates. *S. Afr. med. J.*, **41**, 482.

LEVINE, C. and BLUMBERG, B. S. (1969). Additional specificities of Australia antigen and the possible identification of hepatitis carriers. *Nature*, **221**, 195.

LEVINE, P. H., *et al.* (1971). Elevated antibody titres to Epstein–Barr virus in Hodgkins disease. *Cancer (Philadelphia)*, **27**, 416.

LEVY, L. F. (1968). Porter's neck. *Brit. med. J.*, **2**, 16.

LEVY, L. F., FORBES, J. L. and PARIRENYATWA, T. S. (1964). Epilepsy in Africans. *Cent. Afr. J. Med.*, **10**, 241.

LEVY COMMITTEE (1959). *Report of the Committee of Inquiry on Anthrax 1959*. Cmnd. 846, H.M.S.O.

LEWIS, B., HANSEN, J. D. L., WITTMAN, W., KRUT, L. H. and STEWART, F. (1964). Plasma free fatty acids in kwashiorkor and the pathogenesis of the fatty liver. *Amer. J. clin. Nutr.*, **15**, 161.

LEWIS, E. A. and ANTIA, A. U. (1969). Amoebic colitis: review of 295 cases. *Trans. roy. Soc. trop. Med. Hyg.*, **63**, 633.

LEWIS, E. A. and BOHRER, S. P. (1969). Choledochoduodenal fistula complicating chronic duodenal ulcer in Nigerians. *Gut*, **10**, 146.

LEWIS, M. G. (1967). Possible immunological factors in human malignant melanoma in Uganda. *Lancet*, **2**, 921.

LEWIS, M. G. and JOHNSON, K. (1968). The incidence and distribution of pigmented naevi in Ugandan Africans. *Brit. J. Dermatol.*, **80**, 362.

LEWIS, M. G. and KIRYABWIRE, J. W. M. (1968). Aspects of behaviour and Natural History of malignant melanoma in Uganda. *Cancer (Philad.)*, **21**, 876.

LEWIS, M. G. and PHILLIPS, T. M. (1972). Separation of two distinct tumour-associated antibodies in the serum of melanoma patients. *J. nat. Cancer Inst.*, **49**, 915.

LEWIS, R. A. and JILLY, P. (1966). Haematologic studies in West Africa. *N. Z. med. J. Suppl.*, **65**, 910.

LI, K. H., KAO, J. C. and WU, Y. K. (1962). A survey of the prevalence of carcinoma of the esophagus in North China. *Chin. med. J.*, **81**, 489.

LICHTENBERG, F. V. (1955). Lesions of the intrahepatic portal radicles in Manson's schistosomiasis. *Amer. J. Path.*, **31**, 757.

— (1957). The early phase of endemic bancroftian filariasis in the male: pathological study. *J. Mt Sinai Hosp.*, **24**, 983.

— (1967). Mechanisms of schistosome immunity. In *Bilharziasis* ed. by F. K. Mostofi, p. 286. Springer-Verlag, New York.

LICHTENBERG, F. VON, SMITH, J. H. and CHEEVER, A. W. (1966). The Hoeppli pheno-menon in schistosmiasis; comparative pathology and immunopathology. *Amer. J. trop. Med.*, **15**, 886.

LIDIN-JANSON, G. and STRANNEGÅRD, Ö. (1972). Two cases of Guillain–Barré Syn-drome and encephalitis after measles. *Brit. med. J.*, **2**, 572.

LIEBOW, C. A. A., *et al.* (1946). Tropical ulcers and cutaneous diphtheria. *Arch. int. Med.*, **78**, 255.

LIE-INJO LUAN ENG (1959). Haemoglobin of new-born infants in Indonesia. *Nature (Lond.)*, **183**, 1125.

— (1964). Haemoglobinopathies in East Asia. *Ann. hum. Genet.*, **28**, 101.

LIE-INJO LUHN ENG (1965). Hereditary ovalocytosis and haemoglobin E-ovalocytosis in Malayan aborigines. *Nature (Lond.)*, **208**, 1329.

LIE-INJO LUAN ENG and JO BWAN HIE (1960). A fast-moving haemoglobin in hydrops foetalis. *Nature (Lond.)*, **185**, 698.

LIE-INJO LUAN ENG and SADONO (1958). Haemoglobin O (Buginese X) in Sulawesi. *Brit. med. J.*, **1**, 1461.

LIE INJO LUAN ENG, *et al.* (1962). α-thalassaemia as a cause of hydrops foetalis. *Brit. J. Haemat.*, **8**, 1.

LIE KIAN JOE, *et al.* (1956). *Basidiobolus ranarum* as a cause of subcutaneous mycosis in Indonesia. *Arch. Derm. Syph. (Chic.)*, **74**, 378.

LIJINSKY, W. and EPSTEIN, S. S. (1970). Nitrosamines as environmental carcinogens. *Nature*, **225**, 21.

LIM, S. D. and FUSARO, R. M. (1964). Leprosy. I. β_{2A} and $\beta_2/_M$ immunoglobulins in leprosy sera. *Arch. Derm.*, **89**, 86.

LIM BOO LIAT (1967). *A review of recent studies on Angiostrongylus cantonensis in Malaysia*. SEAMES. The Third Conference on Parasitic Diseases. Abstracts of Papers, p. 109.

LIMBOS, P., FAIN, A. and DE MULDER, P. (1965). Human Coccidiosis caused by *Isospora belli*. A Second Case observed in Belgium. *Trop. geogr. Med.*, *Haarlem.* **17**, 169.

LIN, C. K. and LEI, T. N. (1963). The pathologic anatomy of paragonimiasis. *Chin. med. J.*, **82**, 650.

LINDE, L. M. and ADAMS, F. H. (1963). Prognosis in endocardial fibroelastosis. *Amer. J. Dis. Child.*, **105**, 329.

LINDENBAUM, J. (1965). Malabsorption during and after recovery from acute intes-tinal infection. *Brit. med. J.*, **2**, 326.

— (1969). Intestinal capillariasis. *Ann. intern. Med.*, **70**, 1277.

LINDENBAUM, J., ALAM, A. K. M. J. and KENT, T. H. (1966). Subclinical small-intestinal disease in East Pakistan. *Brit. med. J.*, **2**, 1616.

LINDNER, R. R. (1965). Retrospective X-ray survey for porocephalosis. *J. trop. Med. Hyg.*, **68**, 155.

LINNELL, F. and NORDEN, A. (1954). *Mycobacterium balnei*. A new acid-fast bacillus occurring in swimming pools and capable of producing skin lesions in humans. *Acta tuberc. scand. Suppl.*, **33**, 84.

LIPPI, U., VILLA, A., PAVAN, R. and GUIDI, G. (1971). Anomalous serum protein in hepatocarcinoma and hepatic metastases. *Amer. J. clin. Path.*, **56**, 227.

LISKER, R., RUIZ-REYES, G. and LORIA, A. (1963). Studies on several genetic hematologic characteristics of the Mexican population. IV: The finding of a fast hemoglobin component (hemoglobin Mexico) in an Indian family. *Blood*, **22**, 342.

LLOYD, A., KURBALL, M. and FRASER, G. (1967). Peripheral gangrene in infancy and childhood. *Brit. med. J.*, **1**, 468.

LLOYD, F. P. (1964). Endometriosis in the Negro woman. *Amer. J. Obstet. Gynec.*, **89**, 468.

LÖEHLEIM, H. (1912). Beiträge zur Pathologie der Eingeborenen von Kamerun. *Arch. Schiffs-u. Tropen–hyg.*, **16**, Beihft 9, 637.

LOEFFLER, W. (1936). Endocarditis parietalis fibroplastica mit Bluteosinophilie. *Schweiz. med. Wschr.*, **66**, 817.

LOGAN, L. J., RAPAPORT, S. I. and MAHER, I. (1971). Albinism and abnormal platelet function. *New Engl. J. Med.*, **284**, 1340.

LOGIE, A. W. and SWANSON BECK, J. (1970). *Plasmodium falciparum* in ascitic fluid. *Trans. roy. Soc. trop. Med. Hyg.*, **64**, 829.

LONGBOTTOM, J. L., PEPYS, J. and CLIVE, F. T. (1964). Diagnostic precipition test in aspergillus pulmonary mycetoma. *Lancet*, **1**, 588.

LONTIE, M., *et al.* (1973). Etiology and epidemiology of 474 cases of microbial meningitis observed in Kinshasa (Zaire). *Ann. Soc. belge Méd. trop.*, **53**, 619.

LOPES, C. F. and LAENDER, J. F. (1945). Montenegro skin test in muco-cutaneous leishmaniasis. Negative for yaws. *Brasil-méd.*, **59**, 41.

LOPES DE FARIA, J. (1954). Cor pulmonale in Manson's schistosomiasis. I: Frequency in necropsy material; pulmonary vascular changes caused by schistosome ova. *Amer. J. Path.*, **30**, 167.

LOPES DE FARIA, J. (1954). Pulmonary vascular changes in schistosomal cor pulmonale. *J. Path. Bact.*, **68**, 589.

LOPES DE FARIA, J., BARBAS, J. V., FUJIOKA, T., LION, M. F., ANDRADE E SILVA, U. DE and DÉCOURT, L. V. (1959). Pulmonary schistosomatic arteriovenous fistulas producing a new cyanotic syndrome in Manson's schistosomiasis. *Amer. Heart J.*, **58**, 556.

LOPES DE FARIA, J., CZAPSKI, J., RIBEIRO LEITE, M. O., DE OLIVEIRA PENNA, D., FUJIOKA, T. and DE ULHÔA CINTRA, A. B. (1957). Cyanosis in Manson's schistosomiasis: role of pulmonary schistosomatic arteriovenous fistulas. *Amer. Heart J.*, **54**, 196.

LOPEZ-CORELLA, E., RIDAURA-SANZ, C. and ALBORES-SAARVEDRA, J., (1968). Primary carcinoma of the liver in Mexican adults. *Cancer (Philad.)* **22**, 678.

LORAINE, J. A. (1974). World population situation during 1973. *Lancet*, **1**, 22.

LOTHE, F. (1967). Leukaemia in Uganda. *Trop. geogr. Med.*, **19**, 163.

LOW, G. C. and COOKE, W. E. (1926). A congenital case of kala azar. *Lancet*, **2**, 1209.

LOWE, C. R. (1974). Recent work in cancer epidemiology. An international study of Breast Cancer. *Proc. roy. Soc. Med.*, **67**, 682.

LOWE, C. Y. and MAEGRAITH, B. G. (1970). Electron microscopy of *Entamoeba histolytica* in host tissue. *Amer. J. trop. Med. Parasit.* **64**, 469.

LOWENSTEIN, F. W. (1961). Blood pressure in relation to age and sex in the tropics and subtropics. A review of the literature and an investigation in two tribes of Brazil Indians. *Lancet*, **1**, 389.

LOWENTHAL, M. N. (1967). Peripheral gangrene in infancy and childhood. (Correspondence.) *Brit. med. J.*, **2**, 700.

— (1971). Thyrotoxicosis and thyrotoxic syndromes. *Med. J. Zambia*, **5**, 15.

LOWENTHAL, M. N. and HUTT, M. S. R. (1970). Tropical splenomegaly syndrome in a caucasian in Africa. *Brit. med. J.*, **3**, 262.

LUBOS, M. C., GERRARD, J. W. and BUCHAN, D. J. (1967). Disaccharidase activities in milk-sensitive and celiac patients. *J. Pediat.*, **70**, 325.

LUCAS, A. O. (1964). Pneumococcal meningitis in pregnancy and the puerperium. *Brit. med. J.*, **1**, 92.

LUCAS, A. O., ADENIYI-JONES, C. C., COCKSHOTT, W. P. and GILLES, H. M. (1966). Radiological changes after medical treatment of vesical schistosomiasis. *Lancet*, **1**, 631.

LUCAS, A. O. and MAINWARING, A. R. (1962). Pleural punch biopsy. *Health and Tuber-culosis Conference*. Chest and Heart Association, London. 174.

LUCASSE, C. (1964). Fluorescent antibody test as applied to cerebrospinal fluid in human sleeping sickness. *Bull. Soc. Path. exot.*, **57**, 283.

LUCASSE, C. and HOEPPLI, R. (1963). Immunofluorescence in onchocerciasis. *Z. Tropenmed. Parasit.*, **14**, 262.

LUCIAN, O. (1971). *Lambliaza*. Editura Academiei Republicii Socialiste, Romania, Bucharest.

LUCIO, R. and ALVARADO, I. (1852). *Opúsculo sobre el mal de San Lázaro o elefancíasis de los Griegos*. Murguía, México.

LUGER, A. and SCHMID, E. E. (1961). Immunity of the central nervous system in en-demic syphilis. *Derm. Wschr.*, **143**, 617.

LUGG, J. W. H. and BOWNESS, J. M. (1954). Renal excretion of 17-ketosteroids by members of some ethnic groups living in Malaya. *Nature (Lond.)*, **174**, 1147.

LUISI, A., BERTELLI, A. B., MACHADO, J. C. and ACHE DE FREITAS, J. P. (1965). Linfoma Africano 'em Criancas Brasileiras'. *Rev. Brasil Cirurg.*, **49**, 280.

LUKE, J. L., BOLANDER, R. P. and GROSS, S. (1963). Generalised aspergillosis and asper-gillus endocarditis in infancy. *Paediatrics*, **31**, 115.

LUKES, R. J., BUTLER, J. J. and HICKS, E. B. (1966). Natural history of Hodgkins disease as related to its pathologic picture. *Cancer (Philad.)*, **19**, 317.

LUMSDEN, W. H. R. (1964). Changing patterns of trypanosomiasis research in East Africa. *Trans. roy. Soc. trop. Med. Hyg.*, **58**, 97.

LURIE, A., *et al.* (1969). Platelet life-span and sites of platelet sequestration in Onyalai. *Brit. med. J.*, **4**, 146.

LURIE, H. I. (1963). Five unusual cases of sporotrichose from South Africa showing lesions in muscles, bones and viscera. *Brit. J. Surg.*, **50**, 585.

LUZ, C. C. F. (1969). Experience in the surgical treatment of portal hypertension due to hepatosplenic schistosomiasis. 11th Pan American Congress of Gastro-enterology, San Juan, Puerto Rico.

LUZZATTO, L., ALLAN, N. C. and FLORA, A. DE (1965). Genetic polymorphism of glucose 6-phosphate dehydrogenase. *Biochem. J.*, **97**, 19P.

LUZZATTO, L. and LEWIS, E. A. (1972). Acute erythraemic myelosis in Ibadan. *Dokita*, **4**, 31.

LUZZATTO, L., NWACHUKU-JARRETT, E. S. and REDDY, S. (1970). Increased sickling of parasitized erythrocytes as mechanism of resistance against malaria in the sickle-cell trait. *Lancet*, **1**, 319.

LUZZATTO, L., USANGA, E. A. and REDDY, S. (1969). Glucose-6-phosphate dehydrogenase deficient red cells: resistance to infection by malarial parasites. *Science*, **164**, 839.

LWANGA, D. and WING, A. J. (1970). Renal complications associated with typhoid fever. *E. Afr. med. J.*, **47**, 146.

LYNCH, J. B., VERZIN, J. A. and HASSAN, A. M. (1963). Cancer of the female genital tract in the Sudanese. *J. Obstet. Gynaec. Brit. Cwlth*, **70**, 495.

LYSEK, H. (1974). Epidemiology of ascariasis in man and pig. *Rev. cuba. Med. Trop.*, **26**, 3.

MACCALLUM, F. O., *et al.* (1951). Infective hepatitis studies in East Anglia during the period 1943–47. *Spec. Rep. Ser. med. Res. Counc. (Lond.)*, No. 273, HMSO.

MACCALLUM, P., *et al.* (1948). New mycobacterial infection in man. *J. Path. Bact.*, **60**, 93.

MACCLUER, J. W., NEEL, J. V. and CHAGNON, N. A. (1971). Demographic structure of a primitive population: a simulation. *Amer. J. Phys. Anthrop.* **35,** 193.

MACDONALD, A. and ELMSLIE, W. H. (1967). Serological investigations in suspected brucellosis. *Lancet,* **1,** 380.

MACDONALD, G. (1957). *The Epidemiology and Control of Malaria,* Oxford University Press.

— (1965). The dynamics of helminth infections with special reference to schistosomes. *Trans. roy. Soc. trop. Med. Hyg.,* **59,** No. 5, 489.

MACDONALD, I., HANSEN, J. D. L. and BRONTE-STEWART, B. (1963). Liver, depot and serum lipids during early recovery from kwashiorkor. *Clin. Sci.,* **24,** 55.

MACDONALD, R. (1965). Geographic studies of 'idiopathic haemachromatosis'. *Lab. Invest.,* **14,** 584.

MACDONALD, R. A. and BAUMSLAG, N. (1964). Iron in alcoholic beverages; possible significance for haemochromatosis. *Amer. J. med. Sci.,* **247,** 649.

MACDONALD, R. A. and MALLORY, G. K. (1960). Haemochromatosis and haemosiderosis. *A.M.A. Arch. intern. Med.,* **105,** 686.

MACE, J. W., *et al.* (1973). Magnesium supplementation in Bartter's syndrome. *Arch. Dis. Childh.,* **48,** 485.

MACFARLANE, J. R. and HOLMAN, C. W. (1972). Chylothorax. *Amer. Rev. resp. Dis.,* **105,** 287.

MACFIE, J. W. S. and JOHNSTON, J. E. L. (1913). A note on five cases of porocephaliasis in man from Southern Nigeria. *Lancet,* **2,** 1387.

MACGREGOR, R. R. and REINHART, J. (1973). Person-to-person spread of salmonella: a problem in hospitals. *Lancet,* **2,** 1001.

MACHNICA-ROGUSKA, B. and ZWIERZ, C. (1966). Serological studies on *Taenia saginata. Acta. parasit. pol.,* **14,** 27.

MACKENZIE, R. B., WIEBENGA, N. H. and JOHNSON, K. M. (1963). Hemorrhagic fever in Bolivia: A preliminary report, *7th Int. Congr. trop. Med. Malar., Rio de Janeiro,* Abstracts of Papers, p. 333.

MACKIE, T. T., *et al.* (1946). Observations on tsutsugamushi disease (scrub typhus) in Assam and Burma. Preliminary report. *Amer. J. Hyg.,* **43,** 195.

MACLACHLAN, M. J., RODNAN, G. P., COOPER, W. M. and FENNELL, R. H. (1965). Chronic active ('lupoid') hepatitis: a clinical, serological, and pathological study of 20 patients. *Ann. intern. Med.,* **62,** 425.

MACLEAN, C. M. (1963). Kaposi's sarcoma in Nigeria. *Brit. J. Cancer,* **17,** 195.

MACLEAN, C. M. U. (1958). Blood donor recruitment in Ibadan. *J. trop. Med. Hyg.,* **61,** 311.

MACLEAN, J. D. and KAMATH, K. R. (1970). Infantile scurvy in Malaysia. *Med. J. Malaya,* **24,** 200.

MACLEAN, M. U. (1965). Hospitals or healers: an attitude survey in Ibadan, Nigeria. *Brit. J. prev. soc. Med.,* **19,** 192.

MACNAMARA, F. N. (1954). Isolation of the virus as a diagnostic procedure for yellow fever in West Africa. *Bull. Wld. Hlth. Org.* **11,** 391.

MACNAMARA, F. N., HORN, D. W. and PORTERFIELD, J. S. (1959). Yellow fever and other arthropod-borne viruses. A consideration of two serological surveys made in south western Nigeria. *Trans. roy. Soc. trop. Med. Hyg.,* **53,** 202.

MACSWEEN, Q. N. M. and JACKSON, J. M. (1966). Haemochromatosis. *Scot. med. J.,* **2,** 395.

MCALPINE, D. (1973). Multiple sclerosis. *Brit. med. J.,* **2,** 292.

MCCAFFREY, R. P., *et al.* (1972). Acute haemolysis with Ambilhar treatment in glucose-6-phosphate-dehydrogenase deficiency. *Trans. roy. Soc. trop. Med. Hyg.,* **66,** 795.

MCCARTHY, K., *et al.* (1958). Isolation of virus of measles from three fatal cases of giant cell pneumonia. *Amer. J. Dis. Child.*, **96,** 500.

MCCLATCHIE, S. and MANKU, M. S. (1967). Echinococossis of the orbit. *E. Afr. med. J.*, **44,** 173.

MCCLATCHIE, S. and SAMBHI, J. S. (1971). Amoebiasis of the cervix uteri. *Ann. trop. Med. Parasit.*, **65,** 207.

MCCOLLUM, R. W. (1970). Infectious mononucleosis and the Epstein–Barr virus. *J. infect. Dis.* **121,** 347.

MCCOY, R. C. (1969). Ultrastructural alterations in the kidney of patients with sickle cell disease and the nephrotic syndrome. *Lab. Invest.*, **21,** 85.

MCCRAE, A. W. R., *et al.* (1971). Chikungunya virus in the Entebbe area of Uganda: isolations and epidemiology. *Trans. roy. Soc. trop. Med. Hyg.*, **65,** 152.

MCCULLOUGH, F. S. and BRADLEY, D. J. (1973). Egg output stability and the epidemiology of *Schistosoma haematobium* I. Variation and stability in *Schistosoma haematobium* egg counts. *Trans. roy. Soc. trop. Med. Hyg.*, **67,** 4, 475.

MCFADZEAN, A. J. S. and CHOA, G. H. (1953). Haemolytic anaemia in typhoid fever. *Brit. med. J.*, **2,** 360.

MCFADZEAN, A. J. S. and ONG, G. B. (1966). Intrahepatic typhoid carriers. *Brit. med. J.*, **1,** 1567.

MCFADZEAN, A. J. S., TODD, D. and TSANG, K. C. (1958). Polycythaenia in primary carcinoma of the liver. *Blood,* **13,** 427.

MCFADZEAN, A. J. S. and TSANG, K. C. (1956). Antibody formation in cryptogenetic splenomegaly. I. The response to particulate antigen injected intravenously. *Trans. roy. Soc. trop. Med.*, **50,** 433.

MCFADZEAN, A. J. S. and YEUNG, R. T. T. (1965). Hypoglycaemia in suppurative pancholangiitis due to *Clonorchis sinensis*. *Trans. roy. Soc. trop. Med. Hyg.*, **59,** 179.

— (1966). Acute pancreatitis due to *Clonorchis sinensis*. *Trans. roy. Soc. trop. Med. Hyg.*, **60,** 466.

— (1967). Periodic paralysis complicating thryotoxicosis in Chinese. *Brit. med. J.*, **1,** 451.

— (1969). Further observations on hypoglycaemia in hepatocellular carcinoma. *Amer. J. Med.*, **47,** 220.

MCGILL, P. E. (1971). Thyrotoxicosis in the African. *Brit. med. J.*, **2,** 679.

MCGIVEN, A. R., GHOSE, T. and NAIRN, R. C. (1967). Autoantibodies in ulcerative colitis. *Brit. med. J.*, **2,** 19.

MCGLASHAN, N. D. (1969). Oesophageal cancer and alcoholic spirits in central Africa. *Gut,* **10,** 643.

— (1970). Oesophageal cancer in Northern Iran. *Int. Path.*, July, 50.

MCGOVERN, V. J. (1964). Persistent nephrotic syndrome: A renal biopsy study. *Aust. Ann. Med.*, **13,** 306.

MCGOVERN, V. J. and KARIKS, J. (1966). Liver disease in the territory of Papua-New Guinea: A necropsy study. *Med. J. Aust.*, **2,** 441.

— (1966). Hepatoma in New Britain. *Proc. 9th Int. Cancer Congr., Tokyo*, p. 715.

MCGRATH, J., O'FARRELL, P. T. and BOLAND, S. J. (1940). Giardial steatorrhoea: a fatal case with organic lesions. *Irish J. med. Sci.*, 802.

MCGREGOR, I. A. (1974). Immunity and malaria in man. *Tropical Doctor*, **4,** 104.

MCGREGOR, I. A., *et al.* (1966). Demonstration of circulating antibodies to *Plasmodium falciparum* by gel-diffusion techniques (Correspondence). *Nature (Lond.),* **210,** 1384.

— (1963). Treatment of East African *P. falciparum* malaria with West African human γ-globulin. *Trans. roy. Soc. trop. Med. Hyg.*, **57**, 170.

MCGREGOR, I. A. and BARR, M. (1962). Antibody response to tetanus toxoid inoculation in malarious and non-malarious Gambian children. *Trans. roy. Soc. trop. Med. Hyg.*, **56**, 364.

MCGREGOR, I. A., BILLEWICZ, W. Z. and THOMSON, A. M. (1961). Growth and mortality in children in an African village. *Brit. med. J.*, **2**, 1661.

MCGREGOR, I. A. and GILLES, H. M. (1960). Studies on the significance of high serum gamma-globulin concentrations in Gambian Africans. II. Gamma-globulin concentrations of Gambian children in the fourth, fifth and sixth years of life. *Ann. trop. Med. Parasit.*, **54**, 275.

MCGREGOR, I. A. and SMITH, D. A. (1952). A health, nutrition, and parasitological survey in a rural village (Keneba) in West Kiang, Gambia. *Trans. roy. Soc. Trop. Med. Hyg.*, **46**, 403.

MCGREGOR, I. A. and WILSON, R. J. M. (1971). Precipitating antibodies and immunoglobulins in *P. falciparum* infections in the Gambia, West Africa. *Trans. roy. Socl trop. Med. Hyg.*, **65**, 2, 136.

MCKAY, R. T. (1973). Pineal calcification in Indians and Fijians. *Trans. roy. Soc. trop. Med. Hyg.*, **67**, 214.

MCKINNEY, B. and CRAWFORD, M. A. (1965). Fibrosis in guineapig heart produced by plantain diet. *Lancet*, **2**, 880.

MCLAREN, D. S. (1963). *Malnutrition and the Eye*. Academic Press, New York & London.

— (1966a). A fresh look at protein-calorie malnutrition. *Lancet*, **2**, 485.

— (1966b). The prevention of xerophthalmia. In *Pre-school child malnutrition . . . an international conference on prevention of malnutrition in the pre-school child, Washington, D.C., December 7–11,* 1964, 96–101. Nat. Acad. Sci.—Nat. Res. Coun., Washington.

— (1974). The great protein fiasco. *Lancet*, **2**, 93, 1079.

MCLAREN, D. S., OOMEN, H. A. P. C. and ESCAPINI, H. (1966). Ocular manifestations of vitamin-A deficiency in man. *Bull. Wld Hlth Org.*, **34**, 357.

MCLAREN, D. S. and READ, W. W. C. (1972). Assessment of nutritional status of children. *Lancet*, **2**, 374.

MCLATCHIE, S., WARAMBO, M. W. and BREMNER, A. D. (1969). Myospherulosis: a previously unreported disease? *Amer. J. clin. Path.*, **51**, 699.

MCLEAN, A. E. M. (1966). Enzyme activity in the liver and serum of malnourished children in Jamaica. *Clin. Sci.*, **30**, 129.

MCLEAN, E., BRAS, G. and GYÖRGY, P. (1964). Veno-occlusive lesions in livers of rats fed *Crotalaria fulva*. *Brit. J. exp. Path.*, **45**, 242.

MCLEOD, I. N., WILMOT, A. J. and POWELL, S. J. (1966). Amoebic pericarditis. *Quart. J. Med.*, **35**, 293.

MCLOUGHLIN, M. J. and HOBBS, B. B. (1970). Selective angiography in the diagnosis of hydatid disease of the liver. *Canad. med. Ass. J.*, **103**, 1147.

MCMAHON, N. J. *et al.* (1970). Reed–Sternberg cells in infectious mononucleosis. *Amer. J. Dis. Child.*, **120**, 148.

MCMILLAN, B. and KELLY, A. (1970). *E. polecki* von Prowazek, 1912 in New Guinea. *Trans. roy. Soc. trop. Med. Hyg.*, **64**, 792.

MCSWEEN, R. N. M., *et al.* (1973). Australia antigen and primary biliary cirrhosis. *J. Clin. Path.*, **26**, 335.

MCNAMARA, J. V., *et al.* (1967). Pigment in asexual erythrocytic forms of chloroquine-resistant *Plasmodium falciparum*. *Ann. trop. Med. Parasit.*, **61**, 125.

MADDOCKS, I. and VINES, A. P. (1966). The influence of chronic infection on blood pressure in New Guinea males. *Lancet*, **2**, 262.

MAEGRAITH, B. G. (1948). *Pathological Processes in Malaria and Blackwater Fever.* Blackwell, Oxford.

— (1966). *Pathogenic Processes in Malaria.* Reprinted from *The Pathology of Parasitic Diseases*, Fourth Symposium of the British Society for Parasitology, Blackwell Scientific Publications, Oxford, p. 15.

MAEGRAITH, B. G. and FINDLAY, G. M. (1944). Oliguria in blackwater fever. *Lancet*, **2**, 403.

MAEGRAITH, B. G. and FLETCHER, K. A. (1972). The Pathogenesis of mammalian malaria. *Advanc. Parasit.*, **10**, 49.

MAEKELT, G. A. (1963). Diagnostico de Laboratorio de las trypanosomiasis Americanas. Resumo de Trabalhos. *7th Int. Congr. Med. Trop. Mal.*, Rio de Janeiro.

MAGED, A. and SOLIMAN, L. A. M. (1968). Bilharzial pseudo-calculus of ureter. *J. Urol.*, **99**, 30.

MAGEE, P. N. and BARNES, J. M. (1956). The production of malignant primary hepatic tumours in the rat by feeding Dimethylnitrosamine. *Brit. J. Cancer*, **10**, 114.

MAGNUS, P. VON., et al. (1959). A pox-like disease in cynomongus monkeys. *Acta path. microbiol. scand.*, **46**, 156.

MAHADEVAN, R. (1961). Pancreatic lithiasis: a follow-up study of 17 cases. *Brit. med. J.*, **1**, 626.

MAHMOOD, A., MACINTOSH, D. M. and SHAPER, A. G. (1967). Fibrinolytic activity in the clinical crisis of sickle-cell anaemia. *Brit. med. J.*, **3**, 653.

MAINWARING, A. R. and TOMPKINS, A. B. (1963). Generalised cytomegalic inclusion-body disease in four West African children. *W. Afr. med. J.*, **12**, 123.

MAINZER, F. (1938). Bilharzial asthma. *Trans. roy. Soc. trop. Med. Hyg.*, **32**, 253.

MAIR, N. S. (1968). The laboratory diagnosis of infection with *Pasteurella pseudotuberculosis. Recent Advances in Clinical Pathology*, p. 35. J. & A. Churchill, London.

MAKAR, N. (1957). A note on the pathogensis of cancer in the bilharzial bladder. *Brit. J. Surg.*, **45**, 240.

MAKARI, J. G. (1955). Use of Schultz–Dale test for detection of specific antigen in sera of patients with carcinoma. *Brit. med. J.*, **2**, 1291.

— (1960). Recent studies in the immunology of cancer. III. Detection of cancer antibodies and auto-antibodies by an intradermal reaction, with a view to the detection in human serum of cancer antigens by the Schultz-Dale method. *J. Amer. Geriat. Soc.*, **8**, 16.

MAKI, T. (1961). Cholelithiasis in the Japanese. *Arch. Surg.*, **82**, 599.

MALAMOS, B., FESSAS, PH. and STOMATOYANNOPOULOS, G. (1962). Types of thalassaemia-trait carriers as revealed by a study of their incidence in Greece. *Brit. J. Haemat.*, **8**, 5.

MALAMUD, N., HAYMAKER, W. and CUSTER, R. P. (1946). Heat stroke: a clinico-pathologic study of 125 fatal cases. *Milit. Surg.*, **99**, 397.

MALLORY, F. B. (1911). Cirrhosis of the liver: five different types of lesions from which it may arise. *Johns Hopk. Hosp. Bull.*, **22**, 69.

MALHOTRA, S. L. (1967). Geographical aspects of acute myocardial infarction in India with special reference to patterns of diet and eating. *Brit. Heart J.*, **29**, 337.

MANDOUL, R., DEMARTIAL, L., PESTRE, M. and MOULINIER, C. (1966). La distomatose hepato-biliare a petit douve (a propos d'un nouveau cas). (Hepato-biliary infection with the small fluke (*Dicrocoelium dendriticum*). Report of a Case.) *J. Med. Bordeaux*, **143**, No. 5, 685.

MANN, G. V., SCHAFFER, R. D. and RICH, A. (1965). Physical fitness and immunity to heart disease in the Masai. *Lancet*, **2**, 1308.

MANNHEIMER, E. (1966). Programs for combatting malnutrition in the pre-school child in Ethiopia. In *Pre-school child malnutrition: . . . an international conference on prevention of malnutrition in the pre-school child, Washington, D.C., December 7–11, 1964*, 137. Nat. Acad. Sci.—Nat. Res. Coun., Washington.

MANNING, G. S. and RATANARAT, C. (1970). *Fasciolopsis buski* in Thailand. *Amer. J. trop. Med. Hyg.*, **19**, 613.

MANSON-BAHR, P. E. C. (1961). Immunity in kala-azar *Trans. roy. Soc. trop. Med. Hyg.*, **55**, 550.

— (1963). Variations in the clinical manifestations of leishmaniasis caused by *Leishmania tropica*. 7th *Int. Congr. Trop. Med. Mal., Rio de Janeiro*.

MANSON-BAHR, P. E. C. and CHARTERS, A. D. (1963). Myocarditis in African trypanosomiasis. *Trans. roy. Soc. trop. Med. Hyg.*, **57**, 119.

MANSON-BAHR, P. E. C. and SOUTHGATE, B. A. (1964). Recent research in kala azar in East Africa. *J. trop. Med. Hyg.*, **67**, 79.

MANSOUR, S. E., MEHASEN, A. and EL-ARINY, A. F. (1970). Muscular changes in lepromatous leprosy. *Trans. roy. Soc. trop. Med. Hyg.*, **64**, 918.

MANSSON, T. (1970). Mycobacteria from aquaria. *Brit. med. J.*, **3**, 46.

MANUWA, S. (1971). The challenge of the changing pattern of disease and its implications for the problem of occupational health and Industrial medicine in Nigeria. *Nig. Med. J.*, **1**, 206.

MANUWA, S. L. A. (1928). Notes on a case of porocephalosis. *W. Afr. med. J.*, **2**, 109.

— (1947). Porocephalosis. *Trans. roy. Soc. trop. Med. Hyg.*, **40**, 507.

MARCHETTE, N. J., CARCIA, R. and RUDNICK, A. (1967). *Dengue in Malaya 1965–1967.* SEAMES. The Third Conference on Parasitic Diseases. Abstracts of Papers, p. 34.

MARCIAL-ROJAS, R. A. and FIOL, R. E. (1963). Neurologic complications of schistosomiasis. *Ann. intern. Med.* **59**, 215.

MARGOLIES, M. P. (1951). Sickle cell anemia: a composite study and survey. *Medicine (Baltimore)*, **30**, 357.

MARIGO, C., MULLER, H. and DAVIES, J. N. P. (1969). Survey of cancer in children admitted to a Brazilian charity hospital. *J. nat. Cancer Inst.*, **43**, 1231.

MARINKELLE, C. J. (1973). First finding of *Dipetalonema perstans* in Columbia; filariasis in Columbia III. *Trop. geogr. Med.*, **25**, 51.

MARKS, J. and RICHARDS, M. (1962). Classification of the anonymous mycobacteria as a guide to their significance. *Mth. Bull. Minist. Hlth. Lab. Serv.*, **21**, 200.

MARKS, M. I., LANGSTON, C. and EICKHOFF, T. C. (1970). *Torulopsis glabrata*—an opportunistic pathogen in man. *New. Engl. J. Med.* **283**, 1131.

MARQUES, A. N., *et al.* (1968). Tricuriase retal. *Hospital (Rio de J.)*, **74**, 549.

MARQUEZ, F., REIN, C. R. and ARIAS, O. (1955). Mal del Pinto in Mexico. *Bull. Wld Hlth Org.*, **13**, 299.

MARSDEN, A. T. H. (1958). The geographical pathology of cancer in Malaya. *Brit. J. Cancer*, **12**, 161.

MARSDEN, A. T. H. and REID, H. A. (1961). Pathology of sea-snake poisoning. *Brit. med. J.*, **1**, 1290.

MARSDEN, P. D., *et al.* (1965). An investigation of tropical splenomegaly at Mulago Hospital, Kampala, Uganda. *Brit. med. J.*, **1**, 89.

— (1967). *Splenomegaly in New Guinea.* W.H.O. Mimeographed Document. WHO/Mal/67.593.

MARSHALL, D. and DENEKA, S. I. (1969). Abdominal abscess due to helminthoma of the ascending colon. *Canad. med. Ass. J.*, **100**, 913.

MARSHALL, J. (1964). *Skin Diseases in Africa*. Cape and Transvaal Printers Ltd., Cape Town.

— (1972). The white skin and the sun: The common actinic dermatoses and tumours and a guide to their treatment. *Essays on Tropical Dermatology*, p. 60. Excerpta Medica Foundation, Amsterdam.

MARSHALL, J. D., QUY, D. V. and GIBSON, F. L. (1967). Asymptomatic pharyngeal plague infection in Vietnam. *Amer. J. trop. Med. Hyg.*, **16**, 175.

MARSHALL, R. A. and JANDL, J. H. (1960). Responses to 'physiologic' doses of folic acid in the megaloblastic anemias. *A.M.A. Arch. intern. Med.*, **105**, 352.

MARTIN, L. K. and BEAVER, P. C. (1968). Evaluation of Kato thick-smear technique for quantitative diagnosis of helminth infections. *Amer. J. trop. Med. Hyg.*, **17**, 382.

MARTINEZ-MALDONADO, M., GIROD, C. E., RAMIREZ DE ARELLANO, G. and RAMIREZ, E. A. (1965). Liver cell carcinoma (hepatoma) in Puerto Rico: a survey of 26 cases. *Amer. J. dig. Dis.* (n.s.), **10**, 522.

MARTINI, G. A. (1955). Lebercirrhose bei Morbus Osler, Cirrhosis hepatis teleangiectatica. *Gastroenterologia (Basel)*, **83**, 157.

MARTINI, G. A. and SIEGERT, R. (Eds.) (1971). *Margburg Virus Disease*. Springer-Verlag, New York.

MARTINSON, F. D. (1963). Rhinophycomycosis. *J. Laryng.*, **77**, 691.

— (1967). Corrosive oesophagitis in Nigeria. *J. Nig. Med. Assoc.*, **1**, 16.

— (1967). Primary tuberculosis of the nasopharynx in a Nigerian. *J. Laryng.*, **81**, 229.

MARTINSON, F. D. and CLARK, B. M. (1967). Rhinophycomycosis entomophtorae in Nigeria. *Amer. J. trop. Med. Hyg.*, **16**, 40.

MARVIN, H. N. and AUDU, I. S. (1964). A preliminary study of vitamin E and anaemia of kwashiorkor. *W. Afr. med. J.* (n.s.), **13**, 3.

MASAWE, A. E. J. and GERMAN, G. A. (1972). Neurosyphilis in psychiatric practice in Uganda. *Afr. J. med. Sci.*, **3**, 195.

MASON-BROWNE, N. L. (1974). Rabies. *Tropical Doctor*, **4**, 119.

MASSOUD, J. and NELSON, G. S. (1973). Studies on heterologous immunity in schistosomiasis. B. Observations on cross-immunity to *Ornithobilharzia turkestanicum*, *Schistosoma bovis*, *S. mansoni* and *S. haematobium* in mice, sheep and cattle in Iran. *Bull. WHO*, **44**, 5, Article 2938.

MATHAI, K. V. (1970). Amyotrophic lateral sclerosis and parkinsonism dementia in the Marianas. *Amer. J. trop. Med. Hyg.*, **19**, 151.

MATHAN, V. I., IGNATIUS, M. and BAKER, S. J. (1966). A household epidemic of tropical sprue. *Gut*, **7**, 490.

MATHÉ, G., DAUSSET, J., HERVET, E., AMIEL, J. L., COLOMBANI, J. and BRULE, G. (1964). Immunological studies in patients with placental choriocarcinoma. *J. nat. Cancer Inst.*, **33**, 193.

MATHEW, N. T. and CHANDY, J. (1970). Painful ophthalmoplegia. *J. neurol. Sci.*, **11**, 243.

MATHEWS, J. D., *et al.* (1972). Protein supplementation and enhanced antibody producing capacity in New Guinean school children. *Lancet*, **2**, 675.

MATSUBAYASHI, H. and AKAO, S. (1966). Immuno-electron microscopic studies on *Toxoplasma gomdii*. *Amer. J. trop. Med. Hyg.*, **15**, 486.

MATSUDA, S. (1962). An epidemiologic study of Japanese B encephalitis with special reference to the effectiveness of vaccination. *Bull. Inst. publ. Hlth, Tokyo*, **11**, 173.

MATSUMOTO, S. (1963). Electron microscope studies of rabies virus in mouse brain. *J. Cell Biol.*, **19**, 565.

MATTHEWS, L. J. and TRAUTMAN, J. R. (1965). Clinical and serological profiles in leprosy. *Lancet*, **2**, 915.

MATTERN, P., *et al.* (1965). A study of immunoglobulins in the cerebrospinal fluid in relation to the immuno-fluorescence phenomenon in neurosyphilis and in trypanosomiasis affecting the nervous system. *Méd. Afr. noire*, **12**, 219.

MATTERN, P., *et al.* (1967). Precipitating antibodies in the blood and cerebrospinal fluid of patients suffering from African human trypanosomiasis due to *Trypanosoma gambiense*. *Ann. Inst. Pasteur*, **112**, 105.

MEADOW, S. R. (1968). Infectious hepatitis and stillbirth. *Brit. med. J.*, **1**, 426.

MEDICAL RESEARCH COUNCIL (1958). The determination of the ABO and Rh(D) blood groups for transfusion. *Memor. Med. Res. Coun. (Lond.)*, **36.**

— (1967). Nomenclature of fungi pathogenic to man and animals. Medical Mycology Committee. *Memor. Med. Res. Coun. (Lond.)*, **23.** Her Majesty's Stationery Office, London.

MEHTA, S. K., *et al.* (1972). Small intestinal deficient in pellagra. *Amer. J. clin. Nutr.*, **25,** 545.

MEITAL, V., IZAK, G. and RACHMILEWITZ, M. (1961). L'effect de la grossesse sur la thalassémie. *Nouv. Rev. franc. Hémat.*, **1**, 389.

MELENEY, H. E. (1925). The histopathology of kala-azar in the hamster, monkey, and man. *Amer. J. Path.*, **1**, 147.

MELLGREN, J., ALM, L. and KJESSLER, Å. (1952). The isolation of *Toxoplasma* from the human placenta and uterus. *Acta path. microbiol. scand.*, **30,** 59.

MELTZER, L. E. and BOCKMAN, A. A. (1957). Trichinosis involving the central nervous system. Treatment with corticotropin (ACTH) and cortisone. *J. Amer. med. Ass.*, **164,** 1566.

MENA, I., *et al.* (1967). Chronic manganese poisoning. *Neurology*, **17**, 128.

MENAKANIT, W., MUIR, C. S. and JAIN, D. K. (1971). Cancer in Chiang Mai, North Thailand. *Brit. J. Cancer*, **25,** 225.

MENGEL, C. E., SCHAUBLE, J. F. and HAMMOND, C. B. (1963). Infarct-necrosis of the liver in a patient with S-A hemoglobin. *Arch. intern. Med.*, **111,** 93.

MESSARITAKIS, J., *et al.* (1971). Diabetes following mumps in sibs. *Arch. Dis. Childh.*, **46,** 562.

METSELAAR, D. (1956). Spleens and holoendemic malaria in West New Guinea. *Bull. Wld Hlth Org.*, **15,** 635.

METSELAAR, D., *et al.* (1974). Isolation of arboviruses in Kenya 1966–1971. *Trans. roy. Soc. trop. Med. Hyg.*, **68,** 114.

METZ, J. (1959). Hereditary spherocytosis in the Bantu. *S. Afr. med. J.*, **33,** 1034.

METZGER, I. F., KASE, A. and SMITH, C. W. (1962). Identification of pathogenic fungi in surgical and autopsy specimens by immunofluorescence. *Mycopath. el. Mycolog. Appl.* **17,** 335.

MEYER, H. A. (1973). Acute haemolysis associated with typhoid fever and G-6-PD deficiency. *Lancet*, **1,** 729.

MEYERS, W. M., *et al.* (1974). Distribution of *Mycobacterium ulcerans* infections in Zaire, including the report of new foci. *Ann. Soc. belge Méd. trop.*, **54,** 147.

MIALL, W. E., *et al.* (1962). Factors influencing arterial pressure in the general population in Jamaica. *Brit. med. J.*, **2,** 497.

MIALL, W. E., *et al.* (1972). Longitudinal study of heart disease in a Jamaican rural population: 1. Prevalence with special reference to ECG findings. *Bull. Wld Hlth Org.*, **46**, 429.

— (1972). Longitudinal study of heart disease in a Jamaican rural population: 2. Factors influencing mortality. *Bull. Wld Hlth Org.*, **46**, 685.

— (1972). Longitudinal study of heart disease in a Jamaican rural population: 3. Factors influencing changes in serial electrocardiograms. *Bull. Wld Hlth Org.*, **46**, 695.

MICHAEL, P. (1944). Filariasis among navy and marine personnel: report on laboratory investigations. *Nav. med. Bull.*, **42**, 1059.

MICHAUX, J. L., HEREMANS, J. F. and HITZIG, W. H. (1966). Immunoglobulin levels in cord-blood serum of Negroes and Caucasians. *Trop. geogr. Med.*, **18**, 10.

MIDDLEMISS, H. (1961). *Tropical Radiology.* Heinemann, London.

MIDDLETON, G. D. (1964). Cardiomyopathy of pregnancy. *J. Obstet. Gynaec. Brit. Cwlth*, **71**, 951.

MILIC, A. M. B. (1969). Racial factors in anencephaly. *Amer. J. Obstet. Gynec.*, **104**, 134.

MILLER, A. J., *et al.* (1963). Ventricular endomyocardial changes after impairment of cardiac lymph flow in dogs. *Brit. Heart J.*, **25**, 182.

MILLER, D. S., KEIGHLEY, A. C. and LANGMAN, M. J. S. (1974). Changing patterns in epidemiology of Chrohn's Disease. *Lancet*, **2**, 691.

MILLER, H. (1966). Polyneuritis. *Brit. med. J.*, **2**, 1219.

MILLER, J. R. (1967). Portal hypertension in Nairobi. *E. Afr. med. J.*, **44**, 376.

MILLER, L. H. (1972). The ultrastructure of red cells infected by *Plasmodium falciparum* in man. *Trans. roy. Soc. trop. Med. Hyg.*, **66**, 3, 459.

MILLER, R. W. and BEEBE, G. W. (1973). Infections mononucleosis and the empirical risk of cancer. *J. nat. Cancer Inst.*, **50**, 315.

MILLER, W. S., *et al.* (1963). Stability and infectivity of airborne yellow fever and Rift Valley fever viruses. *Amer. J. Hyg.*, **77**, 114.

MING-CHAI, C. and SHAN-CHI, C. W. (1957). Acute colonic obstruction in *Schistosoma japonicum Chin. med. J.*, **75**, 517.

MIRANDA, R. N. (1963). Faria reaction. (Editorial) *Publicacoes do Centro de Estudos Leprologicos.* Univ. do Parana. **3**, 6.

MISRA, R. C., KASTHURI, D. and CHUTTANI, H. K. (1966). Adult coeliac disease in tropics. *Brit. med. J.*, **2**, 1230.

MISRA, U. K. and VENKITASUBRAMANIAN, T. A. (1964). Serum lipids in leprosy by silicic acid column chromatography. *Int. J. Leprosy*, **32**, 248.

MITCHELL, J. R. (1964). Detection of *Toxocara canis* antibodies with the fluorescent antibody technique. *Proc. Soc. exper. Biol.*, **117**, 267.

MITCHISON, D. A. (1963). The epidemiology of tubercle bacilli. *Scient. Basis Med. ann. Rev.*, 1963, p. 319.

MITRA, K. (1963). A supplement to the results of diet surveys in India 1935–48. *Spec. Rep. Ser. Indian Coun. med. Res.*, No. 25.

MIYAJI, T., IUCHI, I., TAKEDA, I. and SHIBATA, S. (1963). Hemoglobin Shimonoseki ($\alpha_2^{54 \, Arg}\beta^A_2$), a slow-moving hemoglobin found in a Japanese family, with special reference to its chemistry. *Acta haemat. jap.*, **26**, 531.

MIYAKE, M. (1967). The pathology of schistosomiasis in Japan. In *Bilharziasis* ed. F. K. Mostofi, p. 140. Springer-Verlag, New York.

MIYAKE, M., SAITO, M., ENOMOTO, M., SHIKATA, T., ISHIKO, T., URAGUCHI, K., SAKAI, F., TATSUNO, T., TSUKIOKA, M. and SAKAI, Y. (1960). Toxic liver injuries and liver cirrhosis induced in mice and rats through long term feeding with *Penicillium islandicum* Sopp-growing rice. *Acta path. jap.*, **10**, 75.

MIYASAKI, K., *et al.* (1967). A study on the endemic goiter in Madjalengka district of the Republic of Indonesia. *Kobe J. med. Sci.*, **13**, 181.

MIYAZAKI, I. and VAJRASTHIRA, S. (1967). Occurrence of the lung fluke *Paragonimus heterotremus* Chen et Hsia, 1964 in Thailand. (Research Notes.) *J. Parasit.*, **53**, No. 1, 207.

MODAN, B., TULCHINSKY, D. and STEINITZ, R. (1966). An epidemiological study of cancer of the stomach in Israel. *Int. Congr. Cancer, Tokyo*, 713.

MODAN, B., *et al.* (1969). Epidemiological aspects of neoplastic disorders in Israeli migrant population. V. The Lymphomas. *J. nat. Cancer Inst.*, **42**, 375.

MOHAMMED, I. and CARLISLE, R. (1971). Cardiac and renal involvement in Mumps. *W. Afr. med. J.*, **20**, 367.

MOLLISON, P. L. (1967). *Blood Transfusion in Clinical Medicine*. 4th ed. Blackwell, Oxford.

MONATH, T. P. (1974). Lassa fever and Marburg virus disease. *WHO Chron.*, **28**, 212.

MONATH, T. P. and KEMP, G. E. (1973). Importance of non-human primates in yellow fever epidemiology in Nigeria. *Trop. geogr. Med.*, **25**, 28.

MONATH, T. P., *et al.* (1974). Arbovirus studies in Nupeko Forest, a possible natural focus of yellow fever virus in Nigeria. I. Description of the area and serological survey of humans and other vertebrate hosts. *Trans. roy. Soc. trop. Med. Hyg.*, **68**, 30.

MONCADA, G. B. (1963). *Estudios sobre alteraciones del crecimiento y del desarrollo psicológico del síndrome pluricarencial o kwashiorkor*. Editor Grafos, Caracas.

MÖNCKEBERG, F. (1966). Programs for combatting malnutrition in the pre-school child in Chile. In *Pre-school child malnutrition: . . . an international conference on prevention of malnutrition in the pre-school child, Washington, D.C., December 7–11, 1964*, 168. Nat. Acad. Sci.—Nat. Res. Coun., Washington.

MONEKOSSO, G. L. and ASHBY, P. H. (1963). The natural history of an amblyopia syndrome in Western Nigeria. *W. Afr. med. J.*, **12** (n.s.), 226.

MONEKOSSO, G. L. and WILSON, J. (1966). Plasma thiocyanate and vitamin B_{12} in Nigerian patients with degenerative neurological disease. *Lancet*, **1**, 1062.

MONEY, G. L. (1959). Clinical aspects of tropical ataxic neuropathies related to malnutrition. *W. Afr. med. J.*, **8**, 3.

— (1959). Isoniazed neuropathies in malnourished tuberculous patients. *J. trop. Med. Hyg.*, **62**, 198.

MONNET, A., BAYLET, R. and REYNAUD, R. (1952). Contribution a l'étude de l'elimination urinaise des dix-sept cetosteroides neutres chez l'African normal et trypanosomé. *Méd. trop.*, **12**, 307.

MONTEFIORE, D., *et al.* (1963). Trial of type 1 oral poliomyelitis vaccine (Sabin) in Nigerian children. *Brit. med. J.*, **2**, 1569.

MONTENEGRO, M. R., DA SILVA, L. C. and PONTES, J. F. (1958). An evaluation of the problem of hepatic cirrhosis as seen in São Paulo, Brazil. II: Postnecrotic cirrhosis: morphologic aspects. *Gastroenterology*, **34**, 1108.

MONTGOMERY, R. D. (1961). The cause of death in tetanus. *W. Indian med. J.*, **10**, 84.

— (1965). The medical significance of cyanogen in plant foodstuffs. *Amer. J. clin. Nutrition*, **17**, 103.

MONTGOMERY, R. D., *et al.* (1964). Clinical and pathological observations on Jamaican neuropathy. *Brain*, **87**, 425.

— (1973). Post-infective malabsorption: a sprue syndrome. *Brit. med. J.*, **2**, 265.

MONZIOLS, COLLIGNON and ROY, J. (1920). Un cas di'ictère grave suivi de mort et causé chez un sénégalais par le *Porocephalus armillatus* Yman, 1848. *C. R. Soc. Biol. (Paris)*, **83**, 28.

MOORE, D. G. F. (1934). Manioc (kassava) as a native food in Nigeria. *W. Afr. med. J.*, **7**, 97.

MOORE, D. L., *et al.* (1974). An epidemic of chikungunya fever at Ibadan, Nigeria. *Ann. trop. Med. Parasit.*, **68**, 59.

MOORE, G., HOMEWOOD, C. H. and GILLES, H. M. (1975). A comparison of pigment from *S. marooni* and *P. berghei. Ann. trop. Med. Parasit.* **69**, No. 3, (in press).

MOORHOUSE, D. E., *et al.* (1973). Human pulmonary dirofilariasis in Queensland. *Med. J. Aust.*, **2**, 1230.

MORBIDITY AND MORTALITY (1974). Nomenclature of antigens associated with viral hepatitis type B. U.S. Department of Health, Education and Welfare, **23**, 29.

MORE, R. H., MCMILLAN, G. C. and DUFF, G. L. (1946). The pathology of sulfonamide allergy in man. *Amer. J. Path.*, **22**, 703.

MORELL, D. B. and SLATER, E. C. (1946). The fluorimetric determination of riboflavin in urine. *Biochem. J.*, **40**, 652.

MORI, W. (1967). Cirrhosis and primary cancer of the liver: comparative study in Tokyo and Cincinnati. *Cancer*, **20**, 627.

MORLEY, D. (1963). A medical service for children under five years of age in West Africa. *Trans. roy. Soc. trop. Med. Hyg.*, **57**, 79.

MORLEY, D., WOODLAND, M. and MARTIN, W. J. (1963). Measles in Nigerian children. *J. Hyg. (Lond.)*, **61**, 115.

MORONI, M. and SORICE, F. (1966). Contributo delle reasioni di immuno fluorescenza alla diagnosi giologica di idatidosi (The immunofluorescent reaction in the diagnosis of hydatid infection). *G. Mal. infett*, **18**, No. 7, 471.

MORRIS, M. N., *et al.* (1970). Latex agglutination test for invasive amoebiasis. *Lancet*, **1**, 1362.

MORROW, R. H., SAI, F. T. and BARKER, L. F. (1971). Australia antigen and hepatitis in Accra, Ghana. *Brit. med. J.*, **4**, 389.

MORROW, R. H., *et al.* (1968). Unusual features of viral hepatitis in Accra, Ghana. *Ann. int. Med.*, **68**, 1250.

— (1971). Burkitt's lymphoma: a time-space cluster of cases in Bwamba County of Uganda. *Brit. med. J.*, **2**, 491

MOST, H., GELLIN, G. A., YAGER, R., ARON, B., FRIEDLANDER, M. and QUARFORDT, S. (1963). Enterobiasis (pinworm infection): a study of 951 Puerto Rican and 315 non-Puerto Rican children in New York City. *Amer. J. trop. Med. Hyg.*, **12**, 65.

MOSTOFI, F. K. (1966). *The Kidney.* Williams and Wilkins Co., Baltimore.

MOTT, M. G. (1969). Serological studies in infectious mononucleosis. *Brit. med. J.* **4**, 171.

MOURANT, A. E. (1954). *The Distribution of Human Blood Groups.* Blackwell Scientific Publications, Oxford.

MUEHSAM, G. E., PSCHIBUL, F. and SCERBO, J. E. (1964). The natural history of idiopathic cardiomegaly. *Amer. Heart J.*, **67**, 173.

MUGERWA, J. W. (1971). The lymphoreticular system in kwashiorkor. *J. Path.*, **105**, 105.

MUIR, C. S. (1958). Rheumatic heart disease in Singapore. *Trans. roy. Soc. trop. Med. Hyg.*, **52**, 446.

— (1960). Coronary heart disease in seven racial groups in Singapore. *Brit. Heart J.*, **22**, 45.

— (1960). Incidence of congenital heart disease in Singapore. *Brit. Heart J.*, **22**, 243.

— (1962). Male and female genital tract cancer in Singapore. *Cancer*, **15**, 354.

MUIR, C. S. and SHANMUGARATNAM, K. (1966). (Incidence of cancer in) Singapore, Chinese. In *Cancer Incidence in Five Continents*, ed. R. Doll, P. Payne, and J. Waterhouse, Chapter IV, p. 124.

MUKERJEE, N. and KUNDU, S. (1961). The late lepromin reaction in subsided lepromatous cases. *Int. J. Leprosy.*, **29**, 14.

MUKERJEE, S. (1963). Bacteriophage typing of cholera. *Bull. Wld Hlth Org.*, **28**, 337.

MULAS, H. and RODRIGUEZ, R. B. (1964). Amoebic infestation of the female genitalia. *Med. J. Aust.*, **ii**, 179.

MULAY, D. M. (1963). Skin cancer in India. *Nat. Cancer Inst. Monogr.*, **10**, 215.

MULLAN, D. P. and WILLIAMS, N. E. (1965). Left sided amoebic liver abscess with pulmonary involvement, pericarditis and pseudocholinesterase deficiency. *Brit. Med. J.*, **1**, 235.

MULLER, A. S., VALKENBURG, H. A. and GREENWOOD, B. M. (1972). Rheumatoid factor in three West African populations. *E. Afr. med. J.*, **49**, 75.

MULLER, R. L. and TAYLOR, M. G. (1972). The specific differentiation of schistosome eggs by the Ziehl–Neelsen technique. *Trans. roy. Soc. trop. Med. Hyg.*, **66**, 18.

MULLIGAN, H. W. (ed.) (1970). The African trypanosomiases. Allen and Unwin, London.

MULLIGAN, T. O. (1971). Typhoid fever in Ilesha, Western State of Nigeria. *W. Afr. med. J.*, Dec. 358.

MUN, C. T. (1968). Epidemic koro in Singapore. *Brit. med. J.*, **1**, 640.

MUNOZ, N. and CORREA, P. (1970). Arteritis of the aorta and its major branches. *Amer. Heart J.*, **80**, 319.

MURPHY, H. B. M. (1973). Current trends in transcultural psychiatry. *Proc. roy. Soc. Med.*, **66**, 711.

MURRAY, J. F. and LOTHE, F. (1962). *Symposium on Kaposi's Sarcoma*. S. Karger, New York, p. 100.

MURRELL, T. G. C., *et al.* (1966). Pig-bel: enteritis necroticans. *Lancet*, **1**, 217.

MURUGASU, R., and DISSANAIKE, A. S. (1973). First case of schistosomiasis in Malaysia. *Trans. roy. Soc. trop. Med. Hyg.*, **67**, 6, 880.

MUSACCHIO, F. and MITCHELL, N. (1966). Primary renal echinococcosis: a case report. *Amer. J. trop. Med. Hyg.*, **15**, 168.

MUSTAFA, D. (1965). Gross splenomegaly in the Sudan. *J. trop. Med. Hyg.*, **68**, 183.

MWAMBU, P. M. (1973). Importance of cattle as natural reservoir hosts of *T. rhodesiense* and resistance to ethidium (homidium bromide) of *T. brucei* subgroup organisms isolated from cattle. *Trans. roy. Soc. trop. Med. Hyg.*, **67**, 286.

MYERS, J. A. (1959a). The natural history of tuberculosis in the human body. I. The demonstrable primary pulmonary infiltrate. *Amer. Rev. Tuberc.*, **79**, 19.

— (1959b). The natural history of tuberculosis in the human body. II. Longitudinal observations imperative. *Amer. Rev. resp. Dis.*, **80**, 100.

MYERS, J. A. (1961). The natural history of tuberculosis in the human body. III. Tuberculous women and their children. *Amer. Rev. resp. Dis.*, **83**, 558.

— (1962). The natural history of tuberculosis in the human body. IV. Behaviour of tuberculosis among elderly people. *Amer. Rev. resp. Dis.*, **85**, 232.

MYERS, J. A., BEARMAN, J. E. and DIXON, H. G. (1963). The natural history of tuberculosis in the human body. V. Prognosis among tuberculin-reactor children from birth to five years of age. *Amer. Rev. resp. Dis.*, **87**, 354.

MYLINS, R. E. and TEN SELDAM, R. E. J. (1962). Venereal infection by *Entameoba histolytica* in a New Guinea couple. *Trop. geogr. Med.*, **14**, 20.

NAGGAN, L. (1971). Anencephaly and spina bifida in Israel. *Pediatrics*, **47,** 577.

NAI-KUANG, C. and PEN-CHING, C. (1957). Pyloric obstruction and sigimodal fistula due to schistosomiasis. *Chin. med. J.*, **75,** 324.

NA-NAKORN, S. (1959). Haemoglobinopathies in Thailand. In *Abnormal Haemoglobins: Symposium*, p. 357. Blackwell Scientific Publications, Oxford.

NASELL, I. and HIRSCH, W. M. (1973). The transmission dynamics of Schistosomiasis. *Communications on pure and applied mathematics*, **26,** 395.

NASU, T. (1963). Pathology of pulseless disease: a systematic study and critical review of twenty-one autopsy cases reported in Japan. *Angiology*, **14,** 225.

NAUMANN, H. N., *et al.* (1971). Plasma haemoglobin and haemoglobin fractions in sickle cell crisis. *Amer. J. clin. Path.*, **56,** 137.

NAYAK, N. C. and RAMALINGASWAMI, V. (1969). Obliterative portal venopathy of the liver. *Arch. Path.*, **87,** 359.

NAYAK, N. C., VEENA, C., MALAVIYA, A. N., CHANDRA, R. K. (1972). Alpha feto protein in Indian childhood Cirrhosis. *Lancet*, **1,** 68.

NAYEBI, M. (1971). Immunofluorescent technique for diagnosis of *E. histolytica* strains. *Med. Lab. Technol.*, **28,** 413.

NEAFIE, R. C. and PIGGOTT, J. (1971). Human pulmonary dirofilariasis. *Arch. Path.*, **92,** 342.

NEAL, R. A. (1960). Enzymic proteolysis by *Entamoeba histolytica*: biochemical characteristics and relationship with invasiveness. *Parasitology*, **50,** 531.

— (1966). Experimental studies on *Entamoeba* with reference to speciation. In *Advances in Parasitology*, **4.** Academic Press, London.

— (1971). Pathogenesis of amoebiasis. *Gut*, **12,** 483.

— (1972). Virulence of *Entamoeba histolytica*. *Trans. roy. Soc. trop. Med. Hyg.*, **66,** 514.

NEAME, P. B. and PILLAY, V. K. G. (1964). Spontaneous hypoglycaemia, hepatic and renal necrosis following the intake of herbal medicines. *S. Afr. med. J.*, **38,** 729.

NECHELES, T. F., CATES, M., SHEEHAN, R. G. and MEYER, H. J. (1966). Hemoglobin H disease: a family study. *Blood*, **28,** 501.

NEEL, J. V. (1949). The inheritance of sickle cell anemia. *Science, N.Y.*, **110,** 64.

NEGHME, A. and SILVA, R. (1968). Hidatidosis como problema de salud publica en Chile. *Bol. chil. Parasit.*, **23,** 59.

NEIRA, M., *et al.* (1968). Algunos aspectos clinico-radiologicos de la hidatidosis en el nino. *Bol. chil. Parasit.*, **23,** 65.

NELSON, E. R. (1960). Hemorrhagic fever in children in Thailand. Report of 69 cases. *J. Pediat.*, **56,** 101.

NELSON, G. S. (1958). 'Hanging groin' and hernia, complications of onchocerciasis. *Trans. roy. Soc. trop. Med. Hyg.*, **52,** 272.

— (1966). The pathology of filarial infections. *Helminth. Abst.*, **35,** Pt. 4, 311.

NELSON, G. S., GUGGISBERG, C. W. A. and MUKUNDI, J. (1963). Animal hosts of *Trichinella spiralis* in East Africa. *Ann. trop. Med. Parasit.*, **57,** 332.

NELSON, G. S., PESTER, F. R. N. and RICKMAN, R. (1965). The significance of wild animals in the transmission of cestodes of medical importance in Kenya. *Trans. roy. Soc. trop. Med. Hyg.*, **59,** 507.

NEUMANN, M. A., *et al.* (1964). Neuropathological findings in exotic disorders among natives of the Highlands of New Guinea. *J. Neuropath exp. Neurol.*, **23,** 486.

NEVA, F. A. (1970). Amoebic meningoencephalitis—a new disease? *New Engl. J. Med.*, **282,** 450.

NEVA, F. A., MALONE, M. F. and MYERS, B. R. (1961). Factors influencing the intracellular growth of *Trypanosoma cruzi in vitro*. *Am. J. trop. Med. Hyg.*, **10**, 140.

NEVES, J. (1970). In *Esquistossomose mansoni*, ed. Da Cunha. Sarvier, Sao Paulo, Brazil.

NEWELL, K. W. (1966). An epidemiologist's view of leprosy. *Bull. Wld Hlth Org.*, **34**, 827.

NGU, V. A. (1960). Tropical ulcers in Ibadan. *W. Afr. med. J.*, **9** (n.s.), 247.

— (1967). Tropical ulcers. *Brit. med. J.*, **1**, 283.

NGU, V. A. and KONSTAM, P. (1964). Chronic lymphoedema in Western Nigeria. *Brit. J. Surg.*, **51**, 101.

— (1964). Chronic lymphoedema in Western Nigeria. *Brit. J. Surg.*, **51**, 101.

NGU, V. A. and OSUNKOYA, B. O. (1973). The Epstein–Barr virus and Marek's disease. *Afr. J. med. Sci.*, **4**, 37.

NICHOLS, R. L. (1956). The etiology of visceral larva migrans. I: Diagnostic morphology of infective second-stage *Toxocara* larvae. *J. Parasit.*, **42**, 349.

— (1956). The etiology of visceral larva migrans. II: Comparative larval morphology of *Ascaris lumbricoides, Necator americanus, Strongyloides stercoralis* and *Ancylostoma caninum. J. Parasit.*, **42**, 363.

NICHOLS, R. L., *et al.* (1963). Studies on trachoma. II. Comparison of fluorescent antibody, Giemsa, and egg isolation methods for detection of trachoma virus in human conjunctival scrapings. *Amer. J. trop. Med. Hyg.*, **12**, 223.

NICOL, B. M. (1952). The nutrition of Nigerian peasants, with special reference to the effects of deficiencies of the vitamin B Complex, Vitamin A and animal protein. *Brit. J. Nutr.*, **6**, 34.

NIEDERMAN, J. C., EVANS, A. S., SUBRAHMANYAN, M. S. and MCCOLLUM, R. W. (1970). Prevalence, incidence and persistance of EB virus antibody in young adults. *New Engl. J. Med.*, **282**, 361.

NIEDERMAN, J. C., MCCOLLUM, R. W., HENLE, G. and HENLE, W. (1968). Infectious mononucleosis. *J. Amer. med. Ass.*, **203**, 205.

NIGG, CLARA (1963). Serologic studies on subclinical melioidosis. *J. Immunol.*, **91**, 18.

NIKKELS, R. J. (1965). *Neutralisatiereactie in vitro ter bepaling van verworven humorale immuniteit bij toxoplasmosis.* (Thesis.) Sijthoff, Leiden.

NKRUMAH, F. K. (1972). Hereditary elliptocytosis associated with severe haemolytic anaemia and malaria. *Afr. J. med. Sci.*, **3**, 131.

NKRUMAH, F. K. and PERKINS, I. V. (1973). Neurological manifestations of Burkitt's lymphoma in Ghana. *Afr. J. med. Sci.*, **4**, 209.

NOBILI, I., CASCIO, G., COSENTINO, G., COLONNA, V. and PURPURA, R. (1966). Contributo alla diagnosi dell' idatidosi umana mediante la fissazione del complemento e l'emo-agglutinazione condizionata con antigene idatideo criolisato ed ultracentrifugato. (A study of immunological tests for the diagnosis of *Echinococcus* disease. Evaluation of haemagglutination and complement fixation with ultracentrifuged and cryolysed cyst extract.) *Riv. Ist. sieroter. ital.*, **41**, No. 4, 237.

NORMAN, L., SADUN, E. H. and ALLAIN, D. S. (1959). A bentonite flocculation test for the diagnosis of hydatid disease in man and animals. *Amer. J. trop. Med. Hyg.*, **8**, 46.

NORWICH, I. and LIEBERMAN, B. A. (1969). Amoebiasis of the anterior abdominal wall. *S. Afr. Med. J.*, **43**, 1192.

NOUHOUAYI, A. (1967). Les Aspects neurologiques du paludisme a *Plasmodium falciparum*. M.D. Thesis, University of Dakar.

NOURI, L. and AL-RAHIM, K. (1970). Kerosene poisoning in children. *Postgrad. med. J.*, **46**, 71.

NUNEZ ANDRADE, R. (1965). Common dermatological conditions in the tropics with special reference to the Quintana Roo Area, Mexico. *Medicina (Méx.)*, **45**, 25.

NWOKOLO, C. (1955). Endomyocardial fibrosis and other obscure cardiopathies in Eastern Nigeria. *W. Afr. med. J.* (n.s.), **4**, 103.

— (1966). Gastric ulceration in Southern Nigeria. *W. Afr. med. J.* (n.s.), **15**, 210.

— (1967). Ascites in Africa. *Brit. med. J.*, **1**, 33.

NWOKOLO, C., EKPECHI, O. L. and NWOKOLO, U. (1966). New foci of endemic goitre in Eastern Nigeria. *Trans. roy. Soc. trop. Med. Hyg.*, **60**, 97.

NWOKOLO, C. and IKOKU, N. (1967). Pulmonary embolism in Nigeria—the importance of local factors in its aetiology. *J. Nig. Med. Assoc.*, **4**, 45.

NWOKOLO, C. and IMOHIOSEN, E. A. E. (1973). Strongyloidiasis of respiratory tract presenting as 'Asthma'. *Brit. med. J.*, **2**, 153.

NYBOE, J. (1960). The efficacy of the tuberculin test. An analysis based on results from 33 countries. *Bull. Wld Hlth Org.*, **22**, 5.

NYLANDER, P. P. S. (1969). The value of the placenta in the determination of zygosity. *J. Obstet. Gynaec. Brit. Cwlth.*, **76**, 699.

OBASI, O. E. (1964). Gynatrisia in U.C.H. Ibadan. *Dokita*, **6**, 15.

OBEYESEKERE, I. and DE SOYSA (1970). Primary pulmonary hypertension, eosinophilia and filariasis in Ceylon. *Brit. Heart. J.*, **32**, 524.

O'BRIEN, D. D. (1963). Tropical pyomyositis: a manifestation of larva migrans ? *J. roy. Army med. Cps*, **109**, 43.

O'BRIEN, W. and ENGLAND, M. W. J. (1966). Military tropical sprue from south-east Asia. *Brit. med. J.*, **2**, 1157.

O'CONOR, G. T., *et al.* (1972). Ultrastructural survey of primary liver cell carcinomas from Uganda. *J. nat. Cancer Inst.*, **48**, 587.

O'CONOR, G. T. and DAVIES, J. N. (1960). Malignant tumors in African children, with special reference to malignant lymphoma. *J. Pediat.*, **56**, 526.

O'CONOR, G. T., RAPPAPORT, H. and SMITH, G. B. (1965). Childhood lymphoma resembling 'Burkitt tumour' in the United States. *Cancer*, **18**, 411.

— (1965). Childhood lymphoma resembling 'Burkitt tumor' in the United States. *Cancer, N.Y.*, **18**, 411.

ODEKU, E. D., MARTINSON, F. D. and AKINOSI, J. O. (1969). Crainofacial fibrous dysplasia in Nigerian Africans. *Int. Surg.*, **51**, 170.

ODEKU, E. L. (1967). Congenital malformations of the cerebrospinal axis seen in Western Nigeria. *Internat. Surg.*, **48**, 52.

— (1965). Peculiar subgaleal 'inclusion' cysts. *Ghana med. J.*, **4**, 37.

ODEKU, E. L., ADELOYE, A. and OSUNTOKUN, B. O. (1973). The neurological picture of Burkitt's lymphoma in Ibadan. *Afr. J. med. Sci.*, **4**, 119.

ODEKU, E. L., GRANT, I. H. and EKOP, A. C. (1967). Congenital malformations of the cerebrospinal axis seen in Western Nigeria. The spinal meningoceles. *Internat. Surg.*, **47**, 580.

ODEKU, E. L. and JANOTA, I. (1965). Primary spinal cord melanoma and phaeochromocytoma of urinary bladder wall. *Ghana med. J.*, **4**, 113.

— (1967). Intracranial masses—Ibadan. *W. Afr. med. J.*, **16**, 31.

ODEKU, E. L., LUCAS, A. O. and RICHARDS, D. R. (1968). Intramedullary spinal cord schistosomiasis. *J. Neurosurg.*, **29**, 417.

ODURO, K. and SEARLE, J. F. (1972). Anaesthesia in sickle-cell states. *Brit. med. J.*, **4**, 596.

OETTLÉ, A. G. (1962). Skin cancer in Africa. *Nat. Cancer Inst. Monogr.*, No. 10, 197.

— (1964). Cancer in Africa, especially in regions south of the Sahara. *J. nat. Cancer Inst.*, **33**, 383.

— (1965). The aetiology of primary carcinoma of the liver in Africa: a critical appraisal of previous ideas with an outline of the mycotoxin hypothesis. *S. Afr. med. J.*, **39**, 817.

OFORI ATTA, S. B. G. (1958). Intraperitoneal blood transfusion in children in Accra with special reference to the treatment of kwashiorkor. *Arch. Dis. Childh.*, **33**, 202.

OFOSU, F. (1972). The human haptoglobins. *Ghana med. J.*, **11**, 354.

OGILVIE, B. M. (1964). Reagin-like antibodies in animals immune to helminth parasites. (Correspondence.) *Nature (Lond.)*, **204**, 91.

OGILVIE, B. M. and JONES, V. E. (1971). *Nippostrongfus brasiliensis*. A review of immunity and the host/parasite relationship in the rat. *Exp. Parasit.*, **29**, 138.

O'GORMAN, P., ALLSOPP, K. M., LEHMANN, H. and SUKUMARAN, P. K. (1963). Sickle-cell haemoglobin K disease. *Brit. med. J.*, **2**, 1381.

OGUNBA, E. O. (1972). Ecology of human loiasis in Nigeria. *Trans. roy. Soc. trop. Med. Hyg.*, **66**, 743.

OJO, G. O. and PARRATT, J. R. (1966). Urinary excretion of 5-hydroxyindoleacetic acid in Nigerians with endomyocardial fibrosis. *Lancet*, **1**, 854.

OLERNICK, A. (1969). Altered immunity and cancer risk. *J. nat. Cancer Inst.*, **43**, 775.

OLESEN, E. B., *et al.* (1959). Thalassaemia in Libera. *Brit. med. J.*, **1**, 1385.

OLIVER-GONZALEZ, J. and TORREGROSA, M. V. (1944). A substance in animal parasites related to the human isoagglutinogens. *J. infect. Dis.*, **74**, 173.

OLIVER-GONZALEZ, J., RAMOS, F. L. and COKER, C. M. (1955). Serological reactions against egg antigens as an aid in the evaluation of therapy in schistosomiasis. *Amer. J. trop. Med. Hyg.*, **4**, No. 5, 908.

OLIVIER, L. and ANSARI, N. (1967). The epidemiology of bilharziasis. In *Bilharziasis* ed. F. K. Mostofi. p. 8. Springer-Verlag, New York.

OLIVEIRA, M. R. DE, CUTAIT, D. E., BRANCO, P. D., SPERANZINI, M. B., FUJIMURA, I. and CAMPOS, S. DE M. (1963). Obstrução intestinal. I: Volvo do sigmóide; estudo de 107 casos. *Rev. Hosp. Clín. Fac. Med. S. Paulo*, **18**, 469.

OLSEN, L. C., *et al.* (1970). Encephalopathy and fatty degeneration of the viscera in Thai children. *Amer. J. Dis. Child.*, **120**, 1.

— (1971). Encephalopathy and fatty degeneration of the viscera in Northeastern Thailand. *Pediatrics*, **47**, 707.

OLSON, R. A. and JOHNSON, E. H. (1969). Histopathologic changes and small bowel absorption in falciparum malaria. *Amer. J. trop. Med. Hyg.*, **18**, 355.

OLURIN, E. O., AJAYI, O. O. and OSUNKOYA, B. O. (1971). Tuberous Sclerosis. *Brit. J. Urol.*, **43**, 432.

OLURIN, O. (1969). Orbital rhabdomyosarcoma in pregnancy. *Cancer (Philad.)*, **24**, 1013.

— (1970). The aetiology of cortical blindness in Nigeria. *Afr. J. med. Sci.*, **1**, 357.

OLURIN, O. and WILLIAMS, A. O. (1972). Orbito-ocular tumours in Nigeria. *Cancer (Philad.)*, **30**, 580.

OLUWASANMI, J. O. and OSUNKOYA, B. O. (1969). Kaposi's sarcoma in Ibadan. *W. Afr. med. J.*, **18**, 89.

OMER, A., *et al.* (1972). Incidence of G-6-PD deficiency and abnormal haemoglobins in the indigenous and immigrant tribes of the Sudan. *Trop. geogr. Med.*, **24**, 401.

ONI, S. B., OSUNKOYA, B. O. and LUZZATTO, L. (1970). Paroxysmal nocturnal haemo-globinuria. *Blood*, **36**, 145.

ONIFADE, A., AKANDE, E. O. and KOLAWOLE, T. (1970). A case of lithokelyphopedion. *Ghana med. J.*, **9**, 217.

OOMEN, H. A. P. C. (1957). The relationship between liver size, malaria and diet in Papuan children. *Docum. Med. geogr. trop. (Amst.)*, **9**, 84.

OOMEN, H. A. P. C., MCLAREN, D. S. and ESCAPINI, H. (1964). Epidemiology and public health aspects of hypovitaminosis A: a global survey on xerophthalmia. *Trop. geogr. Med. (Amst.)*, **16**, 271.

ORR, I. M., MILLER, A. A. and RUSSELL, J. Y. (1954). Eosinophilic infiltration of the stomach and bowel. *Postgrad. med. J.*, **30**, 485.

OSOBA, A. O. (1972). Mycoplasma in the genito-urinary tract of Nigerians. *Afr. J. med. Sci.*, **3**, 187.

OSTERAAS, G. R., HARDMAN, J. M., BASS, J. W. and WILSON, C. (1971). Neonatal melioi-dosis. *Amer. J. Dis. Child.*, **122**, 446.

OSUNKOYA, B. O. (1966). *Studies on the lymphoreticular and Burkitt tumours in Nigeria*, Ph.D. Thesis, University of Ibadan.

— (1971). The thymus in Birkitt's lymphoma. *J. Nigeria med. Ass.*, **1**, 154.

OSUNKOYA, B. O., NGU, V. A. and MOTTRAM, F. C. (1970). Morphology of Burkitt's lymphoma during regression induced by cyclophosphamide. *Cancer (Philad.)*, **25**, 550.

OSUNKOYA, B. O., OYEDIRAN, A. B. O. and COOKE, A. (1973). Multinucleated giant cells in PHA-stimulated leucocyte cultures of children with measles. *Immunology*, **25**, 737.

OSUNKOYA, B. O., *et al.* (1972). Histopathology of extracardiac tissues in endomyo-cardial fibrosis. *Afr. J. med. Sci.*, **3**, 275.

OSUNTOKUN, B. O. (1968). An ataxic neuropathy in Nigeria—a clinical, biochemical, and electrophysiological study. *Brain*, **91**, 215.

— (1971). Epidemiology of tropical nutritional neuropathy in Nigerians. *Trans. roy. Soc. trop. Med. Hyg.*, **65**, 454.

— (1971). Primary diseases of muscles in Nigerians. *Actualites de Pathologie Neuro-musculaire*, Expansion Scientifique, Paris, 289.

— (1971). Motor nerve conduction in kwashiorkor before and after treatment. *Afr. J. med. Sci.*, **2**, 109.

— (1972). The effects of malnutrition on the development of cognitive functions of the nervous system in childhood. *Trop. geogr. Med.*, **24**, 311.

— (1972). Epidemic ataxia in Western Nigeria. *Brit. med. J.*, **2**, 589.

— (1973). Protein calorie malnutrition and intellect in childhood. A review. *Afr. J. med. Sci.*, **4**, 327.

OSUNTOKUN, B. O. and ODEKU, E. L. (1970). Epilepsy in Ibadan. *Afr. J. Med. Sci.*, **1**, 185.

OSUNTOKUN, B. O., ODEKU, E. L. and ADELOYE, R. B. A. (1969). Non-embolic ischaemic cerebrovascular disease in Nigerians. *J. Neurol. Sci.*, **9**, 361.

OSUNTOKUN, B. O. and OSUNTOKUN, O. (1972). Complicated migrane and haemo-globin AS in Nigerians. *Brit. med. J.*, **2**, 621.

OSUNTOKUN, O., OSUNTOKUN, B. O. and OLURIN, O. (1972). Optic atrophy as a primary presentation in Nigerians. *W. Afr. med. J.*, **21**, 69.

OSUNTOKUN, B. O. and WILLIAMS, A. I. O. (1970). Metal-containing proteins in the Nigerian tropical ataxic neuropathy. *Ghana med. J.*, **9**, 184.

OTSURU, M., *et al.* (1965). Visceral larva migrans of gastro-intestinal tract and its vicinity caused by a larval nematode. *Jap. J. Parasit.* **14**, 542.

OTTO, G. F. (1941). Further observations on the immunity induced in dogs by repeated infections with hookworm, *Ancylostoma caninum. Amer. J. Hyg.*, **33**, 39.

OWOR, R. (1972). Pathology of the liver in chronic pancreatic disease in Ugandan Africans. *Afr. J. med. Sci.*, **3**, 205.

OWUSU, S. K. (1972). Acute haemolysis complicating co-trimoxazole therapy for typhoid fever in a patient with G-6-PD deficiency. *Lancet*, **2**, 819.

— (1972). Absence of glucose-6-phosphate dehydrogenase in red cells of an African. *Brit. med. J.*, **4**, 25.

OWUSU, S. K., *et al.* (1972). Acute reversible renal failure associated with G-6-Pd deficiency. *Lancet*, **1**, 1255.

PACHEO, G., WYKOFF, D. E. and JUNG, R. C. (1960). Trial of an indirect hemagglutination test for the diagnosis of infections with *Clonorchis sinensis. Amer. J. trop. Med. Hyg.*, **9**, 367.

PACHECO-LUNA, R. (1921). Onchocercosis. *Amer. J. Ophthal.*, **4**, 175.

PADMAVATI, S. (1962). Epidemiology of cardiovascular in India. I. Rheumatic heart disease, and II. Ischaemic heart disease. *Circulation*, **25**, 703, 711.

PADMAVATI, S. and PATHAK, S. N. (1959). Chronic cor pulmonale in Delhi: a study of 127 cases. *Circulation*, **20**, 343.

PAGE, E. B., RUCKNAGEL, D. L. and JENSEN, W. N. (1955). Clinical and genetic studies of a new inherited abnormality of haemoglobin characterised by a rapid electrophoretic mobility. *Clin. Res. Proc.*, **3**, 67.

PAHO (1971). Inter-American investigation of mortality in childhood. Provisional Report. P.A.H.O. Washington, D.C. U.S.A.

PAI, K. N. (1967). *Choriocarcinoma*, p. 54. Springer-Verlag, New York.

PAINTER, N. S. and BURKITT, D. P. (1971). Diverticular disease of the colon. *Brit. med. J.*, **2**, 450.

PALMER, C. E. (1953). Tuberculin sensitivity and contact with tuberculosis; further evidence of nonspecific sensitivity. *Amer. Rev. Tuberc.*, **68**, 578.

PALMER, P. E. S. (1962). *Symposium on Kaposi's Sarcoma*. S. Karger, New York, p. 87.

— (1966). Tumoral calcinosis. *Brit. J. Radiol.* (n.s.), **39**, 518.

PALMER, R. L., SERACI, J. E. and THOMAS, B. J. (1962). Histoplasmosis endocarditis. *Arch. int. Med.*, **110**, 359.

PALMER, W. L., KIRSNER, J. B. and RODANICHE, E. C. (1942). Studies on lymphogranuloma venereum infection of the rectum. *J. Amer. med. Ass.*, **118**, 517.

PALTHE, P. M. VAN W. (1950). Tabes dorsalis as a problem of geographical pathology. *Docum. neerl. indones. Morb. trop.*, **2**, 299.

PAN AMERICAN HEALTH ORGANIZATION (1963). II. *Recent arbovirus epidemics in the Americas and information exchange activities*, RES report. 63.1, 25.

DE PAOLA, D. (1962). Pathology of strongyloidiasis. *Bolm Cent. Estud. Hosp. Serv. Estado*, Rio de Janeiro, **14**, 3.

PAPAEVENAGELOU, G. (1974). Biting insects and hepatitis B virus *Trans. roy. Soc. trop. Med. Hyg.*, **68**, 75.

PAPAVASILIOU, C. G. (1965). Tumor simulating intrathoracic extramedullary hemopoiesis: clinical and roentgenologic considerations. *Amer. J. Roentgenol.*, **93**, 695.

PARADINAS, F. J. (1971). Schistosomiasis in a cystic teratoma of the ovary. *J. Path.*, **106**, 123.

PARADINAS, F. J. and WILTSHAW, E. (1972). Neuropsy findings in a case of progressive vaccinia. *J. clin. Path.*, **25**, 233.

PARELKAR, S. N. and STAMM, W. P. (1973). Indirect immunofluorescent staining of trophozoites of *Entamoeba histolytica*. *Trans. roy. Soc. trop. Med. Hyg.*, **67**, 659.

PARENT, M. A. (1973). G-6-PD deficiency in jaundice associated with lobar pneumonia. *Lancet*, **2**, 155.

PARISOT, T. J. and WOOD, E. M. (1960). A comparative study of the causative agent of mycobacterial disease of salmonoid fishes. *Amer. Rev. resp. Dis.*, **82**, 212.

PARK, W. W. (1967). Treatment of choriocarcinoma. (Correspondence.) *Brit. med. J.*, **2**, 52.

PARKER, C. (1970). Cystitis cystica and glandularis. *Proc. roy. Soc. Med.*, **63**, 239.

PARKIN, W. E., *et al.* (1972). Review of current epidemiological literature on viruses of the California arbovirus group. *Amer. J. trop. Med. Hyg.*, **21**, 964.

PARRISH, J. A. (1965). Fiedler's myocarditis. *Brit. Heart J.*, **27**, 458.

PARRY, E. H. O. (1966). Diagnosis and management of heart failure in the young adult African. *Brit. med. J.*, **2**, 1119.

PARRY, E. H. O. and ABRAHAMS, D. G. (1965). The natural history of endomyocardial fibrosis. *Quart. J. Med.*, **36**, 383.

PARTONO, F., *et al.* (1973). Evaluation of thick smear, Knott and membrane filtration methods for demonstrating microfilariae in blood. *Trop. geog. Med.*, **25**, 3, 286.

PATEK, A. J., *et al.* (1969). Sex hormones and susceptibility of the rat to dietary cirrhosis. *Arch. Path.*, **87**, 52.

PATEL, A. K., ZIEGLER, J. L., D'ARBELA, P. G. and SOMERS, K. (1971). Familial cases of endomyocardial fibrosis in Uganda. *Brit. med. J.*, **4**, 331.

PATEL, J. C. and TALWALKAR, M. G. (1968). *Diabetes in the Tropics*, p. iii. Diabetic Assoc. of India, Bombay.

PATEL, Y. C. and BURGER, H. G. A. (1973). Simplified radioimmuno assay for Triiodothyronine. *J. clin. Endocr.*, **36**, 187.

PATERSON, D. E. and JOB, C. K. (1964). Bone changes and absorption in leprosy: a radiological, pathological, and clinical study. In *Leprosy in Theory and Practice*, ed. R. G. Cochrane and T. F. Davey, 2nd ed. p. 425. Wright, Bristol.

PATHAK, U. N. and STEWART, D. B. (1970). Autotransfusion in ruptured ectopic pregnancy. *Lancet*, **1**, 961.

PATRASSI, G. (1965). Primary amyloidosis. *Postgrad. med. J.*, **41**, 247.

PATTANAYAK, S., SINGHA, P. and AROSA, D. D. (1967). *Problems of Communicable Diseases in India*. A review. SEAMES. The First Southeast Asian Regional Seminar on Tropical Medicine. Abstracts of Papers, p. 61.

PAUL, J. R. (1955). Epidemiology of poliomyelitis. *W.H.O. Monogr. Ser.*, No. 26, Geneva, p. 9.

PAUL, J. R., *et al.* (1952). A survey of neutralizing antibodies to poliomyelitis virus in Cairo, Egypt. *Amer. J. Hyg.*, **55**, 402.

PAUL, M. (1963). The riddle of tropical elephantiasis. *Brit. J. Surg.*, **50**, 897.

PAULING, L., ITANO, H. A., SINGER, S. J. and WELLS, I. C. (1949). Sickle cell anemia, a molecular disease. *Science, N.Y.*, **110**, 543.

PAUTRIZEL, R., BAILENGER, J. and CAILLAU, M. (1960). La distomatose. II. Diagnostic serologique. *Rev. Hyg. Méd. soc.* **8**, 618.

PAUTRIZEL, R., BAILENGER, J., DURET, J. and TRIBOULEY, J. (1962). Utilisation d'un antigène distomien délipidé dans le diagnostic allergique de la distomatose à *Fasciola hepatica*. *Revue Immunol. (Paris)*, **26**, 167.

PAVLICA, D. and SAMUEL, I. (1970). Primary carcinoma of the liver in Ethiopia. *Brit. J. Cancer*, **24**, 22.

PAWLOWSKI, Z. and SCHULTZ, M. G. (1972). Taeniasis and cysticercosis (*Taenia saginata*). *Advanc. Parasit.*, **10**, 269.

PAYET, M. and ARMENGAUD, M. (1957). Thrombophlébites cérébrales chez des Africaines recemment accouchés. *Bull. méd. A.O.F.*, **9**, 126.

PAYET, M. and PENE, P. (1955). Les cardiopathies en milieu africain. *Bull. Mém. Éc. prép. Méd. Pharm., Dakar*, **3**, 16.

PAYET, M., PÈNE, P. and SANKALÉ, M. (1966). *Cliniques Africaines*. Gauthier-Villars, Paris.

PAYET, M., *et al.* (1957). 10 fatal cases of amoebic colitis in Africans in Dakar. *Bull. Méd. A.O.F.*, *Dakar*. **2**, 384.

— (1960). La pathologie coranienne chez l'Africain a Dakar. *Bull. Soc. méd. Afr. noire Langue franc.*, **5**, 145.

— (1961). La myocardite primitive du post partum. *Sem. Hôp. Paris.* **37**, 969.

— (1967). Incidence of endomyocardial fibrosis in Africans. *Méd. Afr. noire*, **14**, 53.

PAYMASTER, J. C. (1964). Cancer and its distribution in India. *Cancer, N.Y.*, **17**, 1026.

PAYMASTER, J. C. and GANGADBARAN, P. (1972). Epidemiology of breast cancer in India. *J. nat. Cancer Inst.*, **48**, 1021.

PAYMASTER, J. C., TALWALKAR, G. V. and GANGADHARAN, P. (1971). Carcinomas and malignant melanomas of the skin in Western India. *J. roy. Coll. Surg. Edinb.*, **16**, 166.

PEARSON, J. B. (1963). Carcinoma of the breast in Nigeria. *Brit. J. Cancer*, **17**, 559.

PECK, D. A., LYNN, H. B. and DUSHANE, J. W. (1963). Intussusception in children. *Surg. Gynec. Obstet.*, **116**, 398.

PELLEGRINO, J., POMPEU MEMORIA, J. M. and MACEDO, D. G. (1957). Quantitative aspects of the intradermal test with cercarial antigen in Schistosomiasis. *J. Parasit.*, **43**, No. 3, 304.

PÉNA, C. E. (1967). Deep mycotic infections in Colombia. A clinicopathologic study of 162 cases. *Amer. J. clin. Path.*, **47**, 505.

PENALVER, L. M., RODRIGUEZ, MARIA I., and SANCHO, G. (1956). Human trypanoso-miasis in El Salvador. A preliminary report. I. Epidemiological studies. *Arch. Col. méd. El Salvador.*, **3**, 167.

PENE, P. and SANKALE, M. (1960). La Pellagre. *Méd. Afr. noire*, **7**, 365.

PENMAN, H. C. (1970). Fatal infectious mononucleosis. *J. clin. Path.*, **23**, 765.

PENN, I. (1963). Abdominal aortic aneurysm in the African patient. *Brit. J. Surg.*, **50**, 598.

PENNA, D., *et al.* (1963). Kidney biopsy in human leptospirosis. *Amer. J. trop. Med. Hyg.*, **12**, 896.

PEPLER, W. J. (1955). A study of some of the structural changes of the Bantu aorta. *S. Afr. J. Lab. clin. Med.*, **1**, 203.

PEPLER, W. J. and MEYER, B. J. (1960). A comparative study of South African Bantu and European hearts. *Circulation*, **22**, 14.

PEPLER, W. J. and SIMSON, I. W. (1959). Occlusive disease of the abdominal aorta associated with panarteritis. *A.M.A. Arch. Path.*, **68**, 525.

PEPLER, W. J. and THERON, J. J. (1962). An electron microscopic study of Kaposi's haemangiosarcoma. *J. Path. Bact.*, **83**, 521.

PEREIRA, S. M. and BENJAMIN, V. (1972). Measles in a south Indian community. *Trop. geogr. Med.*, **24**, 124.

PÉREZ-TAMAYO, R. (1958). Diffuse interstitial cirrhosis. *Amer. J. clin. Path.*, **29**, 226.

PERINE, P. L., *et al.* (1971a). Bleeding in louse-borne relapsing fever. I. Clinical studies in 37 patients. *Trans. roy. Soc. trop. Med. Hyg.*, **65**, 776.

— (1971b). Bleeding in louse-borne relapsing fever. II. Fibrinolysis following treatment. *Trans. roy. Soc. trop. Med. Hyg.*, **65**, 782.

— (1972). Benign sickle-cell anaemia. *Lancet*, **2**, 1163.

— (1974). Single-dose Doxycycline Treatment of Louse-borne relapsing fever and epidemic typhus. *Lancet*, **2**, 742.

PERKASH, A., *et al.* (1971). Haemolytic anaemia in Indian childhood cirrhosis. *Arch. Dis. Childh.*, **46**, 46.

PERRINE, R. P. (1967). An obscure myocardiopathy in post partum Saudi Arabs. *Trans. roy. Soc. trop. Med. Hyg.*, **61**, 834.

PERSUAD, T. N. (1967). Foetal abnormalities caused by the active principle of the fruit of *Blighia sapida*. *W. Ind. med. J.*, **16**, 193.

PETCHELAI, B., *et al.* (1973). Autoantibodies in leprosy among Thai patients. *Lancet*, **1**, 1481.

PETERS, D. K. (1974). The Immunological basis of glomerulonephritis. *Proc. roy. Soc. Med.*, **67**, 557.

PETERS, W. (1965). Morphological and physiological variations in chloroquine-resistant *Plasmodium berghei*, Vincke and Lips, 1948. *Ann. Soc. belge Méd.*, **45**, 365.

PETERS, W., FLETCHER, K. A. and STAUBLI, W. (1965). Phagotrophy and pigment formation in a chloroquine-resistant strain of *Plasmodium berghei*, Vincke and Lips. 1948. *Ann. trop. Med. Parasit.*, **59**, 126.

PETERS, W., *et al.* (1973). The chemotherapy of rodent malaria. XVII. Dynamics of drug resistance, part 3. *Ann. trop. Med. Parasit.*, **67**, 143.

PHAM TRONG, TRAN QUY NHU and MARSHALL, J. D., JR. (1967). A mixed pneumonic bubonic plague outbreak in Vietnam. *Milit. Med.*, **132**, 93.

PHILLIPS, C. I. and MACKENZIE, A. D. (1973). Toxocara larval papillitis. *Brit. med. J.*, **1**, 154.

PHILLIPS, I. and WHARTON, B. (1968). Acute bacterial infection in kwashiorkor and marasmus. *Brit. med. J.*, **1**, 407.

PHILLIPS, L. A. (1967). A classification of tetanus. *Lancet*, **1**, 1216.

PHILLIPS, R. S., *et al.* (1970). Immunity to malaria. III. Possible occurrence of a cell-mediated immunity to *Plasmodium knowlesi* in chronically infected and Freund's complete adjuvant-sensitized monkeys. *Exp. Parasit.*, **28**, 2, 339.

PHOON, W. O., *et al.* (1973). Abstracts. 9th International Congress on Tropical Medicine and Malaria, **1**, 168.

PIGGOTT, J., *et al.* (1970). Human ascariasis. *Amer. J. clin. Path.*, **53**, 223.

PIKE, M. C. and MORROW, R. H. (1972). In *Oncogenesis and Herpesviruses*. Ed. P. M. Biggs, G. de The and C. N. Payne. International Agency for Research in Cancer, Lyon, p. 349.

PIMPARKAR, B. D., *et al.* (1970). Gastrointestinal function in ancyclostomiasis. *Trans. roy. Soc. trop. Med. Hyg.*, **64**, 703.

PINDBORG, J. J. (1965). Frequency of oral submucous fibrosis in North India. *Bull. Wld Hlth Org.*, **32**, 748.

PINDBORG, J. J., *et al.* (1968). Prevalence of oral submucous fibrosis among 50,915 Indian villagers. *Brit. J. Cancer*, **22**, 646.

PINKERTON, H., SMILEY, W. L. and ANDERSON, W. A. D. (1945). Giant cell pneumonia with inclusions; lesions common to Hecht's disease, distemper and measles. *Amer. J. Path.*, **21**, 1.

PITNEY, W. R. (1968). The tropical splenomegaly syndrome. *Trans. roy. Soc. trop. Med. Hyg.*, **62**, 717.

PIROSKY, I., *et al.* (1959). *Virosis hemorragica del noroeste Bonaerense*, Instituto Nacional de Microbiologia, Ministerio de Asistencia Social y Salud Publica, Buenos Aires, 216 pp.

PI-SUNYER, F. X., GILLES, H. M. and WILSON, A. M. M. (1965). *Schistosoma haematobium* infection in Nigeria. I. Bacteriological and immunological findings in the presence of schistosomal infection. *Ann. trop. Med. Parasit.*, **59**, 304.

PLANK, S. J. and MILANESI, M. L. (1973). Infant feeding and infant mortality in rural Chile. *Bull. Wld. Hlth. Org.*, **48**, 2 (2997).

PLATT, B. S. (1958). Malnutrition and the pathogenesis of disease. *Trans. roy. Soc. trop. Med. Hyg.*, **52**, 189.

— (1962). Proteins in nutrition. *Proc. roy. Soc., B*, **156**, 337.

— (1966). Protein-calorie deficiency. (Correspondence.) *Lancet*, **2**, 283.

PLATT, B. S., HEARD, C. R. C. and STEWART, R. J. C. (1964). Experimental protein-calorie deficiency. In *Mammalian Protein Metabolism*, ed. H. N. Munro and J. B. Allison, **2**, 445. Academic Press, New York and London.

PLATT, H. S. (1971). Effect of maternal sickle-cell trait on perinatal mortality. *Brit. med. J.*, **4**, 334.

POCOCK, W. A., *et al.* (1965). Left ventricular aneurysms of uncertain aetiology. *Brit. Heart J.*, **27**, 184.

POEN, H. T. and DJOJOPRANATO, M. (1965). The possible etiologic factors of hydatidiform mole and choriocarcinoma: preliminary report. *Amer. J. Obstet. Gynec.*, **92**, 510.

POFFENBARGER, P. L. (1972). Tuberculosis in South Vietnam. *Amer. J. trop. Med. Hyg.*, **21**, 226.

POLDING, J. B. (1956). Some aspects of the epidemiology of *Brucella melitensis* infection. *E. Afr. med. J.*, **33**, 481.

POLIOMYELITIS COMMISSION (1966). Poliomyelitis vaccination in Ibadan, Nigeria, during 1964 with oral vaccine (Sabin strains). *Bull. Wld Hlth Org.*, **34**, 865.

POLISH, S., *et al.* (1962). Idiopathic presinusoidal portal hypertension. *Ann. int. Med.*, **56**, 624.

POLLITZER, R. (1959). Cholera. *W.H.O. Monogr. Ser.* No. 43. Geneva,

POLTERA, A. A. (1972). Pulmonary strongyloidiasis. *Trans. roy. Soc. trop. Med. Hyg.*, **66**, 520.

— (1973). The histopathology of ocular loiasis in Uganda. *Trans. roy. Soc. trop. Med. Hyg.*, **67**, 819.

— (1974). Fatal strongyloidiasis in Uganda. *Ann. trop. Med. Parasit.*, **68**, 81.

POLUNIN, I. (1951). Pineapple dermatosis. *Brit. J. Dermat.*, **63**, 441.

POMERANZ, Y. (1964). Formation of toxic compounds in storage damaged foods and foodstuffs. *Cereal Sci. Today*, **9**, 93.

POOL, R. M. and DUNAVANT, W. D. (1951). Volvulus of the sigmoid colon. *Ann. Surg.*, **133**, 719.

POON-KING, T. (1963). Myocarditis from scorpion stings. *Brit. med. J.*, **1**, 374.

POON-KING, T., HENRY, M. V. and RAMPERSAD, F. (1968). Prevalence and natural history of diabetes in Trinidad. *Lancet*, **1**, 155.

POORTRAKUL, S., WASI, P. and NA-NAKORN, S. (1967). Haemoglobin Bart's hydrops foetalis in Thailand. *Ann. hum. Genet.*, **30**, 293.

PORGES, S. B. (1971). A case of hydatid disease of the thyroid gland. *Med. J. Aust.*, **i**, 641.

PORTERFIELD, J. F. and ZIMMERMAN, L. E. (1962). Rhabdomyosarcoma of the orbit. *Virchows. Arch. path. Anat.*, **335**, 329.

POTDAR, G. G. (1970). Primary reticulum-cell sarcoma of bone in Western India. *Brit. J. Cancer*, **24**, 48.

POTTER, C. W. (1964). Adenovirus infection as anaetiological factor in intussusception of infants and young children. *J. Path. Bact.*, **88**, 263.

POTTER, E. V., *et al.* (1971). Changing types of nephritogenic streptococci in Trinidad. *J. clin. Invest.*, **50**, 1197.

POWELL, L. W. (1967). Idiopathic haemochromatosis. *Brit. med. J.*, **3**, 239.

POWELL, S. J. (1974). Amoebiasis. *Medicine*. A monthly add-on series of practical general medicine: 1972–74. **26**, 1544.

POWELL, S. J., MADDISON, S. E. and ELSDON-DEW, R. (1965). Urinary leucocytes in bilharzia. *S. Afr. med. J.*, **39**, No. 8, 165.

POWELL, S. J. and WILMOT, A. J. (1966). Prognosis in peritonitis complicating severe amoebic dysentery. *Trans. roy. Soc. trop. Med. Hyg.*, **60**, 544.

POWELL, S. J., *et al.* (1965). Amoebic gel-diffusion precipitin-test. Clinical evaluation in amoebic liver-Abscess. *Lancet*, **2**, 602.

— (1966). Cysticercosis and epilepsy in Africans: a clinical and serological study. *Ann. trop. Med. Parasit.*, **60**, 152.

POWER, J. G. P., *et al.* (1969). Lead poisoning in Gurkha soldiers in Hong Kong. *Brit. med. J.*, **3**, 336.

POWER, S. (1946). Funiculitis in British troops in Ceylon. *Lancet*, **1**, 572.

PRANKERD, T. A. J. (1963). The spleen and anaemia. *Brit. med. J.*, **2**, 517.

PRASAD, A. S. and OBERLEAS, D. (1970). Zinc, human nutrition and metabolic effects. *Ann. intern. Med.*, **73**, 631.

PRASASNUK, S. (1974). A case of neuro-otological gnathostomiasis. *Trans. roy. Soc. trop. Med. Hyg.*, **68**, 260.

PRATES, M. D. and TORRES, F. O. (1965). A cancer survey in Lourenço Marques, Portuguese East Africa. *J. nat. Cancer Inst.*, **35**, 729.

PRATHNAP, K., LAU, K. S. and BOLTON, J. M. (1969). Pentastomiasis. *Amer. J. trop. Med. Hyg.*, **18**, 20.

PRATHNAP, K. and GILMAN, R. (1970). The histopathology of acute intestinal amoebiasis: a rectal biopsy study. *Amer. J. Path.*, **60**, 229.

PREECE, M. A., *et al.* (1973). Vitamin-D deficiency among Asian immigrants to Britain. *Lancet*, **1**, 907.

PREHN, R. T. (1972). The role of immunologic mechanisms in carcinogluesis. *U.I.C.C. Bulletin*, p. 3.

PREMATILLEKE, M. N. (1972). Micro-angliopathic haemolytic anaemia associated with a giant haemangioma of the liver. *Postgrad. Med. J.*, **48**, 111.

PRESENT, D. H. and SILTZBACH, L. E. (1967). Sarcoidosis among the Chinese and a review of the world wide epidemiology of sarcoidosis. *Amer. Rev. resp. Dis.*, **43**, 285.

PRETORIUS, P. J. and NOVIS, H. (1965). Nutritional marasmus in Bantu infants in the Pretoria area. Part I: Aetiological factors. *S. Afr. med. J.*, **39**, 237.

— (1965). Nutritional marasmus in Bantu infants in the Pretoria area. Part II: Clinical and pathological aspects. *S. Afr. med. J.*, **39**, 501.

PRIBILLA, W. (1962). Thalassämie-ähnliche Erkrankung mit neuem Minor-Hämoglobin (Hb Köln). In *Haemoglobin Colloquium, Wien*, 31.8.61, ed. H. Lehmann and K. Betke, 73. Thieme, Stuttgart.

PRICE, E. W. (1972). The pathology of non-filarial elephantiasis of the lower legs. *Trans. roy. Soc. trop. Med. Hyg.*, **66**, 150.

— (1974). Endemic elephantiasis of the lower legs—natural history and clinical study. *Trans. roy. Soc. trop. Med. Hyg.*, **68**, 44.

PRICE, E. W. and FITZHERBERT, M. (1965). Cutaneous leishmaniasis in Ethiopia. A clinical study and review of literature. *Ethiopian med. J.*, **3**, 57.

PRIEBE, C. J. and GARBET, R. (1970). Testicular calcification in a 4-year old boy. *Paediatrics*, **46**, 1970.

PRIJYANONDA, B., PRADATSUNDARASAR, A. and VIRANUVATTI, V. (1955). Pulmonary gnathostomiasis. *Ann. trop. Med. Parasit.*, **49**, 121.

PRIMACK, A., VOGEL, C. L. and BARKER, L. F. (1973). Immunological studies in Ugandan patients with hepatocellular carcinoma. *Brit. med. J.*, **1**, 16.

PRINCE, A. M. (1968). An antigen detected in blood during the incubation period of serum hepatitis. *Proc. U.S. Nat. Acad. Sci.*, **60**, 814.

— (1970). Prevalence of serum hepatitis-related antigen (SH) in different geographic regions. *Amer. J. trop. Med. Hyg.*, **19**, 872.

PRINCE, A. M., *et al.* (1970). Immunologic distinction between infectious and serum hepatitis. *New Engl. J. Med.*, **282**, 987.

— (1972). Hepatitis B antigen in wild-caught mosquitoes in Africa. *Lancet*, **2**, 247.

PRINSOLOO, J. G., DEBRUIN, E. J. P. and KRUGER, H. (1971). Comparison of intravenous glucose tolerance tests and serum insulin levels in Kwashiorkor and Pellagra. *Arch. Dis. Childh.*, **46**, 795.

PROCEEDINGS OF THE THIRD CONFERENCE ON THE TOXICITY OF CYCADS (1964). *Fed. Proc.*, **23**, 1333.

PROCTOR, E. M. (1972). Identification of tapeworms. *S. Afr. med. J.*, **46**, 234.

PROSKEY, A. J., *et al.* (1970). Goodpasture's syndrome. *Amer. J. Med.*, **48**, 162.

PRYOR, D. S. (1967a). Tropical splenomegaly in New Guinea. *Quart. J. Med.* (n.s.), **36**, 321.

— (1967b). Splenectomy in tropical splenomegaly. *Brit. med. J.*, **3**, 825.

PRYOR, J. R., BELL, A. J. Y. and PACKHAM, D. A. (1971). Scrotal gangrene after male sterilization. *Brit. med. J.*, **1**, 272.

PSULLEY, J. (1965). Amoebic pericarditis. *Postgrad. med. J.*, **41**, 575.

PULVERTAFT, R. J. V. (1964). Cytology of Burkitt's tumour (African lymphoma). *Lancet*, **1**, 238.

— (1965). A study of malignant tumours in Nigeria by short-term tissue culture. *J. clin. Path.*, **18**, 261.

PUNYAGUPTA, S. (1965). Eosinophilic meningoencephalitis in Thailand: summary of nine cases and observations on *Angiostrongylus cantonensis* as a causative agent and *Pila ampullacea* as a new intermediate host. *Amer. J. trop. Med. Hyg.*, **14**, 370.

PUNYAGUPTA, S. and JUTTIJUDATA, P. (1967). *Hypereosinophilic syndrome with abdominopulmonary involvement, a newly recognised syndrome most likely caused by inapparent infection of gnathostoma.* SEAMES, Third Conference on Parasitic Diseases. Abstracts of Papers, p. 116.

PUNYAGUPTA, S., JUTTIJUDATA, P. and BUNNAG, T. (1967). *Epidemiology of eosinophilic-meningoencephalitis due to Angiostrongylus cantonensis in Thailand.* SEAMES. The Third Conference on Parasitic Diseases. Abstracts of Papers, p. 107.

PUYET, J. H., DOWNS, E. F. and BUDEIR, R. (1963). Nutritional and growth characteristics of Arab refugee children in Lebanon. *Amer. J. clin. Nutr.*, **13**, 147.

QASSAB, K. and AL-KHATEEB, A. K. (1966). Surgical manifestations of ascariasis. *J. Fac. Med. Baghdad* (n.s.), **8**, 62.

QUARCOOPOME, C. O. (1970). Neonatal proptosis. *Ghana med. J.*, **9**, 224.

QUERE, M. A., *et al.* (1963). A statistical study of the frequency and specificity of the ocular complications of onchocerciasis. *Bull. Soc. Méd. Afr. noire Langue franç.*, **8**, 1.

QUISENBERRY, W. B. (1960). Sociocultural factors in cancer in Hawaii. *Ann. N.Y. Acad. Sci.*, **84**, 795.

QUONG, T. L. (1942). The pathology of western equine encephalomyelitis. *Canad. Publ. Hlth J.*, **33**, 300.

DE RAADT, P. (1967). Three serological tests in *T. rhodesiense* infections. *Trans. roy. Soc. trop. Med. Hyg.*, **61**, 137.

RACE, R. R. and SANGER, B. (1962). *Blood Groups in Man*. Blackwell Scientific Publications, Oxford.

RAHMAN, M. A. (1965). Serum protein changes in cholera. *Pak. J. med. Res.*, **4**, 247.

RAHMAN, M. L., *et al.* (1953). Rheumatic fever and rheumatic heart disease in Egypt. *J. Egypt. med. Ass.*, **36**, 611.

RAINE, D. N. (1972). Management of inherited metabolic disease. *Brit. med. J.*, **2**, 329.

RAKOWER, J. and MILWIDSKY, H. (1964). Hydatid pleural disease. *Amer. Rev. resp. Dis.*, **90**, 623.

RAMALINGASWAMI, V. (1964). Perspectives in protein malnutrition. *Nature (Lond.)*, **201**, 546.

RAMALINGASWAMI, V. and PATWARDHAN, V. N. (1949). Diet and health of the South Indian plantation labour. *Indian J. med. Res.*, **37**, 51.

RAMSAY, G. W. ST. C. (1935). Observations on an intradermal test for dracontiasis. *Trans. roy. Soc. trop. Med. Hyg.* **28**, No. 4, 399.

RAMSEY, F. C. (1962). *Trichuris* dysentery syndrome. *W. Indian med. J.*, **11**, 235.

RANNEY, H. M., JACOBS, A. S., BRADLEY, T. B. and CORDOVA, F. A. (1963). A 'new' variant of haemoglobin A_2 and its segration in a family with haemoglobin S. *Nature (Lond.)*, **197**, 164.

RANSOME-KUTI, O., *et al.* (1972). Some socio-economic conditions predisposing to malnutrition in Lagos. *Nig. Med. J.*, **2**, 111.

RAO, S. K. (1974). Malnutrition in the eastern Mediterranean region. *WHO Chron.*, **28**, 172.

RAO, S. N. (1973). Mast cells as a component of the granuloma in Crohn's disease. *J. Path.*, **109**, 79.

RAO, S. S. and MAPLESTONE, P. A. (1940). The adult of *Microfilaria malayi* Brug, 1927. *Indian med. Gaz.*, **75**, 159.

RAO, S. V. (1954). Neurosyphilis—the common types in Hyderabad. *J. Indian med. Ass.*, **24**, 48.

RAO, V. G. and PADMA, M. C. (1971). Some observations on the pathogenicity of *E. histolytica*. *Trans. roy. Soc. trop. Med. Hyg.*, **65**, 606.

RAPER, A. B. (1948). Pigmentation of the tongue. *E. Afr. med. J.*, **25**, 245.

— (1973). Differentiation of iron-deficiency anaemia from thalassaemia trait. *Lancet*, **1**, 778.

RAPER, A. B., AGER, J. A. M. and LEHMANN, H. (1960). Haemoglobin 'Singapore-Bristol': a 'fast' haemoglobin found in infants. *Brit. med. J.*, **1**, 1537.

RAPER, A. B. and DOCKERAY, G. C. (1956). Coenurus cysts in man: five cases from East Africa. *Ann. trop. Med. Parasit.*, **50**, 121.

RAPER, A. B. and LADKIN, R. G. (1950). Endemic dwarfism in Uganda. *E. Afr. med. J.*, **27**, 339.

RATNESAR, V. C., *et al.* (1966). Observations on tropical splenomegaly with hyper-splenic anaemia in Ghana. *Ghana Med.J.*, **5**, 109.

RAY, J. G. and KADULL, P. J. (1965). Agar-gel precipitin-inhibition technique for plague antibody determinations. *Appl. Microbiol.*, **13**, 925.

RAYPORT, M., WISOFF, H. S. and ZAIMAN, H. (1964). Vertebral echinococcosis: report of case of surgical and biological therapy with review of the literature. *J. Neurosurg.*, **21**, 647.

REAY, H. A. J., DIGNAN, A. P. and MAUNDER, C. (1964). Liver abscess caused by adult *Ascaris lumbricoides*. *Brit. med.J.*, **2**, 553.

REBER, E. W. and HOEPPLI, R. (1964). The relationship between macroscopic skin alterations, histological changes and microfilariae in one hundred Liberians with onchocercal dermatitis. *Z. Tropenmed. Parasit.*, **15**, 153.

RECIO, P. M. R. (1965). Amoeboma of the colon. *Dis. Colon. Rect.*, **8**, 205.

REDDY, C. R. R. M., RAO, N. R., ANEES, A. M., REDDY, M. R., MURTHY, D. P. and RAMA-SUBBAIAH, Y. (1970). Non-specific aortitis. *Brit. med.J.*, **1**, 757.

REDDY, C. R. R. M. and SIVARAMAPPA, M. (1968). Guinea-worm arthritis of knee joint. *Brit. med.J.*, **1**, 155.

REDDY, C. R. R. M., SIVAPRASAD, M. D., PARVATHI, G. and CHARI, P. S. (1968). Calcified guinea worm. *Ann. trop. Med. Parasit.*, **62**, 399.

REDDY, C. R. R. M. and VALLI, V. V. (1967). Extradural guinea-worm abscess. Report of two cases. *Amer.J. trop. Med. Hyg.*, **16**, 23.

REDDY, C. R. R. M., *et al.* (1970). Cystic fibrosis of the pancreas in India. *J. trop. Med. Hyg.*, **73**, 59.

REDMOND, A. O. B., *et al.* (1971). The colon in kwashiorkor. *Arch. Dis. Childh.*, **46**, 470.

REED, T. E. (1961). Polymorphism and natural selection in blood groups. *Proc. Conf. Genetic Polymorphism and Geographic variations in Disease*. Greene and Stratton, New York.

REES, J. W. and MEADE, T. W. (1974). Comparison of the modes of spread and the incidence of tuberculosis and leprosy. *Lancet*, **1**, 47.

REES, P. H., *et al.* (1972). Possible role of malaria in the aetiology of the nephrotic syndrome in Nairobi. *Brit. med.J.*, **2**, 130.

REES, R. J. W., WEDDELL, A. G. M., PALMER, E. and PEARSON, J. M. N. (1969). Human leprosy in normal mice. *Brit. med.J.*, **3**, 216.

REID, A. MCK. (1966). Ophthalmology in the tropics: trypanosomiasis (African). In *Manson's Tropical Diseases*, ed. Sir P. H. Manson-Bahr, 16th ed. p. 811. Baillière, Tindall and Cassell, London.

REID, H. A. (1968). Symptomatology, pathology and treatment of landsnake bite in India and South East Asia. In *Venomous Animals and their Venoms*. **1**, 611. Academic Press, U.S.A.

— (1967). Defibrination by *Agkistrodon rhodostoma* venom. *Animal Toxins*, p. 323. First International Symposium on Animal Toxins, 1966.

— (1972). Snakebite. Part I. Clinical Features. Part II. Treatment. *Tropical Doctor*, **2**, 155, 159.

— (1975). Venomous bites and stings. *Tropical Doctor*, **5**, 12.

REID, H. A., GOLDSMITH, H. J. and WRIGHT, F. K. (1967). Peritoneal dialysis in acute renal failure following malaria. *Lancet*, **2**, 436.

REID, H. A. and NKRUMAH, F. K. (1972). Fibrin-degradation products in cerebral malaria. *Lancet*, **1**, 218.

REID, H. A., THEAN, P. C. and MARTIN, W. J. (1963a). Epidemiology of snakebite in North Malaya. *Brit. med.J.*, **1**, 992.

REID, H. A., THEAN, P. C., CHAN, K. E. and BAHAROM, A. R. (1963b). Clinical effects of bites by Malayan viper (*Ancistrodon rhodostoma*). *Lancet*, **1**, 617.

REID, H. A., THEAN, P. C. and MARTIN, W. J. (1963c). Prolonged coagulation defect (defibrination syndrome) in Malayan viper bite. *Lancet*, **1**, 621.

REID, H. A., et al. (1967). Peritoneal dialysis in acute renal failure following malaria. *Lancet*, **2**, 436.

REISS-GUTFREUND, R. J. (1967). The epidemiology of rickettsioses on the Ethiopian high plateau. A six-months' survey from October 1964 to April 1965. *Amer. J. trop. Med. Hyg.*, **16**, 186.

REMINGTON, J. S., JACOBS, L. and KAUFMAN, H. E. (1960). Toxoplasmosis in the adult. *New Engl. J. Med.*, **262**, 180, 237.

RETIEF, F. P. and VANDENPLAS, L. (1970). Platelet function in the Bantu. *Atherosclerosis* **12**, 173.

REYE, R. D. K., MORGAN, G. and BARAL, J. (1963). Encephalopathy and fatty degeneration of the viscera. *Brit. med. J.*, **2**, 749.

REYNOLDS, W. A., WINKELMANN, R. K. and SOULE, E. H. (1965). Kaposi's sarcoma. *Medicine*, **44**, 419.

RHINESMITH, H. S., SCHROEDER, W. A. and MARTIN, N. (1958). The N-terminal sequence of the β chains of normal adult human hemoglobin. *J. Amer. chem. Soc.*, **80**, 3358.

RICHARDS, D. R. (1971). Orthopaedic problems in the tropics. In *Tropical Surgery*, p. 452. McGraw-Hill, London.

RICHMOND, H. G. and GUTHRIE, W. (1964). *Enterobius vermicularis* and the vermiform appendix. *J. Path. Bact.*, **87**, 415.

RICKMAN, L. R. and ROBSON, J. (1970). *Bull. Wld Hlth Org.*, **42**, 4, 650.

RIDER, W. D. and CINADER, B. (1966). Immunotherapy for trophoblastic disease. *Proc. Conf. on Neoplasm (Cancer), Tokyo*, Abstracts, p. 599.

RIDGWAY, A. E. A. (1967). Solar retinopathy. *Brit. med. J.*, **3**, 212.

RIDLEY, D. S. (1956). The complement-fixation test in filariasis. *Trans. roy. Soc. trop. Med. Hyg.*, **50**, 255.

— (1967). The evaluation of drugs for leprosy: bacteriological considerations. *Trans. roy. Soc. trop. Med. Hyg.*, **61**, 596.

RIDLEY, M. J. and RIDLEY, D. S. (1971). Strain techniques and the morphology of *Mycobacterium leprae*. *Leprosy Rev.*, **42**, 88.

RIEDER, R. F. and NAUGHTON, M. A. (1965). Hemoglobin G (Baltimore) a new abnormal hemoglobin, and an additional individual with four hemoglobins. *Bull. Johns Hopk. Hosp.*, **116**, 17.

RIFKIN, H. and THOMPSON, K. J. (1945). Structural changes in early filariasis. *Arch. Path.*, **40**, 220.

RIGAS, D. A., KOLER, R. D. and OSGOOD, E. E. (1955). New hemoglobin possessing a higher electrophoretic mobility than normal adult hemoglobin. *Science, N.Y.*, **121**, 372.

RIJKELS, D. F. (1971). Louse-borne relapsing fever in Ethiopia. *Trop. geogr. Med.*, **23**, 335.

RINGELHANN, B., KONOTEY-AHULU, F. and DODU, S. R. A. (1970). Studies on iron metabolism in sickle-cell anaemia, sickle-cell haemoglobin C disease and haemoglobin C disease using a large volume scintillation counter. *J. clin. Path.*, **23**, 127.

RINGELHANN, B., et al. (1970). A Ghanaian adult, homozygous for hereditary persistence of foetal haemoglobin and heterozygous for elliptocytosis. *Acta haemat.*, **43**, 100.

RIVAS GOMEZ, A. and ALEMAN, C. (1967). Ulcerative colitis in *Strongyloides stercoralis* infections *G.E.N.* (*Caracas*), **21**, 253.

RIVERA, E., *et al.* (1970). Hyperinfection syndrome with *Strongyloides stercoralis*. *Ann. intern. Med.*, **72**, 199.

RIVERA, R. A. (1972). Fatal postpartum amoebic colitis with trophozoites present in peritoneal fluid. *Gastroenterology*, **62**, 314.

RIVEROS, M. and LEBRON, R. F. (1963). Geographical pathology of cancer of the penis. *Cancer*, **16**, 798.

RIVERS, J., *et al.* (1974). Protein requirement. *Lancet*, **2**, 947.

ROBBINS, S. L. (1962). *Pathology*. W. B. Saunders, London.

ROBERTS, W. C., LIEGLER, D. G. and CARBONE, P. P. (1969). Endomyocardial disease and eosinophilia. *Amer. J. Med.*, **46**, 28.

ROBERTS, W. C. and SJOERDSMA, A. (1964). The cardiac disease associated with the carcinoid syndrome. *Amer. J. Med.*, **36**, 5.

ROBERTS, W. C. (1962). The hepatic cirrhosis of cystic fibrosis of the pancreas. *Amer. J. Med.*, **32**, 324.

ROBERTSON, D. H. H. (1963). Human trypanosomiasis in South-East Uganda. A further study of the epidemiology of the disease among fishermen and peasant cultivators. *Bull. Wld Hlth Org.*, **28**, 627.

ROBERTSON, D. H. H. and JENKINS, A. R. (1959). Hepatic dysfunction in human trypanosomiasis. I: Abnormalities of excretory function, seroflocculation phenomena and other tests of hepatic function with observations on the alterations of these tests during treatment and convalescence. *Trans. roy. Soc. trop. Med. Hyg.*, **53**, 511.

ROBERTSON, E. G. (1952). Murray Valley encephalitis: pathological aspects. *Med. J. Aust.*, **1**, 107.

ROBERTSON, J. H. (1960). The significance of intimal thickening in the arteries of the newborn. *Arch. Dis. Childh.*, **35**, 588.

ROBERTSON, J. H. and JACKSON, J. G. (1960). Cardiac aneurysms in Nigeria. *J. Path. Bact.*, **80**, 101.

ROBINSON, A. R., ZUELZER, W. W., NEEL, J. V., LIVINGSTONE, F. B. and MILLER, M. J. (1956). Two 'fast' hemoglobin components in Liberian blood samples. *Blood*, **11**, 902.

ROBINSON, E., SHULMAN, J., BEN-HUR, N., ZUCKERMAN, H. and NEUMAN, Z. (1963). Immunological studies and behaviour of husband and foreign homografts in patients with chorionepithelioma. *Lancet*, **1**, 300.

ROBINSON, G. (1945). A rapid method for detecting the sickle cell trait. *Trans. roy. Soc. trop. Med. Hyg.*, **39**, 264.

ROBINSON, G. L. (1972). The preparation of amoebic extracts and their testing by complement fixation against clinically proved sera. *Trans. roy. Soc. trop. Med. Hyg.*, **66**, 435.

ROBINSON, P. (1942). Relapsing fever in Addis Ababa. *Brit. med. J.*, **2**, 216.

ROBSON, A. (1971). Hydatidiform mole and myperthyroidism. *Brit. med. J.*, **3**, 187.

ROCHE, L., *et al.* (1971). Chronic Salmonellosis and *S. mansoni* infection. *Arch. intern. Med.*, **128**, 254.

ROCHE, M. and LAYRISSE, M. (1966). The nature and causes of 'hookworm anemia' *Amer. J. trop. Med. Hyg.*, **15**, 1032.

ROCHE, M. and PÉREZ-GIMÉNEZ, M. E. (1959). Intestinal loss and reabsorption of iron in hookworm infection. *J. Lab. clin. Med.*, **54**, 49.

ROCHE, P. J. L. (1948). Human dicrocoeliasis in Nigeria. *Trans. roy. Soc. trop. Med. Hyg.*, **41**, No. 6, 819.

RODAN, K. S. and BUCKLEY, J. J. C. (1969). Infection with adult *Toxocara cati*. *Brit. med. J.*, **2**, 188.

RODGER, F. C. (1959). *Blindness in West Africa*. H. K. Lewis, London.

— (1962). A review of recent advances in scientific knowledge of the symptomatology, pathology and pathogenesis of onchocercal infections. *Bull. Wld Hlth Org.*, **27**, 429.

— (1971). Dahlak blindness. *Brit. med. J.*, **4**, 811.

RODGERS, J. B., MALLORY, G. K. and DAVIDSON, C. S. (1964). Massive liver cell necrosis: a retrospective study. *Arch. intern. Med.*, **114**, 637.

ROELSGAARD, E., IVERSEN, E. and BLØCHER, C. (1964). Tuberculosis in tropical Africa. *Bull. Wld Hlth Org.*, **30**, 459.

ROGERS, B. T., KEIR, P. M. and HENDERSON, W. G. (1974). Acute brucellosis with unexpected source. *Brit. med. J.*, **2**, 706.

ROSE, A. W. (1935). Fractional gastric analyses in natives of Nigeria. *W. Afr. med. J.*, **8**, 10.

ROSE, E. F. (1965). Interim report on the survey of cancer of the oesophagus in the Transkei. *S. Afr. med. J.*, **39**, 1098.

ROSE, G., *et al.* (1966). The application of a haemagglutination reaction to the diagnosis of onchocerciasis. *Rev. Hyg. Méd. soc.* **14**, 383.

ROSEMBERG, J., *et al.* (1960). Immunobiologic relation between tuberculosis and leprosy. X. Comparative study of the results of the lepromin test in subjects submitted to serial injections of Mitsuda's antigen and to oral BCG vaccination. *Int. J. Leprosy*, **28**, 271.

ROSEN, E. U. (1971). The controversial role of magnesium in protein–calorie malnutrition. *Amer. Heart J.*, **82**, 1.

ROSEN, L., *et al.* (1962). Eosinophilic meningoencephalitis caused by a metastrongylid lung-worm of rats. *J. Amer. med. Ass.*, **179**, 620.

ROSENBAUM, J. M. and JOHNSTON, C. (1966). Hemobilia with multiple liver abscesses and ascariasis. *Amer. J. Dis. Child.*, **112**, 82.

ROSENBAUM, M. B. (1964). Chagasic myocardiopathy. *Progr. cardiovasc. Dis.*, **7**, 199.

ROSENBERG, E. B., *et al.* (1973). IgM antibodies to red cells and autoimmune anemia in patients with malaria. *Amer. J. trop. Med. Hyg.*, **22**, 2, 146.

ROSENBLATT, G. and STOKES, J. (1963). The epidemiology of rheumatic fever and rheumatic heart disease in temperate versus tropical zones. *Amer. Heart J.*, **65**, 720.

ROSENHEIM, M. L. (1967). Chronic pyelonephritis. *Israeli J. Med. Sci.*, **3**, 93.

ROSENWALD, C. D. (1963). *Annual Report M.O.H.*, Municipal Council of Mombasa 1962.

ROSS, A., *et al.* (1970). Occurrence of an abnormal lipoprotein in patients with liver disease. *Gut*, **11**, 1035.

ROSS, E. J. (1972). Endocrine and metabolic manifestations of cancer. *Brit. med. J.*, **1**, 735.

ROSS, G. W. and KNIGHT, R. (1973). Dietary factors affecting the pathogenicity of *Entamoeba histolytica* in rats. *Trans. roy. Soc. trop. Med. Hyg.*, **67**, 560.

ROSS, H. (1964). Clinical biochemistry and immunology in leprosy—A review. *Leprosy in India*, **36**, 93, 193.

ROSS, O. A. and BUEDING, E. (1950). Survival of *Schistosoma mansoni in vitro*. *Proc. Soc. exp. Biol.*, **73**, No. 2, 179.

ROSS, R. W. (1956). The Newala epidemic. III. The virus: isolation, pathogenic properties and relationship to the epidemic. *J. Hyg.*, **54**, 177.

— (1957). The 'N' factor in resistance to leprosy and its relationship to the lepromin and tuberculin reactions. The doubtful value of BCG in immunization against leprosy. *Rev. bras. leprol.*, S. Paulo. **25,** 85.

ROTTER, R., LUTTGENS, W. F., PETERSON, W. L., STOCK, A. E. and MOTULSKY, A. G. (1956). Splenic infarction in sicklemia during airplane flight: pathogenesis, hemoglobin analysis and clinical features of six cases. *Ann. intern. Med.*, **44,** 257.

ROWLAND, H. A. K. (1963). Neuropathy in Sierra Leone. *J. trop. Med. Hyg.*, **60,** 181.

— (1966). Dyspepsia. duodenitis and hookworm infection. *Trans. roy. trop. Med. Hyg.*, **60,** 481.

ROWLANDS, D. T. and VILTER, C. F. (1960). A study of the cardiac stigmata in prolonged human thiamine deficiency. *Circulation*, **21,** 4.

ROY, S. B., BHATIA, M. L., LAZARO, E. J. and RAMALINGASWAMI, V. (1963). Juvenile mitral stenosis in India. *Lancet*, **2,** 1193.

ROY, S., *et al.* (1970). Comparative evaluation of tests in the diagnosis of pulmonary hydatid cysts. *Trans. roy. Soc. trop. Med. Hyg.*, **64,** 711.

RUCKNAGEL, D. L., PAGE, E. B. and JENSEN, W. N. (1955). Clinical and genetic studies of a new inherited abnormality of hemoglobin characterised by a rapid electrophoretic mobility. *Clin. Res. Proc.*, **3,** 67.

RUCKNAGEL, D. L. (1966). Epidemiologic and Genetic features of leukaemia in the United States. *N.Z. med. J. (Supplement)*, **65,** 869.

RUCKNAGEL, D. L. and LAROS, R. K. (1969). Haemoglobinopathies. Genetics and implications for studies of human reproduction. *Clin. Obstet. Gynaec.*, **12,** 49.

RUDNICK, A., *et al.* (1965). Mosquito-borne haemorrhagic fever in Malaya. *Brit. med. J.*, **1,** 1269.

RUDZINSKA, M. A. and TRAGER, R. W. (1957). Intracellular phagotrophy by malaria parasites: an electron microscope study of *Plasmodium lephurae*. *J. Protozool.*, **4,** 190.

RUOSLAHTI, E., *et al.* (1972). Radio immunoassay of alpha-fetoprotein in primary and secondary cancer of the liver. *J. nat. Cancer Inst.*, **49,** 623.

RUSSELL, A. S. and SCHLAUT, J. W. (1974). HL-A antigens in inflammatory bowel disease. *Lancet*, **1,** 451.

RUSSELL, P. K., AZIZ, M. A., AHMAD, N., KENT, T. H. and GANGAROSA, E. J. (1966). Enteritis and gastritis in young asymptomatic Pakistani men. *Amer. J. dig. Dis.*, **11,** 296.

RUSSELL, P. K., SHUMDERMPADETSUK, S. and PIYARATN, P. (1967). A fatal case of dengue haemorrhagic fever in an American child. *Pediatrics*, **40,** 804.

RUSSELL, P. F., *et al.* (1967). *Practical Malariology*. 2nd edition. Oxford University Press, London.

SABIN, A. B. (1962). Oral poliovirus vaccine, recent results, and recommendations for optimum use. *Roy. Soc. Hlth J.*, **2,** 51.

SABIN, A. B. and FELDMAN, H. A. (1948). Dyes as microchemical indicators of a new immunity phenomenon affecting a protozoon parasite (*Toxoplasma*). *Science, N.Y.*, **108,** 660.

SABIN, T. D. (1970). Preservation of sensation in a cutaneous vascular malformation in lepromatous leprosy. *New Engl. J. Med.*, **282,** 1084.

SACKS, M. I. (1959). Aortic coronary atherosclerosis in the three racial groups in Cape Town. *S. Afr. med. J.*, **33,** 827.

SADRE, M., BASTANFAR, M. and ZIAI, M. (1973). Urinary calculi in Iran. *Trans. roy. Soc. trop. Med. Hyg.*, **67,** 374.

SADUN, E. H. (1955). Studies on *Opisthorchis viverrini* in Thailand. *Amer. J. Hyg.*, **62**, No. 2, 81.

— (1972). The research and development of serologic tests for malaria. *Amer. J. trop. Med. Hyg.*, **21**, 5, (II), 677.

SADUN, E. H., ANDERSON, R. I. and WILLIAMS, J. S. (1961). Fluorescent antibody test for the laboratory diagnosis of schistosomiasis in humans by using dried blood smears on filter paper. *Exp. Parasit.*, **11**, Nos. 2/3, 117.

— (1962). Fluorescent antibody test for the serological diagnosis of trichinosis. *Exp. Parasit.*, **12**, 423.

SADUN, E. H., ANDERSON, R. I. and SCHOENBECHLER, M. J. (1963). A plasma card test for rapid serodiagnosis of schistosomiasis (SPC). *Proc. Soc. exp. Biol.*, **112**, No. 2, 280.

SADUN, E. H., BUCK, A. A., LEED, B. K., MOON, C. H. and BURKE, J. C. (1959). Epidemiologic studies for paragonimiasis and clonorchiasis by the use of intradermal tests. *Amer. J. Hyg.*, **69**, No. 1, 68.

SADUN, E. H. and MAIPHOOM, C. (1953). Studies on the epidemiology of the human intestinal fluke, *Fasciolopsis buski* (Lankester) in Central Thailand. *Amer. J. trop. Med. Hyg.*, **2**, No. 6, 1070.

SADUN, E. H., NORMAN, L. and ALLAIN, D. (1957). The detection of antibodies to infections with the nematode, *Toxocara canis*, a causative agent of visceral larva migrans. *Amer. J. trop. Med. Hyg.*, **6**, 562.

SADUN, E. H., *et al.* (1963). Fluorescent antibody test for the serodiagnosis of African and American trypanosomiasis in man. *J. Parasit.*, **49**, 385.

— (1966). Active and Passive Immunization of chimpanzees infected with West African and Southeast Asian strains of *P. falciparum*. *Research in Malaria, Suppl. to Milit. Med.*, **131**, 1250.

SAFOUH, M. and SHEHATA, A. H. (1965). Hepatic vein occlusion disease of Egyptian children. *J. Pediat.*, **67**, 415.

SAGOE, A. S. (1971). The tropical splenomegaly syndrome in Ibadan. Ph.D. Thesis, University of Ibadan.

SAGOE, A. S. (1970). Tropical splenomegaly syndrome. *Brit. med. J.*, **3**, 378.

SAHA, N. and BANERJEE, B. (1970). A comparative study of serum protein electrophoretic patterns in Indians and Europeans. *Trop. geogr. Med.*, **22**, 53.

SAID, M. E., *et al.* (1969). Visual acuity and field of vision of urban and rural Egyptians. *Publ. Hlth Rep.*, **84**, 955.

SAKAKIBARA, S., *et al.* (1970). Idiopathic post-partum cardiomyopathy. *Amer. Heart J.*, **80**, 385.

SALAH, M. (1938). Mechanisms of oedema in helminthic anaemias. *Trans. roy. Soc. trop. Med. Hyg.*, **31**, 431.

SALAKO, L. A. (1967). Liver function tests in the diagnosis of hepatic amoebiasis. *J. trop. Med. Hyg.*, **70**, 19.

SALAMON, T. (1958). Enlarged parotids and pellagra. *J. trop. Med. Hyg.* **61**, 253.

SALEM, S. N. (1966). Neurological complications of heat-stroke in Kuwait. *Ann. trop. Med. Parasit.*, **60**, 393.

SALEM, S. N. and TRUELOVE, S. C. (1964). Hookworm disease in immigrants. *Brit. med. J.*, **1**, 1074.

SAMS, W. M. and BECK, J. W. (1959). Subcutaneous filarial infections. A report of two additional cases from Florida. *Arch. Derm.*, **79**, No. 3, 294.

SANDERS, V. (1963). Idiopathic disease of myocardium: a prospective study. *Arch. intern. Med.*, **112**, 661.

SANGER, R., RACE, R. R. and JACK, J. (1955). The Duffy blood groups of New York negroes: the phenotype Fy (a-b-). *Brit. J. Haemat.*, **1**, 370.

SANKALE, M. COSTEVEC, A. and RIVOALEN, A. (1958). Contribution à l'étude de la pathologie hypophysaire chez le Noir African. *Bull. méd. A.O.F.*, **3**, 96.

SANSONE, G., PIGA, A. M. and SEGNI, G. (1958). *Il Favismo*, Edizioni Minerva Medica, S.A. Torino.

DI SANT'AGNESE, P. A. and BLANC, W. A. (1956). A distinctive type of biliary cirrhosis of the liver associated with cystic fibrosis of the pancreas; recognition through signs of portal hypertension. *Pediatrics*, **18**, 387.

SANYAL, A. B. and SEN GUPTA, P. C. (1967). Fine structure of *Leishmania* in dermal leishmanoid. *Trans. roy. Soc. trop. Med. Hyg.*, **61**, 211.

SARGEANT, K., SHERIDAN, A., O'KELLY, J. and CARNAGHAN, R. B. A. (1961). Toxicity associated with certain samples of groundnuts. *Nature (Lond.)*, **192**, 1096.

SARVOTHAM, S. G. and BERRY, J. N. (1968). Prevalence of coronary heart disease in an unknown population in N. India. *Circulation*, **37**, 939.

SASEA, B. A. and AMIN, S. P. (1962). *Entamoeba histolytica* in the urine. *Brit. med. J.*, **1**, 157.

SATI, M. H. (1962). Leishmanial enteritis as a cause of intractable diarrhoea and death. *Sudan med. J.* (n.s.), **1**, 216.

SATOKAR, R. S. and LEWIS, R. A. (1954). Plasma protein pattern of Indian students: relation to diet and previous illness. *Indian J. med. Sci.*, **8**, 663.

SAUGRAIN, J. and OUTIN-FABRE, D. (1972). Bilan de vingt années de lutte contre la filariose subpériodique de Bancroft en Polynésia française. *WHO Bulletin*, **46**, 249.

SAUNDERS, S. J. and THATCHER, G. N. (1963). Toxoplasmosis in the adult. *S. Afr. med. J.*, **37**, 1026.

SCHACHER, J. F., SAAB, S., GERMANOS, R. and BOUSTANY, N. (1969). The aetiology of Halzoun in Lebanon. *Trans. roy. Soc. trop. Med. Hyg.*, **63**, 854.

SCHAD, G. A., *et al.* (1973). Arrested development in human hookworm infections: an adaptation to a seasonally unfavourable external environment. *Science*, **180**, 502.

SCHAFFNER, F., *et al.* (1967). Budd chiari syndrome caused by a web in the inferior vena cava. *Amer. J. Med.*, **42**, 838.

SCHENK, E. A., SAMLOFF, I. M. and KLIPSTEIN, F. A. (1965). Morphologic characteristics of jejunal biopsy in celiac disease and tropical sprue. *Amer. J. Path.*, **47**, 765.

SCHERER, W. F., *et al.* (1959). Ecologic studies of Japanese encephalitis virus in Japan, I to IX. *Amer. J. trop. Med. Hyg.*, **8**, 644.

— (1972). Ecologic studies of Venezuelan encephalitis virus in southeastern Mexico. VII. Infection of man. *Amer. J. trop. Med. Hyg.*, **21**, 79.

SCHLESINGER, M. J. and REINER, L. (1955). Focal myocytolysis of the heart. *Amer. J. Path.*, **31**, 443.

SCHMIDT, J. R., *et al.* (1959). Epidemic jungle fever among Okinawan colonists in the Bolivian rain forest. II. Isolation and characterization of Uruma virus, a newly recognized human pathogen. *Amer. J. trop. Med. Hyg.*, **8**, 479.

SCHMIDT, J. *et al.* (1973). Parasitological and epidemiological studies on a small outbreak of histoplasmosis occurring in a rural area of Brasilia, Brazil. *Rev. da Soc. Bras. de Med. Trop.*, **7**, 2, 107.

SCHNEIDER, R. G., ARAT, F. and HAGGARD, M. E. (1964). An inhomogeneous foetal haemoglobin variant (the Texas type). *Nature (Lond.)*, **202**, 1346.

SCHNEIDER, R. G. and HAGGARD, M. E. (1958). Haemoglobin *P* (the 'Galveston' type). *Nature (Lond.)*, **182**, 322.

SCHOENBERG, B. S., BAILAR, J. C. and FRAUMENI, J. F. (1971). Certain mortality patterns of oesophageal cancer in the United States 1930–67. *J. nat. Cancer Inst.*, **46**, 63.

SCHOENTAL, R. (1963). Liver disease and 'natural' hepatotoxins. *Bull. Wld Hlth Org.*, **29**, 823.

SCHOENTAL, R. and MAGEE, P. N. (1959). Further observations on the subacute and chronic liver changes in rats after a single dose of various pyrrolizidine (*Senecio*) alkaloids. *J. Path. Bact.*, **78**, 471.

SCHOFIELD, F. (1964). Changes in haemoglobin values and hepatosplenomegaly produced by control of holoendemic malaria. *Brit. med. J.*, **1**, 587.

SCHOFIELD, F. D., TUCKER, V. M. and WESTBROOK, G. R. (1961). Neonatal tetanus in New Guinea: effect of active immunization in pregnancy. *Brit. med. J.*, **2**, 785.

SCHOFIELD, T. P. C., *et al.* (1968). Leucopenia and fever in the 'Jarisch-Herxheimer' reaction of louse-borne relapsing fever. *Lancet*, **1**, 58.

SCHRIRE, V. (1964). The racial incidence of the less common forms of heart disease at Groote Schuur Hospital, Cape Town 1952–61. *S. Afr. med. J.*, **38**, 598.

SCHRIRE, V. and ASHERSON, R. A. (1964). Arteritis of the aorta and its major branches. *Quart. J. Med.* (n.s.), **33**, 439.

SCHULMAN, S. T. and BEEM, M. O. (1971). A unique presentation of sickle cell disease. *Paediatrics*, **47**, 1019.

SCHUMAN, L. M., CHOI, N. W. and GULLEN, W. H. (1967). Relationship of central nervous system neoplasms to toxo plasma gondii infection. *Amer. J. Pub. Hlth*, **57**, 848.

SCHWARTZ, J. (1952). Atrophia idiopathic (tropica) mucosae oris. (Demonstrated at the 11th International Dental Congress, London, and quoted by Sirsat and Khanolkar, 1962.)

— (1971). African histoplasmosis. (Part 2). In *Human Infection with Fungi, Actinomycetes and algae*, p. 139. Springer Verlag, New York.

SCOTT-EMUAKPOR, M. P. (1970). The problem of post-operative wound sepsis in a city hospital. *J. trop. Med. Hyg.*, **73**, 39.

SCOTTI, T. M. (1955). Basophilic (mucinous) degeneration of the myocardium. *Amer. J. clin. Path.*, **25**, 994.

SCRIMSHAW, N. S. (1964). Ecological factors in nutritional disease. *Amer. J. clin. Nutr.*, **14**, 112.

— (1964). The geographic pathology of thyroid disease. In *The Thyroid*. p. 100. Williams and Wilkins, Baltimore.

SEABURY, J. H. and SAMUELS, M. (1963). The pathogenetic spectrum of aspergillosis. *Amer. J. clin. Path.*, **40**, 21.

SEDACCA, C. M., PERRIN, E., MARTIN, L. and SCHIFF, L. (1961). Polycystic liver: an unusual cause of bleeding esophageal varices. *Gastroenterology*, **40**, 128.

SEFTEL, H. C. (1963). Some medical impressions of India with particular reference to diabetes mellitus and cardiovascular disease. *S. Afr. med. J.*, **38**, 278.

SEFTEL, H. C., ISAACSON, C. and BOTHWELL, T. H. (1960). The relationship between siderosis and diabetes in the Bantu. *S. Afr. J. med. Sci.*, **25**, 89.

SEFTEL, H. C., KEELEY, K. J. and WALKER, A. R. P. (1963). Studies in glycosuria and diabetes in non-white populations of the Transvaal. *S. Afr. med. J.*, **37**, 1213.

SEFTEL, H. C., MALKIN, C., SCHMAMAN, A., ABRAHAMS, C., LYNCH, S. R., CHARLTON, R. W. and BOTHWELL, T. H. (1966). Osteoporosis, scurvy, and siderosis in Johannesburg Bantu. *Brit. med. J.*, **1**, 642.

SEGI, M. (1955). Geographical and racial distribution of cancer of the breast. *Schweiz. Z. allg. Path.*, **18**, 688.

SEITANIDIS, B., *et al.* (1973). Complement levels in beta-thalassaemia major. *Lancet*, **1**, 778.

TEN SELDAM, R. E. J. (1970). Pseudo-malignant cutaneous amoebiasis. *Trop. geogr. Med.*, **22**, 142.

TEN SELDAM, E. J., *et al.* (1966). Childhood lymphoma in the territories of Papua and New Guinea. *Cancer, N.Y.*, **19**, 437.

SELF, J. T., HOPPS, H. C. and WILLIAMS, A. O. (1972). Porocephaliasis in man and experimental mice. *Exper. Parasit.*, **32**, 117.

SELLERS, F. J., KEITH, J. D. and MANNING. J. A. (1964). The diagnosis of primary endocardial fibroelastosis. *Circulation*, **29**, 49.

SELYE, E. (1958). Experimental production of endomyocardial fibrosis. *Lancet*, **1**, 1351.

SELZER, G. and PARKER, R. G. F. (1951). Senecio poisoning exhibiting as Chiari's syndrome: a report on twelve cases. *Amer. J. Path.*, **27**, 885.

SEMPLE, A. B., *et al.* (1954). An outbreak of trichinosis in Liverpool in 1953. *Brit. med. J.* **1**, 1002.

SEN, P. K., KINARE, S. G., KULKARNI, T. P. and PARULKAR, G. B. (1962). Stenosing aortitis of unknown etiology. *Surgery*, **51**, 317.

SENECAL, J., AUBRY, L and FALADE, S (1962). Infectious diseases in the child of pre-school age in Senegal. *W. Afr. Med. J.*, **11**, 93.

SENEWIRATNE, B., *et al.* (1974). Endemic fluorosis in Ceylon. *Trans. roy. Soc. trop. Med. Hyg.*, **68**, 105.

SEN GUPTA, P. C. (1965). Host-parasite relationship in *Leishmania donovani* infection in man. *Parassitologia*, **7**, 1.

SEN GUPTA, P. C. and ADHIKARI, S. L. (1952). Observations on the complement fixation test for kala azar. *J. Indian med. Ass.*, **22**, 89.

SEN GUPTA, P. C. and BHATTACHARJEE, B. (1953). Histopathology of post-kala-azar dermal leishmaniasis. *J. trop. Med. Hyg.*, **56**, 110.

SENNARA, H. (1969). Bilharzial Paraplegia. *J. Bone Jt Surg.*, **51**, 132.

SEPPALA, M. and RUOSLAHTI, E. (1972). Alpha-fetoprotein in abortion. *Brit. med. J.*, **4**, 769.

SERAFINO, X. and CONTE, S. (1960). Sur les techniques 'd'abord direct' dans le mal de Pott. *Bull. Méd. Fac. nat. Med. Dakar.*, **8**, 18.

SERIE, C. (1963). Memorandum on yellow fever in Ethiopia, 1961–1962. *Ethiopian med. J.*, **4**, 206.

SERJEANT, G. R., RICHARDS, R., BARBOR, P. R. H. and MILNER, P. F. (1968). Relatively benign sickle-cell anaemia in 60 patients aged over 30 in the West Indies. *Brit. med. J.*, **3**, 86.

SERPEAU, D., MANNONI, P., DHUMEAUX, D. and BERTHELOT, P. (1971). Hepatitis-associated antigen in human bile. *Lancet*, **2**, 1266.

SEXTON, R. C., EYLES, D. E. and DILLMAN, R. E. (1953). Adult toxoplasmosis. *Amer. J. Med.*, **14**, 366.

SEZI, C. L., *et al.* (1972). A small outbreak of louse typhus in Masaka District, Uganda. *Trans. roy. Soc. trop. Med. Hyg.*, **66**, 783.

SHAFFER, C. F. (1970). Ascorbic acid and atherosclerosis. *Amer. J. clin. Nutrit.*, **23**, 27.

SHAKER, Y. (1966). Thirst fever, with a characteristic temperature pattern in infants in Kuwait. *Brit. med. J.*, **1**, 586.

SHAKIR, A. (1973). Quack stick in the assessment of protein–calorie malnutrition in Baghdad. *Lancet*, **1**, 762.

SHANMUGARATNAM, K. (1961). Liver cancer and cirrhosis in Singapore. *Acta Un. int. Cancr.*, **17**, 888.

SHANMUGARATNAM, K. (1966). *Nasopharyngeal carcinoma.* U.I.C.C. Activities Report.

SHANMUGARATNAM, K. and TYE, C. Y. (1970). Liver cancer differentials in immigrant and local-born Chinese in Singapore. *J. chron. Dis.*, **23**, 443.

SHAPER, A. G. (1960). Chronic pancreatic disease and protein malnutrition. *Lancet*, **1**, 1223.

— (1964). Aetiology of chronic pancreatic fibrosis with calcification seen in Uganda. *Brit. med. J.*, **1**, 1607.

— (1967). On the nature of some tropical cardiomyopathies. *Trans. roy. Soc. trop. Med. Hyg.*, **61**, 458.

— (1972). Seminar on cardiomyopathies. *Postgrad. med. J.*, **48**, 701.

— (1972). Cardiovascular disease in the tropics—IV. Coronary heart disease. *Brit. med. J.*, **4**, 32.

SHAPER, A. G. and LEWIS, P. (1971). Genetic neutropenia in people of African origin. *Lancet*, **2**, 1021.

SHAPER, A. G., *et al.* (1967). Immunological studies in endomyocardial fibrosis and other forms of heart-disease in the tropics. *Lancet*, **1**, 598.

— (1968). Malarial antibodies and autoantibodies to heart and other tissues in the immigrant and indigenous peoples of Uganda. *Lancet*, **1**, 1342.

SHAPIRO, J. L. (1971). The alimentary tract. In *Concepts of Disease*, p. 282. The MacMillan Co., New York.

SHAW, A. F. B. and GHAREEB, A. A. (1938). The pathogenesis of pulmonary schistosomiasis in Egypt with special reference to Ayerza's disease. *J. Path. Bact.*, **46**, 401.

SHEAGREN, I. N., TOBIE, J. E., FOX, L. M. and WOLFF, S. M. (1970). Reticuloendothelial system phagocytic function in naturally acquired human malaria. *J. Lab. clin. Med.*, **75**, 481.

SHEE, J. C. (1963). Myocardial infarction in Southern Rhodesia. *Brit. Heart J.*, **25**, 25

SHEEHAN, H L. (1940). Acute fatty metamorphosis of the liver in pregnancy. *J. Obstet. Gynaec. Brit. Emp.*, **47**, 49.

SHEEHAN, H. L. and MOORE, H. C. (1952). *Renal Cortical Necrosis and the Kidney of Concealed Accidental Haemorrhage.* Blackwell, Oxford.

SHEEHY, T. W., COHEN, W. H. and BRODSKY, J. P. (1963). The intestinal lesion in the initial phase of tropical (military) sprue. *Amer. J. dig. Dis.*, **8**, 826.

SHEEHY, T. W., COHEN, W. C., WALLACE, D. K. and LEGTERS, L. J. (1965). Tropical sprue in North Americans. *J. Amer. med. Ass.*, **194**, 1069.

SHEEHY, T. W., *et al.* (1962). *Gastroenterology*, **42**, 148.

SHEEHY, T. W., PARMLEY, L. F., JOHNSTON, G. S. and BOYCE, H. W. (1968). Resolution time of an amebic liver abscess. *Gastroenterology*, **55**, 26.

SHEIR, Z. M. and ABOUL-ENEIN, E. EL-S. (1970). Demographic, clinical and therapeutic appraisal of heterophyiasis. *J. trop. Med. Hyg.* **73**, 148.

SHEPARD, C. C. (1960). The experimental disease that follows the injection of human leprosy bacilli into foot-pads of mice. *J. exp. Med.*, **112**, 445.

SHEPHERD, J. J. (1967). Quoted by Ahsan and Rahman (1967).

SHERLOCK, S. (1963). *Diseases of the Liver and Biliary System.* 34d ed. Blackwell, Oxford.

— (1968). Chronic cholangitides. *Brit. med. J.*, **3**, 515.

— (1968). Drugs and the liver. *Brit. med. J.*, **1**, 227.

SHERMAN, F. E. and RUCKLE, G. (1958). *In vivo* and *in vitro* cellular changes specific for measles. *Arch. Path.*, **65**, 587.

SHERMAN, I. L. and EICHENWALD, H. F. (1956). Viral hepatitis: descriptive epidemiology based on morbidity and mortality statistics. *Ann. intern. Med.*, **44**, 1049.

SHERMAN, I. W., MUDD, J. B. and TRAGER, W. (1965). Chloroquine resistance and the nature of malarial pigment. *Nature (Lond.)*, **208**, 691.

SHIBATA, S., IUCHI, I., MIYAJI, T., UEDA, S. and TAKEDA, I. (1963). Hemolytic disease associated with the production of abnormal hemoglobin and intraerythrocytic Heinz bodies. *Acta haemat. jap.*, **26**, 164.

SHIBOLET, S., *et al.* (1962). Fibrinolysis and haemorrhages in fatal heatstroke. *New Engl. J. Med*, **25**, 169.

— (1967). Heatstroke: its clinical picture and mechanism in 36 cases. *Quart. J. Med.* (n.s.), **36**, 525.

SHILKIN, K. B., CHEN, B. T. M. and KHOO, O. T. (1972). Rhabdomyolysis caused by hornet venom. *Brit. med. J.*, **1**, 156.

SHILLITO, J. (1964). Carotid arteritis: a cause of hemiplegia in childhood. *J. Neurosurg.*, **21**, 540.

SHIMAZONO, N. and KATSURA, E., eds. (1965). *Review of Japanese literature on beriberi and thiamine*. Vitamin B Res. Comm. of Japan, Kyoto Univ.

SHINNER, J. J. (1963). St. Louis virus encephalomyelitis *Arch. Path.*, **75**, 309.

SHIRAKI, H. (1971). Neuropathology of subacute myelo-optic-neuropathy 'SMON'. *Jap. J. med. Sci. Biol.*, **24**, 217.

SHISHIDO, A. (1964). Strain variation of *Rickettsia orientalis* in the complement fixation test. *Jap. J. med. Sci. Biol.*, **17**, 59.

SHORTT, H. E. and GARNHAM, P. C. C. (1948). The pre-erythrocytic development of *Plasmodium cynomolgi* and *Plasmodium vivax*. *Trans. r. Soc. trop. Med. Hyg.*, **41**, 785.

SHOUSHA, S. and KAMEL, K. (1972). Nitro blue tetrazolium test in children with kwashiorkor with a comment on the use of latex particles in the test. *J. clin. Path.*, **25**, 494.

SHRANK, A. B. (1966). Phrynoderma. *Brit. med. J.*, **1**, 29.

SHWE, T. (1972). Renal involvement in leprosy. *Trans. roy. Soc. trop. Med. Hyg.*, **66**, 26.

SHWE, T. and ZUCKERMAN, V. J. (1972). Australian antigen and antibody in British patients with leprosy. *J. clin. Path.*, **25**, 401.

SIDERYS, H. and VELLIOS, F. (1964). Portal hypertension without cirrhosis or extrahepatic obstruction: report of a case. *Amer. J. Surg.*, **108**, 785.

SIEGERT, R. (1970). The margburg virus (ververt monkey agent). In *Modern Trends in Medical Virology*, p. 204. Butterworths, London.

SIFFERT, G. (1972). Le diagnostic coprologique de la Strongyloidose. *Acta gastro-ent. belg.*, **35**, 499.

SIGURJONSSON, J. (1950). Structure and iodine content of thyrotoxic goitre in Iceland. *Amer. J. Path.*, **26**, 1103.

SILK, M. H., SPENCE, I. M. and GEAR, J. H. S. (1969). Ultrastructural studies of the blood fluke—*Schistosoma mansoni*. The integument. II. The musculature. *S. Afr. J. Med. Sci.* **34**, 1, 11.

SILVERMAN, P. H. (1955). A technique for studying the *in vitro* effect of serum on activated taeniid hexacanth embryos. (Correspondence.) *Nature (Lond.)*, **176**, 589.

SILVERMAN, P. H. and GRIFFITHS, R. B. (1955). A review of methods of sewage disposal in Great Britain, with special reference to the epizootiology of *Cysticercus bovis*. *Ann. trop. Med. Parasit.*, **49**, 436.

SILVESTRONI, E. and BIANCO, I. (1946). Una paticulare anomalia ematologica: 'la microcitemia'. *Minerva med. (Torino)*, **37**, 206.

— (1963). A new variant of human fetal hemoglobin: HbF_{Roma}. *Blood*, **22**, 545.

SILVESTRONI, E., BIANCO, I. and BRANCATI, C. (1963). Haemoglobins N and P in Italian families. *Nature (Lond.)*, **200**, 658.

SIMMONS, W. K. (1970). The plasma amino acid ratio as an indicator of the protein nutrition status. *Bull Wld IIlth Org.*, **42**, 480.

SIMMONS, W. K. and BOHDAL, M. (1970). Assessment of some biochemical parameters related to protein-calorie nutrition in children. *Bull. Wld Hlth Org.*, **42**, 897.

SIMONS, R. D. G. PH. and MARSHALL, J. (1969). *Essays on tropical dermatology.* Excerpta med. (Amst.), p. 283.

SIMPSON, B., *et al.* (1967). Renal function after leptospirosis. *Brit. med. J.*, **3**, 472.

SIMPSON, I. A. and CHOW, A. Y. (1956). The thiamine content of human milk in Malaya. Part II: The effect of the administration of supplementary thiamine on the thiamine level of human milk. *J. trop. Pediat.*, **2**, 69.

SINGER, K., CHERNOFF, A. I. and SINGER, L. (1951). Studies on abnormal hemoglobins. I: Their demonstration in sickle cell anemia and other hematologic disorders by means of alkali denaturation. *Blood*, **6**, 413.

SINGH, A., JOLLY, S. S. and KUMAR, L. R. (1961). Indian childhood cirrhosis. *Lancet*, **1**, 587.

SINGH, A., *et al.* (1966). Spinal cysticercosis with paraplegia (Memoranda). *Brit. med. J.*, **2**, 684.

SINGH, K. S. P., MISRA, S. S. and BHARGAVA, K. P. (1965) 5-Hydroxytryptamine content of cerebrospinal fluid in leprosy. *Nature (Lond.)*, **206**, 206.

SINGH, S., CLIFFORD, P. and PATEL, S. A. (1973). Nervous system involvement in Burkitt's lymphoma in Kenya. *Afr. J. Med. Sci.*, **4**, 187.

SINHA, D. P. and BANG, F. B. (1973). Seasonal variation in signs of vitamin-A deficiency in rural West Bengal children. *Lancet*, **2**, 228.

SINISCALCO, M., BERNINI, L., FILIPPI, G., LATTE, B, MEERA KHAN, P., PIOMELLI, S. and RATTAZZI, M. (1966). Population genetics of haemoglobin variants, thalassaemia and glucose-6-phosphate dehydrogenase deficiency, with particular reference to the malaria hypothesis. *Bull. Wld Hlth Org.*, **34**, 379.

SIRSAT, S. M. and KHANOLKAR, V. R. (1962). Submucous fibrosis of the palate and pillars of the fauces. *Indian J. med. Sci.*, **16**, 189.

SITPRIJA, V., *et al.* (1967). Renal failure in malaria. *Lancet*, **1**, 185.

SKAPINKER, S. (1953). Acute mechanical intestinal obstruction in the Bantu. *S. Afr. med. J.*, **27**, 237.

SKIRROW, M. B. and MAEGRAITH, B. G. (1964). The circulation in malaria. I. Portal angiography in the normal rabbit and monkey (*Macacca mulatta*). *Ann. trop. Med. Parasit.*, **58**, 491.

SLADEN, G. E. and KUMAR, P. J. (1973). Is the xylose test still a worthwhile investigation? *Brit. med. J.*, **3**, 223.

SLAVIN, G., CAMERON, H. MCD. and SINGH, H. (1969). Kaposi's sarcoma in mainland Tanzania. *Brit. J. Cancer*, **23**, 349.

SLAVIN, G., *et al.* (1970). Kaposi's sarcoma in East African children. *J. Path.*, **100**, 187.

SLEEPER, J. C., ORGAIN, E. S. and MCINTOSH, H. D. (1962). Primary pulmonary hypertension: review of clinical features and pathologic physiology with a report of pulmonary hemodynamics derived from repeated catheterization. *Circulation*, **26**, 1358.

SLEISENGER, M. H. (1967). Diseases of malabsorption. In P. B. Beeson and W. M. McDermott, eds., p. 883. *Cecil–Loeb Textbook of Medicine*, 12th ed. W. B. Saunders, Philadelphia.

SLOTWINER, P., SONG, S. K. and ANDERSON, P. J. (1969). Skeletal muscle changes in leprosy. *J. Path.*, **97**, 211.

DE SMET, M. P. (1954). Contributions to the study of thyroid pathology in the Belgian Congo. *Ann. Soc. belge. Méd. trop.*, **34**, 47.

SMETANA, H. F. (1962). Histopathology of experimental yellow fever. *Virchows Arch. path. Anat.*, **335**, 411.

— (1963). The histopathology of drug induced liver disease. *Ann. N.Y. Acad Sci.*, **104**, 821.

SMETANA, H. F., EDLOW, J. B. and GLUNZ, P. R. (1965). Neonatal jaundice: a critical review of persistent obstructive jaundice in infancy. *Arch. Path.*, **80**, 553.

SMETANA, H. F., HADLEY, G. G. and SIRSAT, S. M. (1961). Infantile cirrhosis: an analytic review of the literature and a report of 50 cases. *Pediatrics*, **28**, 107.

SMETANA, H. F. and OLEN, E. (1962). Hereditary galactose disease. *Amer. J. clin. Path.*, **38**, 3.

SMITH, C. E. G. (1951). Haemoglobinuria in typhoid fever treated with chloramphenicol. *Lancet*, **2**, 1020.

SMITH, C. E. G., *et al.* (1974). Arbovirus infections in Sarawak. Serological studies in man. *Trans. roy. Soc. trop. Med. Hyg.*, **68**, 96.

SMITH, D. A. and WOODRUFF, M. F. A. (1951). Deficiency diseases in Japanese prison camps. *Spec. Rep. Ser. med. Res. Counc. (Lond.)*, No. 274.

SMITH, D. H. and THEAKSTON, R. D. G. (1970). Comments on the ultra structure of human erythrocytes infected with *Plasmodium malaraie*. *Ann. trop. Med. Parasit.*, **64**, 433.

SMITH, D. H., *et al.* (1971). Evaluation of the *Dirofilaria immitis* Filarial Skin test antigen in the diagnosis of Filariasis. *Bull. Wld Hlth Org.*, **44**, 771–782.

SMITH, E. W. and TORBERT, J. V. (1958). Study of two abnormal hemoglobins with evidence for a new genetic locus for hemaglobin formation. *Bull. Johns Hopk. Hosp.*, **102**, 38.

SMITH, H., BANNISTER, B. and O'SHEA, M. J. (1973). Cerebrospinal fluid immunoglobulins in meningitis. *Lancet*, **2**, 591.

SMITH, I. H., REYNOLDS, E. S. and VON LICHTENBURG (1969). The integrement of *Schistosoma mansoni*. *Amer. J. trop. Med. Hyg.*, **18**, 28.

SMITH, J. A. (1972). Alpha-foetoprotein: a possible factor necessary for normal development of the embryo. *Lancet*, **1**, 851.

SMITH, J. A., FRANCIS, T. I. and DAVID-WEST, T. S. (1972). Anto antibodies in acute viral hepatitis, yellow fever and hepatocellular carcinoma. *J. Path.*, **109**, 83.

SMITH, J. A., FRANCIS, T. I., EDINGTON, G. M. and WILLIAMS, A. O. (1971). Immunofluorescent localization of human alpha-fetoprotein in foetal and neonatal liver and cultured cells from hepato-cellular carcinoma. *Brit. J. Cancer*, **25**, 343.

— (1971a). Human Alpha-fetoprotein in body fluids. *Brit. J. Cancer*, **25**, 337.

SMITH, J. A., OGUMBA, E. O. and FRANCIS, T. I. (1972). Transmission of Australia Au (1) antigen by culex mosquitoes. *Nature*, **237**, 231.

SMITH, J. H. and LICHTENBERG, F. VON. (1967). The Hoeppli phenomenon in schistosomiasis. II. Histochemistry. *Amer. J. trop. Path.*, **50**, 993.

SMITH, J. H., REYNOLDS, E. S. and VON LICHTENBERG, F. (1969). The integument of *Schistosoma mansoni*. *Amer. J. trop. Med. Hyg.*, **18**, 28.

SMITH, M. G. M., *et al.* (1972). Cell-mediated immune response in chronic liver disease. *Brit. med. J.*, **1**, 527.

SMITH, M. H. (1969). Do intestinal parasites require oxygen ? *Nature (London)*, **223**, 1129.

SMITH, M. J. (1956). Gastric granuloma with eosinophilic infiltration: report of two cases. *Radiology*, **66**, 177.

SMITH, R. and WATERLOW, J. C. (1960). Total exchangeable potassium in infantile malnutrition. *Lancet*, **1**, 147.

SMITH, R. and WRIGHT, A. D. (1963). Gangrene in haemoglobin C trait after exposure to cold. *Lancet*, **2**, 760.

SMITHBURN, K. C., HADDOW, A. J. and MAHAFFY, A. F. (1946). A neurotropic virus isolated from *Aedes* mosquitoes caught in the Semliki forest. *Amer. J. trop. Med.*, **26**, 189.

SMITHBURN, K. C., MAHAFFY, A. F. and PAUL, J. H. (1941). Bwamba fever and its causative virus. *Amer. J. trop. Med.*, **21**, 75.

SMITHBURN, K. C., *et al.* (1957). Studies on arthropodborne viruses of Tongaland. IX. Isolation of Wesselsbron virus from a naturally infected human being and from *Aedes (Banksinella) circumluteolus* Theo. *S. Afr. J. med. Sci.*, **22**, 113.

— (1959). An agent related to Uganda S virus from man and mosquitoes in South Africa. *S. Afr. med. J.*, **33**, 959.

SMITHERS, S. R. (1962). Acquired resistance to bilharziasis. Ciba Foundation Symposium. *Bilharziasis*, p. 239. Churchill, London.

SMITHERS, S. R., TERRY, R. J. and HOCKLEY, D. J. (1969). Host antigens in schistosomiasis. *Proc. roy. Soc. B.*, **171**, 483.

SMITHIES, O. (1955). Zone electrophoresis in starch gels: Group variations in the serum proteins of normal human adults. *Biochem. J.*, **51**, 629.

SNIJDER, J. (1965). Histopathology of pulmonary lesions caused by atypical mycobacteria. *J. Path. Bact.*, **90**, 65.

SODEMAN, W. A. and JEFFERY, G. M. (1966). Primary malarial thrombocytopenia in the rhesus monkey. *Trans. roy. Soc. trop. Med. Hyg.*, **60**, 70.

SOH, C. T. (1969). Clonorchiasis in Kora. *Proc. roy. Soc. B.*, **171**, 219.

SOLTYS, M. A. (1963). Immunity in African trypanosomiasis. *Bull. Wld Hlth Org.*, **28**, 753.

SOMERS, K. (1967). Pericarditis. *Brit. med. J.*, **1**, 423.

SOMERSET, E. J. (1968). In *May and Worth's Manual of Diseases of the Eye*, p. 728, 734. Bailiere, Tindall and Cassell, London.

SONNELAND, J. (1972). The inoperable breast carcinoma. A successful result using zinc chloride fixative. *Amer. J. Surg.*, **124**, 391.

SONNET, J., BRISBOIS, P. and BASTIN, J. P. (1966). Chronic pancreatitis with calcifications in Congolese Bantus. *Trop. geogr. Med.*, **18**, 97.

SOOTHILL, J. F. and HENDRICKSE, R. G. (1967). Some immunological studies of the nephrotic syndrome of Nigerian children. *Lancet*, **2**, 629.

SORNMANI, S. (1969). Schistosomiasis in Thailand: a review. *Proceedings of the 4th S.E. Asian Seminar on Parasitology and Tropical Medicine, Schistosomiasis and other snail-transmitted helminthiasis*, p. 71.

SORNMANI, S., *et al.* (1973). Mekong schistosomiasis. 1. Life cycle of *Schistosoma japonicum*, Mekong strain, in the laboratory. *S.E. Asian J. trop. Med. Pub. Hlth.*, **4**, 2, 218.

SORNMANI, S., *et al.* (1973). A study on the pattern of socioeconomic and health status in relation to parasitic diseases in the inhabitants around Ubolratana Dam in Northeast Thailand. *Southeast Asian J. trop. Med. Pub. Hlth.*, **4**, 421.

SOULSBY, E. J. L. and GILLES, H. M. (1965). Serological studies of *Necator americanus* and *Ascaris lumbricoides* infections in an endemic area. *J. Parasit.*, **51**, 2.

— (1975). *Bull. int. Atomic Energy Agency, Vienna.*

SOUTHGATE, B. A. (1974a). Community diagnosis and management in Bancroftian filariasis. *Trop. Doctor*, **4**, 3.

—(1974b). A quantitative approach to parasitological techniques in Bancroftian filariasis and its effects on epidemology understanding. *Trans. roy. Soc. trop. Med. Hyg.*, **68**, 177.

SOUTHGATE, B. A. and ORIEDO, B. V. E. (1962). Studies in the epidemiology of East African leishmaniasis. I. The circumstantial epidemology of kala-azar in the Kitui District of Kenya. *Trans. roy. Soc. trop. Med. Hyg.*, **56**, 30.

— (1967). Studies in the epidemiology of East African leishmaniasis. 3. Immunity as a determinant of geographical distribution. *J. Trop. Med. Hyg.*, **70**, 1.

SOUTH PACIFIC COMMISSION. Noumea, New Caledonia (1963). The incidence of *Angiostrongylus cantonensis* (Chen) among rats and mollusks in New Caledonia and nearby islands and its possible relationship to eosinophilic meningitis. *Technical Paper No. 139.*

— (1965). Epidemiology of filariasis in the South Pacific. *Technical Paper No. 148.*

SOWA, S., et al. (1965). Trachoma and allied infections in a Gambian village. *Spec. Rep. Ser. med. Res. Coun. (Lond.)*, No. 308.

SPENCE, L., ANDERSON, C. R. and DOWNS, W. G. (1962). Isolation of Ilheus virus from human beings in Trinidad, West Indies. *Trans. roy. Soc. trop. Med. Hyg.*, **56**, 405.

SPILLANE, J. D. (1969). Tropical neurology. *Proc. roy. Soc. Med.*, **62**, 403.

— (1972). The geography of neurology. *Brit. med. J.*, **2**, 506.

— (1973). (Ed.) *Tropical Neurology.* Oxford Univ. Press.

SPINK, W. W. (1956). *The Nature of Brucellosis.* Univ. Minnesota Press, Minneapolis.

SPINK, W. W., HOFFBAUER, F. W., WALKER, W. W. and GREEN, R. A. (1949). Histopathology of the liver in human brucellosis. *J. Lab. clin. Med.*, **34**, 40.

SPÎNU, I., et al. (1963). L'homme comme réservoir de virus dans une épidémie de leptospirose survenne dans la jungle. *Arch. roum. Path. exp.*, **22**, 1081.

SPRINZ, H. (1966). Histopathology of the upper small intestines in typhoid fever. *Amer. J. dig. Dis.*, **2**, 615.

SPRINZ, H., SRIBHIBHADH, R., GANGAROSA, E. J., BENYAJATI, C., KUNDEL, D. and HALSTEAD, S. (1962). Biopsy of small bowel of Thai people, with special reference to recovery from Asiatic cholera and to an intestinal malabsorption syndrome. *Amer. J. clin. Path.*, **38**, 43.

SRICHAIKUL, et al. (1967). Bone-marrow changes in human malaria. *Ann. trop. Med. Parasit.*, **61**, 40.

SRIKANTIA, S. G., SRIRAMACHARI, S. and GOPALAN, C. (1958). A follow-up study of fifteen cases of 'kwashiorkor'. *Indian J. med. Res.*, **46**, 121.

STAMATOYANNOPOULOS, G. and FESSAS, P. (1963). Observations on hemoglobin 'Pylos': the hemaglobin Pylos-hemoglobin S combination. *J. Lab. clin. Med.*, **62**, 193.

— (1964). Thalassaemia, glucose-6-phosphate dehydrogenase deficiency, sickling, and malarial endemicity in Greece: A study of five areas. *Brit. med. J.*, **1**, 875.

STAMM, W. P. (1965). Laboratory aids in the management of some common diarrhoeas in the tropics. *Trans. roy. Soc. trop. Med. Hyg.*, **59**, 712.

— (1966). *Entamoeba Histolytica in Man.* Reprinted from The Pathology of Parasitic Diseases, Fourth Symposium of the British Society for Parasitology. Blackwell Scientific Publications, Oxford, p. 1.

STAMM, W. P., *et al.* (1973). Evaluation of a latex agglutination test for amoebiasis. *Trans. roy. Soc. trop. Med. Hyg.*, **67**, 211.

STANBURY, J. B., *et al.* (1974). Endemic goitre and cretinism: public health significance and prevention. *WHO Chron.*, **28**, 220.

STANFIELD, J. P., HUTT, M. S. R. and TUNNICLIFFE, R. (1965). Intestinal biopsy in kwashiorkor. *Lancet*, **2**, 519.

STANLEY, N. N., ACKRILL, P. and WOOD, J. (1972). Lung perfusion scanning in hepatic cirrhosis. *Brit. med. J.*, **4**, 639.

STEEL, J. M. and MNGOLA, E. N. (1974). Diabetes in Kenya. *Tropical Doctor*, **4**, 184.

STEFANINI, M. (1948). Clinical features and pathogenesis of tropical sprue: observations on a series of cases among Indian prisoners of war in India. *Medicine (Baltimore)*, **27**, 379.

STEIN, A. A., BERGMAN, B. J., COLES, R. M. and SHAPER, A. G. (1965). East African vs American pancreatic and hepatic fibrosis. *Arch. environm. Hlth*, **11**, 669.

STEIN, H. and ISAACSON, C. (1962). Veno-occlusive disease of the liver. *Brit. med. J.*, **1**, 372.

STEINER, I. O. and HUTT, M. S. R. (1972). Vascular changes in the idiopathic peripheral gangrene of the tropics. *Trop. geogr. Med.*, **24**, 219.

STEINER, P. E. (1964). Evolution of research in the etiological types of cirrhotic diseases of the liver, 1931–1961. *Path. et Microbiol.*, **27**, 890.

STEINER, P. E. and DAVIES, J. N. P. (1957). Cirrhosis and primary liver carcinoma in Uganda Africans. *Brit. J. Cancer*, **11**, 523.

STEMMERMANN, G. N. (1967). Strongyloidiasis in immigrants. *Gastroenterology*, **53**, 59.

STEPHEN, S. J. and URAGODA, C. G. (1970). Some observations on oesophageal carcinoma in Ceylon, including its relationship to betel chewing. *Brit. J. Cancer*, **24**, 11.

STEPHENS, J. R. C. (1928). *Porocephalus armillatus*. (Correspondence.) *W. Afr. med. J.*, **2**, 107.

STERN, H. and WILLIAMS, B. M. (1966). Isolation of rubella virus in a case of neonatal giant-cell hepatitis. *Lancet*, **1**, 293.

STERN, R. B., *et al.* (1973). Use of computer-assisted model in diagnosis of drug hypersensitivity jaundice. *Brit. med. J.*, **2**, 767.

STERNER, G., *et al.* (1971). Giardiasis: a problem of current interest in Sweden (Swedish). *Nord. Med.*, **86**, 1343.

STEVENSON, S. (1962). Wild yam (*Dioscorea* sp.) poisoning in Nyasaland. (Correspondence.) *Trans. roy. Soc. trop. Med. Hyg.*, **56**, 438.

STEWART, A. M. (1974). Protein requirement. *Lancet*, **2**, 1026.

STEYN, D. G. (1964). Endemic goitre in the Republic of South Africa and in some neighbouring territories. *The Leech*, **34**, 114.

— (1965). An investigation into cases of suspected poisoning in Africans in Northern Rhodesia. *S. Afr. med. J.*, **39**, 344.

ST. HILL, C. A., FINN, R. and DENYE, V. (1973). Depression of cellular immunity in pregnancy due to a serum factor. *Brit. med. J.*, **3**, 513.

STIRLING, G. A. (1960). Hypertensive disease in Jamaican necropsy material. *Brit. med. J.*, **1**, 1173.

STOCK, F. E. (1946). Collapse of the lung and porocephalosis. *Trans. roy. Soc. trop. Med. Hyg.*, **40**, 101.

STOKER, D. J. (1974). Haemoglobinopathies. *Proc. roy. Soc. Med.*, **67**, 859.

STOTT, G. (1961). Hookworm infection and anaemia in Mauritius. *Trans. roy. Soc. trop. Med. Hyg.*, **55**, 20.

STRACHAN, A. S. (1929). *Haemosiderosis and haemochromatosis in South African natives*. M.D. thesis, Univ. Glasgow.

STRACHAN, R. W. (1966). Pre-pulseless and pulseless Takayasus' arteritis. *Postgrad. med. J.*, **42**, 464.

STRANGWAYS-DIXON, J. and LAINSON, R. (1966). The epidemiology of dermal leishmaniasis in British Honduras. Part III: The transmission of *Leishmania mexicana* to man by *Phlebotomus pessoanus*, with observations on the development of the parasite in different species of *Phlebotomus. Trans. roy. Soc. trop. Med. Hyg.*, **60**, 192.

STRANSKY, E. and DIZON-SANTOS-OCAMPO, P. O. (1958). Clinical rickets in the Philippines (report of 22 cases in Manila). *J. trop. Pediat.*, **4**, 17.

STRASSER, T. and ROTTA, J. (1973). The control of rheumatic fever and rheumatic heart disease. *WHO Chron.*, **27**, 49.

STRICKLAND, G. T. and KOSTINAZI, J. E. (1970). Folic acid deficiency complicating malaria. *Amer. J. trop. Med. Hyg.*, **19**, 910

STRÖM, J. (1951). Toxoplasmosis due to laboratory infection in two adults. *Acta med. scand.*, **139**, 244.

STUART, K. L. (1968). Hypertension in the tropics. *Brit. med. J.*, **1**, 103.

STUART, K. L. and BRAS, G. (1957). Veno-occlusive disease of the liver. *Quart. J. Med.* (n.s.), **26**, 291.

STUART, K. L. and HAYES, J. A. (1963). A cardiac disorder of unknown aetiology in Jamaica. *Quart. J. Med.* (n.s.), **32**, 99.

STUART-HARRIS, SIR C. (1971). Success and failure in human virus diseases. *Brit. med. J.*, **1**, 275.

STUIVER, P. C., *et al.* (1971). Clinical trials of malaria prophylaxis in tropical splenomegaly syndrome. *Brit. med. J.*, **1**, 426.

STURTON, S. D., WEN, H. L. and STURTON, O. G. (1966). Etiology of cancer of the nasopharynx. *Cancer, N.Y.*, **19**, 1666.

STURTON, S. D. *et al.* (1970). Carcinoma of the nasopharynx. *Int. Surg.*, **53**, 1.

SUBRAMANIAM, B. and KULANGRA, A. C. (1967). Incidence of atherosclerotic lesions at Madras, South India. *Brit. Heart J.*, **29**, 333.

SUBRAMANIAN, R. (1949). Symmetrical gangrene. *Indian med. Gaz.*, **84**, 334.

SUJOY, B., *et al.* (1963). Juvenile mitral stenosis in India. *Lancet*, **2**, 1193.

SUKKAR, H. Y., OMER, A. H. S. and AHMED, N. D. (1974). Impaired glucose tolerance in hepatic schistosomiasis. *Trans. roy. Soc. trop. Med. Hyg.*, **68**, 327.

SULLIVAN, J. F. and HEANEY, R. P. (1970). Zinc metabolism in alcoholic liver disease. *Amer. J. clin. Nutrit.*, **23**, 170.

SUN, N. C. and SMITH, V. M. (1966). Hepatitis associated with myocarditis: unusual manifestation of infection with Coxsackie virus group B, type 3. *New Engl. J. Med.*, **274**, 190.

SUN, T. and GIBSON, J. B. (1969). Antigens of *Clonorchis sinensis* in experimental and human infections: an analysis, by gel-diffusion technique. *Amer. J. trop. Med. Hyg.*, **18**, 241.

SUNDHARAGIATI, B., POTHA, U. and HARINASUTA, C. (1967). *Diagnosis of Human Leptospirosis in Provincial hospital of Thailand by dried blood on Filter Paper Method, a Study of 3640 blood specimens*. SEAMES. The Third Conference on Parasitic Diseases. Abstracts of Papers, p. 69.

SUNDHARAGIATI, R., *et al.* (1966). Seasonal incidence of canine leptospirosis in Bangkok. *Trans. roy. Soc. trop. Med. Hyg.*, **60**, 366.

SUNDHARAGIATI, S., BOONPACKNAVIG, S., HARINASUTA, C. and PHOLPOTHI, T. (1966). Human leptospirosis in Thailand. *Trans. roy. Soc. trop. Med. Hyg.*, **60**, 366.

SURI, J. C., DHILLON, H. and GREWAL, H. S. (1964). Active immunization of women in pregnancy for prevention of neonatal tetanus. *Bull. Wld Hlth Org.*, **31**, 349.

SURINGA, D. W. R., BANK, L. J. and ACKERMAN, A. B. (1970). Role of measles virus in skin lesions and Koplik's spots. *New Engl. J. Med.*, **283**, 1139.

SUTHERLAND, J. C., BERRY, A., HYND, M. and PROCTOR, N. S. F. (1965). Placental bilharziasis: report of a case. *S. Afr. J. Obstet. Gynaec.*, **3**, 76.

SUWA, N. (1966). Pathological anatomy of bacillary dysentery in Japan. *Internal. Acad. Path. Kyoto.*

SWANEPOEL, A., SMYTHE, P. M. and CAMPBELL, J. A. H. (1964). The heart in kwashiorkor. *Amer. Heart J.*, **67**, 1.

SWANSON, V. L. and THOMASSEN, R. W. (1965). Pathology of the jejunal mucosa in tropical sprue. *Amer. J. Path.*, **46**, 511.

SWARTZWELDER, J. C., BEAVER, P. C. and HOOD, M. W. (1964). Sparganosis in Southern United States. *Amer. J. trop. Med. Hyg.*, **13**, 43.

SYMMERS, W. ST. C. (1903). Note on a new form of liver cirrhosis due to the presence of the ova of *Bilharzia haematobia*. *J. Path. Bact.*, **9**, 237.

SYMMERS, W. ST. C. (1957). Two cases of eosinophilic prostatitis due to metazoan infestation (with *Oxyuris vermicularis*, and with a larva of *Linguatula serrata*). *J. Path. Bact.*, **73**, 549.

— (1960). Leishmaniasis acquired by contagion. A case of Marital infection in Britain. *Lancet*, **I**, 127.

— (1960). Cytomegalic inclusion disease affecting the parotid gland of an adult. *J. Path. Bact.*, **79**, 406.

— (1969). Primary amoebic meningoencephalitis in Britain. *Brit. med. J.*, **4**, 449.

SYMPOSIUM ON GIARDIASIS (1970). *Indian Practit.*, **23**, 119.

SZEINBERG, A. (1963). In *Genetics of Migrant and Isolate Populations*, ed. E. Goldschmidt, p. 69. Williams and Wilkins, Baltimore.

TADA, I., et al. (1966). Intradermal reactions with *Gnathostoma nipponicum* antigen. *Jap. J. Parasit.*, **15**, 196.

TAILLIEZ, R. and KORACH, S. (1970). Les antigenes de *Fasciola hepatica*. II. Étude immunologique et localisation in situ d'un antigène specifique du genre. *Ann. Inst. Pasteur*, **118**, 330.

TAKAHARA, S. (1952). Progressive oral gangrene probably due to lack of catalase in the blood (acatalasaemia): report of nine cases. *Lancet*, **2**, 1101.

TAKAYASU, M. A. (1908). A case with peculiar changes in the central retinal vessels. *Acta Soc. ophthal. jap.*, **12**, 554.

TAKUCHI, J., et al. (1971). Budd chiari syndrome associated with obstruction of the inferior vena cava. A report of seven cases. *Amer. J. Med.*, **51**, 11.

TALERMAN, A. (1969). Clinico-pathological study of multiple myeloma in Jamaica. *Brit. J. Cancer*, **23**, 285.

TAMIYA, T. (1962). *Recent Advances in Studies of Tsutsugamushi Disease in Japan.* Medical Culture Inc., Tokyo.

TAN, J. S., et al. (1967). *Acute Renal Failure Accompanying Hemorrhagic Fever in the Philippines.* SEAMES. The Third Conference on Parasitic Diseases. Abstracts of Papers, p. 48.

TAN, K. L., TAN, A. Y. O. and WONG, T. T. T. (1972). Necrotizing enterocolitis in young infants. *Clin. pediat. (Philad.)*, **11**, 44.

TANDON, B. N., MATHUR, A. K., MOHAPATRA, L. N., TANDON, H. D. and WIG, K. L. (1965). A study of the prevalence and clinical pattern of non-specific ulcerative colitis in northern India. *Gut*, **6**, 448.

TANDON, B. N., *et al.* (1966). Functional and structural studies of small bowel in Ankylostomiasis. *Brit. med. J.*, **1**, 714.

TANDON, P. N. and BAJPAI, P. C. (1973). The infantile tremor syndrome. In *Tropical Neurology*, ed. J. D. Spillane, p. 114. Oxford University Press, London.

TANEJA, O. P., MALL, M. P. and MITTAL, K. P. (1970). Urological aspects of endemic bladder stones in children. *Aust. N.Z. J. Surg.*, **40**, 130.

T'ANG, F. F., *et al.* (1957). Studies on the etiology of trachoma with special reference to isolation of the virus in chick embryo. *Chin. med. J.*, **75**, 429.

TANPHAICHITR, V., *et al.* (1970). Clinical and biochemical studies of adult beriberi. *Amer. J. clin. Nutr.*, **23**, 1017.

TANSURAT, P. (1961). Cancer of the oral cavity and esophagus in Thais and Chinese. *Acta Un. int. Cancr.*, **17**, 877.

TASHIRO, K. (1924). Clinical, Pathologic-Anatomical and Experimental Studies on 'Plerocercoides Prolifer Iijima (1905), Sparganum Proliferum, Stiles (1906)'. *Mitt. med. Fak. K. Univ. Kyushu*, **9**, 1.

TATARINOV, J. U. (1964). Detection of embryo specific alpha-globulin in the blood sera of patient with primary liver tumour. *Vop. med. Khim.*, **10**, 90.

TAUB, J. (1956). The effect of normal human serum on leishmania. *Bull. Res. Coun. Israel.*, **6E**, 55.

TAUZIN, M. (1972). Aspects cliniques des intoxications par médecine traditionnelle à Tahiti. *Méd. Afr. noire*, **19**, 37.

TAYLOR, J. (1968). The thyroid in Western Nigeria. *E. Afr. med. J.*, **45**, 383, 390.

TAYLOR, J. W. (1963). Cancer in Saudi Arabia. *Cancer, N.Y.*, **16**, 1530.

TAYLOR, R. M., *et al.* (1956). A study of the ecology of West Nile virus in Egypt. *Am. J. trop. Med. Hyg.*, **5**, 579.

TAYLOR-ROBINSON, D. (1971). Mycoplasmas and their pathogenicity. *Proc. roy. Soc. Med.*, **64**, 31.

TEARE, D. (1958). Asymmetrical hypertrophy of the heart in young adults. *Brit. Heart J.*, **20**, 1.

TEE, D. E. N. (1973). Studies with the Makari tumour skin test in the United Kingdom. *Trans. N.Y. acad. Sci.*, **35**, 387.

TEMPLETON, A. C. (1968). Human coenurus infection. A report of 14 cases from Uganda. *Trans. roy. Soc. trop. Med. Hyg.*, **62**, 251.

— (1970). Generalised herpes simplex in malnourished children. *J. clin. Path.*, **23**, 24.

— (1971). Orbital tumours in African children. *Brit. J. Ophthal.*, **55**, 254.

— (1972). Testicular neoplasms in Ugandan Africans. *Afr. J. med. Sci.*, **3**, 157.

TEOTIA, M., TEOTIA, S. P. S. and KUNWAR, K. B. (1971). Endemic skeletal fluorosis. *Arch. Dis. Childh.*, **46**, 686.

TEOTIA, S. P. S. and TEOTIA, M. (1973). Secondary hyperprathyroidism in patients with endemic skeletal fluorosis. *Brit. med. J.*, **1**, 637.

TEUBES, M. N. (1963). Volvulus of the sigmoid colon in relation to the anatomy of the pelvic colon. *S. Afr. med. J.*, **37**, 1151.

THARAVANIJ, S. (1969). Immunity in amoebiasis. In *Proceedings of a Seminar on Filariasis and Immunology of Parasitic Infections, Singapore*, ed. A. A. Sandosham and V. Zaman, p. 22. Singapore and Bangkok.

THENABADU, P. N., FAJASURIYA, A. and WICKREMASINGHE, H. T. (1970). Non-specific arteritis of the aorta and its main branches. *Brit. Heart J.*, **32**, 181.

THERON, J. J., PEPLER, W. J. and MEKOL, R. C. P. M. (1971). Ultrastructure of the liver in Bantu patients with pneumonia and jaundice. *J. Path.*, **106**, 113.

THIJS, A. (1957). Considérations sur les tumeurs malignes des indigènes du Congo belge et du Ruanda-Urundi: à propos de 2,536 cas. *Ann. Soc. belge Méd. trop.*, **37**, 483.

THOMAS, H. O. (1953). Idiopathic gangrene of the scrotum in West Africans. *Brit. J. Urol.*, **25**, 60.

THOMAS, J. B., SIKES, R. K. and RICKER, A. S. (1963). Evaluation of indirect fluorescent antibody technique for detection of rabies antibody in human sera. *J. Immunol.*, **91**, 721.

THOMAS, L. (1971). Mycoplasmas as infectious agents. *Ann. Rev. Med.*, **21**, 179.

THOMAS, M. and JOB, C. K. (1972). Serum atypical pseudocholinesterase and genetic factors in leprosy. *Brit. med. J.*, **3**, 390.

THOMAS, P. K. (1973). Metabolic neuropathy. *J. roy. Coll. Phycns, Lond.*, **7**, 154.

THOMAS, W. A., DAVIES, J. N., O'NEAL, R. M. and DIMAKULANGAN, A. A. (1960). Incidence of myocardial infarction correlated with venous and pulmonary thrombosis and embolism: a geographic study based on autopsies in Uganda, East Africa, and St. Louis, U.S.A. *Amer. J. Cardiol.*, **5**, 41.

THOMAS, A. *et al.* (1971). Le Kwashiorkor de famine (ou de guerre). Reflexions á propos de 1,900 observations. *Presse méd.*, **79**, No. 38 (29), 1681.

THOMPSON, B. and BAIRD, SIR D. (1967*a*). Some impressions of childbearing in tropical areas—I. *J. Obstet. Gynaec. Brit. Cwlth*, **74**, 329.

— (1967*b*). Some impressions of childbearing in tropical areas—II. *J. Obstet. Gynaec. Brit. Cwlth*, **74**, 499.

— (1967*c*). Some impressions of childbearing in tropical areas—III. *J. Obstet. Gynaec. Brit. Cwlth*, **74**, 510.

THOMPSON, O. L., MORELAND, H. J., SMITH, G. W., BOWMAN, B. H., ALEXANDER, M. J. and SCHNEIDER, R. G. (1963). A family with hemoglobin I. *Blood*, **22**, 313.

THOMPSON, R. B., RAU, P. J., ODOM, J. and BELL, W. N. (1965). The sickling phenomenon in a white male without Hb-S. *Acta haemat.*, **34**, 347.

THOMPSON, R. P. H., *et al.* (1970). Cutaneous porphyria due to a malignant primary hepatoma. *Gastroenterology*, **59**, 779.

THOMSON, C., *et al.* (1974). Changes in blood coagulation and fibrinolysis in the nephrotic syndrome. *Quart. J. Med.*, **43**, 399.

THOMSON, J. G. (1961). Cirrhosis of the liver in Europeans, coloureds and native Africans in Cape Town. *Acta Un. int. Cancr.*, **17**, 623.

— (1966). Calcifying collagenolysis (tumoural calcinosis). *Brit. J. Radiol.* (n.s.), **39**, 526.

THONNARD-NEUMANN, E. (1944). Zur Pathogenese der Malaria-Anämie. *Dt. tropenmed. Z.*, **48**, 129.

THORBURN, M. J., MILLER, C. G. and BRAS, G. (1967). Congenital hepatic fibrosis in Jamaican children. *Arch. Dis. Childh.*, **42**, 379.

THORNBURGH, D. B., JOHNSON, C. M. and ELTON, N. W. (1952). The histopathology of cutaneous leishmaniasis in Panama. *Trans. roy. Soc. trop. Med. Hyg.*, **46**, 550.

THORUP, O. A., ITANO, H. A., WHEBY, M. and LEAVELL, B. S. (1956). Hemoglobin J. *Science, N.Y.*, **123**, 889.

TILLETT, H. E. and THOMAS, M. E. M. (1974). Culture of the faeces in the diagnosis of Sonne dysentery: a statistical method for estimating the true isolation rate. *Int. J. Epid.*, **3**, 177.

TINCKLER, L. F. (1966). Fluid and electrolyte observations in tropical surgical practice. *Brit. med. J.*, **1**, 1263.

— (1966). 'Non-incidence' of disease. (Correspondence.) *Brit. med. J.*, **1**, 734.

TOBIE, J. E. and COATNEY, G. R. (1961). Fluorescent antibody staining of human malaria parasites. *Exp. Parasit.*, **11**, 128.

TODD, D. and KAU, P. S. (1965). Anaemia in pregnancy in Hong Kong. *J. Obstet. Gynaec. Brit. Cwlth*, **72**, 738.

TOH, C. C. S. and CHOW, K. W. (1969). Malabsorption syndrome in a patient infected with *Strongyloides stercoralis*. *Ann. trop. Med. Parasit.*, **63**, 493.

TOMPKINS, A. B. (1958). Neonatal tetanus in Nigeria. *Brit. med. J.*, **1**, 1382.

TONDO, C. V., SALZANO, F. M. and RUCKNAGEL, D. L. (1963). Hemoglobin Porto Alegre, a possible polymer of normal hemoglobin in a Caucasian Brazilian family. *Amer. J. hum. Genet.*, **16**, 265.

TOPLEY and WILSON'S *Principles of Bacteriology and Immunity* (1964). 5th edition. Vol. I and II. Edward Arnold, London.

TORRICO, R. A. (1959). Enfermedad de Chagas en Bolivia. *Rev. goiana Med.*, **5**, 375.

TOVEY, F. I. (1974). Geographical distribution of peptic ulcer. *Tropical Doctor*, **4**, 17.

TRAGER, W. (1958). Folinic acid and non-dialysable materials in the nutrition of malaria parasites. *J. exp. Med.*, **108**, 753.

— (1964). Cultivation and physiology of erythrocytic stages of plasmodia. *Amer. J. trop. Med. Hyg.*, **13**, 162.

TRAQUAIR, R. N. (1947). Pyomyositis. *J. trop. Med. Hyg.*, **50**, 81.

TRAUB, R., WISSEMAN, C. L. and AHMAD, N. (1967). The occurrence of scrub typhus infection in unusual habitats in West Pakistan. *Trans. roy. Soc. trop. Med. Hyg.*, **61**, 23.

TRENT, SOPHIE C. (1963). Reevaluation of World War II veterans with filariasis acquired in the South Pacific. *Amer. J. trop. Med. Hyg.*, **12**, 877.

TRIPATHY, J., et al. (1971). Effects of *Ascaris* infection on human nutrition. *Amer. J. trop. Med. Hyg.*, **20**, 212.

TRIPATIZIS, I. and HORST, H. G. (1971). Detection of Australia-SH-antigen in urine. *Nature*, **231**, 266.

TRISHNANANDA, M., et al. (1965). Study on scrub typhus in the jungle of Panasnikhom District, Cholburi Province. *J. med. Assoc. Thailand*, **48**, 642.

TRISHNANANDA, M., et al. (1966). Studies on the vector of *Rickettsia tsutsugamushi* infection in Thailand. *Ann. trop. med. Parasit.*, **60**, 252.

TRONCALE, F. J., et al. (1968). Occurrence of ceroid pigment without malabsorption in Thailand. *Gastroenterology*, **54**, 1122.

TROTTER, M., BROMAN, G. E. and PETERSON, R. R. (1960). Densities of bones of white and negro skeletons. *J. Bone Jt Surg.*, Amer. ed., **42**, 50.

TROUP, J. M., WHITE, H. A., FOM, A. L. M. D. and CAREY, D. E. (1970). An outbreak of Lassa fever on the Jos Plateau, Nigeria, in January-February, 1970. *Amer. J. trop. Med. Hyg.*, **19**, 695.

TROWELL, H. C. (1943). Dimorphic anaemia. *Trans. roy. Soc. trop. Med. Hyg.*, **37**, 19.

— (1960). *Non-infective Disease in Africa*. Edward Arnold, London.

TROWELL, H. C., DAVIES, J. N. P. and DEAN, R. F. A. (1954). *Kwashiorkor*. Edward Arnold, London.

TRUSSELL, R. R., HUTT, M. S. R. and ZEIGLER, O. (1968). Exfoliative cytology in the detection of cervical cancer in Uganda. *Cancer in Africa*, p. 397. East African Publishing House, Nairobi.

TRUSWELL, A. S. and HANSEN, J. D. L. (1969). Fatty liver in protein–calorie malnutrition. *S. Afr. med. J.*, **43**, 280.

TSUBAKI, T., HONMA, Y. and HOSHI, M. (1971). Neurological syndrome associated with clioquinal. *Lancet*, **1**, 696.

TUCHINDA, P. and JAYAVASU, J. (1967). *The Immuno-electrophoretic study of B_{1C}-Globulin in the sera of haemorrhagic fever patients*. SEAMES. The Third Conference on Parasitic Diseases. Abstracts of Papers, p. 48.

TUCHINDA, S., *et al.* (1959). Fast hemoglobin component found in umbilical cord blood of Thai babies. *Pediatrics*, **24**, 43.

TUGWELL, P. (1973). Glucose-6-phosphate dehydrogenase deficiency in Nigerians with jaundice associated with lobar pneumonia. *Lancet*, **1**, 968.

TULLOCH, J. A. (1962). *Diabetes Mellitus in the Tropics*. Livingstone, Edinburgh.

TURK, J. L. and BRYCESON, A. D. M. (1971). Immunological phenomena in leprosy and related diseases. *Advanc. Immunol.*, **13**, 209.

TURK, J. L. and WATERS, M. F. R. (1968). Immunological basis for depression of cellular immunity and the delayed allergic response in patients with lepromatous leprosy. *Lancet*, **2**, 436.

TURNBULL, N. S. (1928). *Porocephalus armillatus*. (Correspondence.) *W. Afr. med. J.*, **1**, 84.

— (1967). Traveller's diarrhoea: a survey of symptoms, occurrence, and possible prophylaxis. *Brit. med. J.*, **4**, 653.

TURNER, G. C., *et al.* (1971). S. H. (Australia) antigen in early life. *Arch. Dis. Child.*, **46**, 616.

TURNER, L. H. (1973). A new look at infective diseases: leptospirosis. *Brit. med. J.*, **1**, 537.

TURNER, L. H. and EDESON, J. F. B. (1957). Studies on filariasis in Malaya: the periodicity of the microfilariae of *Wuchereria malayi*. *Ann. trop. Med. Parasit.*, **51**, 271.

TURNER, P. P. (1962). Pulmonary heart disease in Africans in Mombasa. *E. Afr. med. J.*, **39**, 40.

TURPIE, A. G. G., FORBES, C. D. and MCNICOL, G. P. (1967). Idiopathic gangrene in African children. *Brit. med. J.*, **3**, 646.

UNDIANO, C. (1966). Importance and present-day concepts of the pathogenicity of *Mansonella* infection. *Rev. Fac. Cienc. méd. Univ. Córdoba*, **24**, 183.

UEHLINGER, E. A. (1958). The pathologic anatomy of endemic goitre before the introduction of iodized salt. *Fed. Proc.*, **17** (suppl. 2 Part II), 63.

UNDERHILL, B. M. L. (1964). Salt induced vaginal stenosis of Arabia. *J. Obstet. Gynaec. Brit. Cwlth*, **71**, 293.

URIEL, J., *et al.* (1967). Association de la alpha fetoproteine serique avec l'hepatoma primaire. *C.R. Acad. Sci. (Paris)*, **265**, 75.

URQUHART, G. M., MULLIGAN, W. and JENNINGS, F. W. (1954). Artificial immunity to *Fasciola hepatica* in rabbits. I: Some studies with protein antigens of *F. hepatica*. *J. infect. Dis.*, **94**, 126.

UTIAN, H. L. and HEYMANN, M. A. (1963). Leukaemia in childhood. *S. Afr. med. J.*, **37**, 1295.

UTTLEY, K. H. (1963). The death rate in the age-group 1–4 years as an index of malnutrition in tropical countries. *Trans. roy. Soc. trop. Med. Hyg.*, **57**, 41.

VAHLQUIST, B. (1973). Nutrition: a priority in African development. *Lancet*, **1**, 716.

VAILLANT, H. W., CUMMING, G. T. M. and RICHART, R. M. (1968). An island wide-screening programme for cervical neoplasia in Barbados. *Amer. J. Obstet. Gynec.*, **101**, 943.

VAISH, S. K., IGNATIUS, M. and BAKER, S. J. (1965). Albumin metabolism in tropical sprue. *Quart. J. Med.* (n.s.), **34**, 15.

VAISH, S. K., SAMPATHKUMAR, J., JACOB, R. and BAKER, S. J. (1965). The stomach in tropical sprue. *Gut.*, **6**, 458.

VAIZEY, J. M. (1959). Typhoid at Mulago. *E. Afr. med. J.*, **36**, 65.

VAKIL, B. J., IYER, S. N., TULPULE, A., MEHTA, A. J. and TULPULE, T. H. (1964). Observations on the aetiology and prognosis of tetanus, based on a study of 1852 cases. *J. Indian med. Ass.*, **42**, 203.

VAKIL, B. J., MEHTA, A. J. and DESAI, H. N. (1970). Atypical manifestations of amoebic abscess of the liver. *J. trop. Med. Hyg.*, **73**, 63.

VALMAN, H. B. (1974). Intelligence after malnutrition caused by neonatal resection of the ileum. *Lancet*, **1**, 425.

VAN DEN DRIESSCHE, E. (1973). Primary amoebic meningoencephalitis after swimming in stream water. *Lancet*, **2**, 971.

VANDEPITTE, J. (1959). The incidence of haemoglobinoses in the Belgian Congo. In *Abnormal Haemoglobins: Symposium*, p. 271. Blackwell Scientific Publications, Oxford.

VAN DER GELD, H., et al. (1966). Immunohistological and serological studies in endomyocardial fibrosis. *Lancet*, **2**, 1210.

VAN DER HOEVEN, J. A. and RIJPSTRA, A. C. (1957). Intestinal parasites in the central mountain district of Netherlands New-Guinea. An important focus of *Balantidium coli. Docum. Med. geogr. trop. (Amst.)*, **9**, 225.

VANDERICK, F. X. and MBONYINGABO, P. (1972). La cysticercose humaine au Rwanda. *Ann. Soc. belge Méd. trop.*, **52**, 2, 153.

VAN DER WESTHUYZEN, J. M. (1973). Plasma-T_3 assay in kwashiorkor. *Lancet*, **4**, 965.

VAN ENK, A., LANG, A., WHITE, J. M. and LEHMANN, H. (1972). Benign obstetric history in women with sickle-cell anaemia associated with alpha-thalassaemia. *Brit. med. J.*, **4**, 524.

VAN OYE, E. and BALLION, M. (1950). Faudra-t-il tenir compte d'une nouvelle affection à bacilles acido-resistants en Afrique? *Ann. Soc. belge Méd. trop.*, **30**, 619.

VAN PEENEN, P. D. F., et al. (1973). Dengue type 3 in Indonesia. *Trans. roy. Soc. trop. Med. Hyg.*, **67**, 3, 418.

VAN REEN, R. VALYASEVI, A. and DHANAMITTA, S. (1970). Studies of bladder stone disease in Thailand. *Amer. J. clin. Nutr.*, **23**, 940.

VAN THIEL, P. H. (1960). Comments on a case of *Toxocara* infection in the Netherlands. *Trop. geogr. Med.*, Amsterdam, **12**, 67.

VAN WYMEERSCH, H. and WANSON, M. (1954). *Afmillifer armillatus* infection and its X-ray manifestations. *Ann. Soc. belge Méd. trop.*, **34**, 517.

VARGHESE, P. J. G., et al. (1966). Reported in 'Diabetes in the tropics'. *Brit. med. J.*, **1**, 914.

VASANTHA, L., SRIKANTIA, S. G. and GOPALAN, C. (1970). Biochemical changes in the skin in kwashiorkor. *Amer. J. clin. Nutr.*, **93**, 78.

VAUCEL, M. A., et al. (1963). Répartition de la trypanosomiase africaine chez l'homme et les animaux. *Bull. Wld Hlth Org.*, **28**, 545.

VAUGHAN, J. P., et al. (1970). Chronic idiopathic jaundice in Papua and New Guinea. *Trans. roy. Soc. trop. Med. Hyg.*, **64**, 287.

VEIGA, S. and VAITHIANATHAN, T. (1963). Massive intravascular sickling after exchange transfusion with sickle-cell trait blood. *Transfusion (Philad.)*, **3**, 387.

VEJJAJIVA, A. (1972). In *Tropical Neurology*, quoted by Spillane (1972). Oxford University Press, London.

VELASCO, M., *et al.* (1971). Primary carcinoma of the liver associated with Australia antigen. *Lancet*, **1**, 1183.

VELLA, E. E. (1972). Cholera and vaccine prophylaxis. *Brit. J. Hosp. Med.*, **10**, 255.

— (1974). Rabies. *J. roy. Army med. Cps*, **120**, 80.

VELLA, E. E. and GOODE, D. (1973). Holiday brucellosis. *J. roy. Army med. Cps.*, **119**, 1, 34.

VELLA, F. (1959). Heterogeneity of human foetal haemoglobin: incidence of foetal variants in Singapore. *Nature (Lond.)*, **184**, 272.

— (1973). Thalassaemia in the British. *Brit. med. J.*, **3**, 593.

VELLA, F., AGER, J. A. M. and LEHMANN, H. (1959). New variant of human foetal haemoglobin. *Nature (Lond.)*, **183**, 31.

VELLA, F. and IBRAHIM, S. A. (1961). Thalassaemia in an English and in a German family. *Nature (Lond.)*, **191**, 822.

VELLA, F., WELLS, R. H. C., AGER, J. A. M. and LEHMANN, H. (1958). A haemoglobinopathy involving haemoglobin H and a new (Q) haemoglobin. *Brit. med. J.*, **1**, 752.

VENKATACHALAM, P. S. and PATWARDHAN, V. N. (1953). The role of *Ascaris lumbricoides* in the nutrition of the host: effect of ascariasis on digestion of protein. *Trans. roy. Soc. trop. Med. Hyg.*, **47**, 169.

VENTAKASWAMY, G. (1972). India. *Israel J. med. Sci.*, **8**, 1064.

VENTRUTO, V., BAGLIONI, C., DE ROSA, L., BIANCHI, P., COLOMBO, B. and QUATTRIN, N. (1965). Haemoglobin Caserta: an abnormal haemoglobin observed in a Southern Italian family. *Scand. J. Hameat.*, **2**, 118.

VERDRAGER, J. (1964). Observations on the longevity of *Plasmodium falciparum*: with special reference to findings in Mauritius. *Bull. Wld Hlth Org.*, **31**, 747.

VERHAGEN, A. R. H. B. and KOTEN, J. W. (1967). Psoriasis in Kenya. *Arch. Derm.*, **96**, 39.

VIANNA, N. J., *et al.* (1972). Hodgkin's disease: cases with features of a community outbreak. *Ann. intern. Med.*, **77**, 169.

VICKERMAN, K. (1962). The mechanism of cyclical development in trypanosomes of the *Trypanosoma brucei* subgroup: an hypothesis based on ultrastructural observations. *Trans. roy. Soc. trop. Med. Hyg.*, **56**, 487.

VILLEGAS, A. L., *et al.* (1972). Onchocerciasis in Colombia. Ocular findings in the first observed focus. *Amer. J. trop. Med. Hyg.*, **21**, 944.

VILLELA, E. (1941). Histology of human yellow fever when death is delayed. *Arch. Path.*, **31**, 665.

VIRANUVATTI, V., STITNIMANKARN, T. and TANSURAT, P. (1953). A fatal case of infection with *Fasciolopsis buskii* in Thailand. *Ann. trop. Med. Parasit.*, **47**, 132.

VIRANUVATTI, V., *et al.* (1967). *Percutaneous transheptic cholangiography in opisthorchiasis*. SEAMES, Third Conference on Parasitic Diseases. Abstracts of Papers, p. 134.

VISWANATHAN, R. (1948). Pulmonary eosinophiliosis. *Quart. J. Med.*, **17**, 257.

VOGEL, C. L. and LINSELL, C. A. (1972). International symposium on hepatocellular carcinoma. *J. nat. Cancer Inst.*, **48**, 567.

VOGEL, C. L., *et al.* (1972). Hepatitis associated antigen and antibody in hepatocellular carcinoma. *J. nat. Cancer Inst.*, **48**, 1583.

VOGEL, H. and CREWE, W. (1965). Beobachtungen uber die Lungenegel-Infektion in Kamerun (Westafrika). (Lung Fluke Infection in the Cameroons, West Africa.) *Z. tropenmed. Parasit.*, **16**, No. 2, 109.

VOLLER, A. and BRAY, R. S. (1962). Fluorescent antibody staining as a measure of malarial antibody. *Proc. Soc. exp. Biol.*, **110**, 907.

DE VRIES, A., JOSHUA, H., LEHMANN, H., HILL, R. L. and FELLOWS, R. E. (1963). The first observation of an abnormal haemoglobin in a Jewish family: haemoglobin Beilinson. *Brit. J. Haemat.*, **9**, 484.

WAALER, H. TH. and OECON, C. (1967). *A dynamic model for the epidemiology of tuberculosis.* W.H.O. Mimeographed document. WHO/TB/Techn. Information/67.54).

WADDY, B. B. (1952). Climate and respiratory infections. *Lancet*, **2**, 674.

— (1957). African epidemic cerebro-spinal meningitis. Part I. *J. trop. Med. Hyg.*, **60**, 179.

— (1957). African epidemic cerebro-spinal meningitis. Part II: Cerebro-spinal meningitis in other related African territories. *J. trop. Med. Hyg.*, **60**, 218.

— (1966). Oncocerciasis in the Usambara mountains, Tanzania: the disease, its epidemiology and its relationship to ocular complications. Discussion. *Trans. roy. Soc. trop. Med. Hyg.*, **60**, 727.

WADE, G. and BALL, J. (1957). Unexplained pulmonary hypertension. *Quart. J. Med.* (n.s.), **26**, 83.

WADE, H. H. (1962). Sarcoidosis in the tropics. *Int. J. Leprosy*, **30**, 342.

WADIA, N. H. (1967). Myelopathy complicating congenital atlanto-axial dislocation. *Brain*, **90**, 449.

— (1973). An introduction to neurology in India. In *Tropical Neurology*, ed. J. D. Spillane, p. 25. Oxford University Press, London.

WAHI, P. N., KAPUR, V. L., LUTHRA, U. K. and SRIVASTAVA, M. C. (1966). Submucous fibrosis of the oral cavity. 2: Studies on epidemiology. *Bull. Wld Hlth Org.*, **35**, 793.

WAINWRIGHT, J. (1957). *Coenurus cerebralis* and racemose cysts of the brain. *J. Path. Bact.*, **73**, 347.

— (1957). Siderosis in the African. *S. Afr. J. Lab. clin. Med.*, **3**, 1.

— (1961). Atheroma in the African (Bantu) in Natal. *Lancet*, **1**, 366.

WALDER, B. K., ROBERTSON, M. R. and JEREMY, D. (1971). Skin cancer and immunosuppression. *Lancet*, **2**, 1282.

WALIA, B. N. S., SIDHU, J. K., TANDON, B. N., GHAI, O. P. and BHARGAVA, S. (1966). Coeliac disease in North Indian children. *Brit. med. J.*, **2**, 1233.

WALKER, A. R. P. (1963). Extremes of coronary heart disease mortality in Johannesburg, South Africa. *Amer. Heart J.*, **66**, 293.

WALKER, A. R. P. and WALKER, B. F. (1969). Bowel motility and colonic cancer. *Brit. med. J.*, **3**, 238.

WALKER, D. and JORDAN, W. P. (1968). Tuberculous ulcer of penis. *J. Urol.*, **100**, 36.

WALKER, F. A., HSIA, D. Y. Y., SLATIS, H. M. and STEINBERG, A. G. (1962). Galactosemia: a study of twenty-seven kindreds in North America. *Ann. hum. Genet.*, **25**, 287.

WALKER, G. (1974). The immunology of liver disorders. *Proc. roy. Soc. Med.*, **67**, 566.

WALKER, J. and SPOONER, E. T. C. (1960). Natural infection of the African baboon, *Papio papio*, with the large cell form of histoplasma. *J. Path. Bact.*, **80**, 436.

WALKER, J. S., *et al.* (1973). Involvement of small mammals in the transmission of scrub typhus in Malaysia: Isolation and serological evidence. *Trans. roy. Soc. trop. Med. Hyg.*, **67**, 838.

WALKER, W. and ELLIS, M. I. (1970). Intrauterine transfusion. *Brit. med. J.*, **2**, 223.

WALKER-SMITH, J. A., MCMILLAN, B., MIDDLETON, A. W., ROBERTSON, S. and HOPCROFT, A. (1969). Strongyloidiasis causing small-bowel obstruction in an aboriginal infant. *Med. J. Aust.*, **2**, 1263.

WALLACE, A. F. (1960). Aetiology of the idiopathic hydrocele. *Brit. J. Urol.*, **32**, 79.

WALLACE, C. K., et al. (1966). Classical and El Tor cholera: A clinical comparison. *Brit. med. J.*, **2**, 447.

WALLACE, J., MILNE, G. R. and BARR, A. (1972). Total screening of blood donations for Australia antigen and its antibody. *Brit. med. J.*, **1**, 663.

WALLOOPPILLAI, N. J. and JAYASINGHE, M. S. (1970). Congenital heart disease in Ceylon. *Brit. Heart J.* **32**, 304.

WALSH, J. J., BURCH, G. E., BLACK, W. C., FERRANS, V. J. and HIBBS, R. G. (1965). Idiopathic myocardiopathy of the puerperium (postpartal heart disease). *Circulation*, **32**, 19.

WALTERS, J. H. and SMITH, D. A. (1952). Oedematous beri-beri in Gambian palm wine tappers. *W. Afr. med. J.* (n.s.), **1**, 21.

WALTON, B. C. and CHYU, I. (1959). Clonorchiasis and paragonimiasis in the Republic of Korea. Report on a prevalence survey using intradermal tests. *Bull. Wld Hlth Org.*, **21**, No. 6, 721.

WALZER, P. D., et al. (1971). Giardiasis in travellers. *J. infect. Dis.*, **124**, 235.

WANG, C. I., et al. (1968). Cystic fibrosis in an oriental child. *New Engl. J. Med.*, **279**, 1216.

WAPNICK, A. A., BOTHWELL, T. H. and SEFTEL, H. (1970). The relationship between serum iron levels and ascorbic acid stores in siderotic Bantu. *Brit. J. Haemat.*, **19**, 271.

WARD, J. S. (1972). *Yellow Fever in Latin America: A Geographical Study*. Published by the Centre for Latin American Studies, University of Liverpool, Monograph Series No. 3.

WARLEY, M. A., BLACKLEDGE, P. and O'GORMAN, P. (1968). Lead poisoning from eye cosmetics. *Brit. med. J.*, **1**, 117.

WARREN, K. S. (1969). Intestinal obstruction in urinary *Schistosomiasis japonica*. *Gastroenterology*, **57**, 697.

— (1972). The immunopathogenesis of schistosomiasis. A multidisciplinary approach. *Trans. roy. Soc. trop. Med. Hyg.*, **66**, 3, 417.

WARSHAW, J. B. and SPACH, M. S. (1965). Takayasu's disease (primary aortitis) in childhood: case report with review of literature. *Pediatrics*, Springfield, **35**, 620.

WARTMAN, W. B. (1947). Filariasis in American armed forces in World War II. *Medicine (Baltimore)*, **26**, 333.

WASI, C., WASI, P. and THONGCHAROEN, P. (1971). Serum-immunoglobulin levels in thalassaemia and the effects of splenectomy. *Lancet*, **1**, 237.

WASI, P., et al. (1967). Haemoglobin E and α-thalassaemia. *Brit. med. J.*, **4**, 29.

WASSERMAN, H. P. (1965). The circulation of melanin—its clinical and physiological significance. *S. Afr. med. J.*, **39**, 711.

WATERLOW, J. C. (1948). Fatty liver disease in infants in the British West Indies. *Spec. Rep. Ser. med. Res. Coun. (Lond.)*, No. 263.

— (1959). Protein nutrition and enzyme changes in man. *Fed. Proc.*, **18**, 1143.

— (1971). Enzyme changes in malnutrition. *J. clin. Path.*, **24**, suppl. 4, 75.

— (1973). Nutrition and the developing brain. *Lancet*, **1**, 425.

— (1973). Note on the assessment and classification of protein energy malnutrition in children. *Lancet*, **2**, 87.

— (1974). Evolution of kwashiorkor and marasmus. *Lancet*, **2**, 712.

— (1974). Some aspects of childhood malnutrition as a public health problem. *Brit. med. J.*, **4**, 88.

WATLER, D. C. (1960). Congenital heart disease in Jamaica. *W. Indian med. J.*, **9**, 194.

WATLER, D. C., BRAS, G. and BROOKS, S. E. N. (1961). The incidence of malignant neoplasms in Jamaica. *Path. Microbiol.*, **24**, 698.

WATSON, H. J. C. (1973). The epidemiology of human sleeping sickness in the Lambwe Valley, South Nyanza, Kenya. *Bull. Wld Hlth Org.*, **47**, 6, Article 2956.

WATSON, J. M. and KERIM, R. A. (1956). Observations on forms of parasitic pharyngitis known as 'Halzoun' in the Middle East. *J. trop. Med. Hyg.*, **59**, 147.

WATSON, K. C. and LAURIE, W. (1955). Cerebral coenuriasis in man. *Lancet*, **2**, 1321.

WATSON, P. G. and GAIRDNER, D. (1968). Tric agent as a cause of neonatal eye sepsis. *Brit. med. J.*, **3**, 527.

WATSON-WILLIAMS, E. J. (1965). Herediatry persistence of foetal haemoglobin and β-thalassaemia in Nigerians. *Abnormal Haemoglobins: Symposium*. Ibadan. Blackwell Scientific Publications, Oxford.

WATSON-WILLIAMS, E. J. and ALLAN, N. C. (1968). Idiopathic tropical splenomegaly syndrome in Ibadan. *Brit. med. J.*, **4**, 793.

WATSON-WILLIAMS, E. J. and FLEMING, A. F. (1966). Isolated malabsorption of Vitamin B_{12} causing megaloblastic anaemia and hyperpigmentation in a Nigerian. *Blood*, **28**, 770.

WATT, J. M. and BREYER-BRANDWIJK, M. G. (1962). *The Medicinal and Poisonous Plants of Southern and Eastern Africa*. 2nd ed. Livingstone, Edinburgh.

WATTEN, R. H., KUNTZ, R. E. and LIU, H. Y. (1960). Use of purified antigens for Detection of *Paragonimus westermani* and *Clonorchis sinensis* in peoples of Hsinchu Hsien, Taiwan (Formosa). *J. Formosan med. Ass.*, **59**, No. 6, 364.

WATTEN, R. H., *et al.* (1972). Clinical studies of capillariasis Philippinensis. *Trans. roy. Soc. trop. Med. Hyg.*, **66**, 828.

WATTS, R. W. E. (1973). Oxaluria. *J. roy. Coll. Phycns.*, *Lond.*, **7**, 161.

WEATHERALL, D. J. (1964). Hemoglobin J (Baltimore) coexisting in a family with hemoglobin S[1]. *Bull. Johns Hopk. Hosp.*, **114**, 1.

— (1964). The relationship of hemoglobin of unusual genetic interest. *Blood*, **21**, 675.

WEATHERALL, D. J. and BOYER, S. H. (1962). Evidence for the genetic identity of alpha-chain determinants in hemoglobins A, A_2, and F. *Bull. Johns Hopk. Hosp.*, **111**, 143.

WEATHERALL, D. J. and GLEGG, J. B. (1974). *The Thalassaemia Syndromes*. Blackwell Scientific Publications, Oxford.

WEAVER, A. L. and SPITTELL, J. A., JR. (1964). Lathyrism. *Mayo Clinic Proc.* **39**, 485.

WEBB, J. F. and SIMPSON, B. (1966). Tropical sprue in Hong Kong. *Brit. med. J.*, **2**, 1162.

WEBB, J. K. G., JOB, C. K. and GAULT, E. W. (1960). Tropical eosinophila. Demonstration of microfilariae in lung, liver and lymph-nodes. *Lancet*, **1**, 835.

WEBB, W. R. and HERRING, J. L. (1962). Pericarditis due to histoplasmosis. *Amer. Heart J.*, **64**, 679.

WEBBE, G. (1965). Natural trends in snail populations in relation to control of bilharziasis in East Africa. *E. Afr. med. J.*, **42**, No. 11, 605.

WEBBER, T. H. and HANSHAW, J. B. (1962). Urologic and clinical observations on cytomegalic inclusion disease. *New Engl. J. Med.*, **266**, 1233.

WEDDERBURN, N. (1970). Effect of concurrent malarial infection on development of virus-induced lymphoma in BALB/C mice. *Lancet*, **2**, 1114.

WEEREKOON, L. (1972). Ocular leprosy in West Malaysia. *Brit. J. Ophthal.*, **56**, 106.

WEINBERG, M. and PARVU, M. (1908). Diagnostic de l'échinococcose par la recherche des anticorps spécifiques. *C. R. Soc. Biol.*, **65**, 562.

WEINMAN, D. (1963). Problems of diagnosis of trypanosomiasis. *Bull. Wld Hlth Org.*, **28**, 731.

WEINSTEIN, P. P. (1958). Some projected uses for the axenic cultivation of helminths. *Amer. J. trop. Med. Hyg.*, **7**, 1.

WEINSTEIN, P. P., KRAWCZYK, H. J. and PEERS, J. H. (1954). Sparganosis in Korea. *Amer. J. trop. Med. Hyg.*, **3**, 112.

WEIR, J. M., WASIF, I. M., HASSAN, F. R., ATTIA, S. M., KADU, M. A. (1952). An evaluation of health and sanitation in Egyptian villages. *J. Egypt. publ. Hlth Ass.*, **27**, 55.

WEISS, D. W. (1973). Current aspects of tumour immunology. *Israeli J. med. Sci.*, **9**, 205.

WEISS, H. J., *et al.* (1969). Afibrinogenaemia in man following the bite of rattlesnake. *Amer. J. med.*, **47**, 625.

WEISS, S. and WILKINS, R. W. (1937). The nature of cardiovascular disturbances in nutritional deficiency states (beriberi). *Ann. intern. Med.*, **11**, 104.

WEISS-CARMINE, S. (1957). Die Endocarditis parietalis fibroplastica mit Bluteosinophilie (Löffler) und ihre Stellung im Rahmen der Parientalendokardfibrosen. *Schweiz. med. Wschr.*, **87**, 890.

WEITZ, B. (1963). The antigenicity of some African trypanosomes. In *Immunity to Protozoa*, eds. P. C. C. Garnham, A. E. Pierce and I. Roitt. Blackwell Scientific Publications, Oxford.

WELLER, T. H. and HANSHAW, J. B. (1962). Virologic and clinical observations on cytomegalic inclusion disease. *New Engl. J. Med.*, **266**, 1233.

WELLS, R. (1958). Anaemia in Singapore—an analysis of 1,046 cases. *Trans. roy. Soc. trop. Med. Hyg.*, **52**, 431.

WELTY, R. F., LUDDEN, T. E. and BEAVER, P. C. (1963). Dirofilariasis in man: report of a case from the State of Washington. *Amer. J. trop. Med. Hyg.*, **12**, 888.

WEMAMBU, S. N. C., TURK, J. L., WATERS, M. F. R. and REES, R. J. W. (1969). Erythema nodosum leprosum. *Lancet*, **2**, 933.

WÉRY-PASKOFF, S., *et al.* (1974). The fluorescent antibody test in the serological diagnosis of amoebiasis. Possible epidemiological application. *Ann. Soc. belge Méd. trop.*, **54**, 65.

WESSEL, H. U., SOMMERS, H. M., CUGELL, D. W. and PAUL, M. H. (1965). Variants of cardiopulmonary manifestations of Manson's schistosomiasis: report of two cases. *Ann. intern Med.*, **62**, 757.

WHALEN, G. C., *et al.* (1969). Intestinal capillariasis. A new disease in man. *Lancet*, **1**, 13.

WHALLEY, P. J., *et al.* (1964). Sickle cell trait and pyelonephritis, in pregnancy. *J. Amer. med. Assoc.*, **189**, 903.

WHARTON, B. (1970). Hypoglycaemia in children with kwashiorkor. *Lancet*, **1**, 171.

WHARTON, B., HOWELLS, G. and PHILLIPS, I. (1968). Diarrhoea in kwashiorkor. *Brit. med. J.*, **4**, 608.

WHARTON, B. A., *et al.* (1969). The myocardium in kwashiorkor. *Quart. J. Med.*, **38**, 107.

WHITAKER, J. A., *et al.* (1967). Hematologic response to vitamin E in the anemia associated with protein-calorie malnutrition. *Amer. J. clin. Nutr.*, **20**, 783.

WHITCOMB, M. E., *et al.* (1970). Interstitial fibrosis after *Pneumocystis carinii* pneumonia. *Ann. intern. Med.*, **73**, 761.

WHITE, G. B. B., LASHEEN, R. M., BAILLIE, M. B. and TURNER, G. C. (1971). Comparison of three serological methods for the detection of hepatitis-associated antigen. *J. clin. Path.*, **24**, 8.

WHITE, H. A. (1972). Lassa fever. A study of 23 hospital cases. *Trans. roy. Soc. trop. Med. Hyg.*, **66**, 390.

WHITE, J. M. and DACIE, J. V. (1971). The unstable hemoglobins. *Progress in Hematology*. I, p. 69. Heinemann, London.

WHITEHEAD, R. G. (1964). Rapid determination of some plasma aminoacids in subclinical kwashiorkor. *Lancet*, **1**, 250.

— (1965). Hydroxyproline creatinine ratio as an index of nutritional status and rate of growth. *Lancet*, **2**, 567.

WHITEHEAD, R. G., *et al.* (1973). Serum-albumin concentration and the onset of kwashiorkor. *Lancet*, **1**, 63.

WHITTLE, H. C., *et al.* (1973). Scabies, pyoderma and nephritis in Zaria, Nigeria. *Trans. roy. Soc. trop. Med. Hyg.*, **67**, 349.

WHITTLE, H. C., *et al.* (1973). Allergic complications of meningococcal disease. *Brit. med. J.*, **2**, 733.

— (1974). Rapid bacteriological diagnosis of pyogenic meningitis by latex agglutination. *Lancet*, **2**, 619.

WICKS, A. C. B. and JONES, J. J. (1973). Insulinopenic diabetes in Africa. *Brit. med. J.* **1**, 773.

WICKS, A. C. B., *et al.* (1971). Endemic typhoid fever. *J. med. Quart.* **40**, 341

WIDDELL, A. G. M., PALMER, E. and REES, R. J. W. (1970). The fate of mycobacterium leprae in CBA mice. *J. Path.*, **108**, 77.

WIDE, L., ROOS, P. and GEMZELL, C. A. (1961). Immunological determination of human pituitary luteinizing hormone. *Acta endocr., Copenh.*, **37**, 445.

WIENER, A. S. (1942). The Rh factor and racial origins. *Science*, **96**, 407.

WIG, K. L., *et al.* (1962). Prevalence of coronary atherosclerosis in Northern India. *Brit. med. J.*, **1**, 510.

WIJERS, D. J. B. (1958). Factors that may influence the infection rate of *Glossina palpalis* with *Trypanosoma gambiense*. I. The age of the fly at the time of the infected feed. *Ann. trop. Med. Parasit.*, **52**, 385.

WILDER, H. C. (1950). Nematode endophthalmitis. *Trans. Amer. Acad. Ophthal. Otolaryng.*, 99.

— (1952). *Toxoplasma* chorioretinitis in adults. *A.M.A. Arch. Ophthal.*, **48**, 127.

WILLAERT, E. (1974). Primary amoebic meningo-encephalitis. A selected bibliography and tabular survey of cases. *Ann. Soc. belge. Méd. trop.*, **54**, 429.

WILLETT, K. C. (1965). Some observations on the recent epidemiology of sleeping sickness in Nyanza region, Kenya, and its relation to the general epidemiology of Gambian and Rhodesian sleeping sickness in Africa. *Trans. roy. Soc. trop. Med. Hyg.*, **59**, 374.

WILLIAMS, A. O. (1966). Haemoglobin genotypes, ABO blood groups, and Burkitt's tumour. *J. Med. Genetics*, **3**, 177.

— (1967). Pathology of schistosomiasis of the uterine cervix due to *S. haematobium*. *Amer. J. Obstet. Gynaec.*, **98**, 784.

— (1967). Melanotic ameloblastoma (Progonoma) of infancy showing osteogenesis. *J. Path. Bact.*, **93**, 545.

— (1969). Atherosclerosis in the Nigerian. *J. Path.*, **99**, 219.

WILLIAMS, A. O. and ALMEIDA, J. D. (1972). Hepatitis associated (Australia) antigen in Nigerians. *Amer. J. trop. Med. Hyg.*, **21**, 473.

WILLIAMS, A. O., LAGUNDOYE, S. B. and BANKOLE, M. A. (1970). Sacrococcygeal teratoma in Nigerian children. *Arch. Dis. Childh.*, **45**, 110.

WILLIAMS, A. O., LAWSON, E. A. and LUCAS, A. O. (1971). African histoplasmosis. *Arch.
Path.*, **92**, 306.

WILLIAMS, A. O., MARTINSON, F. D. and ALLI, A. F. (1968). Rhabdomyosarcoma of the
upper respiratory tract in Ibadan, Nigeria. *Brit. J. Cancer*, **22**, 12.

WILLIAMS, A. O. and OSOTIMEHIN, B. (1970). Autopsy study of measles in Ibadan,
Nigeria. *Ghana med. J.*, March 13–27.

WILLIAMS, A. O. and OSUNTOKUN, B. O. (1969). Peripheral neuropathy in tropical
(nutritional) ataxia in Nigeria. *Arch. Neurol.*, **21**, 475.

WILLIAMS, C. D. (1933). A nutritional disease of childhood associated with a maize
diet. *Arch. Dis. Childh.*, **8**, 423.

— (1946). Rickets in Singapore. *Arch. Dis. Childh.*, **21**, 37.

WILLIAMS, E. (1973). Brucellosis. *Brit. med. J.*, **1**, 791.

WILLIAMS, J. E. and IMLARP, S. (1972). Susceptibility of rodents to Japanese encephalitis virus. *Bull. Wld Hlth Org.*, **46**, 854.

WILLIAMS, J. F., LOPEZ ADAROS, H. and TREJOS, A. (1971). Current prevalence and
distribution of hydatidosis with special reference to the Americas. *Amer. J. trop.
Med. Hyg.*, **20**, 224.

WILLIAMS, R., PARSONSON, A., SOMERS, K. and HAMILTON, P. J. S. (1966). Portal hypertension in idiopathic tropical splenomegaly. *Lancet*, **1**, 329.

WILLIAMS, R. C., CATHCART, E. S., CALKINS, E., FITE, G. L., BARBA RUBIO, J. and COHEN,
A. S. (1965). Secondary amyloidosis in lepromatous leprosy: possible relationships
of diet and environment. *Ann. intern Med.*, **62**, 1000.

WILLIAMSON, J. (1963). The chemical composition of trypanosomes. *Proc. 16th Int.
Congr. Zool.*, **4**, 189.

WILLIS, A. J. P., and NWOKOLO, C. (1966). Steroid therapy and strongyloidiasis.
Lancet, **1**, 1396.

WILLMOT, F. C. and ROBERTSON, G. W. (1920). Senecio disease, or cirrhosis of the liver
due to senecio poisoning. *Lancet*, **2**, 848.

WILMOT, A. J. (1962). *Clinical Amoebiasis*. Blackwell Scientific Publications, Oxford.

WILLS, V. G. and WATERLOW, J. C. (1958). The death-rate in the age-group 1–4 years
as an index of malnutrition. *J. trop. Pediat.*, **3**, 167.

WILSON, A. H. (1915). Notes of two cases of *Porocephalus armillatus* infection occurring in man. *A. med. Rep. Sth. Nigeria*, 1913, 71.

WILSON, J. (1972). Keynote address. *Israel J. med. Sci.*, **8**, 1032.

WILSON, R. J. M., MCGREGOR, I. A. and WILSON, M. E. (1973). The stability and frac-
tionation of malarial antigens from the blood of Africans infected with *Plasmodium
falciparum*. *Int. J. Parasit.*, **3**, 4, 511.

WILSON, S. and THOMPSON, A. E. (1964). A fatal case of strongyloidiasis. *J. Path. Bact.*,
87, 169.

WILSON, T. (1961). Filariasis in Malaya—a general review. *Trans. roy. Soc. trop. Med.
Hyg.*, **55**, 107.

WILSON, V. C. L. C., *et al.* (1972). Human cocnurosis—the first reported case from
Ghana. *Trans. roy. Soc. trop. Med. Hyg.*, **66**, 4, 611.

WING, A. J., *et al.* (1971). Urinary pH values in African, Asian and European subjects
in Kampala. *Afr. J. Med. Sci.*, **2**, 329.

WINKLER, P. G., *et al.* (1973). Differences in the severity of physical signs in the right
and left eyes of patients with trachoma in Syria and Burma. *Bull. Wld Hlth Org.*,
47, 177.

WINSLOW, D. J. (1971). *Mycetoma in Human Infection with Fungi, Actinomycetes and Algae*, ed. R. D. Barker, p. 589. Springer Verlag, New York.

WINTER, S. T. (1954). The incidence of rickets in Israeli infants: a clinical and radiological study. *Acta med. orient.*, **13**, 91.

WINTROBE, W. M. (1961). *Clinical Haematology.* 5th ed. Kimpton, London.

WISEMAN, R. A. (1967). *Acanthocheilonema perstans.* A cause of significant eosinophilia in the tropics: comments on its pathogenicity. *Trans. roy. Soc. trop. Med. Hyg.*, **61**, 667.

WISEMAN, R. A. and LOVEL, T. W. I. (1969). Human infection with adult *Toxocara cati.* *Brit. med. J.*, **3**, 454.

WISEMAN, R. A. and WOODRUFF, A. W. (1971). Toxocariasis in Africa and Malta. *Trans. roy. Soc. trop. Med. Hyg.*, **65**, 439.

WOKES, F., BADENOCH, J. and SINCLAIR, H. M. (1955). Human dietary deficiency of vitamin B_{12}. *Am. J. clin. Nutr.*, **3**, 375.

WOLLF, H. L. (1971). A quantitative approach to epidemiology and control of cholera. *Bull. Soc. Path. exot.*, **64**, 582.

WOLFF, J. W. (1954). *The Laboratory Diagnosis of Leptospirosis.* Charles C. Thomas, Springfield, Illinois.

WONG HOCK BOON, ANG POON LIAT and GHAZALI ISMAIL (1973). Dengue haemorrhagic fever in children in Singapore in the 1973 outbreak. I. General features and criteria for shock and pre-shock. *J. Singapore Paed. Soc.*, **15**, 2, 46.

WONG, P. C. (1964). Anonymous mycobacteria isolated from clinical specimens in Hong Kong. *J. trop. Med. Hyg.*, **67**, 100.

WONG, W. M. (1964). Studies on microfilaremia in dogs. II. Levels of microfilaremia in relation to immunologic responses of the host. *Amer. J. trop. Med. Hyg.*, **13**, 66.

WOODFIELD, D. G. (1972). An antigen and antibody in cord and maternal serum. *Brit. med. J.*, **3**, 763.

WOODROW, J. C., NOBLE, R. L. and MARTINDALE, J. H. (1964). Haemoglobin H disease in an English family. *Brit. med. J.*, **1**, 36.

WOODRUFF, A. W. (1964). Infection with animal helminths. *Brit. med. J.*, **1**, 1001.

— (1968). Helminths as vehicles and synergists of microbial infections. *Trans. roy. Soc. trop. Med. Hyg.*, **62**, 446.

— (1970). Toxocariasis. *Brit. med. J.*, **3**, 663.

WOODRUFF, A. W., *et al.* (1963). Onchocerciasis and the eye in Western Uganda. *Trans. roy. Soc. trop. Med. Hyg.*, **57**, 50.

WOODRUFF, A. W., *et al.* (1966a). Onchocerciasis in the Usambara Mountains, Tanzania: the disease, its epidemiology and its relationship to ocular complications. *Trans. roy. Soc. trop. Med. Hyg.*, **60**, 695.

WOODRUFF, A. W., *et al.* (1966b). Onchocerciasis in Guatemala. A clinical and parasitological study with comparisons between the disease there and in East Africa. *Trans. roy. Soc. trop. Med. Hyg.*, **60**, 707.

WORINGER, F., TULASNE, R. and TRENSZ, F. (1961). Large ulceration with paratubercular bacilli (*Mycobacterium ulcerans*). *Bull. Soc. franç. Derm. Syph.*, **68**, 325.

WORKING GROUP (1965). Working group on asbestosis and cancer. *Arch. Environm. Hlth*, **11**, 221.

WORLD HEALTH ORGANIZATION TUBERCULOSIS CHEMOTHERAPY CENTRE (1961). An investigation of household contacts of open cases of pulmonary tuberculosis amongst the Kikuyu in Kiambu, Kenya. *Bull. Wld Hlth Org.*, **25**, 831.

WORLD HEALTH ORGANIZATION (1962). Poliomyelitis in the Eastern Mediterranean Region. *W.H.O. Chron.*, **16**, 91.

— (1962). Problems of leukaemia. *W.H.O. Chron.*, **16**, 399.

— (1964). W.H.O. expert committee on smallpox. *Wld Hlth Org. techn. Rep. Ser.* No. 283.

— (1964). Soil-transmitted helminths: report of a W.H.O. expert committee on helminthiases. *Wld Hlth Org. tech. Rep. Ser.*, No. 277.

— (1964). Joint F.A.O./W.H.O. expert committee on brucellosis, fourth report. *Wld Hlth Org. tech. Rep. Ser.*, No. 289.

— (1965). Cardiomyopathies. *Bull. Wld Hlth Org.*, **33**, 257.

— (1965). Diabetes mellitus. *Wld Hlth Org. tech. Rep. Ser.*, No. 310.

— (1965). Hypovitaminosis A and the eye. (Notes and news.) *W.H.O. Chron.*, **19**, 197.

— (1965). W.H.O. expert committee on bilharziasis. Third report. *Wld Hlth Org. tech. Rep. Ser.*, No. 299.

— (1965). Bibliography of hookworm disease (Ancylostomiasis) 1920–1962, W.H.O. Geneva.

— (1966). Plague in 1965. *Wkly epidem. Rec.*, **41**, 362.

— (1966). Malnutrition in early childhood. *W.H.O. Chron.*, **20**, 83.

— (1966). W.H.O. expert committee on leprosy, third report. *Wld Hlth Org. tech. Rep. Ser.*, No. 319.

— (1966). W.H.O. expert committee on rabies. Fifth report, Geneva. *Wld Hlth Org. tech. Rep. Ser.*, No. 321.

— (1966). W.H.O. expert committee on onchocerciasis. Second Report. Geneva. 29 June–5 July 1965. *Wld Hlth Org. tech. Rep. Ser.*, No. 335.

— (1967). Arbo viruses and human disease. *Wld Hlth Org. tech. Rep. Ser.*, No. 369.

— (1967). Current problems in leptospirosis research. Report of a W.H.O. Expert Group. *Wld Hlth Org. tech. Rep. Ser.*, No. 380.

— (1967). The Cardiomyopathies. *W.H.O. Chron.*, **21**, 411.

— (1967). *World Health Statistics Annual.* Vol. 1. Vital Statistics and Causes of Death—Geneva.

— (1967). Requirements of vitamin A, thiamine, niacin: report of a riboflavine and joint F.A.O./W.H.O. expert group, Rome, Italy, 6–17 September 1965. *Wld Hlth Org. tech. Rep. Ser.*, No. 362; *F.A.O. Nutr. Mtg Rep. Ser.*, No. 41.

— (1967). Urbanization and public health *W.H.O. Chron.*, **21**, 428.

— (1968). Food poisoning by insecticides in Arabia. *W.H.O. Chron.*, **22**, 131.

— (1970). Fluorides and human health. Monograph series No. 59.

— (1971). Primary immunodeficiencies. *Pediatrics*, **47**, 927.

— (1972). Yellow Fever. *W.H.O. Chron.*, **26**, 60.

— (1972). Paracoccidiomycosis. Scientific Publication No. 254.

— (1972). Trace Elements and Cardiovascular Diseases. *W.H.O. Chron.*, **26**, 51.

— (1972). Nutrition: A review of the W.H.O. Programme—I. *W.H.O. Chron.*, **26**, 160.

— (1972). Nutrition: A review of the W.H.O. Programme—II. *W.H.O. Chron.*, **26**, 195.

— (1973). Prevention of blindness. *W.H.O. Chron.*, **27**, 21.

— (1973). Plague in 1972. *Wkly epidem. Rec.* **13**, 141.

— (1973). Pathogenic mechanisms in dengue haemorrhagic fever: report of an international collaborative study. *Bull. Wld Hlth Org.*, **48**, 117.

— (1973). Expert Committee on Rabies. *Wld Hlth Org. techn. Rep. Ser.*, No. 523.

— (1973). Viral Hepatitis. *Tech. Rep. Ser.*, 512.

— (1973). Epidemiological surveillance and control of cerebrospinal meningitis in Africa. *W.H.O. Chron.*, **27**, 347.

— (1973). Yellow fever. *Bull. Wld. Hlth. Org.*, **49**, 106.

— (1974). Dengue Haemorrhagic Fever in Thailand. *Wkly. epidem. Rec.*, **49**, 133.

— (1974). Louse-Borne Typhus in 1973. *Wkly. epidem. Rec.*, **49**, 149.

— (1974). Cardiovascular diseases: (1) Care and prevention. *W.H.O. Chron.*, **28**, 55.

— (1974). Cardiovascular diseases: (2) Care and prevention. *W.H.O. Chron.*, **28**, 116.

— (1974). Cardiovascular diseases: (3) Care and prevention. *W.H.O. Chron.*, **28**, 190.

— (1974). Malnutrition and mental development. *W.H.O. Chron.*, **28**, 95.

— (1974). Recent work on virus diseases. *WHO Chron.*, **28**, 410.

— (1974). WHO Expert Committee on Malaria—Sixteenth Report. *Techn. Rep. Ser.* 549.

WORLLEDGE, S., LUZZATTO, L., OGIEMUDIA, S. E., LUZZATTO, P., and EDINGTON, G. M. (1968). Rhesus immunization in Nigeria. *Vox Sang.*, **14**, 202.

WRIGHT, C. A., SOUTHGATE, V. R. and KNOWLES, R. J. (1972). What is *schistosoma intercalatum* Fisher 1934? *Trans. roy. Soc. trop. Med. Hyg.*, **66**, 28.

WRIGHT, D. H. (1963). Cytology and histochemistry of the Burkitt lymphoma. *Brit. J. Cancer*, **17**, 50.

WRIGHT, D. H., BELL, T. M. and WILLIAMS, M. C. (1967). Burkitt's tumour; A review of clinical features, treatment, pathology, epidemiology, entomology, and virology. *E. Afr. Med. J.*, **44**, 51.

WRIGHT, D. H. and STANFIELD, J. P. (1967). Enteritis necroticans in Uganda. *J. Pediat.*, **71**, 264.

WRIGHT, G. P. (1955). The neurotoxins of *Clostridium botulinum* and *Clostridium tetani*. *Pharmacol. Rev.*, **7**, 413.

WRIGHT, J. M. D. (1973). Autoantibodies in leprosy. *Lancet*, **2**, 40.

WYATT, G. B. (1974). Diphtheria. *Tropical Doctor*, **4**, 110.

WYATT, G. B. and MATTHEW, G. K. (1972). Prevalence of umbilical herniae in African preschool children. *Trans. roy. Soc. trop. Med. Hyg.*, **66**, 508.

WYNDER, E. L., *et al.* (1973). Epidemiology of cancer of the pancreas. *J. nat. Cancer Inst.*, **50**, 645.

WYNDHAM, C. H. (1961). Applied physiological research in the South African gold mining industry. *Proc. 7th Cwlth Min. Metall. Congr.*, Johannesburg.

YAMAGATI, S., *et al.* (1964). Studies on clonorchiasis in Miyagi Prefecture. I. Infection of *Clonorchis* in general inhabitants. *Japanese J. Parasit.*, **13**, 112.

YAMAOKA, K., KAWAMURA, K., HANADA, M., SEITA, M., HITSUMOTO, S. and OOYA, L. (1960). Studies of abnormal haemoglobins. *Jap. J. hum. Genet.*, **5**, 99.

YARDLEY, J. H., TAKANO, J. and HENDRIX, T. B. (1964). Epithelial and other mucosal lesions of the jejunum in giardiasis: jejunal biopsy studies. *Bull. Johns Hopk. Hosp.*, **115**, 389.

YASE, Y. (1970). Neurologic disease in the Western Pacific islands with a report on the focus of amyotrophic lateral sclerosis found in the Kii peninsula, Japan. *Amer. J. trop. Med. Hyg.*, **19**, 155.

YAWSON, G. I., HUNTSMAN, R. G. and METTERS, J. S. (1970). An assessment of techniques suitable for the diagnosis of sickle-cell disease and haemoglobin C disease in cord blood samples. *J. clin. Path.*, **23**, 533.

YEH, S. (1966). Some geographical aspects of the most common diseases in Taiwan. *Internat. Path.*, **7**, 24.

YEH, T. F. (1959). Primary carcinoma of the liver. *Chin. med. J.*, **79**, 538.

YEUNG LAIWAN, A. A. C. (1971). Australia antigen in acute and chronic liver disease. *Lancet*, **2**, 470.

YONG, W. K. (1973). Indirect fluorescent antibody technique with microfragments of *W. bancrofti*. *Trans. roy. Soc. trop. Med. Hyg.*, **67**, 3, 338.

YOUSSEF, A. F., FAYAD, M. M. and SHAFEEK, M. A. (1970). Bilharziasis of the Cervix Uteri. *J. Obstet. Gynaec. Birt. Cwlth*, **77**, 847.

YUE, P. C. K. (1974). Recurrent pyogenic cholangitis in children. *Aust. New Zeal. J. Surg.*, **44**, 53.

ZAHER, M. H. and EL DEEB, A. A. (1969). Bilharzial urethritis cystica. *J. Urol.*, **101**, 870,

ZAMAN, V. (1964). Studies on the immobilization reaction in the genus *Balantidium*. *Trans. roy. Soc. trop. Med. Hyg.*, **58**, 255.

— (1965). The application of fluorescent antibody test to *Balantidium coli*. *Trans. roy. Soc. trop. Med. Hyg.*, **59**, 80.

— (1972). Use of impregnated filter paper strips for staining malaria parasites. *Trans. roy. Soc. trop. Med. Hyg.*, **66**, 5, 810.

ZAMAN, V. and COLLEY, F. C. (1972). Ultrastructural study of penetration of macrophages by *Toxoplasma gondii*. *Trans. roy. Soc. trop. Med. Hyg.*, **66**, 781.

ZAMAN, V. and GOH, T. K. (1969). Toxoplasmic antibodies in various ethnic groups in Singapore. *Trans. roy. Soc. trop. Med. Hyg.*, **63**, 884.

ZELEDON, R. (1974). *Epidemiology, Modes of transmission and Reservoir Hosts of Chagas' Disease*. Ciba Foundation Symposium 20 (new series). Associated Scientific Publishers, Amsterdam.

ZERPA, F., HIRSCHHAUT, E., FERRER, A., CAPRILES, M. A. and DUBOIS, E. (1966). Takayasu's disease (primary aortitis): report on two cases in children. *Pediatrics*, Springfield, **38**, 637.

ZIEGLER, J. L. and STUIVER, P. C. (1972). Tropical splenomegaly syndrome in a Rwandan Kindred in Uganda. *Br. med. J.*, **3**, 79.

ZIGAS, V. (1973). Effect of kuru on pregnancy. *Trop. geogr. Med.*, **25**, 262.

ZIGAS, V. and BENFANTE, R. J. (1972). Human toxoplasmosis: an evaluation of current progress. *Trop. geogr. Med.*, **24**, 1.

ZIGAS, V. and GAJDUSEK, D. C. (1957). Kuru: Clinical study of a new syndrome resembling paralysis agitans in natives of the Eastern Highlands of Australian New Guinea. *Med. J. Aust.*, **2**, 745.

ZIMMERMAN, H. M. (1946). The pathology of Japanese B encephalitis. *Amer. J. Path.*, **22**, 965.

ZIPPIN, C., LUM, D. and HOM, P. (1966). *Epidemiology of Cancer of the Nasopharynx*, p. 722. Tokyo.

ZUCKERMAN, A. (1963). *Immunity in Malaria with Particular Reference to Red-cell Destruction in Immunity to Protozoa*. Blackwell Scientific Publications, Oxford.

ZUCKERMAN, A. J., TAYLOR, P. E., BIRD, R. G. and RUSSELL, S. M. (1971). The Australia antigen in fibrinogen and other fractions of human plasma. *J. clin. Path.*, **24**, 2.

ZUCKERMAN, S. S. and HIBBARD, J. S. (1945). Clinicopathologic study of early filariasis with lymph node biopsies. *Nav. med. Bull.*, **44**, 27.

ZUIDEMA, P. J. (1959). Ulcerative colitis in an Indonesian. *Trop. geogr. Med.*, **11**, 246.

— (1959). Cirrhosis and disseminated calcification of the pancreas in patients with malnutrition. *Trop. geogr. Med.*, **11**, 70.

ZUIDEMA, P. J. and MEUWISSEN, J. H. E. (1966). Malaria ovale. *Bull. Soc. Path. exot.*, **59**, 668.

Index

Abnormal haemoglobin diseases, 415, *et seq.*
(*see* haemoglobin for individual types)
blood transfusion and, 431
classification, 420, 447
diagnosis, 421, 422
electrophoresis, 418, 424, 767
family studies in, 425
finger printing, 418
inheritance of, 419, 424
laboratory tests in, 766, *et seq.*
nomenclature, 416
ABO blood groups, 475
(*see also* blood groups)
cancrum oris and, 515
cross matching tests, 769
haemolytic disease of the newborn, 488, 568
Abortion:
kidney in, 634
and malaria, 32
and pelvic angiography, 650
Absidia, 275
Acanthocheilonema:
perstans, 141
microfilaria of, 123
streptocerca:
life cycle, 140
microfilaria of, 123
Acatalasaemia, and cancrum oris, 515
Accidental haemorrhage, kidney in, 634
Aceylaninum, and larva migrans, 144
Achondroplasia, 714
Acid fast bacilli, in mycobacterial skin
ulcers, 729
Ackee poisoning, 558
Actinomyes bovis, 276
israelii, 276
Actinomycosis, 276, 543
Active juvenile cirrhosis, 556
Acute tubular necrosis, 634
in blackwater fever, 464
in cholera, 316
massive liver cell necrosis and, 586
Acute yellow atrophy of the liver, 585
Adamantinoma, 535
Addisonian anaemia, 404, 407
Addison's disease, 661
in malaria, 30
Adenolymphocoele, in onchocerciasis, 138
Adrenal gland, 660
Addisonian syndrome in South American
trypanosomiasis, 47
amoebiasis, 70

Adrenal gland: *continued*
amyloidosis, 723
Burkitt tumour, 506, 661
dengue viruses and, 225
diseases of, 660
haemorrhage in C.S.M., 604
histoplasmosis and, 286
Kaposi's sarcoma, 705
in kwashiorkor, 679
in malaria, 30
necrosis in heatstroke, 734
normal in tropics, 660
and strongyloidiasis, 107
and toxoplasmosis, 86
tumours of, 661
visceral leishmaniasis and, 57
Aedes:
and filariasis, 122
aegypti and dengue viruses, 224
and yellow fever, 220
africanus and yellow fever, 220
simpsoni and yellow fever, 220
Aflatoxin, 559
in Indian childhood cirrhosis, 575
African histoplasmosis, 286
African siderosis, 570
African trypanosomiasis, 35
Age pyramid in tropics, 3
Ainhum, 738
Air embolism, complication of blood
transfusion, 488
Alastrim, 238
Albinism, 703, 744
basal cell carcinoma in, 702
malignant melanoma in, 708
squamous cell carcinoma in, 702
tyrosinase and, 703
Albright's disease, 715
Alcoholism:
and cirrhosis, 553
and hepatitis, 553
and osteoporosis, 571
and peripheral neuritis, 382
and siderosis, 571
and the heart, 380
and the liver, 553
Aleppo boil, 58
Aleutian mink disease, 249
Algae, 142
Alkaptonuria, 688
Alimentary system, 513, *et seq.*
tumours of, 539
Allergy and blood transfusion reactions, 485

Alpha-feto protein, 592
  Australia antigen and, 579, 593, 597
  gastric cancer and, 593
  in Indian childhood cirrhosis, 575
  liver cell cancer and, 592, 597
  liver cell dysplasia and, 594
  pregnancy and, 592
  pyridoxine deficiency and, 593
  testicular cancer and, 592
Amanita and liver disease, 559
Amaurotic familial idiocy, 602
Ameloblastoma, 535
American spotted fevers, 212
Amoebiasis, 64, *et seq.*
  diagnostic pathology, 73, 74
  diet and, 66
  epidemiology, 65
  liver abscess, complications, 73
  liver in, 71
  malignancy and, 74
  meningoencephalitis, 77
  pathology, 67
  pregnancy and, 68
  reservoir hosts, 66
  ulcerative post-dysenteric colitis, 71
  venereal, 70
Amoeboma, 70
Amyloidosis, 723, *et seq.*
  diagnosis, 724
  familial Mediterranean fever and, 740
  leprosy and, 312
  localized, 723
  in myelomatosis, 723
  and pulmonary hypertension, 375
  renal vein thrombosis, 723
  tuberculosis, 394
Amyotrophic lateral sclerosis, 608
  pathology of, 609
Anaemia, 404
  aetiology, 404
  blood transfusion in, 487
    exchange, 487
    packed cells and diuretics, 487
  dimorphic, 411
  gram-negative organisms and, 296
  haemolytic, 414
    classification, 414
    hereditary intracorpuscular defects and, 412
    malaria and, 18, 20, 23
    oroya fever and, 337
  heart and, 379
  hookworm infection and, 94
  in cirrhosis, 549
  iron deficient, 406
  in kwashiorkor, 674
  megaloblastic, 407
    diagnosis, 409
    diphyllobothriasis and, 208
    folic acid deficiency, 408
    in hookworm infection, 94
    pyridoxine deficiency in, 409
    vitamin B_{12} deficiency, 409

Anaemia: *continued*
  in pregnancy, 412
  and symmetrical gangrene, 387
  in tropical splenomegaly syndrome, 494
  tuberculosis and, 397
Anaesthesia:
  and malaria, 30
  in sickle-cell anaemia, 433
  and sickle-cell trait, 429
Anchovy sauce pus, in amoebiasis, 74
Ancylostoma:
  braziliense, and larva migrans, 144
  caninum,
    and larva migrans, 144
    and visceral larva migrans, 105
  duodenale, life cycle, 92
Anencephaly, 601, 602
Aneurin (*see* Thiamine), 380
Aneurysm:
  apex of left ventricle in South American trypanosomiasis, 48
  in arteritis of obscure aetiology, 386
  syphilitic, 385
  tuberculosis and, 398
  ventricular, 366
Angiomatoids, in schistosomiasis, 170
Angiostrongyliasis, 118
Angiostrongylus cantonensis, life cycle, 118
Annular subvalvular left-ventricular aneurysm, 366, *et seq.*
  diagnosis, 370
  heterotopic bone in, 368
  heterotopic marrow in, 368
  pathogenesis, 367
Anopheles:
  darlingi, 10
  funestus, 10
  gambiae, 10
  punctulatus, 10
Anorectal disease, 526
  malignant melanoma, 707
Anthrax, 332
  pathology, 333
Antibodies, blood group, 476
  detection of, 480
Antihaemophilic globulin, 471
Anuria, in blood transfusion reactions, 486
Aortic arch syndrome, 384
Appendicitis, 519
  in ascariasis, 101
  in balantidiasis, 90
  in enterobiasis, 113
  schistosomiasis and, 163, 519
  in trichuriasis, 112
Appendix:
  amoebiasis and, 70
  Burkitt tumour and, 506
  carcinoid tumour of, 519
  in schistosomiasis, 162
Arboviruses, 216
  group A, 217, 218
  group B, 217, 219

Arboviruses: *continued*
  group C, 217, 227
  classification of, 217
  vectors of, 217
Arcus Senilis, 745
Arenavirus group, 229
Argemone mexicana, and the heart, 374
  glaucoma and, 746
Argentaffin cells, 541
Argentaffinomas, 541
Argentinian haemorrhagic fever, 228
Arias-Stella phenomenon, 738
Ariboflavinosis, 514
Arrow poisons, 374
Arsenic:
  and the heart, 374
  and skin cancer, 704
Arteries, 383
  see Atherosclerosis
  coronary in new born, 383
  cystic myxomatous degeneration, 384
Arteritis:
  affecting the carotid artery, 387
  giant-cell, 385
  of obscure aetiology, 384
    hypertension in, 386
    necropsy findings, 386
    thrombosis of aorta in, 386
  temporal, 385
Arthritis, 716
  acute tropical, 716
  chylous, 128
  dracontiasis and, 143
  dysentery, bacillary and, 330
  loiasis and, 132
  onchocerciasis and, 136
  rheumatoid, 716
  typhoid, 327
Asbestosis, 391
Ascariasis, 98, *et seq.*
  diagnosis, 103
  epidemiology, 99
  immunity in, 99
  intestinal obstruction in, 101
  jaundice in, 102
  larval migration, effects of, 100
  liver abscess in, 102
  Loeffler's syndrome, 100
  malabsorption in, 99
  ova, quantitative count, 757
Ascaris lumbricoides, 98
  and visceral larva migrans, 105
  A. suis, and visceral larva migrans, 105
  A. suum, 99
Ascites:
  Burkitt tumour, 506
  chylous in filariasis, 128
  in endomyocardial fibrosis, 365
  in tuberculosis, 397
  portal hypertension and, 550
Aspergillosis, 273
Aspergillus flavus, 275
  liver disease and, 559

Aspergillus flavus: *continued*
  fumigatus, 273
  niger, 273
Asteroid body, 401
  in sporotrichosis, 284
Asthma, 376, 390
Atherosclerosis, 377
  aortic, 377
  cerebral, 377
  cirrhosis and, 551
  coronary, 377
  and pulmonary hypertension, 375
  pulmonary in schistosomiasis, 175
Auberger blood group system, 475
Australia antigen, 577, 578
  biliary cirrhosis and, 561
  blood donors and, 480
  blood transfusion and, 578
  cirrhosis and, 555, 579
  detection, 580
  Down's syndrome and, 598
  Hodgkin's disease and, 598
  Indian childhood cirrhosis and, 575
  kidney and, 618
  leprosy and, 598
  leukaemia and, 598
  liver carcinoma and, 597
  liver cell dysplasia and, 594
  massive liver cell necrosis and, 586
  mosquitoes and, 579
  nomenclature, 580
  renal disease and, 618
  subtypes, 578
Autoimmune disease, 710
  incidence in tropics, 713
Autotransfusion, 484
Avian malaria, 12

Babesiosis, 34
Baboons, and schistosomiasis, 149
Bacillary dysentery, 328
Bacillus:
  anthracis, 332
  pyocyaneus and amoebic liver abscess, 72
  whitmori, 339
Baghdad boil, 58
Balantidiasis, 88
  diagnosis, 90
  epidemiology, 88
  pathology, 90
Balantidium coli, life cycle, 88
Bananas, serotonin content, 541
Banti's syndrome, 497
Bartonella bacilliformis, 337
Bartonellosis, 337
Bartter's syndrome, 382
Basal cell carcinoma, 702
  in albinism, 702
  arsenical dermatitis, 704
  rarity in pigmented races, 702
Basidiobolus, 292
B.C.G. vaccination, in leprosy, 298
Bedsoniae, 242

Bell's palsy, 613
Bengal splenomegaly, 492
Beri beri, 380, *et seq.*
    adult, 684
    and alcoholic heart disease, pathology,
       382
    C.N.S. changes in, 685
    heart disease in infants, 382
    infantile, 684
Beta glucuronidase, and carcinoma of the
    bladder, 167
Betel nut, and oral cancer, 534, 536
Big spleen disease, 492
Bile ducts,
    cancer of, 598, 599
    Caroli's disease, 599
    clonorchiasis and, 185
    congenital dilatation, 588
Bilharzioma, 168
Biliary cirrhosis of the liver, 556, 561
Biliary mud, in clonorchiasis, 185
Bilious remittent fever, 20
Bilirubin:
    metabolism in malaria, 25
Blackwater fever, 463
    kidneys in, 464
    pathogenesis, 463
    pathology, 463
    urinary changes, 465
Bladder:
    amoebiasis, 70
    calcification in schistosomiasis, 156, 165
    calculi and, 636
    cancer and *Schistosoma haematobium*
      infection, 165
    cystitis, 639
    cystitis cystica, 158
      glandularis, 158
    filling defects in schistosomiasis, 157
    malakoplakia, 639
    polyps and schistosomiasis, 157
    in schistosomiasis, 156
    stone disease in children, 636
    tumours of, 166
Blastomyces dermatitidis, 279
Blastomycosis:
    cheloidal, 290
    North American, 279
    South American, 281
Blighia sapida, and ackee poisoning,
    558
Blindness, 742
    onchocercal, 134
Blister beetles, 724
Blood:
    despatch of samples, 777
    parasites, stain for, 758, 759, 760
    thick film preparation, 759
    thin film preparation, 760
Blood donors:
    abnormal haemoglobins and, 482
    anaemia and, 482
    brucellosis and, 481

Blood donors: *continued*
    Chagas disease and, 481
    danger of O group, 480
    filariasis and, 481
    G-6-PD and, 482
    haemoglobin content and, 482
    infectious hepatitis and, 480
    leishmaniasis and, 481
    malaria and, 481
    recruitment, 474
    selection, 482
    syphilis and, 481
    thalassaemia and, 482
    trypanosomiasis and, 481
    venesection, 483
    yaws and, 481
Blood groups, 475
    A and stomach cancer, 538
    ABO groups, 475, 477
    antibodies, 476
      detection, 480
    Auberger system, 475
    Cartwright system, 475
    compatibility tests, 771
    Diego system, 475
    Duffy system, 475
    I system, 475
    Kell system, 475
    Kidd system, 475
    Lewis system, 475
    Lutheran system, 475
    MNss system, 475
    P system, 475
      and hydatid disease, 205
    Rhesus system, 478
    Sutter antigen, 480
Blood transfusion, 474, *et seq.*
    air embolism, 488
    allergic reactions, 485
    in anaemia, 487
    auto transfusion, 484
    blood, storage, 483
    citrate toxicity, 485, 488
    compatibility tests, 480, 471
    complications, 484
    cross matching, 771
    defibrination syndrome, 485
    donor selection, 482
    equipment, 485
    exchange transfusion, 487
    grouping, 770
    incidence of reaction, 485
    intraperitoneal transfusion, 483
    investigation of reactions, 486
    O group and, 773
    oliguria and, 486
    packed cells, 487
    potassium toxicity, 488
    sickle-cell trait and, 431
    siderosis and, 488
    techniques, 769
    thrombophlebitis and, 488
    venesection, technique, 488

Blood vessels, and aspergillosis, 275
Bolivian haemorrhagic fever, 228
Bone, 714
  in Burkitt tumour, 504, 512
  changes in sickle-cell disease, 436, 444
  congenital disorders, 714
  Ewing's tumour 715
  fibrous dysplasia, 714
  fractures, 714
  giant cell tumour of, 715
  heterotopic, 719
  hydatid disease and, 203
  Kaposi's sarcoma, 705
  lesions in sickle-cell disease, 444
  neuroblastoma, 512
  osteomyelitis, 714
  reticulum cell sarcoma simulating Burkitt
    tumour, 512
  salmonella and sickle-cell disease, 446
  surgery in sickle-cell disease, 436
  tumours of, 714
Bone marrow:
  biopsy, 778
  blood transfusion by, 483
  brucellosis and, 332
  Burkitt tumour, 505
  embolism, 441
  malaria, 26
  marrow and peripheral blood barrier,
    24
  puncture, 777
  siderosis, African and, 572
  in tuberculosis, 397
  in typhoid fever, 325
Bornholm disease, 717
Borrelia:
  duttoni, 343
  recurrentis, 344
  vincenti:
    cancrum oris and, 516
    morphology, 516
    tropical ulcer and, 726
Botulism, 318
Bouton d'Orient, 58
Brain, 601, et seq.
  amoebic abscess, 70
  Burkitt tumour, 504
  chorion carcinoma and, 648
  coenurus and, 209
  cortical blindness, 747
  hyperpyrexia, 23
  malaria, cerebral, 21
  in massive liver cell necrosis, 586
  in South American trypanosomiasis,
    49
  in sparganosis, 211
  in toxocariasis, 105
  in toxoplasmosis, 84, 86
  trypanosomes in, 39
  tuberculoma, 603
Brazilian blastomycosis, 281
Break-bone fever, 224
Breast, 650

Breast: continued
  benign mammary dysplasia, 652
  Burkitt tumour, 506
  carcinoma of, 651
  conditions affecting, 650
  elephantiasis of, 115
  and filariasis, 126
  tuberculosis, 398
Brilliant cresyl blue dye test, G-6-Pd,
  method, 768
Brill-Zinsser disease, 212
Bronchiectasis, 390
Bronchopneumonia, 390
Bronzed diabetes, 569
Brucella abortus, 330
  melitensis, 330
  suis, 330
Brucellosis, 330
  in blood transfusion, 481
  diagnostic pathology, 332
  liver disease and, 560
Brugia malayi: 122
  diagnostic methods, 759, 765
  geographical distribution, 124
  life cycle, 124
  microfilaria of, 123
Brunn's nests, 158
  in ureters in schistosomiasis, 159
Budd-Chiari syndrome, 565
Buffer solutions, 763
Bulinus, 149
Bunostomum phlebotomum, and larva migrans, 144
Bunyamwera virus, 227
Burkitt tumour, 500, et seq.
  clinical presentation, 504
  cytology, imprint, 509
  diagnosis, 510
  EB virus and, 502
  emperipolesis, 510
  epidemiology, 501
  histiocyte, imprint cytology, 509
  histochemistry, 509
  histopathology, 507
  immunology of, 503
  and leukaemia, 473
  lymphocytic transformation in, 502
  malaria and, 502, 503
  neuroblastoma and, 509
  organ distribution, 504
  pathology, 504
  phase contrast microscopy, 509
  radiological findings, 512
  retinoblastoma and, 509
  sickle-cell trait and, 503
  tissue culture, 509
  Wilm's tumour and, 510
'Burning feet' syndrome, 685, 688
Burse-Buschke's disease, 289
Bursitis, 716
Buruli ulcer: 729
Bwamba virus, 228
Byssinosis, 2

C reactive protein, in leprosy, 266
Calabar swellings, 132, 141
Calcification:
 dystrophic, 719
 metastatic, 719
Calcifying collagenolysis, 719
Calcinosis circumscripta, 719
 localizata, 719
 universalis, 719
Calcium:
 gluconate, and citrate toxicity, 488
 metabolism:
  classifications of disorders, 718
  deranged in tumoral calcinosis, 719
Calculi:
 renal, in schistosomiasis, 160, 636
 vesical, 160, 636
 ureteric, in schistosomiasis, 160
 urethral, in schistosomiasis, 160
California group viruses, 217
Cancer (see Malignant disease), 690
 altered immunological status and, 498, 713
Cancrum oris, 515
Candida albicans, 270
Candidiasis, 270, 514
Capillaria philippinensis, 144
Capillariasis, 144
Caraparu, 217
Carbon monoxide poisoning, 374
Carbon tetrachloride:
 kidney and, 634
Carcino-embryonic antigen, 698
Carcinoid tumour, and endomyocardial fibrosis, 358
Carcinoid syndrome, 358, 541
Carcinoma of the liver, 589, et seq.
 (see liver, primary liver cell carcinoma)
Cardiomegaly, idiopathic, 351
Carotid arteritis, 387
Carpal fusions, 714
Carrion's disease, 337
Cartilage, tumours of, 715
Cartwright blood group system, 475
Casoni test, 205
Cassava:
 goitre and, 657
 neuropathy and, 610
Cataract, 746
Cat scratch disease, 247
Cats:
 and gnathostomiasis, 120
 and larva migrans, 144
 and sparganosis, 210
 and Toxocara catis, 103
Caustic soda and oesophagitis, 518
Central nervous system, 601, et seq.
 acute symptoms in schistosomiasis, 153
 in angiostrongyliasis, 119
 beri-beri and, 685
 brucellosis and, 331
 Burkitt tumour, 505
 calcification in toxoplasmosis, 86

Central nervous system: continued
 changes in alcoholism, 382
 changes in beri-beri, 382, 685
 changes in Veld sore, 728
 cirrhosis and, 552
 congenital malformations, 601
 cysticercosis and, 199
 demyelinating neuropathy, 610
 endemic syphilis, 340
 in heat disorders, 735
 hydatid disease and, 204
 Kaposi's sarcoma, 704
 in kwashiorkor, 680
 and malaria, 21
 malignant melanoma, 707
 neuropathic syndrome of uncertain origin, 610
 paragonimiasis and, 193
 phycomycosis and, 275
 pinta, 341
 poliomyelitis and, 261
 polyneuritic leprosy, 306
 rabies and, 234
 in Schistosoma haematobium infection, 176
 in sickle-cell disease, 443
 in trichinellosis, 116
 trypanosomiasis, 39
 tuberculosis, 396
 tumours of, 614
 and typhoid fever, 327
 vascular diseases of, 606
Cerebral calcification, cytomegalic inclusion disease and, 262
Cerebral malaria, 20
Cerebrospinal fluid:
 Angiostrongylus cantonensis in, 118
 Burkitt tumour cells in, 507
 in hydatid disease, 203
 in loiasis, 132
 in meningococcal meningitis, 605
 in paragonomiasis, 193
 in pneumococcal meningitis, 603
 in Schistosoma haematobium infection, 176
 in Schistosoma japonicum and S. mansoni infections, 176
 in toxoplasmosis, 87
 in trichinellosis, 115
 in trypanosomiasis, 38
 in tuberculous meningitis, 396
Cerebro vascular disease, 606
Ceroid, 532
Cervix: 646
 in amoebiasis, 70
 carcinoma of, 646
 in schistosomiasis, 162, 647
 tuberculosis, 398
Cestodes, 194
Chagas cardiopathy, 48
Chagas Disease, 42
 (See also Trypanosomiasis, South American)
 in blood transfusion, 481

Chancroid, 338
Charcot's joints, 716
Charcot-Leyden crystals:
  in angiostrongyliasis, 118
  in ascariasis, 100
  in enterobiasis, 113
  paragonimiasis and, 192
  in schistosomiasis, 155
  sparganosis and, 211
Cheloidal blastomycosis, 290
Cheilomastix mesnili, 69
Cheilosis, 514
Chickenpox, 241
Chiclero ulcer, 59
  pathology, 59
Chikungunya virus, 218, 224
Childhood mortality, 4
Children,
  cancer in, 709
Chloramphenicol, in G-6-PD deficiency, 460
Chlorpromazine, and liver disease, 557
Cholangitis: 600
  in ascariasis, 102, 600
  clonorchiasis and, 184, 599
  fascioliasis and, 189
Cholecystitis:
  acute, in ascariasis, 102
  Ascaris lumbricoides and, 600
  Schistosoma haematobium infection and, 164
  typhoid and, 325
Cholelithiasis, in sickle cell anaemia, 432, 441
Cholera, 314
  diagnostic pathology, 317
  Vibrio cholerae, 314
Choleraic malaria, 20
Cholergan, 317
Chorioadenoma destruens, 647
Choriocarcinoma, 647
  immunological factors, 647
  pathology, 648
Chorioretinitis, in toxoplasmosis, 85
Chromoblastomycosis, 282
Chromomycosis, 282
Chromosomes: 602
  Burkitt tumour, 503
  in leukaemia, 473
Chronic active hepatitis, 584
Chronic venous congestion, in spleen, 492
Chrysops, and loiasis, 131
Chutta cancer, 535
Chylothorax, 391
Chyluria in filariasis, 128
Circulatory system, 348, *et seq.*
Circumcision, and penile cancer, 640, 691
Circumoval test, in schistosomiasis, 179
Cirrhosis, 545, *et seq.*
  African siderosis and, 570
  age, sex, social class, 552
  alcohol and, 553
  anaemia in, 549

Cirrhosis: *continued*
  Australia antigen and, 555, 579
  Banti's syndrome and, 497
  biliary, 561
  central, 562
  clay pipe-stem, 169
  coma in, 549
  cryptogenic, 556, 584
  cystic fibrosis and, 567
  dietary toxic factors and, 557 *et seq.*
  fructose intolerance, 567
  galactosaemia, 566
  geographical distribution, 552
  gynaecomastia in, 596
  haemochromatosis, 570
  hypersensitivity, 556
  idiopathic tropical splenomegaly syndrome and, 496
  Indian childhood cirrhosis, 574
  juvenile, active, 584
  lungs and, 552
  macronodular, 542
  malaria and, 29, 556
  malnutrition and, 553, 555
  massive liver cell necrosis and, 585
  micronodular, 542
  mixed, 549
  neonatal hepatitis and, 543, 568
  parasites and, 555
  pericellular, 565
  porphyria and, 567
  portal, 546
    hypertension, 550
  postnecrotic, 547
  primary liver cell carcinoma and, 589, 594
  sarcoidosis and, 560
  sickle-cell disease and, 440
  ulcerative colitis and, 561
  viral infections and, 554
  Wilson's disease and, 566
  yellow fever and, 223
Citrate toxicity, in blood transfusion, 488
Cladosporiosis epidermica, 266
Cladosporium, 282
  werneckii Horta, 266
Climatic bubo, 244
Clonorchiasis, 182
  cholangiocellular carcinoma of the liver and, 185
  diagnostic pathology, 186
  epidemiology, 183
  pathology, 183
  S. typhi and, 322
Clonorchis sinensis, life cycle, 182
Clostridia species and gas gangrene, 318
Clostridium botulinum, 318
Clostridium tetani, 319
  welchii, and intestinal disease, 319, 520
Cobalt and cirrhosis, 557
Coccidioidis immitis, 277
Coccidioidomycosis, 277
Coeliac disease, 531

Coenuris cerebralis, 209
Coin lesion, 140
  histoplasmosis and, 285
Cold growing organism and blood transfusion, 487
Colon, 525
  carcinoma and schistosomiasis, 169
  intussusception, 524
  megacolon, 46, 523
  perforation, 526
  tumours of, 540
  ulcerative colitis, 521
  ulcerative post dysenteric colitis, 71
  volvulus, 523
Colorado tick fever, 217
Colour blindness, 613
Complement, 618
Congenital annular constriction of the
  digits, 738
Congenital disease,
  rubella and, 251
Congenital dislocation of the hip, 714
Congenital spherocytic anaemia with
  haemoglobin S, 422
Conjunctivitis, inclusion, 244
Convulsions,
  children and, 601
Cooleys anaemia, 454
Coomb's test:
  indirect blood grouping, 480
  indirect, method, 771
Copper and kwashiorkor, 674
Copper sulphate, method for haemoglobin
  estimation, 482
Coronary artery disease, 377
  anastomotic pattern and, 378
  geographical distribution, 377
  schistosomiasis and, 165
  ventricular aneurysms and, 367
Cor pulmonale, 374, *et seq.*
  geographical distribution, 376
  idiopathic pulmonary hypertension, 375
  in schistosomiasis, 175
  in sickle-cell anaemia, 433, 441
Corynebacteria diphtheriae, 313
  veld sore and, 728
Councilman lesion, 222, 585
Cow's urine poisoning, 558
Coxiella burneti, 212
Coxsackie virus, 259, 717
Coxsackie B virus, 371
Creeping eruption, 144
  (*see also* larva migrans)
  in gnathostomiasis, 121
  in strongyloidiasis, 101
Crigler-Najjar syndrome, 568
Crimean-Central Asian, haemorrhagic
  fever, 217
Crohn's disease, 521
Crossmatching, 769
Crotalaria, 558, 563
  crispata, 563
    Kimberley horse disease and, 563

Crotalaria: *continued*
  dura, cause of 'jagsiekte', 563
  fulva, 558
  retusa, 563
    Kimberley horse disease and, 563
Cryptococcal infection, 605
Cryptococcosis, 289
Cryptococcus neoformans, 269, 289
Cryptogenic splenomegaly, 492
Culex:
  and filariasis, 122
  tarsalis, 218
Culicoides spp., 140
  austini, 140
  grahami, 140
Cushing's syndrome, 661
Cutaneous larva migrans, 144
Cyanogenetic glycosides and tropical
  neuropathy, 610
Cyanotic syndrome, 176
Cycas circinalis L.:
  liver disease and, 559
  possible toxicity of, 608
Cyclops:
  Diphyllobothrium latum and, 207
  dracontiasis and, 142
  gnathostomiasis and, 120
  sparganosis and, 210
Cysteine, and massive liver necrosis, 585
Cysticercosis, 194, 198
  diagnostic pathology, 201
  epidemiology, 198
  pathology, 199
Cysticercus bovis, 196, 199
  cellulosae, 196, 198
Cystography in schistosomiasis, 156
Cytomegalic inclusion disease, 262
  pancreatic calcification and, 665
Cytomegalovirus infection, 262
Cytosiderosis, 570

Dactylitis,
  in sickle-cell anaemia, 432
Darling's disease, 285
Defibrination syndrome:
  incompatible blood and, 485
  liver cell carcinoma and, 591
  malaria and, 26
  in meningitis, 604
Delacroixia coronata, 294
Delhi boil, 58
Demyelinating neuropathy, 610
Dengue, 224
  viruses, pathology, 224
Dental caries, 514
Depigmentation,
  onchocerciasis and, 138
Dermatitis: see skin 748
Dermatomycosis furfuracea, 266
Desert rheumatism, 277
Desert sore, 728
Desiccators, 776
Dhoti cancer, 704

Diabetes mellitus: 662
  classification of, 662
  haemochromatosis and, 569
  kidney in, 626, 634
  pathology of, 663
  siderosis, African and, 571
Diarrhoeal diseases, 6
Dicrocoeliasis, 190
Diego blood group system, 480
Dientamoeba fragilis, 77
Dihydroxyphenylalamine (DOPA), in albinism, 703
Dimercaprol in G-6-PD deficiency, 460
Dimorphic anaemia, 411
Dipetalonema perstans, 141
  microfilaria of, 123
Diphyllobothriasis, 207
  epidemiology, 207
  pathology, 208
Diphyllobothrium latum, life cycle, 207
Diphtheria, 313, 728
  blood groups in, 476
  cutaneous, 728
  myocarditis, 372
Dipylidiasis, 210
Dipylidium caninum, life cycle, 210
Dirofilaria:
  conjunctivae, 140
  immitis, 131, 140
  louisanensis, 140
  magalhaesi, 140
  repeus, 140
Dirofilariasis, 140
Disseminated lupus erythematosis, liver disease and, 556
  renal disease and, 634
Diverticular disease, 525
Diverticulitis, 519, 539
Dogs:
  and gnathostomiasis, 120
  and hydatid disease, 202
  and larva migrans, 144
  and sparganosis, 210
  and Toxocara canis, 103
  rabies in, 233
Donovan bodies, 336
Donovania granulomatosis, 336
Donovanosis, 336
Dracontiasis, 142
  diagnostic pathology, 143
  epidemiology, 142
  pathology, 143
Dracunculiasis, 142
  (see Dracontiasis)
Dracunculus medinensis, life cycle, 142
Drepanidotaenia lanceolata, life cycle, 208
Drug resistance, 296
Dubin-Johnson syndrome, 568
Duffy blood group system, 475
Duodenal ulcer, 518
Duodenitis in hookworm infection, 97
Durand-Nicolas-Favre disease, 244

Dwarfism:
  renal disease and, 622
  in Schistosoma japonicum and S. mansoni infections, 173, 177
  skin lesions and, 752
  in tropical splenomegaly syndrome, 497
Dysentery, bacillary, 328
  pathology, 329
  Shigella spp., 328

Ear, and enterobiasis, 144
Eastern equine encephalitis virus, 218
Echinococcus:
  granulosus, life cycle, 201
  multilocularis, life cycle, 201
  oligaettas, life cycle, 201
Echo virus, 259
  in pericarditis, 383
Electron microscopy:
  albinism, 703
  embedding technique, 779
  Kaposi's sarcoma, 705
  leishmaniasis, 51
  malarial parasite, 11
Electrophoresis, paper, method, 767
Elephantiasis, 129
  and Acanthocheilonema perstans, 129
  and Acanthocheilonema streptocerca, 130
  Ethiopian cutaneous leishmaniasis and, 61
  in filariasis, 129
  and Loa loa, 130
  lymphogranuloma venererum and, 130, 246
  malignant disease and, 130
  and Onchocerca volvulus, 130
  in onchocerciasis, 138
  pathology, 130
  of penis in schistosomiasis, 130, 160
  prototothecosis and, 142
  pyogenic infection and, 130
  in schistosomiasis, 130
  silica and, 129
  streptocerciasis and, 140
  tuberculosis and, 130, 395
Elliptocytosis, 459
Emetine and the heart, 374
Emperipolesis, Burkitt tumour, 510
Encephalitis:
  Eastern equine virus and, 218
  herpes simplex and, 254
  Japanese virus and, 226
  measles and, 248
  mumps and, 249
  Murray valley virus and, 219
  St. Louis virus and, 225
  tick-borne viruses and, 226
  typhus and, 215
  Venezuelan virus and, 218
  Western equine virus and, 218
Encephalocoele, 601
Encephalopathy and fatty degeneration of the viscera, 607
Endemic syphilis, 341

Endocardial fibroelastosis, 356
Endocarditis, bacterial, 348, 372
Endocrine glands, 653 *et. seq.*
Endocrines:
  cancer and, 699
Endolimax nana, 77
Endometriosis, 644
Endometritis:
  syncytial, 649
  tuberculous, 357, 398
Endomyocardial fibrosis, 357, *et seq.*
  cardiac cirrhosis in, 365
  diagnosis, 365
  embolism in, 365
  oxygen desaturation of the arterial blood
    in, 365
  pathology, 359
Entamoeba:
  coli, 77
  hartmanni, cystic, 65
  histolytica, 65
    cysts of, 75
    enzymes in, 64
    life cycle, 64
    staining in faeces, 612
  polecki, 78
Enteritis necroticans, 319, 520
Enterobiasis, 112
  diagnosis, 775
  diagnostic pathology, 114, 775
  epidemiology, 112
  pathology, 113
Enterobius vermicularis,
  life cycle, 112
Enteroviruses, 259
Enthacrynic acid in exchange transfusion,
  485
Entomophthora coronata, 294
Eosinophilia, 405
  tropical, 383
Eosinophilic granuloma of the intestine, 522
Eosinophilic lung, 383
Eosinophils, 405
Epidemic dropsy, 374
Epididymis:
  and ascariasis, 101
  and filariasis, 126
  non-filarial, 126
  in schistosomiasis, 162
  tuberculosis of, 398
Epilepsy, idiopathic, 606
Epstein Barr virus, 253, 255
  Burkitt tumour and, 502
  Hodgkin's disease and, 499
  infectious mononucleosis and, 255
  nasopharyngeal cancer and, 402
Epulides, 534
Erisipela de la costa, 139
Ergotism, 559
Erythema nodosum leprosum, 308
Erythema nodosum, 398
Erythraemic myelosis, 474
Erythrasma, 266

Erythroblastosis foetalis, 488, 568
Erythrocyte:
  age in malarial infection, 11
  antigen antibody complexes, 490
  effects of stasis in spleen, 491
  glucose deprivation, 492
  hypersplenism, changes in, 491
  inclusion bodies in Haemoglobin Zurich
    disease, 453
  lysolecithins, 492
  in malaria, 15–17
  osmotic fragility, *see* osmotic fragility, 491
  potassium in hypersplenism, 491
  sedimentation rate, 405
  sodium in hypersplenism, 435
Escherichia coli, and amoebic liver abscess,
  72
Espundia, 61
Essential hypertension, 376
Esthiomene, 244
Ethiopian cutaneous leishmaniasis, 61
European blastomycosis, 289
Eustachian tube and ascariasis, 102
Eustoma rotundatum, and eosinophilic
  granuloma of intestine, 522
Ewing's tumour:
  Burkitt tumour, smear radiological ap-
    pearances, 512
  incidence, 715
Exchange blood transfusion, 487
  and citrate toxicity, 488
  in haemolytic disease of the newborn, 488
  and potassium toxicity, 488
  in prematurity, 488
Eye, 742, *et seq.*
  albinism and, 744
  brucellosis and, 330
  coenurus cysts and, 209
  cysticercosis and, 199
  cytomegalic inclusion disease and, 262
  gnathostomiasis and, 121
  inclusion conjunctivitis, 244
  leprosy and, 310
  loiasis and, 132
  malignant melanoma, 707
  in onchocerciasis, 134, 139
  in sickle-cell disease, 433, 436
  smallpox and, 239
  sparganosis and, 211
  in toxocariasis, 104, 105
  in toxoplasmosis, 85
  and trichinellosis, 116
  in trypanosomiasis, 41
  tuberculosis and, 395
  tumours of, 745
  and Vitamin A deficiency, 682

Face, tuberculosis of, 398
Factor VII, 471
Factor VIII, 471
Faeces, 753
  examination of, concentration methods,
    754

Faeces: *continued*
filtration-Ninhydrin method, 755
flotation in brine, 755
glycerol sedimentation, 611
iodine and, 754
ova counts, quantitative, 757
ova in, 762
protozoa, 753
saline and, 753
saline sedimentation, 755
staining of amoebae, 756
staining methods, 756
preservation of, 757
transmission of, 777
Faget's sign, 221
Fallopian tube, 644
amoebiasis, 70
conditions affecting, 644
in enterobiasis, 113
in schistosomiasis, 162
tuberculosis, 397, 398
Familial Mediterranean fever, 740
Fanconi syndrome, 687
Far Eastern encephalitis, 226
Faria reaction in leprosy, 299
Fasciola gigantica, life cycle, 188
  hepatica, life cycle, 188
Fascioliasis, 188
diagnostic pathology, 189
epidemiology, 188
pathology, 188
Fasciolopsiasis, 180
diagnostic pathology, 181
epidemiology, 180
Fasciolopsis buski, life cycle, 180
Fat embolism, 441
Favism, 461
Favus, 267
Fernandez reaction in leprosy, 299
Fertility, 3
Fetal haemoglobin, 416, 425
  α chain in, 416
  γ chain in, 416
abnormal forms, 425
alkali resistant haemoglobin in, 423
detection of, 426
distribution in erythrocytes, 423
estimation of, 766
hereditary persistence of, 426
High F gene and β-thalassaemia, 427
High F gene and C, 427
High F gene and S, 427
and malaria, 427
Norfolk form, 418
Fetal mortality, and malaria, 32
Fibrin, in malaria, 17
cerebral, 23
Fibrinogen:
in the defibrination syndrome, 485
Fibrinolysis and pulmonary embolism, 388
in coronary artery disease, 377
splenectomy, 497
Fibroblastic parietal endocarditis, 372

Fibrous dysplasia, 534, 714
Field's stain, 763
Fievre boutonneuse, 212
FIGLU excretion in kwashiorkor, 672
FIGLU excretion test, 411
Filariases, classification, 122
Filariasis, 122
Bancroftian, 122
in blood transfusion, 481
chyluria in, 128
diagnostic methods, 759
diagnostic pathology, 130
in endomyocardial fibrosis, 357
epidemiology, 122
hydrocele in, 129
Malayan, 122
pathology, 125
periodicity of microfilaria, 124
in pyomyositis, tropical, 718
scrotum, gangrene of, 643
Timor microfilaria, 125
tropical eosinophilia and, 399
Finger clubbing, 549
Fish and gnathostomiasis, 120
Fluorescent antibody test, 765
Fluorosis, 514, 722
Folic acid deficiency, 408
in chronic anaemia, 379
in dimorphic anaemia, 411
in hookworm infection, 94
in pregnancy, 412
in malaria, 25
Food poisoning, 519
Formalin, preservation of tissues, 774
Formiminoglutamic acid (FIGLU) excretion test, 411
Formol ether, concentration method, 755
Forssman antibody, 259
Fournier's gangrene of scrotum, 643
Frei test, 246
Fructose intolerance, 567
Fungal diseases, 264, *et seq.*
dimorphic, 265
filamentous, 264
Imperfecti, 264
morphology of, 264
nomenclature, 265
superficial, 265, 775
systemic, 268
pathological classification, 269
staining of, 268
Funiculitis and filariasis, 126
Furazolidone in G-6-PD deficiency, 460
Fusarium sporotrichoides and aleukia, 559
Fusiformis fusiformis:
cancrum oris and, 516
tropical ulcer and, 726

Galactosaemia, 566, 602
Gall bladder, 599
in amoebiasis, 72
in ascariasis, 98

Gall bladder: *continued*
  carcinoma of, 600
  clonorchiasis and, 184
  diseases of, 599
  fascioliasis and, 188
  in opisthorciasis, 187
  in trichinellosis, 116
  in typhoid fever, 324
  in schistosomiasis, 164
Gall stones, 600
  in β thalassaemia, 455
  cirrhosis and, 551
  rarity in tropics, 561
  in sickle-cell disease, 441
Gambian trypanosomiasis, 35
  (*See* also trypanosomiasis, Gambian)
Gandy-Gamma bodies, 438
Ganglia, 716
Gangrene:
  breast, skin of, 650
  gas, 318
  in haemoglobin C trait, 435
  scrotum, skin of, 643
  in sickle-cell anaemia, 432
  symmetrical, 387
Gastric ulcer, 518
Gastroenteritis:
  malaria and, 31
Gaucher's disease, hypersplenism, 602
Genetics, 8
Genu valgum, 714
German measles, 251
Germiston virus, 228
Giant cells:
  arteritis and, 385, 386
Giardia lamblia, 78
Giardiasis, 78
  diagnosis, 81
  epidemiology, 79
  life cycle, 78
  pathology, 80
Giemsa's stain, 763
  microfilaria and, 764
Gilbert's syndrome, 568
Gilchrist's disease, 279
Glandular fever, 255
Glaucoma, 746
  onchocerciasis and, 135
Glomerulonephritis, 616, *et seq.*
  acute diffuse proliferative, 619
  chronic, 622
  classification, 619
  Ellis type I, 617
  Ellis type II, 617
  end stage kidney, 622
  focal, 623
  lobular glomerulitis, 625
  malaria and, 619
  membranous, 626
  proliferative, 625
  rapidly progressive, 621
  subacute, 621
  terminology of glomerular lesions, 617

Glossina, trypanosomiasis and, 35
Glossina morsitans, and *Trypanosoma rho-
    desiense*, 35
  pallidipes and *Trypanosoma rhodesiense*, 35
  palpalis, and *Trypanosoma gambiense*, 35
  tachinoides and *Trypanosoma gambiense*,
    35
Glucose-6-phosphate dehydrogenase (G-6-
    PD) deficiency, 460
  in ABO haemolytic disease of the new-
    born, 478
  drugs in, 460
  favism, 462
  haemolytic anaemia in, 460
  hazard in blood transfusion, 482
  hepatitis and, 583
  hereditary non spherocytic haemolytic
    anaemia types, 460
  in infections, 391, 461
  inheritance, 460
  and malaria, 462, 469
  and malarial anaemia, 467
  'Negro' type, 460
  and neonatal jaundice, 462
  non-Negro type, 460
  partial enzyme deficiency type, 460
  screening methods, 768
  starch gel in, 460
  tests for, 462
Glucuronyl transferase, liver disease and,
    568
Glycogen-storage disease, 379
Gnathostoma spinigerum, life cycle, 120
Gnathostomiasis, 120
Goats, brucellosis and, 330
Goitre, endemic, 655
Gonadotrophin, malignant trophoblastic
    disease and, 648
Gonorrhoea, 639
Goodpasture's syndrome, 620, 621
Gout, 714
Gram-negative organisms, 296
Granuloma multiforme, 313
Granuloma venereum, 336
Groundnut, *Aspergillus flavus* and, 560
Group A arboviruses, 217
Group C arboviruses, 217
Guama group viruses, 217
Guarnieri bodies, 240
Guaroa virus, 228
Guinea-worm, 142
Gynatresia, 645
Gynaecomastia, 595, 650
  in cirrhosis, 551
  leprosy and, 311
  pathology of, 595

H antigen, 475
Haemagogus, yellow fever and, 219
Haematuria:
  in schistosomiasis, 156
  in sickle-cell trait, 429
Haemochromatosis, 569

Haemoglobin:
  copper sulphate method of estimation, 482
  despatch of samples, 768
  electrophoresis of, 421, 424, 767
  haptoglobins and, 414
  normal structure, 416
  normal values, 7
  paper electrophoresis, method, 767
  solubility test, 768
  'unstable' form, 453
Haemoglobin A, 416, et seq.
  α chain, 417
  β chain, 417
  C, G. and GC in one individual, 420
  (normal), structure of molecule, 416
Haemoglobin Aegina, 426
Haemoglobin Alexandra, 426
Haemoglobin A₂; 416, 425
  abnormal forms, 425
  α chain, in 425
  in acute malaria, 456
  in β thalassaemia, 425
  δ chain in, 425
  Flatbush, 425
  in hereditary persistence of foetal haemo-
    globin, 425
  in the Negro, 425
  in thalassaemia minor, 425
Haemoglobin Bart's, 415, 421, 457
  in haemoglobin H disease, 459
  sickling and, 428
Haemoglobin Beilenson, 452
Haemoglobin C, 416, 419
  AC, 434
  α chain, 418
  β chain, 418, 434
  CC, 435
  CF, 435
  CS, 436
  (see sickle-cell disease)
  C thalassaemia, 435
  C trait, 435
  diagnosis, 435
  incidence, 434
  lysine substitution, 418, 434
  and malaria, 467
  and other abnormal haemoglobins, 435
  and target cells, 435
Haemoglobin Caserta, 452
Haemoglobin D, 418, 446
  AD, 447
  α chain, 446
  β chain, 446
  DD, 447
  diagnosis, 447
  DS, 447
  D-thalassaemia, 447
  geographical distribution, 447
  target cells and, 447
Haemoglobin δ₄, 425
Haemoglobin E, 415, 420, 421, 447
  AE, 447

Haemoglobin E: continued
  β chain, 447
  diagnosis, 449
  EE, 447
  E and ovalocytosis, 447
  E thalassaemia, 447
  geographical distribution, 447
  and malaria, 449, 468
  and target cells, 447
  in West Africa, 420
Haemoglobin F (fetal), 416, 423, 425 et seq.
  abnormal forms of, 426
  alkali resistant haemoglobin in, 426, 766
  α chain, 425
  conditions in which increased, 426
  diagnosis, 426
  distribution in erythrocytes, 426
  FC, 427
  FS, 427
  estimation of, 766
  γ chain, 425
  hereditary persistence of, 426
  and malaria, 468
  minor components of, 426
  Norfolk form, 452
  normal, 425
Haemoglobin Flatbush, 425
Haemoglobin G, 418, 450
  α chain, 450
  β chain, 450
  diagnosis, 450
Haemoglobin Galveston, 426
Haemoglobin H (β₄), 457
  brilliant cresyl blue test, 423, 768
  diagnosis, 459
  disease, 458
  geographical distribution, 458
  inclusion bodies in, 768
  pregnancy and, 458
Haemoglobin Hopkins I and II, 452
Haemoglobin I, 450
Haemoglobin I C, 450
Haemoglobin J, 450
Haemoglobin K, 450
Haemoglobin Koln disease, 453
Haemoglobin L, 451
Haemoglobin Lepore, 452
Haemoglobin M, 451
Haemoglobin Mexico, 453
Haemoglobin N, 451
Haemoglobin Norfolk, 452
Haemoglobin O, 451
Haemoglobin P, 451
Haemoglobin Porto Alegre, 452
Haemoglobin Q, 451
Haemoglobin Roma, 426
Haemoglobin S, 416, 418, 419, 427, et seq
  α chain, 427
  AS, 429, et seq.
    diagnosis, 431
    geographical distribution, 429
    inheritance, 419
    and malaria, 466

Haemoglobin S, AS: *continued*
  pathology, 429
  sickling mechanism, 427, 428
  sickling test, 428
  valine substitution, 418
  viscosity of blood, 428
  β chain, 418
  SF, 427, 434
    SS, *see* sickle-cell anaemia, 431
    diagnosis, 434
Haemoglobin St. Mary's disease, 453
Haemoglobin Seattle disease, 453
Haemoglobin Shimonoseki, 452
Haemoglobin Stanleyville I and II, 452
Haemoglobin Texas, 426
Haemoglobin Ube-I disease, 453
Haemoglobin Zurich disease, 453
Haemoglobinuria, in blackwater fever, 464
Haemolysin, in blood transfusion reactions, 485
Haemolytic anaemia:
  see also) Anaemia, haemolytic, 414
  autoimmune, 489
  drugs and, 460
  G-6-PD deficiency, 460
  in heatstroke, 736
Haemolytic disease of the newborn, 488
  ABO incompatibility, 478
  assessment of severity, 489
  intra-uterine transfusion, 484
  rhesus incompatability in, 479
  therapy, 489
Haemophilia, 471
  joints and, 716
Haemophilus ducreyi, 338
Haemorrhagic disease of the newborn, 471
Haemorrhagic disorders, 469
Haemorrhagic fever, 224
  Junin virus and, 224
Haemorrhoids, 526
Haemosiderin:
  in African siderosis, 570
  in haemochromatosis, 569
  in malaria, 26
  in urine, 465
Haemosiderosis, 568
  in sickle-cell disease, 440
Haemozoin (*see* malaria, pigment), 18
Halbersaedter-Prowazek bodies, 264
Halzoun:
  Fasciola hepatica and, 188
  Limnatis nilotica and, 188
Hanging groin in onchocerciasis, 138
Haptoglobins, 414
Hartmanella, 77
Hashimoto's disease, 654
  and active juvenile cirrhosis, 584
Heat-unstable haemoglobin disease, 453
Heart, 348, *et seq.*
  alcoholic heart disease, 380
  amyloidosis, 723
  in anaemia, 379

Heart: *continued*
  annular subvalvular left ventricular aneurysms, 366
  and ascariasis, 102
  bacterial endocarditis, 372
  beri-beri, 380
  brown atrophy, 348, 379
  Burkitt tumour, 505
  carcinoid syndrome in, 358, 542
  cardiopathy, 351
  Chagas disease, 46
  in citrate toxicity, 488
  congenital heart disease, 365
  cor pulmonale, 374
  cryptogenic heart disease, 351
  cysticercosis and, 199
  diphtheritic myocarditis, 372
  dirofilariasis and, 140
  endocardial fibroelastosis, 356
  endomyocardial fibrosis, 357
  Fiedler type myocarditis, 371
  giant cell myocarditis, 371
  heart muscle disease, 351
  hydatid disease and, 205
  5-hydroxytryptamine in, 358
  idiopathic cardiomegaly, 351
    diagnosis, 355
    infarction in, 355
    occurring in late pregnancy and the puerperum, 355
    pathogenesis, 352
  idiopathic cardiomyopathy, 351
  idiopathic familial heart disease, 349
  intracardiac post-operative thrombosis, 355
  in kwashiorkor, 678
  Loeffler's disease, 373
  and loiasis, 132
  measles and, 250
  metabolic disorders, 379
  metastatic tumour, 382
  myocardiopathies, classification of, 349
  myocardiosis, 351
  normal values, 348
  nutritional heart disease, 351
  obstruction cardiomyopathy, 349
  palm wine-tappers heart, 381
  parasitic myocarditis, 372
  primary myocardial disease, 351
  primary tumours, 382
  sarcoidosis, 382
  in schistosomiasis, 165
  secondary tumours of, 382
  in sickle-cell anaemia, 433
  in South American trypanosomiasis, 46
  syphilitic myocarditis, 372
  thrush breast, 348
  thyrotoxic heart disease, 348
  toxic myocarditis, 373
  in toxocariasis, 105
  in toxoplasmosis, 84
  in trichinellosis, 116
  Trypanosoma cruzi, 48

Heart: *continued*
in tuberculosis, 378
tuberculous myocarditis, 372
tumours of, 382
viral myocarditis, 371
Heat disorders, 734
Heat stroke, 735
Hecht, giant cell pneumonia of, 250
Heidenhain's stain, 756
Heinz bodies:
in haemoglobin Zurich disease, 453
in heat unstable haemoglobin disease, 453
Heliotropium, 558, 563
Helminthic diseases, 91 *et seq.*
Helminths, faeces examination, 753
Henoch—Schonlein purpura, 470
Heparin, in the defibrination syndrome, 425
Hepatitis:
active chronic, 584
alcoholic acute, 553
cholestatic and drugs, 557
cholestatic type, 583
comparison of infectious hepatitis and homologous serum jaundice, 582
chronic aggressive, 584
chronic persistent, 584
liver cell cancer and, 597
lupoid, 584
plasma cell, 584
'post-hepatitis syndrome', 584
viral type A, 577
viral type B, 578
Hepatitis associated antigen,
see Australia antigen, 578
Hepatitis B antigen,
see Australia antigen, 578
Hepatolenticular degeneration, 566, 612
Herbal medicine, 558
Hereditary persistence of foetal haemo-globin, 426
Hereditary spherocytosis, 459
Hernia:
inguinal, 642
umbilical, 513
Herpes simplex, 253
Herpes viruses, 253
Epstein-Barr virus, 253, 255
H. ateles, 253
H. hominis, 253
H. saimiri, 253
H. simiae, 253
H. suis, 253
Herpes zoster, 241
Heterophyes heterophyes, life cycle, 181
Heterophyiasis, 181
Hirschsprung's disease, 513
Histidinaemia, 602
Histochemistry:
amyloidosis, 724
Burkitt tumour, 510
lymphosarcoma, 510
reticulum cell sarcoma, 510

Histopathology:
preservation of tissue for, 774
Histoplasma capsulatum, 285
differentiation from *Leishmania tropica*, 64
duboisii, 286
Histoplasmosis, 285
African, 286
Hodgkins disease, 498, 499
and brucellosis, 332
Hoeppli phenomenon in schistosomiasis, 154
Homologous serum jaundice,
see Viral hepatitis type B, 576
Hookworm infection, 7, 91
anaemia and, 94
diagnostic pathology, 97
epidemiology, 92
folic acid deficiency in, 95
hypoalbuminaemia in, 95
immunity, 93
malabsorption in, 97
ova, quantitative counts, 757
pulmonary reactions and, 94
Hunter's disease, 602
Hurler's disease, 602
Hyaline membrane, 390
malaria and, 31
Hydatid disease, 201
anti-P antibody in, 205
blood group P, antibody in, 205
diagnostic pathology, 205
epidemiology, 202
pathology, 201
Hydatid sand, 203
Hydatidiform mole, 647, 648
Hydrocele:
in filariasis, 129
and *Loa loa*, 129
and loiasis, 132
and *Mansonella ozzardi*, 129
and *Onchocerca volvulus*, 129
Hydrocephalus, 601
Hydronephrosis, 635
in schistosomiasis, 160
Hydrops foetalis:
in ABO incompatibility, 488, 568
in α thalassaemia, 457
5-hydroxyindolacetic acid, 541
5-hydroxytryptamine, 541
and endomyocardial fibrosis, 358
in leprosy, 312
Hymenolepis diminuta:
epidemiology, 208
life cycle, 208
nana:
epidemiology, 208
life cycle, 208
Hypernephroma, 638
Hyperpyrexia, 735
malaria, 20
Hypersplenism, 490
brucellosis and, 330

Hypersplenism: *continued*
  causes of splenic 'pooling', 491
  in chronic liver disease, 549
  definition, 490
  'pooling', effects of, 491, 492
  primary, 491
  in *Schistosoma japonicum* and *S. mansoni* infections, 173
  secondary, 491
  spleen in, 491
  splenectomy in, 492
  in visceral Kala-azar, 54
Hypertension, 328, 527, 376
  in arteritis of obscure aetiology, 386
  kidney in, 616
  schistosomiasis and, 160
Hypertensive heart disease, 376
Hypertrophic osteoarthropathy, 549
Hypogammaglobulinaemia, 711
Hypoglycaemia:
  in liver cell carcinoma, 591
  plant alkaloids and, 558
  in trypanosomiasis, 37
Hypophosphatasia, 687
Hypoprothrombinaemia:
  in liver disease, 471
  vitamin K deficiency, 471
Hyposthenuria, 616
  in sickle-cell trait, 429, 430
Hypothermia, 671

Idiopathic multiple haemorrhagic sarcoma, 704
Idiopathic splenomegaly, 492
Ihesha virus, 227
Ilheus virus, 219
Immunity:
  malaria, 15
    humoral, 15
    pregnancy, 32
    racial, 16
  malarial pigment distribution in liver, 28
Immunoglobulins: 710
Immunology, 710
  cell mediated immunity in, 711
  diseases of immune origin, 711
Inclusion conjunctivitis, 244
Indian childhood cirrhosis (ICC), 574
  pathology, 575
Infant mortality and malnutrition, 1
Infantile tremor syndrome, 608
Infantilism in idiopathic tropical spleno-megaly syndrome, 497
Infectious hepatitis,
  see Viral hepatitis type A, 576
Infectious mononucleosis, 255
Infertility in schistosomiasis, 160
Influenza, 371
  blood groups in, 476
Insect bites, thrombocytopenia, 471
Intestinal obstruction, 523
  ascariasis, 101
  in enterobiasis, 113

Intestinal obstruction: *continued*
  herniae and, 523
  ileus and peritonitis, 523
  intussusception, 524
  mesenteric thrombosis, 523
  porocephalus, 739
  pyloric stenosis, 523
  Schistosoma japonica and, 523
  in *Schistosoma japonicum* infection, 168
  in *Schistosoma mansoni* infection, 168
  in strongyloidiasis, 107
  tuberculosis and, 523
  volvulus, 523
Intestine:
  anthrax and, 333
  Brown bowel syndrome, 532
  in Burkitt tumour, 506
  carcinoma and, 539
  and *Clostridium welchii* infection, 318
  in enterobiasis, 112
  eosinophilic granuloma, 522
  Kaposi's sarcoma, 704
  large:
    in balantidiasis, 90
    Burkitt tumour, 506
    cancer, incidence in tropics, 539
    classification of tumours, 540
  malaria and, 31
  paragonomiasis and, 191
  perforation, 525
    amoebiasis and, 526
    ascariasis and, 101, 526
    idiopathic, 101, 526
    peptic ulcer and, 525
    tuberculosis and, 526
    typhoid and, 526
  in *S. haematobium*, 162
  in South American trypanosomiasis, 46
  in strongyloidiasis, 108
  in trichinellosis, 116
  typhoid fever and, 323
Intussusception, 524
  in ascariasis, 101
  Burkitt tumour, 504
  in *Schistosoma haematobium* infecton, 163
  in *Schistosoma japonicum* infection, 169
  in *Schistosoma mansoni* infection, 169
Iodamoeba butschlii, 77
  death from, 77
Iodides, purpura, 470
Iodine:
  goitre and, 655
Iron deficiency anaemia, 406
Ischio rectal abscess:
  in enterobiasis, 114
  in *Schistosoma mansoni* and *S. japonicum* infections, 169
Isospora belli, 82
  hominis, 82
Isosporiasis, 82
Itaqui, 217
Ixodes persucaltus, 226
  rincus, 226

Jagsiekte, Crotalaria in, 563
Japanese encephalitis virus, 226
Japanese river fever, 213
Japanese seven-day fever, 345
Jaundice:
    liver function tests in, 582
Jaw bones, Burkitt tumour, 504
Jejunal biopsy:
    in cholera, 316
    in coeliac disease, 531
    in giardiasis, 80
    in haemochromatosis, 570
    in hookworm infection, 97
    in kwashiorkor, 679
    in strongyloidiasis, 107
    tropical sprue, 531
    in tropics, 532
    in tuberculosis, 396
    in typhoid fever, 323
Jigger flea, 741
Joints, 715
    amoebiasis, 70
    amyloidosis, 724
    brucellosis and, 332
    in dracontiasis, 143, 716
    in onchocerciasis, 136
    pain in sickle-cell anaemia, 432
    pain in sickle-cell disease, 444
    in Schistosoma haematobium infection, 165
    suppurative arthritis in loiasis, 132
Junin virus, 228
Juvenile motor neurone disease, 607
Juxta articular nodes in the treponematosis, 342

Kala-Azar, 52
    (See also visceral leishmaniasis)
    African, 53
    associated with a canine reservoir, 53
    hypersplenism, 490
    Indian, 53
Kangri cancer, 703
Kaposi's sarcoma, 704
    pathology, 705
Katayama syndrome, 153, 154
Kell blood group system, 475
Keloid, 731
    sarcomatous change in, 732
Kemerovo, 217
Kerandel's sign, 37
Keratitis, measles and, 250
    in trypanosomiasis, 41
Keratoacanthoma, rarity in coloured races, 702
Keratomalacia, 683
Keratomycosis nigricans palmaris, 266
Kernicterus, 462
    and G-6-PD deficiency, 462
    infection and, 602
    in prematurity, 489
Khaini cancer, 535
Khan test, 342
Kidd blood group system, 475

Kidney, 616, et seq.
    abortion and, 634
    abscess and, 635
    accidental haemorrhage and, 634
    acute tubular necrosis, 634
    amoebiasis, 70
    amyloidosis, 724
    blackwater fever and, 463, 634
    in blood transfusion reactions, 486
    in Burkitt tumour, 506
    carbon tetrachloride and, 634
    cholera and, 317
    cirrhosis, 552
    complement in, 618
    congenital anomalies of, 616
    cortical necrosis, 635
    crush injury in, 634
    in diabetes mellitus, 626, 634
    glomerulonephritis, 616
    Goodpasture's syndrome, 620
    haemolytic anaemia and, 634
    in heatstroke, 736
    hydatid disease and, 205
    hydronephrosis, 160, 635
    hypertension, essential and, 616
    hypokalaemia and, 634
    immunology and, 618
    in incompatible blood transfusion, 634
    in kwashiorkor, 680
    lipoid nephrosis, 624
    in leptospirosis, 346
    liver disease and, 634
    in lupus erythematosis, 617
    magnesium deficiency and, 381
    malaria, pathology, 29, 30
        renal failure in, 18
    malarial nephrosis, 627
    massive liver cell necrosis and, 587
    mercury and, 634
    minimal change, 624
    myoglobinuria and, 634
    nephrotic syndrome and, 623
    normal function, 616
    pyelonephritis, 635
        chronic, 622
    pyonephrosis, 635
    renal vein thrombosis in amyloidosis, 724
    in schistosomiasis, 176
    senile arteriosclerotic, 616
    shock and, 634
    in sickle-cell anaemia, 433
    sickle-cell disease and, 441
    and sickle-cell trait, 430
    in strongyloidiasis, 107
    sulphonamides and, 634
    in toxocariasis, 105
    in trichinellosis, 116
    tuberculosis, 398, 621, 635
    tubular necrosis, acute in malaria, 29
        in blackwater fever, 464
    tubules, affections of, 634
    tumours of, 638
    in typhoid fever, 326

Kidney: *continued*
  uric acid precipitates, 634
  yellow fever and, 221
Kimberley horse disease, 563
Klebsiella rhinoscleromatosis, 732
Klinefelter's syndrome, 596
Knott's method, 765
Kulschitsky, argentaffin cells, 541
Kuru, 262
Kveim test, 401
Kwashiorkor, 669
  alimentary tract and, 678
  anaemia in, 674
  carbohydrates and, 672
  central nervous system in, 680
  cirrhosis and, 553
  clinical presentation, 670
  electrolytes in, 674
  endocrine glands and, 679
  essential amino acids in, 671
  fat metabolism and, 673
  folic acid deficiency and, 672
  heart in, 678
  hypothermia in, 671
  kidneys in, 680
  liver in, 676
  liver function tests in, 673
  lungs in, 680
  malaria and, 674
  metabolic effects, 671
  pancreas in, 675
  plasma proteins and, 671
  post mortem findings, 675
  reticulo-endothelial system in, 681
Kyasanur forest disease, 227
Kyphoscoliosis and pulmonary hypertension, 375
Kyphosis, tuberculous, 395

Lactase deficiency, 533
Lagochilascaris minor, in pyomyositis, tropical, 718
Larva migrans, cutaneous, 144
  visceral, 104
Larynx:
  carcinoma of, 403
  leprosy and, 304
Schistosoma haematobium infection and, 164
  smallpox and, 239
  tuberculosis of, 394
Lassa fever, 229
  diagnosis, 232
  pathology, 230
Lathyrism, 612
Lead poisoning, 742
Leber cells, 244
Leeches and Halzoun, 189
Leishman-Donovan body, 51
Leishmania, culture method, 765
Leishmania braziliensis, mucocutaneous leishmaniasis, 61
  donovani, 50
    visceral leishmaniasis, 52

Leishmania braziliensis: *continued*
  guyanensis, 50
  mexicana, 50
  peruviana, 50
  pifanoi, 50
  tropica, 50
Leishmaniasis: 49
  and blood transfusion, 481
  blood transfusion transmitted, 52
  classification, 50
  culture, 64
    method, 765
  cutaneous, 58
    chiclero ulcer, 59
    Ethiopian, 61
    leishmaniasis tegumentaria diffusa, 60
    lupoid, 61
    muco-cutaneous, 61
    oriental sore, 58
    Uta, 60
  diagnostic methods, 759
  epidemiology, 52
  geographical distribution, 53
  life cycle, 49
  marital transmission, 49
    pathology, 54
  post-Kala-azar dermal leishmaniasis, 52, 57
  reservoir hosts, 53
  recivida, 50
  tegumentaria diffusa, 60
  visceral, *See* visceral leishmaniasis, 52
Leishmanoma, in African Kala-azar, 53
Leishman's stain, 762
Lepromin test, B.C.G. vaccination and, 299
Leprosy, 297
  amyloidosis and, 312
  bone changes in, 309
  borderline, 306
  classification, 298
  diagnostic pathology, 312
  dimorphous, 306
  endocrine glands in, 312
  epidemiology, 297
  erythema nodosum leprosum, 308
  eye in, 304, 310
  globi, 303
  gynaecomastia, 311, 596
  immunology, 299
  indeterminate, 301
  lepra cells, 303
  lepromatous, 302
  lepromin test, 299
  liver in, 309
  Lucio phenomenon, 307
  masked, 307
  muscle in, 312
  Myco. leprae, 297
  nose in, 304
  pathology, 301
  polyneuritic, 306
  progressive lepra reaction, 308

Leprosy: *continued*
  reactional states, 308
  and sickle cell trait, 429
  skin, 751
  testes, 311
  tuberculoid, 304
  Virchow cells, 303
Leptospira, 345
  bataviae, 345
  cunicula, 345
  grippotyphosa, 345
  icterohaemorrhagiae, 345
Leptospirosis, 345
Letterer-Siwe's disease, measles virus and, 251
Leucopenia: 8
  hypersplenism, 490
  in malaria, 25
  in megaloblastic anaemia, 411
  in tuberculosis, 397
Leukaemia, 472
  Burkitt tumour, 512
  chronic lymphatic, 474
    and malaria, 27
  chronic myeloid, 474
  geographical distribution, 472
  hypersplenism, in, 490
  measles virus and, 251
  rarity of acute in children, 472
  types of, 473
Leukaemoid reaction, 474
  alkaline phosphatase in, 474
  in brucellosis, 332
  in toxoplasmosis, 85
  in tuberculosis, 397
  in visceral Kala-azar, 55
Leukoplakia, bladder and schistosomiasis, 158
Lewis blood group system, 479
  antibodies in incidence in Negroes, 479
Linguatula serrata, 739
Lipocalcinogranulomatosis, see tumoral calcinosis, 719
Lipofuscin:
  in haemochromatosis, 569
  heart and, 379
  hepatitis, and, 583
Lipotropic factors, 673
Liver, 542, *et seq.*
  abscess of, 543
    in amoebiasis, 72
    in ascariasis, 100, 102
    in clonorchiasis, 184
    in *Schistosoma japonicum* infection, 171
  active juvenile cirrhosis, 584
  African siderosis, 570
  alkaloids and, 558
  amyloidosis, 723
  ascariasis, 100
  Banti's syndrome, 497
  biliary infection in fascioliasis, 188

Liver: *continued*
  brucellosis and, 332
  Budd-Chiari syndrome, 565
  Burkitt tumour, 506
  carcinoma, 589
  cirrhosis, *see* cirrhosis, 545
  clay pipe-stem fibrosis, 169
  clonorchiasis and carcinoma, 185
  cystic fibrosis, 567
  disease and citrate toxicity, 488
  disease, classification, 544
  drugs and, 557
  fascioliasis and, 188
  fatty, acute in pregnancy, 587
  filariasis and, 128
  function tests in jaundice, 582
  galactosaemia, 566
  giant-cell hepatitis, 568
  granulomatous lesions, 555
  haemochromatosis, 570
  heatstroke and, 736
  hepatitis, amoebic, 72
    infectious, 577
  hepatolenticular degeneration, 566
  homologous serum jaundice, 578
  hydatid disease, 204
  Indian childhood cirrhosis, 574
  Kaposi's sarcoma, 705
  kidney in, 634
  kwashiorkor and, 676
  leprosy and, 309
  malaria and, 27, 556
  massive liver-cell necrosis, 585
    in schistosomiasis, 171
  mesenchymal tumours of, 599
  mycotoxins and, 559
  neonatal conditions, 543
  opisthorchiasis and, 187
  pigment in malaria, 27
    in schistosomiasis, 171
  pipe-stem fibrosis, 169
  portal hypertension, 550
  Q fever and, 213
  Schistosoma haematobium, 164
    japonicum and *S. mansoni*, 169
  secondary tumours, 599
  sickle-cell anaemia and, 440
  stellate fibrosis, 553, 676
  strongyloidiasis and, 109
  toxocariasis, and 105
  toxoplasmosis and, 86
  tropical splenomegaly syndrome and, 495
  trypanosomiasis, 39
  tuberculosis, 398
  tumours of, 588, *et seq.*
    alpha-feto protein and, 592
    Australia antigen and, 579
    cholangiocellular carcinoma, 185, 598, 599
    classification, 588
    hepatocellular and mixed carcinoma, 598

Liver, tumours: *continued*
    liver-cell carcinoma, 589
      aetiology, 593
      age and, 596
      cirrhosis and, 594
      geographical distribution, 593
      hypoglycaemia and, 591
      oestrogenization and, 595
      polycythaemia and, 591
      sex, 595
      toxic factors in, 596, 597
      viral hepatitis and, 597
    typhoid fever and, 324
    veno-occlusive disease, 562
    visceral leishmaniasis and, 56
    yellow fever and, 221
Loa loa:
    life cycle, 131
    microfilaria of, 123
Loboa loboi, 290
Lobo's disease, 290
Loefflerella whitmori, 339
Loefflers disease, 373
    eosinophilic myocarditis in, 373
Loeffler's syndrome, 100
    in strongyloidiasis, 107
Loiasis, 131
    diagnostic pathology, 132
    epidemiology, 131
    pathology, 132
Louping ill, 226
Lucio phenomenon, in leprosy, 307
Lumpy jaw, 276
Lung, 390, *et seq.*
    abscess, 390
      amoebiasis and, 73
    actinomycosis, 276
    African histoplasmosis, 286
    anthrax and, 333
    asbestosis, 391
    ascariasis and, 98, 102
    ascaris pneumonia, 99, 100
    aspergillosis and, 273
    bronchitis, 375
      malarial, 31
    in Burkitt tumour, 505
    cancer, cigarette smoking, 536
      low incidence in tropics, 403
    chorion carcinoma and, 648
    coccidioidomycosis, 277
    cor pulmonale, 375
    cryptococcosis, 289
    dirofilariasis and, 140
    emphysema, 375, 391
    eosinophilia, tropical, 383
    in filariasis, 128
    giant-cell pneumonia, 250
    histoplasmosis, 285
    in hookworm infection, 94
    hyaline membrane, 390
    hydatid disease, 204
    in larva migrans, 144
    lobar pneumonia, 391

Lung: *continued*
    Loeffler's syndrome, 100
    marrow embolism in sickle-cell disease, 441
    measles, 250
    North American blastomycosis, 279
    paragonimiasis and, 192
    phycomycosis, 275
    Pneumocystis carinii, 88
    porocephalus, 739
    pulmonary embolism, 388
      hypertension, 374
    respiratory distress syndrome, 390
    sarcoidosis, 401
    in *Schistosoma haematobium* infection, 153, 164, 173
    in strongyloidiasis, 109, 110
    in toxocariasis, 105
    in toxoplasmosis, 85
    in trichinellosis, 116
    trypanosomiasis and, 39
    tuberculosis, 391
    tumours of, 403
    in typhoid fever, 326
    veno-occlusive disease of, 376
    whooping cough, 390
Lupoid hepatitis, 584
    leishmaniasis, 61
Lupus erythematosis:
    cells, active juvenile cirrhosis and, 584
    disseminated, 617
    kidney in, 626
Lutheran blood group system, 475
Lutz-splendore-Almeida's disease, 281
Lymph node puncture, 778
Lymphangiography in filariasis, 129
Lympho-epithelioma, 403
Lymphocyte transformation:
    in biliary cirrhosis, 561
    Burkitt tumour and, 502
    in kwashiorkor, 670
    leprosy and, 299
    malaria and, 15
    measles and, 249
    tropical splenomegaly syndrome and, 497
    viral hepatitis B and, 561
Lymphocytosis in tropical splenomegaly syndrome, 497
Lymphoedema, see elephantiasis, 129
Lymphogranuloma inguinale, 244, 526
    venereum, 244
Lymphoreticular tumours, 498
    classification, 500
    parasites and, 498
Lymphosarcoma, 499
    Burkitt tumour, 500
    histochemistry, 510
Lysol, suicide and, 518
Lyssa bodies, 236

Machupo virus, 228
Madelung's deformity, 714
Madrid virus, 217

Madura foot, 271
Magnesium:
  bladder stone disease and, 637
  in cirrhosis, 674
  hypomagnesaemia in alcoholism, 381
  in kwashiorkor, 674
Malabsorption: 526
  in capillariasis, 144
  classification, 526
  giardiasis and, 80
  in hookwork infection, 97
    pancreatic calcification and, 665
    strongyloidiasis and, 109
    tuberculosis, 396
Malaria, 10
  and abnormal haemoglobins, 465
  adrenals in, 30
  in adults, 14
  algid, 20, 31
  anaemia, 18, 20, 23
    brain in, 22
    haematological findings, 25
    mechanism of, 23
  antibodies, in, 19
    tropical splenomegaly syndrome, 493
  avian, 12
  blockade of reticuloendothelial system, 19
  blood film, preparation, 759
  and blood transfusion, 481
  bone marrow in, 26
  brain, pathology, 21
  cerebral, 20
  in children, 14, 26, 33
  choleraic, 20
  cirrhosis and, 556
  coagulation factors, 25
  congenital, 33
  cryptozoic schizonts, 11
  diagnosis, 33
  differentiation of species, 34
  endemicity, measurement, 14
  epidemiology, 12
  fibrin, 17, 23
  first infection, 14
  fluorescent antibody techniques, 16
    method, 765
  gamma globulin, therapeutic effect, 15
  and G-6-PD, 462, 469
  gel diffusion technique, 16
  genetic aspects of immunity, 465
  geographical distribution, 10
  haemoglobin breakdown in, 23
  and haemoglobin C, 467
    E, 468
    F, 468
    S, 466
  haemosiderin in, 18
  and the heart, 31
  hepatic failure, 20
  host/parasite relationship, 18
  hyperpyrexia, 20
  immunity, cellular, 15

Malaria, immunity: continued
    developing, 15
    humoral, 15
    and neonate, 13
    racial, 16
  immunosuppression in, 503
  inherited factors and immunity, 16
  kidney, 18, 619
    pathology, 29
  life cycle, 11
  liver and cirrhosis, 29
    fibrosis, 29
  liver function tests in, 29
  liver, pathology, 27
    pigment distribution and immunity, 28
  lungs in, 20, 31
  malignancy and, 503, et seq.
  malnutrition and, 19
  mitochondria, 19
  morbidity, 13
  mortality in, 13
  necropsy findings, 20
  neonate and, 13
  nephrosis and, 617, 627
  in non-immune, 20
  parasite rates, 14
    counts, 765
  in partially immune, 20
  pathology, 17
    effect of parasite, 17
  pigment, 12, 18
    composition of, 18
    histochemistry, 18
    in kidney, 29
    in liver, 28
    in polymorphonuclear, 25
  placenta in, 32
  Plasmodium falciparum, 10
  pre-erythrocytic cycle, 11
  and pregnancy, 32
  proliferative nephritis, 29
  pulmonary oedema, 20, 31
  pyrexia, 17
  racial factors, 16
  relapse, 12
  relationship with other infections, 19
  renal failure in, 20
  reticulocytosis in, 25
  reticuloendothelial system, 23
  rhesus factor and, 469
  shock in, 20
  spleen, pathology, 27
    rates, 14
    rupture of, 27
  splenectomy in, 27
  splenic smear in, 27
  stable, 13
  staining procedures, 762
  stains for, 758
  stellate fibrosis of the liver in, 676
  steroids in, 30
  and stress, 30
  and symmetrical gangrene, 387

Malaria: *continued*
  and thalassaemia, 468
  tubular necrosis, 29
  unstable, 13
  vectors, 10
Malarial nephrosis, 627
Malarial parasite:
  electron microscopy, 11
  erythrocytic cycle, 11
  exo-erythrocytic cycle, 11
  metabolism of, 12
    in erythrocyte, 12
  schizonts, 11
  sporozoites, 11
Malassezia furfur, 266
Mal del morado, 139
Malignant disease, 690
  amoebiasis and, 74
  in children, 709
  endocrine disturbance in, 699
  immunological aspects, 697
  neurological complications in, 699
  in the tropics, 690
    age, rarity in older groups, 693
    age specific rates, 695
    common tumours in, 702
    environmental factors, 691
    histopathology, 701
    incidence, 691
    indirect standardization, 695
    racial factors, 690
    sociological factors, 690
Malignant trophoblastic disease, 647
  pelvic angiography, 649
  urinary gonadotrophin in, 650
Malnutrition, 668
  in adults, 682
  causative factors, 668
  cirrhosis and, 553, 555
  imbalance or kwashiorkor, 669
  liver-cell cancer and, 596
  and malaria, 20
  overnutrition, 668
  protein-calorie malnutrition of early
    childhood, 669
  trichuriasis and, 112
  undernutrition or marasmus, 681
Manganese:
  poisoning, 602
Manic depressive psychosis, 615
Mansonella ozzardi, 141
  microfilaria of, 123
Mansonioides and filariasis, 122
Marasmic, kwashiorkor, 669
Marasmus, 681
Marble bone disease, 714
Marek's disease, 253
Marfan's syndrome, 716, 720
Margburg virus disease, 252
Marituba virus, 217
Marrow:
  heterotopic in annular subvalvular left-
    ventricular aneurysm, 368

Marrow: *continued*
  paravertebral masses, 455
  pulmonary embolism, 441
Massive liver cell necrosis, 583, 585
  pathology, 586
Maurer's clefts, malaria, 23
Maxillary sinus:
  carcinoma of, 402
Mayaro virus, 217
Measles, 248
  giant cell pneumonia and, 250
  kwashiorkor and, 250
  pathology, 248
Meconium ileus, 664
Megacolon, 524
  in trypanosomiasis, South American, 47
Megaloblastic anaemia, 407
  differentiation of B_{12} and folic acid
    deficiency, 411
Megaoesophagus, 517
  trypanosomiasis, South American and, 47
Meischer's tubes, 87
Melania spp., paragonomiasis and, 191
Melanin:
  in haemochromatosis, 569
  oral cavity, 514
  physiology of, 703
  staining properties, 709
Melanocytes:
  in albinism, 703
  in Whites, Negroes and Albinos, 708
Melanoma: 707
  in albinism, 703
  incidence, 708
  histopathology, 709
Melanosis coli, 532
Melioidosis, 339
Menarche, 644
Meninges, Burkitt tumour, 504
Meningitis:
  amoebic, 77
  in ascariasis, 101
  (cerebrospinal) meningococcal, 604
  cryptococcosis and, 289
  enteroviruses and, 259
  eosinophilic in angiostrongyliasis, 118
    in gnathostomiasis, 121
  pneumococcal, 603
  porocephalus, 739
  and trichinellosis, 116
  tuberculous, 396
  typhus, scrub and, 214
Meningococcal septicaemia, purpura in, 604
Meningocoele, 601
Meningo-encephalitis:
  Acanthamoeba spp. and, 77
  trypanosomiasis, South American and, 47
Mental deficiency, 602
Mental disease, 615
Mepacrine, in G-6-PD deficiency, 460
Mercury:
  kidney and, 634
  purpura and, 470

Mesothelioma, 391
Metagonimiasis, 181
Metagonimus yokagawai, life cycle, 181
Methaemalbumin, 463
 in malaria, 26, 33
Methionine, massive liver necrosis and, 585
Metropathia haemorrhagica, 644
Microcephaly, cytomegalic inclusion
 disease and, 262
Microfilaria, diagnostic table, 123
Microfilariae:
 concentration method, 759, 765
 diagnostic methods, 759
 staining of, 764
Microscopes, protection in tropics, 775
Microsporium audouini, 267
Microsporosis nigra, 266
Migraine:
 sickle cell trait and, 430
Mikulicz cells, in rhinoscleroma, 733
Milk intolerance, 533
Minimal change kidney, 624
Mitsuda reaction, 300
 lucio phenomenon and, 307
 in progressive lepra reaction, 309
Mkar disease, 313
MNSs blood group system, 475
Molybdenum:
 cirrhosis and, 557
 oesophageal cancer and, 536
Monckeberg sclerosis, 384
Mongolism, 602
Monkey pox, 239
Monkeys, malaria, 17
Mononucleosis, infectious and toxoplasmo-
 sis, 83
Montenegro reaction, 64
Morquio's disease, 602
Morula cell, 38
Mountain sickness, 375
Mucocutaneous leishmaniasis, 61
Mucor, 275
 diabetes mellitus and, 663
Mucormycosis, 275
 cerebral, 605
Mucoviscidosis, 664
Multiceps multiceps, life cycle, 209
Multiple sclerosis, 609
 measles and, 249
Mumps, 247
 and endocardial fibroelastosis, 356
 pancreatic calcification and, 665
Murray valley encephalitis, 217
Murutucu, 217
Muscles, 716
 amyloidosis, 726
 biopsy, 717
 cysticercosis and, 199
 dermatomyositis, 717
 myasthenia gravis, 717
 paragonomiasis and, 193
 pyomyositis, tropical, 718
 sarcosporidiosis, 87

Muscles: *continued*
 in toxocariasis, 105
 in toxoplasmosis, 85
 and trichinellosis, 116
 tumours of, 717
Muscular system, in leprosy, 312
Myasis, 741
Mycetomas, 271
Mycobacteria, 296
 anonymous, 297
Mycobacterial skin ulcers, 729
Mycobacterium balnei, 297, 729
 johnei, 297
 leprae, 297
 tuberculosis, bovine strain, 392, 394
 isoniazid resistance, 392
 virulence, 392
 ulcerans, 297, 729
Mycoplasmas, 339
Mycosis:
 superficial, 265
 systemic, and see Fungi, systemic, 268
Mycotoxins, liver disease and, 559
Myelitis:
 in *Schistosoma haematobium* infection, 165
 transverse, in paragonomiasis, 191
Myeloma, 499, 711
Myelomatosis, amyloidosis in, 724
Myocarditis, 371, *et seq.*
Myocytolysis:
 in endomyocardial fibrosis, 362
 in idiopathic cardiomegaly, 353
Myoglobinuria, 634
 tetanus and, 717
Myospherulosis, 295

Naegleria, 77
Naevus, junctional, 703
Nairobi sheep disease, 217
Nakiwogo, 217
Naphthalene, in G-6-PD deficiency, 460
Nasal cavity:
 and enterobiasis, 115
 polypi in mucocutaneous leishmaniasis,
 61
 in rhinophycomycosis, 294
 rhinoscleroma and, 732
 rhinosporidiosis and, 290
Nasopharyngeal carcinoma, 402
Nass, and oral cancer, 535
Necator americanus:
 and larva migrans, 144
 life cycle, 92
 and visceral larva migrans, 105
Necrotising enterocolitis, 520
Negishi virus, 226
Negri bodies, 236
Neisseria meningitides, 604
Nematodes, 91, *et seq.*
Neonatal jaundice (*See also* haemolytic
 disease of the newborn), 488
 and G-6-PD deficiency, 462

Neonatal jaundice: *continued*
and prematurity, 488
and vitamin K overdosage, 488
Neonate:
alimentary conditions, 513
Australia antigen and, 579
C.N.S. lesions, 601
congenital heart disease, 365
congenital renal lesions, 616
congenital toxoplasmosis, 86
coronary arteries in, 384
cytomegalic inclusion disease and, 262
endocardial fibroelastosis, 356
gamma globulin in, 13
gastric ulcer and, 518
G-6-PD deficiency and, 462, 635
haemoglobin E and, 447
F and, 416, 425
S and, 432
haemolytic disease of the newborn, 488
haemophilia and circumcision, 471
jaundice, 568, 635
liver disease and, 543
malaria in, 13
malaria, therapeutic effect of umbilical cord serum, 15
malarial deaths, 33
meconium ileus, 513
mortality, 4
pyloric stenosis, 513
respiratory conditions in, 390
tetanus and, 320
thalassaemia and, 457
Neoplasms, in the tropics, 690
Nephritis, 616, *et seq.*
(*see* glomerulonephritis and kidney)
Nephrotic syndrome, 623
amyloidosis, 723
causes of, 621
chronic glomerulonephritis and, 626
lobular glomerulitis and, 625
malarial nephrosis, 627
membrano-proliferative G.N., 625
membranous glomerulonephritis and, 626
mercury and, 624
minimal change kidney, 624
proliferative glomerulonephritis and, 625
renal vein thrombosis and, 627
Nepuyo, 217
Nerves:
Bell's palsy, 613
Burkitt tumour, 504
in lepromatous leprosy, 303
malaria, effects on, 20
polyneuritis, 613
retrobulbar neuritis, 613
in tuberculoid leprosy, 304
tumours of, 614
Nervous system, 601
cancer and, 699

Neuroblastoma, 709
and Burkitt tumour, 509, 512
phase contrast microscopy, 509
radiological findings, 512
secondary of bone simulating Burkitt tumour, 512
Neuropathic syndrome of uncertain origin, 610
Neurosyphilis, 603
Niacin deficiency, 686
Niemann–Pick's disease, 602
Nitrofurantoin in G-6-PD deficiency, 460
Nitrofurazone in G-6-PD deficiency, 460
Nitrosamine:
nasopharyngeal cancer and, 402
oesophageal cancer and, 536
Nocardia asteroides, 270
braziliensis, 270, 272
caviae, 270
minutissima, 266
Nocardiosis, 270
North American blastomycosis, 279
Nutritional siderosis, 571

Oesophagostoma, 145
Oesophagus, 517
cancer of, 536, 691
corrosive oesophagitis, 518
stricture of, 512
trypanosomiasis, South American and, 47
varices, 171, 549, 551
Oestrogens:
cirrhosis and, 551
gynaecomastia and, 595
liver cancer and, 595
nasopharyngeal cancer and, 401
Omsk haemorrhagic fever, 230
Onchocerca caecutiens, 133
volvulus, life cycle, 133
microfilaria of, 123
Onchocerciasis, 133
and blindness, 134
diagnostic pathology, 139
elephantiasis in, 138
epidemiology, 133
Erisipela de la Costa, 134, 139
Mal morado, 134, 139
ocular lesions in, 134, 139
pathology, 136
Onyalai, 470
O'Nyong-Nyong virus, 217
Ophthalmoplegia, 748
Opisthorchiasis, 186
carcinoma of liver and, 187
diagnostic pathology, 187
epidemiology, 187
pathology, 187
Opisthorchis felineus, life cycle, 186
viverrini, life cycle, 186
Oporonchi virus, 228
Optic atrophy, 747

Oral cavity, 514
  carcinoma of, 534
  Chutta cancer, 535
  Khaini cancer, 535
  malignant melanoma, 708
  pigmentation and, 514
  South American blastomycosis and, 282
  tuberculosis, 396
  tumours of, 534
Oral submucous fibrosis, 514
Oriboca, 217
Oriental sore, 58
Oroya fever, 337
  salmonellosis, 338
Ossa, 217
Ossifying fibroma, 534
Osteoarthritis, 715
Osteogenesis imperfecta, 714
Osteomalacia, 687
  malabsorption and, 531
  renal disease and, 687
Osteomyelitis, 714
  brucellosis and, 331
  haemoglobin S and, 446
  smallpox and, 240
  typhoid fever and, 327
Osteoporosis, 721
Ova, concentration methods, 754
  quantitative counts, 757
Ovary, 643, et seq.
  amoebiasis, 70
  Burkitt tumour, 506
  conditions affecting, 643
  hydatid disease, 205
  in schistosomiasis, 162, 177
  tuberculosis, 398
Oxaluria, 637
Oxyhaemoglobin, preparation of, 766

P blood group, 475
P blood group system, in hydatid disease, 205
Paget's disease, 714
Palate, Burkitt tumour, 506
Palmar erythema, in cirrhosis, 551
Pamaquine, in G-6-PD deficiency, 460
Pancreas, 664
  Burkitt tumour, 506
  calcification of, 665
  carcinoma of, 665
  clonorchiasis and, 185
  cystic fibrosis, 664
  diseases of, 664
  in haemochromatosis, 570
  in kwashiorkor, 675
  in massive liver cell necrosis, 587
  and Schistosoma haematobium infection, 164
  in Schistosoma japonicum and S. mansoni infections, 169
  in schistosomiasis, 177
  in trichinellosis, 116

Pancreatitis:
  and ascariasis, 101, 665
  chronic in cirrhosis, 551
Pantothenic acid, 688
Paracoccidioidal granuloma, 281
Paracoccidioides brasiliensis, 281
Paradenitis nostras, 244
Paragonimiasis, 190
  epidemiology, 191
  pathology, 191
Paragonimus africanus, 190
  heterotremus, 190
  siamensis, 190
  westermani, life cycle, 190
Paraplegia:
  in β thalassaemia, 454
  in Burkitt tumour, 504
  dracontiasis and, 143
  lathyrism and, 612
  in schistosomiasis, 176
  trauma and, 714
  tuberculous, 396
Parasitic infection, 6
Parathyroid gland, 653
  fluorosis and, 722
Paravertebral abscesses, tuberculous, 395
Paravertebral lesions, Burkitt tumour, 455
Parkinsonism—dementia complex, 608
  pathology of, 609
Parotid gland, 516
  in cirrhosis, 551
Parotitis:
  dysentery, bacillary in, 328
  in typhoid fever, 327
Pasteurella:
  P. pestis, 334
  P. pseudotuberculosis, 335
  P. tularensis, 335
Pathological specimens:
  transmission of, 776
Paul–Bunnell test, 258
Pavassan virus, 226
Pediculus humanus:
  typhus and, 212
  in relapsing fever, 344
Pellagra, 686
Pendah sore, 58
Penicillin, purpura, 470
Penicillium islandicum, 559
  liver disease and, 559
Penis, 640
  cancer of, 640, 691
  elephantiasis of, 138
    due to schistosomiasis, 159
  koro, 640
  venereal disease and, 640
Pentaquine, in G-6-PD deficiency, 460
Peptic ulcer, 518
  cirrhosis and, 551
Perforation, 525
  intestinal, in ascariasis, 101
  in typhoid fever, 324

Pericarditis:
  amoebic, 73
  in annular subvalvular left-ventricular
    aneurysm, 367
  constrictive, 383
  in dracontiasis, 143
  idiopathic, 383
  in leptospirosis, 346
  pneumococcal, 383
  pyogenic, 383
  rheumatic, 383
  tuberculous, 383
  uraemic, 383
  viral, 383
Pericardium, 383
  anaemia and, 383
  β thalassaemia and, 454
  Burkitt tumour, 504
  endomyocardial fibrosis and, 383
  hydropericardium, 383
  idiopathic cardiomegaly and, 383
  tumours of, 383
Periodontal disease, 514
  and Burkitt tumour, 502
Peripheral neuritis, diabetes mellitus and,
  663
Peritonitis:
  amoebiasis and, 70
  ascariasis and, 101
  enterobius and, 113
  in schistosomiasis, 168
  'silent' in cirrhosis, 551
  in trichuriasis, 111
  tuberculous, 396
Pernicious anaemia:
  and gastric cancer, 538
  rarity of, 713
Phaeochromocytoma, 661
Pharynx, leeches and, 189
Phenacetin:
  in G-6-PD deficiency, 460
  purpura, 470
Phenazone in G-6-PD deficiency, 460
Phenylanamine in kwashiorkor, 671
Phenylhydrazine, in G-6-PD deficiency, 460
Phenylthiocarbamide, taste and, 657
Phialophora, 282
Phlebotomus argentipes:
  in Indian Kala-azar, 52
  chinensis, and Kala-azar associated with a
    canine reservoir, 53
  longipalpis in Kala-azar associated with a
    canine reservoir, 53
  martini, in African Kala-azar, 53
  migonei, muco-cutaneous leishmaniasis,
    61
  orientalis, in African Kala-azar, 53
  papatasii, 58
  passoai, muco-cutaneous leishmaniasis, 61
  perniciosus in Kala-azar associated with a
    canine reservoir, 53
  pessoanus, 59
    chiclero ulcer, 59

Phlebotomus argentipes: continued
  sergenti, 58
  whitmani, muco-cutaneous leishmaniasis,
    61
Phlebotomus fever viruses, 228
Phlegmasia alba dolens, 388
Phlyctenular keratitis, 395
Phrynoderma, 751
Phycomycosis, 275
Phytohaemagglutinin and Burkitt's tumour,
  502
Phytohaemagglutinin, 710
  measles and, 249
Piedra:
  black, 266
  white, 267
Piedraia hortae, 266
Pig:
  brucellosis and, 330
  fasciolopsiasis and, 180
  and gnathostomiasis, 120
  and trichinellosis, 115
Pigbel, 319
Pineal gland, 602
Pinealoma, 614
Pinta, 341
Pinworm, diagnosis of, 775
Pironella conica, heterophyiasis and, 181
Piroplasms, 34
Pithomyces chartarum, liver disease and, 559
Pituitary gland, 659
  tumours of, 660
Pityriasis nigra, 266
  versicolor, 266
Placenta:
  and bilirubin excretion, 488
  cytomegalic cells and, 262
  malaria and, 32
  passage of antibodies, 476
Plague, 334
  bacillus, relation to blood group O, 476
  diagnostic pathology, 335
Plantains:
  and endomyocardial fibrosis, 357
  serotonin content, 541
Plantar keratosis and ainhum, 738
Plasmodium:
  differentiation of species, 10
  berghei, chloroquine resistance, 18
  falciparum, 10
    age of erythrocyte, 10
    algid malaria, 18
    central nervous system, pathology of, 21
    chloroquine resistant strains, pigment
      in, 18
    chronic renal disease, 29
    death, 20
    East African strain, 16
    erythrocytic cycle, 11
    exoerythrocytic cycle, 11
    liver in, 27
    nephritis in, 29, 619
    nephritis, proliferative in, 29, 619

Plasmodium, *falciparum*: *continued*
  pathology, 20
  renal biopsy in, 29
  renal failure in, 29
  knowlesi, 17
  lophurae, 12
  malariae, 10
    age of erythrocyte, 11
    erythrocytic cycle, 11
    exoerythrocytic cycle, 11
    kidney in, 29
    mortality, 20
    nephrosis and, 627
    pathology, 20
    renal disease, 20
    tropical splenomegaly syndrome, 20, 492
  ovale, 10
    erythrocytic cycle, 11
    exoerythrocytic cycle, 11
    mortality, 20
    pathology, 20
  vivax, 10
    age of erythrocyte, 11
    death, 20
    erythrocytic cycle, 11
    exoerythrocytic cycle, 11
    Negroes, U.S.A., 16
    pathology, 20
    West Africa, absence of, 16
Platelets:
  coronary disease and, 378
Pneumococcal meningitis, 603
Pneumocystis carinii, 88
Pneumonia:
  blood groups in, 476
  haemoglobin S and, 429
  lobar pneumonia, 391
  jaundice in, 391
Poisoning, 741
  kerosine, 390
  lead, 742
  lysol, 518
  manganese, 602
Poliomyelitis, 259, 260
  pathology, 261
Polyarteritis nodosa and symmetrica gangrene, 387, 621
Polycythaemia:
  liver-cell carcinoma and, 591
  vera, 474
    and pulmonary hypertension, 375
Polydactyly, 714
Polyneuritis, 613
Polyposis coli, 539
Porcephalus armillatus, 739
  moniliformis, 739
Porocephalus, 739
Porphyria, 567
Portal hypertension, 550
  classification of, 550
  fascioliasis and, 189
  idiopathic, 550

Portal hypertension: *continued*
  in schistosomiasis, 171
  in tropical splenomegaly syndrome, 497
Portal vein thrombosis, in schistosomiasis, 172
Post Kala-azar dermal leishmaniasis, 57
Potassium:
  in kwashiorkor, 674
  toxicity, in blood transfusion, 488
Pregnancy: 737
  alpha-feto protein and, 592
  amoebiasis and, 68
  anaemia in, 412
  Burkitt tumour, 506
  dimorphic anaemia in, 412
  ectopic in schistosomiasis, 162
  foetal haemoglobin in, 426
  folic acid in, 412
  and haemoglobin E, 447
    H disease, 458
  kidney in, 634
  pneumococcal meningitis and, 603
  hepatitis and, 577, 583
  immunity and malaria, 30
  immunological status in, 648
  iron deficiency anaemia in, 412
  liver, fatty, acute in, 587
  malaria in, 32
  malarial anaemia in, 32
  malarial infection in, 413
  massive liver cell necrosis and, 585, 586
  pelvic angiography and, 650
  and pneumococcal meningitis, 603, 648
  pulmonary marrow embolism in sickle cell disease, 441
  pyelonephritis and sickle cell trait, 429
  renal cortical necrosis, 635
  rhabdomyosarcoma and, 717
  in sickle-cell anaemia, 434
  in sickle-cell disease, 436
  sickle-cell disease, marrow infarction, 436
  sickle-cell disease, sequestration crisis, 436
  sickle-cell thalassaemia in, 456
  smallpox and, 240
  thalassaemia minor in, 455
  toad test and, 650
  in tropical splenomegaly syndrome, 497
  tuberculosis in, 399
  vitamin B$_{12}$ in, 412
Priapism in sickle cell anaemia, 433
Primary liver cell carcinoma, 589
Primaquine, in G-6-PD deficiency, 460
Probenecid, in G-6-PD deficiency, 460
Progressive muscular atrophy, 607
Proptosis, 748
Prostate, 640
  benign hyperplasia, 641
  cancer, low incidence in tropics, 641
  carcinoma of, 641
  in schistosomiasis, 160, 641
  tuberculosis, 398, 641
Prostatitis, in enterobiasis, 113, 114
Protein, dietary, 5

Proteus:
  OXK, 216
  OX2, 216
  OX19, 216
Protothecosis, 142
Pruritis ani:
  enterobiasis and, 113
Psittacosis-lymphogranuloma viruses, 242
Pseudomonas pseudomallei, 339
Pseudo-tumour, 169
Pterygium, 745
Pulmonary embolism, in sickle cell disease,
  388, 442
Pulmonary hypertension:
  chorioncarcinoma and, 649
  idiopathic, 374
  in sickle cell disease, 442
Pulseless disease, 384
Pure haemoglobin C disease, 435
Purpuras, 470
  classification, 470
  non thrombocytopenic, 470
  snake bite and, 471
Pyelonephritis, 635
  acute, in schistosomiasis, 160
  chronic, 622
    in schistosomiasis, 160
Pyomyositis, tropical, 105, 718
  Lagochilascaris minor in, 718
Pyonephrosis, 635
  in schistosomiasis, 160
Pyridoxine:
  kwashiorkor and, 675
Pyridoxine deficiency, 688
  liver cell cancer and, 593
  urinary calculi and, 637
Pyrrolizidine, liver disease and, 563
Pyruvate kinase deficiency, 489

Q fever, 213
Quartan malarial nephrosis, 627
Queensland tick typhus, 212
Quinidine, in G-6-PD deficiency, 460
Quinine:
  in G-6-PD deficiency, 460
  purpura, 470
Quinocide, in G-6-PD deficiency, 460

Rabies, 233
  diagnostic pathology, 236
  epidemiology, 233
  pathology, 234
  Sellers' technique, 774
  suspected, procedure in, 237
  virology, 234
Rectal stricture, 245
  caustics and, 526
  schistosomiasis and, 526
Rectum:
  fistulae in amoebiasis, 70
  haemorrhoids, 526
  prolapse, malnutrition and, 526
  in schistosomiasis, 162, 168

Rectum: *continued*
  stricture of, 246
  tumours of, 540
Reduviid bug:
  in *Trypanosoma cruzi* infection, 42
  in *Trypanosoma rangeli* infection, 43
Reed-Sternberg cell:
  infectious mononucleosis and, 258
Regional ileitis, 521
Reiter's disease, 716
Relapsing fevers, 342
  Borrelia duttoni, 343
  louse borne, 343
    Borrelia recurrentis, 344
    Ornithodorus moubata, 343
  tick borne, 343
Renal cortical necrosis, 635
  accidental haemorrhage and, 635
  burns and, 635
Renal failure:
  acute, 634
  in *Plasmodium falciparum* malaria, 29
Renal papillary necrosis:
  drugs and, 635
  sickle-cell disease and, 441
Renal vein thrombosis:
  amyloid and, 723
Reovirus, 259
Reticuloendothelial system:
  'blockade', 15
  blockade in aetiology of neoplasms, 697
  'crowding out' phenomena, 19
  hyperplasia and splenic 'pooling', 490
  neoplasms of, 498
Reticulum cell sarcoma, 499
  Burkitt tumour of bone simulating, 512
Retina, lesions in sickle-cell disease, 433
Retinoblastoma, 614
  Burkitt tumour, 509, 512
  cytology, 509
  phase contrast microscopy, 509
Retrolental fibroplasia, 746
Retropharyngeal abscess, tuberculous, 395
Retrobulbar neuritis, 613
Reye's disease, 607
Rhabdomyosarcoma, 403, 717
Rhesus blood group system, 478
Rhesus factor, emergency grouping
  methods, 771
Rhesus incompatibility, differentiation from
  ABO haemolytic disease of the newborn,
  478
Rhesus negative gene, and malaria, 469
Rhesus system: 478
  CDE/cde antigens, 478
  DU antigen, 479
  incidence of Rh negative gene, 479
Rheumatic fever:
  active juvenile cirrhosis and, 584
  and endomyocardial fibrosis, 358
Rheumatic heart disease, 371
  chorea, 372
  and endomyocardial fibrosis, 358

Rheumatoid arthritis, 713
  active juvenile cirrhosis and, 584
Rhino-entomophthoromycosis, 294
Rhinophycomycosis, 294
Rhinoscleroma, 732
Rhinosporidiosis, 290
Rhinosporidium seeberi, 290
Rhizopus, 275
Riboflavine deficiency, 685
Rice water stools, 316
Rickets, 686
  renal, 687
Rickettsia akari, 212
  australis, 212
  conori, 212
  mooseri, 212
  orientalis, 214
  prowazeki, 212
  rickettsi, 212
  siberica, 212
  tsutsugamushi, 212, 214
Rickettsial diseases, 212
  classification of, 212
  Q fever, 213
  typhus, 213
Rickettsialpox, 212
Rift valley fever, 228
Rochalimaea quintana, 212
Romana's sign, 43
Romanowsky stains, 762
Rose spots, 327
Rotor syndrome, 568
Rubella, 251
Rubeola, 248
Russell body, 733
Russian spring summer encephalitis, 226

St. Louis encephalitis virus, 225
Saline, normal, 769
Salivary gland:
  Burkitt tumour, 506
  tumours, 535
  virus, 262
Salmonella, 321, *et seq.*
  in bone in sickle-cell trait, 429
  in *Schistosoma mansoni* infection, 173
Salmonella typhi, amoebic liver abscess and,
  72
Salmonellosis, oroya fever and, 338
Sandy patches, bladder in schistosomiasis,
  158
Sarcoidosis:
  incidence in tropics, 401
  liver disease and, 561
Sarcocystis lindemanni, 87
Sarcosporidiosis, 87
Sasswood tree, liver disease and, 560
Scalp, tuberculosis of, 398
Schaumann body, 401
Schistosoma, bovis, 145
  capense, 145
  curassoni, 145

Schistosoma: *continued*
  haematobium, 145
    bladder in, 156
    and bladder cancer, 165
    blood forming, organs and, 165
    and calcification of bladder, 165
    and carcinoma of the liver, 171
    cervix and, 162
    diagnostic pathology, 177
    egg load in, 147
    filtration-Ninhydrin method, 755
    gastrointestinal tract and, 162
    geographical distribution, 145
    and hypertension, 160
    kidney in, 160
    life cycle, 146
    liver in, 164
    lung and, 164
    other organs affected, 165
    ova, quantitative count, 766
    pathology, 155
    pigment, 148
    reproductive organs in, 160
    snail hosts, 149
    ureters in, 159
  intercalatum, 145
  japonicum, 145
    carcinoma of the colon and, 169
    and carcinoma of the liver, 171
    central nervous system and, 176
    cirrhosis of the liver in, 172, 556
    diagnostic pathology, 177
    faeces, examination of, 753
    genitourinary system and, 176
    geographical distribution, 146
    life cycle, 146
    liver in, 169
    lungs in, 173
    ova in faeces, 753
    ova, quantitative count, 757, 766
    pathology, 168
    reservoir hosts, 150
    reticulo-endothelial system in, 173
    snail hosts in, 149
    spleen in, 173
  mansoni, 145
    and carcinoma of the liver, 171
    central nervous system and, 176
    cirrhosis of liver in, 171, 556
    cyanotic syndrome, 176
    diagnostic pathology, 177
    egg load in, 147
    faeces, examination of, 753
    genito-urinary system and, 176
    geographical distribution, 145
    life cycle, 146
    liver in, 169
    lungs in, 173
    ova in faeces, 753
    ova, quantitative count, 757, 766
    pathology, 168
    reticulo-endothelial system in, 173
    salmonella infection in, 173, 322

Schistosoma, mansoni: *continued*
    snail hosts in, 149
    spleen in, 173
    Ziehl-Neelsen stain, 154
  matthei, 145
  rhodaini, 150
Schistosomiasis, 145
  age, influence of, 150
  calculi and, 160
  and central nervous system, 605
  classification of stages of infection, 153
  digest method of counting ova in tissues, 766
  epidemiology, 148
  immunity in, 151
  intensity of infection and, 151
  kidney in, 160, 176
  liver cell cancer and, 171
  liver cirrhosis and, 171, 556
  lymphomas and, 175
  nutrition and, 150
    and therapy, 150
  pathogenesis of, 152
  pigment in, 148
  and portal hypertension, 171
  and pulmonary hypertension, 175
  reservoir hosts, 150
  Salmonella typhi infection and, 159, 322
  snail hosts in, 149
  stage of established infection, 154
  stage of invasion, 152
  stage of late effects, 154
  stage of maturation, 152
  typhoid and, 176, 326
Schizophrenia, 615
Schumm's test, 464
Schwann cells, Kaposi's sarcoma, 707
Scleroderma:
  and calcinosis universalis, 719
  and pulmonary hypertension, 375
Scorpion stings, 725
Scrapie, 249
Scrotum:
  calcinosis circumscripta in onchocerciasis, 136
  elephantiasis of, 128, 129, 138
  gangrene of, 126, 643
  paragonomiasis and, 191
  schistosomiasis and, 159
Scurvy, 470
  osteoporosis in, 721
Sea-snake, pathology, 726
Sellers' technique, 774
Seminal vesicles in schistosomiasis, 160
Semisulcospira, metagonimiasis and, 181
Senecio, 558, 563
  disease in man, 563
Sequestration crises, and blood transfusion, 482
Serotonin, 167, 541
Sheehan's syndrome, 660
Shigella species, 328

Shock:
  gram-negative organisms and, 296
  kidney in, 634
  in malaria, 20
Siberian tick typhus, 212
Sickle-cell anaemia, 431, 432
  anaesthesia in, 433
  Burkitt tumour and, 503
  clinical aspects, 432
  diagnosis, 434
  duodenal ulceration and, 432
  exchange transfusion in, 433
  folic acid deficiency, 432
  and malaria, 432, 466
  pathology, 437
  solubility test in, 768
Sickle-cell disease, 431, 436
  and blood transfusion, 482
  bone changes in, 436, 444
  bone marrow emboli, 436
    infarction, 436
  the central nervous system, 436, 443
  and cholelithiasis, 441
  and cirrhosis, 441
  diagnosis, 436
  the heart, 443
  kidney in, 441
  the liver, 440
  lungs in, 441
  marrow embolism, 441
  pathology, 437
    of sequestration crisis, 438
  and pulmonary embolism, 441
  and pulmonary hypertension, 441
  SD disease, 431
  SE disease, 431
  SF, 431
  SG disease, 431
  S Hopkins II, 431
  SJ disease, 431
  SK disease, 431
  sequestration crisis, 436, 438
  sequestration crisis and splenic 'pooling', 491
  S Stanleyville II, 431
  SP, 431
  the spleen, 438
Sickle-cell trait, 429
  anaesthesia in, 429
  and blood transfusion, 430, 482
  diagnosis, 431
  erythrocyte fragility, 431
  haematuria in, 429
  hookworm anaemia, 429
  hyposthenuria, 430
  incidence, 429
  kidney in, 430
  leprosy, 429
  and liver, 429
  pathology, 429
  pneumonia, 429
  pyelonephritis in pregnancy, 429
  and salmonella infection, 429

Sickle-cell trait: *continued*
  sickling in, 431
  splenic abscess, 429
    infarction, 429
  sudden death in, 429
  target cells in, 431
  and typhoid fever, 429
Sickling test, 766
Siderofibrotic nodules:
  in tropical splenomegaly syndrome, 495
  in sickle-cell disease, 439
Siderosis:
  African, 570
  haemolytic, 574
  and osteoporosis, 721
  transfusional, 574
Simbum group viruses, 228
Simmond's disease, 660
Simulium fly, 133
  callidium, 133
  damnosum, 133
  metallicum, 133
  naevi, 133
  ochraceum, 133
  and onchocerciasis, 133
Skin, 748, *et seq.*
  albinism, 703
  adnexal tumours of, 703
  African Kala-azar, 49
  basal-cell carcinoma, 702
  beetle dermatitis, 724
  cancer of, 702, *et seq.*
  cheloidal blastomycosis, 290
  chromomycosis, 282
  dwarfism and, 752
  elephantiasis and, 130
  Espundia, 61
  fungi, superficial, 265, *et seq.*
  granuloma multiforme, 313
  histoplasmosis, 285
    African, 286
  keratoacanthoma, 702
  larva migrans, 144
  leishmaniasis, 58, *et seq.*
  leprosy, 297, *et seq.*
  lichen planus, 751
  lupus vulgaris, 398, 750, 751
  melanoma, 707
  mycetoma, 271
  North American blastomycosis, 279
  occupational dermatoses, 750
  onchocerciasis, 137
  Oriental sore, 58
  post-Kala-azar dermal leishmaniasis, 57
  prickly heat, 751
  in *Schistosoma haematobium* infection, 152, 165
  smallpox, 240
  snip method, 759
  sporotrichosis, 284
  squamous-cell carcinoma, 703
  subcutaneous phycomycosis, 292
  treponematoses, 340, *et seq.*

Skin: *continued*
  tuberculosis and, 398, 750
  ulcers:
    Chiclero, 59
    mycobacterial, 728
    tropical, 726
    veld sore, 728
  Uta, 59
  velvet leg, 752
  verruga peruana, 337
Slow virus infections, 262
Small intestine, Burkitt tumour, 506
Smallpox, 238
  diagnostic pathology, 241
  epidemiology, 238
  pathology, 239
  vaccination, and leprosy, 308
  vaccine, and the heart, 376
  virus-relation to A antigen, 476
Snails, hosts in schistosomiasis, 146
Snake bite, 725
  pathology, 725
  thrombocytopenia, 471
Snuff:
  and carcinoma of the maxillary sinus, 402
  and nasopharyngeal carcinoma, 402
Soft chancre, 338
Solar retinopathy, 747
South American blastomycosis, 281
South American trypanosomiasis, 42
  (*See also* Trypanosomiasis, South American)
South-East-Asian haemorrhagic fever, 224
Sparganosis, 210
  epidemiology, 210
  pathology, 211
Sparganum mansoni, life cycle, 210
  proliferum, life cycle, 210
Spider naevi, in cirrhosis, 551
Spina bifida, 602, 714
Spinal cord:
  and ascariasis, 101
  Burkitt tumour, 504
  diseases of, 601, *et seq.*
  and malaria, 21
  schistosomiasis, 176
  trauma, 714
  tuberculosis, 395
  viral infections, 216, *et seq.*
Spirochaetal jaundice, 345
Spleen, 489
  abscess, primary of, 498
  abscess in sickle-cell anaemia, 432
  abscess in sickle-cell trait, 429
  amoebiasis, 498
  amyloidosis, 723
  brucellosis, 330
  Burkitt tumour, 504
  calcification in sickle-cell disease, 439
  in chronic venous congestion, 491
  cysts of, 498
  extra sinusoidal circulation, 492
  in filariasis, 125

Spleen: *continued*
in hereditary non-spherocytic anaemia, 491
hydatid disease and, 205
in hypersplenism, 490
infarction in sickle cell trait, 429
intrasinusoidal circulation, 492
malaria, 27
  indices in, 14
  pathology, 27
  rupture in, 27
neoplasms of, 498
relapsing fever and, 344
rupture, 173
schistosomiasis and, 165, 173
in sickle-cell disease, 432, 438
siderofibrotic nodules in schistosomiasis, 173
  in sickle-cell disease, 438
splenomegaly causes of, 490
in tropical splenomegaly syndrome, 495
in toxoplasmosis, 86
trypanosomiasis, 38
tuberculosis, 397
in typhoid fever, 325
in visceral leishmaniasis, 56
weight, 489
Splenectomy:
hypersplenism, 492
indications for, 492
malaria, and, 27
malarial infection following, 497
Piroplasmosis following, 497
pneumococcal infection following, 497
streptococcal infection following, 497
in tropical splenomegaly syndrome, 495, 497
Splenomegalie Algerienne, 492
Spondylitis, active juvenile cirrhosis and, 584
Spondylosis, cervical, 606
Spondweni virus, 217
Sporothrix schenckii, 284
Sporotrichosis, 229, 284
Sprue, tropical, 528
Sputum:
amoebae in, 75
ascaris larvae in, 101
aspergillosis in, 274
Blastomyces dermatitidis in, 281
coccidiodomycosis and, 278
Cryptococcus neoformans in, 289
examination for parasites, 391, 775
Histoplasma capsulatum in, 285
hydatid disease and, 205
larvae of strongyloides in, 110
ova in schistosomiasis, 176
paragonimiasis, 191
toxocara larvae in, 105
Squamous-cell carcinoma, 703
arsenical dermatitis, 704
Dhoti cancer, 704
Kangri cancer, 703

Staphylococcus aureus, in pyomyositis, tropical, 718
Steatorrhoea, 526
Stillbirth, malaria and, 31
Still's disease, 713
Stoll's method, 757
Stomach:
amoebiasis, 70, 73
Burkitt tumour, 506
carcinoma, 537
eosinophilic granuloma, 522
lymphomas, 539
peptic ulcer, 518
polyps, 539
and *Schistosoma haematobium* infection, 165
in *Schistosoma japonicum* and *S. mansoni* infections, 169
trypanosomiasis, South American and, 46
tuberculosis, 397
Stomatitis, 514
vesicular, 259
Streptocerciasis, 140
and elephantiasis, 140
String test, 81, 111
Strongyloides spp:
and larva migrans, 144
stercoralis, 104
  life cycle, 106
  and visceral larva migrans, 104
Strongyloidiasis, 105, *et seq.*
autoinfection in, 106
diagnostic pathology, 110
epidemiology, 106
malabsorption in, 107
pathology, 107
Subacute myelo-optico neuropathy, 610
Subacute sclerosing panencephalitis, 249
Subcutaneous phycomycosis, 292
Sudden death, in sickle-cell trait, 429
Sulphonamides:
in G-6-PD deficiency, 460
and the heart, 373
Sulphones, in G-6-PD deficiency, 460
Sulphuric acid, oesophagitis and, 517
Summer grippe, 259
Swamp fever, 345
Sweat gland carcinoma, in albinism, 703
Swimmers granuloma, 728
itch, in schistosomiasis, 152
Symmetrical gangrene, 387
Synovia, tumours of, 714
Syphilis, 340
in arteritis of obscure aetiology, 385
in blood transfusion, 481
congenital, liver in, 565
false biological tests in, 342
oral cavity and, 514
pericellular cirrhosis, 565
and symmetrical gangrene, 387
Systemic lupus erythematosis, 617

Tabes dorsalis, 340, 603
Tacaribe, 228
Tacaribe group viruses, 228
Taenia saginata, life cycle, 194
  solium, life cycle, 194
Taeniasis, 194
  diagnostic pathology, 197
  epidemiology, 197
  pathology, 197
Takayasu's disease, 384
Talipes equinovarus, 714
Tanapox, 241
Tape worm:
  dog, 209
  dwarf, 208
  fish, 207
Target cells, 405
  in haemoglobin C trait, 435
  in haemoglobin E, 447
  in pure haemoglobin C disease, 435
  in sickle-cell anaemia, 434
  in sickle-cell trait, 431
  in β thalassaemia, 454
  β thalassaemia minor and, 455
Tay Sach's disease, 612
Temporal arteritis, 385
Tenosynovitis, 716
Testes, 642, *et seq.*
  amoebiasis, 70
  atrophy in cirrhosis, 551
  Burkitt tumour, 506
  in filariasis, 126, 129
  leprosy, 311
  in schistosomiasis, 162
  tuberculosis of, 398, 642
  tumours of, 643
  and typhoid fever, 326
Testis:
  calcification and, 643
  onchocerciasis and, 139
Tetanus, 319
  diagnostic pathology, 321
  neonatal, 320
  sickle-cell disease and, 321
  in sickle-cell trait, 429
Thai haemmorhagic fever, 230
Thalassaemia, 453, *et seq.*
  and blood transfusion, 482
  and malaria, 468
  α thalassaemia, 453, 457
  characteristics of, 457, 458
  hydrops foetalis in, 457
α-thalassaemia$_1$/α-thalassaemia$_2$/haemo-
  globin E disease, 459
α and β thalassaemia, differential diagnosis,
  459
β thalassaemia, 453
  anaemia in, 454
  autopsy findings, 455
  haemoglobin A$_2$ in, 454
    C, 456
    D, 456
    E, 456

β thalassaemia, haemaglobin A$_2$ in: *continued*
  F in, 445
  G, 456
  J, 456
  N, 456
  S, 434, 456
  heart in, 455
  incidence, 454
  inheritance of, 454
  major, 454
  minor, 455
    thalassaemia minima, 455
  paraplegia in, 455
  red cell inclusions, 454
  skeletal changes in, 454
Thiamine deficiency, 380, 684
  pathology, 684
Threadworm, diagnosis of, 775
Thrombocytopenia:
  drugs in, 470
  essential, 470
  in heatstroke, 736
  hypersplenism, 490
  in malaria, 26
  in tropical splenomegaly syndrome, 492
Thrombophlebitis, 388, *et seq.*
  complication of blood transfusion, 488
  multiple idiopathic, 389
Thrombosis, kwashiorkor and, 388, 675
  venous, 388
Thrush, 514
Thymus gland, 653
  Burkitt tumour and, 504, 506
  kwashiorkor and, 653
  measles and, 653
Thyroid, 654
  Burkitt tumour, 506
  carcinoma, incidence of, 658
  classification of diseases, 656
  goitre, aetiology of, 655
    endemic, 655
    pathology of, 657
  goitrogens, 657
  Hashimoto's disease, 654
  liver disease and, 561
  periodic paralysis and, 654
  in South American trypanosomiasis, 43
  thyroiditis, acute, 654
  thyroxine synthesis, 655
  tumours of, 658
Thyrotoxicosis, 379, 654
  chorioncarcinoma and, 649
Tick borne encephalitis, 226
  viruses, 226
Timor microfilaria, 125
Tinea capitis, 267
  corporis, 268
  flava, 266
  nigra, 266
  versicolor, 266
Tonsil, Burkitt tumour, 506
Torres bodies, 223
Torulopsis glabrata, 295

Torulosis, 289
Toxocara canis, life cycle, 103
  catis, life cycle, 103
Toxocariasis, 103
  and ascariasis, 101, 105
  diagnostic pathology, 105
  epidemiology, 104
  pathology, 104
Toxoplasma gondii, 82
Toxoplasmosis, 82
  acquired, 83
  congenital, 86
  diagnosis, 87, 759
  epidemiology, 82
  immunology, 83
  organ distribution, 84
  serological tests, 87
  staining reactions, 84
Trachoma, 242
  clinico-pathology of, 243
  diagnostic pathology, 244
Transfusional siderosis, 574
  and haemochromatosis, 574
Traveller's diarrhoea, 520
Trematodes, 145, *et seq.*
Trench fever, 212
Treponema carateum, 340
  pallidum, 340
  pertenue, 340
Treponematoses, 340
  diagnosis, 342
  Kahn test, 342
Treponema pallidum immobilization (T.P.I.)
  test, 342
  Venereal Disease Research Laboratories
  (V.D.R.L.) flocculation test, 342
Tric agents, 242
Trichinella spiralis, life cycle, 115
Trichinellosis, 114
  diagnostic pathology, 117
  epidemiology, 115
  pathology, 115
Trichomonas hominis, 81
  vaginalis, 81
Trichomycosis axillaris, 267
Trichophyta mentagrophytes, 267
Trichosporon beigelii, 267
Trichuriasis, 111
  diagnostic pathology, 112
  epidemiology, 111
  pathology, 111
Trichuris trichiura, life cycle, 111
Trigeminal neuralgia, 613
Trinitrotoluene, in G-6-PD deficiency, 460
Trombicula akamushi, 214
  deliensis, 214
  pallida, 214
  scutellaris, 214
Tropical amblyopia, 610
Tropical cryptogenic splenomegaly, 492
Tropical eosinophilia, 399
  Acanthocheilonema perstans and, 141
  diagnosis, 401

Tropical eosinophilia: *continued*
  and filariasis, 128
Tropical phlebitis, 389
Tropical pulmonary eosinophilia, 383
Tropical splenomegaly syndrome, 492
  antimalarial therapy in, 497
  definition, 492
  diagnosis, 497
  dwarfism, 497
  epidemiology, 493
  haematological findings, 494
  liver in, 495, 550
  and malaria, 493
  pathology, 494
  Plasmodium malariae, 493, 496
  rarity in South African Bantu, 493
  spleen in, 495
  splenectomy in, 494, 497
  ulcers, leg, 497
Tropical sprue, 528
  diagnostic pathology, 532
  jejunal biopsy in, 531
Tropical thrombophlebitis, and symmetrical gangrene, 388
Tropical ulcers, 320, 726
Trychophyta aubrum, 268
Trychophyta faviforme, 268
  floccosum, 268
  rubrum, 268
  schoenleini, 267
  verrucosum, 267
  violaceum, 267
Trypanosoma cruzi, 42
  diagnostic methods, 42
  leishmania forms, 44
  life cycle, 42
    pseudocysts, 45
    reservoir hosts, 43
  gambiense, endotoxin from, 40
    life cycle, 35
  rangeli, 43
  rhodesiense, animal reservoirs, 36
    life cycle, 35
Trypanosomes, concentration method, 765
Trypanosomiasis, 35
  African, cerebrospinal fluid in, 41
    diagnosis, 42
    epidemiology, 36
    immunology, 36
    life cycle, 35
  blood, examination of, 758
  and blood transfusion, 481
  and central nervous system, 39
  concentration techniques in blood, 765
  Gambian, central nervous system
    changes, 39
    reticulo-endothelial system in, 38
  Rhodesiense, 41
    pathology, 41
  South American, brain in, 46
    cardiopathy in, 46
    congenital form, 43
    diagnostic pathology, 49

Trypanosomiasis, S. American: *continued*
  epidemiology, 42
  heart in, 48
  pathology, 43
Tryptophan, 167, 541
Tsetse fly, see Glossina spp. 35
Tsutsugamushi disease, 213
Tuberculosis, 391, *et seq.*
  abdominal, 397
  adult type, 394
  alimentary tract, 396
  alkaline phosphatase in leucocytes, 397
  anaemia in, 397
  in annular subvalvular left-ventricular
    aneurysm, 367
  amyloidosis in, 394
  'anonymous' mycobacteria and, 399
  ascitic fluid in, 397
  of blood forming organs, 397
  bone, 395
  bone marrow in, 397
  breast, 398
  bronchiectasis, 393
  bronchopneumonia, 393
  calcification, 393
  central nervous system, 396
    tuberculoma, 396
  cervix, 398
  childhood form, 393
  destroyed lung, 394
  diagnosis, 395, 399
  empyema, 394
  endometritis, 398
  of epididymis, 398
  epidemiology, 392
  fallopian tubes, 397, 398
  geniturinary tuberculosis, 398
  Ghon focus, 393
  intestinal fistulae in, 397
  joints, 395
  kidney and, 398
  larynx, 394
  leucopenia in, 397
  leukaemoid reaction, 397
  in liver, 398
  lupus vulgaris, 398
  lymphatic glands, 394
  lymphoedema, 395
  malabsorption syndrome, 396
  meningitis, 396
  miliary form, 393
  myelofibrosis in, 398
  nasopharyngeal, 394
  oral cavity, 396
  ovary, 398
  paraplegia, 395
  paravertebral abscesses, 395
  pericarditis, 383
  peritonitis, 396
  phylctenular keratitis, 395
  pleural effusion, 394
    punch biopsy, 394
  in pregnancy, 399

Tuberculosis: *continued*
  of prostate, 398
  renal, 398
  retropharyngeal abscess, 395
  scalp, 398
  skin, 750
  spine, 395
  spleen, 397
  splenic puncture in, 397
  steroid therapy, 394
  stomach, 396
  stricture of intestine, 396
  of testicle, 398
  thrombosis of calf veins, 388
  tuberculin test, 392
Tuberous sclerosis, 607
Tularaemia, 335
Tumbu fly (external myiasis), 741
Tumoral calcinosis, 719
Tunga penetrans, 741
Twinning, 738
Typhoid fever, 321
  blood groups in, 476
  diagnostic pathology, 328
  and G-6-PD deficiency, 323
  rose spots, 327
  and sickle-cell trait, 429
Typhus:
  epidemic, 213
  flea borne, 213
  louse-borne, 213
  mite borne, 213
  murine, 213
  scrub, 213
    pathology, 214
  Weil-Felix reaction, 216
Tyrosinase, albinism, 703
Tyrosine, in kwashiorkor, 672

Uganda S-M 336 virus, 217
Ulcer:
  Bairnsdale, 729
  Buruli, 729
  Kakerifu, 729
  Kasongo, 729
  leg, in idiopathic tropical splenomegaly
    syndrome, 497
  Mycobacterium ulcerans and, 729
  Orebro, 729
  in sickle-cell anaemia, 433
  tropical, 726
    malignant change in, 728
    phagedenic diagnosis, 727
      Borrelia vincenti and *Fusobacterium
        fusiformis* in, 727
Ulcerative colitis, 521
  active juvenile cirrhosis and, 584
  amoebiasis and, 71
  carcinoma and, 521, 539
Uncinaria stenocephala and larva migrans,
  144
Unstable haemoglobin diseases, 453

Uraemia:
  in arteritis of obscure aetiology, 386
  pericarditis in, 383
  purpura in, 471
Urea, normal levels in blood, 616
Ureter, 638
  calculi and, 638
  diseases of, 638
  reflux in schistosomiasis, 159
  stricture in schistosomiasis, 159
  ureteritis cystica, 159
    glandularis, 159
  in schistosomiasis, 159
Urethra:
  amoebiasis and, 70
  gonorrhoea and, 639
  inclusion conjunctivitis and, 244
  in schistosomiasis, 159
  stricture and bladder cancer, 167
  stricture of, 639
  in *T. vaginalis* infection, 82
  urethritis, non-gonococcal, 640
Urine:
  cytomegalic cells in, 262
  enzymes and carcinoma of the bladder, 167
  Erlich's aldehyde reagent and 5-hydroxy-indol acetic acid, 541
  larvae of *strongyloides* in, 110
  Leishmania donovani in, 56
  ova concentration method, 755
  protein selectivity, 624
Urolithiasis, 636
Uta, 60
Uterus, 644
  carcinoma of, 647
  in enterobiasis, 113
  fibroids and, 644
  hydatid disease, 205
  infection of, 644
  prolapse of, 644
  rupture of, 644
  sarcoma of, 644
  in schistosomiasis, 162
  tuberculosis, 398
Uvulectomy, 514

Vaccinia, 238, 711
Vagina, 645
  amoebiasis and, 63
  chorion carcinoma and, 645, 648
  infections of, 645
  paragonomiasis and, 191
  schistosomiasis and, 162
  tumours of, 645
  Trichomonas vaginalis in, 82
Vaginitis in enterobiasis, 113
Varicella, 241
Varicocele in filariasis, 128
Variola major, 238
  minor, 238

Veins, 387
  haemorrhoids, 388
  phleboliths, 388
  pulmonary embolism, 388
  thrombosis, 388
  tropical phlebitis, 389
  varicocele, 388
  ulcers, 388
Veld sore, 728
  Corynebacterium diphtheriae, 728
Venereal disease, amoebiasis, 70
Venereal Disease Research Laboratories
  flocculation test (V.D.R.L.), 342
Venesection:
  in blood transfusion, 483
Venezuelan equine encephalitis virus, 217
Veno-occlusive disease: 562
  aetiology, 563
  Crotalaria fulva, 563
    retusa, 563
  pathology, 564
Venomous bites, 724
  stings, 724
Verruga peruana, 337
  pathology, 338
Vesico-vaginal fistula, 636
  lymphogranuloma venereum and, 245
  vesical calculi and, 636
Vesicular stomatitis viruses, 217
Vibrio cholerae: 314
  diagnosis, 317
Vibrio El Tor:
  carrier state, 315
  diagnosis, 317
  epidemiology, 315
Village surveys, 1
Viral diseases, 216
Viral hepatitis type A, 576
  comparison with type B, 581
  epidemiology, 577
  pathology, 581
  pregnancy and, 577
Viral hepatitis type B, 576
  Australia antigen and, 577
  comparison with A, 581
  excess blood group O in, 583
  mosquito transmission, 579
  pathology, 581
Viral infections and G-6-PD deficiency, 461
Viral meningo-encephalitis, 605
Visceral larva migrans, 103
  due to *Ascaris lumbricoides*, 105
  due to *Ascaris suis*, 105
  due to *Necator americanus*, 105
  due to *Strongyloides stercoralis*, 105
Visceral leishmaniasis:
  African Kala-azar, 53
  anaemia in, 54
  gastro-intestinal tract, 56
  immunity, 54
  Indian Kala-azar, 53
  Kala-azar associated with a canine reservoir, 53

Visceral leishmaniasis: *continued*
  liver in, 56
  pathology, 54
  reticulo-endothelial system in, 55
  staining of parasite in tissue, 55
Vitamin A, 682
  bladder stone disease and, 637
  in kwashiorkor, 670
  and oral cancer, 534
Vitamin B, 684
  and symmetrical gangrene, 387
Vitamin B_1 (thiamine), 684
Vitamin B_{12}, 409
  in malabsorption syndrome, 529
  in pregnancy, 412
  in tropical sprue, 531
Vitamin C, 688
Vitamin D, 686
Vitamin E, 688
  kwashiorkor and, 674
  massive liver-cell necrosis and, 586
Vitamin K, 471, 688
  and liver disease, 550
  in G-6-PD deficiency, 460
Vitamin deficiencies, 482
  folic acid, 408
  niacin, 686
  pantothenic acid, 688
  pyridoxine, 688
  riboflavine and, 685
  thiamine, 684
Volvulus, 523
  ascariasis and, 101
Von Willebrand's disease, 471
Vulva, 645
  circumcisional operations, 645
  elephantiasis of, 128, 129, 138
  native medicines and, 646
  in schistosomiasis, 160
  tumours of, 646

Warthin-Finkeldy cells, 248
Waterhouse–Friderichsen syndrome, 604
Weil-Felix reaction, 216
Weil's disease, 345

Wesselsbron virus, 217
Western equine encephalitis virus, 218
West Nile virus, 217
Whipworm, *see* trichuriasis, 111
Whooping cough, 390
Widal reaction, 328
Wilm's tumour, 638
  Burkitt tumour, 510, 512
Wilson's disease, 566, 612
Winterbottom's sign, 37
Wood smoke, and nasopharyngeal carcinoma, 402
Wound sepsis, 296
Wuchereria bancrofti:
  diagnostic methods, 759
  geographical distribution, 124
  life cycle, 124
  microfilaria of, 123
Wuchereria bancrofti var. *Vauceli*, 125

Xenopsylla cheopis 212
  plague and, 334
Xerophthalmia, 745
Xerosis, 683
Xg blood group system, 475

Yam poisoning, 559
Yaws, 341
  in blood transfusion, 481
Yeasts, 264
Yellow fever, 219
  diagnostic pathology, 223
  epidemiology, 220
  liver in, 222
  pathology, 221
Yersinia pestis, 334

Zenkers degeneration, 327
Ziehl-Neelsen stain, in schistosomiasis, 154
Zinc, 689
  cirrhosis and, 561
  gastric cancer and, 538
  sulphate flotation method, 754
Zollinger Ellison syndrome, 667

Gift of H. M. Gilles (Rhodes Scholar,
1946-1951, BSc, 1952)